PATHOLOGY

for the PHYSICAL THERAPIST ASSISTANT

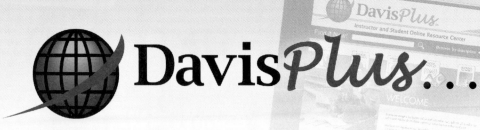

Online Resource Center

Davis*Plus* is your online source for a wealth of learning resources and teaching tools, as well as electronic and mobile versions of our products.

STUDENTS

Unlimited Free access.
No password.
No registration.
No fee.

INSTRUCTORS

Upon Adoption.
Password-protected library of title-specific, online course content.

Visit http://davisplus.fadavis.com

WELCOME CLINICAL SCENARIOS INTERACTIVE MEDIA MOBILE PRODUCT LEARNING ACTIVITIES E-EDITION

Explore more online resources from F.A. Davis...

DAVIS'S DRUG GUIDE.com
powered by
Unbound Medicine®

www.drugguide.com
is Davis's Drug Guide Online, the complete Davis's Drug Guide for Nurses® database of over 1,100 monographs on the web.

Taber's Online
powered by
Unbound Medicine®

www.tabersonline.com
delivers the power of Taber's Cyclopedic Medical Dictionary on the web. Find more than 60,000 terms, 1,000 images, and more.

Davis PT NETWORK

www.davisptnetwork.com
is the PT community's source for online continuing education, social networking, professional information, and more.

---

www.fadavis.com

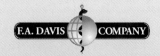

PATHOLOGY

for the PHYSICAL THERAPIST ASSISTANT

Penelope J. Lescher, PT, MA, MCSP

Associate Professor and Interim PTA
Program Director and Chair
Mount Aloysius College
Cresson, Pennsylvania

Member of Chartered Society of
Physiotherapy (Bachelor's equivalent)
Leeds School of Physical Therapy
Yorkshire, United Kingdom
Master of Arts, College of Notre Dame,
Baltimore, Maryland

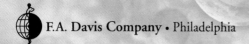
F.A. Davis Company • Philadelphia

F. A. Davis Company
1915 Arch Street
Philadelphia, PA 19103
www.fadavis.com

Printed in the United States of America

Last digit indicates print number: 10 9 8 7 6 5 4 3 2 1

Publisher: Margaret M. Biblis
Acquisitions Editor: Melissa A. Duffield
Manager of Content Development: George W. Lang
Developmental Editor: Jill Rembetski
Art and Design Manager: Carolyn O'Brien

As new scientific information becomes available through basic and clinical research, recommended treatments and drug therapies undergo changes. The author(s) and publisher have done everything possible to make this book accurate, up to date, and in accord with accepted standards at the time of publication. The author(s), editors, and publisher are not responsible for errors or omissions or for consequences from application of the book, and make no warranty, expressed or implied, in regard to the contents of the book. Any practice described in this book should be applied by the reader in accordance with professional standards of care used in regard to the unique circumstances that may apply in each situation. The reader is advised always to check product information (package inserts) for changes and new information regarding dose and contraindications before administering any drug. Caution is especially urged when using new or infrequently ordered drugs.

Library of Congress Cataloging-in-Publication Data
Lescher, Penelope J.
  Pathology for the physical therapist assistant / Penelope J. Lescher.
      p. ; cm.
  Includes bibliographical references and index.
  ISBN 978-0-8036-0786-6 (alk. paper)
  1. Physiology, Pathological. 2. Physical therapy assistants. I. Title.
  [DNLM: 1. Pathology. 2. Physical Therapy Modalities. QZ 4]
  RB113.L47 2011
  616.07--dc22
                                                                      2010053692

For my husband Jerry, who has been my support and cheerleader through the years of writing this text, and to all my co-workers and fellow educators, relatives, friends, and students, who have patiently endured my eccentricities.

Pathology for the Physical Therapist Assistant is a comprehensive pathology text uniquely designed for physical therapist assistant (PTA) education and practice. As PTAs graduate and enter clinical practice it will continue to be a reference volume. The impetus to write this book was the lack of a specific text for pathology related to PTA practice. As a PTA program director and educator for the past 15 years with a specialization in teaching the pathology content of the program, I became acutely aware that none of the pathology texts available were really appropriate for the PTA students. The required knowledge level of pathology for the PTA is less than that of the physical therapist, but different from other associate degree–level health care workers. The aim of this book is to highlight the most important information and diagnoses relevant for the PTA student and practitioner and fill the gap as far as pathology content for PTA associate degree programs. The content of the text includes, but is not restricted to, that required by "a normative model of physical therapist assistant education" published by the APTA.

This 14-chapter book was designed to facilitate use in a 15-week semester of a pathology course or to use each chapter as stand-alone content within PTA programs where the pathology content is spread throughout the curriculum. The features of this book are designed to assist student learning, encourage critical thinking, and ensure the appropriate knowledge of pathology required for both passing the national licensing examination and functioning within the clinic. Each chapter and many sections have a heading called "Why does the physical therapist assistant need to know about. . .," which helps to focus the reader on the importance of the content for practice. An understanding of the relevance of information for PT practice and PTA work makes the study of a subject more interesting. Each chapter begins with the anatomy and physiology of the body system as a review of the normal system prior to learning about the pathology. Throughout the text the relationship between the PTA and the physical therapist is emphasized and the "scope of work" of the PTA is delineated. Careful consideration has been given to the scope of work of the PTA, although this does not mean that tests and measures and specific diagnostic procedures are not described in the text where relevant. PTAs need to be able to read the patient chart and understand the meaning of

physical therapy and medical tests. Reference to the *Guide for Physical Therapist Practice* is emphasized in each chapter and *Guide* language is used throughout the text. The use of medical terminology is consistent with explanations within the text of the meaning of medical terms as well as inclusion of each term within the extensive glossary at the back of the book. Some of the specific terms and words relevant to the PTA are listed at the beginning of each chapter as "key terms," bolded within the text, and included in the glossary. The extensive use of tables, lists, information boxes, and illustrations gives the chapters a more easily understandable format. Many tables are provided to make the content more understandable for the reader and are particularly useful for more complicated content.

Some of the other unique features of this book include:

- Each chapter has a distinct focus on a specific body system.
- Chapter outlines provide an easy method for students and faculty to find content.
- The anatomy and physiology of the specific body system is described as a review for the PTA prior to discussion regarding the pathology of that system.
- Physical therapy interventions are included for all appropriate pathological conditions.
- Tables, lists, and information boxes facilitate student learning and break up the text, making for easier reading.
- Specific content related to precautions and contraindications for certain patient diagnoses related to physical therapy practice help to focus students on clinical practice issues.
- Medical tests are described as they relate to the pathology of the body system.
- Specific boxes for "geriatric considerations" in each chapter help to make the chapter content relevant to clinical practice.
- "It happened in the clinic" boxes in each chapter relate real-life situations within the clinic that provide interesting insights into physical therapy practice for students regarding chapter content.
- The use of an icon within the text enables students and faculty to immediately identify pediatric content.

- Inclusion of a list of useful Web sites pertaining to the chapter content encourages students to further research topics and make use of professional-level sources of information.
- References for each chapter include those from scientific literature and professional sources to ensure accuracy of information.
- Case studies at the end of each chapter assist students to apply the knowledge gained from the chapter to increase the clinical relevance of the information and to provide talking points within class.

- Review questions for each chapter allow for student self-testing, homework assignments, or team projects.

This text was never intended to provide detailed physical therapy interventions for people with specific diagnoses or manifestations of the disease process, but the inclusion of content more specific to practice for the PTA hopefully makes this a useful addition to texts for PTA education.

Penny Lescher

ACKNOWLEDGMENTS

The task of thanking all those who have helped me during the writing of this text is a difficult one since so many people have helped along the way. Writing this book has truly been an enormous project made easier by all the help and encouragement I have received. Many people encouraged me to write a pathology text, especially all my fellow PTA educators throughout the country. Particular thanks go to Pam Ritzline PT, EdD, for all her help with the content editing; David C. Thomas, PT, MGA, my fellow PTA educator and friend in Maryland, for his help in reviewing initial writing of the cardiopulmonary chapter and writing test questions; Alan Brownlie, PhD, Associate Professor of English at Anne Arundel Community College, for his help in re-directing my grammatical construction; and my friend and colleague

Amy Murphy, PT, for her assistance with writing test questions for the instructor's manual.

Particular thanks go to all the people at F. A. Davis for their encouragement and patience. To Jean Francois Vilain, retired publisher, for making my dream of writing this text a reality and Margaret M. Biblis, publisher, for continuing to believe the text would be completed. To Melissa Duffield, my patient publishing editor; Jill Rembetski, my developmental editor; Peg Waltner, developmental editor and all those who were instrumental in helping me achieve my goal of writing and publishing this book.

And finally many thanks to all the PTA students who have inspired me to write this text. Without their enthusiasm and zest for learning I would never have started this endeavor.

Wendy D. Bircher, PT, EdD
Director, Physical Therapist Assistant Program
San Juan College
Farmington, NM

Leila Darress, PT, MHSA
Director, Physical Therapist Assistant Program
Indian River Community College
Fort Pierce, FL

James W. Farris, PT, PhD
Associate Professor, Physical Therapy Program
Arkansas State University
Jonesboro, AR

Diana N. Ploeger, PT, MEd
Coordinator and Associate Professor, Physical
Therapist Assistant Program
Salt Lake Community College
Salt Lake City, UT

Pamela D. Ritzline, PT, EdD
Director and Assistant Professor, Physical
Therapist Assistant Program
University of Indianapolis
Greenwood, IN

Julie A. Toney, PT, MPH
Physical Therapy Program
University of Findlay and Promedica Health
System
Toledo, OH

Christopher H. Wise, PT, MS, OCS, FAAOMPT, MTC, ATC
Physical Therapy Department
Widener University
Chester, PA

Jane E. Worley, PT, MS
Director, Physical Therapist Assistant Program
Lake Superior College
Duluth, MN

CONTENTS

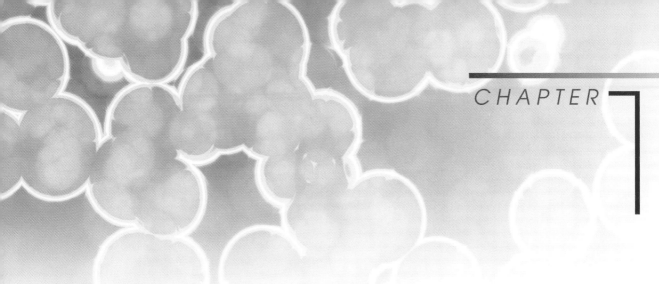

Inflammation and Healing

LEARNING OBJECTIVES

After completion of this chapter, students should be able to:

- Describe the anatomy and physiology of the cell.
- Describe the physiological mechanisms of injury at the cellular level, including necrosis and the inflammatory response.
- Describe the physiology of cellular and tissue repair.
- Identify the phases of wound healing.
- Explain the complications of wound healing.
- Analyze how physical therapy can be used to reduce inflammation and facilitate wound healing.
- Describe the healing process for bone, ligaments, tendons, and muscle.
- Discuss various pain-control theories.

CHAPTER OUTLINE

KEY TERMS

Acute on chronic inflammation
Adhesions
Autolytic débridement
Cardinal signs of inflammation
Débridement
Disuse atrophy
Edema
Endogenous opiates
Eschar
First intention healing
Gate Control Theory of pain
Granulation tissue
Heterotopic calcification/ ossification
Hypertrophic scarring
Ischemia
Keloid scarring
Palpation
Pus
Second intention healing

Introduction

In this first chapter, several basic concepts are introduced that are crucial to the knowledge base of the physical therapist assistant. Although these topics may seem unrelated to the study of pathology, they are nevertheless important as an introduction. Understanding the anatomy and physiology of the human body is required before studying pathology to make accurate comparisons between the normal and abnormal states. This chapter focuses on normal cell anatomy and physiology, cell injury, tissue injury, the process of inflammation, the healing of tissues, and the subject of pain. Inflammation is a key concept in physical therapy because all injuries—whether to cells, tissues, or body organs—result in the inflammatory process. Inflammation is a necessary initiator of the healing process, and pain is the product of both injury and inflammation. Thus, what at first may seem different topics are combined into a chapter that develops the basic concepts necessary to understanding the subject of pathology in the human body.

Why Does the Physical Therapist Assistant Need to Know About Normal Cell Anatomy and Physiology?

The physical therapist assistant (PTA) should be knowledgeable about normal cellular physiology and the effects of changes in that physiology. The PTA needs to be able to communicate knowledgeably and effectively with the physical therapist (PT), other health-care providers, and patients regarding the appearance of tissues and presenting signs and symptoms. Although selection of interventions is determined by the PT at the initial examination evaluation and reexamination, the PTA must be able to make decisions regarding ongoing therapy. If cellular and tissue changes occur which require intervention by the PT, then the PTA must know when to alert the supervising PT to these changes in patient status. If treatment is not effective, the PTA must know when to discuss this with the supervising PT and how to provide rationale for possible change of treatment. The PTA must also be familiar with the indications, contraindications, and precautions for the treatment of many pathological conditions. Effective patient care depends on the knowledge and expertise of all those providing treatment.

Normal Cell Anatomy and Physiology

Understanding the normal functions and cell structure of the healthy human body is an essential part of trying to understand pathology, or the abnormal state. Although the PT examines the patient and establishes the plan of care, the PTA must understand how the body reacts to certain stimuli at the cellular level to ensure use of the correct physical therapy intervention and facilitate the healing process. The following discussion of normal cell biology is merely a review for the PTA. For further information, the PTA should consult a physiology text.

Most cells within the human body have a nucleus and cytoplasm (Fig. 1-1) and are surrounded and contained within the plasma membrane (Fig. 1-2). The exceptions to this rule are mature red blood cells and platelets, which do not have a nucleus. Many cells in the body are specialized for specific functions but retain these common traits.

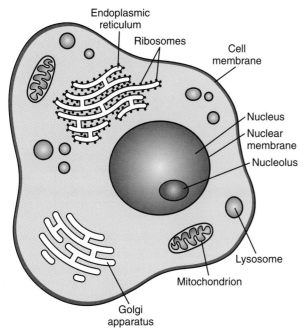

FIGURE 1.1 The cell.

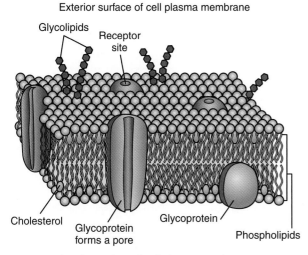

FIGURE 1.2 The cell plasma membrane.

Nucleus

The nucleus contains nucleic acids and nuclear proteins. Nucleic acids include deoxyribonucleic acid (DNA) and ribonucleic acid (RNA). Some types of RNA are found in the cytoplasm of the cell and some in the nucleolus or the nucleus, but DNA is located in the nucleus. DNA is aggregated with other proteins called histones, forming strands of chromatin. These histones are positively charged proteins that help bind the negatively charged DNA into smaller units that fit within the nucleus of the cell. The chromatin plays a role in strengthening DNA so that cell mitosis and meiosis can take place.[1] Several differences between DNA and RNA exist. RNA consists of a single-stranded helix, whereas DNA has a double-helix structure. The sugar in DNA is deoxyribose (no oxygen molecule), and that of RNA is ribose. Both DNA and RNA are composed of any of five nitrogen bases. Two are the purines adenine and guanine, and three are the pyrimidines thymine, cytosine, and uracil. Of the five, only uracil is specific to RNA. The molecules of RNA are smaller than those of DNA and are found in the cytoplasm of the cell. Functionally, DNA acts as the store house for genetic information. The function of RNA depends on its type. Of the many types of RNA, three of the most important are ribosomal RNA (rRNA), messenger RNA (mRNA), and transfer RNA (tRNA).[2] Ribosomal RNA (rRNA) is found in the cytoplasm of the cell within the ribosomes where synthesis of proteins occurs. The ribosomes actually consist of approximately 60% rRNA, and the other 40% is protein. Messenger RNA (mRNA) is a nucleic acid that acts as a messenger service taking information from the DNA to the ribosomes. Transfer RNA (tRNA) is a transport system that takes amino acids to the ribosomes for the development of proteins.[3] A special organelle exists within the nucleus called a nucleolus, which is the location of the synthesis of three of the types of RNA.[4]

During mitosis, when cells divide, the chromatin changes into chromosomes. DNA is the library of genetic material that is unique for each individual person. This genetic material is altered within each organ to enable differing body functions. Although the genetic material in cells within the kidney will be the same as that within a strand of hair, the functions of the cells in each case are quite different.

Cytoplasm

Cytoplasm consists of a ground substance called hyaloplasm, which is composed mainly of water. All cells within the body contain cytoplasm in varying amounts. More cytoplasm is present in mature cells than in embryonic or tumor cells. The higher the degree of specialization of the cell, such as those in the liver, the higher the cytoplasmic content of the cell, and the greater the number of organelles within the cytoplasm. Organelles contained within the cytoplasm include mitochondria, endoplasmic reticulum (ER), ribosomes, the Golgi apparatus, and lysosomes (Table 1-1). In muscle, there are other specialized organelles, such as the myofilaments of myosin and actin. A plasma membrane (outer wall of the cell) surrounds the cytoplasm of each cell.

Plasma Membrane

The plasma membrane is composed of a mixture of proteins, lipids, and carbohydrates. The inner surface of the cell is continuous with the ER. The outer surface of the cell may have cilia, projections through the cell membrane that enable certain specialized cells, such as those lining the respiratory system to move secretions or cells such as sperm. The plasma membrane protects the cell and acts as the medium through which the cell reacts to its environment (refer to Fig. 1-1).

Under normal circumstances, the cell is in a state of homeostasis (equilibrium) with its environment. This means that the cell's oxygen needs are met, and waste products are excreted from the cell. This state of homeostasis depends on the correct balance of minerals, such as sodium, potassium, calcium, and iron, within the cell, which are essential for normal cell health. When this state of homeostasis is challenged, the cell responds in several ways. If the change is minimal, the cell will recover, but if the trauma to the cell is too great, the cell will necrose (die).

Cell Injury

Cells have the ability to adapt to changes in their environment. When a cell is exposed to a stimulus, changes, or

Table 1.1 Cytoplasmic Organelles and Their Functions

CYTOPLASMIC ORGANELLE	LOCATION	COMPONENTS	FUNCTION
Mitochondria	Cytoplasm; more prolific in highly specialized organs, such as kidney, liver, nerves; numbers in a cell vary from a few hundred to several thousand	Double membrane—inner membrane has folds of cristae	Main cell energy producers Energy produced is stored as Adenosine triphosphate (ATP) Aerobic cell respiration (requiring oxygen) Turn glucose into CO_2 and water through processes of glycolysis (breakdown of glucose into pyruvic acid) and oxidation of pyruvic acid into CO_2 and water
Endoplasmic reticulum (ER)	Between nuclear and cell membranes	Rough ER—ribosomes on its surface Smooth ER—no ribosomes	Transport system within the cell; eg, for proteins synthesized on rough ER and lipids by smooth ER
Ribosomes	Surface of rough ER Free floating in cytoplasm	Proteins and ribosomal RNA	Protein synthesis; turn information within the mRNA into polypeptides to produce energy
Golgi apparatus	Cytoplasm	Stacks of flat membranous sacs	Carbohydrate synthesis; processes proteins synthesized in the ER into carbohydrates; produces lysosomes
Lysosomes	Cytoplasm; round bodies produced by the Golgi apparatus	Single membrane structure; contain many enzymes such as proteases and lipases	Digestion of material ingested into the cell or of damaged tissue; "cleanup crew" (phagocytosis)

injury can be either reversible or irreversible. In the reversible type, the cell will usually recover from injury, but in the irreversible type, the cell will either experience apoptosis (programmed cell death) or necrosis (death). Depending on the extent of damage to the plasma membrane, repair may be possible, or necrosis of the cell may occur.

Cell Injury—Reversible

Reversible cell injury occurs when damage to the cell is mild or short in duration, in which case the cell can overcome the damage (see Fig. 1-3). Reversible cell injury may result from **hypoxia** (reduction of oxygen to the cell for brief periods of time) or anoxia (loss of oxygen). Such

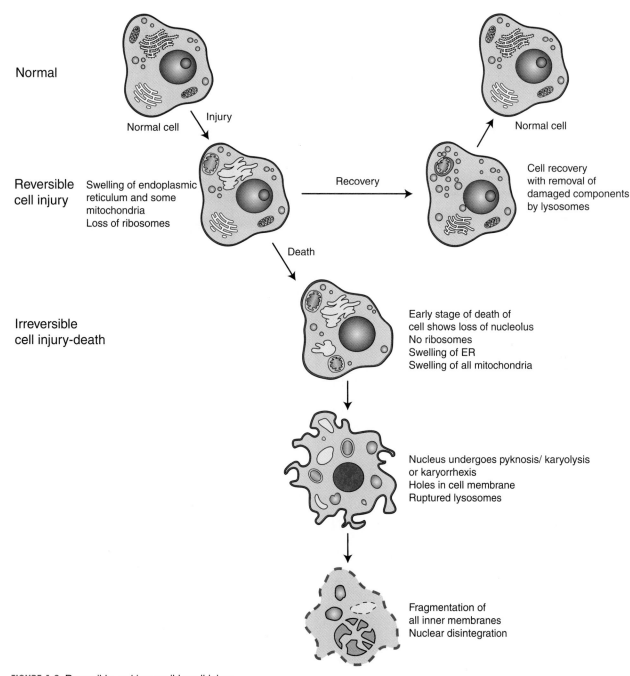

Normal

Normal cell

Injury

Reversible cell injury

Swelling of endoplasmic reticulum and some mitochondria
Loss of ribosomes

Recovery

Normal cell

Cell recovery with removal of damaged components by lysosomes

Death

Irreversible cell injury-death

Early stage of death of cell shows loss of nucleolus
No ribosomes
Swelling of ER
Swelling of all mitochondria

Nucleus undergoes pyknosis/ karyolysis or karyorrhexis
Holes in cell membrane
Ruptured lysosomes

Fragmentation of all inner membranes
Nuclear disintegration

FIGURE 1.3 Reversible and irreversible cell injury.

brief periods of reduction of oxygen result in **edema** (swelling) of the cytoplasm in the cell. Edema is caused by water passing into the cell through the selectively semipermeable cell membrane. When the oxygen supply to the cell is reduced, the normal pumping mechanism of the cell, which is performed by the enzyme adenosine triphosphatase (ATPase), is restricted. ATPase is a sodium/chloride pump and normally pumps sodium (Na+) ions out of the cell together with chloride (Cl–) ions to maintain an optimal cell environment (see Fig. 1-4). The normal concentration of Na+ and Cl– is lower inside than outside the cell, and the potassium levels are higher within the cell. When deprived of oxygen, the pump is disturbed, and Na+ and Cl– ions flood into the cell. Water then passes through the semipermeable plasma membrane into the cell, resulting in dilution of the concentration of these ions, which prevents severe damage to the cell. This engorgement of the cell causes changes in cell function, including lowered energy production by the mitochondria. The mitochondria also become swollen and begin to produce energy through

anaerobic (without oxygen) glycolysis, which produces lactic acid. The ER becomes damaged, and the nucleus has to muster its defenses to survive. When the nucleus remains intact, the cell will recover.

Examples of such reversible damage include some muscle injuries and, to a lesser degree, muscle fatigue. A muscle cramp results in a buildup of lactic acid in the muscle due to the process of anaerobic glycolysis in the muscle cells. The actual mechanism of a muscle cramp is unknown, but various theories include electrolytic imbalance, dehydration, mechanical issues, and interference with neural control. The muscle cells produce lactic acid in response to injury, and the buildup of lactic acid within the cell causes pain. The pain acts as a warning sign to the individual to protect the muscle and usually results in the prevention of irreversible cell damage.

Other types of reversible cell adaptation to stimuli occur that are desirable, such as hypertrophy, hyperplasia, and metaplasia. Hypertrophy of a muscle occurs in response to exercise. Atrophy is also a reversible cell adaptation in response to disuse. Some of the irreversible cell adaptations include anaplasia, dysplasia, dyscrasia, carcinoma in situ, and various types of necrosis. All of these are detailed in the following sections.

Cell Injury—Irreversible

All cells have a normal "shelf life," similar to products in a grocery store, which varies with the type of cell. This normal death of cells is due to a programmed death cycle called apoptosis. When a healthy cell is damaged beyond repair, necrosis occurs. Necrosis may occur as a result of major injury to cells caused by toxins, severe anoxia, or direct trauma, which damage the nucleus of the cell and cause the plasma membrane to rupture. The nucleus is essential for cell life, and without it the cell dies. Three types of nucleus damage are pyknosis, karyorrhexis, and karyolysis[5] (also see Fig. 1-5).

- **Pyknosis**—chromatin becomes condensed and shows on electromicroscopy as a dark area
- **Karyorrhexis**—fragmentation of the nucleus
- **Karyolysis**—nuclear structure dissolves

Table 1-2 displays several causes of cell injury and necrosis, including hypoxia, which occurs when cells are deprived of sufficient oxygen for short periods of time. If the cell is healthy prior to oxygen deprivation and is only deprived of oxygen for a short time, the cell or tissue may recover. However, recovery may not occur if the cell was not healthy initially. Anoxia is complete loss of oxygen to the tissues and results in the death of those cells or tissues

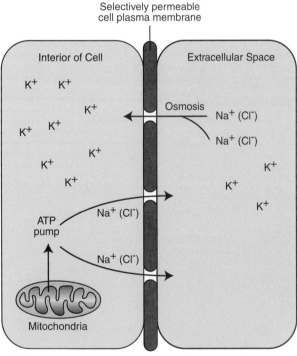

FIGURE 1.4 Sodium pump. Sodium ions (Na+) are higher in concentration in the extracellular spaces than in the cell. Thus, NA+ ions continually try to pass into the cell, together with chlorine ions (CL–), through the process of osmosis. Potassium ions (K+) are higher in concentration inside the cell. The sodium pump is driven by ATPase and shunts Na+ out of the cell to maintain homeostasis.

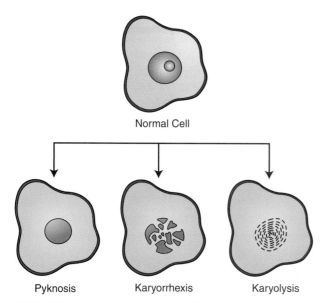

Normal Cell

Pyknosis   Karyorrhexis   Karyolysis

FIGURE 1.5 Pyknosis, karyorrhexis, and karyolysis.

if it occurs for more than a matter of a few minutes. **Ischemia,** or lack of blood supply to an area of tissue or part of an organ, can cause injury or cell death. In many cases, ischemic tissue is capable of recovery; in contrast, infarction is cell death, and no recovery is possible in these cells. Because blood supply is the means through which oxygen reaches the tissue, this has the same effect as anoxia. Toxicity is another factor in cell injury and occurs in many forms. Toxic effects in cells can be caused by high levels of toxic metals, such as lead or mercury; pathogens such as bacteria, viruses, or parasites; or toxic levels of chemicals, including medicines. In addition, toxicity can be caused by substances that the body needs to function normally, such as sodium and glucose if these substances are found in too high a concentration.

NECROSIS

Necrosis (death of cells) occurs naturally in apoptosis when cells die because they have reached the limit of their programmed life. Autolysis is the term used for disintegration of cells within a dead body or organism as a result of loss of respiration and thus oxygen to the tissues. Necrosis of cells in a living body is a response to abnormal stimuli. Knowledge of the types of necrosis is of importance to the PTA when working with wounds. Necrosis occurs in several forms, such as liquefactive, coagulative, caseous, and fat necrosis.

Liquefactive necrosis occurs when cells die and become liquid. Infarcts in the brain most often cause liquefaction of brain tissue, forming a cavity with a liquid center. This process is precipitated by leukocytes, which release lytic enzymes that break down the cells into liquid form to eliminate them. If the appearance of the liquid is yellow, it is called **pus.** Pus consists of leukocytes and dead cell debris.

Coagulative necrosis is so called because the cytoplasm has a coagulated appearance. The cells retain a clear outline, but their nuclei disintegrate. This often occurs in the heart in response to a myocardial infarct (MI) when the cells experience anoxia (lack of oxygen). Coagulative necrosis often becomes liquefactive.

Table 1.2   **Causes of Cell Injury**

CAUSE	MECHANISM	RESULT
Hypoxia	Reduced oxygen, eg, suffocation, pneumonia, anemia	Short periods—reversible damage Tissue dependent: heart cells more resilient than brain cells
Anoxia	Complete lack of oxygen	Prolonged—irreversible damage
Toxicity	Direct—heavy metals such as mercury Indirect—excessive amounts of certain drugs or chemical compounds that are inhaled and cause toxic substances to be formed inside the body	Death of cells if in large enough concentration; may be organ specific and depends on the dose/concentration of the substance taken
Pathogens—bacteria, viruses	Bacteria produce toxins Some are directly cytopathic	Toxins may kill cells in certain parts of the body
Ischemia	Loss of blood supply to an area	Death of cells due to lack of oxygen transfer from blood supply

Gangrene is the result of infected coagulative necrotic tissue (see Figure 1-6). The resulting inflammation causes a liquefactive process called wet gangrene. When this turns to a dry, blackened mass of necrotic tissue, it is known as dry gangrene. PTAs commonly see dry gangrene in the distal lower extremities of clients with peripheral vascular disease (PVD) and diabetes. The condition may also occur in the residual limb of the person with lower extremity amputation as a result of poor circulation.

Caseous necrosis is a type of coagulative necrosis that occurs in tuberculosis (TB). Patients with TB form granulomas in the lung (lumps or foci of granular material) in which the center of the granuloma becomes cheese-like in consistency (Latin: *caseum* = cheese).

Fat necrosis occurs in fat tissue due to special lipolytic enzymes that only act on fat. One of the most common examples occurs after a motor vehicle accident (MVA) in which the seat belt ruptures the pancreas, and the pancreatic enzymes degrade the adjacent fat into fatty acids and glycerol.

Dystrophic calcification is a process of hardening or calcification of necrotic tissues that occurs in arteries, heart valves, and certain tumors as a result of too much calcium production. Such calcification can also occur in cancer, in which case it is called metastatic calcification.

Heterotopic calcification, or heterotopic ossification, is the development of bone in areas where it is not normally found, such as in muscles and fascia. This may occur in cases of posttrauma, such as specific muscle trauma, traumatic brain injury, spinal cord injury, or following myocardial infarction (MI). Heterotopic calcification is most frequently found in muscles and soft tissue in the areas of the hip, knee, or shoulder.[6] The formation of bone within muscle results in reduced function of the structure involved.

Cellular Responses to Damage or Stimuli

Changes in cells of either reduction or increase in size or number occur as a result of external stimuli. Some of these changes are reversible, and others, such as metaplasia, are irreversible. Review Table 1-3 for a comparison of the various types of growth changes of cells.

ATROPHY

Atrophy is a reduction in the size of cells, resulting in a reduced size of tissue or organs (Fig. 1-7). The PTA is often concerned with muscle atrophy in clients due to

Table 1.3 **Types of Growth Changes of Cells**

TYPE	CHARACTERISTICS
Atrophy	Reduction in cell size
Hypertrophy	Increase in cell size
Hyperplasia	Increase in number of cells
Involution/hypoplasia	Decrease in number of cells
Metaplasia	Change of cell from one type to another

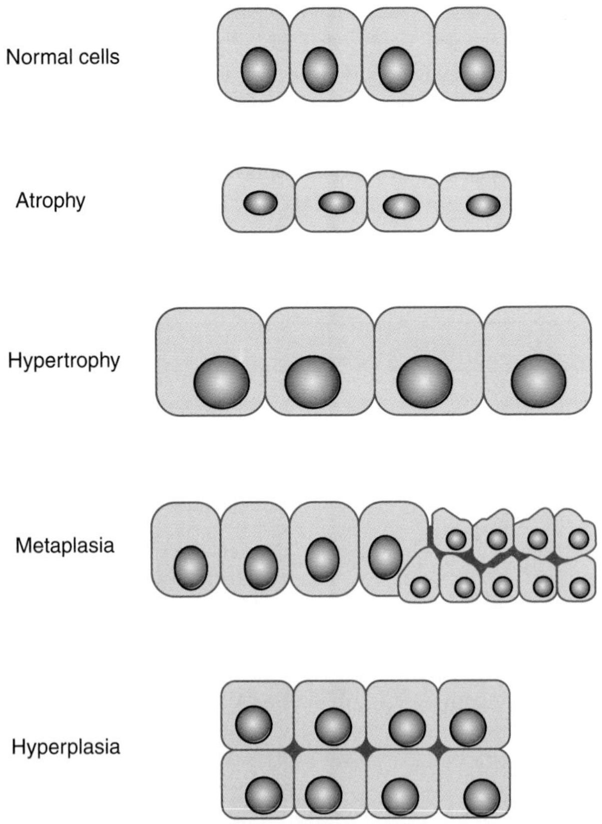

Normal cells

Atrophy

Hypertrophy

Metaplasia

Hyperplasia

FIGURE 1.7 Abnormal cellular growth patterns: atrophy, hypertrophy, hyperplasia, metaplasia.

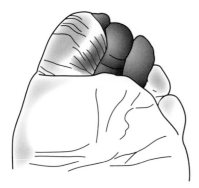

FIGURE 1.6 Gangrene of toes.

inactivity called **disuse atrophy.** Atrophy occurs after protracted periods of enforced immobilization, such as after a fracture or a prolonged illness. Disuse atrophy is usually reversible. The PTA assists clients to regain muscle strength, bulk, and endurance after these episodes of immobility or inactivity. Other types of atrophy include physiological aging of the brain, which results in reduced size, and osteoporosis of the bones. Pathological atrophy occurs because of lack of nutrition as in cancer or malnutrition. Senile dementia is a form of brain cell atrophy. In many cases, the pathological types of atrophy may not be reversible.

HYPERTROPHY

Hypertrophy is an increase in the size of the individual cells, resulting in an increased size of tissues and organs. An example is hypertrophy of the left ventricle of the heart in response to hypertension (high blood pressure). Heart striated muscle cells are unable to divide, so they respond to the need to work harder by increasing in size. This increase in individual cell size increases the overall size of the heart.

HYPERPLASIA

Hyperplasia is an increase in the number of cells within a tissue or organ. An example includes male benign prostate disease (benign fibroadenoma), in which the walls of the prostate gland hypertrophy and cause restriction of the ureter with associated interference with micturition (passing urine). Other examples include hyperplasia of the uterus during pregnancy caused by hormonal changes and hyperplasia of a kidney in response to surgical removal or disease of the other kidney. Hyperplasia also occurs as a result of friction on the skin, which produces calluses and corns. Hyperplastic polyps within the intestine are common with no known etiology (cause), but these can become neoplastic (cancerous) and are usually surgically removed as a precaution.

INVOLUTION AND HYPOPLASIA

Involution and hypoplasia are both names for a reduction in the number of cells within a tissue or organ. However, involution usually refers to the return to normal size of an organ, as when the uterus returns to normal size after delivery of a baby, and also pertains to the process of infolding of structures during fetal development to form such structures as the bladder and other hollow organs. In contrast, hypoplasia more often refers to the abnormal reduction in size of an organ that occurs as an abnormality of the developmental process of the fetus.

METAPLASIA

In metaplasia, cells change from one type into another. For example, the columnar cells of the bronchial mucosa of the respiratory system change into stratified squamous epithelium cells in response to smoke irritation in the bronchi. Another example of metaplasia is the transition within tissue that takes place when a tendon graft is used to replace the anterior cruciate ligament. Over time, the graft tissue takes on the histological properties of a ligament rather than the original tendon.[7–8]

When tissue becomes cancerous, as in carcinoma in situ, the changes in cells lead to loss of function of the tissue, which is referred to as anaplasia, rather than metaplasia. Another term applied to tissue changes is dysplasia in which the tissue develops abnormally in utero. The term dyscrasia is sometimes used to indicate disease, especially as in plasma cell dyscrasias such as multiple myeloma, amyloidosis, and other immune or blood diseases.[9]

Why Does the Physical Therapist Assistant Need to Know About Inflammation?

The treatment of inflammation is basic to physical therapy. All injuries and illnesses cause inflammation of body cells, tissues, and organs. Because the PTA works with people with inflammation resulting from many diseases and injuries, a detailed knowledge of the inflammatory process is essential to understanding the treatment interventions provided at each stage of inflammation. A sound knowledge of the basics also is essential to be able to speak knowledgeably to the PT and the physician. Knowledge of the basic principles of inflammation also helps when explaining to patients the reasons for the advice and treatment to gain compliance with a home program of management and exercises.

Inflammation

Inflammation is the body's response to injury. Short-term inflammation is both necessary and desirable after injury because it promotes healing of tissues and allows the return of the tissue to the normal state of homeostasis. Any living tissue in the body will react in a typical way to injury with the four **cardinal signs of inflammation:** heat (Latin: *calor*), redness (*rubor*), swelling (*tumor*), and pain (*dolor*). These cardinal signs have been recognized since Roman times when Celsus, a Roman physician, wrote about them.[10] In physical therapy, five cardinal signs of inflammation are referred to, with the addition of loss of function of the tissue. The inflammatory response acts both to isolate the injured area and to resolve the problem. Inflammation can be acute or chronic. Additionally, in rehabilitation, **acute on chronic**

inflammation is frequently seen, which is an acute injury superimposed on a preexisting chronic state of inflammation. Acute inflammation is of sudden onset and short duration. When this process continues for more than a short time, it becomes chronic inflammation, which can last for considerable periods, up to months or even years. Acute on chronic inflammation is often seen in ankle sprains. When an ankle is sprained and healing is not complete, a state of chronic inflammation exists. When a further sprain occurs, the inflammatory process starts again, and acute inflammation is added to the already chronic inflammatory state of the ankle. The mechanisms of inflammation are complicated but are important for the PTA to understand because of the implications for physical therapy intervention.

Causes of the Inflammatory Response

Causes of the inflammatory response are varied. Skin abrasions; burns; cuts; trauma from direct blows or accidents; sunburn; chemical burns; infective organisms such as bacteria, viruses, fungi, and protozoa; chemicals including medicines; and foreign bodies are all possible initiators of inflammation.

When tissue such as skin is damaged, the mast cells and platelets release chemicals that affect the surrounding tissues. Histamine, bradykinin, serotonin, and prostaglandins are some of these chemical mediators of inflammation. Histamine is a protein released by damaged platelets, basophils, and mast cells[11] within seconds of tissue damage. First, however, an immediate *vasoconstriction* of the tissue is noted, sometimes as an area of lighter colored skin, due to lack of blood in the immediate area, and then a weal (red mark) starts to appear as the result of histamine release. Histamine causes transudation, increased blood vessel permeability that allows blood cells and fluid to leak into the extracellular and interstitial spaces. As a result of transudation, *vasodilation* occurs, the red effect and edema (swelling) of the skin. The effect of histamine lasts for about 30 minutes because the cells quickly produce histaminase, which neutralizes the histamine and helps to prevent extensive tissue damage. The release of fluids into the interstitial spaces causes edema. The effects of this histamine-mediated inflammation are hyperemia (redness or rubor), edema (swelling or tumor), and mild warmth (calor).[12]

Following this initial phase of inflammation, congestion of the dilated vessels occurs due to slowing of blood flow, which results in erythrocytes forming rouleaux or stacks. White cells attach to the epithelium, causing a pavementing effect and, in combination with the action of the platelets, produce clotting. Bradykinin is a plasma protein with similar effects to those of histamine, including vasodilation of blood vessels,[13] but it reacts more slowly, hence the term bradykinin (Greek: *brady* = slow). Bradykinin prolongs the inflammatory response and causes pain, the fourth cardinal sign of inflammation. The roles of cytokines and fibrin are described in the sections on healing and immunopathology.

CELLS INVOLVED IN THE INFLAMMATORY RESPONSE

Increased permeability of the blood vessel walls secondary to the inflammatory response can last several days. The transudate, mainly composed of water and a few blood cells, collects in the extracellular and interstitial spaces, causing edema.[14,15] Another process occurs called diapedesis in which cells cross the vessel walls into the affected tissue, forming an exudate that, unlike transudate, is rich in protein and inflammatory cells. Most of the cells initially contained in exudate are polymorphonuclear leucocytes (PMNs) closely followed by eosinophils, and after about 48 hours, monocytes, macrophages, platelets, basophils, lymphocytes, and plasma cells appear (see Table 1-4). Exudate can be of various consistencies, including serous (watery) as in burns, fibrinous with a thick, gluelike consistency, purulent (containing pus), or hemorrhagic (containing blood).[16]

Polymorphonucleocytes

Polymorphonucleocytes, or polymorphonuclear leucocytes (PMNs), also known as neutrophils, are white blood cells with multiple segmented nuclei, which are mobile and phagocytic (amoeba-like) and ingest the bacteria and cell debris in the area of the inflammation (Fig. 1-8). PMNs release proteins called cytokines, which increase the inflammatory response. Cytokines stimulate the hypothalamus and cause systemic effects such as fever. The PMNs only last about 2 to 4 days and are thus part of the acute phase of inflammation.

Eosinophils

Eosinophils are white blood cells (leukocytes), which are so called because they stain pink with eosin. These cells appear approximately 2 to 3 days after the PMNs. Eosinophils are mobile but slower moving than PMNs and are phagocytic, bacteriocidal (kill bacteria chemically), and have a single nucleus with two lobes.[17] Eosinophils contain chemicals that are toxic to bacteria and parasites. These cells are present in respiratory allergic reactions such as asthma and can also be found in chronic inflammation.

Monocytes and Macrophages

Monocytes are white blood cells produced by the myeloid stem cells, which are precursors of macrophages. After these cells are approximately 24 hours old, they mature

Table 1.4 **Cells of Inflammation**

CELL TYPE	DESCRIPTION	FUNCTION
Polymorphonucleocytes (PMNs; also known as neutrophils)	White blood cells Multiple segmented nuclei Mobile cells—amoeba-like Only live approximately 2 days and thus are part of acute inflammatory response	Phagocytic—ingest cell debris/foreign material from injured site Migrate to area of injury to engulf debris Release cytokines, which stimulate a systemic response of fever by affecting the hypothalamus
Eosinophils	White blood cells Mobile—slower moving than PMNs and arrive at inflammation site 2–3 days after PMNs Single nucleus Present in chronic inflammation	Phagocytic Bacteriocidal—give off chemicals that kill bacteria and parasites
Monocytes	White blood cells Precursors to macrophages	Develop into macrophages
Macrophages (histiocytes)	White blood cells Differentiated from monocytes	Phagocytic
Platelets (thrombocytes)	Fragments of cytoplasm	Release serotonin at site of damaged tissue which causes vasoconstriction of the damaged blood vessels Form rouleaux which help in blood clotting mechanism Release histamine and plasma proteins that facilitate clotting
Basophils	White blood cells	Precursors of mast cells Contain histamine which is released during inflammatory response

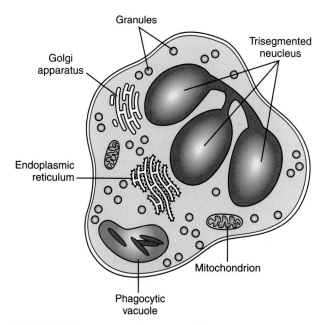

FIGURE 1.8 Polymorphonuclear neutrophils.

Labels: Granules, Golgi apparatus, Endoplasmic reticulum, Phagocytic vacuole, Trisegmented neucleus, Mitochondrion

into macrophages[18] and enter various tissues of the body. Macrophages or histiocytes are larger than PMNs and are also phagocytes. They are the main scavenger cells of the immune system.[19] The macrophages arrive at the inflammation site around Day 4, and because these cells live a long time, they are present in chronic inflammation. The macrophages produce cytokines, which in turn stimulate an increase in the inflammatory response.

Platelets

Platelets, or thrombocytes, are fragments of cells produced in bone marrow[20] from cells called megakaryocytes.[21] They circulate in the blood system for about 10 days and are not true cells because they have no nucleus. Platelets release platelet factor, which starts the clotting process of blood and the formation of connective tissue essential for the healing process. The release of serotonin by the platelets adds to this clotting mechanism by causing vasoconstriction of damaged blood vessels that helps to seal the damaged blood vessels and thus reduce blood loss (see Chapter 2 for further details). Platelets are active components of inflammation, appearing especially in the first phases.

Basophils

Basophils are white blood cells that play a part in chronic inflammation. They are the precursors of mast cells and produce histamine and platelet activating factor in the immune response.[22]

Lymphocytes and Plasma Cells

Lymphocytes and plasma cells play a part mainly in chronic inflammation; more important, they serve as part of the immune system. Both of these cell types are described in Chapter 2.

Classification of Inflammation

As briefly discussed earlier in this chapter, inflammation may be subdivided into different categories, including acute, subacute, chronic, and acute on chronic. In addition, the difference between transudate and exudate should be understood. Transudate is a watery fluid that can build up in the tissues, especially in extracellular spaces, as a result of fluid passing through the cell membranes of the blood vessels in response to changes in pressure gradients. This occurs secondary to hypertension, which causes an increase in hydrostatic pressure across the blood vessel walls, and there is a leakage of water and perhaps a few proteins and cells from the vessels into the surrounding tissues. However, hypertension does not change the selective permeability of the vessel walls, and therefore most cells are unable to pass through. Transudate can create edema of the tissues. In contrast, exudate is the fluid buildup that occurs as a result of the inflammatory process. Exudate also can cause edema but consists of water, proteins, and many of the cells of inflammation previously described. The inflammatory process changes the selective permeability of the vessel walls, resulting in passage of the inflammatory cells into the interstitial and extracellular spaces. Several types of inflammation are detailed in Table 1-5.

ACUTE INFLAMMATION

Acute inflammation lasts anywhere from a few hours to several days.[23] In some cases, the area affected remains hot or warm to **palpation** (touch) for several days. This heat may subside somewhat, and the injury is then termed subacute inflammation. Acute inflammation may also reoccur. The presence of acute inflammation is at least a precaution and usually a contraindication for most physical therapy interventions. During this phase, active exercise, most electrical stimulation techniques, ultrasound, and other heat modalities are contraindicated. The exception to this rule may be interferential electrical stimulation.

SUBACUTE INFLAMMATION

The term "subacute inflammation" is sometimes used to refer to the phase of inflammation that starts after resolution of the immediate acute inflammation, in most cases during the first 24 hours postinjury. However, the subacute phase can last from a few hours to several weeks and may or may not turn into chronic inflammation. This subacute phase is actually part of the acute phase. Sometimes the inflammation subsides during this phase when factors that caused the inflammation are removed or resolved. In this stage, there may still be some heat, erythema, and edema in the area of injury, but it will have subsided from the acute phase. This phase is of importance to the PTA because at this point modalities and PT intervention can be initiated. After the extreme heat, pain, and edema begin to subside, the PT and PTA can start to provide modalities to further reduce the effects of the inflammatory process.

CHRONIC INFLAMMATION

Chronic inflammation can be a sequel to the acute and subacute phases, occur as a result of prolonged healing of the acute and subacute stages, or be chronic from the onset. Tuberculosis (TB) is considered a chronic inflammatory condition from the onset. If the inflammation does not resolve within a few days, the tissue is considered to be in a chronic inflammatory state. In certain cases in which the inflammation subsides during the subacute phase, there may not be a chronic inflammatory phase. In other cases, there may not be an acute phase. The initial injury may not be severe enough to produce an acute response. If a low-grade irritant is present, then the area may go straight into a chronic inflammatory response. Problems that occur due to chronic inflammation have implications for physical therapy interventions. Chronic inflammation is more likely to result in considerable scar tissue within the connective tissues[24] and interferes with the function of the tissue involved. The role of physical therapy intervention in such cases is to reduce the amount of scar tissue formation and improve the function of the area. Interventions such as heat modalities, ultrasound, electrical stimulation, active range of motion and isometric exercises, massage, and mobilization can help improve tissue, joint, and muscle function during rehabilitation after injury.

ACUTE ON CHRONIC INFLAMMATION

In physical therapy, a pattern of acute on chronic inflammation is often observed. Acute on chronic inflammation occurs when an injury never fully heals and the area is

Table 1.5 **Types of Inflammation**

TYPE	EXAMPLES	CHARACTERISTICS
Serous	Burns Skin paper cuts Skin abrasions	Clear fluid exudate containing few inflammatory cells as seen in a blister after a burn
Fibrinous	Bacterial pneumonia Strep throat	Exudate contains a lot of fibrin

Purulent	Streptococcal infections
	Abscesses
	   Sinus
	   Fistula
	   Empyema
		Pus producing areas of inflammation
		Infection usually indicated by yellow or greenish exudate
		Abscesses localized within a tissue or organ
		Abscess may have a sinus—a cavity that drains to the surface of the body, allowing the pus to drain from the infected abscess
		Fistula may form—abnormal cavity or tunnel that forms joining together two previously existing cavities or connecting a hollow organ with the skin surface
		Empyema—accumulation of pus in a cavity

Ulcerative	Diabetic skin ulcers on lower extremities secondary to peripheral vascular disease, causing poor circulation Intestinal and stomach ulcers	Local areas of skin ulceration (wounds) usually on the lower extremities; usually in persons with peripheral vascular disease or diabetes Ulcers may occur on the epithelial linings of the stomach or small or large intestines
Pseudomembranous	Diphtheria Colitis	Inflamed areas in bronchi that become covered with a membrane that can close off the bronchi and produce suffocation if not treated Pseudomembranous inflammation of the colon
Granulomatous	Sarcoidosis in lungs Syphilis TB lungs	Granulomas formed within selective tissue. Walled off, encapsulated areas of inflammatory tissue In tuberculosis, these granulomas may show up on chest X-ray as an area of white, dense matter within the lung tissue; these tuberculosis granulomas may remain in the lung indefinitely, but if they remain encapsulated, they are not dangerous

reinjured. Acute on chronic inflammation also occurs in chronic inflammatory diseases when an acute exacerbation takes place. Other examples include acute respiratory infections in a person with a chronic lung disease, acute exacerbations of chronic diseases such as multiple sclerosis, and cases of low back pain in which the original injury has not healed correctly or fully and an additional injury produces an acute inflammatory response in addition to the chronic problem. Another example is a sprained ankle in which the ligaments and tendons are not fully healed, adhesions are present, and the ankle is resprained, resulting in an acute response superimposed on the chronically inflamed state of the ankle tissue. One

of the major factors in the resprain of ankles arises from adhesion formation in the tissues secondary to the original injury that are susceptible to reinjury. One aim of PT intervention is therefore to minimize the formation of adhesions during intervention for the original injury.

Physical Therapy Treatment for Inflammation

The inflammatory process occurs with all injuries and open wounds. The following physical therapy intervention is described for closed injuries only. Interventions for open wounds are described later in this chapter.

Some simple rules apply when dealing with a part of the body that is inflamed. *If it is hot, cool it down. If it is cool, heat it up. Never* heat an area that is already hot. This could cause a drastic increase in temperature and lead to irreversible tissue damage. The general adage is to use ice in the first 24 hours (acute stage) after injury, but if the area remains hot or warm to the touch, it is acceptable to continue to use ice on the area. A study by Bleakley et al in 2004 showed that there is insufficient evidence-based research to conclude the efficacy of the use of ice. The use of ice is according to experience and anecdotal evidence of practice.[25] Some people do, however, respond better to ice than heat at all stages of their recovery. Because ultrasound produces thermal effects, it is contraindicated for acute inflammation. Interferential therapy, but no other form of electrical stimulation, may be used to treat an acute area. If asked whether it is safe to use electrical stimulation on an acute joint or injury, it is always safest to say no and then qualify it with the possibility of interferential therapy. The acronym RICE is used for inflammation management meaning <u>R</u>est, <u>I</u>ce, <u>C</u>ompression, and <u>E</u>levation. Rest allows the body's healing processes to occur and relieves pain. In a weight-bearing limb, this means no weight bearing, and in an upper extremity, this could mean using a sling to rest the injured arm. In severe cases such as fracture, a cast may be used; a splinting device can be used for a bad sprain. Ice helps to reduce pain and edema, compression controls edema, and elevation assists with edema control and may reduce pain as well as stimulate venous and lymphatic drainage.

In the subacute phase, after the first 24 hours, if the area is not warm to the touch with erythema (red in appearance), then physical therapy may include such modalities as electrical stimulation for edema reduction, pain control and reduction of inflammation, nonthermal ultrasound to stimulate the healing process, and gentle active range of motion exercises as tolerated by the patient. If the area affected remains warm to the touch with an erythema, continue to apply cold packs to the area.

If the chronic stage of inflammation develops, types of PT intervention can include any modality such as electrical stimulation to stimulate healing and reduce pain; ultrasound to break down scar tissue, mobilize tissue, and reduce pain; and exercise as appropriate. Transverse friction massage may also be necessary to mobilize the area and release scar tissue to improve function. This is not an all-inclusive list of interventions. Consult a physical modalities textbook to determine the parameters for electrical stimulation and ultrasound suitable for specific conditions.

Why Does the Physical Therapist Assistant Need to Know About the Healing Process?

The process of healing is necessary for all types of pathological conditions to return the human body to functional levels. Encouraging and enhancing the normal physiological healing process is one of the main aims of physical therapy interventions. Without an understanding of the stages of healing of body tissues, the PTA cannot relate to specific physical therapy interventions that can enhance the healing process and return patients to their fully functional capacity. The ability to identify delays in the healing process also assists the PTA in appropriate communication with the supervising PT and physician.

A large part of physical therapy practice is involved with stimulating the healing process of body tissues. Whether damage to tissues results from disease, injury, illness, or surgery, the PTA will work with many people who have tissue injury. An understanding of the normal and complex process of tissue healing is essential to determine which physical therapy interventions are appropriate at a particular stage of tissue healing. Recognizing when the healing process has been compromised is also important so that specific physical therapy interventions can be used to stimulate the healing process.

Healing

HINTS ON THE USE OF THE GUIDE TO PHYSICAL THERAPIST PRACTICE (1-1)

Skin wounds fall within various areas of the *Guide to Physical Therapist Practice*

Preferred Practice Pattern: "Integumentary" 7.

- 7A practice pattern, "primary prevention/risk reduction for integumentary disorders" (p. 589): patients at risk for developing skin wounds due to factors such as reduced skin sensation or reduced physical activity
- 7B "impaired integumentary integrity associated with superficial skin involvement" (p. 601): patients with Stage 2 pressure ulcers, superficial burns, and vascular disease due to venous or arterial insufficiency and diabetes

- 7C "impaired integumentary integrity associated with partial-thickness skin involvement and scar formation" (p. 619): if skin involvement is more extensive, as in partial thickness burns, Stage 2 pressure ulcers, surgical wounds, among others

- 7D "impaired integumentary integrity associated with full-thickness skin involvement and scar formation" (p. 637): patients with full-thickness skin lesions such as frostbite, burns, vascular ulcers, and Stage 3 pressure ulcers

- 7E "impaired integumentary integrity associated with skin involvement extending into fascia, muscle, or bone and scar formation" (p. 655): patients with problems that extend deeper than the skin into the muscle, fascia, and bone

Remember that patients may have other comorbid conditions that place them in other practice patterns such as those involved with cardiac or musculoskeletal conditions.

(From the American Physical Therapy Association, 2003. *Guide to physical therapist practice*, revised 2nd edition. Alexandria, VA: APTA. Used with permission.)

Wound healing is classified into two categories.[26] **First intention** (or primary intention) **healing**[27] is healing of a clinical or surgical wound or of a skin-penetrating injury with clear, clean margins that have not become separated or that can be closed using sutures, staples, or Steristrips. Examples of such wounds might be a knife or paper cut. **Second intention healing** is delayed healing of a surgical wound or healing of a nonsurgical wound. Second intention healing can also include healing of a wound that has a loss of skin or where the subcutaneous tissue has been exposed too long to enable closing of the wound through use of stitches, staples, or Steristrips. Wounds in which there is loss of a significant amount of tissue also fall within this category. This method also covers the healing of venous stasis ulcers and pressure ulcers. Healing takes place as the result of the inflammatory process. Some wounds may never heal, whereas others heal quickly. Many factors are involved in determining the rate of healing of a wound. Understanding which cells assist in healing and what their individual functions are in relation to the process is important for the PTA. Some areas of the body, such as the skin, heal quickly. Tissues of the heart and brain were once thought to be unable to regenerate, but recent findings suggest that new tissue starts to generate in the areas of loss and revascularization of tissue occurs in cases of ischemia.[28,29] With the

recent scientific work with stem cells, the possibilities of renewal of tissues in the heart, brain, and spinal cord are even more encouraging.[30,31] However, if there is necrosis of heart or neuronal cells, there is likely to be permanent damage to these structures, resulting in varying degrees of loss of function depending on the location and extent of the injury.

Cells Involved in the Healing Process

Some of the key cells involved in the healing process include leucocytes (PMNs), myofibroblasts-angioblasts, and fibroblasts. As described earlier in the chapter, the PMNs play a role in the initial phases of healing. PMNs are among the first cells to arrive at the injury site to start the cleanup of damaged cells. PMNs live for a few days at the most, and then the macrophages take over. These macrophages are present both in chronic inflammation and in the healing wound. The macrophages produce chemicals such as cytokines that stimulate the healing process by acting on the myofibroblasts, fibroblasts, and angioblasts. In bone healing, the PMNs also stimulate the osteoblasts.[32]

MYOFIBROBLASTS

Myofibroblasts are cells with a mixture of properties similar to those of smooth muscle cells (myo) and fibroblasts. Because the cells have similar contractile properties to those of muscle, they play a part in the contraction of the wound during the initial phases of healing. This holds the wound together and allows a network of epithelial cells to gather and cover the affected area.

ANGIOBLASTS

Angioblasts are precursors of blood vessels. These cells enable the macrophages and other phagocytic cells to reach the wound and remove necrotic tissue, such as the scab. In a larger open wound, they form a red dotted effect in the wound bed called **granulation tissue** (see Fig. 1-9). The appearance of granulation tissue in the base of a wound indicates that the wound is healthy and healing.

FIBROBLASTS

Fibroblasts produce fibrin and collagen (fibronectin). The fibrin acts as a sticky mesh across the wound to bind the cells together, forming a network of fibers across the wound and holding the entire wound together. Collagen is the basic structure of the network that forms across the wound to strengthen the healing area and is known as connective tissue. Collagen is composed of protein molecules and is found throughout the body in all tissues and organs. Many types of collagen exist, but four main types are of significance in physical therapy: Types I through IV.[33]

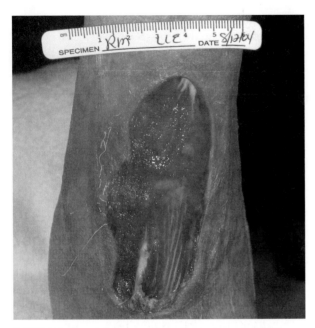

FIGURE 1.9 Granulation tissue in the base of a wound. From Sussman, C., & Bates-Jensen, B. M. (2001). *Wound care: a collaborative practice manual for physical therapists and nurses,* 2nd edition. Gaithersburg, MD: Aspen, Plate 8, color plate p. 3. Reproduced with permission.

Each type of collagen serves a different purpose (see Table 1-6). Normal skin contains a lot of both Type I and Type III collagen, giving it elasticity and strength. The proportions of types of collagen in skin change over the life span.[34] In most cases, normal tissue is composed of several types of collagen fibers, the Type I fibers providing tensile strength to skin, and the Type III giving it the resistance to friction. The first type to form in the wound is similar to Type III collagen. Type III collagen contains thin strands, which give body tissues strength and flexibility. Type III collagen forms the initial scar tissue of a wound. This collagen is the one that provides a network of fibers across the wound to support the underlying healing blood vessels and cells. As the wound matures, the Type III collagen is replaced by Type I collagen. Type I collagen forms the scar tissue, which replaces the original skin. Type I collagen is fairly strong but lacks the elasticity of the original skin.[35,36]

Types of Healing

Healing takes place in one of two ways, either through the process of regeneration of tissue that was minimally damaged or a process of repair in which the original tissue is replaced with scar tissue. In reversible cell injury, as previously described, the process of healing is through regeneration. The cells recover and are replaced with cells of the same type that were damaged. This process is achieved through cell mitosis of the involved organ or tissue.

Irreversible cell injury in most tissues and organs results in repair with fibrous connective tissue. In this process, tissues that have undergone necrosis are replaced by tissue that is not the same as the original tissue. When replaced in this way, there is a loss of function of the tissue because the cells no longer have the functional properties of the ones they replace, and the result is a fibrosis. Cirrhosis of the liver is an example of fibrosis. This replacement of original tissue by fibrotic connective tissue

Table 1.6 **Types of Collagen**

TYPE	STRUCTURE	LOCATION	FUNCTION
Type I	A thick bundle of protein fibers that mixes with other types of collagen	Tendons, bones, mature scar tissue	Provides strength
Type II	Thin filaments	Cartilage	Flexibility and strength
Type III	Thin filaments with cross-bridges of disulfide molecules	Wound healing in initial scarring Skin and blood vessels	Supports the developing blood vessels in the base of a wound in initial stages of healing Pliability and strength
Type IV	Protein mass not fibers	Basement membranes throughout the body	Provides an attachment for the cells of epithelium and endothelium when mixed with other proteins

is called scarring. Scar tissue is never as strong as the original tissue and remains a weak area throughout a person's life. When scar tissue is fully formed, it has approximately 70% to 80% of the strength of the original tissue[37,38] and has a good blood supply.[39] Skin wounds are commonly treated in physical therapy and follow two types of healing as previously described: namely, fibrous connective tissue repair or regeneration. In addition, a surgical wound usually heals by first intention if no complicating factors are present. If complicating factors exist, healing will take place through second intention.

In fibrous connective tissue repair, a specific sequence of events occurs that leads to scarring of the area involved (see Fig. 1-10). This scar tissue, or fibrosis, has a different appearance and function to that of the original tissue. When damage to tissue is too extensive to allow for first intention healing, the sequence of repair in this healing by second intention through fibrous connective tissue repair is as follows:

1. **Contraction of the wound (proliferative phase)**
   In the proliferative phase, contraction of the wound is an attempt to make the wound smaller and minimize the effect of the wound. Myofibroblasts, stimulated by chemicals such as bradykinins and epinephrine,[40] gather around the wound and cause shrinking of the edges of the wound in much the same way as when the strings of a jewelry pouch are pulled to close the bag.

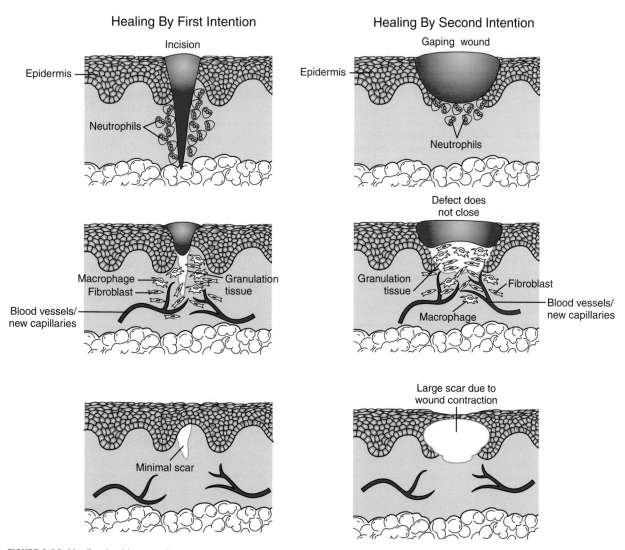

FIGURE 1.10 Healing in skin wounds.

During this contraction process, the phagocytes, especially macrophages, remove necrotic tissue from the area of the wound. A scab forms over the open wound due to the coagulation of blood seeping from the wound. This scab is part of the necrotic tissue eventually removed by the macrophages; however, the formation of granulation tissue occurs beneath the protection of this scab. The scab prevents dehydration of the wound bed, keeping the environment moist for healing to take place. The scab also helps to protect the granulation tissue in the wound from damage due to friction or trauma.

2. **Formation of granulation tissue (part of the proliferative phase)**

   When the wound is clean, granulation tissue in the form of fibronectin is formed from fibrin present in the exudate, myofibroblasts, and the newly contracting tissue.[41] Blood vessels start to grow beneath the wound and produce buds protruding into the wound bed, which become the base of the granulation tissue. This tissue is delicate and easily damaged. Protection of the wound at this stage is important.

3. **Organization**

   Organization of the tissue then occurs due to the action of fibroblasts. Deposition of fibrin occurs throughout the wound, which leads to the next phase of healing.

4. **Scar tissue**

   Scar tissue is the result of the healing process. Scar tissue consists mainly of Type III collagen fibers produced by the fibroblasts, which gradually turn into Type I collagen fibers over time. The bed of granulation tissue provides the nutrition for this network of collagen.

5. **Remodeling of the scar tissue (maturation phase)**

   Remodeling of the scar tissue takes place in the final maturation phase of healing. During this phase, the wound loses its red appearance and becomes visually more like the original tissue, even though it does not have the same structure. The fibrous tissue scar can take up to 18 months to become fully healed.[42]

First intention healing follows the same phases as second intention healing. The total process takes between 3 and 6 weeks; however, initial closing of the wound occurs within 7 to 10 days. The advantage of a first intention healed wound is that there is minimal scar tissue formation and, thus, minimal disruption to function within the area affected.

In cases in which the wound heals by second intention, there is a larger wound and thus more extensive scar tissue. The same phases occur in both types of skin healing, but the second intention will take longer to heal fully.

In some cases, extensive wounds may never fully heal. In cases of large wounds, the body may be unable to close the wound, and medical intervention may be required to graft it. Second intention wounds are usually treated in physical therapy.

Delayed healing is caused by many factors. Delayed healing can occur during the first intention process or as a result of an extensive wound caused by injury that heals through second intention. Factors causing delayed wound healing are as follows:

- **Location of the wound:** Skin wounds generally heal well barring any other problems. Damage to heart tissue resulting in infarction of the tissue can remodel with the development of fibrous connective tissue. Wounds situated over joints may not heal well if they are not immobilized.

- **Excessive movement:** Excessive movement of the edges of the wound prevents or interferes with wound healing. If there is movement of the edges of the wound, it will not be able to organize and will not heal as quickly. If the wound is sutured, the edges will be held together assisting the healing process. Wounds situated over joints are particularly vulnerable to motion, and the area needs to be immobilized to allow healing to take place effectively.

- **Foreign bodies:** Foreign bodies in the wound such as dirt will prevent the wound healing.

- **Size of the wound:** Smaller wounds heal faster than large ones.

- **Infections:** The presence of infection in the wound prevents healing. The body's normal defense mechanisms prevent a wound from healing and trapping the infection inside the body. Some patients unfortunately acquire infections while in the hospital and have to be placed on antibiotic therapy. Such infection is called a nosocomial infection, meaning that it is acquired in the hospital or health care facility and was not present in the patient before hospitalization.

- **Age:** The age of the patient may affect healing. The healthy individual, whether young or old, heals at the normal rate. The very young may be susceptible to infections because of their immature immune systems. Elderly persons with an underlying disease process may also heal slowly.

- **Circulatory conditions:** The perfusion rate of the tissues (amount of circulation within the wound area) affects the rate of healing. In a limb with impaired circulation, such as in a patient with diabetes or peripheral vascular disease, healing may be delayed or even prevented. Certain more vascular areas of the body, such as the face and hands heal faster than other areas of the body.

- **Nutritional status:** Patients' nutritional status affects the rate of healing. Malnutrition or lack of certain vitamins and minerals will slow down or stop the rate of healing.
- **Interference by the patient:** If the patient constantly "picks" at the wound and keeps it open, this can also delay the healing process. In addition, not taking care of the wound can result in infection and delayed healing.
- **Medications:** Certain medications interfere with the healing of wounds, such as use of corticosteroids and anticoagulants such as warfarin (Coumadin).

It Happened in the Clinic

A 30-year-old male admitted to the hospital with dehydration and extensive open wounds on the dorsum of both hands was referred to PT. After evaluation, he was treated with whirlpool therapy to débride the partially necrotic areas on the open wounds. He progressed well with BID treatments and was discharged home. The wounds had contracted by 40%, the wound bed had granulation tissue, and there were no necrotic areas. The exudate was minimal, and the patient was referred for outpatient PT treatment for whirlpool and dressings. The first day he arrived in the outpatient PT department, 3 days after discharge, the wound on the dorsum of the left hand had heavy exudate and was larger than on discharge; the surrounding skin was inflamed. On questioning, the patient admitted he had been "shooting up" (injecting illicit drugs) straight into the wounds on both hands since returning home. He had received drug counseling in the hospital, but had returned to his usual routine upon discharge. The PT referred the patient back to the physician for follow-up.

Complications of Wound Healing Other Than Delayed Healing

Scar tissue formation is a natural by-product of the healing process but has its problems. As described previously, the function of scar tissue does not mimic that of the original tissue, so the affected area experiences loss of function. Two forms of skin scarring that can be a problem are **keloid scarring** and **hypertrophic scarring.** A keloid scar is often an unsightly raised area of scar tissue on the skin that spreads beyond the borders of the original wound, resulting from the formation of excessive amounts of granulation tissue and thus too much collagen

production (see Fig. 1-11). Certain individuals seem to be more prone to keloid scarring than others. Unfortunately, cosmetic surgery may remove the keloid, but the surgery itself may stimulate further keloid formation in susceptible individuals in up to 50% of cases.[43] Recent advances in the use of interferon injections into wounds and the use of laser therapy on existing keloid scars seem to offer promise of future improvements.[44] Keloid scars may continue to grow after healing of the wound. Some individuals may develop excess collagen tissue, resulting in a hypertrophic scar. These scars are not keloid but are thick, can be unsightly, and may interfere with function, especially if located round the area of a joint. Hypertrophic scars, unlike keloids, remain within the boundary of the original wound.[45] Hypertrophic scarring is frequently found in persons who have been burned.

Contractures (shortening of soft tissue structures, leading to reduction of joint motion) may occur due to the formation of **adhesions.** An adhesion is scar tissue that connects structures together that are not normally linked. An example would be when a tendon is injured and heals and adhesions form that bind the tendon to an adjacent muscle. This situation can result in the inability of the tendon to glide over the muscle, resulting in a loss of

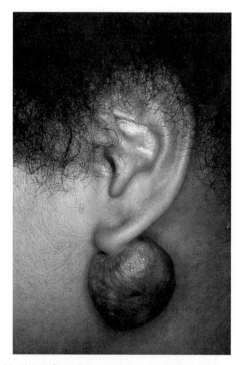

FIGURE 1.11 Keloid Scar. Reprinted with permission from Goldsmith, L. A., Lazarus, G. S., Tharp, M. D. (1997). *Adult and pediatric dermatology. A color guide to diagnosis and treatment.* Philadelphia: F. A. Davis, p. 162.

function of the involved muscles and perhaps restriction of motion of the associated joints. An example of this type of scarring is when the long head of the biceps brachii is injured and becomes adhered to its tendon sheath, resulting in a loss of shoulder flexion and pain in the affected area.

Fibrosis, or scar tissue formation within a hollow organ of the body, can have drastic results. Examples include fibrosis of the lung tissue and of the liver. In both cases, the fibrosis interferes with the function of the organ. Stenosis, or narrowing of the organ, can occur, which may impair function. In extreme cases, this can result in occlusion of the organ, causing a blockage of the area, for instance, in the intestine. This condition can be life threatening and may occur after surgery. A further result of scar tissue is extreme shortening of the tissue known as cicatrization. If this occurs in skin after a burn, it can affect joint motion because motion relies on the mobility of the skin and soft tissue structures surrounding the joint.

Dehiscence is a fairly rare problem that can occur after surgical closing of a wound. With dehiscence, the wound bursts open before it is fully healed as a result of too much tension on the wound or, more often, as a result of lack of sufficient healthy tissue surrounding the wound. Although not common, it sometimes occurs in abdominal wounds in the elderly population or in those whose immune system is compromised. Dehiscence also occurs in the residual limb following amputation in some patients with compromised circulation resulting from diabetes.[46]

Special Aspects Regarding Pressure Ulcers

Pressure ulcers, sometimes known as decubiti, are caused when constant pressure is placed on the skin over an area of bony prominence. This usually occurs in the immobile elderly or in those unable to move because of spinal cord injury or muscle inactivity. If a person is unable to move or has impaired skin sensation in an area, pressure on an area of skin may go undetected. In such cases, the tissues beneath the skin may necrose before the skin breaks down. Pressure ulcers are a significant problem in nursing homes and long-term care facilities and in persons unable to detect pain due to pressure on the skin. Under normal circumstances, a person constantly shifts weight to prevent skin pressure over bony prominences. When sitting in a chair or lying in bed, a person usually moves around because of discomfort. In individuals without adequate skin sensation or those unable to move, pressure builds up on the skin and underlying tissues overlying bony prominences and causes compression of tissues. The compression on the area prevents the circulation from supplying needed oxygen to the tissues, and the tissues start to necrose. Such breakdown can occur as quickly as within 1 hour of constant pressure on an area. In many cases of pressure ulcers, the area of skin affected may be small, but the damage to underlying muscle, fat, and other tissue may be extensive. Persons with an underlying disease process are more susceptible to skin breakdown than those in an otherwise healthy state. Shearing forces created by sliding the skin over bed linens may increase the risk of skin breakdown, especially in the sacrum. In the presence of moisture, such as when a person is incontinent of urine, the problem is compounded by maceration of the tissues. When skin is soaked in moisture for prolonged periods, it becomes soft and more liable to break down. The macerated tissue appears white, wrinkled, and is soft to the touch.[47] Keeping the individual dry and free from sweat, urine, and wound exudate helps to prevent skin breakdown. Hyperemia on the skin may occur after prolonged periods of constant pressure on an area of skin. The amount of time that it takes to cause pressure damage to the skin and underlying tissues varies with the physiological state of the tissues of the individual. A person with a compromised circulatory system may be unable to tolerate even short periods of constant pressure on a specific area without causing some damage. A general rule of thumb is that an immobile person needs to be turned onto a different area of the body at least every 2 hours. In individuals with compromised circulation, the turning may need to be done every 30 minutes. If pressure is relieved soon enough to prevent pressure damage to the skin and underlying tissues, the skin will usually return to normal color within approximately 1 hour. As a general rule, a person should never be placed in a position that puts pressure on an already reddened area of skin. If constant pressure is exerted on an area for over 2 hours, ischemia is likely to occur.[48] If the ischemia is not too severe, the area of tissue may recover in up to 36 hours. However, in persons with poor circulation and skin condition, the time it takes for areas of the skin to become ischemic may be much shorter.[49] When the ischemia is severe, necrosis of the tissue will occur. With necrosis, the skin over the area loses its normal color and becomes darker or gray. In some cases, this necrosis will progress to a pressure ulcer. A pressure ulcer can be caused by a person lying or sitting in one position for a prolonged period of time or by an excessive amount of pressure in a shorter period of time. Warning signs of too much pressure may be a discoloration or reddening of the skin that does not disappear within an hour.

Any area of skin that overlies a bony area can be susceptible to pressure. However, the main areas of the body affected by pressure ulcers are the sacrum, greater trochanter of the femur, heel, malleoli of the ankles, and ischial tuberosity. In some cases, there may be breakdown of the ears, nose, scapulae, ribs, and elbows. If a patient is placed prone for long periods of time, areas of the face and patellae may be affected. Pressure ulcers are classified into four stages as described in Table 1-7.

Wound healing for pressure ulcers follows the same principles as those for other wounds. Pressure must be relieved from affected tissues if the wound is to heal. Further details regarding risk assessment, prevention and management of the patient with pressure ulcers is contained in Chapter 14.

Physical Therapy Intervention for Wounds

The PT and PTA are frequently members of the wound-care team in a hospital or nursing home setting. The PT and PTA can utilize many types of intervention to treat wounds healing through second intention. Interventions include, but are not limited to, ultrasound to the wound bed and surrounding area, electrical stimulation to the wound bed and/or surrounding area, use of whirlpool treatments to débride wounds, and the application of suitable dressings to facilitate the healing process. Research has proved that wounds heal best in a moist environment.[50] The wound should be neither too wet nor too dry, and the choice of appropriate dressings cannot be underestimated. The PTA should be able to recognize the phases of wound healing and the appropriate modality or intervention for each phase to be able to provide the optimal intervention to promote wound healing. The PTA also needs to be able to know when to alert the supervising PT when the current intervention is no longer appropriate for the phase of wound healing and requires a change of the plan of care by the PT. **Débridement** of a wound is the removal of necrotic tissue so that the underlying tissue can heal (see Figure 1-12). **Eschar** is a special type of necrotic tissue that is hard, black or brown, and leathery in texture. A wound will not heal until all necrotic tissue is removed. Sharp débridement is performed with instruments such as a scalpel, scissors, or tweezers. Chemical débridement is the use of pharmaceutical débriding agents. Mechanical débridement can be performed with the use of wet or dry dressings. When the dressing is removed, it pulls necrotic tissue away with it. **Autolytic débridement** is achieved with the use of occlusive dressings. When the dressing is removed after several days, the necrotic tissue is also removed. Autolytic débridement should not be used for dry gangrene or other very dry wounds. Both the PT and PTA must be able to recognize necrotic tissue and distinguish tendon tissue from connective tissue, or the results can be devastating. This level of wound care is a specialty and should not be undertaken lightly. Sharp débridement procedures require constant reevaluation and are beyond the scope of work of the PTA. Postgraduation courses are necessary for the PTA to become further educated in other kinds of wound débridement procedures.

Table 1.7 Stages of Pressure Ulcers

STAGE	CHARACTERISTICS
Stage I	Intact skin
	Skin temperature warmer or cooler than surrounding area
	Pain, discomfort of itching in the area
Stage II	Some skin breakdown (partial thickness skin loss)
	Blister
	Injury to epidermis and/or dermis
Stage III	Skin breakdown (Full thickness skin loss)
	Necrosis of subcutaneous fat layers
	A surface ulcer is visible as a crater in the skin
Stage IV	Skin breakdown (Full thickness skin loss)
	Necrosis of subcutaneous fat, fascia, muscle, joint structures and even bone
	Tunneling and undermining of tissue may occur (the wound may extend further than apparent under the skin around the area)

Adapted from Sussman, C., & Bates-Jensen, B. M. (2001). *Wound care: A collaborative practice manual for physical therapists and nurses*, 2nd edition. Gaithersburg, MD: Aspen, p. 331.

GERIATRIC CONSIDERATIONS

An elderly patient with open wounds on the lower extremities due to venous insufficiency may not be able to handle dressing changes independently. If the wounds are heavily exudating, this can be a problem. An occlusive dressing, which does not have to be changed every day, may be an option so that the dressing changes can be performed in the outpatient PT department every few days. An alternative is to have the patient attend PT every other day or every third day and have a home health nurse or PT visit on the other days. Occasionally a family member may be able to help with dressing changes, but this is frequently not possible. In addition, the patient may not be as mobile because of pain in the affected leg. This increases the risk of reduced circulation and the recovery time for the wound to heal. An ambulatory assistive device may be necessary during the recovery phase to encourage the patient to walk, and circulatory exercises should be taught. The physician's instructions regarding weight-bearing status should be followed.

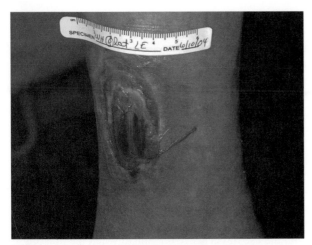

FIGURE 1.12 Wound with necrotic tissue. From Sussman, C., & Bates-Jensen, B. M. (2001). *Wound care: a collaborative practice manual for physical therapists and nurses,* 2nd edition. Gaithersburg, MD: Aspen Publishers, plate 29, color plate p. 9. Reproduced with permission.

Knowing when to intervene in the wound-healing process is especially important for the PTA to understand. Application of an inappropriate dressing over a granulating wound could result in damage to the wound and delayed healing. Conversely, continuing to treat a wound with necrotic tissue present without attempting to remove the tissue could also delay healing. A detailed description of types of wound dressings is not pursued in this book; however, some basic principles apply. If the wound is very wet with an excessive amount of drainage, the dressing should facilitate moisture absorption. Use of an alginate dressing is useful for such wounds. These dressings are made from seaweed and are very absorbent and biodegradable. The alginate dressing absorbs excess moisture from the wound to keep the wound moist but not wet. The alginate becomes a gel when moisture is absorbed, and this can be gently washed away from the wound with water without risk of damaging the granulating wound bed. If the wound is dry or has minimal exudate, a hydrocolloid dressing may be used. These dressings fall into categories of occlusive (keep moisture out) or semiocclusive dressings. Occlusive dressings are waterproof from the outside and inside so that moisture is retained within the wound, maintaining a good environment for healing. These dressings do not need to be changed every day and do not damage the tissue when removed. Hydrocolloid dressings are ideal when a wound is granulating and no longer requires débridement. Other types of dressings are used during the phase that requires débridement, including wet-to-dry and wet-to-wet methods. Such dressings should be used with great care because their removal may also remove healing tissue from the wound.

Some examples of modalities for stimulation of wound healing include:

- **Electrical stimulation:** The use of galvanic and pulsed monophasic currents using the negative electrode as the active can stimulate wound healing. The polarity is often changed after the first few treatment sessions to simulate the varying changes in the normal polarity of healing wounds. Use of biphasic current is increasing in popularity subsequent to recent positive research findings. Specific protocols may be found in Sussman and Bates-Jensen's (2001) *Wound Care: A collaborative practice manual for physical therapists and nurses.*[51]

- **Ultrasound (US):** US may be used on open wounds during the acute inflammatory phase (unlike in the acute inflammatory phase of an injury) to stimulate the progression into the proliferative phase of wound healing.[52] During the proliferative phase, US stimulates the production of granulation tissue and may also assist with the contraction of the wound. In addition, US stimulates the circulation, reduces pain, and may assist in edema reduction.

- **Pulsatile lavage:** Pulsatile lavage is a method of using water under pressure to cleanse and débride a wound simultaneously, especially when used with the suction option. Suction is applied at the same time to assist with the débridement. Recently, this has become a popular tool for physical therapists, particularly in the hospital setting. A wide variety of application tips are available for the machines to provide selected pressure to wound beds, sinuses, and tunnels. Although these machines are used for debridement and stimulation of tissue, it is important to select the appropriate pressure to prevent damage to surrounding healing tissue. Sussman and Bates-Jensen reported findings from a study by Haynes et al that showed some promising findings in reduction of length of healing times regarding the use of pulsatile lavage in the treatment of open wounds.[53] Because each patient has a separate treatment tip for the machine, there is reduced possibility of cross-infection.

- **Short-wave diathermy (SWD):** Both continuous and pulsed SWD (PSWD) can be used in wound healing. SWD uses electromagnetic and induction effects to heat body tissues. PSWD provides the electromagnetic effects with reduced thermal output. As Sussman and Bates-Jensen pointed out, there is little research evidence regarding the efficacy of SWD for wound care.[54] However, the use of SWD does produce heat, and heating is known to stimulate perfusion rates of tissues. Care should be taken not to use thermal SWD on anyone with compromised circulation.

- **Ultraviolet radiation (UV):** Ultraviolet light wave bands are divided into A, B, and C, namely UVA, UVB, and UVC. UVC is the shorter wave-band UV light used to destroy bacteria. Although UV radiation has been used for wound healing for a long time, Sussman and Bates-Jensen (2001)[55] reported recent findings indicating that the efficacy of UVC radiation for infected wounds is more evident than the use of other wavelengths of ultraviolet light. Original calculations of UV dosage relied on the erythemal dose patch test on the inner aspect of the arm of the patient. A more recent "UVC treatment algorithm"[56] is now recommended for calculating the length of exposure required.

- **Whirlpool:** Whirlpools are used in many outpatient and inpatient PT departments. The use of whirlpool for wound care is currently under reconsideration because of potential damage to healing granulation tissue and the possibility of cross-infection. The PTA should know when using a whirlpool is an advantage for wound healing. A high agitation level directed at the wound may be used during the initial stages of wound care to assist with loosening of necrotic tissue through the mechanical débridement effects provided by the agitation of the whirlpool. After granulation tissue forms in the wound, care must be taken not to damage the sensitive tissue, and thus it is advisable to discontinue whirlpool therapy.[57] The thermal effects of the warm water help to increase the tissue perfusion of the area, have an anesthetic effect on pain, speed healing, and make tissues more resistant to infection.[58] The temperature of the water used is determined by the circulatory status of the affected limb, remembering not to overheat areas that have poor circulation. Whirlpool tends to be overused, and careful consideration should be given to the required effects on the wound. *Caution:* All whirlpool equipment should be cleaned effectively and monitored regularly for bacterial count. The possibility of cross-infection and maceration of tissues are risk factors in the use of the whirlpool for open wounds. Placing the limb in a dependent position may also increase the risk of additional edema. Bactericidal solutions can be added to the whirlpool water but should be chosen selectively and used only on wounds that are infected or that require débridement. If such solutions contain iodine, patients who are allergic to iodine may have an extreme allergic reaction.

- **Vacuum-assisted closure (VAC):** VAC is a comparatively recent treatment modality approved by the Food and Drug Administration in 1995. The electrical modality applies a negative pressure (below atmospheric pressure) to the wound through a foam pad electrode placed directly on the wound bed. Effects of the VAC include reduction of edema, increased rate of healing, increased blood flow, stimulation of granulation tissue growth, and facilitation of closure of the wound.[59]

Bone Healing

Although this is not an orthopedic text, the PTA needs to understand the different types of healing of tissues within the body. In this way, the PTA can compare the similarities and differences of healing of various tissues.

Bone consists of a matrix mixed mainly with calcium and phosphate salts. The matrix is approximately 90% collagen fibers, and the rest is a ground substance composed of fluid and the proteoglycans, hyaluronic acid, and chondroitin sulphate. The collagen fibers of the matrix give bone its tensile strength and its resistance to breakage along its length. The collagen fibers form along the regions of stress of the bone, creating a series of trabeculae, which act much as a series of steel pipes placed together. A 1-inch steel pipe can be bent quite easily, but if several 1-inch steel pipes are placed together, it is almost impossible to bend them. This is known as increasing the tensile strength of a material. The arrangement of collagen fibers in the bone creates a similar mechanism to increase bone strength. The resistance of bone to damage from compressive forces is provided by the calcium salts in the bone. The collagen fibers are stimulated by weight bearing on long bones and by the use of muscles. Such stresses on the bone increase the organization of the collagen along the length of the bones and increase the strength of the bone. In pathological conditions such as osteoporosis, the number of collagen fibers is reduced, the fibers have a less organized structure, and there are fewer calcium salts. The combination of these factors creates a honeycomb-type matrix in the bones that makes them more susceptible to fracture.

Under normal circumstances, osteoblasts form collagen fibers, and osteoclast cells absorb collagen. When the bone is in a state of equilibrium, these cells work in harmony to maintain a balance within the bone. New bone is formed constantly within the body. Most cells in the body have a natural life span and are replaced by new cells under a normal physiological process.

When a bone is fractured, the osteoblasts go into overtime to promote healing (see Fig. 1-13). Three distinct phases are recognized in bone healing: an initial inflammatory response that lasts about 1 to 2 weeks, a reparative phase that can last several months, and a

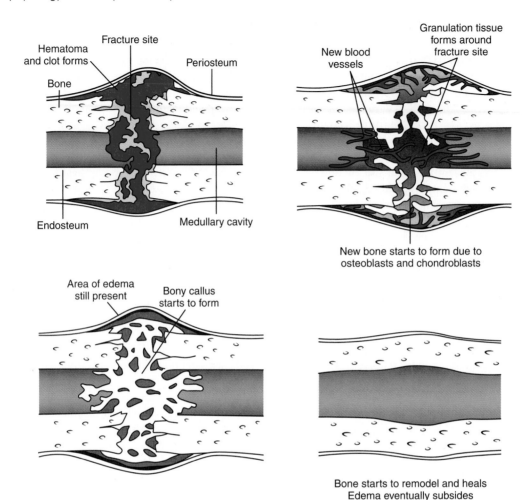

FIGURE 1.13 Stages of bone healing.

remodeling phase that may last for a few years.[60] In the inflammatory phase, hemorrhage at the fracture site results in the formation of a hematoma, or internal bruise, then granulation tissue is laid down as a result of the hematoma. Any necrotic tissue is removed by the phagocytes during this phase. During the reparative phase, the granulation tissue forms a soft callus (lump) to bridge the gap in the bone, and the osteoblasts gather in the area to produce new bone and a hard callus. Toward the end of this phase, the fracture site becomes more stable. The callus forms an enlargement on the bone, which is gradually reshaped through the remodeling phase to the original shape of the bone. The basic sequence of events in the first 24 to 48 hours after injury is similar to that of acute soft tissue inflammation. The callus in bone is equivalent to a scar in soft tissue. For the bone to heal correctly, there must be good alignment of the bone ends, minimal motion

(some movement may be beneficial) of the bone ends to allow the callus to form, and absence of infection. Fixation of the fracture site may be necessary in the form of external splinting or internal pinning and plating, in cases of displacement of bone ends.

The average length of time for long bones to become stable enough to allow weight bearing varies, but it is generally accepted practice that it takes 6 to 12 weeks for the lower extremity and 4 to 8 weeks for fractures of the upper extremity. Length of healing time will vary according to factors of circulation, age, general health, and nutrition, much as for soft tissue healing. Each patient will be evaluated by the physician, and guidelines will be provided to the PT and PTA for weight-bearing status. The PTA should remember not to place too much stress on the bone until it is healed sufficiently to withstand these stresses without interfering with the healing mechanism of the fracture. This includes muscle actions that produce a torque on the healing bone ends. Complications of bone healing include delayed union, nonunion, and malunion or poor alignment of bone ends, resulting in reduced function. Delayed union may be caused if too much motion is present at the fracture site. Physical therapy initiated too soon can cause delayed union, so the PT and PTA must be aware of the physician's orders and follow them carefully. A fine line exists between too much activity and too little, because some activity and gradual, progressive weight bearing stimulate the healing process. Determination of the appropriate weight-bearing status is provided by the PT in conjunction with the physician. Cases of nonunion are caused by poor blood supply to the fracture site, infection, or such severe soft tissue damage that the tissue lies between the bone ends. Malunion results when the bone ends heal in poor alignment. Causes of nonunion or malunion include an inadequate length of time for immobilization, poor choice of the type of immobilization used, or patient noncompliance with the physician's orders. Types of fractures and fixation devices are beyond the scope of this book, and the PTA should consult an orthopedic text for further information.

Ligament Healing

Ligaments are structures composed mainly of connective tissue that attach bone to bone across joints and act to stabilize joints. Ligaments do not contract like muscle tissue, and so when damaged they may either tear partially or completely. The term "sprain" is used when talking about a ligamentous injury. Classification of a ligamentous injury depends on the amount of damage or number of ligament fibers damaged and the amount of instability in the joint as a result of the injury. Grading for ligament injuries is Grade I (mild or first degree), Grade II (moderate or second degree), and Grade III (severe or third degree) when the ligament is completely ruptured.[61] Alternative classification can be used in which a partial tear is Grade I, a full tear is Grade II, and a tear that involves bone avulsion is a Grade III. In a Grade I injury, some local tenderness and swelling occur at the site of injury due to damage of ligamentous fibers; however, there is no instability of the joint. In a Grade II sprain, there is considerable damage to the ligament with many torn fibers, which results in some joint instability. In Grade III sprains, total severance of the ligament occurs, either where it attaches to the bone or along its length. Surgical repair may be performed for Grade III injuries to restore the stability of the joint involved, such as a ruptured cruciate ligament of the knee. In some cases, as in a medial collateral ligament

rupture of the knee, it may be sufficient to immobilize the joint for several weeks.[62] However, surgery may be impossible if the person is medically unsuitable or may be declined if the person feels able to live with the joint laxity.

Slight variations occur in the grading scales for ligamentous injuries in different parts of the body. In inversion ankle sprains, the grading system is adjusted as follows:

First-degree sprain = a single ligament rupture (anterior talofibular ligament)
Second-degree sprain = Two ligament rupture (anterior talofibular and fibulocalcaneal ligaments)
Third degree sprain = Three ligaments ruptured (anterior talofibular, posterior talofibular and fibulocalcaneal ligaments) [63]

Within the knee, a similar grading system to the Grade I, II, and III is used. The addition of a ligamentous laxity scale is often used for the knee. An example is one devised by Hughston[64] in which a mild instability is noted as a 1+, a moderate instability as a 2+, and a severe instability as a 3+ when compared with the intact limb.

The healing mechanism is similar to that of soft tissue; however, the rate of healing depends on the location of the ligament and the blood supply available. Phase I healing of ligaments lasts up to 48 hours after injury, Phase II from 48 to 72 hours, and Phase III lasts about a year.[65] Even a year or more postinjury, a ligament may only achieve about 50% of its original strength.[66] The criteria for healing are much the same as for bone in that the ligament needs to be protected during the healing process and also needs some stress placed on it to make the scar tissue form in a functional way. Protective braces, joint immobilizers, and taping can be helpful during the healing process. Specific ligament injuries and treatment protocols are detailed in orthopedic texts.

Muscle and Tendon Healing

The usual terminology for damage to muscle and tendon tissue is a strain, although the terms "pull" and "tears" are also used. Such a strain may be the result of muscle pulls related to repetitive microtrauma to the muscle, overstretching of the muscle, incorrect exercise routines, or secondary to a direct or indirect muscle pull. In some cases, the musculotendinous junction is damaged, and in others the belly of the muscle is damaged. Healing in muscle tissue follows the previously described sequence for the inflammatory response. Muscle has a high level of blood and nerve supply, so it heals with scar tissue formation. Unfortunately, the scar tissue may interfere with the function of the muscle, by reducing the extensibility of the muscle tissue. Tears to the muscle or tendon are usually incomplete, but rupture can occur. Because of the contractile nature of muscle, if it is severed, the muscle will recoil into a shortened position and form a "bump" that can be seen and palpated on the surface of the skin. An example of a ruptured muscle is a ruptured Achilles tendon in which the gastrocnemius and soleus muscles form a lump on the posterior superior aspect of the lower leg. Such an injury requires rapid surgical intervention to reattach it; otherwise, the whole muscle will shorten and lose its extensibility, making it difficult to obtain full range of motion at the ankle once repaired.[67] Tendon healing tends to be slow with need for periods of rest and controlled activity. The PTA should consult an orthopedic text for details of specific muscle and tendon injuries and the appropriate PT intervention.

In rare cases, in an orthopedic injury such as a fracture of the tibia in the lower leg, a compartment syndrome may occur.[68,69] This injury is a potentially dangerous situation in which edema occurs within a fascial compartment of the limb as a result of damage to the muscle. The fascia is not elastic, and therefore the edema is contained within the compartment, and pressure is exerted on the nerves and blood vessels within it. This problem requires immediate surgical release of the fascia so that permanent damage to the neurovascular bundle does not occur.[70]

Why Does the Physical Therapist Assistant Need to Know About Pain?

Pain is a subjective patient complaint, the perception of which is particular to the individual. Pain is precipitated by disease and injury. Because the PTA works with people who have pain for many different reasons, the physiological and neurological processes involved in the perception of pain must be understood. The understanding of the pain response allows the PTA to have a rationale for the use of specific physical therapy interventions and to empathize with patients experiencing pain. The ability to explain the mechanism of pain to patients is helpful in gaining their compliance for home programs of exercise and self-care.

Pain

Pain is the body's natural way of warning about a potential problem. Pain occurs after injury to any bodily structure containing nociceptors (pain nerve endings) such as skin, joints, and visceral organs[71] and can be manifested either locally at the injury site or in a site distant to that of the injury through referred pain. Referred pain is felt within the area of skin supplied by the same nerve root as that supplying the injured area. This concept accounts for the mechanism that causes a myocardial infarct to be felt as pain in the left arm and left upper chest, rather than over the area of the heart itself. The mechanism of referred pain is not fully understood. Some theories suggest that referred pain is the result of a reflex feedback mechanism between overstimulated nociceptors in deep structures, neurons in the dorsal horn of the spinal cord, and nociceptors in muscles.[72] Nociceptors are found in skin, joints, muscles, tendons, and deep viscera. Several types of nociceptors exist. Mechanical nociceptors are triggered in response to contact with a sharp object. Heat and cold nociceptors respond when the temperature becomes dangerously hot (over 45°C) or too cold (below 18°C).[73] Chemical nociceptors are triggered in response to the release of histamine or other by-products of inflammation, and polymodal nociceptors respond to other types of stimuli likely to damage the body. A total body response to trauma results in the "fight-or-flight" reaction. This response is a survival reflex that stimulates the person to prepare to get away from the problem causing the pain. In the inflammatory response previously described, pain is produced by the release of histamine, bradykinin, serotonin, and prostaglandins at the site of the injury. Pain produces a reaction in the muscles that causes spasm. Muscle spasm acts to provide a splinting mechanism, preventing the affected area from moving. In some cases the edema, which is secondary to the inflammatory response, can cause pain through direct pressure on nerves. In such cases, relief of the edema also reduces the pain.

Pain is a subjective experience and is influenced by past experience, cultural factors, level of fatigue, psychological factors such as anxiety and emotional factors, and genetics.[74,75] Scientists still do not fully understand the mechanism of the perception of pain. Pain receptors triggered by a stimulus send signals along A-delta fibers, which are myelinated and thus transmit at a fast rate. These A-delta fibers cause the localized sensation of sharp or pricking type pain that is often felt when a sharp object is touched. The C fibers are unmyelinated and thus transmit impulses more slowly and are responsible for producing a more prolonged burning type of sensation, which is less localized. The A-delta and C fibers transmit impulses from the painful stimulus to the brain via the dorsal root ganglia of the spinal cord. The stimulus has to reach the brain for the individual to "feel" the pain.[76] The ascending tract in the spinal cord responsible for the transmission of pain signals is the spinothalamic tract. Because the sensations of dull and sharp, and hot and cold are transmitted along the same spinothalamic tract, the PTA can test whether a patient can detect hot and cold by testing the skin sensation for sharp and dull stimuli. The body can control some of its own pain by the release of endogenous opiates. Relaxation techniques, exercise, electrical stimulation, and even laughter can stimulate production of endogenous opiates by the body.

Classification of pain is separated into acute and chronic. Acute pain occurs as the result of injury, infection, or a disease process and can be compounded by psychological stress. After the cause is treated, the pain usually diminishes or disappears. Chronic pain is, however, a different mechanism and may or may not respond to treatment. The complex interaction of psychological and physiological factors in chronic pain is still not fully understood.[77]

Pain Control Theories

Knowledge of the body's production of **endogenous opiates** is a useful tool for the PT and PTA. Techniques can be used to increase these naturally occurring substances and thus alter the pain experience. The benefit of this approach is that such techniques are noninvasive, meaning they do not involve putting anything into the body, such as medications. Techniques used in physical therapy to stimulate the production of endogenous opiates include,

but are not limited to, relaxation techniques, intensive exercise programs that can be performed at home, and electrical stimulation modalities such as transcutaneous electrical nerve stimulation (TENS), which can also be provided for home use.

Another theory of pain used to develop PT intervention strategies is the **Gate Control Theory.** This theory was first formulated by Melzack and Wall in 1965[78] and underwent modifications by them in 1978[79] and 1983.[80] Melzack and Wall stated that for a pain impulse to be perceived by the brain, the number of pain impulses had to outnumber the pain inhibiting factors to open the "Gate" to the brain to send impulses registering pain. Out of this theory arose the idea that psychological factors play a large role in whether the brain registers pain. Biofeedback mechanisms are thought to be effective in modulating the patient's response to pain on the basis of the Gate Control Theory and by providing volitional (voluntary) control over the perception of pain. Biofeedback enables patients to take control of their own pain perception and experience.

Physical Therapy Interventions

The PT and PTA treat both acute and chronic pain. Acute pain typically resolves once an injury is rehabilitated. The concentration of the PT intervention should be on resolution of the problem, which in turn takes care of the pain. Chronic pain, however, is less easily understood and is often difficult to treat (see Table 1-8). Many

Table 1.8 **Causes of Chronic Pain**

CAUSATIVE MECHANISM	TYPE OF PROBLEM	CLINICAL EXAMPLE
Chemical	Tissue irritation from by-products of inflammation	Skin burn causes release of prostaglandins, which in turn cause more pain
Mechanical	Nerve entrapment at a bony or ligamentous channel	Carpel tunnel syndrome—entrapment of the median nerve in the carpel tunnel Entrapment of a spinal nerve at the intervertebral foramina
Nerve regeneration	Nerves cut as a result of trauma or surgery	As a severed peripheral nerve regenerates, the end of the nerve is acutely sensitive and even painful because of discharge from the peripheral nerve fibers
Abnormally overactive protective reflexes	The reflexes that protect the body against damage may go into overdrive and cause excessive muscle spasm associated with chronic pain; normally spasm reduces after the acute phase of an injury It is not fully understood why this mechanism does not shut off	If muscle spasm occurs for a prolonged period (eg, spasm in the piriformis muscle in the buttock), there may be pressure on nerves and blood vessels, causing pain from nerve compression and possibly ischemia (lack of oxygen to tissues) due to pressure on blood vessels

physical therapy techniques can be used to treat both acute and chronic pain. In acute pain, the first line of intervention is to eliminate the cause, if possible. Next is to reduce the swelling associated with the inflammatory response and promote healing of the tissue by the use of RICE (described earlier in this chapter). After the acute phase, interventions can progress to appropriate subacute modalities including, but not limited to, heat, electrical stimulation, ultrasound, traction, and progressive exercises. As the injury heals, the pain usually decreases in proportion to the stage of the healing process. If the pain does not resolve and seems to be inconsistent with the usual length of time needed for healing, it can be considered chronic in nature, and a different approach may be required by the PT and PTA.

Patients experiencing chronic pain may require intervention from a team of professionals including physician, physician's assistant, nurse practitioner, psychologist, PT/PTA, occupational therapist (OT), certified occupational therapy assistant (COTA), and social worker. The perception of pain varies according to many factors. Cultural differences can affect the way individuals perceive pain.[81] If the patient is from a culture that denies the existence of pain or discourages verbalizing the existence of pain, the intervention may be much more difficult. In addition, such patients may take much longer to seek help, and the pain may have become deep-seated and more difficult to treat. Biofeedback techniques may be used to help patients redirect their perceptions of pain and help them cope with long-standing pain. The PT and PTA can help in this process by using biofeedback mechanisms, teaching relaxation techniques, correcting posture, teaching the use of electrical modalities such as TENS (which can be provided for home use), providing instruction in the use of ice or heat at home, and developing exercise programs that help to strengthen and create endurance that have a positive effect on pain. The emphasis relies on teaching patients to manage their own pain. Physical therapy techniques such as myofascial release, massage, mobilization, and manipulation may be used, but it is important that the patient not become too dependent on PT intervention. The patient must understand that chronic pain, although very real, may be difficult to eliminate completely. Goals should be developed with the patient so that the PT and patient are in agreement with the expected and desired outcomes of the therapy from the start. Patient expectations for treatment outcomes are often too high. Writing a contract signed by the patient and the therapist can help to set guidelines for expected treatment outcomes and may prevent, or at least reduce, patient disappointment by setting realistic goals. The effects of chronic pain cannot be overemphasized. Many patients with chronic diseases such as arthritis are in constant pain, and this can lead to depression and abuse of medications, or use of recreational drugs and alcohol. One of the most discouraging things for patients to experience is when a health care professional does not believe they are in pain. The PTA should always listen to the patient but not allow the person to dwell on the negative more than necessary. One thing PTs/PTAs can provide to their patients is hope, and this plays a major part in the rehabilitation of those with chronic pain.

Pain Assessment

As already stated, pain is a subjective phenomenon. The perception of pain is purely the level of pain perceived by the individual patient. The PTA cannot see or feel the pain in another person, and thus pain assessment is not considered an objective finding. The pain in one individual cannot be compared with that of another. Tools that are used in pain measurement such as visual analog scales[82] (Fig. 1-14) and the McGill Pain Questionnaire[83,84] are an attempt to make the pain as objective as possible.

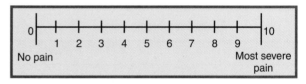

FIGURE 1.14 Visual analog scale. Instruction to patient: Mark on the line where your pain is with 0 being no pain and 10 being the highest possible pain.

CASE STUDY 1.1

A 50-year-old woman presents with a cut on her right forearm, which she sustained 1 hour earlier when chopping vegetables for the evening meal.

1. What is the PTA likely to observe in the area of the cut regarding the inflammatory process?

2. Describe the mechanisms at the cellular level of each of the observations that you noted.

CASE STUDY 1.2

A 60-year-old woman with a history of arthritis in the right knee is receiving an intervention at the PT clinic. She has had numerous sessions of physical therapy with little or no success, and her main complaint now is pain, which prevents her from playing golf. X-rays indicate that the knee is not affected enough to require joint replacement. The PT has reevaluated the client and decided interventions are necessary to address the chronic pain. The client has a good basic exercise program, which she indicates she has followed faithfully at home.

1. Describe some strategies the PTA can teach the patient to use at home in addition to the existing basic exercise program.

2. What modalities should the PTA provide for this patient at home, and what instructions should be given for safe use of the equipment? (The PTA student will probably only be able to answer this question if modalities have been covered in class. Consult a modalities text for further information.)

3. What general advice should the PTA give to the patient?

4. How would the PTA explain the two theories of pain to a client in terms he or she can understand? (Try explaining these theories to a member of your family or a friend who does not already know them.)

STUDY QUESTIONS

1. Describe the cell structures that are general to most cells in the body, as well as the function of each component part.

2. List the types of cell injury.

3. Describe each type of cell injury.

4. Describe the various types of growth changes that can occur in cells.

5. Describe three causes of cell or tissue necrosis.

6. Name three causes of inflammation.

7. List the four cardinal signs of inflammation and the additional factor included in rehabilitation.

8. For each of the four cardinal signs of inflammation, describe the cellular mechanisms involved.

9. Describe the difference between acute and chronic inflammation.

10. Explain the role of PMNs in the inflammatory process.

11. List the cells involved in the inflammatory process, and state each type of cell's role in the process.

12. List four chemicals released during the inflammatory response that can cause pain.

13. Discuss ways in which physical therapy intervention can be used to reduce inflammation.

14. Describe the Pain Gate Theory through diagram or a short paragraph so that a nonmedical family member can understand it.

15. Describe the acronym "RICE" to another person in terms that a layperson can understand and give the reasons for the use of this in treatment.

16. Describe the similarities and differences of the healing processes in skin, tendons, and bone.

17. Describe the phases of wound healing.

18. List the possible causes of delayed healing of a wound.

19. Describe a physical therapy intervention to promote wound healing.

20. List the four stages of a pressure ulcer and the associated characteristics.

21. Describe which patients are most at risk of developing pressure ulcers.

● USEFUL WEB SITES

Access Excellence @ the National Health Museum
http://www.accessexcellence.org

Go to "Graphics Gallery" to view useful graphics depicting cell functions, including the molecular structure of DNA and RNA.

Kimball's Biology Pages
http://biology-pages.info

This site provides basic cell physiology and biology information from a past biology professor with a doctorate from Harvard University.

● REFERENCES

[1] Kimball, J. W. (2007). The nucleus. *Kimball's biology pages.* Retrieved 3.22.07 from http://users.rcn.com/jkimball.ma.ultranet/BiologyPages/N/Nucleus.html

[2] Kimball, J. (2006). Kimball's biology pages home page. Retrieved from http://users.rcn.com/jkimball.ma.ultranet/BiologyPages/W/Welcome.html

[3] Petty, Y. (2002). DNA tutorial. Retrieved 2.20.07 from www.ncc.gmu.edu/dna/rna.htm

[4] Kimball, J. W. (2006). Kimball's biology pages home page. Retrieved 2.20.07 from http://users.rcn.com/jkimball.ma.ultranet/BiologyPages/W/Welcome.html

[5] Burgoyne, L. A. (1999). The mechanisms of pyknosis: hypercondensation and death. *Exp Cell Res* 10:248: 214–222. Retrieved 2.20.07 from http://www.ncbi.nlm.nih.gov/entrez/query.fcgi?cmd=Retrieve&db=PubMed&list_uids=10094828&dopt=Abstract

[6] O'Sullivan, S. B., & Schmitz, T. J. (2007). *Physical rehabilitation,* 5th edition. Philadelphia: F. A. Davis, p. 909.

[7] Arnoczky, S. P., Tarvin, G. B., & Marshall, J. L., (1982). Anterior cruciate ligament replacement using patellar tendon. An evaluation of graft revascularization in the dog. *J Bone Joint Surg Am.* 64:217–224.

[8] Affagnini, S., De Pasquale, V., Reggiani, L. M., Russo A, Agati P, Bacchelli B, & Marcacci M. (2007). *Knee* 14:87–93.

[9] Miller-Keane Encyclopedia and dictionary of medicine, nursing, and allied health, 6th edition. (1997). Philadelphia: W. B. Saunders, p. 489.

[10] MedicineNet.com. Definition of inflammation. Retrieved 2.21.07 from http://www.medterms.com/script/main/art.asp?articlekey=3979

[11] Messer, W. S., Jr. (2000). Histamine synthesis. Retrieved 2.21.07 from http://www.neurosci.pharm.utoledo.edu/MBC3320/histamine.htm

[12] MedicineNet.com. Definition of inflammation. Idem.

[13] Endocrine and metabolic disorders: carcinoid tumors. Carcinoid syndrome. Merck Manuals Online Medical Library for Healthcare Professionals. (2005). Retrieved 2.21.07 from http://www.merck.com/mmpe/print/sec12/ch161/ch161b.html

[14] MedicineNet.com. Definition of transudate. Retrieved 2.21.07 from http://www.medterms.com/script/main/art.asp?articlekey=9901

[15] Taber's cyclopedic medical dictionary, 20th edition. (2005). Philadelphia: F. A. Davis, p. 2228.

[16] Ibid., p. 765.

[17] MedicineNet.com. Definition of eosinophil. Retrieved 2.21.07 from http://www.medterms.com/script/main/art.asp?articlekey=3268

[18] Taber's cyclopedic medical dictionary, 20th edition. (2005). Idem, p. 1380.

[19] Monocyte disorders. Merck Manuals Online Medical Library for Healthcare Professionals. (2003). Retrieved 2.21.07 from http://www.merck.com/mmhe/sec14/ch174/ch174f.html

[20] Taber's cyclopedic medical dictionary, 20th edition. (2005). Idem, p. 1686.

[21] Hematology and oncology: thrombocytopenia and platelet dysfunction. Merck Manuals Online Medical Library for Healthcare Professionals. (2005). Retrieved 2.21.07 from http://www.merck.com/mmpe/sec11/ch133/ch133a.html

[22] Components of the immune system. Merck Manuals Online Medical Library for Healthcare Professionals (2005). Retrieved 2.21.07 from http://www.merck.com/mmpe/sec13/ch163/ch163b.html

[23] Goodman, C. C., Boissonnault, W. G., & Fuller, K. S. (2003). *Pathology: implications for the physical therapist,* 2nd edition. Philadelphia: W. B. Saunders, p. 130.

[24] Ibid., p. 139.

[25] Bleakley, C., McDonough, S., & MacAuley, D. (2004) . The use of ice in the treatment of acute soft-tissue injury: a systematic review of randomized controlled trials. *Am J Sports Med* 32:1, 251–261.

[26] U.S. Department of Health and Human Services. *AHCPR supported clinical practice guidelines for wound treatment.* Retrieved 2.21.07 from http://www.ncbi.nlm.nih.gov/books/bv.fcgi?rid=hstat2.chapter.5124

[27] Mercandetti, M., & Cohen, A. J. (2005). Wound healing, healing and repair. eMedicine. Retrieved 2.21.07 from http://www.emedicine.com/plastic/topic411.htm

[28] Kajstura, J., Leri, A., Castaldo, C., Nadal-Ginard, B., & Anversa, P. (2004). Myocyte growth in the failing heart. *Surg Clin North Am* 84:161–177.

[29] Hamada, H., Kim, M. K., Iwakura, A., Ii, M., Thorne, T., Qin, G., et al. (2006). Estrogen receptors alpha and beta mediate contribution of bone marrow-derived endothelial progenitor cells to functional recovery after myocardial infarction. *Circulation* 114: 2261–2270.

[30] Bernreuther, C., Dihné, M., Johann, V., Schiefer, J., Cui, Y., Hargus, G., et al. (2006). Neural cell adhesion molecule L1-transfected embryonic stem cells promote functional recovery after excitotoxic lesion of the mouse striatum. *J Neurosci* 26:11532–11539.

[31] Yano, S., Kuroda, S., Shichinohe, H., Seki, T., Ohnishi, T., et al. (2006). Bone marrow stromal cell transplantation preserves gammaaminobutyric acid receptor function in the injured spinal cord. *J Neurotrauma* 23:1682–1692.

[32] Enoch, S., & Harding, K. (2003). Wound bed preparation: the science behind the removal of barriers to healing. *Wounds* 15:213–229.

[33] Goodman, C. C., Boissonault, W. G., & Fuller K. S. (2003). *Pathology: implications for the physical therapist,* 2nd edition. Philadelphia: Saunders, p. 141.

[34] McCulloch, J. M., Kloth, L. C., & Feedar, J. A. (1995). *Wound healing: alternatives in management,* 2nd edition. Philadelphia: F. A. Davis, p. 23.

[35] Ibid., p. 19.

[36] Sussman, C., & Bates-Jensen, B. M. (2001). *Wound care: a collaborative practice manual for physical therapists and nurses,* 2nd edition. Gaithersburg, MD: Aspen Publishers, p. 40.

[37] Goodman, C. C., Boissonnault, W. G., & Fuller, K. S. (2003). *Pathology: implications for the physical therapist,* 2nd edition. Philadelphia: Saunders, p. 144.

[38] Gogia, P. P. (1995). *Clinical wound management.* Thorofare, NJ: Slack, p. 5.

[39] Sussman, C., & Bates-Jensen, B. M. (2001). Idem, p. 296.

[40] McCulloch, J. M., Kloth, L. C., & Feedar, J. A. (1995). Idem, p. 38.

[41] Sussman, C., & Bates-Jensen, B. M. (2001). Idem, p. 39.

[42] Goodman, C. C., Boissonnault, W. G., & Fuller, K. S. (2003). Idem, p. 144.

[43] Chapman, M. S. (2001). Promising dermatologic therapies: imiquimod may prevent recurrence of keloid scars after surgery. Retrieved 2.22.07 from http://www.medscape.com/viewarticle/423106

[44] Chapman, M. S. (2001). Promising dermatologic therapies: imiquimod may prevent recurrence of keloid scars after surgery. Ibid.

[45] Tanzi, E. L., & Alster, T. S.(2004). Laser treatment of scars. Retrieved 2.22.07 from http://www.medscape.com/viewarticle/467347

[46] Pattison, P. S., Gordon, J. K., Muto, P. M., Mallen, J. K., & Hoerner, J. (2005). Case report: using dual therapies—negative pressure wound therapy and modified silicone gel liner—to treat a limb

postamputation and dehiscence. *Wound*. Retrieved 2.22.07 at http://www.medscape.com/viewarticle/513366

[47] Sussman, C., & Bates-Jensen, B. M. (2001). Idem, p. 96.

[48] Maklebust, J., & Sieggreen, M. (2000). *Pressure ulcers: guidelines for prevention and management*, 3rd edition. Springhouse, PA: Springhouse, p. 21.

[49] Maklebust, J., & Sieggreen, M. (2000). *Pressure ulcers: Guidelines for prevention and management*, 3rd edition. Idem, p. 42.

[50] Enoch, S., & Harding, K. (2003). Wound bed preparation: the science behind the removal of barriers to healing. *Wounds* 15:213–229.

[51] Sussman, C., & Bates-Jensen, B. M. (2001). Idem.

[52] Ibid., p. 603.

[53] Haynes, L. J. Handley, C. & Brown, M. H. (1994). Comparison of Pulsavac and sterile whirlpool regarding the promotion of tissue granulation, p. 643. In ibid.

[54] Sussman, C., & Bates-Jensen, B. M. Idem, p. 558.

[55] Ibid., pp. 582-587.

[56] Ibid., p. 589.

[57] Ibid., p. 622.

[58] Ikeda, T., Tayefeh, F., Sessler, D. I., Kurz, A., Plattner, O., Petschnigg, B., et al. (1998). Local radiant heating increase subcutaneous oxygen tension. *Am J Surg* 175:33–37. Cited in ibid., p. 624.

[59] Sussman, C., & Bates-Jensen, B. M. Idem, p. 282.

[60] Hoppenfeld, S., & Murthy, V. L. (2000). *Treatment and rehabilitation of fractures*. Philadelphia: Lippincott Williams & Wilkins, pp. 2–5.

[61] Shankman, G. A. (2004). *Fundamental orthopedic management for the physical therapist assistant*, 2nd edition. St. Louis, MO: Mosby, p. 139.

[62] Malone, T. R., McPoil, T., & Nitz, A. J. (1997). *Orthopedic and sports physical therapy*, 3rd edition. St. Louis, MO: Mosby, p. 149.

[63] Shankman, G. A. (2004). Idem, pp. 260–261.

[64] Hughston, J. (1993). Knee ligaments: injury and repair. Cited in ibid., p. 292.

[65] Shankman, G. A. (2004). Idem, p. 139.

[66] Ibid., p. 139.

[67] Haraldson, S., & Blasko, B. (2001). Ruptured tendon. Retrieved 3.19.07 from http://www.emedicine.com/aaem/topic384.htm

[68] Shankman, G. A. (2004). Idem, p. 272.

[69] Paula, R. (2006). Compartment syndrome: extremity. Retrieved 3.19.07 from http://www.emedicine.com/EMERG/topic739.htm

[70] Shankman, G. A. (2004). Idem, p. 272.

[71] Paice, J. A. (2002). Controlling pain: understanding nociceptive pain. *Nursing* 32:74–75.

[72] Giamberardino, M. A. (2003). Referred muscle pain/hyperalgesia and central sensitization. *J Rehabil Med* 41:85–88.

[73] Carver, A., (2006), Pain: neurobiology of pain. *ACP Medicine Online*. Retrieved 2.22.07 from http://www.medscape.com/viewarticle/534650

[74] Ayded, M. (2002). Some foundational problems in the scientific study of pain. *Philosophy Sci* 69:265–283.

[75] Pridmore, S., Oberoi, G., & Samilowitz, H. (2002). Pain from many inputs. *Australas Psychiatry* 10:51–53.

[76] Wheeler, A. H. (2004). Myofascial pain disorders. *Drugs* 64:45–62.

[77] Dallel, R., & Voisin, D. (2001). Towards pain treatment based on the identification of the pain-generating mechanisms. *Eur Neurol* 45:126–132

[78] Melzack, R., & Wall P. D. (1965). Pain mechanisms: a new theory. *Science* 150:971.

[79] Wall, P. D. (1978). The gate control theory of pain mechanism: an examination and restatement. *Brain* 101:2.

[80] Melzack, R., & Wall, P. D (1983). *The challenge of pain*. New York: Basic Books.

[81] Main, C. J., & Spanswick, C. C. (2000). Pain management: an interdisciplinary approach. Edinburgh, United Kingdom: Churchill Livingstone.

[82] Duncan, G. H., Bushnell, M. C., & Lavigne, G. J. (1989). Comparison of verbal and visual analog scales for measuring the intensity and unpleasantness of experimental pain. *Pain* 37:296–303.

[83] Melzack, R. (1975). The McGill Pain Questionnaire: major properties and scoring methods. *Pain* 1:277–299.

[84] Melzack, R., & Raja, S. N. (2005). The McGill Pain Questionnaire: from description to measurement. *Anesthesiology* 103:199–202.

CHAPTER 2

Immunopathology, Neoplasia, and Chromosome Abnormalities

LEARNING OBJECTIVES

After completion of this chapter, students should be able to:

- Describe the physiological mechanisms of the immune response.
- Identify the role vaccination plays in defense against infectious disease.
- State the causes, classification, and medical treatment for neoplasias.
- Compare benign and malignant tumors.
- Determine the implications of neoplasia for physical therapy interventions.
- Become familiar with various chromosome abnormalities and genetically linked diseases.
- Identify the impact of antibiotic-resistant infections and emerging infections on the future of health care.
- Determine the role of the physical therapist/physical therapist assistant in providing physical therapy interventions for patients with hereditary conditions.

CHAPTER OUTLINE

Introduction
Immunopathology
   Cells of the Immune Response
Hypersensitivity Reactions
   Type I Hypersensitivity
   Type II Hypersensitivity
   Type III Hypersensitivity
   Type IV Hypersensitivity
   Vaccination
   Effects of Exercise on the Immune Response

KEY TERMS

Anaphylactic shock/response
Angiogenesis
Antibiotic-resistant bacteria
Antimicrobial medications
Broad-spectrum antibiotics
Carcinogenesis
Epinephrine
Hemolytic diseases of the newborn
Hydrocephalus
Hypotonia
Immune complex reaction
Immunoglobulins
Meningocele
Myelomeningocele
Neonatal intensive care unit (NICU)
Neonatal respiratory distress
   syndrome
Nosocomial infections
Spina bifida occulta

CHAPTER OUTLINE (continued)

Introduction

This chapter provides descriptions of many of the basic physiological, cellular, and genetic components of the disease process. At first glance, it may seem as if the topics are unrelated to each other, but an understanding of how the immune system works and the role genetics plays are basic concepts of disease. The first section of the chapter is focused on immunopathology and includes the immune response, hypersensitivity reactions, vaccinations, and infections. The second part of the chapter focuses on basic genetics and the part it plays in genetic and hereditary chromosome diseases, developmental diseases, and genetically linked diseases; it includes details of specific diseases within these categories.

Why Does the Physical Therapist Assistant Need to Know About Immunopathology?

Physical therapist assistants (PTAs) need to understand the mechanisms of immunopathology for both their own and their patients' protection. The body's natural immunity to infections protects people against infectious diseases through the development of antibodies to that disease. When working with people with compromised immune systems who are less able to fight off infections, the PTA must take additional care to prevent these patients from contracting infections.

Although standard/universal precautions should be used when working with all patients, some of the additional precautions taken with people who are extremely susceptible to infections may include treating them within their own hospital room or keeping them away from other patients. In addition, sometimes the immune system goes into overdrive, causing severe allergic reactions to a substance such as latex, or the allergic response can elicit certain conditions such as allergic asthma. The signs and symptoms of such allergic reactions may be exhibited during physical therapy sessions, and an understanding of these responses may alert the PTA to these issues before the situation becomes a danger to patients. Vaccinations are a method of prodding the body into developing antigens to diseases. As members of the health care team, all PTAs must demonstrate immunity to certain diseases for their own protection and that of their patients. Knowledge of the way the body develops these antibodies is essential for understanding how the human body protects itself against diseases.

Immunopathology

The body has an innate immunity (natural immunity system) that resists infections. The constituents of this innate protection include the skin, mucous membranes, and bactericidal substances found in tears, the nose, and the intestinal tract. A secondary immune response, or acquired immunity, develops in the body as a result of exposure of the body to antigens. An antigen is a stimulus such as an irritant or chemical that elicits an immune response.[1] The body's immune response recognizes foreign particles or chemicals. After a stimulus is recognized as foreign, the immune system is activated to destroy the antigen. Antibodies—proteins specific to the antigen—are formed, which help to fight current and future intrusions by that particular antigen. Each antibody is specific to one antigen.[2] In people with compromised immune systems or babies with immature immune systems, the ability to fight off infections or intrusions is either reduced or absent.

Cells of the Immune Response

The cells involved in the immune system are primarily the T and B lymphocytes. The various types of T and B lymphocytes are described in this section.

LYMPHOCYTES

Lymphocytes are white blood cells that develop from stem cells. Lymphocytes have large, round nuclei and a small amount of cytoplasm. Two types of lymphocytes are the primary cells of the immune system, T lymphocytes and B lymphocytes. The T lymphocytes develop within the bone marrow but mature within the thymus, and the B lymphocytes both develop and mature within the bone marrow[3] or in the liver in the fetus.[4] Once mature, both types of lymphocytes also migrate to the lymph glands, spleen, bronchi, and intestinal mucous membranes. In general, the T lymphocytes act on the tissues in a local way, and the B lymphocytes produce antibodies that are transmitted through the circulatory system and have a distant effect on tissues.[5]

T lymphocytes are the most common. T lymphocytes actually migrate to parts of the body where infection or damage is recognized and have a local effect on the cells.[6] Types of T lymphocytes include helper T cells and cytotoxic T cells. The helper T cells are responsible for stimulating the action of B lymphocytes and macrophages during the immune reaction to antigens and assist the B lymphocytes to produce antibodies by the release of chemical substances called cytokines.[7] Macrophages are white blood cells that use phagocytosis (engulfing of foreign particles) to destroy bacteria, foreign particles, and parasitic organisms. Cytotoxic T cells actually kill infected cells. Some of the cytotoxic T lymphocytes are known as T suppressor cells, which attack, and attempt to destroy, tumor cells and cells infected with viruses. The T suppressor cells may also be responsible for

preventing antibody formation to the body's own tissues. Other cytotoxic T cells are called natural killer (NK) cells. These NK cells are the first-line response in the attack against tumor cells and virus-infected cells. Basically, the T lymphocytes recognize intruders and set out to destroy them.

The B lymphocytes produce **immunoglobulins** known as antibodies. The three most important immunoglobulins for the PTA to know about are immunoglobulin (Ig)E, IgG, and IgM. IgG and IgM are activated after an immunization.[8] Immunization stimulates the initial production of immunoglobulin to a disease, and if the body subsequently comes into contact with the disease antigen, an overproduction of the antigen occurs that enables the body to fight the disease successfully. IgG goes into attack mode when the body is exposed to a disease or virus after immunization has occurred. IgG become more active when the body is exposed to an antigen for a second or subsequent time. Each infective organism stimulates the production in the body of a separate type of antibody unique to that organism. The antibodies combine with the antigen and immobilize them. IgE is the immunoglobulin active in allergic reactions[9] and is described within the hypersensitivity sections of this chapter (see Table 2.1).

Hypersensitivity Reactions

The following section details the types of hypersensitivity reaction and provides examples for each type. The types of hypersensitivity include Type I hypersensitivity, known as immediate or anaphylactic reactions; Type II, hypersensitivity, which results in antibody production; Type III hypersensitivity, or immune complex reactions; and Type IV hypersensitivity, also known as delayed response or cell mediated hypersensitivity.

Type I Hypersensitivity

Type I hypersensitivity reactions are also known as immediate, or anaphylactic, reactions.[10] Examples of Type I hypersensitivity reactions include conditions such as bronchial asthma, allergic rhinitis (hay fever allergy), atopic dermatitis (eczema), and anaphylactic shock (see Fig. 2-1). Refer to Chapter 8 for details about atopic dermatitis and eczema. In these conditions, the hypersensitivity reaction sets off the IgE immunoglobulins in response to sensitivity of the B lymphocytes to a causative irritant, such as pollen. IgE immunoglobulins are produced by plasma cells. When IgE is released, it

Table 2.1 **Hypersensitivity Reactions**

HYPERSENSITIVITY REACTION	EXAMPLES	CHARACTERISTICS	INTERVENTION
Type I—allergy	Hay fever	Sneezing, itching, runny nose	Antihistamine medications, desensitization therapy
	Food allergies	Nausea/vomiting, diarrhea, skin rash (hives) that can be in the pharynx and cause airflow obstruction	Antihistamine medications, desensitization therapy
	Anaphylactic shock	Generalized itching, difficulty breathing, redness/hives on skin, edema of face, hands, feet, dizziness, weakness, panic leading to loss of consciousness if not treated	Epinephrine injection
Type II—Cytotoxic	Intrinsic—autoimmune diseases	Body attacks its own tissues as in rheumatoid arthritis, in which the body attacks the joints and some organs	Described in Chapter 6
	Extrinsic—hemolytic disease of the newborn	RH-negative mother develops antibodies to fetus with RH-positive blood so that next fetus with RH-positive blood is attacked by the antibodies; infant will need blood transfusion at birth or may die	Mother given anti-D factor after first birth to prevent her developing antibodies to rhesus factor
	Extrinsic—blood transfusion incompatibility	Type A blood has antibodies to B; If Type B blood given to Type A, antigen/antibody reaction destroys red blood cells of recipient	Ensure patients are blood typed before transfusion; complete blood transfusion if given wrong type blood
Type III—Immune complex	Glomerulonephritis, rheumatoid arthritis	Antigen/antibody combine to form a complex that is deposited in blood vessel walls and causes destruction of tissue	
Type IV—Delayed	Mantoux test	T lymphocytes already sensitized to TB produce a delayed skin reaction when the antigen is injected under the skin	Positive skin reaction indicates antibodies to TB are present; does not necessarily mean the person has TB
	Perfume sensitivity	Local skin response with inflammation	Avoid use of offending agent
	Latex sensitivity	Local skin response with inflammation, open sores	Avoid skin contact with latex products

links with receptors on the mast cells, causing a Type I hypersensitivity reaction. Mast cells are floating cells found in tissues that are formed in the bone marrow and contain histamine. During both inflammation and immune reactions, mast cells release the histamine into the affected area. The mast cells' release of histamine mediates an inflammatory reaction in the tissues. Mast cells also release secondary substances that further the inflammatory response. These substances are prostaglandins and leukotrienes, as well as proteins such as cytokines and enzymes.[11]

Bronchial Asthma

Bronchial asthma affects approximately 17 million people in the United States.[12] Many of those affected are children. Asthma is a condition that lasts throughout a person's life, although some people outgrow asthma as they become adults.

Etiology. Bronchial asthma can result from several factors, and methods are underway to classify the various types.[13] When asthma is caused by an allergic reaction, it

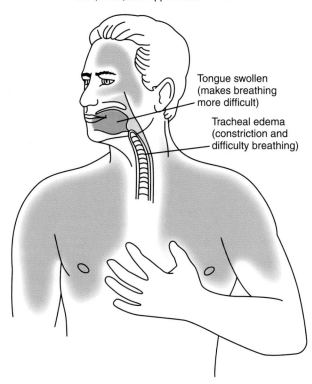

Edema and purplish/red coloration of skin in upper trunk, face, neck, and upper arms

Tongue swollen (makes breathing more difficult)

Tracheal edema (constriction and difficulty breathing)

FIGURE 2.1 A person experiencing anaphylactic shock.

is classified as a Type I hypersensitivity reaction. Large numbers of natural killer (NK) T lymphocytes have been found in the respiratory tract of patients with asthma, indicating that these probably play a significant role in the allergic reaction process.[14] One of the allergens that can cause an asthma episode is exercise. People with exercise-induced asthma are sensitive to the changes in humidity and temperature of the atmosphere. During intense exercise when breathing takes place through the mouth instead of the nose, the cold or hot external air is directly inhaled into the lungs and elicits an allergic response resulting in an asthma episode. Extremely cold air seems to be the most responsible as an allergen. Activities such as running, skiing, and outdoor sports performed in winter are most likely to cause asthmatic episodes.[15]

Signs and Symptoms. The characteristic signs and symptoms of asthma are coughing with wheezing and production of mucous in the bronchi. During an asthma episode, the bronchioles go into spasm, effectively closing the lumen of the tubes and preventing air exchange. The inflammation within the walls of the bronchioles causes a buildup of fluid that cannot be expelled until the spasm in the bronchioles is reduced. Difficulty breathing can be distressing for the patient and must be controlled by medications (see Medical Intervention).

Prognosis. Asthma is distressing and in severe cases can cause death, but usually it can be controlled with medications. Death can result from the person not initiating intervention quickly enough or not responding to the intervention.

Medical Intervention. The physician must decide what will be the most effective treatment for asthma in each patient. A referral to physical therapy may be part of the plan. Determining the allergen that precipitates allergic asthma is helpful so that the patient can avoid exposure to these allergens, if possible. Daily inhaled corticosteroids are often used to control asthma symptoms.[16] Beta-adrenoceptor agonists (β-agonists) are another form of medication used for asthma that cause bronchodilation of the inflamed airways, thus relieving breathing difficulties.[17]

Physical Therapy Intervention. Breathing exercises and general exercise have been shown to be effective in reducing the need for medications for people with asthma.[18] Physical therapy techniques for improving breathing patterns, as well as teaching self-monitoring of airway health by using a peak flow meter and effective deep-breathing exercises can be beneficial for all ages.[19] Relaxation training for all age groups can also reduce the panic associated with an acute asthma episode. Instruction in the use of appropriate warm-up and cool-down before exercise or sports can decrease the onset of exercise induced asthma.

Allergic Rhinitis

Allergic rhinitis is common in the United States, with approximately 39 million people affected,[20] or 20% of the population.[21] Symptoms of allergic rhinitis often start in early childhood and continue throughout the person's life span, although symptoms can occur at any age.[22]

Etiology. Allergic rhinitis (hay fever) may be caused by reaction to tree and grass pollen or other antigens such as animal dander, molds, or dust.[23,24] The overactive immune system develops antibodies to the allergen. The pollen reaction may be caused by a generally high pollen count in the air or may be due to specific types of pollen such as evergreen or ragweed pollen. After the allergic reaction is stimulated, the released histamine sets in motion the process of inflammation, which results in the signs and symptoms of allergic rhinitis.

Signs and Symptoms. The characteristic signs and symptoms of allergic rhinitis include sneezing, runny nose, edema of the nasal mucous membranes and the conjunctiva of the eye, coughing, sore throat, headache, and skin rashes with itching.[25]

Prognosis. Allergic rhinitis can cause some quality-of-life issues but is not usually life threatening.[26] People who are allergic to specific allergens should attempt to avoid them to decrease or prevent the onset of symptoms.

Medical Intervention. Allergy testing may be performed through the use of skin tests or blood tests to determine the cause of the allergic reaction.[27] Medical treatment options include the use of antihistamine medications of varying intensities and length of action and the use of corticosteroid inhalers or injections. Decongestants may also be helpful.[28]

Physical Therapy Intervention. No physical therapy intervention is indicated for allergic rhinitis. However, the clinical manifestations of this condition may affect a person's ability to participate in physical therapy.

Anaphylactic Shock (Anaphylaxis)

Anaphylactic shock or anaphylaxis is a systemic Type I hypersensitivity reaction (see Fig. 2-1). The anaphylactic response can occur in any age group and in all populations.

Etiology. An anaphylactic response is produced upon exposure to an allergen, which results in the release of huge amounts of histamine into the general circulatory system. The histamine causes vasodilation of the blood vessels and a drop in blood pressure. For such a reaction to occur, the body must have previously been exposed to an allergen or antigen to develop sensitivity. The most commonly recognized allergen is a bee sting.[29] When working in a hospital setting, PTAs may see an anaphylactic response to the dyes used in radiographic techniques, to anesthetics used in surgery,[30] or to the use of antibiotics

or other medications.[31,32] Some people may develop such a response to certain foods such as peanuts, seafood, or eggs.

Signs and Symptoms. The characteristic signs and symptoms of anaphylactic shock are edema in the larynx, bronchi, and lungs, resulting in closing of the airways and breathing difficulties. The onset of these symptoms can be rapid, often within minutes of exposure to the irritant. The airway may be occluded altogether, causing asphyxiation (suffocation) if the anaphylactic shock is not treated. Spasm in the bronchi and pulmonary edema can result in major circulatory symptoms, including very low blood pressure, which places the body in a state of "shock." Gastrointestinal symptoms are also common, such as pain in the abdomen, severe muscle cramping, nausea, diarrhea, and vomiting.[33] The person may collapse, be unable to breathe, and lose consciousness.[34] Other symptoms include rapid and weak pulse, dizziness, weakness, warmth, redness, and edema of the skin of the face, neck, upper chest and arms, and urticaria (hives)[35] (see Fig. 2-1).

Prognosis. If treated, the condition usually resolves. Severe anaphylactic reactions can be fatal if treatment is not provided or if the person does not respond to the intervention.

Medical Intervention. Anaphylactic shock is treated by an injection of **epinephrine** (adrenalin), which stimulates the heart and reduces the effects of the allergen. Individuals who have a history of anaphylactic shock are recommended to carry an epinephrine kit or epi-pen with them at all times[36] so that they can self-administer a dose of epinephrine if they are exposed to the offending allergen and start to exhibit the symptoms of anaphylactic shock. When emergency medical attention is available in severe cases of anaphylaxis, the injection or injections of epinephrine may need to be followed up with intravenous epinephrine, oxygen therapy, and use of oral antihistamines.[37]

Physical Therapy Intervention. No physical therapy is indicated for anaphylactic shock. The person with suspected anaphylactic shock should be monitored for vital signs, cardiopulmonary resuscitation provided as needed, and the emergency medical system (EMS) activated. When awaiting the EMS services, the person should be kept warm and positioned in supine with the lower extremities elevated above the level of the heart.

It Happened in the Clinic

A young female physical therapist was having lunch and eating a piece of quiche in the hospital where she worked. Coworkers noted that the PT was becoming flushed and asked if she was feeling ill. The person felt fine and continued to eat her lunch. After 10 minutes, she started to feel strange and returned to the PT department, where she noted she was extremely red, almost purple, in the face, upper chest, and arms and was starting to become edematous in the same areas. She immediately went to the emergency room (ER), was intercepted by a transporter, and rushed in a wheelchair to the ER. On arrival at ER, she experienced difficulty breathing. She was transferred to a bed, injected with epinephrine, and an IV of epinephrine was started. Relief of symptoms occurred within a few seconds, and a subsequent antihistamine medication was administered orally. The patient was kept in the ER for an additional 30 minutes and released to return to work with instructions to return immediately to ER if the symptoms resumed. The PT experienced anaphylactic shock, a Type I hypersensitivity reaction, in this case thought to be due to an allergic reaction to eggs. **Note:** Patients who have experienced anaphylactic shock are advised to carry an epinephrine kit at all times in case of future occurrences. In this case, the PT was fortunate that she was working in a hospital at the time of onset of symptoms.

Type II Hypersensitivity

Type II hypersensitivity reactions are the result of antibodies that react with antigens within the body's own tissues. The antigens can be either extrinsic (external) or intrinsic (internal). Such reactions are known as cytotoxic because the antigens are toxic to cells. The intrinsic antigens include certain proteins and RNA and DNA. In the autoimmune diseases, it is such antigens that cause destructive damage to the body. Extrinsic antigens include drugs and chemicals. No scientific explanation exists as to what causes the body to react to, and destroy, its own tissue as if it were a foreign substance. Physical therapists and PTAs treat people with many of the conditions resulting from Type II hypersensitivity such as rheumatoid arthritis, systemic lupus erythematosus, diabetes mellitus, multiple sclerosis, myasthenia gravis, and Reiter's syndrome, all of which are discussed in later chapters.

Blood transfusion incompatibility is an example of a Type II hypersensitivity. Type A blood contains antigens to A on the red blood cells and anti-B antibodies.[38] Type B blood contains antigens to B on the red blood cells and anti-A antibodies. If Type A blood is given to a Type B recipient, an antibody antigen reaction destroys the red blood cells of the person with type B blood.

Another type II hypersensitivity reaction is **hemolytic disease of the newborn** (HDN). This disease is similar to the result of a blood transfusion that is incompatible with the recipient blood type. In HDN, if the baby is rhesus (RH) or D positive, having the antigens to factor D, and the mother is RH or D negative, without the antigens to factor D, the baby and maternal blood may mix through the placental vessels during birth.[39] This does not affect the firstborn baby because the birth occurs before the mother has a chance to develop antibodies in response to the D factor in the baby's blood.[40] If a second baby is also RH or D positive, the fetus may be in considerable danger because the mother has developed antibodies in response to the D factor, which destroy the baby's red blood cells, causing severe anemia. If these babies survive to full term, they may have to receive a blood transfusion at birth, which does not contain the antibodies. Many of the fetuses with this problem do not mature to full term and may spontaneously abort because of the buildup of antibodies. Prevention of this problem can be achieved by giving the mother an anti-D immunoglobulin injection immediately after the first birth.[41] This injection of anti-D prevents the maternal system from producing antibodies to factor D.

Type III Hypersensitivity

This type of hypersensitivity is known as an **immune complex reaction.** The antigens and antibodies combine to form a complex, which becomes embedded in certain tissue, such as blood vessel walls. The complex causes an inflammatory response and results in tissue destruction. Examples of such a reaction occur in glomerulonephritis[42] (inflammation of the kidney glomeruli), systemic lupus erythematosus (SLE), and rheumatoid arthritis.

Type IV Hypersensitivity

A Type IV response is a delayed response hypersensitivity also known as cell mediated hypersensitivity.[43] The T lymphocytes become sensitive to the presence of antigens and produce a delayed response when exposed to that antigen. Certain tests such as the PPD test, used to check for the presence of antibodies to tuberculosis (TB), rely on this type of reaction.[44] When the antigen for TB is injected under the skin of the forearm, a delayed inflammatory reaction in the form of a local skin response occurs within a couple of days. A positive reaction producing an area of inflamed skin over a specified diameter indicates that the person has been previously exposed to the antigen and has produced antibodies. A skin reaction does not, however, mean that the person actually has active TB but merely that the person has been exposed to it and has produced antibodies to the disease. In some countries, a bacille Calmette-Guerin (BCG) vaccine is administered to children that stimulates antibodies to TB, often resulting in a positive PPD test.[45]

Another example of Type IV hypersensitivity is an allergic reaction to direct contact with certain chemicals in perfumes, soaps and cosmetics, metals present in jewelry, plant toxins found in poison oak, poison ivy and poison sumac, and latex, causing contact dermatitis. Latex products are used extensively in health care, and latex sensitivity is an increasing problem. Studies have shown that as many as 17% of health care workers are sensitive to latex products.[46] Latex gloves can cause a local skin reaction on the hands and wrists, which can lead to sores. Individuals with this direct contact sensitivity must use nonlatex products when working in the health care environment. In some cases, individuals develop sensitivity to latex when they have not previously been affected. Latex sensitivity falls within the Type IV hypersensitivity reaction but in some cases can also be a Type I reaction, resulting in anaphylactic shock.[47] Sensitivity to latex products and perfumes is relevant to the practice of physical therapy. If PTAs or their patients are allergic to latex, the PTA must ensure that no latex is used during treatment. PTAs who are allergic to perfumed products may need to ask their patients to refrain from using any scented products, including hair gels and sprays, especially when performing hands-on intervention techniques. Rejection of organ transplants also falls under the Type IV hypersensitivity category.[48]

Vaccination

Vaccination, or immunization, is a way to establish resistance to disease by introducing the body to certain antigens that elicit the immune response and cause the body to create antibodies to the antigen responsible for the disease. These antigens are administered to the body by mouth or injection. A vaccine contains either dead or very weak antigen or a synthetic compound that mimics the effects of the antigen, so that it does not actually cause the disease when administered but stimulates the body to produce antibodies to the antigen. After the antibodies are produced, they are able to fight off attacks from the actual disease. Many vaccines are given to children and adults to help prevent acquisition of the disease. Vaccinations include those against rubella (German measles), rubeola (measles), mumps, varicella (chicken pox), poliomyelitis, hepatitis B, influenza, diphtheria, tetanus and pertussis (DTaP vaccine), hepatitis A and B, and polio.[49] Vaccination is important for health care workers, including PTAs, to protect themselves from these diseases, because as health care providers, they are at higher risk of coming in contact with them.[50] Before receiving a vaccine, people may have a blood titer taken to determine whether they already have antibodies to the disease in their blood. The level of antibody present in the blood required to be able to fight off the disease varies with the disease. Prior infection or contact with the disease does not necessarily mean that a person is immune to it. In some cases, vaccination is required even though the person has previously been infected with the disease. The use of the blood titer for antibodies is recommended by the Centers for Disease Control and Prevention (CDC). After vaccination for a particular disease, a blood titer determines whether the person has converted (produced antibodies to the disease). Some persons never actually "convert" by producing antibodies to the disease after vaccination that are detectable by a blood titer test, and the decision to revaccinate must be made by the physician. Booster vaccinations are required for certain diseases because the antibody level in the blood diminishes over time.

Vaccines for different diseases are constantly developed and reviewed in the United States by the Advisory Committee on Immunization Practices (ACIP) of the CDC. In 2006, the ACIP recommended approval of a herpes zoster (shingles) vaccine for people aged over 60 years.[51] In 2007, the ACIP approved a vaccine against the genital human papillomavirus (HPV). Extensive trials of the vaccine demonstrated that it reduced the risk of several strains of the HPV.[52] HPV is responsible for causing cervical cancer, some types of genital warts, and vaginal and vulvar cancer. It is estimated that approximately 6.2 million people in the United States are infected each year with the HPV. The general vaccination will help to reduce these numbers.[53] Recent controversy has arisen over the proposal for mandatory HPV vaccination for young girls within several states in the United States.

Effects of Exercise on the Immune Response

New evidence is emerging to prove that moderate exercise actually does boost the immune system, and intense exercise stimulates the increase of the natural killer T cells in the body.[54] Exercise stimulates the production of white blood cells that assist the body in fighting off infection.[55]

Evidence indicates that a healthy person fights infection better than one who has another disease. Regular exercise seems to play a role in the ability to fight infections. Research has also shown that exercise stimulates the body to produce endorphins, which are natural opiates produced by the body to diminish the effects of pain[56] that may also reduce the effects of depression and improve sleep patterns.[57]

Why Does the Physical Therapist Assistant Need to Know About Infection?

PTAs treat many people who are susceptible to infection, and thus the PTA must be aware of the beneficial effects of regular hand washing to help prevent the spread of infection from one person to another. The PTA must practice sterile technique, when appropriate, for wound care cases and understand the need to follow standard/universal precautions when working with all patients. Unless the PT and PTA have an understanding of the methods of transmission of infective agents, they cannot help to reduce the risk of spread of infection to patients and each other.

Many types of infectious agents exist that can affect the body in various ways. Some diseases, such as rubella, have been suppressed by vaccination, but comparatively new diseases have become a problem, such as the human immunodeficiency virus (HIV). A continual battle within the medical profession is taking place to find new ways to combat the spread of these diseases. Several kinds of organisms are responsible for the spread of infection. It is important that PTAs understand how infection is spread and ways in which they may prevent the spread, as much as possible.

Nosocomial infections, or health care–associated infections,[58] are infections that patients acquire while in the health care setting that they did not have before they entered the hospital or health care facility (refer to Chapter 10 for further details about nosocomial infections). According to the CDC (2006), these health care–associated infections cause "2 million infections, 90,000 deaths, and $4.5 billion in excess health care costs annually"[59] in the United States. The CDC also developed guidelines for health care workers on hand washing in 2002.[60] PTAs can help to reduce the nosocomial infection rate by washing their hands before and after treating a patient, before and after using rubber gloves, before and after eating, and after using the bathroom. The role that hand washing plays in reducing the spread of infection cannot be stressed strongly enough.

Infections

Infections may be endogenous (already within the body) or exogenous (from a source outside the body). Diseases that are spread from one person to another are considered to be infectious or contagious. Infectious or contagious diseases can be spread through the air into the bronchial system, directly onto open wounds, through contact with body fluids, by ingesting the infective agent in food or drinks, or from direct contact with the pathogenic organism. Infective agents include bacteria, viruses, and fungi. Another mechanism of transmission is via a vector, such as an insect. Diseases spread by insects include Lyme disease, plague, West Nile virus, and yellow fever.[61] Parasitic diseases are caused by parasites that enter the body directly from infected water; through the skin, as in the case of the nematode that causes filariasis;[62] through the mouth, as in the protozoan that causes giardiasis;[63] or via an insect vector such as the *Anopheles* mosquito, which transmits the plasmodium parasite that causes malaria.[64]

Types of Microorganisms

Bacteria are unicellular (one cell) organisms with no mitochondria and a single chromosome.[65] Some bacteria can live outside living tissue, but others can only live within the tissue of a host (see Fig. 2-2). Bacteria occur in various shapes and sizes and are named according to their appearance. Some of the more common are the bacilli, which are rod shaped; the cocci, which are spherical; and the spirilla, which have curved outer walls.[66] When the bacteria combine with each other into groups they acquire a name dependent on that grouping. Some examples are streptococci, which combine in chains, and staphylococci, which combine in clusters. Bacteria have an external cell wall, which provides resistance to damage. Some bacteria have an additional defense of a coating of sticky, slimy material that makes them difficult to engulf by phagocytosis, or the action by neutrophils, monocytes, and macrophages of engulfing and destroying bacteria. The bacterial cell membrane is inside the cell wall and is selectively permeable, like that of a human cell. The selective permeability to substances depends on the type of bacteria. Bacteria contain DNA and RNA unique to the specific bacteria. Some bacteria can move because of a tail-like mechanism called a flagella, whereas other bacteria such as *Clostridium tetani*, which causes tetanus,[67] produce spores that can survive high temperatures and chemicals such as bleach, which would normally destroy other bacteria. This type of bacteria is more difficult to destroy. The *C. tetani* bacteria can live in the soil in spore form for many years waiting for a suitable host (a person to infect). Some bacteria are normally present in areas of the body such as the nose and intestines and do not cause infection unless they find their way into an area where they should not be or multiply to an extent that the body is unable to handle.

Viruses need a living host to survive and reproduce (see Fig. 2-3). Unlike bacteria, viruses contain either RNA or DNA. After the virus finds a host cell, it invades it and uses it to provide the energy and nutrients needed for it to reproduce.[68] The host cell is destroyed, and the virus reproduces and infects other cells. One factor that makes viruses dangerous is that they mutate (change) rapidly, and thus any immunity built up against them also has to change. That is why the influenza virus is so difficult to fight. An influenza vaccination will only protect against certain strains of the influenza virus and because the virus constantly mutates and new strains are produced that may not be susceptible to the antibodies produced by the vaccination.

Fungi are molds or yeasts. These require moisture and warmth to reproduce and are most often found on the skin or on mucous membranes. Because fungi thrive in warm, moist environments, they may be found in areas of the body that are prone to sweating. A common fungal infection is caused by the tinea pedis fungus, which causes athlete's foot.[69]

Development of Infection

The infective agent has to overcome many human body defense mechanisms for a person to develop an infection. The person or host has a natural defense and must be susceptible to the infection. The immune system, previously described, must fail to resist the infection. It may be that the individual has another illness, which is taxing the immune system and reducing the ability to fight off the

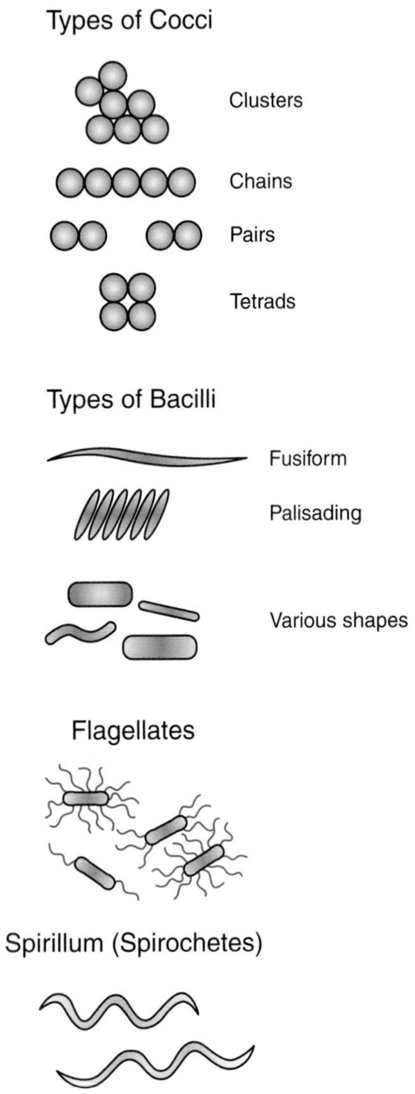

Types of Cocci

Clusters

Chains

Pairs

Tetrads

Types of Bacilli

Fusiform

Palisading

Various shapes

Flagellates

Spirillum (Spirochetes)

FIGURE 2.2 Bacteria.

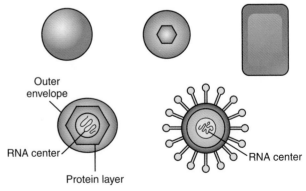

Outer envelope

RNA center

Protein layer

RNA center

FIGURE 2.3 Viruses come in many shapes and sizes.

infection. In other cases, the infecting organism may be resilient and present in high concentrations, making it difficult for the human body to overcome.

The transmission of an infection can be considered a cycle of events. The infective agent has to enter the host through a portal of entry from a source such as an open wound, an insect, a contaminated needle, inhalation through the respiratory tract, contaminated food, or sexual contact. Prevention of this initial contact can be achieved in many cases through adequate teaching of methods to prevent disease transmission. In the PT setting, use of standard precautions, sterile technique when dressing wounds, and frequent hand washing play a major role in the reduction of the spread of infection. Standard precautions, or universal precautions, are defined as the precautions taken by health care workers with all patients when there is a possibility of contact with blood or body fluids, excretions, or mucous membranes. In practice, standard precautions are often used when working with all patients to prevent infection of either the patient from the health care provider or the health care provider from the patient, as well as to prevent transmitting infectious agents from one patient to another. These guidelines are recommended by the CDC.[70] Precautions include the use of regular hand washing and the use of gloves, gowns, masks, and eye protection whenever indicated. Hand washing is the primary preventive measure to decrease the spread of infectious or harmful agents. The use of gloves is the most common. Gowns, masks, and eye protection should be used if there is danger of blood or bodily fluids splashing onto the care provider. The PTA is referred to the U.S. Department of Labor, Occupational Safety and Health Administration (OSHA) Bloodborne pathogens and needlestick prevention OSHA standards at http://www.osha.gov[71] for further details on standard/universal precautions. The guidelines can also be found in the appendix of *Taber's Cyclopedic Medical Dictionary*, 20th edition (F. A. Davis, 2005).

After an infection has invaded the body, it may be a few days or even weeks before observable signs and symptoms of the disease are apparent or detectable. The period of time between contact with the infection and initial onset of symptoms is known as the incubation period. The infective organism must multiply and settle in a particular site in the body to reproduce. Characteristic signs and symptoms of an infection may include general body fatigue, headaches, diarrhea or constipation, a skin rash, severe pain in a specific area, abscesses with purulent drainage, and inflammation of specific areas. An example of inflammation in response to a disease process is manifested as edema of the bronchial mucosa in a throat infection.

Treatment of Infection

To treat an infection, the physician must determine a diagnosis. This is usually achieved by taking a blood, urine, or tissue sample, creating a culture of the infective agent, and examining it in the laboratory. After the infection is identified, a suitable medication can be chosen for treatment. Certain medications act on specific bacteria, and thus diagnosis of the causative agent is necessary to provide effective treatment. The medications used to combat infections fall into various types. **Antimicrobial medications** include antibiotics, antivirals, and antifungals. Each type of medication is used to fight a specific type of infective agent. Of the antibacterials, the bacteriocidals act to destroy the organism, and the bacteriostatic medications reduce the rate of reproduction of the bacteria so that the immune system can destroy the infective organism. A **broad-spectrum antibiotic** is used to destroy a wide range of types of bacteria.

Antibiotic-resistant bacteria are becoming more common. Commonly occurring resistant bacteria include methicillin-resistant *Staphylococcus aureus* (MRSA), vancomycin-resistant *Enterococcus* (VRE),[72] vancomycin-intermediate *S. aureus* (VISA), multidrug-resistant TB (MDR TB), drug-resistant *Streptococcus pneumoniae* (DRSP), glycopeptide-intermediate *S. aureus,* resistant gram-negative *pseudomonas,* and a resistant form of *Neisseria gonorrhoeae*. The CDC has a special task force to monitor these antimicrobial-resistant bacteria.[73] According to the CDC (2007), data shows that antimicrobial-resistant infections are increasing: "In 1974, MRSA infections accounted for two percent of the total number of staph infections; in 1995 it was 22%; in 2004 it was some 63%."[74]

Recent studies suggest that prescribing antimicrobial medications to children for minor infections increases antimicrobial-resistant bacteria for the whole population.[75] Completing the entire prescription of antibiotic drugs during an infection is extremely important. Often patients stop taking antibiotics once they start to have diminished symptoms, thinking that the infection has resolved. If the entire prescription is not taken, the bacteria strains that are susceptible to the antibiotic are killed, but the stronger, more resilient parts of the infective agent are not killed; thus, the remaining strain develops a resistance to the antibiotic received.[76] Transmission of the resistant bacteria results in resistance to the antibiotic in the next host. When these bacteria migrate to a new host, the antibiotic does not work against this new strain of bacteria.[77]

The factors affecting the antimicrobial-resistant bacteria problem are extensive and include the following:

- Overprescription of antibiotics for conditions that do not require antibiotic intervention, including viral infections that do not respond to antibiotics such as colds and influenza
- The incorrect prescription or dosage of antibiotics
- Prescription of an antibiotic not specific to the bacterial infection
- Failure of patients to follow the prescribed dosage, including not completing the length of time the medication should be taken
- Purchase of antibiotics from mail-order businesses that enable patients to take the medications without a physician's recommendation
- The use of antibiotics in food animals, resulting in increased resistance in humans via consumption of the meat[78]
- Antibacterial agents sprayed on fruits and vegetables, which increases the importance of washing fruit and vegetables before eating

According to the CDC the medical community is concerned that this problem will become worse if steps are not taken to reduce the risks. The medical community has started to become more vigilant in its prescription of antibiotics, seeking alternative methods of treatment for minor infections. In addition, microbiology testing of tissue samples, blood, wound exudate, and other body fluids is recommended to identify the specific infective organism so that an infection-specific antimicrobial medication may be prescribed.

Several factors increase this risk of resistant bacteria within health care settings, including the advanced general age of the patients, severity of the illness, or having many patients undergoing invasive procedures, increasing the likelihood of transmission of infection in a situation where many infections exist.[79] Before a prescription is given, a culture should be taken and analyzed to determine which antimicrobial medication is most appropriate for treatment of the specific organism. Medically prescribed antimicrobial medications should be taken as directed by the physician, and the complete prescription should be finished.

The implications for the future of health care regarding antimicrobial-resistant organisms are enormous because a constant fight is necessary to develop more potent antibiotics to combat the resistant strains of bacteria. Bacteria and viruses are becoming more and more resistant to the available antimicrobial medications, necessitating stronger medications to be developed. The medical field is running out of options, and these resistant strains of microorganisms are creating a difficult problem for the future of medicine. The resultant emerging infections are likely to be a major medical challenge in the 21st century.

Why Does the Physical Therapist Assistant Need to Know About Neoplasia and Oncology Treatments?

The implications of neoplasias and oncology treatments for physical therapy interventions are many. According to the American Cancer Society, projected statistics for 2007 indicate that cancer will overtake heart disease as the number one cause of death in the United States. However, the news is not all bleak because cancer deaths rose steadily between 1930 and 2005 in the United States, but a reduction in overall numbers of deaths from cancer was noted in 2006. Reduction in the actual number of deaths was attributed to reduced deaths from lung and bronchi cancer in men.[80] Estimates for 2007 are that 26% of cancer cases in women will involve the breast and 29% of cases in men will involve the prostate. Lung and bronchi cancers are projected to account for 15% of cases in both men and women.[81] However, the percentage of deaths from cancer are expected to remain proportionately higher in lung and bronchi cases. Advances in the treatment available for cancer, and the early detection and diagnosis of tumors, have improved the survival rate for most types of cancer.

The evaluating PT must be aware of the possibility of tumors and their effects on the body. Primary tumors in bone can cause fractures, and primary or metastatic tumors in joints can cause abnormal "empty" end feels in the joints. Occasionally a soft tissue injury is misdiagnosed, and a tumor may actually be causing the pain and dysfunction. Malignant tumors may or may not be painful. A red flag for the PT and PTA would be if a patient does not respond as expected to a particular PT treatment regimen. A referral back to the treating physician for further tests is indicated under such circumstances.

Neoplasia

Neoplasia is the term used for production of neoplasms (malignant/cancerous tumors). The study of neoplasia is called oncology. A tumor, or new growth beyond the normal, may be classified as benign or malignant (see Table 2-2). A benign tumor is a growth that is self-limiting in size and does not necessarily spread. A malignant (cancerous) tumor grows uncontrollably and has the potential to spread to other tissues. The process of development of a cancerous tumor is called **carcinogenesis,** and the progression of growth of malignant tumors is termed the metastatic cascade. For a tumor to grow, it has to resist the attack from the immune system previously described—in particular, T lymphocytes, macrophages, and the NK cells. It also has to undergo **angiogenesis** (development of its own blood supply). Malignant tumors are invasive and usually destroy the tissue in which they develop and may metastasize (spread) to other areas of the body. Such tumors can be life threatening depending on where they are located and how aggressive they are. Benign tumors usually have the suffix "oma," and the prefix describes the tissue of origin. An osteoma[82] is a benign tumor in bone. Malignant tumors have a suffix of "sarcoma" or "carcinoma," again using a prefix of the tissue of origin. An osteosarcoma[83] is a malignant tumor of bone. Exceptions to this rule do occur, and specific tumors may be named for the person who first described them, such as Ewing's sarcoma, Kaposi's sarcoma (see Fig. 2-4), Burkitt's lymphoma, and Hodgkin's disease (see Table 2-3 for the names of some tumors and their locations and classifications).

Table 2.2   **Characteristics of Benign and Malignant Tumors**

CHARACTERISTIC	BENIGN TUMORS	MALIGNANT TUMORS
Appearance of cells	Similar to cells of host tissue	Cells "undifferentiated"—do not look like host tissue cells
Rate of growth	Slow	Fast
Metastases (spread)	None, remains localized	Yes, readily metastasizes
Appearance of tumor surface	Smooth (often encapsulated); well-defined borders; noninvasive	Irregular—not encapsulated; invasive
Vascularity	Little to no vascularity	High vascularity
Recurrence	Rare	Recur readily

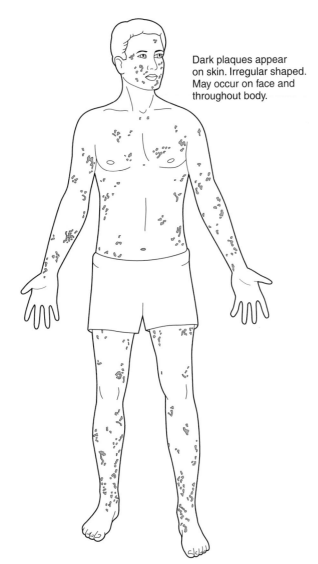

Dark plaques appear on skin. Irregular shaped. May occur on face and throughout body.

FIGURE 2.4 Kaposi's sarcoma.

Metastasis of a malignant tumor occurs through several means. The process involves the relocation of cancerous cells from the primary tumor to another area of the body, which then becomes an area of secondary cancerous tumors.[84] Metastasis can occur via the blood or lymphatic systems[85] or by "seeding," in which a cancerous cell breaks off from the original tumor and is transmitted through a body cavity, where it lodges elsewhere and starts to develop another tumor at a distant site. A malignancy that metastasizes to another area is still named for the site of the source of the neoplasia. Breast cancer cells that metastasize to bone are still breast cancer cells.[86]

Tumors tend to grow at a more accelerated rate than normal tissue and replace the original tissue cells. After the tumor becomes resident in an area, the original function of the host tissue becomes nonfunctional. The cells of a young tumor are similar to those of the host tissue and are classified as Grade I, but as the tumor becomes more advanced, the cells are known as "undifferentiated" in that they do not resemble the tissue of the host cells. Such tumors may progress through Grades II and III to a Grade IV. A Grade IV tumor is more invasive, likely to develop quickly, and is more life threatening.

Carcinogens

Carcinogens are causes of cancer and are classified as exogenous and endogenous. Exogenous factors are those that are external to the body and include physical, chemical, and viral agents. The National Institutes of Health 11th National Toxicology Report on Carcinogens lists numerous substances that are known to be carcinogenic and even more that are under investigation.[87] Some of the more common known carcinogens include asbestos dust; the chemical hydrocarbons found in gasoline, tar, and cigarettes; and high levels of x-ray and atomic radiation. Some physical carcinogens such as radiation from the sun may cause exposure to damaging levels of ultraviolet light that elicit cancerous changes in the skin. Certain RNA and DNA viruses have also been isolated as carcinogens. Both types of viruses transform the genetic makeup of the cell, causing it to become cancerous. Examples of DNA viruses include HPV, which can cause malignant tumors, especially of the cervix, vagina, and vulva. The Epstein-Barr virus (EBV), which is very common, can cause Burkitt's lymphoma, a lymphatic system cancer.[88]

Endogenous factors that can cause cancer include genetic tendencies passed down through the generations that reside in the chromosomes. These genetic factors do not necessarily mean that the individual will develop a particular cancer, but they may indicate a higher risk of developing it. Identification of genetic markers can help in the fight against breast, colon, and ovarian cancers that seem to have a familial association. After a genetic marker for a particular cancer is identified, more regular testing can be performed to provide early diagnosis of cancerous lesions.

Risk Factors for Malignant Tumors

Many risk factors exist for the development of malignant tumors. Some risk factors can be avoided, and others cannot. In some cases, there is a history of a certain type of

Table 2.3   **Some Tumors and Their Locations/Classifications**

TUMOR	LOCATION/TISSUE OF ORIGIN	CLASSIFICATION
Chondroma	Cartilage	Benign
Chondrosarcoma	Cartilage	Malignant
Osteoma	Bone	Benign
Osteosarcoma	Bone	Malignant
Lipoma	Fat cells	Benign
Liposarcoma	Fat cells	Malignant
Kaposi's sarcoma	Skin/mucous membranes	Malignant
Melanoma	Skin/melanocyte cells which synthesize melanin	Malignant
Hodgkin's disease	Lymph tissue	Malignant
Leukemia	White blood cells in bone marrow	Malignant
Burkitt's lymphoma	Lymph tissue	Malignant
Meningioma	Meninges of brain and nerves	Benign
Glioma	Nerve tissue	Malignant
Leiomyoma	Smooth muscle cells	Benign
Leiomyosarcoma	Smooth muscle cells	Malignant
Rhabdomyoma	Striated muscle cells	Benign
Rhabdomyosarcoma	Striated muscle cells	Malignant

cancer in a person's family, which increases the individual's tendency to develop the disease. Physician and patient knowledge of the patient's family history can help to determine suitable testing procedures for early identification of problems.[89] Breast cancer is a prime example of a hereditary risk factor. A high incidence of breast cancer in the family can alert the individual to have regular mammography tests, which are radiographic tests, for early detection of a tumor and to perform regular self-breast examinations (see Fig. 2-5 for an illustration of breast cancer). Another hereditary risk factor is colon cancer in the family. Colonoscopy, a procedure in which a flexible fiber-optic tube is passed via the rectum into the colon, can detect signs of colon cancer. Individuals who have a family history of such cancers can have these procedures performed more regularly at the advice of their family physician to detect any abnormalities early enough to

receive treatment and thus increase the chances of recovery from the invasive tumor. Factors such as age cannot be changed, but additional proactive tests can be performed for cancers that are known to be age-related. Prostate cancer is more prevalent in older men. Screening for prostate cancer can be performed during annual physical examinations to detect signs of the problem. Early detection is usually the key to successful treatment of any malignant tumor.

Controllable risk factors exist for the development of malignant tumors. Controllable risk factors include smoking, which can cause lung cancer; overexposure to the sun, which can cause skin cancer; promiscuity, which can cause cancer of the cervix; and high levels of fat in the diet, which is thought to increase the risk of colon cancer. Smoking causes approximately 90% of all lung cancers, and a person who smokes has 13.3 times more risk of

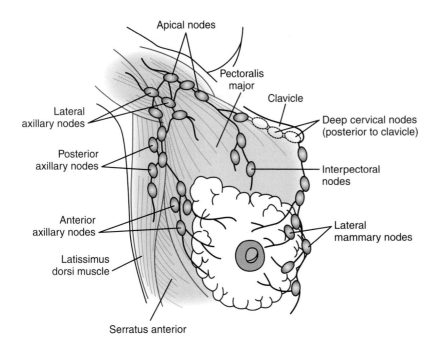

FIGURE 2.5 Common sites of lymphatic nodes affected by breast cancer.

developing lung cancer than someone who does not smoke.[90] Knowledge of some of the warning signs of cancer can alert the PT and PTA to refer the patient to the physician (see Box 2-1).

Incidences of different types of cancer vary worldwide. A higher incidence of both breast cancer and testicular cancer in North America, Australia, Western Europe, and Scandinavia has been found to be greater than in other parts of the world. However, the incidence of cervical cancer is lower in these countries than other parts of the world.[91] Various factors are thought to be responsible, including dietary habits, smoking, and pollution levels. The incidence of lung cancer is directly related to the incidence of smoking in a given population,

---

Box 2.1   Warning Signs for Cancer May Include:

- A skin lesion or sore that does not heal
- A mole or wart that suddenly starts to alter in size or shape
- Any unusual bleeding from the cervix or rectum
- Changes in bladder or bowel habits, such as habitual diarrhea or constipation when previously not noted
- A persistent cough or voice changes
- A lump within the tissue not previously recognized, such as in the breast, testicle, or skin
- Any such changes should prompt a visit to the physician.

GERIATRIC CONSIDERATIONS

Many older patients with end-stage neoplasia are referred to physical therapy for mobility training and exercises. Some patients may be under the care of hospice in the home setting. Emphasis should be placed on improving the quality of life for such patients, as it would be with a younger person in the same situation. Particular consideration should be given to ensuring the patient is as comfortable as possible during the treatment session and requesting the nurse or physician to have the patient take pain medications, if appropriate, before the treatment session. The physical therapy schedule may have to be planned to occur after pain medications have been administered. In some cases, the PTA may have to instruct the care providers how to use a mechanical lift for transferring the patient from the bed to a chair. In all cases, care should be taken to avoid overfatiguing the patient, bearing in mind that the goal of treatment is to improve function and quality of remaining life.

and although deaths from lung cancer are declining in North America and parts of Western Europe, they are increasing in Eastern Europe and other countries where smoking is increasing.[92] Skin cancer is more prevalent in hot climates, and prostate cancer is more prevalent in the elderly. Because the general life expectancy is increasing in the Western world, more cases of prostate cancer are being reported.

Treatment Interventions for Cancer

Medical interventions for cancer include chemotherapy, radiation, and surgery depending on the location, type, and stage of the cancerous tissue. If the tumor is diagnosed when small and localized, surgery may be performed to remove the whole tumor. Sometimes chemotherapy or radiation treatment is administered after surgery to ensure that the cancerous tissue is eliminated. In such cases, chemotherapy is known as prophylactic (preventive) treatment. In cancers such as leukemia, which involve blood cells, chemotherapy may be the only choice of treatment possible.[93] Side effects of chemotherapy and radiation can, however, include production of another form of cancer in some cases. If a cancer has already spread, chemotherapy and radiation therapy may be used palliatively to attempt to prolong life by reducing the size of the tumor and the metastases. Palliative treatment relieves the symptoms and prolongs life but does not cure. These treatments may require weekly visits to the hospital and can be exhausting and debilitating for the patient. In such cases, physical therapy intervention can assist in increasing endurance and strength to counteract some of these side effects. New procedures are constantly being developed for the treatment of cancer. An option for treatment of prostate cancer is insertion of a "seed" (brachytherapy) of a radioactive pellet in, or near, the prostate.[94] The use of this "seed" of radioactive material minimizes the more systemic side effects of prolonged chemotherapy and radiation therapy. Another comparatively new treatment is the CyberKnife, which has enabled treatment of difficult-to-reach tumors (not in the brain) with high doses of radiation that target the tumor very specifically without damage to the surrounding tissues.[95] A similar type of treatment with the Gamma Knife is used for tumors within the brain.[96] Both the Cyber Knife and the Gamma Knife use multiple rays of radiation in a three-dimensional pattern that converge on the tumor to destroy the cancerous cells. Other types of therapy for cancer are proton therapy,[97] intensity-modulated radiation therapy (IMRT),[98] and external beam therapy (EBT).[99]

The side effects of radiation therapy depend on the intensity of radiation administered and the length of time a person undergoes treatment.[100] More common side effects include damage to the skin and epithelial tissues, resulting in hair loss and inflammation of the skin, and damage to the mucous membranes of the intestines and mouth with associated diarrhea, vomiting, nausea, and mouth ulcers. Most side effects of radiation therapy are local to the treatment area, so not all symptoms will be experienced in each case.[101] Most patients become fatigued and can be depressed when undergoing radiation therapy. The full effects of radiation intervention may not be apparent until several weeks or even months after the exposure; however, most symptoms caused by the radiation therapy resolve gradually.[102] In some instances, radiation therapy treatment for cancer can result in fibrosis of connective tissue in the area radiated, causing restriction of adjacent joint range of motion (ROM). Recent advances in radiation therapy treatment have reduced the possibility of such side effects, but in rare cases, the treatment of breast cancer may cause a "frozen" shoulder due to scarring of the skin over the breast. Such restriction of joint motion requires physical therapy intervention and diligent gentle stretching of the affected tissue by the patient.[103] The development of scarring as a result of radiation therapy can predispose the person to lymphedema of the affected upper extremity.

Chemotherapy is a complicated process. The oncology physician determines what kind of medication will effectively attack the particular type of malignant cells. A combination of medications is often given at one time.[104] These medications interfere with the cycle of carcinogenesis. Some medications act to reduce the reproduction of malignant cells, others slow down the metabolism of the cells, and others inhibit the development of angiogenesis (new blood vessels that feed the tumor).[105] Examples of some chemotherapy medications are shown in Table 2-4. The problem with chemotherapy is that it is nonselective, so normal cells are affected as well as the cancerous ones. Side effects are similar to those of radiotherapy and include vomiting, intestinal problems, and hair loss. Patients benefit from psychosocial support during and after the oncology treatment. In many cases, a combination of chemotherapy and radiation therapy is used in the treatment of malignancy. Involvement of the entire medical oncology team including the oncology physician, general practitioner physician, physician assistant, nurse

Table 2.4 **Examples of Chemotherapy Medications With Their Classification**

MEDICATION	TYPE OF MEDICATION	USES	OF SPECIAL NOTE
Adriamycin	Antibiotic chemotherapy medication (one of the older chemotherapy medications)		Adriamycin, bleomycin, vincristine, and dacarbazine are collectively known as ABVD; often used in combination to treat Hodgkin's lymphoma
Bleomycin	Antibiotic chemotherapy and antimitotic	General use; also in testicular cancer and lymphoma[235]	
Vinblastine or vincristine	Antimitotic (prevents cell division of tumor)[236]	Used to treat lymphoma and leukemia as well as in combination with other chemotherapy medications for other cancers[237]	
Dacarbazine	Nonspecific anticancer that increases alkalinity of malignant cells to destroy them[238]	Used especially to treat Hodgkin's disease and malignant melanoma[239]	
Bevacizumab	Inhibits angiogenesis (formation of new blood vessels)	Used in combination with other medications in the treatment of solid tumors and colon cancer[240]	

practitioner, oncology nurse, social worker, psychologist, dietician, PT/PTA, and OT/COTA can make a major difference in the outcome of the treatment.

PHYSICAL THERAPY INTERVENTION

Physical therapy interventions are frequently indicated for people with neoplasia. Although the PT interventions may not relate directly to the actual neoplasia, mobility, strengthening, endurance, and aerobic exercises may be appropriate. PT is commonly indicated for patients postmastectomy (excision of breast) to help increase or maintain full range of motion of the shoulder and prevent, or reduce the risk of, edema or lymphedema of the upper extremity. Patients who have lymphedema postmastectomy receive lymphedema treatment from a specialized team of PT, OT, and physician. Many patients postmastectomy do not use their arm and thus develop adhesive capsulitis (frozen shoulder). Intervention with physical therapy can reduce the incidence of adhesive capsulitis. After a lobectomy (excision of a lung lobe), the PT and PTA can provide postural drainage and breathing exercises to assist with the recovery of lung tissue expansion and vital capacity. When treating patients with bone metastases, it is important to avoid applying resistance to the bones because of the possibility of fractures. Some patients undergoing chemotherapy and radiation therapy are referred for physical therapy to assist in increasing endurance,

strength, and aerobic fitness as a counter to the side effects of the cancer treatment.

Patients in the end stage of oncology are frequently referred for physical therapy through the hospice system. Intervention may include improving quality of life for the patient by teaching strengthening and endurance exercises, working on independent gait with an appropriate assistive device, providing modalities to reduce pain such as a transcutaneous electrical nerve stimulation (TENS) unit and heat, and teaching strategies to reduce fatigue and conserve energy. Teaching techniques for lifting, transferring, and maintaining joint mobility to care providers is an important function of the PT and PTA. This may include teaching the use of a mechanical lift in the home or demonstrating the use of a gait belt. Teaching correct body mechanics to care providers is important to prevent injury during the patient's illness.

Knowledge of the side effects produced by chemotherapy and radiation therapy can help the PTA determine when to avoid pushing the patient to do exercises. Working with patients with oncological problems can be psychologically difficult for the PTA. Many patients discuss issues with their PT and PTA that they would not discuss with anyone else. When working with patients with cancer, the PTA should avoid trying to answer questions beyond their scope of work and should refer the patient to the PT or the physician for specific answers to medical topics.

It Happened in the Clinic

A 54-year-old male was attending the outpatient clinic for a strained left elbow of unknown etiology. The PT evaluated the patient and determined that he had a ligamentous sprain and commenced treatment with heat, ultrasound, electrical stimulation, massage, and exercises. The patient was seen for six treatment interventions over a period of 2 weeks with no significant improvement, and the pain continued to be a problem on motion. By this time, the patient was exhibiting some atypical signs and symptoms, such as an empty-end feel in the joint, pain at rest and on motion, and inability to obtain relief of pain in any position. The patient was referred back to the treating orthopedist, and it was determined on magnetic resonance imaging that the patient had metastases in the elbow from a tumor in the lungs and was in the end stage of the disease process. The patient subsequently received chemotherapy and radiation therapy for the condition. Of note in this scenario is that if something does not seem right and the patient is not responding to treatment, a referral should be made back to the physician. In the case of the PTA, the PT should be consulted if treatment efficacy is not as expected.

Why Does the Physical Therapist Assistant Need to Know About Chromosome Abnormalities and Genetic and Hereditary Diseases?

Individuals with many of the diseases and conditions caused by chromosome abnormalities, whether hereditary or spontaneous genetic mutations, are treated in physical therapy clinics. The associated orthopedic, neurological, and developmental problems exhibited by these individuals can be reduced through physical therapy intervention. Much of the work with children involves educating the parents and caregivers about management of the problem and highlighting rehabilitation concepts to promote functional activity and improve quality of life. Many individuals with these diseases will require physical therapy intervention intermittently throughout their lives.

Genetic and Hereditary Chromosome Diseases

This section describes genetic and hereditary chromosome diseases the PT and PTA might encounter in practice. The content begins with an overview of the normal chromosome, before presenting examples of different kinds of genetic and hereditary diseases.

The Normal Chromosome

The normal human cell consists of 46 chromosomes (23 pairs). Twenty-two pairs are called autosomes, and one pair is called the sex chromosomes (see Fig. 2-6). The autosomes are of various shapes and are numbered according to their size and shape. The 23rd pair of sex chromosomes in males are XY and in females XX. The X chromosome is inherited from the mother, and the Y from the father. In the female child, each parent contributes an X chromosome. Cells of the body have 23 pairs of chromosomes except for the egg in the female and the sperm in the male, which each have only 23 chromosomes. When the egg is fertilized by the sperm, the resultant zygote has the required 23 pairs made up of a

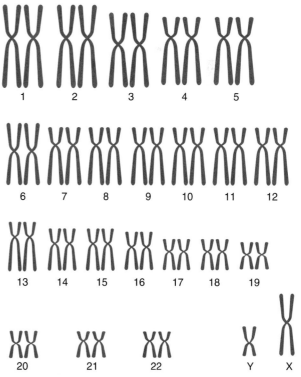

FIGURE 2.6 Normal complement of chromosomes

combination of maternal and paternal chromosomes. The genes contained within the chromosomes are sequences of deoxyribonucleic acid (DNA) containing specific information responsible for different cell functions. Each person has a different genetic arrangement called a genotype, making them unique, except for identical twins who have the same genotype. Ribonucleic acid (RNA) within the cell provides the communication mechanism with DNA during cellular protein synthesis.

HINTS ON USE OF THE GUIDE TO PHYSICAL THERAPIST PRACTICE 2-2

Most **genetic diseases** that require physical therapy intervention and premature infants have neuromuscular involvement. The most common patterns from the *Guide to Physical Therapist Practice* associated with such conditions are the "Neuromuscular" Practice Patterns 5

- 5B—Impaired neuromotor development

   Includes diagnoses such as birth trauma, fetal alcohol syndrome, prematurity, and other genetic disorders described in this chapter

- 5C—Impaired motor function and sensory integrity associated with nonprogressive disorders of the central nervous system—congenital origin or acquired in infancy or childhood

   Includes cerebral palsy, hydrocephalus, meningocele, prematurity, and traumatic brain injury when sustained during infancy or childhood.

   Premature infants may also fall under Cardiovascular/Pulmonary Practice Pattern 6

- 6G—Impaired ventilation, respiration/gas exchange, and aerobic capacity/endurance associated with respiratory failure in the neonate.

(From the American Physical Therapy Association, 2003. *Guide to physical therapist practice*, revised 2nd edition. Alexandria, VA: APTA. Used with permission.)

Overview of Genetic and Hereditary Chromosome Diseases

Several kinds of genetic and hereditary diseases exist. Some occur from traits passed on from the parents, and some occur due to mutations of the DNA sequencing in the genes during meiosis (division) of the cells into eggs and sperm. In DNA mutations that occur during meiosis, some are linked to the X or Y chromosome and are thus inherited by the resulting fetuses depending on whether they are male or female. If the defect is in a single gene, there are three possible types of inheritance known as autosomal recessive, autosomal dominant, and X-linked. Gregor Johann Mendel, an Austrian monk, studied traits in garden peas and was the first person to identify these methods of inheritance in the 19th century. In an autosomal dominant situation, the factor is inherited from one parent only, and each child has a 50% chance of inheriting the factor or trait. Occasionally disorders caused by an autosomal dominant gene may occur spontaneously in the egg or sperm and thus are not actually inherited but are due to a mutation during the fertilization process. In cases of spontaneous mutation of the genes, other children of the same couple will not be affected by the genetic defect. Diseases or disorders caused by autosomal dominance tend to have a total body effect. Examples of autosomal dominant diseases include Marfan's syndrome, a disorder of connective tissue that affects bones and the cardiovascular system (see Chapter 5); Huntington's disease, a neurological condition that takes effect in midlife (see Chapter 7); and osteogenesis imperfecta, a disease causing brittle bones (see Chapter 5). Autosomal recessive conditions are more common than autosomal dominant. The autosomal recessive conditions require the transmission of the same mutant genetic factor from each parent to cause a manifestation in a child. Under the Mendelian rules, children have a 25% risk of acquiring the genetic factor from their parents if both parents carry the trait.[106] Such conditions tend to occur more frequently when there is intermarriage within a community or population. Intermarriage increases the likelihood that both parents will have the same genetic mutation to pass on to their offspring. Disorders of this type include sickle-cell disease (sickle-cell anemia) and cystic fibrosis (see Chapter 4). X chromosome–linked disorders are manifested only in males because they are examples of recessive traits. The male has only one X chromosome; thus the trait is able to dominate. If the trait is passed on to the female, she will be a carrier but will not exhibit the disease. Examples of X-linked disorders include Duchenne's and Becker's muscular dystrophy (see Chapter 6), Fragile-X syndrome, and hemophilia A and B.

Some chromosome abnormalities are due to the effect of teratogens, a chemical or other agent that causes birth abnormalities by affecting the normal growth of the fetus (see Table 2-5). Rubella is a major cause of birth defects, especially retardation secondary to microcephaly (a small brain) in the fetus (see Fig. 2-7). The highest risk to the fetus occurs if the mother contracts rubella during the first trimester of pregnancy. Potential mothers should be

Table 2.5 **Exogenous Teratogens and Their Possible Effects on the Fetus**

TYPE OF EXOGENOUS TERATOGEN (EXTERNAL TO THE BODY)	EXAMPLE	EFFECTS
Physical	X-Rays	Birth defects
Chemical	Medications—thalidomide (sleeping pill taken in late 1950s by pregnant women)	Malformation of limbs (shortened or missing)
Chemical	Alcohol	Fetal alcohol syndrome—growth and mental retardation with low IQ, altered facial features may occur
Microbial	Toxoplasma, rubella, cytomegalovirus, herpes virus, Epstein-Barr virus, varicella, leptospira	TORCH syndrome—internal organ defects of brain, heart, lungs, spleen, liver; mental retardation, neurological problems
Microbial	Rubella (German measles)	Microcephaly (small brain) with associated mental retardation, heart defects
Microbial	Toxoplasmosis, cytomegalovirus	Brain abnormalities in basal ganglia and lateral ventricles (hydrocephalus), small eyes

provided immunity to rubella to protect the fetus. Other examples of teratogens include alcohol use (see Fig. 2-8); known teratogenic prescription and over-the-counter legal medications and illicit drug use by the mother during pregnancy; various types of virus, including syphilis and cytomegalovirus (CMV); and many types of infectious diseases.[107,108] (See Chapter 10 for details of syphilis and CMV.) Some of these teratogens cause a syndrome of defects known as TORCH. This acronym stands for the causative agents of the syndrome, which are toxoplasma, rubella, CMV, and the herpes virus. The "O" covers other viruses such as varicella and EBV. Characteristics of TORCH include mental retardation, neural defects, eye defects, and problems with heart, lungs, spleen, and liver.[109,110]

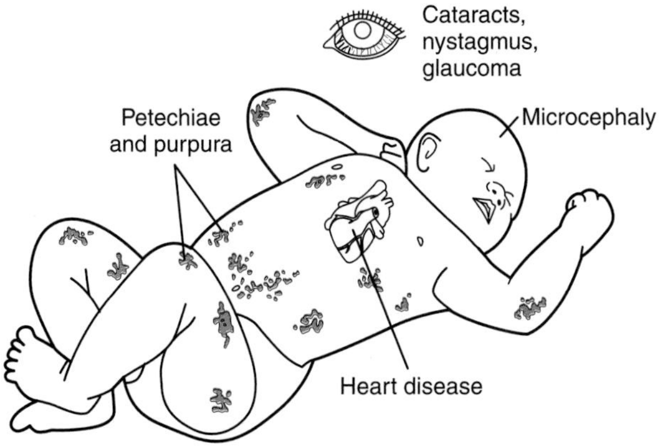

Cataracts, nystagmus, glaucoma

Petechiae and purpura

Microcephaly

Heart disease

FIGURE 2.7 Signs and symptoms of congenital rubella syndrome.

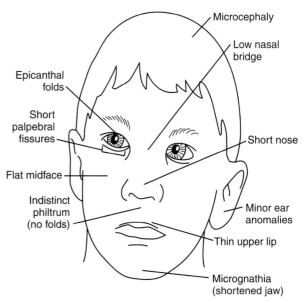

Microcephaly

Low nasal bridge

Epicanthal folds

Short palpebral fissures

Flat midface

Indistinct philtrum (no folds)

Short nose

Minor ear anomalies

Thin upper lip

Micrognathia (shortened jaw)

FIGURE 2.8 Signs and symptoms of fetal alcohol syndrome.

Chromosome Abnormalities

Some chromosomal abnormalities occur as a result of an anomaly during the division of cells within the zygote and are not due to traits passed on from a parent. Such abnormalities may result from breakage of a chromosome with resultant recombination in a different pattern causing an abnormal sequencing of the DNA (see Fig. 2-9). This may lead to an extra chromosome (trisomy) or only one chromosome (monosomy). When these cells divide, they can produce a mosaic effect with joining of the wrong parts of the chromosomes to each other. Other types of abnormality associated with breakage of chromosomes include translocation, deletion, inversion, and ring chromosomes. Translocations occur when part of a chromosome is transferred to another chromosome. A Robertsonian translocation occurs when one of the five acrocentric chromosomes (the centromere is situated close to the end of the chromosome) 13, 14, 15, 21, and 22 has a fusion of the long arms. Some people are carriers for this type of translocation with no symptoms, and in others the condition results in such disorders as Patau's syndrome with translocation of chromosomes 13 and 14, or Down syndrome with translocation of chromosomes 21 and 22.[111]

Deletions are loss of a part of a chromosome. Inversion occurs when there is a break in two places and the chromosome reconnects in the wrong order. A ring chromosome is the result of a breakage in the chromosome and the two ends joining together to form a ring.

DETECTION OF CHROMOSOME ABNORMALITIES

Several prenatal tests can be performed to detect abnormalities of the fetus. These tests can be achieved by taking blood samples of the mother or amniotic fluid samples through amniocentesis (withdrawal of amniotic fluid by a needle placed through the maternal abdominal wall into the amniotic sac). The science involved in detecting fetal abnormalities continues to evolve. Some diseases such as the neural tube defect spina bifida can be detected by the presence of enzymes in the blood during a maternal serum alpha-fetal protein (MSAFP) test. The MSAFP test is usually performed during the 15th to 18th week of pregnancy.[112] Ultrasound scanning of the mother's abdomen can also detect some abnormalities. An amniocentesis test in which a sample of amniotic fluid is taken via a needle through the mother's abdomen may also be performed.[113] Since the development of the MSAFP test, amniocentesis is not performed as frequently. In some cases, chromosome analysis is performed to screen for potential abnormalities. Before conception of a child, couples can be given genetic counseling. Both potential parents provide a blood sample and have a chromosome analysis performed. This can be particularly useful for those with a family history of certain genetic abnormalities. Detection of a possible genetic abnormality may give the couple choices regarding family planning and information about the risks involved with pregnancy.

Chromosome Abnormality Conditions

This section presents some of the most common chromosome abnormality conditions that may be seen by the PT and PTA in practice.

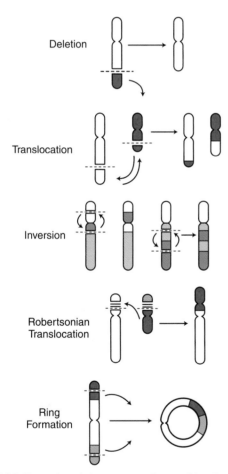

FIGURE 2.9 Examples of chromosome abnormalities due to breakage and rearrangement. a) Deletions are loss of a part of a chromosome. b) Translocations occur when part of a chromosome is transferred to another chromosome. c) Inversion occurs when there is a break in two places and the chromosome reconnects in the wrong order. d) Robertsonian translocation occurs when the breakage is close to the centromere of the chromosome. e) A ring chromosome is the result of a breakage in the chromosome and the two ends joining together to form a ring.

Deletion

Translocation

Inversion

Robertsonian
Translocation

Ring
Formation

Down Syndrome (Trisomy 21) ⊕

Down syndrome is one of the more common chromosome abnormalities, with an incidence of approximately 1 in every 660 to 800 births.[114,115] Most children with Down syndrome are born to older mothers.

Etiology. Down syndrome is the result of a trisomy on chromosome 21 in approximately 95% of all cases (see Figure 2-10). Parents are genetically healthy, but in many cases, the mother is older. When mothers are approximately 25 years of age, there is a 1:1250 chance of having a child with Down syndrome; when the mother reaches the age of 40, the risk increases to 1:100.[116] Recommendations by the American College of Obstetricians and Gynecologists (ACOG) in early 2007 suggest that all pregnant women receive screening for Down syndrome, including the MSAFP blood test and a "nuchal translucency" ultrasound scan.[117]

Signs and Symptoms. The characteristic signs and symptoms of a child with Down syndrome include varying degrees of mental retardation, flattened facial characteristics, loose skin on the neck, a Simean crease on the palm

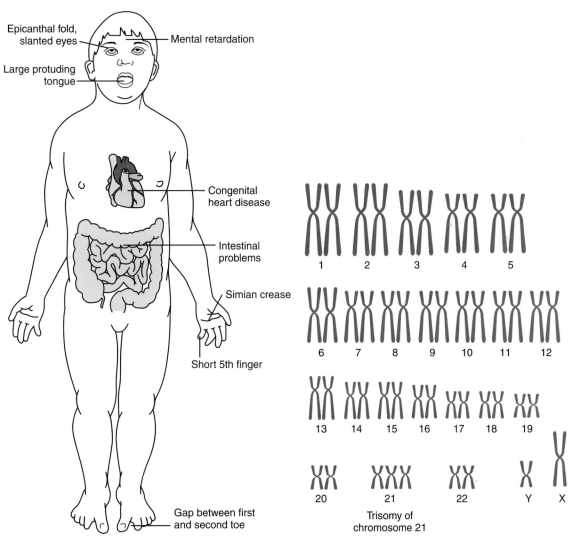

FIGURE 2.10 Down syndrome and associated karyotype showing trisomy of chromosome 21.

of the hand (a single palm line), underdeveloped intestines (e.g., stenosis), developmental dysplasia of the hip (DDH), atlantoaxial subluxation, congenital heart defects, hypotonia (low muscle tone), and hearing deficits. Children with Down syndrome do not necessarily have all of these signs and symptoms. These children are more susceptible to heart problems and infections[118] than children without Down syndrome, and have an increased risk of developing leukemia.[119]

Prognosis. The life expectancy of a person with Down syndrome has increased greatly over the past few years. Individuals with Down syndrome often live into their 50s, have jobs, and marry. The degree of mental retardation has a large bearing on the mental abilities of people with Down syndrome. Early intervention with rehabilitation services, including physical therapy, assists with the cognitive and physical development of children with Down syndrome. However, individuals with Down syndrome tend to prematurely age, have multiple medical problems, and are prone to dementia.[120]

Medical Intervention. Medical intervention begins before and during pregnancy with the diagnosis of birth defects and genetic counseling. Children with Down syndrome require the same follow-up physician visits as any other child. Because of the increased risk of infections and other medical problems, more visits to the physician may be necessary. Recent findings have resulted in the recommendation of intake of folic acid supplements for women before and during pregnancy because of the beneficial effects for prevention of birth defects.[121]

Physical Therapy Intervention. The hypotonia, or flaccidity of the muscles, predisposes children with Down syndrome to several problems that may require physical therapy intervention. PT can help to stimulate more normal tone in the muscles through early childhood intervention. Infants with Down syndrome are prone to developmental dysplasia of the hip (DDH), formerly termed congenital dislocation of hips, resulting from lax ligaments and low tone of hip musculature. Instability at the atlantoaxial joint is also common in children with Down syndrome. These problems can be identified and monitored by PT. Intermittent intervention to teach the family techniques to stimulate the neurological and motor development of the infant can be beneficial.

Fragile X Syndrome ☺

Fragile X syndrome, also called Martin-Bell syndrome, is a sex-linked recessive disorder that can be detected through DNA testing. The name of the condition is derived from the characteristic fragile section of the X chromosome. The incidence of the genetic abnormality is estimated to be between 1:3,500 and 1:8,900 males.[122]

Etiology. A fragile section on the X chromosome known as FMRI is transmitted from the parent to the child.[123] This condition can become worse from one generation to the next as the fragile site becomes increasingly more fragile.

Signs and Symptoms. The main characteristic of fragile X syndrome in males is mental retardation with associated learning difficulties. Males with the condition may also have facial characteristics that include an elongated face and large ears. Females with the syndrome tend to be less severely affected than males. Fragile X syndrome is one of the recognized causes of autism, with approximately one third of males with fragile X syndrome diagnosed with autism.[124,125] Other symptoms can include seizure disorders, tactile defensiveness (dislike of touch), reduced attention span, speech disorders, cognitive delay, connective tissue abnormalities,[126] and varying degrees of attention deficit-hyperactivity disorder (ADHD).[127]

Prognosis. The life expectancy for individuals with Fragile X syndrome is normal. Older adults with the disorder and individuals who are carriers for the disorder tend to develop fragile X–associated tremor/ataxia syndrome (FXTAS), which can cause severe tremors that interfere with day-to-day functional activity, symptomatically similar to Parkinson's disease.[128]

Medical Intervention. A team approach to the intervention for the child with fragile X syndrome is required. The physician monitors the child for all medical conditions and provides medications as needed especially for behavioral manifestations of the disorder.[129] Referral is made by the physician to any necessary therapeutic services, such as the speech and language pathologist, OT, PT, and social worker.[130] In older individuals with this syndrome, PT intervention may be required to alleviate the FXTAS symptoms of tremor and ataxia.[131]

Physical Therapy Intervention. Physical therapy intervention is determined on an individual basis after a full evaluation from the PT. Early childhood intervention is important from infancy to assist in the stimulation of motor development and cognitive development. The rehabilitation team comprises PT, OT, speech and language pathologist, in consultation with the physician.

Klinefelter Syndrome (47 X-X-Y syndrome) ⊛

Klinefelter Syndrome is a chromosomal abnormality affecting males. The incidence is approximately 1:500–1,000 male births and is more of a risk for mothers over age 35.[132]

Etiology. Klinefelter syndrome affects only males and is caused by the presence of an additional X chromosome.

Signs and Symptoms. The characteristic signs and symptoms of Klinefelter syndrome include abnormalities of the sexual organs, such as small testes and enlarged mammary glands. Individuals with the syndrome tend to be tall with long limbs and a short body and are infertile.[133] If the syndrome is characterized by more than one additional X chromosome, mental retardation is likely.[134]

Prognosis. The life expectancy of individuals with Klinefelter syndrome is normal; however, an increased risk of several comorbid conditions exists such as lung disease, osteoporosis, autoimmune diseases, depression, and attention deficit-hyperactivity disorder.[135]

Medical Intervention. The physician may prescribe male hormone therapy with testosterone to assist in the normal development of the male sexual characteristics.

Physical Therapy Intervention. No physical therapy is indicated for individuals with Klinefelter syndrome.

Patau Syndrome ⊛

Patau syndrome is a rare chromosomal disease. The incidence of Patau syndrome is approximately 1 in 5,000 live births.[136]

Etiology. In most cases, Patau syndrome results from a trisomy of chromosome 13.

Signs and Symptoms. Infants with Patau syndrome have microcephaly (small brain) with severe mental retardation, polydactyly (extra fingers and toes), kidney abnormalities, cardiac defects, eye defects, hypotonia, and cleft lip and palate (see Fig. 2-11).[137] Children with this condition often have "rocker-bottom" feet, which makes it difficult for them to walk with a normal gait pattern.[138]

Prognosis. The prognosis of infants with Patau syndrome is poor. Most children do not survive beyond 3 days of age, and many of them die within a few months of birth.[139] About 1 in 20 children with Patau syndrome survive 6 months, and a few children survive until the teen years. The causes of mortality are usually the effects of severe neurological impairments, brain malformations, and cardiopulmonary complications.[140]

Medical Intervention. Medical intervention is largely in the pre-pregnancy phase for genetic counseling and for medical management of the infant. Children with Patau syndrome are monitored in the same way as other children, although they may require more frequent physician visits. Medical intervention depends on the severity of the

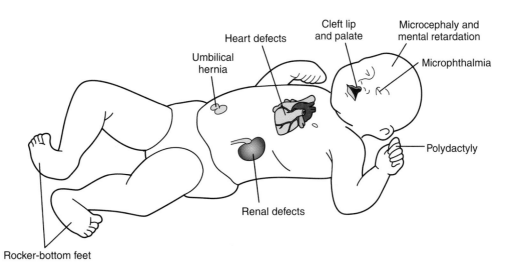

FIGURE 2.11 Signs and symptoms of Patau syndrome

child's condition. If cardiac abnormalities exist, prophylactic antibiotics are required before dental work.[141]

Physical Therapy Intervention. Physical therapy intervention may be needed for children with Patau syndrome to assist with the stimulation of motor development and provide positioning and seating advice in the home and, in some cases, in school.

Turner Syndrome ⊕

Turner syndrome is a chromosomal condition affecting females. The incidence of Turner syndrome is approximately 1 in 2,500 live births.[142]

Etiology. Turner syndrome is caused by a total or partial lack of the X chromosome. The cause of the genetic abnormality is not known.[143]

Signs and Symptoms. The characteristic signs and symptoms of Turner syndrome include inhibition of growth resulting in a short stature, a short neck, a wide chest with nipples spaced far apart, abnormalities of the kidneys, aorta, and heart, nonfunctioning ovaries, failure to develop secondary sexual characteristics such as breasts and pubic hair, and infertility (see Figure 2-12). A high incidence of Type 2 diabetes, high blood pressure, and thyroid dysfunction are noted in individuals with Turner syndrome.[144]

Prognosis. Individuals with Turner syndrome have varying degrees of symptoms. Life expectancy is usually normal.

Medical Intervention. The administration of growth hormone and estrogen has proved to help normal growth and sexual maturity for some individuals with Turner syndrome.[145]

Physical Therapy Intervention. Physical therapy is not indicated for individuals with Turner syndrome unless they have an orthopedic problem.

Why Does the Physical Therapist Assistant (PTA) Need to Know About Developmental Diseases and Birth Injuries?

Physical therapy interventions such as neurodevelopmental therapy are used for children and adults with a variety of developmental diseases and birth injuries. The resulting neuromuscular deficits caused by many of these conditions require interventions to stimulate the normal developmental process. To work with children with these developmental diseases and birth defects, the PTA requires an understanding of the associated pathology.

Developmental Diseases/Birth Injuries

This section covers some of the developmental diseases and birth defects that affect both children and adults seen by the PT and PTA. Prematurity is included in this section because of its impact on the development of the neuromuscular system.

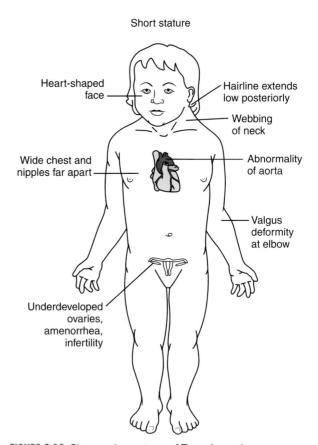

Short stature

Heart-shaped face

Hairline extends low posteriorly

Webbing of neck

Wide chest and nipples far apart

Abnormality of aorta

Valgus deformity at elbow

Underdeveloped ovaries, amenorrhea, infertility

FIGURE 2.12 Signs and symptoms of Turner's syndrome

Cerebral Palsy ⊛

The term cerebral palsy (CP) is a global term and covers many types of problems that involve some level of impairment of the immature neuromotor system. Discussion within the medical field is currently ongoing regarding the use of the term "cerebral palsy." In most cases a more specific diagnosis related to the actual etiology (cause) of the neurological deficit is recommended. The term cerebral palsy is still used with an additional descriptor indicating the etiology of the condition, if one is known. In general, the term cerebral palsy applies to any injury of the central nervous system caused by congenital abnormalities, prenatal trauma, or postnatal trauma such as traumatic brain injury or meningitis up to the age of 2 years old. The effects of the condition continue throughout life and result in various degrees of motor deficits. The main types of cerebral palsy recognized are spastic, athetoid, ataxic, and mixed. In the United States, there are between 2.5 and 4.2 cases of CP for every 1,000 births.[146] The National Institutes of Health (2007) estimated that there are more than 800,000 children and adults in the United States living with CP.[147] This number has changed little during the past few decades.[148]

Etiology. CP is the result of damage to the infant brain before, during, or immediately after birth. Causes can include hypoxia in the uterus, brain abnormalities, congenital genetic defects, mechanical trauma, and hypoglycemia (low sugar levels). Anoxia, traumatic brain injury, and meningitis can also cause neurological damage postnatally. Many people with CP are affected by congenital genetic defects that occur during early development of the fetus. A cerebrovascular accident (CVA) may occur in the fetus as a result of clots in the placenta or intracranial hemorrhage. Maternal hypertension or pelvic inflammatory disease may increase the risk of the fetus having a CVA. Infections in the mother during pregnancy such as toxoplasmosis, rubella (German measles), CMV, and herpes increase the risk of brain damage. Other risk factors for having an infant with cerebral palsy include maternal exposure to toxic substances during pregnancy; a baby with a very low birth weight (less than 1,500 grams);[149] infant jaundice that remains untreated; seizures in the infant; mothers with mental retardation, seizures, or thyroid abnormalities; and breech presentations at birth (feet first delivery).[150] Other causes in the infant can include seizures that occur immediately after birth, respiratory or circulatory problems before birth resulting in lack of blood supply and oxygen to the brain, head injuries after birth, or infections after birth such as bacterial meningitis. [151]

Signs and Symptoms. CP is not progressive as far as brain involvement is concerned, but as children grow, they are likely to experience difficulties in function related to development patterns. The signs and symptoms of cerebral palsy vary widely depending on the area of the brain affected. The symptoms range from unilateral hemiparesis or hemiplegia to bilateral spastic diplegia or diparesis affecting both lower extremities, spastic quadriplegia or quadriparesis affecting all limbs, hypertonicity (increased muscle tone) to hypotonicity (low muscle tone), and ataxia (poor balance and depth perception) to nonataxia. Some children may have dyskinetic CP with athetoid slow, involuntary writhing movements. Some infants with CP will have some level of mental retardation, and 40% will have seizures. Many will exhibit development delay.[152] A 2008 study by Hagglund and Wagner (2008) with 547 children with CP showed that across all types of cerebral palsy, children had increased hypertonicity in the gastrocnemius/soleus up to age 4 years and then the hypertonicity started to reduce each year up to 12 years.[153] Other signs and symptoms may include the development of scoliosis (S-shaped spinal curve) or increased kyphosis (thoracic spine) or lordosis (lumbar spine). Vision, speech, and hearing deficits also are common in children with cerebral palsy. Abnormal skin sensation and incontinence may be present.[154] Some of the symptoms that may develop as a result of the cerebral palsy are depression, osteopenia (reduced bone density), or osteoporosis (severe loss of bone density), resulting from inactivity and non–weight bearing, and postimpairment syndrome consisting of fatigue, pain, weakness, arthritis, and overuse syndromes.[155]

Prognosis. No cure exists for cerebral palsy, but children and adults with cerebral palsy do not necessarily have severe disabilities. The condition is not progressive, and with adequate medical and therapeutic intervention, many people can lead functional lives. Some children may be functionally limited if they have experienced brain damage. Many physical disabilities resulting from CP can be overcome with the use of assistive devices and orthoses and the help of physical and occupational therapy.

Medical Intervention. Prevention of CP is difficult because the causes are so varied. Accidents resulting in head injuries to young children can be minimized by the use of car seats and helmets when riding bicycles and supervising bathing. Mothers can protect themselves against rubella with vaccination. The diagnosis of CP may be made immediately after birth if the motor disorders are severe or may not be noticeable until the infant shows delayed motor development. The diagnosis is confirmed by performing computed tomography (CT) scans or magnetic resonance imaging (MRI) of the brain or cranial ultrasound. The medications used depend on the specific characteristics of the condition. Some infants require anti-seizure medications to prevent further brain damage. Muscle relaxants may be prescribed for infants with hypertonicity (spasticity). In older children, severe spasticity may cause pain, and analgesics may be needed. In children with severe spasticity accompanied by joint contractures and soft tissue shortening, surgery may be performed to "release" the tight muscles and tendons.[156,157] Injections into hypertonic muscles with botulinum toxin (BT-A) may allow stretching to be performed more easily and with less pain. Intrathecal baclofen may be delivered to the spinal column through a pump implanted in the abdomen to reduce hypertonicity.[158] In some children, the severe spasticity may cause joint problems as a result of contractures, and orthopedic surgery may be required. Another surgical approach for children with severe spasticity is a selective dorsal rhizotomy in which the posterior spinal cord roots are severed.[159] A team approach to management of children with cerebral palsy is essential. Members of the medical team may include the physician, orthopedist, psychologist, behavioral therapist, social worker, physical therapist, occupational therapist, and speech and language pathologist. The teacher in the school must be included to ensure optimal handling and management of the child during classes.

Physical Therapy Intervention. PT and PTA involvement as part of the team approach for these children is important. Physical therapy, occupational therapy, and sometimes speech and language pathology may be required for children with cerebral palsy.[160] Children may be seen in the home, the physical therapy clinic, or the school setting for physical therapy intervention. The management of children with CP depends on the specific characteristics of the individual person. Children with hypertonicity may require orthotic devices to help manage the joint position and prevent muscle and joint contractures. Walkers, crutches, wheelchairs, and canes are all possible assistive devices. In children with associated speech difficulties, communication aids may be necessary, and these include computers with special controls, alphabet boards, and word boards. A variety of types of physical therapy intervention may be indicated depending on whether children have hypertonicity (high muscle tone), hypotonicity (low muscle tone), or ataxia (uncontrolled movement). PT intervention may include exercises to improve

function and increase strength, passive and active stretching of involved muscles, ambulation training, and teaching home programs, seating positions, and patient handling to care providers. Involvement of the PT after surgery is crucial for the long-term success of muscle releases to ensure the muscle is stretched and the release is maintained by the patient and the family. The use of adaptive equipment and orthotics such as ankle foot orthoses (AFO) to correct for drop foot and provide a good ankle position for functional ambulation may be useful. Other interventions may include relaxation exercises and aquatherapy. The techniques for providing interventions for children with CP may include, but are not limited to, constraint-induced therapy, neurodevelopmental therapy (NDT), proprioceptive neuromuscular facilitation (PNF), and stretching and strengthening exercise programs.[161] (Refer to Chapter 7 for details of these techniques.)

The early diagnosis of children with CP enables early therapeutic intervention and teaching of home programs to care providers to help improve outcomes. The role of the PT and PTA in the school system is to enhance the participation of the child in the education process and may include seating adaptations and other adaptive equipment needs, as well as specific physical therapy provided after orthopedic surgery. Controversy exists regarding the frequency of therapy sessions. Some studies have shown that the main aspect of physical therapy intervention is the monitoring of children and teaching of the family, with no significant difference in outcome noted whether children are seen every week or intermittently.[162] The frequency of physical therapy intervention is determined by the evaluating physical therapist. Most children will require intermittent physical therapy interventions throughout the school years. Within the school system seating adaptations may be required to allow children to participate in the education process. Children with severe disorders may require wheelchairs, and these must be refitted as children grow. The orthotist, physical therapist, and occupational therapist will work together to ensure appropriate assistive devices for children with CP. Physical therapy intervention is especially helpful for stretching of the muscles after surgical release to prevent soft tissues from tightening again. Feedback provided by the physical therapist to the physician can assist in adjusting medications to ensure optimum stretching is achieved.

Erb's Palsy

Erb's palsy is a paralysis of the upper extremity resulting from a traction injury to the brachial plexus during birth.[163] Other names for Erb's palsy are brachial palsy,

Klumpke paralysis, and Erb-Duchenne paralysis. Erb's palsy can affect different nerve root levels between C5 and T1. The number of cases of Erb's palsy has reduced in recent years because of advances in obstetric (pregnant mother and fetus) care.

Etiology. The cause of Erb's palsy arises from a traction injury, which may include breach births (child born feet first or one arm first), babies with high birth weight, and forceps or vacuum suction deliveries.

Signs and Symptoms. In Erb's palsy, the arm is held in shoulder adduction and internal rotation with pronation of the forearm, known as a "waiter's tip" position. Another variant of the palsy is Klumpke's palsy, which involves the lower levels of the brachial plexus and causes paralysis of the intrinsic muscles of the hand (those completely within the hand) and the wrist flexors, resulting in functional problems of the hand. Some children have complete paralysis of the arm. Damage to the brachial plexus can also be caused in an infant or young child by someone pulling on the arm forcefully. This kind of Erb's palsy is sometimes called "nursemaid's palsy."

Prognosis. The prognosis of Erb's palsy depends on the degree of injury to the nerve. Most cases of Erb's palsy resolve without any intervention, but some cases result in permanent loss of function to the involved arm.

Medical Intervention. In cases of Erb's palsy that do not heal, surgery may be necessary. The most common surgeries are forms of microsurgery (performed with use of a microscope), such as a nerve graft or a nerve transfer.[164]

Physical Therapy Intervention. When providing intervention for children with Erb's palsy, the PT and PTA may use various strategies depending on the level of involvement of the injury. Interventions may include soft tissue techniques, electrical stimulation, aquatherapy, splinting for functional positioning, exercises, and teaching passive, active, and active assisted range of motion to the family. The goals of PT intervention are the prevention of contractures at the elbow and shoulder, facilitation of active motion at the shoulder, elbow, and hand and restoration or promotion of functional motion. In addition, retaining as normal a pattern of motion at the shoulder as possible and prevention of shoulder subluxation are important.[165]

Prematurity ☺

Although prematurity is not a birth injury, it is included in this section because of the implications for physical therapy management of children born prematurely.

Etiology. In more than half of the babies born prematurely, the cause is unknown.[166] Other known causes of premature births include lack of sufficient blood supply to the fetus that cause premature contractions and an early delivery, infections in the mother, the presence of more than one fetus that overstretches the uterus, and placental displacement from the wall of the uterus.[167] Other causes of premature delivery include preeclampsia, substance abuse by the mother, maternal diabetes or heart disease, and poor maternal nutrition.[168] The normal length of pregnancy is 37 to 42 weeks, which allows time for the normal development of the fetus to what is called full term. If an infant is born before the 37th week of pregnancy, or with a birth weight below 2,500 g, the child is considered to be premature.[169] If the infant is born after 42 weeks, this is considered postterm. In most cases, premature infants are mature enough to survive with some additional medical monitoring. The medically accepted age of a viable fetus is 24 weeks. Before 24 weeks, the internal organs of a fetus are not developed sufficiently to allow for survival outside the uterus.[170] As medical science advances, the age of fetus viability may change.

Signs and Symptoms. Infants born before the 34th week of pregnancy have more complications than those born after the 34th week. Such complications can include respiratory distress syndrome and intraventricular hemorrhage in which there is bleeding within the brain.[171] Premature infants may be delayed in their motor development but will usually catch up to normal levels within the first year. Some infants who are born with extremely low birth weight and are considered to be immature experience more problems. A common problem in the immature infant is **neonatal respiratory distress syndrome,** also called pulmonary hyaline membrane disease. This is a condition caused by the immature nature of the fetal lungs. Fetal lung maturation occurs in the latter part of pregnancy with surfactant levels only becoming apparent at approximately 34 weeks of gestation.[172] A fetus under 34 weeks old tends to lack lung development. This condition is responsible for many neonatal deaths. The condition is due to lack of surfactant in the lungs. Normally surfactant reduces the surface tension of the lungs and enables the alveoli to inflate and the lungs to expand, but when surfactant is lacking, the lungs are unable to expand.

In addition to the lack of lung expansion, scar tissue forms, which further restricts the lung tissue and prevents the lungs from expanding. This condition can be a cause of restrictive lung disease. Infants born prematurely with this problem require an artificial respirator to enable them to breathe until they are mature enough to start producing surfactant. Because the infant is not fully developed, functional and anatomical deficiencies are common. Another problem in premature babies is atresia (lack of development) of the esophagus, which means that the esophagus is not connected with the stomach and may require surgical connection for the infant to eat by mouth. Sometimes the esophagus will grow and connect naturally to the stomach as the infant matures in the **neonatal intensive care unit** (NICU). Until this occurs, feeding is performed through intravenous feeding or a gastric tube into the stomach. In other cases, the atresia must be surgically corrected.[173]

Prognosis. The prognosis for premature infants is generally good. With adequate care, these infants live normal lives, although they may be slightly motor delayed. If an infant is born 6 weeks prematurely, it should be considered that the child is 6 weeks younger than the actual birth date when looking at the motor development level of the child.

Medical Intervention. If the birth weight is below 1,500 g, the infant will need to be medically monitored in a NICU. Surgery to connect the esophageal atresia may be required. A respirator may be necessary for those infants with neonatal respiratory distress syndrome.

Physical Therapy Intervention. PTs and PTAs may be involved in the treatment of neonates in the NICU. Intervention may include facilitation of breathing techniques, teaching handling techniques to parents, positioning of the infant, and movement facilitation. Sometimes premature infants are tactile defensive, and PTs and PTAs may need to work on decreasing this condition. Positioning is important because many premature infants lie supine, and thus their limbs are placed in a retracted or extended position. These infants may have difficulty bringing their hands to the midline position as they mature if they are not encouraged to flex their limbs. Because immaturity means that muscles are also underdeveloped, the role of the PT is important. Many of these infants will require PT and OT intervention after discharge from the hospital because of delay in motor function.

Rhesus Disease/Hemolytic Disease of the Newborn ☸

Rhesus disease, also called hemolytic disease of the newborn, is the result of incompatibility of the blood types of the mother and infant. The incidence of this condition is 10.2 per 10,000 births.[174]

Etiology. As noted earlier in the chapter, rhesus disease or hemolytic disease of the newborn is caused by rhesus incompatibility of the maternal blood to that of the fetus. In a mother with rhesus negative (Rh–) blood who has a fetus with rhesus positive (Rh+) blood, the maternal and fetal blood mix during the first birth, which causes the mother to develop antibodies to the Rh+ blood of the child. This does not affect the first child because the mother has not developed the antibodies during the first pregnancy. If the second child is also Rh+, the mother will have developed antibodies to Rh+ and will reject (spontaneously abort) the fetus.[175]

Signs and Symptoms. In some cases of rhesus incompatibility, the mother will spontaneously abort the fetus because of the antibody reaction. In other instances, the newborn may have hydrops fetalis and be anemic, have breathing problems, and suffer from severe lung, liver, and heart problems. Many infants with hydrops fetalis do not survive.[176] Hydrops fetalis is a condition in which edema builds up in the fetus. Rhesus incompatibility causes immune hydrops fetalis in which the mother's antibodies attack the blood cells of the fetus and destroy them causing severe anemia. In nonimmune hydrops fetalis the edema is caused by other diseases or pathological conditions such as heart and lung defects, liver disease, chromosomal abnormalities and birth defects, or infections.[177] In some cases, the mother does not develop the antibodies to the rhesus protein during the first birth, and there are no problems during the second birth.

Prognosis. Complications of rhesus incompatibility can include death of the fetus or newborn from such conditions as hemolytic disease and hydrops fetalis. In such severe cases, complete blood transfusion of the newborn may be needed. In most cases, the blood types of the mother and father are known, and the rhesus negative mother can be injected with anti-D factor immediately after the birth of the first child to prevent the formation of antibodies to the rhesus factor.[178]

Medical Intervention. The problems associated with rhesus incompatibility can be prevented by injecting the

mother within 12 hours of the first birth with anti-D immunoglobulin (RhoGAM), which prevents the development of antibodies to the Rh+ blood of any future fetus.
Women at risk for rhesus incompatibility must be closely
monitored by a physician during and after pregnancy to
ensure the health of the newborn.

Physical Therapy Intervention. Physical therapy is not
usually associated with rhesus babies. However, the infant
may require respiratory physical therapy treatment in the
NICU. If complications such as bilirubin encephalopathy
occur in infants with hemolytic disease of the newborn
brain, damage can occur that may affect motor development.[179] The rehabilitation team is involved with the early
intervention to stimulate motor development.

Scoliosis ⊕

Scoliosis is an abnormal lateral curvature of the spine that
affects approximately 2% of the U.S. population.[180] Girls
are affected more often than boys.[181]

Etiology. Scoliosis can be either structural or functional.
Structural scoliosis can be congenital (acquired at
birth), which is thought to be transmitted as an autosomal dominant chromosomal characteristic, or idiopathic, without a known cause. Most cases of scoliosis
are of unknown cause. Structural scoliosis causes a permanent change in the spine, and the curve does not alter
when the person moves. Functional scoliosis is often
caused by pain or poor posture and does not affect the
structure of the spine. In functional scoliosis, if the person moves, the scoliosis appears to change configura-
tion. Many cases of scoliosis are mild and do not cause
any problems.[182] Other causes of scoliosis include osteopathic (bone abnormalities), neuropathic due to a
neurological condition such as spinal cord injury, or
myopathic as a result of a muscle disorder such as muscular dystrophy.[183]

Signs and Symptoms. The curvature of the spine in scoliosis is usually exhibited as a curve to the right in the thoracic spine and to the left in the lumbar spine. One shoulder may appear higher than the other, and the waistline
may be asymmetrical. Rotation of the spine also occurs,
and thus rotation of the chest cavity causing abnormalities
of the ribs and disturbed breathing patterns. Increased
kyphosis of the thoracic spine and increased lordosis of
the lumbar spine are generally noted with severe cases of
scoliosis.

Prognosis. The prognosis of patients with scoliosis varies
with the degree of severity of the curvature. Severe scoliosis can be limiting for breathing and activity levels. A
marked curvature of the spine can reduce the capacity of
the thoracic cavity, thus reducing the possible volume of
the lungs and lowering endurance to levels of activity. The
reduction of lung capacity causes increased susceptibility
to upper respiratory infections.

Medical Intervention. Individuals with a mild case of
scoliosis require only monitoring with physical examinations. If the degree of curvature is greater than
20 degrees, the physician may recommend the use of a
body brace to prevent the curve from progressing. When
the curvature is greater than 40 or 45 degrees, the physician may recommend surgery to prevent further increases of the curvature.[184] Severe cases of structural
scoliosis often require surgical intervention after puberty
for fusion of parts of the spine. The placement of a
Harrington rod along the spine is one method that helps
to maintain the spine in position while the bones fuse.
Another method of fixation of the spine enables the
reduction of the kyphosis component of the scoliosis
through use of a system of hooks and rods with "pedicle
screws" along the length of the lumbar and thoracic
spines.[185] An alternative surgery for some cases of scoliosis is a thoracoscopic anterior instrumentation technique to fuse several sections of the spine. This surgery
requires temporarily deflating one lung but is less invasive on the spine than other techniques.[186]

Physical Therapy Intervention. Functional scoliosis
caused by pain or poor posture can be improved with
physical therapy intervention. Postural awareness and
appropriate exercises can assist in resolving the postural
problems and restoring a more normal alignment of the
spine. Physical therapy intervention for those patients
with structural scoliosis is aimed at ensuring adequate
function of the cardiovascular and respiratory systems.
The PT will often monitor the child every 6 months
during growth to evaluate for the possible need for
spinal orthoses. Several studies have shown the efficacy
of respiratory intervention techniques on individuals
who have had spinal surgery for correction of scoliosis.[187,188] The use of electrical stimulation to weak
muscles and resistance exercises is under review for
efficacy in the intervention for scoliosis. A study by
Mooney and Brigham (2003) showed some promising
results with use of resisted exercises for adolescents
with scoliosis.[189]

It Happened in the Clinic

Jimmy was an 11-year-old with spina bifida. He was born with a defect at the level of the thoracic 9, 10, and 11. The spinal defect was closed immediately after birth, but damage to the spinal cord had already occurred during birth resulting in loss of movement of the lower extremities and lack of bowel and bladder control. Jimmy was seen in the physical therapy clinic for consultations when he needed a new wheelchair. On this occasion, Jimmy had grown 10 inches in height since the last wheelchair fitting 2 years earlier and was starting to develop a scoliosis with some mid and lower back pain after sitting in his chair at school all day. He had well-developed upper extremity strength and was using a light-weight sport wheelchair with a hard seat and memory foam cushion insert. No additional back support was in use. After consultation with the orthotist and the family, it was decided to order a new light-weight sport wheelchair with a slightly higher back so that a molded firm-back support could be added to the chair with wings to maintain Jimmy's spine in a better position. The firm seat and cushion were augmented by a lap strap to ensure correct positioning in the chair. Although this additional weight would mean extra effort for Jimmy when propelling the chair, he had sufficient upper-extremity strength to manage the change. Once the wheelchair was delivered and the molded back support crafted by the orthotist, Jimmy found he was able to tolerate sitting in the wheelchair for longer periods throughout the day without experiencing back pain. At follow-up in 3 months, the scoliosis had not worsened, and the back pain had resolved.

Spina Bifida ⊛

The term "spina bifida" includes several types of neural tube defects in the development of the spinal column, including **spina bifida occulta, meningocele,** and **myelomeningocele** (see Fig. 2-13). In spina bifida, the spinal column fails to close during the first month of pregnancy and results in various degrees of malformation of part of the spine. This is one of the most common forms of birth defects in the United States.[190] According to the CDC, the U.S. incidence of spina bifida in 2004 was 19.56 for every 100,000 live births; in 2005, this number was reduced to the lowest recorded number of 17.96 per 100,000 live births.[191] People of Caucasian and Hispanic descent are more at risk of having children with spina bifida than African Americans.[192]

Etiology. The specific etiology of spina bifida is unknown. A combination of genetics and environment are considered responsible for the defect. Multiple genes are under scientific investigation connected with the condition. The risk for having an infant with spina bifida is known to be increased by as much as 20% to 50% in mothers who have had a previous pregnancy with a child with spina bifida. Family history of the condition also increases the risk; however, 95% of all people with spina bifida have no family history of the condition.[193] Other risk factors include maternal conditions, such as insulin-dependent diabetes and obesity; maternal use of anti-seizure medications during pregnancy; maternal exposure to high temperatures during the first month of pregnancy as a result of hot tub and sauna use or a high fever; and paternal (father) exposure to Agent Orange, a defoliating agent used in warfare. The use of 0.4 mg of folic acid by the mother before and during pregnancy has been found to reduce the risk of having an infant with spina bifida by up to 75%.[194,195,196] Folic acid is a B vitamin found in orange juice and leafy green vegetables. Some of these nutritional concerns are eliminated or reduced as the population becomes more aware of good nutrition and use of supplemental vitamins.

Signs and Symptoms. The signs and symptoms of children with spina bifida depend on the type of defect present. As noted earlier, there are three general types of spina bifida: spina bifida occulta (the mildest form), meningocele, and myelomeningocele. A myelomeningocele is the severest form of spinal bifida. In this form, the meninges and spinal cord protrude through the spinal defect and the opening in the skin. Damage to the neural tissue is often sustained during birth, and nerve damage is usually extensive. Paralysis occurs distal to the spinal lesion, bowel and bladder dysfunction are evident, and hydrocephalus, seizures, learning disabilities, multiple medical problems, and infections such as meningitis are common.[197]

Spina bifida occulta is not visible to the eye, but a defect occurs in the development of the vertebral arch. Children with spina bifida occulta may not exhibit any signs or symptoms, and the diagnosis may not be made until a spinal radiograph is taken for other reasons. At birth, skin covers the spinal cord defect, and it may not be noticed. Occasionally, signs of the presence of spina bifida occulta include a tuft of hair, a birth mark, or a dimple over the area of the spinal defect.

In **meningocele,** the meninges (coverings of the brain and spinal cord) of the spine protrude through the opening in the vertebra, but the spinal cord remains intact.

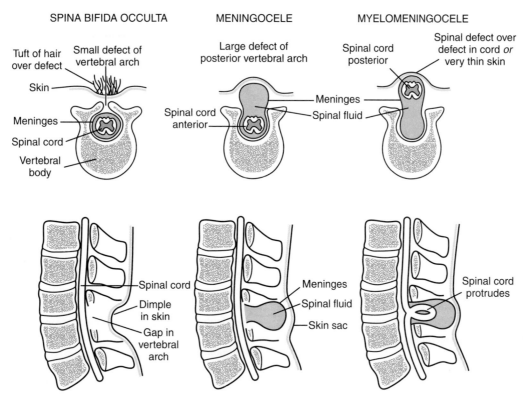

| SPINA BIFIDA OCCULTA | MENINGOCELE | MYELOMENINGOCELE |

FIGURE 2.13 Examples of spina bifida include spina bifida occulta, meningocele, and myelomeningocele.

Minimal damage is sustained to the neural system, particularly if the spinal defect is closed immediately after birth. A **meningomyelocele** is characterized by both the meninges and spinal cord protruding through the vertebral defect and the skin.[198] All these defects are more common in the lumbar spine but may also occur in the sacral, thoracic, and cervical spines. Babies with spina bifida, especially those with meningomyelocele, have varying degrees of neurological involvement depending on the severity of the defect. At birth, the skin is surgically closed, but in severe cases, there are certain to be some neurological problems.[199] Damage to the neural tissue is often sustained during birth and nerve damage is usually extensive.[200] Some of the problems experienced by children with spina bifida include **hydrocephalus** (buildup of fluid in the brain), which requires surgery. The hydrocephalus is sometimes caused by Chiari II malformation.[201] Chiari II malformation is the descent of parts of the brainstem and cerebellum into the spinal canal, which can also result in difficulties with swallowing and breathing, as well as upper extremity weakness due to cervical peripheral nerve compression.[202] **Hypotonia** in the trunk muscles (low tone), slowed postural reflexes, flaccid (limp to minimal or no tone) or spastic (high tone) paralysis

of the lower extremities, and bowel and bladder dysfunction are also common symptoms of spina bifida. Deformities of the musculoskeletal system may also exist, such as scoliosis, dislocated hip, joint contractures, and talipes equinovarus (clubfoot). Less frequently, there may be mental retardation, especially in cases where the hydrocephalus is a marked feature of the condition. However, most individuals with spina bifida are of normal intelligence.[203] Individuals with spina bifida have other problems associated with lower extremity paralysis, such as pressure ulcers on the sacrum, ischium, and other bony prominences due to lack of sensation. Bowel and bladder incontinence is associated with a high risk of urinary and alimentary tract infections. Because bowel and bladder control is from the sacral S2–4 level, most affected children have problems with these functions.

Prognosis. No cure exists for spina bifida. The prognosis of children with this disorder depends on the extent of the neurological damage. Some infants die shortly after birth if the symptoms are severe with marked hydrocephalus and extensive neurological damage. Many children live into adulthood with a normal life expectancy as the result of prompt diagnosis, medical care, and surgical closure of the defect. However, most children with spina bifida will have some form of permanent paralysis below the level of the spinal lesion.[204]

Medical Intervention. The diagnosis of spina bifida is usually determined prenatally (before birth). In some mild cases, the diagnosis may be made postnatally (after birth). During the second trimester of pregnancy, a maternal blood sample is tested for levels of alpha-fetoprotein (MSAFP screening), and a fetal ultrasound is performed. If the levels of alpha-fetoprotein (AFP) are high, a neural tube defect such as spina bifida may be suspected, although levels of AFP are higher when more than one fetus is developing. Further testing by amniocentesis may then be performed to confirm the diagnosis. In amniocentesis, a small amount of amniotic fluid is removed by needle from the amniotic sac for further laboratory testing. Prenatal testing will not always show the severity of the spinal defect. Postnatal testing for spina bifida includes the use of magnetic resonance imaging or computed tomography scan.[205]

The medical management for infants with spinal defects includes surgery to close the spinal defect, which takes place within 72 hours of birth. A cesarean birth may help to prevent further damage to the spinal cord if spina bifida is diagnosed. In cases in which the infant has hydrocephalus, the prompt placement of a shunt reduces the risk of brain damage.[206] The sooner the surgical closure is completed, the less is the risk of neural damage. Recent advances in surgical interventions enable the closure of spinal cord defects of the fetus in utero (while still in the uterus). This procedure is still experimental according to the National Institutes of Health.[207] Although there are risks involved for both the mother and the fetus, results of this surgical technique are promising. Existing neurological defects cannot be reversed, but the early intervention of closing the spinal lesion during gestation seems to improve the physical and mental outcomes of the child by reducing the complications associated with hydrocephalus.[208] Children with spina bifida require ongoing medical treatment throughout their lives. Parents may be helped by joining support groups and are usually offered genetic counseling.[209]

Physical Therapy Intervention. Physical therapy intervention may be indicated on an intermittent, long-term basis for consultation for assistive and adaptive devices, wheelchair prescription, and positioning advice. There is generally surgical insertion of a shunt soon after birth to drain the excess spinal fluid from the brain in hydrocephalus, and the PTA must be aware of the location of the shunt on the head. The shunt tubing lies superficially beneath the skin on the side of the head, so care must be taken not to damage it during handling of the infant. With successful insertion of shunts, most children with spina bifida do not have mental retardation. However, the PTA should watch for signs of increased head size, indicating the shunt is not working properly. PT intervention includes seating management so that the child can participate in school and be as mobile and independent as possible. A power chair may be necessary if there is reduced upper-extremity strength. Initial evaluation by a PT is performed to determine the level of motor involvement and then monitoring of progress as the child grows. Because most of these children lack muscle control or have low muscle tone, they are prone to scoliosis. The PT and PTA are also involved with teaching the family how to assist the infant with appropriate exercises and perform passive range of motion (PROM) to joints. Instruction regarding prevention of pressure ulcers is important because children with spina bifida have no sensation in the lower body and lower extremities and are thus unable to detect when to move their body to prevent pressure areas. Because many of these children are not able to bear weight through their legs, they are more likely to experience spontaneous fractures due to osteoporosis and may be prone to dislocated hips; thus care must be taken when performing PROM not to force the joints or overstretch ligaments and muscles.[210] In some cases the use of reciprocal walkers can enable the child to "walk" and reduce the risk of osteoporosis. If the child is unable to walk with an assistive device, a standing frame can be used to facilitate weight bearing through the lower extremities. Children with spina bifida may require Lofstrand crutches, walkers, wheelchairs, braces, and orthoses. As the child grows, these items must be reordered with measurements taken for fitting of devices.[211] Education on watching for increased head size is important as well. Parents and caregivers should watch for signs of malfunction of the shunt. Any complaints from the child of headache, dizziness, or observation of an increase in head size warrant a trip to the pediatrician.

Why Does the Physical Therapist Assistant Need to Know About Genetically Linked Diseases?

People with many of the diseases associated with genetically inherited traits have neuromuscular or joint manifestations and require physical therapy intervention. Familiarity with the mechanisms of these diseases is important for the PTA. These diseases affect people throughout the life span and may require intermittent physical therapy intervention during phases of exacerbation.

Genetically Linked Diseases

This section describes some of the genetically linked diseases that are caused by inherited genetic traits most frequently observed in physical therapy.

Hemophilia ⊛

Hemophilia is a rare disorder of the clotting mechanism of the blood. The disease affects males exclusively, with females being carriers of the trait. Hemophilia affects all populations throughout the world with an incidence in males of 1 in 5,000 to 10,000 births.[212] In the United States, about 18,000 people are affected by the disease, and approximately 400 babies are born each year with hemophilia.[213]

Etiology. Hemophilia A, caused by lack of or deficient amounts of Factor VIII clotting agent, accounts for approximately 80% to 90% of all cases in the United States. The other 10% to 20% of people with hemophilia have hemophilia B, caused by the lack or deficiency of clotting factor XI.[214] Cases of hemophilia vary from mild to severe. Hemophilia is usually caused by a sex-linked autosomal recessive trait. Although the disease is known to be hereditary, occasionally someone with no previous family history will have hemophilia. In this situation, the assumption is that the gene mutates.

Signs and Symptoms. The severity of the bleeding disorder depends on the amount of clotting factor present in the blood. Persons with hemophilia have blood that does not clot as quickly as individuals without the disorder, and consequently, a small injury can result in internal bleeding, such as hemarthrosis (bleeding into a joint), intestinal bleeding, or bleeding into the brain. In some people, bleeding into a joint causes arthritis related to hemophilia. During activity, signs of bleeding into a joint may include joint effusion (swelling), severe pain and tenderness, muscle spasms, and stiffness of the joint. Bleeding can also occur into a muscle with the associated symptoms of swelling and pain. Bleeding into the brain causes

symptoms similar to those of a stroke, such as vision problems, motoric difficulties, and disorientation and requires immediate medical intervention.

Prognosis. The prognosis for people with hemophilia is generally good with adequate medication and medical care. Many people with hemophilia have undergone multiple blood transfusions, and as a result may have hepatitis or HIV infections. The blood supply from donors is now screened for these diseases, but if transfusions were received in the early 1980s, recipients were at a greater risk of acquiring HIV or hepatitis from contaminated blood or plasma.

Medical Intervention. Treatment with clotting factor isolated from blood plasma is used after injury to assist the clotting mechanism. In people with severe hemophilia, the clotting factor may be administered regularly as a prophylactic measure to prevent ongoing problems, such as hemorrhage.

Physical Therapy Intervention. The significance for the PTA is in understanding the precautions needed when treating patients with hemophilia. Many individuals experience hemarthrosis (bleeding into the joint) with resulting arthritis. Bleeding into the muscles can cause severe pain and contractures.[215] The slightest trauma may cause severe bruising and prolonged bleeding in the person with hemophilia but might go unnoticed in a healthy individual. When assisting a patient with hemophilia for gait reeducation, suitable assistive devices should be selected carefully. Axillary crutches should be used with caution because of possible pressure in the axilla with resultant bruising. Overexertion with exercise in a person with a severe case of hemophilia may cause bleeding.

Muscular Dystrophy ⊛

Many types of muscular dystrophy (MD) have been identified. The two main types are Duchenne's (DMD) and Becker's (BMD) muscular dystrophy.

Etiology. DMD and BMD are caused by an X-linked recessive chromosomal trait affecting males and, rarely, females. The mother is the carrier of the gene in two thirds of the cases, but the other third are due to spontaneous mutations of the gene responsible for the production of dystrophin. The disease affects the production of dystrophin, a protein responsible for normal muscle function.[216] DMD is the more severe type of MD affecting 1 in 3,300 male births.

Signs and Symptoms. Characteristic signs and symptoms of DMD include severe, progressive muscle atrophy starting in the lower extremities and progressing to the trunk and upper extremities. In the early stages, children exhibit pseudohypertrophy of the gastrocnemius muscles from the deposit of fatty tissue and additional connective tissue in place of the muscle, and tightness in the tibialis anterior and peroneal muscles, resulting in toe walking.[217,218] Children with DMD have great difficulty walking and running and often lose their balance. Patients with DMD and BMD demonstrate proximal muscle weakness in both the lower and upper extremities before developing weakness in the distal muscles. They show signs of increased lumbar lordosis as a result of weakness in the hip extensors and may have a Trendelenburg gait pattern progressing to a gluteus medius gait as the hip abductors become weaker. In the Trendelenburg gait pattern, the weakness of the hip abductors prevents the maintenance of the upright body over the lower extremity during the stance phase of the gait pattern resulting in the pelvis dipping to the unaffected side. As the weakness progresses, a gluteus medius gait pattern develops in which the person actually side bends the trunk over the affected side in an attempt to fix the hip and compensate for the lack of abductor strength. Children with DMD tend to have a specific way of getting up from the floor in the early stages of the disease, which is called the Gower's maneuver.[219] In this maneuver, the child goes on to the hands and feet and then "walks" the hands up the legs to stand up. Most children with DMD need a power wheelchair for at least part of the day by the time they reach school age and are unable to walk somewhere between the ages of 7 to 12 years.[220] DMD eventually progresses and affects the muscles of respiration, causing breathing difficulties and requiring the use of a respirator. The onset of scoliosis due to the lack of muscle support adds to the respiratory problems by reducing the volume of the thoracic cavity and the inability to expand the lungs fully on inhalation.

Prognosis. The life expectancy for patients with DMD is in the late teens to early adulthood. The life expectancy for individuals with BMD is midlife.

Medical Intervention. Many children with DMD have progressively worsening scoliosis resulting from muscle weakness and may require surgery to correct the spine and assist breathing. Breathing assistance with a respirator and oxygen may be necessary in the later stages of the disease. Parents and care providers are usually referred for counseling. The Muscular Dystrophy Association (http://www.mdausa.org) can also provide valuable information and support for patients and their families.

Physical Therapy Intervention. Physical therapy for children with DMD includes breathing exercises and balance and strengthening exercises, ensuring that the child does not become fatigued. Wheelchair and seating prescription is essential to minimize deformities and assist in providing a position that enables the chest to expand as much as possible. The use of power chairs is often necessary to provide optimal mobility for the child at home and at school. The PT and PTA must teach care providers lifting and transfer techniques to minimize injury for both the child and the care provider. Mobility for these children is essential, and the PT and PTA are involved with advising classroom teachers in daily management to enable the child to participate in the classroom. Home visits by the rehabilitation team to instruct the parents and caregivers in adaptations and accommodations are important, and the use of standers at home and in school helps to stretch leg muscles. Aquatherapy is of enormous benefit for these children. The goal of physical therapy is to keep the child functioning at the highest level possible for as long as possible. Another important note is that these children can now do many things that were not possible even in the recent past. Some go canoeing, and even rappelling, in their wheelchairs.

Sickle Cell Disease ☺

Sickle cell disease is a term that covers several types of inherited abnormalities of hemoglobin within the erythrocytes causing anemia. Sickle cell disease is common worldwide, affecting millions of people, especially in black and Hispanic populations throughout the world and in parts of the Mediterranean. In the United States, approximately 70,000 to 80,000 people have sickle cell disease. One in 12 African Americans carry the trait for sickle cell disease, and 1 in 500 black babies have sickle cell disease.[221] Another type of anemia is thalassemia, which is common in people of Mediterranean, African, and southern Asian descent.

Etiology. Sickle cell disease is an autosomal recessive hereditary, chronic disease in which both parents must pass on the trait to the offspring.

Signs and Symptoms. Sickle cell disease causes anemia due to the rupture of erythrocytes, which release hemoglobin into the plasma of the blood. The erythrocytes are thus unable to transport oxygen through the body to where it is needed. The disease is characterized by crises, which are periods when blood flow and oxygen delivery are unable to reach the vital organs and cells of the body. Symptoms during a crisis may include fever and pain in the joints and abdomen. A crisis can be precipitated by many factors, such as an infection, emotional problems, heat or cold, fatigue, physical exercise, trauma, or pregnancy. A crisis can be life threatening for the patient.[222] Complications associated with sickle cell disease that the PTA must be aware of include stasis ulcers of the ankles, feet and hands, pulmonary problems, neurological symptoms including seizures, and gastrointestinal complaints. Many of these problems are caused by clots of the sickle-shaped blood cells that lodge in the blood vessels of major organs and cut off vital oxygen supply to tissues. Most patients are in severe pain during crisis.

Prognosis. No cure exists for sickle-cell disease and a crisis of the disease can cause death. Death most frequently occurs as the result of thrombus formation.

Medical Intervention. Constant medical attention is needed for patients with sickle cell disease to reduce the risk of crisis. Vitamin supplements of folic acid and use of analgesics for pain are often prescribed.[223] Bone marrow transplant is performed for a few patients. Total joint arthroplasties may be necessary when joints are destroyed by the disease process, and kidney dialysis is necessary for those with kidneys affected by the disease.[224]

Physical Therapy Intervention. The PT and PTA may be involved in treatment of patients with the condition and should be aware of the possible problems with thrombus formation. Listening to the patient is essential because the onset of a crisis may be anticipated through past experience by the patient. Pain control and management may be part of the PT treatment. Because extremes of cold and heat can cause a crisis, these should be avoided if the PT treatment is being performed for a primary orthopedic injury or musculoskeletal problem. Awareness of the signs and symptoms of sickle cell disease is important for the therapist when providing intervention for other conditions when the patient has the disease. Overexertion and stressful situations should be avoided with the patient to reduce the risk of precipitating a crisis.

Spinal Muscular Atrophy ⊛

Other names for spinal muscular atrophy (SMA) include floppy infant syndrome, Werdnig-Hoffman disease, and Kugelberg-Welander disease.[225] SMA progressively affects the anterior horn cells of the spinal cord. The disease affects one child in 15,000 births, and the genetic defect is carried by 1 in 80 people.[226]

Etiology. SMA is an autosomal recessive hereditary neuromuscular disorder. The faulty genes responsible for SMA have been identified as SMN1 and SMN2 (survival of motor neuron).[227,228]

Signs and Symptoms. Children with SMA exhibit progressive spinal muscular atrophy affecting all skeletal muscles. The degeneration of the anterior horn cells of the spinal cord results in hypotonia (low tone/floppy) and weakness with scoliosis, respiratory, and feeding problems. These children tend to have bloated looking abdomens as a result of the necessity for diaphragmatic breathing patterns.[229] Children with SMA have normal intelligence levels.

Prognosis. SMA is the most common genetic cause of infant mortality.[230] No known current cure exists for this disease. In severe cases, life expectancy is between 3 to 7 years and may be less if the child has severe respiratory problems.

Medical Intervention. Medical intervention involves the diagnosis of the condition and providing medical continuity and referral for appropriate therapies. The advances in genetic coding are offering possibilities for future treatment of the inherited diseases.

Physical Therapy Intervention. Physical therapy intervention can help with improving function and providing seating advice where appropriate.

Tetralogy of Fallot ⊛

Tetralogy of Fallot (TOF) is a congenital heart disease. About 3,000 babies are born with TOF each year in the United States.[231]

Etiology. The cause of TOF is partially genetic but may also be due to other factors including maternal rubella infection, maternal diabetes, and maternal alcohol and drug abuse during pregnancy. Many cases of TOF have an unknown etiology.

Signs and Symptoms. TOF consists of four heart defects, including pulmonary stenosis, a defect in the ventricular septum, hypertrophy (enlargement) of the right ventricle, and a defect causing the aorta to be open into both ventricles.[232] The defects within the heart cause a mixing of oxygenated and deoxygenated blood often resulting in cyanosis of the lips, fingertips, and ears. [233]

Prognosis. The prognosis for children with TOF is generally good if heart surgery is performed to correct the heart defects. Some individuals may have heart arrhythmias or heart valve problems later in life.[234]

Medical Intervention. Children with TOF undergo surgery to rectify the heart defects. The care of a cardiologist is advisable due to the increased risk of arrhythmias in later life. Further heart surgery is necessary for some patients with TOF.

Physical Therapy Intervention. The PT and the PTA may be involved with the general exercise protocols needed during recovery from heart surgery of children with TOF.

CASE STUDY 2.1

A 40-year-old female client is seeking physical therapy after right simple mastectomy subsequent to a malignant mass in the breast 1 week earlier. The physician has ordered postmastectomy protocol for the patient, and the PT has performed an initial evaluation, which indicates the patient has limited range of motion in the right shoulder secondary to surgery with weakness of right upper extremity muscles and some pain in the right upper extremity. The PT has delegated the treatment of this client to the PTA.

1. What exercises would the PTA institute for this patient?

2. What precautions would the PTA have to consider? Pay specific attention to the motions the PTA thinks would be particularly affected by the surgery.

3. How would the PTA progress the exercise program within the plan of care developed by the PT over the next month?

4. What are the warning signs the PTA needs to be aware of that would require alerting the PT?

5. What modalities, if any, might the PTA use?

6. Develop a home program for the patient.

STUDY QUESTIONS

1. Explain to a neighbor who has no knowledge of immunology or science why he or she should take a complete course of antibiotics even if the individual starts to feel better after the first few days.

2. Discuss with another student or PTA the implications for the future of bacteriocidal-resistant bacteria.

3. Describe the roles of T and B lymphocytes in the immune response.

4. Explain to another person how vaccination works and the mechanisms of antibodies and antigens in this process.

5. Describe the mechanism of anaphylactic shock at a cellular level and include the signs and symptoms and possible causes of the problem.

6. List three conditions that are examples of a Type I hypersensitivity reaction.

7. Describe the four types of immune response.

8. List three types of exogenous teratogens.

9. Describe angiogenesis.

10. Discuss the staging of malignant tumors and the relevance to the outcome for the patient.

11. Discuss two methods of metastasis of a malignant tumor.

12. Describe three types of chromosome abnormalities that can result in a birth defect. For each type, give an example of a resulting abnormality.

13. What are two types of muscular dystrophy?

14. Describe the pathology of muscular dystrophy.

15. Discuss the physical therapy intervention that may be indicated for a patient with Duchenne's muscular dystrophy.

16. Consider what type of ambulatory assistive device the PTA would provide to a 40-year-old male client with hemophilia who has sustained a fracture of the right femur and has to be non-weight-bearing for the next 6 weeks. Give reasons for your choice of device and think about the precautions needed. Also think about specific instructions the PTA needs to give to the patient.

17. List four characteristics of sickle cell disease.

18. Describe the etiology and characteristics of Erb's palsy.

USEFUL WEB SITES

American Heart Association
http://www.americanheart.org

Centers for Disease Control and Prevention
http://www.cdc.gov

Cystic Fibrosis Foundation
http://www.cff.org

Emory University (2006): Cancer Quest.
http://www.cancerquest.org
Oklahoma State University College of Veterinary Medicine

Fox, J. C. Veterinary clinical parasitology images
http://www.cvm.okstate.edu/~users/jcfox/htdocs/clinpara/Index.htm
This site includes interesting images of parasites.

March of Dimes
http://www.marchofdimes.com/professionals/professionals.asp
Includes information regarding genetics, birth defects, and pregnancy care with a section of the site specific to interested medical professionals

Medscape from WebMD
http://www.medscape.com/medscapetoday
Users must register with this website to receive a password, but it is free and provides up-to-date professional articles regarding all types of medical research.

Muscular Dystrophy Association
http://www.mda.org

National Hemophilia Foundation
http://www.hemophilia.org
Search under Researchers and Healthcare Providers, then within the Physical Therapists Working Group for resources and images.

National Institutes of Health, National Institute of Child Health & Human Development
http://www.nichd.nih.gov
Search under Publications and then Health Information for information on all childhood development diseases and infectious diseases.

Organization of Teratology Information Specialist
http://otispregnancy.org/otis_about_us.asp

Spinal Muscular Atrophy Foundation
http://www.smafoundation.org

Spina Bifida Association of America
www.spinabifidaassociation.org

United States National Library of Medicine, National Institutes of Health
http://sis.nlm.nih.gov/
This website details many aspects of medicine and pathology.

World Oncology Network (WON)
http://www.worldoncology.net/carcinogenesis.htm.
A site that provides links to a variety of professional oncology resources throughout the world.

REFERENCES

[1] Little, F. F. (2005). *Medline Plus Medical Encyclopedia.* Retrieved 3.24.07 from http://www.nlm.nih.gov/medlineplus/ency/article/002224.htm

[2] Accetta, D. (2006). Antibody. *Medline Plus Medical Encyclopedia.* Retrieved 3.24.07 from http://www.nlm.nih.gov/medlineplus/ency/article/002223.htm

[3] Kimball, J. W. (2006). B cells and T cells. *Kimball's biology pages.* Retrieved 3.24.07 from http://users.rcn.com/jkimball.ma.ultranet/BiologyPages/B/B_and_Tcells.html

[4] Alberts, B., et al (2002). Lymphocytes and the cellular basis of adaptive immunity. *Molecular biology of the cell*, 4th edition. Garland Science. Retrieved on 3.24.07 from http://www.ncbi.nlm.nih.gov/books/bv.fcgi?rid=mboc4.section.4422

[5] Ibid.

6 Ibid.

7 Ibid.

8 Kimball, J. W. (2006). Antigen receptors. *Kimball's biology pages.* Retrieved 3.24.07 from http://users.rcn.com/jkimball.ma.ultranet/BiologyPages/A/AntigenReceptors.html

9 Kimball, J. W. (2006). Allergies. *Kimball's biology pages.* Retrieved 3.24.07 from http://users.rcn.com/jkimball.ma.ultranet/BiologyPages/A/Allergies.html#immediate

10 Ghaffar, A. (2006). Hypersensitivity reactions. Chapter 17 in *Immunology.* Microbiology and immunology on-line. School of Medicine, University of South Carolina. Retrieved on 3.24.07 from http://pathmicro.med.sc.edu/ghaffar/hyper00.htm

11 Holmes, N. (1999). Hypersensitivity and chronic inflammation. Retrieved 3.24.07 from http://www-immuno.path.cam.ac.uk/~immuno/part1/lec13/lec13_97.html

12 Medscape Today. (n.d.) Asthma Resource Center. Retrieved on 3.24.07 from http://www.medscape.com/resource/asthma

13 Green, R. H., Brightling, C. E., & Bradding, P. (2007). The reclassification of asthma based on subphenotypes. *Curr Opin Allergy Clin Immunol* 7:43–50.

14 Akbari, O., et al (2006). Role of natural killer cells in bronchial asthma. *N Engl J Med* 354:1117–1129.

15 eMedicineHealth, WebMD (2005). Exercise induced asthma. Retrieved 7.27.07 from http://www.emedicinehealth.com/exercise-induced_asthma/article_em.htm

16 Boulet, L.-P. (2004). Once daily inhaled corticosteroids for the treatment of asthma. *Curr Opin Pulm Med.* Retrieved 3.24.07 from http://www.medscape.com/viewarticle/466827

17 Klabunde, R. E. (2007). Beta-adrenoceptor agonists (β-agonists). *Cardiovascular pharmacology concepts.* Retrieved 3.24.07 from http://cvpharmacology.com/cardiostimulatory/beta-agonist.htm

18 Barcley, L., & Vega, C. (2006). Breathing Exercises Similar to Nonspecific Exercises in Reducing Need for Beta-Agonists in Asthma. *Medscape Medical News.* Retrieved 3.24.07 from http://www.medscape.com/viewarticle/535790

19 Lotz, T. (2005). Developing an asthma action plan. *Medscape Pulmonary Medicine.* Retrieved 3.24.07 from http://www.medscape.com/viewarticle/511131

20 Nguyen, Q. A. (2007). Allergic rhinitis. *eMedicine Specialties, Otolaryngology and Facial Plastic Surgery.* Retrieved 3.25.07 from http://www.emedicine.com/ent/topic194.htm

21 Becker, J. M. (2007). Allergic rhinitis. *eMedicine Specialties, Pediatrics, Allergy and Immunology.* Retrieved 3.25.07 from http://www.emedicine.com/ped/topic2560.htm

22 Ibid.

23 *Medline Plus* (2006). Allergic rhinitis. Retrieved 3.25.07 from http://www.nlm.nih.gov/medlineplus/ency/article/000813.htm

24 Becker, J. M. (2007). Ibid.

25 Medline Plus. (2006). Ibid.

26 Nguyen, Q. A. (2007). Ibid.

27 Allergic rhinitis. (2006). *Medline Plus.* Retrieved 03.25.07 from http://www.nlm.nih.gov/medlineplus/ency/article/000813.htm

28 *Medline Plus.* (2006). Ibid.

29 Emergency care and consumer health. Severe allergic reaction (anaphylactic shock). (2005). *eMedicineHealth.* Retrieved 3.26.07 from http://www.emedicinehealth.com/severe_allergic_reaction_anaphylactic_shock/page4_em.htm

30 Kaufman, D. A. (2006). Anaphylaxis. *Medline Plus Medical Encyclopedia.* Retrieved 3.24.07 from http://www.nlm.nih.gov/medlineplus/ency/article/000844.htm

31 Krause, R. S. (2006). Anaphylaxis. *E-medicine from WebMD.* Retrieved 3.24.07 from http://www.emedicine.com/EMERG/topic25.htm

32 Gomes, E. R., & Demoly, P. (2005). *Curr Opin Allergy Clin Immunon* 5:309–316. Retrieved 3.04.07 from http://www.medscape.com/viewarticle/508375?rss

33 Kaufman, D. A. (2006). Ibid.

34 Lieberman, P., et al. (2005). The diagnosis and management of anaphylaxis: an updated practice paradigm. *J Allergy Clin Immunol* 115:S490.

35 Krause, R. S. (2006). Anaphylaxis. *E-medicine from WebMD.* Retrieved 3.24.07 from http://www.emedicine.com/EMERG/topic25.htm

36 Kaufman, D. A. (2006). Ibid.

37 Lieberman, P., et al. (2005). Ibid., p. S492.

38 Nanda, R. (2005). Transfusion reaction. *MedlinePlus.* Retrieved 3.26.07 from http://www.nlm.nih.gov/medlineplus/ency/article/001303.htm

39 Salem, L. (2005). RH incompatibility. *eMedicine from WebMD.* Retrieved 3.26.07 from http://www.emedicine.com/emerg/topic507.htm

40 Dean, L. (2007). Blood groups and red cell antigens. National Library of Medicine, National Center for Biotechnology Information. Retrieved 3.26.07 from http://www.ncbi.nlm.nih.gov/books/bv.fcgi?rid=rbcantigen.chapter.ch4

41 Salem, L. (2005). RH incompatibility. *eMedicine from WebMD.* Retrieved 3.26.07 from http://www.emedicine.com/emerg/topic507.htm

42 Mushnick, R. (2005). Glomerulonephritis. *MedlinePlus.* National Institutes of Health. Retrieved 3.26.07 from http://www.nlm.nih.gov/medlineplus/ency/article/000484.htm

43 Ghaffar, A. (2006). Ibid.

44 Centers for Disease Control and Prevention, Division of Tuberculosis Elimination. (n.d.). Tuberculosis. Retrieved 3.26.07 from http://www.cdc.gov/nchstp/tb/faqs/qa_latenttbinf.htm#Latent1

45 Ibid.

46 Behrman, A. J., & Howarth, M. (2005). Latex allergy. *eMedicine from WebMD.* Retrieved 03.26.07 from http://www.emedicine.com/emerg/topic814.htm

47 Asthma Foundation New South Wales (2005). Hypersensitivity reaction type IV. *Virtual Allergy Centre.* Retrieved 3.26.07 from http://www.virtualallergycentre.com/diseases.asp?did=769

48 Ibid.

49 Centers for Disease Control and Prevention (2007). National immunization program. Retrieved 03.27.07 from http://www.cdc.gov/nip/menus/vaccines.htm#flu

50 Centers for Disease Control and Prevention (2007). National immunization program. Retrieved 3.27.07 from http://www.cdc.gov/nip/menus/vaccines.htm#flu

51 Advisory Committee on Immunization Practices, Centers for Disease Control and Prevention. (2006). Retrieved 3.27.07 from http://www.cdc.gov/nip/recs/provisional_recs/zoster-11-20-06.pdf

52 Markowitz, L. E., et al (2007). Quadrivalent human papillomavirus vaccine: recommendations of the advisory committee on immunization practices (ACIP). Centers for Disease Control and Prevention. Retrieved 3.27.07 from http://www.cdc.gov/mmwr/preview/mmwrhtml/rr56e312a1.htm?s_cid=rr56e312a1_e

53 Markowitz, L. E., et al (2007). Ibid.

54 Nemet, D., Mills, P. J., & Cooper, D. M. (2004). Effect of intense wrestling exercise on leucocytes and adhesion molecules in adolescent boys. *Br J Sports Med* 38:154–158.

55 Woods, J., et al (2000). Special feature for the Olympics: effect of exercise on the immune system: exercise induced modulation of macrophage function. *Immunol Cell Biol* 78:545–553.

56 Mayo Clinic (2007). Chronic pain: exercise can bring relief. Retrieved 3.27.07 from http://www.mayoclinic.com/health/chronic-pain/AR00017

57 Artal, Michal. (1998). Exercise against depression. *Physician Sportsmed* 26. Retrieved 3.27.07 from http://www.physsportsmed.com/issues/1998/10Oct/artal.htm

58 Centers for Disease Control and Prevention (2006). Healthcare-associated infections. Retrieved 3.28.07 from http://www.cdc.gov/ncidod/dhqp/healthDis.html

59 Ibid.

60 Centers for Disease Control and Prevention (2002). Hand hygiene guidelines fact sheet. Retrieved 3.28.07 from http://www.cdc.gov/od/oc/media/pressrel/fs021025.htm

61 Centers for Disease Control and Prevention (2007). National Center for Infectious Diseases, Division of Vector-Borne Infectious Diseases. Retrieved 3.28.07 from http://www.cdc.gov/ncidod/dvbid

62 Centers for Disease Control and Prevention (2007). Filariasis, parasites and health. Retrieved 3.28.07 from http://www.dpd.cdc.gov/dpdx/HTML/Filariasis.htm

63 Centers for Disease Control and Prevention (2004). Giardiasis, parasites and health. Retrieved 3.28.07 from http://www.dpd.cdc.gov/dpdx/HTML/Giardiasis.htm

64 Centers for Disease Control and Prevention (2005). Malaria. Retrieved 3.28.07 from http://www.cdc.gov/malaria/clinicians.htm

65 Kimball, J. W. (2007). Properties of bacteria. *Kimball's biology pages.* Retrieved 3.28.07 from http://users.rcn.com/jkimball.ma.ultranet/BiologyPages/E/Eubacteria.html

66 Kimball, J. W. (2007). Classification of bacteria. *Kimball's biology pages.* Retrieved 3.28.07 from http://users.rcn.com/jkimball.ma.ultranet/BiologyPages/E/Eubacteria.html

67 Kimball, J. W. (2007). Firmicutes. *Kimball's biology pages.* Retrieved 3.28.07 from http://users.rcn.com/jkimball.ma.ultranet/BiologyPages/E/Eubacteria.html

68 Kimball, J. W. (2007). Viruses. *Kimball's biology pages.* Retrieved 3.28.07 from http://users.rcn.com/jkimball.ma.ultranet/BiologyPages/V/Viruses.html#negative_ssRNA

69 Robbins, C. M., & Foster, K. W. (2005). Tinea pedis. Specialties, dermatology, fungal infections. *eMedicine by WebMD.* Retrieved 3.28.07 from http://www.emedicine.com/derm/topic470.htm

70 Centers for Disease Control and Prevention (2007). Infection control in healthcare settings. Retrieved 3.28.07 from http://www.cdc.gov/ncidod/dhqp/index.html

71 U.S. Department of Labor, Occupational Safety and Health Administration (2001). Bloodborne pathogens and needlestick prevention. OSHA guidelines. Retrieved 3.28.07 from http://www.osha.gov/SLTC/bloodbornepathogens/standards.html

72 Rice, L. B. (2001). Emergence of vancomycin-resistant enterococci. *Emerging Infect Dis* 7. Centers for Disease Control and Prevention. Retrieved 8.07.07 from http://www.cdc.gov/ncidod/eid/vol7no2/rice.htm

73 Centers for Disease Control and Prevention (2007). *Antimicrobial Resistance Interagency Task Force 2006 annual report.* Retrieved 8.07.07 from http://www.cdc.gov/drugresistance/actionplan/2006report/index.htm

74 Centers for Disease Control and Prevention (2006). MRSA in healthcare settings. Retrieved 3.28.07 from http://www.cdc.gov/ncidod/dhqp/ar_mrsa_spotlight_2006.html

75 Barclay, L., & Vega, C. (2007). Antibiotic prescribing increases antibiotic resistance in individual children in primary care. *Med Gen Med eJournal.* Retrieved 08.08.07 from http://www.medscape.com/viewarticle/560620?src=mp

76 Centers for Disease Control and Prevention (2006). About antibiotic resistance. Retrieved 2.28.07 from http://www.cdc.gov/drugresistance/community/anitbiotic-resistance.htm

77 Ibid.

78 Centers for Disease Control and Prevention (2006). Antibiotic/antimicrobial resistance. Retrieved 8.07.07 from http://www.cdc.gov/drugresistance/

79 Centers for Disease Control and Prevention (2001). Campaign to prevent antimicrobial resistance in healthcare settings. Retrieved 3.28.07 from http://www.cdc.gov/drugresistance/healthcare/problem.htm

80 American Cancer Society (2007). Research milestones 2000–2007. Retrieved 7.27.07 from http://www.cancer.org/docroot/RES/content/RES_1_1X_Research_Milestones_from_2000-2002.asp?sitearea=RES

81 American Cancer Society (2007). Statistics for 2007. Retrieved 7.27.07 from http://www.cancer.org/docroot/STT/stt_0.asp

82 Khan, A. N. (2005). Osteoid osteoma. *eMedicine from WebMD.* Retrieved 3.28.07 from http://www.emedicine.com/radio/topic498.htm

83 DeGroot, H., III (n.d.). Osteosarcoma. Retrieved 3.28.07 from http://www.bonetumor.org/tumors/pages/page15.html

84 Emory University (2006). Metastasis. *Cancer Quest.* Retrieved 3.29.07 from http://www.cancerquest.org/index.cfm?page=408#

85 Matsui, W. (2006). Metastasis. *Medline Plus.* Retrieved 3.28.07 from http://www.nlm.nih.gov/medlineplus/ency/article/002260.htm

86 Emory University (2006). Ibid.

87 U.S. Department of Health and Human Services, Public Health Service, National Toxicology Program. (n.d.). *Report on carcinogens,* 11th edition. Retrieved 09.26.10 from http://ntp.niehs.nih.gov/ntp/roc/toc11.html

88 Huang, H., & Aguilar, L. (2005). Burkitt lymphoma. *eMedicine from WebMD.* Retrieved 3.29.07 from http://www.emedicine.com/med/topic256.htm

89 Goodman, C. C., Boissonnault, W. G., & Fuller, K. S. (2003). *Pathology: implications for the physical therapist,* 2nd edition. Philadelphia: Saunders, p. 240.

90 Maghfoor, I., & Perry, M. (2005). Lung cancer, non-small cell. *eMedicine from WebMD.* Retrieved 03.29.07 from http://www.emedicine.com/med/topic1333.htm

91 Mackay, J., et al (2007). *The cancer atlas.* American Cancer Society. Retrieved 3.29.07 from http://www.cancer.org/docroot/AA/content/AA_2_5_9x_Cancer_Atlas.asp

92 Ibid. Retrieved 3.29.07 from http://www.cancer.org/downloads/AA/CancerAtlas13.pdf

93 Rizzo, T., & Cloos, R. (2002). Chemotherapy. *Healthline.* Retrieved 3.29.07 from http://www.healthline.com/galecontent/chemotherapy-2

94 Familydoctor.org. (n.d.). Prostate cancer treatment options. Retrieved 3.29.07 from http://familydoctor.org/264.xml

95 CyberKnife Center, St. Catherine's Hospital, Chicago, IL. (n.d.). How does CyberKnife work? Retrieved 3.29.07 from http://www.comhs.org/CyberKnife/work.asp

96 Radiological Society of North America. (n.d.). Gamma Knife. Retrieved 3.29.07 from http://www.radiologyinfo.org/en/info.cfm?PG=gamma_knife&bhcp=1

97 Radiological Society of North America. (n.d.). Proton therapy. Retrieved 3.29.07 from http://www.radiologyinfo.org/en/info.cfm?PG=protonthera&bhcp=1

98 The American College of Radiology, Radiological Society of North America. (n.d.). Intensity-modulated radiation therapy. Retrieved 3.29.07 from http://www.radiologyinfo.org/en/info.cfm?PG=imrt

99 The American College of Radiology, Radiological Society of North America. (n.d.). External beam therapy. Retrieved 3.29.07 from http://www.radiologyinfo.org/en/info.cfm?pg=ebt

100 American Cancer Society. (n.d.). Radiation therapy effects. Retrieved 3.29.07 from http://www.cancer.org/docroot/MBC/MBC_2x_RadiationEffects.asp

101 Ibid.

102 Ibid.

103 Singletary, S. E. (2005). Breast cancer radiation therapy: treatment overview. *WebMD.* Retrieved 3.29.07 from http://www.webmd.com/breast-cancer/radiation-therapy-overview

104 National Cancer Institute, U.S. National Institutes of Health (2004). Bevacizumab (Avastin™) for treatment of solid tumors. NCI fact sheet. Retrieved 3.30.07 from http://www.nci.nih.gov/cancertopics/factsheet/AvastinFactSheet

105 Ibid.

106 U.S. National Library of Medicine. (2007). Autosomal recessive. *Genetics Home Reference.* Retrieved 3.30.07 from http://ghr.nlm.nih.gov/handbook/illustrations/autorecessive;jsessionid=C818BF6EAA994692797045D697E96BAD

107 March of Dimes (2007). Retrieved 3.30.07 from http://www.marchofdimes.com/professionals/professionals.asp

108 Organization of Teratology Information Specialists (2007). Retrieved 3.30.07 from http://otispregnancy.org/otis_about_us.asp

109 Zimmerman, L., & Reef, S (2002). Congenital rubella syndrome. *VPD Surveillance Manual*, 3rd edition, chapter 12. Retrieved 7.26.07 from http://www.cdc.gov/vaccines/pubs/surv-manual/downloads/chpt12_rub_crs.pdf

110 O'Leary, D. (2003). West Nile virus disease in pregnancy. Centers for Disease Control and Prevention, Division of Vector-Borne Infectious Diseases. (n.d.). Retrieved 7.26.07 from http://www.cdc.gov/ncidod/dvbid/westnile/conf/pdf/OLeary_2_04.pdf

111 Rare Chromosome Disorder Support Group (2005). Robertsonian translocations. Retrieved 3.11.2010 from http://www.rarechromo.org/information/Other/Robertsonian%20Translocations%20FTNW.pdf

112 University of Rochester Medical Center. (n.d.). Maternity information. *Strong Health.* Retrieved 3.30.07 from http://www.stronghealth.com/services/womenshealth/maternity/testing.cfm

113 Robertson, A. (2006). Amniocentesis. *Medline Plus.* U.S. National Library of Medicine, National Institutes of Health. Retrieved 3.30.07 from http://www.nlm.nih.gov/medlineplus/ency/article/003921.htm

114 Sondheimer, N. (2005). Down syndrome. *Medline Plus.* U.S. National Library of Medicine, National Institutes of Health. Retrieved 3.30.07 from http://www.nlm.nih.gov/medlineplus/ency/article/000997.htm

115 Centers for Disease Control and Prevention (2006). Birth defects. Retrieved 3.30.07 from http://www.cdc.gov/ncbddd/bd/faq1.htm#CommonBD

116 March of Dimes (2007). Birth defects and genetics: Down syndrome. Retrieved 3.30.07 from http://www.marchofdimes.com/pnhec/4439_1214.asp

117 Ibid.

118 Ibid.

119 Sondheimer, N. (2005). Ibid.

120 National Institutes of Health, National Institute of Child Health & Human Development (2006). Facts about Down syndrome. Retrieved 3.30.07 from http://www.nichd.nih.gov/publications/pubs/downsyndrome.cfm

121 Centers for Disease Control and Prevention (2005). Folic acid home. Retrieved 3.30.07 from http://www.cdc.gov/ncbddd/folicacid/index.htm

122 MedicineNet.com (2008). Fragile X syndrome: how many people are affected by fragile X syndrome? Retrieved 09.26.10 from http://www.medicinenet.com/fragile_x_syndrome/page4.htm

123 Belmonte, M. K., & Bourgeron, T. (2006). Fragile X syndrome and autism at the intersection of genetic and neural networks. *Nat Neurosci* 9:1221–1225. Retrieved 4.02.07 from http://www.fragilex.org/BelmonteNatureNeuroscienceNov20061.pdf

124 U.S. National Library of Medicine (2007). Fragile X syndrome. *Genetics Home Reference.* Retrieved 4.02.07 from http://ghr.nlm.nih.gov/condition=fragilexsyndrome

125 Rogers, S. J., Wehner, E. A., & Hagerman, R. (2001). The behavioral phenotype in fragile X: symptoms of autism in very young children with fragile X syndrome, idiopathic autism, and other developmental disorders. *Dev Behav Pediatr* 22:409–417. Retrieved 04.02.07 from http://www.fragilex.org/rogers-autism-paper2001.pdf

126 Hagerman, R. J., & Hagerman, P. (2002). *Fragile X syndrome: diagnosis, treatment, and research*, 3rd edition. Baltimore: Johns Hopkins University Press. Retrieved 04.02.07 from http://www.fragilex.org/html/infancy.htm

127 Harris-Schmidt, G. (2007). Behavior characteristics in children. *The National Fragile X Foundation.* Retrieved 04.02.07 from http://www.fragilex.org/html/behavior.htm

128 The National Fragile X Foundation. (2007). Fragile X-associated tremor/ataxia syndrome. Retrieved 4.02.07 from http://www.fragilex.org/html/fxtas.htm

129 Hagerman, R. J., & Hagerman, P. (2002). Ibid. Retrieved 4.02.07 from http://www.fragilex.org/html/medicalpharm.htm

130 The National Fragile X Foundation. (2007). Infancy: occupational and physical therapy. Retrieved 4.02.07 from http://www.fragilex.org/html/otpt.htm

131 Greco, C. M., et al. (2006). Neuropathology of fragile X-associated tremor/ataxia syndrome (FXTAS). *Brain* 129:243–255. Retrieved 4.02.07 from http://www.fragilex.org/2006_Greco_Brain.pdf

132 Kirmse, B. (2006). Klinefelter syndrome. *Medline Plus.* U.S. Library of Medicine, National Institutes of Health. Retrieved 4.02.07 from http://www.nlm.nih.gov/medlineplus/ency/article/000382.htm

133 Ibid.

134 Chen, H. (2005). Klinefelter syndrome. *eMedicine.* Retrieved 4.02.07 from http://www.emedicine.com/PED/topic1252.htm

135 Kirmse, B. (2006). Ibid.

136 Sondheimer, N. (2005). Trisomy 13. U.S. National Library of Medicine, National Institutes of Health, *Medline Plus.* Retrieved 3.30.07 from http://www.nlm.nih.gov/medlineplus/ency/article/001660.htm

137 Ibid.

138 Kugler, M. (2005). Patau syndrome (trisomy 13). *About Rare Diseases.* Retrieved 3.30.07 from http://rarediseases.about.com/od/rarediseasesp/a/patau05.htm

139 Sondheimer, N. (2005). Ibid.

140 Best, R. G., & Stallworth, J. (2006). Patau syndrome. *E-medicine from WebMD.* Retrieved 7.26.07 from http://www.emedicine.com/ped/topic1745.htm

141 Ibid.

142 National Institute of Child Health & Human Development (2004). Clinical features of Turner syndrome. Retrieved 3.30.07 from http://turners.nichd.nih.gov/ClinFrIntro.html

143 Turner Syndrome Society of the United States. (n.d.). Retrieved 3.30.07 from http://www.turner-syndrome-us.org/resource/faq.html

144 National Institute of Child Health & Human Development (2004). Ibid.

145 Turner Syndrome Society of the United States. Ibid.

146 March of Dimes (2004). Cerebral palsy fact sheet. Retrieved 4.21.07 from http://search.marchofdimes.com/cgi-bin/MsmGo.exe?grab_id=0&page_id=152&query=cerebral%20palsy&hiword=PALS%20PALSEY%20cerebral%20palsy%20

147 National Institute of Neurological Disorders and Stroke, National Institutes of Health (2007). Cerebral palsy: hope through research. Retrieved 4.21.07 from http://www.ninds.nih.gov/disorders/cerebral_palsy/detail_cerebral_palsy.htm#88113104

148 Ibid.

149 Centers for Disease Control and Prevention (2004). Cerebral palsy. Department of Health and Human Services, National Center for Birth Defects and Developmental Disabilities. Available from http://www.cdc.gov/ncbddd/dd/cp3.htm#common

150 National Institute of Neurological Disorders and Stroke (2008). Cerebral palsy: hope through research. Available from http://www.ninds.nih.gov/disorders/cerebral_palsy/detail_cerebral_palsy.htm#126913104

151 National Institute of Neurological Disorders and Stroke (2008). NINDS cerebral palsy information page. Available from http://www.ninds.nih.gov/disorders/cerebral_palsy/cerebral_palsy.htm

152 National Institute of Neurological Disorders and Stroke (2008). Cerebral palsy: hope through research. Ibid.

153 Hagglund, G., & Wagner, P. (2008). Development of spasticity with age in a total population of children with cerebral palsy. *BMC Musculoskelet Disord* 9:150.

154 National Institute of Neurological Disorders and Stroke (2008). Cerebral palsy: hope through research. Ibid.

155 Ibid.

156 National Institute of Neurological Disorders and Stroke (2008). NINDS cerebral palsy information page. Ibid.

157 Bishay, S. N. (2008, March). Short-term results of musculotendinous release for paralytic hip subluxation in children with spastic cerebral palsy. *Ann R Coll Surg Engl* 90:127–132.

158 National Institute of Neurological Disorders and Stroke, National Institutes of Health (2007). Ibid.

159 National Institute of Neurological Disorders and Stroke, National Institutes of Health (2007). Cerebral palsy: hope through research. Selective dorsal rhizotomy. Retrieved 4.21.07 from http://www.ninds.nih.gov/disorders/cerebral_palsy/detail_cerebral_palsy.htm#88113104

160 Anttila, H., et al (2008). Effectiveness of physical therapy interventions for children with cerebral palsy: a systematic review. *BMC Pediatr* 8:14.

161 Scholtes, V. A., et al (2008). Lower limb strength training in children with cerebral palsy—a randomized controlled trial protocol for functional strength training based on progressive resistance exercise principles. *BMC Pediatr* 8:41.

162 Christiansen, A. S., et al (2008). Intermittent versus continuous physiotherapy in children with cerebral palsy. *Dev Me Child Neurol* 50:290–293.

163 Rauch, D. (2006). Brachial palsy in newborns. *Medline Plus*. Retrieved 04.21.07 from http://www.nlm.nih.gov/medlineplus/ency/article/001395.htm

164 Mayo Clinic. (n.d.). Erb's palsy treatment in children at Mayo Clinic. Retrieved 4.21.07 from http://www.mayoclinic.org/brachial-plexus/erbs-palsy.html

165 Goodman, C. C., Boissonnault, W. G., & Fuller, K. S. (2003). Ibid., p. 862.

166 March of Dimes. (2009). Premature birth. Retrieved 4.21.07 from http://www.marchofdimes.com/prematurity/21191_5582.asp

167 March of Dimes. (2005). Why do women deliver early? Retrieved 4.21.07 from http://www.marchofdimes.com/prematurity/21191_5582.asp

168 Marshall, I. (2006). Premature infant. *Medline Plus*. Retrieved 4.21.07 from http://www.nlm.nih.gov/medlineplus/ency/article/001562.htm

169 Ibid.

170 British Medical Association (2005). Abortion time limits, fetal viability. Retrieved 7.27.07 from http://www.bma.org.uk/ap.nsf/Content/AbortionTimeLimits~Factors~viability

171 March of Dimes. (2006). Premature birth: newborn complications. Retrieved 4.21.07 from http://www.marchofdimes.com/prematurity/21191_6342.asp

172 Moses, S. (2007). Fetal lung maturity. *Family Practice Notebook*. Retrieved 7.27.07 from http://www.fpnotebook.com/OB75.htm

173 Marshall, I. (2006). Ibid.

174 Wagle, S., & Deshpande, P. G. (2010). Hemolytic disease of newborn. *eMedicine from WebMD*. Retrieved 09.26.10 from http://emedicine.medscape.com/article/974349-overview

175 Moise, K. J. (n.d.). The process of alloimmunization. *University of North Carolina Department of Obstetrics and Gynecology*. Retrieved 4.21.07 from http://www.med.unc.edu/obgyn/MaternalFetalMedicine/RHdisease.html

176 Greene, A. (1999). How to determine and manage Rh incompatibility. Retrieved 4.21.07 from http://www.drgreene.com/21_580.html

177 University of Virginia Health System (2004). High risk new born, hydrops fetalis. Retrieved 7.27.07 from http://www.healthsystem.virginia.edu/uvahealth/peds_hrnewborn/hydrops.cfm

178 Moise, K. J. (n.d.). The process of alloimmunization. *University of North Carolina Department of Obstetrics and Gynecology*. Ibid.

179 Wagle, S. (2006). Hemolytic disease of the newborn. *eMedicine from WebMD* Retrieved 7.27.07 from http://www.emedicine.com/ped/topic959.htm#section~differentials

180 American Academy of Orthopaedic Surgeons (2000). Scoliosis. Retrieved 4.02.07 from http://orthoinfo.aaos.org/brochure/thr_report.cfm?Thread_ID=14&topcategory=Spine

181 Mayo Clinic. (2005). Scoliosis: definition. Retrieved 4.02.07 from http://www.mayoclinic.com/health/scoliosis/DS00194

182 American Physical Therapy Association. (n.d.). Scoliosis. Retrieved 4.02.07 from http://www.apta.org/AM/Template.cfm?Section=Home&TEMPLATE=/CM/HTMLDisplay.cfm&CONTENTID=20446

183 Ibid.

184 Mayo Clinic (2007). Scoliosis treatment. Retrieved 04.02.07 from http://www.mayoclinic.com/health/scoliosis/DS00194/DSECTION=8

185 Bridwell, K. (2005). Idiopathic scoliosis: options of fixation and fusion of thoracic curves. *Spine Universe*. Washington University School of Medicine, St. Louis, MO. Retrieved 4.02.07 from http://www.spineuniverse.com/displayarticle.php/article614.html

186 Betz, R., Clements, D. H., & Balsara, R. K. (2006). Thoracoscopic anterior instrumentation. Advances in the management of idiopathic adolescent scoliosis. *Spine Universe*. Retrieved 4.02.07 from http://www.spineuniverse.com/displayarticle.php/article498.html

187 Bayer, B., et al (2004). The short term effects of an exercise programme as an adjunct to an orthosis in neuromuscular scoliosis. *Prosthet Orthot Int* 28:273–277.

188 Dos Santos, A., Stirbulov, R., & Avanzi, O. (2006). Impact of a physical rehabilitation program on the respiratory function of adolescents with idiopathic scoliosis. *Chest* 130:500–505.

189 Mooney, V., & Brigham, A. (2003). The role of measured resistance exercises in adolescent scoliosis. *Orthopedics* 26:167–171.

190 U.S. National Library of Medicine, National Institutes of Health (2009). Spina bifida. *MedlinePlus*. Retrieved 09.26.10 from http://www.nlm.nih.gov/medlineplus/spinabifida.html

191 Centers for Disease Control and Prevention (2009). Trends in spina bifida, United States, 1991–2005. National Center for Health Statistics, Division of Health and Nutrition Examination Survey. Retrieved 09.26.10 from http://www.cdc.gov/Features/dsSpinaBifida/

192 Spina Bifida Association of America (2009). Genetics and spina bifida. Retrieved 09.26.10 from http://www.spinabifidaassociation.org/site/c.liKWL7PLLrF/b.2664425/apps/s/content.asp?ct=3822567

193 March of Dimes (2006). Spina bifida fact sheet. Retrieved 4.21.07 from http://search.marchofdimes.com/cgi- bin/MsmGo.exe?grab_id=0&page_id=165&query= spina%20bifida&hiword=SPINAL%20SPINE%20bifida%20spina%20

194 Spina Bifida Association of America (2009). Ibid.

195 National Institute of Child Health and Human Development, National Institutes of Health. (2007). Neural tube defects. Retrieved 4.02.07 from http://www.nichd.nih.gov/health/topics/neural_tube_defects.cfm

196 Oakley, G. P. (2007). When will we eliminate folic acid–preventable spina bifida? *Epidemiology* 18:367–368.

197 Mayo Clinic Staff (2009). Spina bifida. Mayo Foundation for Medical Education and Research (MFMER). Retrieved 09.26.10 from http://www.mayoclinic.com/print/spina-bifida/DS00417/DSECTION=all&METHOD=print

198 Liptak, G. S. (2006). Brain and spinal cord defects. *Merck Manuals Online Medical Library for Health Professionals*. Retrieved 4.02.07 from http://www.merck.com/mmhe/sec23/ch265/ch265h.html

199 Spina bifida. *Merck Manuals Online Medical Library for Health Professionals* (2005). Retrieved 4.02.07 from http://www.merck.com/mmpe/sec19/ch292/ch292c.html?qt=spina%20bifida&alt=sh

200 Mayo Clinic Staff (2009). Ibid.

201 National Institute of Neurological Disorders and Stroke (2007). Spina bifida fact sheet. Retrieved 4.21.07 from http://www.ninds.nih.gov/disorders/spina_bifida/detail_spina_bifida.htm#86053258

202 Ibid.

203 Ibid.

204 Ibid.

205 Ibid.

206 *Merck Manuals Online Medical Library for Health Professionals* (2005). Ibid.

207 National Institute of Neurological Disorders and Stroke, National Institutes of Health (2007). Ibid.

208 Ibid.

209 Mayo Clinic Staff (2009). Ibid.

210 Goodman, C. C., Boissonnault, W. G., & Fuller, K. S. (2003). Ibid., p. 844.

211 Mayo Clinic Staff (2009). Ibid.

212 National Hemophilia Foundation. Hemophilia A. Retrieved 4.22.07 from http://www.hemophilia.org/NHFWeb/MainPgs/MainNHF.aspx?menuid=180&contentid=45&rptname=bleeding

213 U.S. National Library of Medicine, National Institutes of Health. (2007). Hemophilia. *Medline Plus*. Retrieved 4.22.07 from http://www.nlm.nih.gov/medlineplus/hemophilia.html

214 National Heart, Lung and Blood Institute, National Institutes of Health, U.S. Department of Health and Human Services (2006). What is hemophilia? Retrieved 4.22.07 from http://www.nhlbi.nih.gov/health/dci/Diseases/hemophilia/hemophilia_what.html

215 Goodman, C. C., Boissonnault, W. G., & Fuller, K. S. (2003). Ibid., p. 549.

216 National Institute of Neurological Disorders and Stroke, National Institutes of Health (2007). NINDS Muscular dystrophy information page. Retrieved 4.22.07 from http://www.ninds.nih.gov/disorders/md/md.htm

217 Muscular Dystrophy Association (2006). Facts about Duchenne and Becker muscular dystrophies. Retrieved 4.22.07 from http://www.mda.org/publications/fa-dmdbmd-what.html

218 Goodman, C. C., Boissonnault, W. G., & Fuller, K. S. (2003). Ibid., p. 848.

219 Muscular Dystrophy Association (2006). Ibid.

220 Ibid.

221 U.S. National Library of Medicine, National Institutes of Health (2007). Sickle cell disease. Retrieved 3.11.10 from http://ghr.nlm.nih.gov/condition=sicklecelldisease

222 Hart, J. A. (2005). Sickle cell anemia. *Medline Plus*. U.S. Library of Medicine, National Institutes of Health. Retrieved 4.21.07 from http://www.nlm.nih.gov/medlineplus/ency/article/000527.htm

223 Hart, J. A. (2005). Sickle cell disease treatment. *Medline Plus*. U.S. National Library of Medicine and National Institutes of Health.

Retrieved 4.21.07 from http://www.nlm.nih.gov/medlineplus/ency/article/000527.htm#Treatment

224 Ibid.

225 Goodman, C. C., Boissonnault, W. G., & Fuller, K. S. (2003). Ibid., p. 855.

226 Oleszek, J. L. et al. (2008). Kugelberg Welender spinal muscular atrophy. *EMedicine from WebMD*. Retrieved 09.26.10 from http://emedicine.medscape.com/article/306812-overview

227 Spinal Muscular Atrophy Foundation (2006). SMA is scientifically "solvable." Retrieved 4.22.07 from http://www.smafoundation.org/science_research.asp

228 Monani, U. R. (2005). Spinal muscular atrophy: a deficiency in a ubiquitous protein; a motor neuron-specific disease. *Neuron* 48:885–896

229 Wang, C. H., Finkel, R. S., Bertini, E. S., Schroth, M., Simonds, A., & Wong, B. et al. (2007). Concerns statement for standard of care in spinal muscular atrophy. *J. Child Neurol*, 22(8), 1027-1049, p. 1040.

230 Monani, U. R. (2005). Ibid.

231 National Institute of Neurological Disorders and Stroke, National Institutes of Health, U.S. Department of Health and Human Services (2006). What is tetralogy of Fallot? Retrieved 4.22.07 from http://www.nhlbi.nih.gov/health/dci/Diseases/tof/tof_what.html

232 American Heart Association (2007). Tetralogy of Fallot. Retrieved 4.22.07 from http://www.americanheart.org/presenter.jhtml?identifier=11071

233 National Heart, Lung and Blood Institute, National Institutes of Health, U.S. Department of Health and Human Services (2006). Ibid.

234 American Heart Association (2007). Ibid.

235 American Cancer Institute (2004). Bleomycin. Retrieved 3.30.07 from http://www.cancer.org/docroot/CDG/content/CDG_bleomycin.asp

236 American Cancer Institute (2004). Vincristine. Retrieved 3.30.07 from http://www.cancer.org/docroot/CDG/content/CDG_vincristine.asp

237 Ibid.

238 American Cancer Institute (2004). Dacarbazine. Retrieved 3.30.07 from http://www.cancer.org/docroot/CDG/content/CDG_dacarbazine.asp

239 Ibid.

240 National Cancer Institute (2004). Bevacizumab combined with oxaliplatin-based chemotherapy prolongs survival for previously treated patients with advanced colorectal cancer. Retrieved 3.30.07 from http://www.nci.nih.gov/newscenter/pressreleases/BevacizumabOxaliplatin

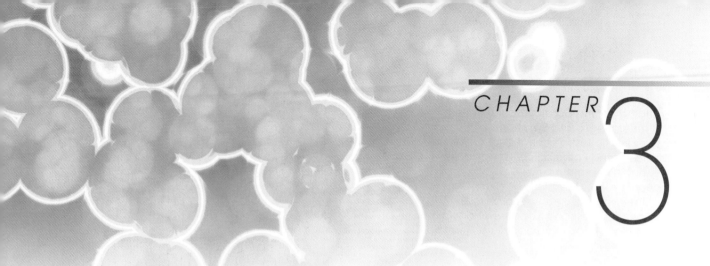

CHAPTER 3

Cardiovascular Pathologies

CHAPTER OUTLINE (continued)

Introduction

This chapter combines all the content regarding the circulatory system. The initial topics include an overview of the cardiovascular system and a view of its general pathology, as well as the signs and symptoms associated with disease of this system. Major pathological conditions of the heart are accompanied by a description of the diagnostic tests performed on people with heart conditions. The vascular system, including arterial, venous, and lymphatic diseases, is delineated together with the role of physical therapy interventions in the management of people with cardiac and vascular diseases.

Why Does the Physical Therapist Assistant Need to Know About the Anatomy and Physiology of the Cardiovascular System?

The intervention for patients with cardiovascular pathologies is a large part of physical therapy practice. The anatomy and physiology of the cardiovascular system is complex. Many factors affect the physiological response of the heart, including exercise. To understand how to monitor patients receiving physical therapy interventions, the PTA must have a basic concept of how the systems usually work. The normal values of the vital signs and the body's response to activity are crucial aspects of participation in treatment intervention for the patient with any cardiovascular pathology.

Anatomy and Physiology of the Cardiovascular System

This section provides an overview of the structures, functions, and physiology of the cardiovascular system.

The Heart

The heart is a double-sided muscular pump that circulates oxygenated and deoxygenated blood round the body. Located between the lungs in the mediastinum the heart lies with its apex pointing downward toward the diaphragm slightly left of center. The heart is enclosed in three pericardial membranes. The outer fibrous pericardium extends onto the diaphragm and blood vessels entering and exiting the heart. The middle parietal pericardium is a serous membrane and lines the fibrous pericardium. The

pericardial membrane, which clothes the heart itself, is known as the visceral pericardium or epicardium. Serous fluid lies between the parietal and visceral pericardia to reduce friction by allowing the membranes to slide over each other when the heart beats.

The four chambers of the heart are composed of cardiac muscle or myocardium. The internal surface of the chambers is smooth and lined with squamous epithelial cells, making up the endocardium layer (see Fig. 3-1). The four chambers are the right and left atria in the upper part divided by the interatrial septum, and the right and left ventricles in the lower part divided by the interventricular septum. The role of the atria is to receive blood, and that of the ventricles to pump out blood.

The right atrium receives deoxygenated blood via the superior and inferior venae cavae (singular: vena cava). The superior vena cava collects deoxygenated blood from the upper body, and the inferior vena cava collects it from the lower body (see Fig. 3-2). Both venae cavae empty into the right atrium and then into the right ventricle via the tricuspid valve. This valve is so called because it has three cusps or sections. The valve prevents backflow of blood into the right atria when the right ventricle contracts.

The right ventricle receives deoxygenated blood from the right atrium and contracts to pump this blood to the lungs for reoxygenation via the pulmonary artery through

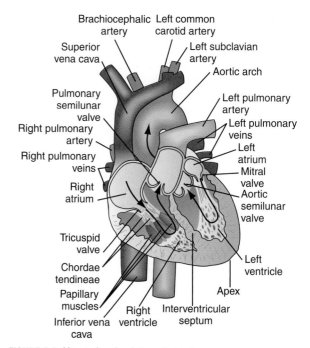

FIGURE 3.1 Heart showing internal structures.

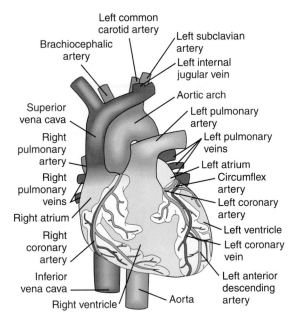

FIGURE 3.2 Heart showing major blood vessels.

the pulmonary semilunar valve (see Fig. 3-1). This valve prevents backflow of blood into the right ventricle. The pulmonary artery is the only artery in the body that carries deoxygenated blood. The role of the various heart valves in preventing backflow of blood into areas previously exited should be understood, because loss of function of these valves is responsible for various heart diseases and conditions, which are described later in the chapter. Additionally, there are bands of fibrous connective tissue called chordae tendinae in the right ventricle that extend from papillary muscles inside the right ventricle to the tricuspid valve and prevent the tricuspid valve opening when the right ventricle contracts. The tricuspid valve is tethered by the chordae tendinae in much the same way that the spokes of an umbrella prevent an umbrella from turning inside out.

The left atrium is the receiving chamber for newly oxygenated blood from the lungs via the pulmonary veins. Again the term is an anomaly because these veins carry oxygenated blood. The blood passes into the left ventricle via the mitral valve otherwise called the bicuspid valve, because it has two cusps. This valve prevents back-flow of blood into the left atrium when the left ventricle contracts. Chordae tendinae anchor the mitral valve in the same way as in the right ventricle.

The left ventricle has thick muscular walls, which enables blood to be pumped into the aorta and round the body. The aortic semilunar valve is located at the junction of the aorta and the left ventricle and prevents backflow of blood into the ventricle.

Neural Control of the Heart

The functions of the heart are controlled by the cardiac control center in the medulla of the brain. Receptors in the walls of the aorta and carotid arteries called baroreceptors monitor changes in blood pressure and send impulses to the medulla that stimulate the sympathetic and parasympathetic nervous systems to adjust the rate and force of contractions in the heart. Sympathetic intervention produces tachycardia (increased heart rate) and also increases the degree of contraction of the heart muscle. Parasympathetic intervention via the vagus nerve causes bradycardia (slowing down of the heart rate). Receptors in the heart respond to these impulses and are also responsible for the reactions to other factors, such as epinephrine and fever.

Nerve Conduction System of the Heart

Nerve control of the heart is essential for stimulation of the muscle to cause contractions in a logical and effective rhythm. No actual nerves exist in the cardiac muscle, but there are discs between cardiac fibers that quickly transmit nervous impulses and allow the whole heart to react as a single muscle when an impulse is received. Chaos would result within the heart if each cardiac muscle fiber reacted individually to nerve impulses. The usual origin of nervous impulses to the rest of the heart is from the sinoatrial (SA) node located in the right atrium. This SA node is known as the pacemaker because it sets the pace of contraction of the heart. The normal pace set is called the sinus rhythm and is approximately 70 beats per minute. This rate is affected by external factors, such as release of epinephrine in response to stress, or by the autonomic nervous system, resulting in a speeding up of the rhythm. Impulses start at the SA node, spread over the surface of the atria causing contraction of the atria, and pass to the atrioventricular (AV) node in the base of the right atrium. The impulses pause slightly at the AV node and then pass into the ventricle through the bundle of His (AV bundle) to the Purkinje network, which stimulates both ventricles to contract.

The conduction of electrical impulses through the heart enables it to be monitored by an electrocardiogram (ECG). When electrodes are attached to the skin, the electric impulses of the heart can be recorded (see Fig. 3-3). Atrial contraction is demonstrated by depolarization of the P wave, ventricular contraction by the large wave of depolarization in the ventricles or QRS wave. The third wave, or T wave, shows the repolarization of the ventricles

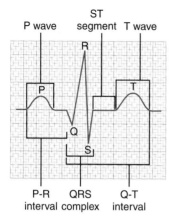

FIGURE 3.3 Electrocardiogram (ECG) showing normal data.

during the recovery phase of the heartbeat. Because the normal graph produced on the ECG by the heart contraction is readily recognized, it is possible to detect abnormalities of the heart through the graph tracings. Such abnormalities are called arrhythmias and are used diagnostically for detecting heart diseases.

Coronary Circulation

The heart requires a circulatory system for nourishment of the heart muscle. This is provided by the right and left coronary arteries, which branch from the ascending aorta. The left coronary artery branches into the left anterior descending or interventricular artery and the left circumflex artery circles around the heart. The right coronary artery branches into the right marginal artery and the posterior interventricular artery. The right and left coronary arteries anastomose (connect) at various points where they lie close to each other. The ability of these vessels to anastomose facilitates the formation of a **collateral circulation,** which can reduce the risks of blockage of heart vessels by giving an alternative blood supply to areas of heart muscle. As a general rule, the right coronary artery supplies the right side of the heart and part of the inferior aspect of the left ventricle and the posterior interventricular septum. The left coronary artery circumflex portion supplies the left atrium and parts of the walls of the left ventricle. The left anterior descending portion of the left coronary artery supplies the anterior walls of the ventricles and the anterior septum. The network of arterioles and capillaries formed by these arteries that supply the heart muscle empty directly into the coronary sinus, which then returns the deoxygenated blood into the right atrium. Failure of the coronary vessels causes ischemia to areas of heart muscle, the mechanism of which is described later in the chapter.

Cardiac Cycle

The cardiac cycle is the normal alternating rhythm of contraction and relaxation of the heart muscle. Diastole is the relaxation phase and systole the contraction phase. In diastole, both atria fill with blood while the AV valves are closed. Atrial pressure rises and opens the atrioventricular valves, causing blood to flow into the ventricles. Systole begins with atrial contraction squeezing all the blood from the atria into the ventricles, causing the ventricles to be full. The next part of systole is when the ventricles start to contract, the pressure of blood in the ventricles closes the atrioventricular valves, and the atria relax. Next, the ventricles contract, causing increased pressure within the ventricles, which opens the aortic and pulmonary valves and pushes blood into the aorta and the pulmonary artery. After the blood has passed into the aorta and pulmonary artery, the aortic and pulmonary valves close, and diastole or relaxation is resumed.

Heart Sounds

The closing of valves within the heart during the cardiac cycle creates heart sounds. These can be heard using a stethoscope placed against the chest wall. The listening, called auscultation, must be performed in a quiet room so that the heart sounds can be heard more easily. Two websites where the PTA can listen to both normal and abnormal heart sounds are provided, because it is much easier when these sounds are heard rather than simply described.[1,2] Practice is necessary to detect the heart sounds. PTAs should be familiar with normal heart sounds so that detection of the abnormal is possible. The main sounds are a "lubb," when the atrioventricular valve closes at the start of ventricular systole, known as the first heart sound or S1. This is followed by a "dupp," second heart sound or S2, caused by closure of the semilunar valves at ventricular diastole (see Table 3-1). A third heart sound (S3) is normal in children ☻ and young adults, but a sign of abnormality if heard in adults over age 40. When the heart valves are not functional and allow leaking of blood back into the compartment from which the blood exited, there is a strange sound called a murmur, which can sound like a whooshing noise. The sound is difficult to describe until one has heard it. One of the more common abnormal heart sounds is in aortic stenosis in which there is scarring of the aortic valve that resists blood flow into the aorta, causing turbulence, which can be heard as a loud murmur. Another is in mitral valve regurgitation, when the blood flows backward through the mitral valve into the left atrium during systole, causing a "swishing" sound. See Table 3-2 for abnormal heart sounds. If the

Table 3.1 **Normal Heart Sounds**

SOUND	AUSCULTATION SITE	WHAT YOU ARE HEARING	OF INTEREST	NORMAL OR ABNORMAL
First heart sound (S1), "Lubb"	Cardiac apex, intersection of the mid clavicular line with the fifth intercostal space	Closing of the tricuspid and mitral valves (atrioventricular valves)	Can be heard loudly after exercise due to tachycardia	Normal in both adults and children ⏏
Second heart sound (S2), "Dupp"	Either side of the upper portion of the sternum; the left side for the pulmonary vein and the right for the aorta	Closing of semilunar valves in aorta and pulmonary vein; the end of ventricular systole	May also be heard at the cardiac apex, but may be very faint	Normal in both adults and children ⏏
Third heart sound (S3)	Cardiac apex with person in left side lying	Filling of ventricles in early diastole when the tricuspid and mitral valves open	Difficult to hear in the normal heart	Normal in children, adolescents, and young adults; abnormal in adults over 40 ⏏

stethoscope is placed over the apex of the heart, the point of maximum impulse (PMI), this sound may be heard in individuals with this problem. The surface-marking location of the apex of the heart is at a point where a line running toward the abdomen from the midpoint of the clavicle meets the fifth intercostal space.[3] This point is where the first heart sound can also be heard most strongly. PTAs are not expected to be able to detect the various abnormal heart sounds and associate them with pathologies, but they should know what the normal heart sounds like so that they can alert the PT if they suspect a deviation from the normal.

Pulse

Pulse is the heart rate in beats per minute. The pulse is taken by placing the tips of two or three fingers over an artery where it lies fairly superficial and over a firm area of bone or tissue. The thumb should not be used to take pulse because it has a pulse of its own. The most usual sites for taking pulse readings are the radial pulse at the wrist, the brachial pulse in the upper arm on the medial aspect just posterior to the biceps brachii muscle, or in the antecubital fossa at the elbow. Another pulse important for the PTA is the dorsalis pedis (pedal pulse) on the dorsum of the foot. Palpation of the dorsalis pedis is necessary to detect intact blood supply to the foot when treating wounds in the distal lower extremity. Pulse irregularities felt during ventricular systole may be a weak or thready pulse difficult to detect or a bounding pulse, which is very strong. If the pulse is weak, it may be possible to block or occlude the

artery completely by pressure of the fingers. Irregularities of rhythm of the pulse can occur, which may be predictable irregularities or unpredictable irregularities. Such irregularities are known as arrhythmia and dysrhythmia. Any abnormality of the pulse reading may indicate a problem that should be referred to the treating physician. PTAs take pulse readings on patients before, during, and after a PT intervention session and need to be well versed in the possible abnormalities to report them to the physician and the supervising physical therapist. Apical pulse is measured directly over the heart, and a **pulse deficit** occurs when the apical pulse is a different rate from the radial or peripheral pulse. Any of these noted abnormalities should be documented and referred to the PT and the physician immediately.

Cardiac Output

Cardiac output (CO) is the amount of blood pumped out by a ventricle in a 1-minute period. The cardiac output depends on heart rate (HR) and stroke volume (SV), which is the amount pumped from one ventricle during one contraction. The resting cardiac output is approximately 5 liters per minute and can be expressed by the following equation:

$$CO = SV \times HR = 70 \times 70 = 4,900 \text{ mL}$$

During exercise or when the body is under stress or has an infection, the cardiac output is increased. Changes during exercise are due to the increased volume of venous blood returning to the heart, stretching the heart and causing

Table 3.2 **Abnormal Heart Sounds**

SOUND	AUSCULTATION SITE	WHAT YOU ARE HEARING	ASSOCIATED PATHOLOGIES	OF INTEREST
Third heart sound, ventricular gallop, (S3); a faint sound	Cardiac apex with person in left side lying	Filling of ventricles in early diastole when the tricuspid and mitral valves open; Heard after S2	In adults: left ventricular failure, tachycardia, mitral valve regurgitation, congestive heart failure	A normal heart sound in children, adolescents, and young adults; 🔔 best heard using the bell side of the stethoscope
Fourth heart sound, atrial gallop, (S4); a dull sound	Cardiac apex with person supine or sitting	Ventricles filling after atrial contraction; heard before S1	Left ventricular hypertrophy, chronic hypertension, cardiomyopathy, myocardial infarction	Abnormal in both children and adults 🔔
Murmurs	Cardiac apex with person supine or sitting	Turbulent blood flow causing vibrations	Associated with cardiac pathologies when Grade III or more	The loudness of the murmur generally denotes the severity because it indicates the amount of turbulence of blood flow in the heart:
a. Systolic murmurs	Cardiac apex with person supine or sitting	Heard between S1 and S2 during systole		Grade I = faint sound, very difficult to hear
b. Diastolic murmurs	Cardiac apex with person supine or sitting	Heard between S2 and S1 during diastole		Grade II = faint, but easier to hear
c. Continuous murmurs	Cardiac apex with person supine or sitting	Heard through both S1 and S2 during diastole		Grade III = moderate loudness
				Grade IV = loud and vibratory (called a "thrill")
				Grade V = very loud with a "thrill"
				Grade VI = extremely loud and can be heard without a stethoscope
Pericardial friction rub, squeaky sound[57]	Cardiac apex with person supine or sitting	Rubbing of the heart against an inflamed pericardium	Pericardial disease due to infections, myocardial infarction, trauma, tumors	

the muscle to contract more fully. To adapt to changes in demand, the heart has to have reserve energy known as cardiac reserve, which enables it to increase output by up to 5 times normal levels. One disease in which the cardiac output is increased is hyperthyroidism, in which metabolism increases in the tissues and cardiac output increases to meet the increased need. When heart tissue is badly damaged, such as in valve damage or damage to heart muscle, there is a decrease in cardiac output, and output may not be able to meet the needs of the body for oxygen transmission. Cardiac diseases are discussed later in the chapter.

Blood Pressure

Blood pressure (BP) is a reading of the pressure exerted against the walls of the peripheral or systemic arteries. A normal resting blood pressure reading is approximately 120/80 mm Hg in a healthy young adult. The high number is the systolic pressure created by the force of contraction of the left ventricle as it forces blood out of the heart via the aorta. The lower number is the diastolic pressure, which occurs when the ventricles are relaxed. The usual method of measuring blood pressure is through pressure on the brachial artery in the upper arm using a stethoscope and sphygmomanometer attached to an inflatable cuff. The **pulse pressure** is the difference between systolic and diastolic pressure readings. The importance of taking frequent blood pressure and other vital sign readings in physical therapy practice cannot be overemphasized. When working with patients or clients who have cardiac or vascular pathologies, these readings taken regularly during rehabilitation and exercise programs ensure safety of the patient and appropriate referral by the PTA to the PT, nurse, or physician.

Blood pressure varies with cardiac output and the peripheral resistance of blood vessels. Other factors are blood volume and viscosity (thickness), the rate of venous return, force of heart contractions, and the elasticity of arteries. Peripheral resistance is the amount of force, which acts against the flow of blood through vessels. The resistance increases when the lumen or hole in the blood vessels is small, for example, the diameter is decreased or there is an obstruction within the blood vessels. Under normal circumstances, changes in blood flow can be adjusted through control of constriction or dilation of blood vessels. The medulla, as previously described, controls the heart but also controls distribution of blood and vasoconstriction of blood vessels throughout the body. The medulla responds to positions of the body and stimuli from hormones such as epinephrine and norepinephrine. Antidiuretic hormone (ADH) increases blood volume and elevates blood pressure. Epinephrine and norepinephrine increase vasoconstriction by affecting receptors in arterioles of the skin and viscera. Epinephrine also acts on receptors in the heart, increasing the force and rate of contraction.

Blood Vessels

This section includes descriptions of the main blood vessels including the arteries, veins, capillaries, and lymphatic vessels.

ARTERIES

Arteries are blood vessels that carry oxygenated blood from the heart to the rest of the body, the exception being the pulmonary artery, which carries deoxygenated blood from the heart to the lungs (see Fig. 3-4). The pulmonary artery is called an artery because it exits the heart, taking blood away from the heart, as does the aorta. Arteries are largest closer to the heart and become arterioles as they reach the peripheral extremities and join with the capillaries for oxygen exchange to the tissues (see Fig. 3-5). The interconnection of arteries is called anastomosis and is a safety mechanism in case of blockage to one artery. The connection of arteries enables blood to be pumped to vital organs and the peripheral areas when there is reduction in

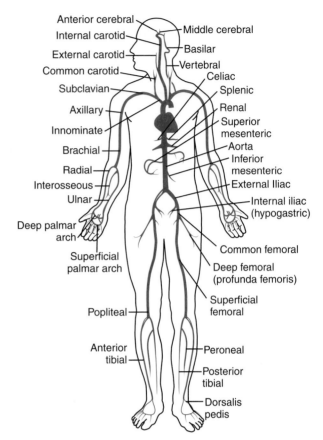

FIGURE 3.4 Systemic arteries, anterior view.

blood flow in one artery. The arterial system acts like a beltway round a major city, which has arteries into the city and also around the city, with alternative routes into the city. The three layers of artery walls are the inner endothelium, called tunica intima, which is composed of squamous epithelium, the middle smooth muscle layer of tunica media, and the fibrous outer layer of tunica externa. The outer layer of the artery provides strength to prevent rupture of the artery from pressure when the blood is pumped from the heart. The muscular layer enables the artery to undergo the constriction and dilation required for control of blood pressure in response to stimuli from the medulla and the autonomic nervous system.

VEINS

Veins are the vessels that carry deoxygenated blood from the tissues back to the heart (see Fig. 3-6). The exception is the pulmonary vein, which carries oxygenated blood from the lungs to the heart. The pulmonary vein is so called because it enters and brings blood to the heart, as do the superior and inferior venae cavae. Veins also have

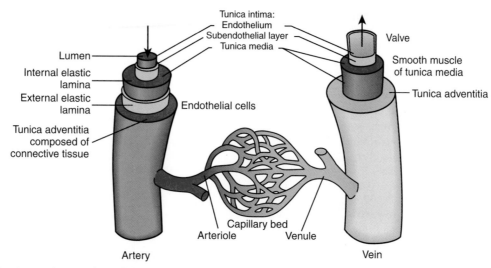

FIGURE 3.5 Structure and connections of the vessels of the arterial and venous systems.

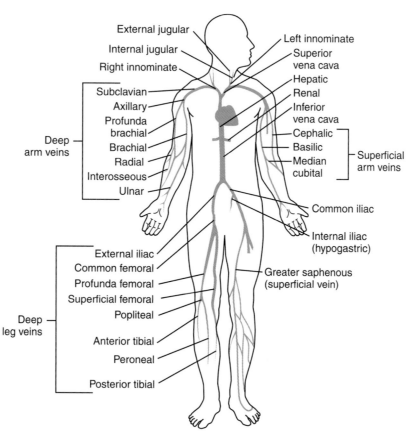

FIGURE 3.6 Anterior view of the venous system.

anastomoses to provide alternative routes for the blood to return to the heart. The walls of veins are thinner than those of arteries. They consist of the same three layers, but the inner layer forms valves to prevent the backflow of blood. Because the lower extremity veins have to overcome the effects of gravity, there are a large number of valves in the veins of the lower extremity. The middle muscular layer of tissue in the vein is thin, allowing for constriction of the vein under extreme circumstances, such as severe blood loss by the body.

CAPILLARIES

Both venous and arterial systems end in a system of capillaries at the tissue level where oxygen is diffused into the tissues from the arterial blood and the carbon dioxide is diffused back to the veins for transport back to the heart (refer to Fig. 3-4). Several factors stimulate the flow of blood across the cell membranes at the capillary and arteriole level. The hydrostatic pressure in the interstitial (between cells) fluids, when high, tends to move fluid from the tissues into the blood vessels. The hydrostatic pressure in the capillaries, controlled by blood pressure, which when higher than the interstitial pressure allows blood to enter the tissues. The capillary oncotic pressure, created by the presence of proteins inside the blood vessels, causes retention of fluid within the blood vessels and prevents excess transfer of blood into the tissues. An interstitial oncotic pressure assists the transfer of blood from the blood vessels into the tissues. These factors ideally work together to supply the necessary nutrients and oxygen where they are needed by the tissues and to remove the partially deoxygenated blood from the tissues.[4]

Lymphatic System

The lymphatic system is a network of lymph vessels, lymph nodes, and lymphatic tissue that includes the spleen, thymus, and tonsils, all of which play a part in the body's immune system (see Fig. 3-7). The spleen is located just beneath the diaphragm in the left upper abdomen. The spleen produces lymphocytes and monocytes after birth, whereas before birth, it produces red blood cells. Antibodies are produced by the plasma cells of the spleen, and macrophages act as phagocytes for pathogens and unwanted foreign matter. The thymus is located adjacent to the thyroid gland in the upper chest and produces T cells (see Chapter 2). The function of the lymphatic system is to recirculate any excess interstitial fluid back into the blood to prevent buildup of excess fluid in the tissues, which may cause edema. The lymph nodes and tissues also act as a defense mechanism to prevent foreign or unwanted material from entering the blood circulation. The

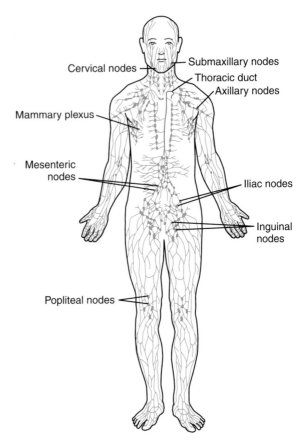

FIGURE 3.7 Anterior view of lymph vessels and the major groups of lymph nodes.

lymph nodes are filter beds for the body. This explains why lymph nodes occasionally become swollen during an infection because they attempt to filter out offending organisms from the body. Major groups of lymph nodes are located in the axilla, neck, and inguinal regions (see Fig. 3-7).

Lymph fluid is similar to blood plasma but contains a higher level of lymphocytes. The lymph vessels are dead-ended vessels, which take in fluid from the interstitial spaces when pressure in the spaces builds up. Lymph vessels have valves preventing backflow similar to those of veins. The lymph vessels on the right side of the body empty into the right lymphatic duct and thence to the right subclavian vein. All other lymphatic vessels empty into the thoracic duct, which empties into the left subclavian vein. The lymphatic system of vessels follows the direction and location of the venous system, and lymphatic nodes lie adjacent to all the venous and lymphatic vessels throughout the body to act as filters for unwanted materials in body fluids (see Fig. 3-8).

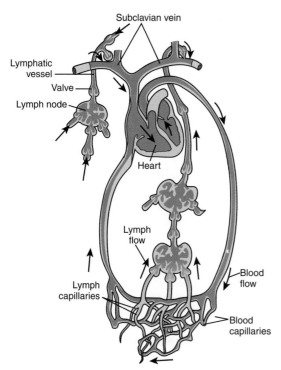

Subclavian vein

Lymphatic vessel

Valve

Lymph node

Heart

Lymph flow

Blood flow

Lymph capillaries

Blood capillaries

FIGURE 3.8 Relationship of lymphatic vessels to the cardiovascular system.

Pathology of the Cardiovascular System

Patients with cardiac pathology conditions can fall into various patterns in the *Guide to Physical Therapist Practice,* as indicated in the box on hints for use of the *Guide.* Depending on the characteristics of the disease exhibited by the patient the practice pattern may be within the cardiovascular-pulmonary patterns in Pattern 6. However, there may be some crossover with the musculoskeletal (Pattern 4) and integumentary (Pattern 7) patterns due to impaired posture, impaired muscle performance, edema, ischemia, and decreased levels of activities, which would fall under these practice patterns. When looking at the *Guide to Physical Therapist Practice,* the PTA needs to determine which impairments the patient exhibits and which pattern seems to be the most appropriate. Many patients with cardiovascular disorders have multiple diagnoses and thus may also fall under several patterns. During intervention for the cardiac problem, the patient may follow the guidelines for that particular pattern and then after recovery from the problem may be more accurately placed within a different pattern.

Why Does the Physical Therapist Assistant Need to Know About Pathology of the Cardiovascular System?

When working with patients with cardiac pathologies, the PTA must be familiar with the normal heart function as well as the abnormal. PTAs need to be able to recognize the symptoms of patients with cardiovascular disorders to alert the PT when there is an additional problem. Such signs and symptoms include atrial fibrillation, cyanosis, dyspnea, edema, fatigue, heart block, intermittent claudication, pain, palpitations, premature ventricular contractions (PVCs), reduced ejection fraction, syncope, and ventricular fibrillation. If treatment is not going as planned, fast recognition and intervention is necessary with these potentially medically unstable individuals. The usual involvement of the PTA in cardiac rehabilitation is during the later stages when the patient is more medically stable and thus does not require constant reevaluation. Details of all tests, surgery, and symptoms should be made available to the PTA.

HINTS ON THE GUIDE TO PHYSICAL THERAPY PRACTICE

The cardiovascular diseases fall into the *Guide to Physical Therapist Practice,* Cardiovascular/Pulmonary Preferred Practice Pattern 6.

- 6A "Primary prevention/risk reduction for cardiovascular/Pulmonary disorders" (p. 465): includes those patients with a family history of heart disease or other risk factors, such as smoking, obesity, or a sedentary lifestyle
- 6B "Impaired aerobic capacity/endurance associated with deconditioning" (p. 475): may be involved if a patient is exhibiting reduced endurance to activity, shortness of breath, and inability to perform simple tasks at work and home without an increased perceived exertion level
- 6C "Impaired ventilation, respiration/gas exchange, and aerobic capacity/endurance associated with airway clearance dysfunction" (p. 489): may be involved after cardiothoracic surgery
- 6D "Impaired aerobic capacity/endurance associated with cardiovascular pump dysfunction or failure" (p. 505): this is an obvious pattern for many patients

(Continued)

with cardiac diseases and includes diagnoses such as cardiomyopathy, ventricular arrhythmias, myocardial infarction, coronary artery disease, hypertensive heart disease, and heart valve disorders

- 6F – "Impaired ventilation and respiration/gas exchange associated with respiratory failure" (p. 539): This pattern is associated mainly with patients who have had cardiothoracic surgery and have resultant problems with impaired gas exchange, dyspnea, and reduced vital capacity

(From the American Physical Therapy Association. (2003). *Guide to physical therapist practice, revised 2nd edition.* Alexandria, VA: APTA. Used with permission.)

The PTA should read the PT evaluation, treatment notes, and patient medical history carefully before working with these patients. Blood pressure, pulse, respirations, and even temperature should be taken before, during, and after each treatment session or as required by the supervising PT (see Table 3-3 for the normal adult heart values). The **rate-pressure product (RPP)** is the heart rate multiplied by the systolic blood pressure.

Rate-Pressure Product (RPP) = HR × Systolic BP

This is a 5-digit figure with the last two numbers not used. The number gives an indication of the aerobic exercise condition of the patient. As the aerobic fitness of the patient improves, the RPP value is reduced. The PT will take the

Table 3.3 **Normal Adult Heart Values**

CARDIAC TERM	NORMAL VALUES	WHAT IT MEASURES	OF INTEREST	CHANGES
Cardiac output (CO)	4–5 L/min in adults	The amount of blood pumped from both ventricles in 1 minute	Depends on intact neural control of heart, sufficient perfusion of the heart (enough oxygen supply to heart muscle), and the ability of the heart muscle to contract	CO is altered when the heart rate and the stroke volume change
Cardiac index (CI)	2.5 to 3–5 L/min/m² in adults	The cardiac output expressed in relationship to the size of the individual	CI is used often in clinical practice because it gives a better indication of how efficiently the heart is working	If a person is small and has a CI of 3 L/min, this would indicate a better heart contraction efficiency than someone who is large and has a CI of 3 L/min
Central venous pressure (CVP) (Hemodynamic value)	0–8 mm Hg	Pressure exerted by the blood in one of the deep large veins such as the internal jugular or subclavian	May be found in the cardiac patient's medical chart if a right heart catheterization has been performed	
Ejection fraction (EF)[58]	55%–75%	The ratio between the SV and the preload; measures the ability of the heart to contract	Will be found in the patient's medical chart	The higher the percentage, the better the heart is contracting
Heart rate (HR)	60–100 bpm	Number of times the heart beats each minute	Should be checked often for the patient with a cardiac pathology during PT intervention	Lower than 60 bpm = bradycardia; higher than 100 bpm = tachycardia
Pulmonary artery pressure (PA) (hemodynamic value)	Systolic = 20–25 mm Hg; diastolic = 6–12 mm Hg	Pressure exerted by the blood in the pulmonary artery	May be found in the cardiac patient's medical chart if a right heart catheterization has been performed (Note the higher values of arterial versus venous pressures)	

Table 3.3 **Normal Adult Heart Values—cont'd**

CARDIAC TERM	NORMAL VALUES	WHAT IT MEASURES	OF INTEREST	CHANGES
Pulmonary capillary wedge pressure (PCWP) (hemodynamic value)	6–12 mm Hg	In effect, measures the pressure in the left ventricle at the end of the diastole and indicates the health of the left ventricle	May be found in the cardiac patient's medical chart if a right heart catheterization has been performed	
Stroke volume (SV)	0.5–1 L per heartbeat	The amount of blood pumped from the heart in one contraction	Depends on preload (amount of blood in ventricles after diastole), the contraction of the ventricles, and afterload (the amount the left ventricle has to contract to force blood into the aorta)	SV increases with greater heart contraction and greater preload values; SV decreases if afterload increases

RPP into consideration when developing an exercise protocol for the patient with a cardiac condition or deconditioning. PTAs need to monitor the RPP so that they can tell if the patient is responding well to treatment. If the RPP goes up rather than down, there may be a problem that requires referral back to the PT for reevaluation. Subjective data should be documented carefully, including any deviations from the usual between the last PT intervention session and the current one and any symptoms during or immediately after treatment. Perceived rate of exertion (PRE) is a subjective monitoring technique used in cardiac rehabilitation when patients become familiar enough with their response to exercise to be able to determine a safe level of intensity of activity. The PRE is based on a **Rating of Perceived Exertion (RPE)** developed by Borg (see Table 3-4). Borg's RPE scale runs from 6 to 20, defining 6 as no exertion at all and 20 as maximal exertion. Using this scale, or a similar one, patients can give an indication of their perceived exertion during different activity levels. The monitoring of the perceived rate of exertion by the PTA is helpful because the PRE is often indicative of the patient's status. Exercise programs need to be adapted in accordance with the perceived rate of exertion as well as with objective data. Objective data such as vital signs and any observed signs exhibited by the patient should be documented, as well as the PT intervention provided and the patient's response to the intervention. In addition, any precautions taken or discussions with the PT regarding suspicious signs or symptoms should be documented in the patient chart.

General Signs and Symptoms of Cardiac Disease

The general signs and symptoms of cardiac diseases include atrial fibrillation, cyanosis, dyspnea, edema, fatigue,

Table 3.4 **The Borg Rate of Perceived Exertion Scale**

6	No exertion at all
7	
8	Extremely light
9	Very light
10	
11	Light
12	
13	Somewhat hard
14	
15	Hard (heavy)
16	
17	Very hard
18	
19	Extremely hard
20	Maximal exertion

heart block, intermittent claudication, pain, palpitations, PVCs, reduced ejection fraction, syncope, and ventricular fibrillation. All of these are explained in this section.

ATRIAL FIBRILLATION

Atrial fibrillation is an abnormal, involuntary contraction of the atria muscle, which causes an arrhythmia of the heart and a reduction of contraction of the ventricles. The irregularity is caused by too many stimuli to the atrium, which causes an involuntary, rapid quivering of the atrial myocardium, resulting in ineffective pumping of blood into the ventricles. The atrial myocardium goes into a state of trembling and is unable to function. Atrial fibrillation is detected through an ECG. The immediate treatment for atrial fibrillation is the use of anti-arrhythmic drugs. Digitalis is then used on a regular basis to slow down the atrial contractions and thus restore them to functional contraction. Many cardiac diseases cause atrial fibrillation, including hypertension, rheumatic heart disease, and cardiomyopathy, and all conditions can result in serious problems, such as cardiac failure. Other causes of atrial fibrillation include thyrotoxicosis, and those people who are in withdrawal from overuse of alcohol. If the PTA suspects that the patient is in atrial fibrillation, the supervising PT should be consulted immediately. In severe cases, when the patient becomes unconscious, cardiopulmonary resuscitation (CPR) may be required and the emergency medical system activated. PTAs are rarely alone with acute cardiac patients. In the inpatient or outpatient setting instances of atrial fibrillation may occur and the PTA needs to be familiar with the procedure for activating the emergency medical system in that particular work setting.

CYANOSIS

Cyanosis is either central or peripheral. Central cyanosis occurs more with pulmonary diseases in which there is an oxygen saturation level of less than 80%, meaning there is poor oxygen uptake by the tissues (see Chapter 4). In central cyanosis the lips, tongue, ears, and other mucous membranes have a bluish tinge. Peripheral cyanosis is associated more with cardiac diseases in which there is low cardiac output. Indications of peripheral cyanosis include blueness in the fingertips, nail beds, toes, and the nose. When the area is warmed, these areas of peripheral cyanosis tend to resolve, whereas the central cyanosis does not resolve unless the oxygen perfusion rate is increased through the use of oxygen therapy. The implications for the PTA of central cyanosis in a patient are limited exercise tolerance. A pulse oximeter should be used during treatment sessions to ensure adequate oxygenation of the tissues during activity. Levels should be above 95% unless otherwise specified by the physician. Monitoring of the oxygen perfusion level and the use of supplemental oxygen makes the treatment of the patient with cyanosis more complex for the PTA. In many settings, the PTA would not be designated to treat such patients alone.

DYSPNEA

Dyspnea (shortness of breath), particularly dyspnea on exertion (DOE), is often associated with heart conditions but is also exhibited with allergic responses such as asthma (see Chapter 4) and in people who are obese or in poor physical condition. If dyspnea symptoms are severe or occur at rest, patients should be referred to a physician, regardless of whether they happen to be a cardiac patient. Many kinds of dyspnea are due to pulmonary problems, and these are discussed in Chapter 4. The PTA needs to carefully observe the patient for signs of dyspnea during

PT interventions and require periods of rest if necessary. Consultation with the PT should be performed if there is any doubt about the dyspnea. Particular attention should be given to those patients who suddenly begin having dyspnea symptoms who have never exhibited them before.

EDEMA

Edema is a side effect of cardiac disease. Edema is usually manifested as swelling of the hands, feet, ankles, and abdomen and is often accompanied by shortness of breath, dyspnea, and fatigue. If all these symptoms occur together, there is a high probability of a cardiac disease such as congestive heart failure (CHF), and patients will probably be placed on an ECG during their exercise regimen. The PTA may be involved with the treatment of these patients as part of the cardiac rehabilitation team.

FATIGUE

Fatigue is a symptom that must be closely monitored in the patient with a cardiac condition. When the patient becomes fatigued during exercise, it can certainly be a result of weak muscles or some pulmonary problem, which is discussed in Chapter 4, but may also be part of the cardiac disease process. If the fatigue occurs with other symptoms previously described such as dyspnea, headache, chest pain, or arrhythmias, it is probably due to the cardiac condition, and the exercise or activity should be stopped immediately, the patient instructed to rest, and the PT consulted. The PTA is part of the cardiac rehabilitation team, and it is usual, and advisable, that there is a PT immediately available when working with these patients.

HEART BLOCK

Heart block occurs when the normal neurological impulses that stimulate the heart to contract are interrupted. A complete heart block occurs when the impulses do not reach the ventricles, causing the heart to "skip" a beat. The ventricles have the ability to contract on their own without the nerve impulses, but the beats are much slower at about 40 beats per minute (BPM), and this is not sufficient for the heart to pump the circulation. During a heart block episode, the person may become unconscious. Causes of this condition may be ischemic heart disease or a too-high dose of digitalis. Patients with this condition usually must have a cardiac pacemaker surgically inserted to regulate their heart rhythm. Three degrees of heart block are recognized: the complete or third-degree block just described, the second-degree block in which electrical impulses are occasionally obstructed, and the first-degree block in which electrical impulses are slowed but do not interfere with the heart contraction. In cases of patients who become unconscious, the PTA should contact the PT, nurse, or physician immediately, and initiate CPR and the emergency medical system when necessary.

INTERMITTENT CLAUDICATION

Intermittent claudication is a symptom of arterial disease that can be associated with cardiac conditions. This condition occurs most often as a result of disease in the popliteal artery and causes severe pain in the calf during walking activities, exercise, or prolonged standing. Rest alleviates the pain, but as the disease process progresses, the symptoms become worse and occur more frequently. The pain of intermittent claudication is due to insufficient blood supply to the muscles affected by the diseased artery. The iliac and femoral arteries may also be involved, affecting glutei, quadriceps, and anterior tibial muscles. The PTA may encounter this symptom with patients and needs to understand the mechanism involved. Certain exercises involving alternate elevation of the affected leg and lowering into a dependent position have been shown to offer some relief to patients. These are known as Buerger-Allen exercises and are thought to stimulate the development of collateral circulation in the legs (see Box 3-1).

Improvement is measured by a reduction in time for the skin to return to normal color after elevation and dependent positioning. The PTA should use a watch to measure the time for each section of the maneuver and note them in the chart.

PAIN

Pain in patients with cardiac conditions can be felt in referred areas such as the left shoulder as well as over the left and central chest areas and into the left neck and jaw. The heart is supplied by nerves from the fifth and sixth cervical spinal segments, and thus pain in the heart can be transferred to dermatomes (areas of skin supplied by a nerve root) supplied by the same nerve supply. The dermatome for C5 lies over the deltoid muscle. Conversely, there are several types of chest pain, which may have other causes. These include gallbladder disease and trigger point areas. Examples of types of pain experienced by those having a heart attack include sharp, shooting pain into the left shoulder, pain shooting into the neck and shoulder, pain in the neck and jaw, pain over the area of the heart, pain that feels like a band tightening around the chest, central chest pain, indigestion acid reflux–like pain, and other milder types of pain. In many cases, there may be no pain associated with a heart attack. Gallbladder disease can also mimic heart pain by causing central chest pain. Because the PTA is not expected to diagnose symptoms, any type of pain should be cause for concern. If in doubt about origins of pain in a patient with cardiac problems, the PTA should immediately consult the PT. Any change in pain distribution should be carefully documented and also reported to the PT.

PALPITATIONS

Palpitations are largely a lay term and difficult to describe. They are arrhythmias or deviations from the normal heart rhythm. A person may describe a pounding of the heart or a sudden awareness of the heart changing beat pattern. People are not normally aware of their heart beating, but when it beats more rapidly or more strongly, they may become acutely aware of these changes. Palpitations may occur with serious conditions such as coronary artery disease (CAD) or less serious ones such as mitral valve incompetence. They can occur as part of the normal physiological response to stress and after intake of caffeine. They can also occur due to use of certain medical or nonmedical drugs. If the PTA is in doubt regarding the complaint of palpitations by the patient, the PT should be consulted.

PREMATURE VENTRICULAR CONTRACTIONS

Arrhythmias are abnormalities in the rhythm of the heart caused by a ventricular lesion. They are potentially life threatening and require immediate attention from the physician. **Premature ventricular contraction (PVC)** is the most common arrhythmia and is characterized on the ECG by a premature beat of the ventricle. PVCs are seen within the normal population after caffeine use, smoking, anxiety, or drinking alcohol. PVCs are also evident on ECG after a myocardial infarction (MI) or in other cardiac conditions that cause ischemia of heart tissue, such as CAD or CHF. A reduced ST segment is seen on ECG after cardiac ischemia (see the section on ECG). Conversely, with an acute infarct of the heart, there is an elevated ST segment. If the ST segment remains elevated, it may indicate a ventricular aneurism. PTAs are unlikely to detect a PVC during PT interventions. An unusual sound may be detected on taking vital signs including pulse and

---

Box 3.1 **Routine for Buerger-Allen Exercises**

1. Elevate legs at 45° angle, with legs well supported, for 2 minutes or until blanching (paling) of the skin of affected leg(s) occurs.
2. Sit on edge of bed with legs down (dependent position) for 3 minutes or until skin turns bright red.
3. Lie down with legs in horizontal position until skin returns to normal color, approximately 5 minutes.
4. Repeat the first three steps five times each session.
5. Repeat the entire routine three times per day.

blood pressure, in which case the PT should be consulted. Many patients are aware that they have PVCs and may be under the supervision of a physician.

REDUCED EJECTION FRACTION

In pathologies where cardiac muscle function is affected, there is a reduction in the ability of the heart to pump blood to the body. The reduction in effectiveness of the left ventricle reduces the ejection fraction of the heart and consequently reduces the ability of the patient to perform aerobic activities. Pathologies in which a reduced ejection fraction may be a significant factor include CHF, hypertension, CAD, and MI. When treating patients with a reduced ejection fraction (see Table 3-3), the PTA needs to adapt the pace of the exercise and activity program to suit the needs of the patient. The patient should be carefully monitored for signs of fatigue and dyspnea and allowed to rest as frequently as necessary. Increasing activity endurance in these patients may be difficult because of the reduced functional pumping ability of the heart.

SYNCOPE

Syncope is caused by reduction of oxygen to the brain that results in feelings of light-headedness or episodes of fainting. When it is caused by a cardiac condition such as an arrhythmia or CAD, it is called cardiac syncope. Headaches are another common symptom caused by the lack of blood circulation to the brain in syncope. If the PTA is working with a patient who faints or experiences periods of light-headedness or headaches, the PT, nurse, or physician should be alerted immediately. In many cases, the symptom is transitory, but the patient should be referred to a physician for diagnosis. The usual recommendation for patient safety is that the treatment session be discontinued for that day and the patient be required to see the physician before returning for further PT intervention. All such incidents should be recorded in the patient treatment note, and if the patient fell as a result of fainting, an incident report should be completed following the medical facility guidelines.

VENTRICULAR FIBRILLATION

Ventricular fibrillation is serious and leads to complete loss of muscle contractions in the heart. This phenomenon occurs in MI and, if not treated immediately, will result in death. The heart muscle is kick-started by use of a defibrillation machine, which stops the heart and starts it again. This electrical shock given to the heart aims to override the abnormal rhythm, stop the heartbeat, and stimulate a return to the normal rhythm. All medical personnel including PTAs are required to be educated in the administration of CPR and the defibrillator machine. The PTA should initiate the emergency medical system in cases when the heart stops and perform CPR in the interim, using the defibrillator machine if needed. Newer defibrillators are equipped with automatic sensors that give instructions for use and detect whether defibrillation is actually required, so there is a minimal possibility of administering an electric shock to someone who does not need one.

Diagnostic Tests Performed for Cardiac Patients

This section describes some of the most commonly used tests that are performed on people with suspected cardiac conditions.

CARDIAC CATHETERIZATION AND ANGIOGRAPHY

Cardiac catheterization, also known as cardiac angiography, is an invasive (entering the body) procedure performed to determine a diagnosis for patients with suspected cardiac pathologies. Cardiac catheterization can show how severe the coronary artery disease (CAD) is and whether there is valve disease, an aneurysm, myocardial infarction, or pericardial disease. The procedure is performed in a special laboratory or radiology department. A catheter is inserted through the brachial or femoral artery and passed into the vessels of the heart. A contrast fluid is used that can be seen on special x-ray equipment and narrowing of blood vessels can be observed.

ECHOCARDIOGRAPHY

This is performed using a diagnostic ultrasound machine (not the type used in PT). Echocardiography is a noninvasive procedure meaning it does not put anything into the body. A reading is taken of the heart and coronary blood vessels by bouncing sound waves off the heart at different angles and recording it on a screen, the pictures can then be printed out. Echocardiography can detect many things including the size of the heart, valve function, the thickness of the walls of the heart, coronary artery disease (CAD), and ischemia of the heart muscle.

ELECTROCARDIOGRAM

An ECG is a recording of the heart rhythm on paper or computer taken by placing electrodes that measure electrical potentials in the heart. A standard ECG uses 12 leads: six on the chest and six on the limbs. The ECG measures heart rhythm and rate and can indicate hypertrophy and infarction of heart muscle. Graph paper used in an ECG has 1-mm^2 divisions, and by setting the speed of the paper feed, the heart rate can be calculated. The PTA does not need to know detailed facts about reading an ECG, but several key terms should be understood. Cardiac muscle has certain characteristics different from other muscle. Electrical impulses are given off by heart muscle without the input of a nerve. An impulse set off at the SA node is rapidly spread to other muscle cells because heart muscle is a good conductor of electrical impulses. When the heart muscle contracts, it is called depolarization and shows up on the ECG graph as an upward curve. As the wave of contraction spreads from the SA node to the left atrium, the atrial depolarization is seen on the ECG as the "P" wave. The impulse spreads to the AV node, which makes the impulse pause for one tenth of a second to allow the atria to push blood into the ventricles. This is seen on the graph as a straight line after the P wave and is called the atrial kick. The P wave and the line are called the P-R segment. The impulses then pass into the ventricles, and this ventricular contraction can be seen on the graph as the **QRS complex.** The QRS complex is different depending on which electrode is being read. After this, there is a pause known as the ST segment, which is another flat line on the graph. During this flat line, the ventricle is repolarizing and preparing for another contraction. The T wave follows the ST segment and represents the repolarization of the ventricles (see Table 3-5).

Certain characteristics should be constant on the ECG graph. A P wave is normally a rounded, upward curve and is present before each QRS complex. The ST segment should always follow the QRS complex, and the T wave comes last. The ST segment and the P-R interval should be on the same horizontal line on the graph paper. In a normal sinus rhythm, the sequence of events of one cycle depicted on the graph, the Q-T interval between the start of the QRS complex and the end of the T wave, is 0.32 to 0.40 seconds. The P-R interval is 0.12 to 0.20 seconds. All QRS complexes are the same and last from 0.04 to 0.10 seconds and heart rate is 60 to 100 beats per minute (see Fig. 3-3).

Some basic differences for common heart abnormalities are depicted in changes in these characteristics of the normal sinus rhythm. **Sinus tachycardia** is demonstrated as a heart rate of more than 100 beats per minute and **sinus bradycardia** as less than 60 bpm.[5, 6] In more serious problems, there are changes in the wave patterns or irregular patterns. In atrial flutter, the P wave is affected, giving the appearance on the graph of several spikes. In atrial fibrillation, there are no P waves. This makes sense because atrial contraction forms the P wave, and when the atria are in fibrillation, they do not contract. In heart blocks, the P-R interval is longer than normal. In ventricular arrhythmias, patterns called premature ventricular complexes or contractions (PVCs) are found. PVCs are caused by ectopic areas of depolarization other than the SA or AV nodes and create a widened QRS wave on the graph. The PVCs can be frequent, in groups of a few at a time, or isolated incidences. In ventricular fibrillation, the graph becomes a series of irregular spikes with no real normal pattern. To gain more information on ECG readings, consult a cardiopulmonary text and visit Stephen Gerred and Dean Jenkin's ECG library at http://www.ecglibrary.com [7]

HOLTER MONITORING

Holter monitoring is usually performed for 24 hours but sometimes longer. A Holter monitor is an ECG with leads attached to a portable unit that continuously monitors heart rhythm to diagnose certain problems, such as shortness of breath, arrhythmias, and dizziness. Patients wear the monitor while performing regular daily activities and may have a tape recorder so that they can report those activities. The results of the graph are transferred to a readable report, which is analyzed and used to determine whether the patient is able to continue activity. The PT interprets ECG readings to develop a suitable level of exercise program for the patient. The PTA is not expected to be able to read the printed graph.

LABORATORY STUDIES (BLOOD AND URINE)

Certain enzymes are released into the blood when myocardial necrosis occurs after an MI. The presence of these enzymes in the blood can help with diagnosis. Some of these enzymes are creatine phosphokinase (CPK), lactic dehydrogenase (LDH), and aspartate aminotransferase (AST). The PTA should be able to recognize the names of these enzymes that may be found in the medical chart.

A **complete blood count (CBC)** indicates several things to the physician. The hemoglobin (Hgb) levels have a bearing on the amount of oxygen transported around the body. Levels of hemoglobin in a normal healthy male are 14 to 18 grams per 100 mL of blood. The level for females is slightly lower. If the Hgb level is low, the heart must

Table 3.5 **Characteristics of Electrocardiogram Graph With Associated Activity**

CHARACTERISTIC	CAUSE
P wave	Depolarization (contraction) of atria
Atrial kick	Atria push blood into ventricles
P-R interval	Start of P wave to start of QRS complex
QRS complex	Depolarization of ventricles
ST segment	Ventricles prepare to repolarize
T wave	Ventricles repolarize
Premature ventricular complexes	Ectopic (not SA or AV node) areas of depolarization in ventricles

work harder to increase cardiac output so that enough hemoglobin will reach areas of the body to provide oxygen transfer. The hematocrit (HCT) measures the percentage of cells in the blood and thus the viscosity (thickness) of the blood. If the HCT level is high, it could slow down the rate of flow of blood because of the high viscosity. The range of normal hematocrit levels is 40% to 54% in males and 37% to 47% in females. If HCT levels are high, there is a higher risk for clot formation because of the slower speed of the blood flowing through the vessels. In such a case, anticoagulant therapy may be prescribed by the physician, with regular checks of HCT levels to ensure they remain within normal ranges. Normal white blood cell count (WBCC) is 6,000 to 8,000 per cubic millimeter of blood. A high white blood cell count (WBCC) of more than 10,000 per microliter is called leukocytosis and indicates the presence of infection in the body. A lowered level of white blood cells is called leukopenia.

Electrolyte levels in the blood are monitored for the patient with cardiac problems. Sodium (Na+), potassium (K+), and carbon dioxide (CO_2) are the most important. If these levels are not within normal range, they can cause serious problems. High potassium levels can cause reduction in heart muscle contraction, and high levels can produce heart arrhythmias. Increases in blood lipid levels are a risk factor for CAD. Ratios of high density lipoproteins (HDL) and low density lipoproteins (LDL) are important, with risk increasing as the ratio of total cholesterol to HDL increases, and also as the level of LDL ("bad" cholesterol) increases above 160 mg/dL (milligrams per deciliter) or above 130 mg/dL for those people with more than two known risk factors for heart and stroke problems.[8] According to the American Heart Association, levels of HDL should be above 40 mg/100 mL.[9] Another useful test measures the rate of clotting of the blood, which is determined by the prothrombin time. This measures the time it takes for the blood to clot. Blood urea nitrogen (BUN) and creatinine tests are also performed. Normal BUN levels are from 8 to 18 mg/dL per deciliter of blood.[10] If this level is high, it can indicate heart or kidney failure. Blood creatinine levels should be below 1.5 mg/dL of blood. The ratio of these two tests indicates a problem if the BUN:creatinine ratio is over 15.

POSITRON EMISSION TOMOGRAPHY

Positron emission tomography (PET) scan is a nuclear technique that requires special equipment. The PET scan measures blood flow in the heart and other types of metabolism. This procedure is expensive and used for evaluation of the heart without the need for stress testing. Heart rate is increased by use of medications. A PET may be used in cases in which exercise stress testing is not possible as a result of patient inactivity levels or immediately after an MI.

STRESS TEST

The stress test is a type of exercise testing used to evaluate patients with both cardiac and respiratory problems. A stress test may be given to patients if they are having chest pain; are known to have CAD, arrhythmias, or hypertension; or as a general assessment before giving an exercise program. The test is usually performed under the direction of a physician with emergency facilities on hand in case the patient has an MI during the test. The physician determines what level of heart rate the patient should obtain during the test, usually 70% or 75% of predicted maximal heart rate (PMHR), and electrodes are placed on the chest to monitor the heart rate through a machine that can print a diagram of the heart rhythm. Such tests are usually performed with the patient on a treadmill or bicycle. However, a chemically induced stress test may be performed on those patients who are unable to tolerate moderate levels of exercise. A low-level stress test may be performed by the physical therapist on cardiac rehabilitation patients. The risks involved with this test preclude the PTA from performing these procedures. Constant evaluation is required for the cardiac patient that is beyond the scope of practice of the PTA. The PTA may, however, be involved as part of the cardiac rehabilitation team. Details of stress testing are beyond the scope of this book.

Why Does the Physical Therapist Assistant Need to Know About Disorders and Pathological Conditions of the Heart?

Because the normal physiological response of the heart is complex, the response is even more complex with a heart that is diseased. In many cases, the PTA will be part of the team working with people with heart conditions. Understanding the basic pathology of cardiovascular diseases is essential to be able to work with patients with such conditions safely and effectively. The importance of a timely response with patients with cardiac pathologies and the referral back to the supervising PT with any suspected problems is essential.

Disorders and Pathological Conditions of the Heart

Pathological conditions of the heart refer to those conditions associated with the functioning—or malfunctioning—of the heart. Many of these diseases cause systemic effects on the body, as described in this section.

Angina Pectoris

Angina is acute ischemic chest pain. In 2006, the prevalence of cases of angina pectoris in the United States was 10.2 million, and only 20% of cases of MI occurred in people with a prior history of angina pectoris.[11]

Etiology. Angina pectoris is chest pain caused by ischemia to myocardium and is related to arteriosclerotic heart disease.

Signs and Symptoms. The pain of angina pectoris tends to be severe and sharp in nature. Angina pectoris is of sudden onset and often occurs as a result of overexertion, emotional stress, or exposure to extremes of temperature or high humidity. Because the pain is from the heart, it is felt either in the upper chest area or as referred pain in the neck, shoulder, or left arm. Angina is caused by transient ischemia of myocardial tissue.

Prognosis. People may live for many years with angina pectoris. If the condition becomes severe, heart bypass surgery may be performed. In some cases, angina can lead to a heart attack, but it is not usually a direct cause of death. Medical monitoring of the condition is essential.

Medical Intervention. Rest or the use of a vasodilator such as nitroglycerin relieves angina pain. The nitroglycerin is dissolved under the tongue and acts almost instantaneously to relieve pain. In some people, the nitroglycerin is administered through an adhesive patch on the skin that provides a slow-acting, continuous dose through the skin. If a patient takes the oral medicine and one pill does not work, another one is taken after about 3 minutes. A general rule is that if the pain is not relieved with a third pill, the patient needs to seek medical help immediately.[12] The PT and PTA are not allowed to administer drugs, but if patients know they have angina, they will usually carry nitroglycerin with them at all times. When they have an angina attack, they will know to administer a pill immediately. The PTA should be aware of a patient having a history of angina because many of those having PT for reasons other than heart disorders may have angina.

Nitroglycerin needs to be kept in a tightly closed glass container because exposure to the air degrades the medicine. Severe cases of angina pectoris may require coronary bypass surgery or percutaneous transluminal coronary artery angioplasty, which are described later in the chapter.

Physical Therapy Intervention. Physical therapy is not usually indicated for patients with angina pectoris, but because many patients have this condition, it may be a comorbid diagnosis for other disorders. PTAs should make sure they know the medical background of the patients with whom they are working so that they know how to respond if there is a change in status during PT intervention. Of note is that nitroglycerin pills cause quite severe headaches in many patients, and physical therapy may not be able to continue after an angina attack. If the patient complains of chest pain during PT intervention, the PTA should have the person rest immediately and seek help from the supervising PT or the patient's nurse or physician. The PTA should note onset of pain during treatment in the patient's chart, together with the response to the complaint indicating the follow-up performed to ensure patient safety.

Aortic Atherosclerosis

Aortic atherosclerosis is a "silent" disease. Plaque builds up in the aorta with rarely any outward signs or symptoms.

Etiology. The etiology and risk factors for aortic atherosclerosis are the same as those for other forms of the disease; however, aortic aneurysms have a familial tendency, and it is advisable for people with a family history of the problem to be checked medically. Aortic atherosclerosis is found mostly in older men. After age 50, most people have some degree of atherosclerosis in the aorta.

Signs and Symptoms. Frequently no symptoms are associated with this problem. In the mild form of aortic atherosclerosis, there are fatty deposits with some fibrotic plaques and minimal atheromas. Progression of the disease, however, may cause almost complete obliteration of the aorta due to massive deposition of atheromas. A danger also exists that emboli will form from the atherosclerotic aorta. The aorta becomes rigid with calcification (aortic calcification), rough on its interior, and has a very small lumen. At this stage, the aorta becomes unable to adjust to the normal changes in the cardiac cycle and, together with the small lumen of the aorta, causes hypertension. Frequently an aneurysm develops in the aorta due to the pressure of blood from the heart. The most common site for an aortic aneurysm is in the abdominal aorta.

Prognosis. As noted earlier, these aneurysms are often termed "silent" because there are no symptoms involved. Sometimes they may be discovered when the person undergoes a medical examination, and in such a case, they be surgically repaired. More often, however, the person is unaware of the existence of the aneurysm, and it can spontaneously rupture, usually causing death.

Medical Intervention. Medical intervention follows the same path as previously described for atherosclerosis. Surgical repair of aortic aneurysm may be performed if the condition is discovered.

Physical Therapy Intervention. No physical therapy is provided directly for this condition; however, the presence of an aortic aneurysm is a contraindication for heavy weight-lifting exercises that increase the pressure on the aorta. The problem is that neither the patient nor the therapist is usually aware that there is an aneurysm. An exercise program may be instituted after surgical repair of aneurysms for return of the patient to normal activity levels.

Atherosclerosis and Arteriosclerosis

Atherosclerosis literally means hardening of the arteries. **Arteriosclerosis** is hardening of the walls of the smaller arterial vessels, called arterioles, found in the extremities of the limbs and in body organs. When located in the arteriole walls, this hardening causes an increased resistance to the flow of blood within the vessels and changes blood pressure. In both cases, it is the narrowing and thickening of the walls of the arteries/arterioles that causes a reduction of the lumen (the channel through the vessel). The thickening of the vessel walls is accompanied by loss of elasticity, flexibility, and contractility. This is largely due to deposition of fatty, cholesterol plaques on the interior wall of the artery (see Fig. 3-9).

Atherosclerosis is common throughout the Western world and causes most of the deaths from MI and ischemic heart disease. Incidence of the disease in Asia, Africa, and South America, is much less than in the West. The United States has a 6 times higher rate of death from ischemic heart disease than Japan. More than 8 million Americans, approximately 12% to 20% of the population over 65, have peripheral arterial disease, which is an indicator for atherosclerosis. This is probably a low estimate for the numbers of people in the United States with atherosclerosis. The over-40 age group seems to be more prone to the problem, with an increased risk with age. Men are more prone to the disease until age 70, when the risk levels out equally between men and women.[13]

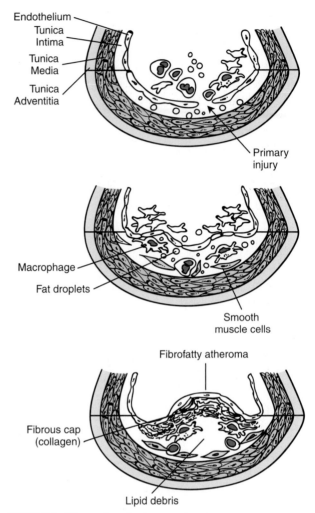

FIGURE 3.9 Atherosclerosis of a vessel

Etiology. Atherosclerosis is caused by changes in the walls of the arteries. Such changes can be due to high blood pressure over a prolonged period of time, diabetes, and cigarette smoking.[14] Many of the causes of atherosclerosis can be controlled by smoking cessation, reducing intake of cholesterol in the diet, reducing intake of saturated fats found in animal products, and keeping hypertension under control. Risk factors for the disease include age, sex, and heredity, as well as lifestyle (see Table 3-6). Strong evidence of a family tendency to

Table 3.6 **Risk Factors, Location, and Associated Problems of Atherosclerosis**

RISK FACTORS	LOCATION	ASSOCIATED PROBLEMS
Smoking Age Sex (men more than women under age 70)	Coronary arteries (heart)	Congestive Heart Failure Angina pectoris Myocardial infarction Cardiac aneurysm/rupture
Heredity Obesity	Cerebral arteries (brain)	Cardiovascular disease Cardiovascular Accident
Diabetes mellitus (uncontrolled) Hypertension (uncontrolled)	Aorta	Renal artery atherosclerosis Aortic aneurysm Hypertension
Hypercholesteremia/hyperlipidemia Hypothyroidism	Peripheral arteries (peripheral vascular disease) Renal arteries (kidney) Intestinal arteries	Intermittent claudication Gangrene (wet and dry) Arterial insufficiency ulcers End-stage renal failure Small and large intestine ischemia

develop the problem exists, with high levels of cholesterol or hypercholesterolemia running in families.[15] Sometimes the risk level for developing atherosclerosis is combined with a hereditary tendency for developing diabetes, hypertension, and hypothyroidism (underactive thyroid). Acquired risk factors are those that involve lifestyle choices. Smoking is known to be a major factor in development of the condition. The plaques in atherosclerotic medium and large arteries consist of lipids (fats) with high levels of cholesterol and cholesteryl esters. A relationship has been determined between the level of blood cholesterol and the development of cardiovascular disease.[16] High levels of LDL increase the risk of plaque formation, whereas high levels of HDL seem to reduce the risk.[17] HDL participates in transport of cholesterol to the liver for excretion. Hypertension, diabetes mellitus, familial hypercholesterolemia, and hypothyroidism all increase the risk for the disease. Minor factors contributing to the risk for the disease include lack of exercise, obesity, and use of oral contraceptives. Multiple risk factors increase the likelihood for developing the disease, but even those with no risk factors may develop it. All that is currently known is that people can reduce their risk by reducing acquired risk factors.

Because of the deposition of plaques, the arteries become narrowed, hardened, and inflexible with less ability to contract and relax in response to needs of the circulatory system. The plaques (atheromas) project into the lumen of the artery causing partial or total obstruction. The mechanism for development of the disease is complex and not fully understood. An inflammatory process may be set off by an injury to the inner wall (endothelium) of the artery caused by toxins, cigarette smoke, viruses, hypoxia (too little oxygen), turbulent blood flow, high levels of cholesterol in the blood, or several of these acting together. The inflammation causes increased permeability of the endothelium of the vessel and also causes monocytes to stick to the walls. Macrophages multiply at the site, and platelets build up. Smooth muscle cells change into foam cells that have a fatty consistency. These foam cells absorb cholesterol and eventually form the plaques that narrow the lumen of the arteries. The macrophages absorb the lipid contents of the dead smooth muscle cells and then also turn into foam cells. The repair of the damage to the endothelium forms scarring, which leads to the hardening aspect of the disease. The walls of the artery actually become calcified when released lipids absorb calcium salts, and these are deposited in the atheromas and the fibrous scar tissue.

In later stages of the disease, thrombosis of the atheromas may occur, with subsequent emboli in which a section of the atheroma breaks off and travels through the arterial system. If such an embolus blocks an essential artery to the heart, lung, or brain, it can cause death.

Atherosclerosis may be found in any artery but is more prevalent in several major areas of the body, including the vessels of the heart and brain, and in the aorta and vessels of the extremities. When the disease is located in the coronary arteries that supply nutrients to the heart muscle, it is called coronary atherosclerosis, CHD, or CAD. Refer to the section on ischemic heart disease. Clinical manifestations of CHD include congestive heart failure, angina pectoris, and MI, all previously described.

Signs and Symptoms. No outward signs and symptoms may occur with this disease. The first signs of the condition may be when a deep venous thrombosis occurs, perhaps causing pain in the limb. Another sign is of a cerebrovascular accident in which a clot becomes lodged in the vessels of the brain. A thrombus may also lodge in the blood vessels of the lungs.

Prognosis. The prognosis of atherosclerosis depends on many factors. If the sclerosis is situated in arteries that supply major organs such as the brain, heart, and lungs, there is the potential for a clot to form and interrupt blood supply to these organs, causing ischemia, severe injury, or death. If diagnosed early, medical and surgical procedures can be performed to improve the prognosis.

Medical Intervention. Physicians often prescribe use of a daily low dose of aspirin to reduce the clotting properties of blood for patients with arteriosclerosis. The American Heart Association recommends use of aspirin to help prevent or treat MI and for those people at high risk of developing cardiac conditions, such as those with arteriosclerosis.[18]

Surgical intervention may be required for severe cases of atherosclerosis. If the carotid arteries are affected, causing reduced blood flow to the brain, a carotid **endarterectomy** may be performed. In this procedure, a section of the artery is replaced by a vessel removed from the leg, such as the saphenous vein, and a stent may be inserted to keep the vessel patent (open). A similar procedure can be used for other arteries affected by atherosclerosis. Another procedure is a bypass, in which the blocked artery is bypassed by grafting of a disease free vessel to either side of the blockage. These procedures are performed for the coronary arteries that supply blood to the heart tissue and also in the lower extremities, such as in a femoral artery bypass. In such cases, veins from the patient's body are used to replace, or bypass, the diseased artery.

Physical Therapy Intervention. No physical therapy is indicated for atherosclerosis or arteriosclerosis. However, many patients who receive physical therapy services will have this condition, either diagnosed or undiagnosed. The PTA needs to understand the disease process to recognize any complications that may occur while treating patients such as clot formation.

Cardiac Arrest and Myocardial Infarction

Cardiac arrest is the sudden stopping of the heart. The estimated incidence of MI is 565,000 new cases and 300,000 repeat attacks in a year.[19]

Etiology. Cardiac arrest can be the result of various factors, including a MI, a loss of blood to the heart secondary to a systemic shock or injury causing massive loss of blood, or some traumatic event such as electric shock or drowning. Predisposition to MI includes factors such as heredity, age, obesity, smoking, hypertension, diabetes mellitus, sedentary lifestyle, and high cholesterol and triglyceride levels.

Signs and Symptoms. The main area of the heart involved in a MI is the left ventricle. Some signs and symptoms may indicate an impending MI, but in many cases, there are no warning signs. In some cases, there will be signs such as dyspnea, angina, or tachycardia. In most cases, the onset is sudden, with symptoms of tachycardia or bradycardia, shut down of the respiratory system with no breathing observable, possible pain in the chest and/or neck, and left arm described as "crushing," sweating, pallor, nausea, rapid pulse, and loss of consciousness. Many MI incidents are not accompanied by pain and are termed silent myocardial infarction.

Prognosis. There are various possible outcomes of MI. Some patients recover with minimal to moderate problems, whereas others die. In 2003, the average age of onset for a MI was 65.8 years for men and 70.4 years for women.[20] According to the figures published by the American Heart Association, 25% of men and 38% of women will die within 1 year of having an MI, and 50% of those who died due to heart disease had no prior warning of a heart condition.[21] Death is caused by several factors, including rupture of the infarcted (necrotic) area of the heart, ventricular fibrillation (previously described), backup of blood in the peripheral or pulmonary venous circulation, and cardiac shock.

Medical Intervention. CPR is necessary for the patient to breathe, and compression over the heart is necessary to stimulate the circulation mechanically and maintain vital systems until an emergency medical services (EMS) team is available. The EMS team, as described earlier in the chapter, may perform defibrillation. Speed of reaction is essential because irreversible brain damage occurs after the first 3 minutes. All health care personnel are required to be trained in CPR to respond to such incidents. The PTA should remember that it is not always possible to save the life of the patient. CPR provided quickly merely increases the chances of survival for the patient. Further treatment for MI includes rest, oxygen, anticoagulants such as aspirin and warfarin, pain medications, thrombolytic agents (dissolve the thrombus/clot), and a progressive exercise and activity rehabilitation program. Medical improvements in the treatment of MI have helped to reduce the mortality rate in this disease. The key to survival, as with many pathologies, is speed of treatment.

When there is only a small area of ischemia, the heart recovers more rapidly. A temporary loss of function of the affected heart muscle may occur due to reduced circulation, but this recovers. When a large area of heart muscle is affected, there are several problems. The central area of ischemic tissue becomes necrotic almost immediately within the first few hours after MI. The area surrounding the MI is nonfunctional. Further away from the site of the MI, the muscle contracts very weakly because of the effects of ischemia. Healing of heart tissue is similar to that of skin. The central area of ischemic tissue dies with enlargement of the necrotic area over the next few days. Collateral circulation develops to supply the area of heart muscle around the necrotic area, and by 3 weeks after MI, the area around the infarction is either functional or has died. The dead muscle tissue is replaced by fibrous scar tissue, which will eventually contract in size over a period of about 1 year, and the rest of the heart hypertrophies to make up for the lost tissue function. The heart recovers either fully or partially. Complications that can occur after a MI include cardiac shock, heart infarct rupture, venous system backup, and ventricular fibrillation.

Physical Therapy Intervention. PTAs may have to perform CPR in the clinical situation and should be familiar with the procedure. All health care professionals are required to pass the CPR certification for health care providers.

Cardiac Shock, Cardiac Failure, Heart Failure

Cardiac shock, cardiac failure, and heart failure are all terms used for the same condition. This condition occurs when some cardiac muscle is weak and some is not working at all. The heart is unable to pump blood to the extremities, the peripheral tissue (furthest away from the heart) becomes ischemic, and there is cardiac failure. A rule of thumb is that cardiac shock/failure will develop when more than 40% of the left ventricle becomes infarcted. Recent statistics based on data from 2003 show that diabetes is the greatest risk factor for cases of heart failure. The risk also increases with age, with the highest percentage of cases in the over 75 age group. According to the American Heart Association publication "Heart Disease and Stroke statistics: 2006 Update," deaths due to heart failure increased by 20.5% between 1993 and 2003. In addition, more than 57,000 deaths were attributed to cardiac failure in 2003.[22]

Cardiomyopathy

Cardiomyopathy is not one disease but a group of diseases affecting the heart, all of which are serious and can lead to the need for heart replacement surgery. When the heart muscle or myocardium is damaged, it may hypertrophy or dilate.

Etiology. The causes of cardiomyopathy include heart attacks; alcoholism; long-term, severe hypertension; systemic lupus erythematosus (SLE); celiac disease; end-stage renal disease; and viral infections.

Signs and Symptoms. In dilated cardiomyopathy, the heart muscle is thinner than usual. In hypertrophic cardiomyopathy, there is thickening of the myocardium, particularly in the left ventricle. In restrictive cardiomyopathy, the heart is unable to expand because of deposition of fibrous or amyloid tissue. Signs and symptoms include dyspnea, cough, heart palpitations (awareness of a loudly beating heart), lower extremity **dependent edema** or just edema (dependent edema occurs when the legs are hanging down), **ascites** (abdominal edema), angina chest pain, dizziness and light-headedness, low daily urine output, changes in mental alertness, appetite loss, and general deconditioning.

Prognosis. The outcome for this condition depends on the cause and severity of the disease and whether it responds to drug therapy. Cardiomyopathy is a serious, chronic problem and can get progressively worse. Serious complications of the disease include heart failure and arrhythmia.

Medical Intervention. Diagnosis of this condition is performed through the use of coronary angioplasty, echocardiogram, chest computed tomography and MRI scans, electrocardiogram, and blood tests such as a complete blood count, blood chemistry, and tests for the presence of cardiac enzymes. Medications used for treatment of the condition depend on the cause of the condition and may include the use of diuretics (to remove fluid), vasodilators, and beta blockers, which slow down heart rate. Recent developments include the use of a special biventricular pacemaker. This is a serious condition and may require heart replacement.

Physical Therapy Intervention. Physical therapy is not indicated in this condition unless physical deconditioning occurs and therapy can help to improve quality of life.

Congestive Heart Failure

In CHF the heart is no longer able to pump enough blood to meet the body's needs. Two types of CHF exist: right and left ventricular failure (see Table 3-7).

Etiology. Causes of CHF include a previous myocardial infarction, heart valve incompetence, hypertension over a prolonged period, or very low or very high heart rate.

Signs and Symptoms. Left heart failure results in pulmonary edema, and right ventricular failure results in peripheral edema evident in the lower legs. In right ventricular failure, there is a backup of the venous system, causing peripheral edema and ascites (abdominal edema). Blood stagnates and causes extra resistance for venous blood returning to the heart. Peripheral edema is obvious, with swelling of the legs, ankles, and feet, particularly at the end of the day. This kind of edema is called dependent edema because it is caused when the legs are in a dependent (hanging down) position. Venous congestion also causes enlargement of the liver, with resultant pain under the right lower ribs. Venous pressure in abdominal vessels causes edema in the abdomen. If there is failure of the left ventricle, there is acute pulmonary edema, which is life threatening. Pleural effusion occurs, causing dyspnea that is apparent on exertion in mild cases but present all the time in severe cases. Other results of the impaired heart function include functional breakdown of major organs due to lack of oxygen. Patients become readily fatigued and lethargic, become short of breath often with a cough, and develop renal failure with **oliguria** (reduced urine formation), which in turn causes sodium and water retention, leading to **anasarca** (general body edema).

Prognosis. Patients with CHF tend to develop progressive multiorgan and heart failure, often succumbing to pneumonia. Death is frequently a result of these complications.

Medical Intervention. A program that includes a balanced diet, exercise and activity interspersed with periods of adequate rest, and medications such as angiotensin converting enzyme (ACE) inhibitors, beta blockers, digitalis, vasodilators, and diuretics will likely be prescribed by the

Table 3.7 **Causes and Effects of Congestive Heart Failure**

TYPE OF HEART FAILURE	CAUSES	SYMPTOMS/EFFECTS
Right-sided	Right ventricle infarction Stenosis of pulmonary valve Pulmonary disease (e.g., cor pulmonale)	Dependent edema of lower extremities Edema of abdomen (ascites) and enlargement of spleen (splenomegaly) Pain in right lower ribs due to enlargement of liver Reduced cardiac output Flushing of face, distended neck veins, headaches
Left sided	Left ventricular infarction Stenosis of aortic valve Hypertension Hyperthyroidism	Reduced cardiac output Pulmonary edema Dyspnea Central cyanosis (lips, tongue, ears) Renal failure, oliguria (low urine output), increased water and sodium retention Cough and shortness of breath with rales
Both left and right sided		Fatigue and dyspnea Low tolerance to activity and cold due to decreased cardiac output Tachycardia

physician. Beta blockers and digitalis help to increase the pumping ability of the heart; ACE inhibitors and vasodilators dilate blood vessels and reduce the resistance to blood flow, thus reducing the pumping effort needed by the heart; and diuretics help the body to expel the excess water and salt built up in the body as edema.[23] In more severe cases, a heart transplant may be considered.

Physical Therapy Intervention. Physical therapy intervention may be indicated for increasing strength and endurance to activity, as well as for gait reeducation with a suitable assistive device.

GERIATRIC CONSIDERATIONS

Rehabilitation for the elderly patient with cardiovascular disease must proceed with caution. There may be comorbid conditions such as arthritis that slow down the rehabilitation process. Hospital stays may be longer and more home health physical therapy may be required before the patient is ready to attend outpatient cardiac rehabilitation. There may also be transport difficulties in getting to the rehabilitation facility, and social work may need to become involved to obtain transport. On the positive side, older patients tend to be more compliant with physical therapy and medical instructions.

Endocarditis

Endocarditis is a bacterial infection of the lining of the heart, including the heart valves, that can lead to cardiac failure. Endocarditis usually occurs in people who have had some prior damage to heart valves or who are born with heart-valve defects. The mitral valve is most commonly affected.

Etiology. The major bacteria causing this disease are *Staphylococcus* and *Streptococcus*. In cases of endocarditis found in people addicted to drugs, there may be the presence of mixed types of infective agents due to use of infected needles. In individuals who are immunosuppressed, such as those undergoing anticancer treatments, gram-negative bacteria or fungi may be responsible.

Signs and Symptoms. The outward characteristic signs and symptoms of endocarditis include fever, which may be of sudden or slow onset, coupled with weakness. Pathologically, bacteria attach themselves to the valves of the heart, eroding the surface of the valve and causing breakdown of the connective tissue. This roughened tissue then attracts fibrin and platelets deposited from the blood, and projections filled with bacteria grow from the valves. The valves become inflamed, perhaps ulcerated, and deformed in shape and stop performing their normal function. The projections that form on the valves can become broken off and start to circulate in the blood supply. These fragments contain bacteria and, when they circulate to other parts of the body, spread the infection further. Bacterial endocarditis may also result in splinter hemorrhages in the nails of the feet and hands (see Fig. 3-10).

Prognosis. As with many diseases, early diagnosis and medical treatment is the key to a successful outcome. Complications that can occur if the heart valves are damaged include atrial fibrillation, thrombus formation, stroke due to emboli traveling to the brain, and renal disease. Other organs such as the lungs may be damaged if an embolus causes ischemia.[24]

Medical Intervention. Treatment with antibiotics usually resolves the infection, but heart valves may remain deformed and in some cases must be replaced surgically. The use of preventive antibiotics before dental work and certain surgeries such as those to the intestinal, urinary, and respiratory tracts is recommended to reduce the risk of infection.

Physical Therapy Intervention. Physical therapy intervention is not usually indicated unless there is physical deconditioning associated with the disease process.

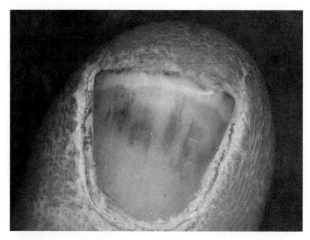

FIGURE 3.10 Bacterial endocarditis showing splinter hemorrhages in the nail. Reprinted with permission from Goldsmith, L. A., Lazarus, G. S., and Tharp, M. D. (1997). *Adult and pediatric dermatology. A color guide to diagnosis and treatment.* Philadelphia: F.A. Davis Company, p. 535.

Heart Infarct Rupture

An infarct in the heart is an area of necrotic tissue resulting from loss of blood supply, also termed a cardiac aneurysm. After a large MI, there is a danger that the area of infarct may rupture if it is large enough. During each heart contraction, the infarcted area is stretched, and if it is thin, it may eventually rupture. Blood then escapes into the pericardial cavity, causing external pressure on the heart and death of the patient due to loss of cardiac output.

Hypertension and Hypertensive Heart Disease

Hypertensive heart disease falls within the *Guide to Physical Therapist Practice* Preferred Practice Pattern 6 for cardiovascular and pulmonary conditions. If a patient has comorbid conditions, other practice patterns may also be involved.

Hypertension is a condition in which the normal blood pressure exceeds a certain amount. Hypertension does not take into account the raising of blood pressure through increased activity levels, which is considered normal raising of blood pressure that returns to normal at rest. Hypertension can be classified as mild, moderate, or severe and is either essential (primary) or secondary.

Etiology. Primary or essential hypertension occurs in approximately 90% of those with hypertension (Frownfelter, 2006, p. 521).[25] This means there is no known cause for the condition. Factors involved may include heredity, diet, and occupation or lifestyle issues. Some major causes of secondary hypertension, which is due to another disease process, include kidney disease, adrenal tumors (which require surgical removal), psychological factors, and some drugs such as painkillers and oral contraceptives.

Signs and Symptoms. According to Centers for Disease Control and Prevention (CDC) November 2006 data, adult hypertension exists when the systolic blood pressure is 140 mm Hg or higher or the diastolic blood pressure is 90 mm Hg or higher. The CDC also defines a state of prehypertension as a systolic blood pressure between 120 and 139 mm Hg or a diastolic pressure of between 80 and 89 mm Hg.

Prognosis. Hypertension is a risk factor for many other serious complications such as heart disease, atherosclerosis, angina pectoris, heart failure, eye damage and blindness, and kidney disease. Many people have hypertension and are unaware of the fact. The importance of regular medical checkups cannot be underestimated. Early diagnosis of hypertension can reduce most of the side effects of the condition.

Medical Intervention. The usual treatment for cases of essential hypertension is with diet modification and antihypertensive drugs. A rare form of essential hypertension is called malignant hypertension, also called labile hypertension, which indicates that it does not respond well to any form of intervention and can remain dangerously high. Malignant hypertension is usually of sudden onset and can cause necrosis of the small arteries. Benign hypertension is the term used for a prolonged history of hypertension, and this can cause fibrosis of the small arteries. The remaining 10% of patients with hypertension

It Happened in the Clinic

A 40-year-old man status post severe myocardial infarct (MI) was on the intensive care unit (ICU). On Day 2, he was prescribed physical therapy by the physician, and after evaluation, exercises were initiated in bed. The patient was impatient and wished to do more exercise, but the PT insisted he work within his tolerance and take notice of his feelings of shortness of breath and fatigue. By Day 3, the patient was assisted to sit bedside in a chair under instructions from the physician. The physician requested the patient to be treated in the physical therapy department, but the patient was extremely fatigued. The PT decided to see the patient in his room. The patient managed to ambulate only 10 feet and was extremely fatigued. On the fourth day, the patient was a little better, vital signs were stable, and he was insistent to nursing staff that he be transported to the PT department in a wheelchair. Upon arrival in the PT department, the patient was noted to be cyanotic and was returned immediately to bed. This patient subsequently died on Day 8. The importance of this scenario is that if the PT or PTA works with a patient and the signs and symptoms indicate a problem, particularly with a patient with cardiac pathology, he or she should refer the patient back to the physician immediately. Younger cardiac patients tend to be impatient and not compliant with protocols. It is important for the PT and PTA to emphasize the need for caution not to overexert and to follow instructions closely. In this particular case, the MI was so severe that the patient would not have survived in any case. It is important for PTAs to understand that not all patients can be helped, not all will recover, and, above all, PTAs should not blame themselves.

have a disease process or medication causing the problem. This type is termed secondary hypertension, and treatment of the causative disease will usually resolve the problem.

Complications of Hypertension. Cardiomegaly (enlargement of the heart) is one of the side effects of hypertension on the body due to hypertrophy of the left ventricle, which can also lead to myocardial fibrosis. Another name for this total process is hypertensive heart disease. Hypertrophy of the left ventricle leads to poor pumping ability of the heart, creating a back pressure that increases the pressure in the pulmonary artery and causes hypertrophy of the right ventricle. As previously described, the results of right ventricular failure are severe. The total effects on the heart from the right ventricular hypertrophy are known as **cor pulmonale.** Hypertension increases the development of atherosclerosis and can speed up the process of cardiac atherosclerosis involving the coronary arteries. Hypertensive encephalopathy causes changes in vessels within the brain, leading to cerebral ischemia. Such changes often cause alterations in mental status ranging from forgetfulness to extensive dementia. Severe damage with rupture to arteries in the brain can lead to hypertensive strokes, which have wide-ranging neurological effects. Early detection of hypertension is important to minimize the effects on the body. Another complication of hypertension is its effect on the retinal arteries. These changes can result in blindness. Regular eye examinations are recommended, especially for those with a family history of hypertension, because an eye exam can detect early stages of hypertensive disease.

Physical Therapy Intervention. Although physical therapy is not prescribed for hypertension, the PTA will treat patients with high blood pressure as a comorbid diagnosis. The importance of checking blood pressure and other vital signs prior, during, and after treatment is extremely important for these patients.

Ischemic Heart Disease

Ischemic heart disease is the most common cause of death in the United States.[26] Ischemic heart disease is really a group of diseases including angina pectoris, acute MI, sudden cardiac arrest and death, and chronic ischemic heart disease accompanied by CHF. According to the American Heart Association (2010),[27] there are approximately 4 million people in the United States who have silent ischemic heart disease, meaning there is no associated pain with the episode. This means that there are many

people who could have a sudden heart attack without ever knowing they have a problem with the heart.

The PTA should remember to concentrate on the functional impairments of the patient when determining the practice pattern in the *Guide to Physical Therapist Practice* that best fits with the type of PT intervention needed.

Etiology. In all these conditions, the heart is deprived of blood supply because of damage or inefficiency of the coronary circulation that supplies blood to the muscle of the heart. Such problems may be caused by a clot that blocks a coronary artery, thus cutting off circulation to a section of heart muscle, or by atherosclerosis (hardening and thickening of the vessel walls) of the coronary vessels, causing a reduction of blood supply to the muscle and resulting in reduced heart function. A clot causes a sudden MI, whereas coronary atherosclerosis may cause a gradual decline in function of the heart with a progressive disease process.

Signs and Symptoms. When the blood supply is cut off, the heart muscle dies because of anoxia, causing an MI that can result in cardiac arrest, as described later in the chapter. In such cases, there is often the associated pain in the chest, or referred pain into the neck, left shoulder, and jaw. In some cases, there is no pain experienced with an ischemic episode that causes a heart attack. Shortness of breath, sweating, and feelings of uneasiness or panic may occur. If the blood supply to the heart is temporarily reduced, there is pain, usually in the chest, which is called angina pectoris.

Prognosis. Collateral circulation in the coronary arteries is an important factor in survival with coronary artery disease (CAD). In those individuals with atherosclerosis that develops over a prolonged period, there is gradual formation of a collateral or alternative circulation between the smaller arteries that allows the blood to bypass the larger arteries and continue to meet the needs of the cardiac muscle. With MI, there is a sudden cutoff of the blood to the heart, possibly due to a clot blocking one of the coronary vessels, and there is no collateral circulation to supply the affected heart muscle. Within about 24 hours of MI, the smaller vessels start to enlarge to take over the function of the larger vessel. If the area of damage to the heart from the MI is not too great, the individual will recover. If a large portion of the heart is damaged, the individual may not survive. In persons with atherosclerosis of the coronary arteries in which collateral circulation develops, there may also be eventual atherosclerosis of the collateral circulation, leading to cardiac failure, especially in the older population.

Medical Intervention. If an ischemic episode is suspected, the patient will be placed on a 24-hour ECG Holter monitor to check for heart irregularities.[28] Another possible diagnostic intervention is an exercise stress test. The underlying cause of the ischemia is determined, and the patient may be placed on a regime of daily low-dose aspirin or other anticoagulant therapy. In severe cases, cardiac bypass surgery may be required.

Physical Therapy Intervention. Physical therapy intervention includes a progressive cardiac rehabilitation program, starting with treatment during the initial hospitalization and progressing through the rehabilitation process, which may last several months.

Myocarditis

Myocarditis is an inflammation of the myocardium (muscle) of the heart. The condition is comparatively rare.

Etiology. Myocarditis is a disease of the myocardium caused by viruses or by parasites such as *Toxoplasma* or *Trypanosoma*. Myocarditis can also be caused as a result of diseases such as poliomyelitis, influenza, and rubella and through exposure to chemicals. Myocarditis may also be a symptom of autoimmune disease.[29]

Signs and Symptoms. Many signs and symptoms are associated with myocarditis. These include mild fever, joint pain and edema, chest pain similar to that of a heart attack, heart murmurs, tachycardia, lower extremity edema, and reduced urine output. Patients are also often unable to lie supine because of shortness of breath.[30] Pathologically, the parasites or viruses cause inflammation, which in turn attracts T lymphocytes that secrete cytokines to kill the virus or parasite but that also further damage the heart muscle cells.

Prognosis. Many patients recover fully, but some may have heart failure, pericarditis, or cardiomyopathy.[31]

Medical Intervention. This disease is often difficult to treat effectively. Medical tests performed for diagnosis include an electrocardiogram, chest x-ray, and echocardiogram to determine whether there is an increase in size of the heart or fluid around the heart. The blood tests performed are usually white blood cell count, red blood cell count, and a blood culture to detect infection.

Physical Therapy Intervention. Physical therapy intervention is not indicated for this condition.

Pericarditis

Pericarditis is inflammation of the pericardium that often occurs in association with myocarditis.

Etiology. Pericarditis may be caused by a virus or bacteria, as a result of open heart surgery, or as a sequel to radiation therapy. Pericarditis may also occur in certain rheumatoid related connective tissue diseases, such as systemic lupus erythematosus and rheumatoid arthritis.

Signs and Symptoms. Characteristic signs and symptoms include chest pain, which may radiate into the neck, shoulder or back, as well as dyspnea and fever.

Prognosis. The recovery rate is usually good for bacterial pericarditis once antibacterial medications are administered. The condition often takes time to resolve if it results from surgery or radiation treatment.

Medical Intervention. If the pericarditis is caused by a bacterial infection, the physician will prescribe an appropriate antibacterial drug. When the condition is caused by surgery or radiation, the inflammation takes time to resolve, and anti-inflammatory medications may be prescribed.

Physical Therapy Intervention. Physical therapy is not indicated for this condition.

Rheumatic Heart Disease and Rheumatic Fever

Rheumatic fever is not as prevalent in Western countries because of the existence of antibiotic drugs. However, it remains a problem in developing countries.

Etiology. Rheumatic fever is one of the precursors of mitral valve disease. This disease results in an acute fever caused by a streptococci throat infection.

Signs and Symptoms. The characteristics of rheumatic fever include multiple painful joints associated with fever and cold or sore throat symptoms. Occasionally a skin rash is present. The joints most commonly affected are the knees, feet and ankles, shoulders, elbows, hands, and neck.

Prognosis. The general prognosis is good with the use of antibiotic and antimicrobial drugs. Some patients, however, tend to develop heart valve disease and carditis in later life.[32]

Medical Intervention. Diagnosis of rheumatic fever is often difficult. Medical management includes the use of antibiotics such as penicillin to cure the infection, bed rest, and anti-inflammatory medications such as salicylates. In cases in which heart failure results from the rheumatic fever, heart-valve transplant may be required.[33]

Physical Therapy Intervention. Physical therapy is not indicated in this condition.

NOTE: *The congenital heart condition Tetralogy of Fallot is covered in Chapter 2.*

Valve Diseases

As previously described, many heart-valve problems are a result of endocarditis. Three major types of heart-valve problems include stenosis, insufficiency, and prolapse. Stenosis means narrowing and in a valve refers to inability to open fully due to scarring from a previous disease process. If a valve does not open as fully as it should, it means that the chamber of the heart providing the "push" for blood through the valve has to work extra hard to keep the cardiac output constant, and this puts stress on the heart muscle. Insufficiency, or regurgitation, is caused by the valve failing to close fully after blood has passed through. This results in backflow of the blood into the previous heart chamber and will result in increased heart size in response to the extra work required. Prolapse of the mitral valve is fairly common and involves enlargement of the cusps of the valve that project into the left atrium.

Etiology. Mitral valve problems are often genetically inherited. Any of the valve problems create an increased workload for the heart and predispose a patient to heart infections and may ultimately lead to heart failure.

Signs and Symptoms. Many cases of heart-valve problems are mild and the patient does not have any symptoms. The main symptoms associated with heart-valve disease are dyspnea (shortness of breath) and fatigue. An enlarged heart may be apparent on x-ray due to the extra workload required of the heart. In advanced stages of mitral stenosis, atrial fibrillation may develop. Mitral valve insufficiency usually occurs as a result of valve prolapse. Heart failure can occur in advanced cases of valve disease, and symptoms can include swollen ankles toward evening, night dyspnea, greater than usual fatigue, or unexplained increases in weight.

Prognosis. Many people have mitral valve problems, and unless serious, may not require any treatment. In severe cases, surgical replacement may be performed. Occasionally, more advanced cases may result in heart failure.

Medical Intervention. Heart valves can now be surgically replaced with animal-derived prostheses known as bioprosthetic valves or mechanical synthetic valves. Approximately 65,000 heart valves are replaced in the United States every year. The Biocor stented tissue valve is an example of one type of artificial valve replacement used in Europe for more than 20 years and approved by the U.S. Food and Drug Administration in 2005. Complications from prosthetic valves can include deterioration that can result in stenosis of the valve, thrombus production, and emboli formation. However, the long-term trials performed in Sweden using the Biocor valve have been promising, with minimal complications. Anticoagulant therapy is provided for all valve-replacement patients. Patients with valve replacements are more prone to infections affecting the heart valves and also may develop leaks in the valves causing regurgitation. Patients with valve incompetence are recommended to take prophylactic antibiotics before dental work to prevent the possibility of bacteria from the teeth entering the bloodstream and causing infection of the heart valves.

Physical Therapy Intervention. Mild heart valve problems do not usually prevent a person from participating in exercise. If patients start coughing after vigorous exercise, it could mean they have pulmonary congestion resulting from valve disease, and the PTA should stop the exercise. If a patient has weakness, fatigue, and becomes pale, the PTA should also stop the exercise session. In any of these instances, the PTA should consult the supervising PT.

Venous System Backup. This occurs when the heart is unable to pump as much blood as usual through the body, and blood collects in the vessels of the peripheral circulation and the lungs. This backup increases the pressure in both left and right atria and increases capillary pressures in the lungs. Some patients develop edema in the lungs after a MI and die within a few hours of onset of the edema.

Ventricular Fibrillation. Although ventricular fibrillation has been described, there are some specifics that occur after MI. The danger periods for this after myocardial infarction are within 10 minutes of the development of infarction and then about 1 hour later. The possibility of ventricular fibrillation several days after infarction also exists. The theory of why this occurs is that the injury to the heart muscle creates a disturbance in the electrical polarity of the heart tissue that makes it transmit confusing messages to the normal heart tissue producing ventricular fibrillation. One such example is premature ventricular contractions.

Why Does the Physical Therapist Assistant Need to Know About Cardiac Surgeries and Rehabilitation?

PTAs work as part of the health care team with many people who have had cardiac surgery. Understanding cardiac surgery procedures enables PTAs to determine some of the side effects of the surgeries and be better prepared for participation in the rehabilitation process. Knowledge of the muscles and tissues involved during the surgery can help to highlight those areas of the body that require specific interventions as designated in the plan of care developed by the supervising PT.

Cardiac Surgeries and Cardiac Rehabilitation

Patients who have heart disease or other cardiac problems frequently undergo surgery and subsequent rehabilitation as part of their treatment. This section describes some of the most common types of both cardiac surgeries and the rehabilitation provided for patients who have undergone surgery.

Coronary Artery Bypass Graft

After the coronary artery is completely occluded or beyond the point where an angioplasty is thought to be helpful, a coronary artery bypass graft (CABG) may be performed. (The CABG is often referred to as a "cabbage" in medical circles.) This surgery requires opening of the chest cavity to enable the coronary vessels to be replaced and bypassed. The donor vessels used for the procedure are the saphenous veins in the leg or the internal mammary artery. The new piece of vessel is joined to the occluded coronary artery above and below the occlusion to provide a bypass for the blood and restore arterial oxygenated blood supply to the heart muscle. Another procedure performed on arteries such as the carotid, femoral, or popliteal is an **endarterectomy.** This is the surgical removal of the lining of an artery with replacement using a donor vessel.

Heart Transplant

The first heart transplant in a human was performed by Dr. Christian Barnard in 1967 in South Africa. Approximately 2,000 per year are now performed in the United States.[34] Most modern transplants use a human heart as a donor, although attempts have been made to use hearts of nonhuman primates. Transplants are either orthotopic in which the patient's heart is replaced or heterotopic in which the donor heart is placed next to the existing heart and connected to it. To be considered for a heart transplant, an adult patient usually has to have end-stage CAD or cardiomyopathy (heart failure). In children, the main reasons for heart transplantation are congenital heart diseases and cardiomyopathy. Because there is a shortage of donor hearts, candidates for transplantation are screened carefully on the basis of criteria developed by the Committee on Heart Failure and Cardiac Transplantation of the Council on Clinical Cardiology of the American Heart Association. The main factors considered when deciding whether a transplant is in the best interests of the patient are the chances of survival, that the quality of life would be improved, and relief of symptoms would be likely achieved.[35] Postsurgical complications include rejection of the new heart by the patient. To prevent this from occurring, the patient is placed on immunosuppressive drugs. Infection is another complication. Physical therapy may be requested for early mobility and exercises on Day 2 or 3 after surgery. Chest PT may be ordered while the patient is still in the intensive care unit.

Open Heart Surgery

The term open heart surgery is used for any procedure in which the heart must be opened to provide access for surgical intervention. Valve replacements or repairs are performed for all the heart valves but most commonly for the mitral valve. Although a description of all types of open heart surgery is beyond the scope of this text, some aspects of this procedure must be considered.

The surgical incision for opening of the chest cavity for heart surgery is usually through a median sternotomy incision. The incision runs from the sternal notch to below the xiphoid process. Sternal retractors (a kind of vice) are used to open the sternum so that surgery can be performed. PTAs are likely to see the incision if they work in cardiac rehabilitation or may even work with patients immediately after the procedure in the acute care setting. Care must be taken to support the sternal incision, with a pillow or pressure, when performing coughing or huffing techniques for airway clearance. The patient must also be careful when getting in and out of bed when a strain may be put on the incision. An audible click in the sternum indicates that there is too much motion at the incision site, which could interfere with, or prolong healing. Driving a car is usually contraindicated for the first 6 weeks after surgery to protect the sternal incision site. Heavy lifting is not advisable after open heart surgery because of the strain it places on the sternum. On discharge, most patients will enter a cardiac rehabilitation program for increasing strength, endurance, and aerobic capacity.

Pacemaker Insertion

Patients with ischemic heart disease, heart block, disturbances of the SA node, arrhythmias due to myocardial infarction, or post cardiac surgery temporary arrhythmias may require a cardiac pacemaker. The cardiac pacemaker takes over the function of the SA node in the heart when it is not functioning correctly. A conductive lead is attached to the heart muscle by passing it along the cephalic vein and into the right atrium, and the pacemaker is usually located under the skin overlying the upper left chest wall. Pacemakers can be unipolar or bipolar with two conductive leads to the heart. Most pacemakers use lithium batteries, which last up to 10 years, and then the pacemaker needs to be replaced. Some pacemakers are temporary measures, and others are required permanently. On-demand pacemakers only send an electrical impulse when they detect the heart has failed to do so, whereas fixed-rate pacemakers send out continuous impulses. The on-demand pacemakers are more efficient because they do not compete with the natural impulses of the heart. Cardiac pacemakers are a contraindication for treatment with electrical stimulation. Physical therapy departments should have a notice attached to the main entrance door stating that machines are in use that may interfere with the function of pacemakers.

Percutaneous Transluminal Coronary Artery Angioplasty

Percutaneous transluminal coronary artery angioplasty (PCTA) is performed on coronary vessels with atherosclerosis when the artery is not completely occluded. A catheter is advanced to the coronary artery, usually via the femoral artery, and a balloon at the end of the catheter is inflated at the site of the problem area. The pressure from the balloon is intended to widen the lumen of the artery. The procedure is repeated using progressively larger catheters until the lumen at the area of partial obstruction is expanded. Another type of this procedure is called a directional coronary arthrectomy in which a cutting blade is inserted with the catheter and actually cuts away some of

the atheromatous material to enlarge the lumen of the artery. These procedures are now being performed using laser surgery. Another option is to insert a stent (a mesh of metallic substance) with the catheter. The stent keeps the artery open once it has been opened up by the angioplasty procedure. Risks are involved with the procedure such as rupture or perforation of the artery. This procedure is also used with arteries in other locations such as a popliteal artery bypass.

Why Does the Physical Therapist Assistant Need to Know About Arterial Diseases?

People with arterial diseases are often seen in the physical therapy clinic for the treatment of associated conditions such as **arterial insufficiency ulcers.** People with arterial diseases require specific precautions during physical therapy interventions to prevent exacerbation of their condition. Knowledge of the mechanisms of arterial disease and the precautions and contraindications for interventions are therefore necessary when working with patients with these conditions to ensure safe and effective treatment.

Arterial Diseases

The arterial diseases described in this section are characterized by pathology to the actual arterial blood vessels. This pathology frequently causes systemic changes within the body pertinent to physical therapy practice. See Chapter 8 for discussion regarding arterial insufficiency ulcers.

Arteritis

Arteritis is also called giant cell arteritis and cranial or temporal arteritis because of its effect on the arteries of the head and temples. The term vasculitis refers to any vessel that is inflamed and can be a part of several types of pathological conditions. Giant cell arteritis is often associated with polymyalgia rheumatica.[36]

Etiology. The condition involves inflammation of the arteries of unknown origin.

Signs and Symptoms. The onset of symptoms is fast, with severe headaches and pain extending into the face, neck, and occipital area; tenderness particularly in the temples; and possible fever. Vision may be affected, causing blurred vision, double vision, and sometimes blindness. Arteritis is mainly found in adults over 50.[37]

Prognosis. The prognosis varies depending on the severity of the condition. Permanent damage to vision may be experienced. In cases in which thrombosis results, there is a higher risk of death if the thrombus blocks an artery of the brain, heart, or lungs.

Medical Intervention. Diagnosis is determined through a sedimentation rate blood test, which demonstrates above-normal values and possibly by a biopsy of the temporal artery. Anti-inflammatory drugs to reduce the risk of blindness are prescribed for arteritis by the physician, particularly the use of corticosteroids.[38]

Physical Therapy Intervention. Physical therapy is not indicated in this condition.

Cerebrovascular Disease

Atherosclerosis in the arteries of the brain or the carotid artery that leads to the brain is termed cerebrovascular disease (CVD). This is a major cause of stroke or cerebrovascular accident (CVA). Stroke is the third leading cause of death in the United States according to 2006 statistics published in 2010.[39] Over 795,000 people have a stroke each year in the United States and more than 4.4 million people in the United States are survivors of a CVA.[40]

Etiology. Cerebrovascular disease is mainly a disease of older people and involves atherosclerosis of the cerebral arteries and carotid arteries. Risk factors for the disease include those that cannot be controlled, such as age, gender, and family history. Some risk factors can be controlled, such as exercise levels, obesity, hypertension, and high LDL cholesterol levels.[41]

Signs and Symptoms. The mechanism of disease is the same as for other areas of the body, involving either a slow damage to the vessels with deposition of atheromas or a sudden occlusion of vessels due to a thrombus breaking off and forming an embolus, which occludes a cerebral artery. Ischemia of the brain leads to ischemic stroke or cerebrovascular accident (CVA). Early signs of atherosclerosis of the affected arteries can manifest as transient ischemic attacks (TIA) in which there is a transient weakness of one side of the body or changes in speech or skin sensation. When prolonged ischemia occurs, there is oxygen deprivation to part of the brain. Results of the disease will depend on where the damage occurs in the brain.

Prognosis. The prognosis depends on the severity of the condition. If atherosclerosis of the cerebrovascular vessels is diagnosed before a stroke occurs, some treatments are now available. After a stroke has occurred, a patient's recovery will depend on the extent and location of the cerebrovascular accident in the brain. This is discussed in Chapter 7 on neurological disorders.

Medical Intervention. Diagnosis of atherosclerosis of the cerebral and carotid arteries can be determined by magnetic resonance imaging, angiography, and Doppler ultrasound. Medical management is through recommendations for lifestyle changes, including weight loss (if appropriate), increased levels of exercise, and use of cholesterol-lowering drugs such as statins.[42] Other medical interventions include control of hypertension and diabetes. If the carotid arteries are affected with atherosclerosis, a carotid endarterectomy may be performed to replace the diseased carotid vessels and prevent, or reduce the risk, of onset of complications such as a stroke.

Physical Therapy Intervention. In atherosclerosis of the cerebrovascular system, physical therapy may be involved with development of exercise programs for the patient. The role of the PT and PTA in intervention for the patient who has had a stroke is extensive. This is discussed further in Chapter 7 on neurological disorders.

Patent Ductus Arteriosus ⊛

The ductus arteriosus is a vessel that connects the pulmonary artery to the aorta in the fetus. Usually this vessel closes soon after birth, but in some cases, it does not, and this can cause congestive heart failure. Patent ductus arteriosus (PDA) is one of a group of congenital heart defects that can affect a baby. Tetralogy of Fallot was discussed in Chapter 2; another congenital defect is a ventricular septal defect (VSD) in which the dividing wall between the two ventricles does not close fully.

Peripheral Vascular Disease

Peripheral vascular disease (PVD) is the term used for atherosclerosis of the peripheral arteries, mainly of the lower extremities. PVD is common in the elderly population, especially those with diabetes mellitus, hypertension, or hyperlipidemia.

Etiology. Total body atherosclerosis may occur. Atherosclerosis of the renal (kidney) arteries is often associated with aortic atherosclerosis because the renal arteries branch directly from the aorta. The term also applies, however, to atherosclerosis of the arteries supplying the major abdominal organs, including the kidneys and intestines. Involvement of the peripheral arteries of the lower extremities may be particular to those arteries or may be a side effect of the involvement of the abdominal cavity organs. A history of trauma to the lower leg that did not fully heal may also be present.

Signs and Symptoms. Narrowing of the renal arteries causes hypoperfusion, resulting in under nourishment of the kidneys, and thus kidney function is reduced. The results are hypertension, reduced output of urine, and concentration of sodium in the kidney, which causes damage to the organ. When atherosclerosis affects the arteries supplying the intestine, there is ischemia of the small and large intestines. Slow-onset chronic ischemia causes gastrointestinal symptoms such as constipation and malabsorption problems, with progressively increasing severity of these symptoms. The blood vessels most often involved in atherosclerosis are the femoral and popliteal arteries affecting the muscles of the leg. On exertion, intermittent claudication occurs due to insufficient blood supply to the muscles (previously described). If the smaller arteries are involved in the distal part of the lower extremities and occlusion occurs, then the tissue undergoes gangrene (necrosis/death). (Refer to Chapter 1 for further details regarding gangrene.)

Prognosis. Atherosclerosis of the renal vessels is one of the factors leading to end-stage renal failure, a life-threatening condition. In severe occlusion of the arteries to the intestines, there is infarction of the intestine, which is serious and can cause death. However, in many cases, peripheral vascular disease can be controlled and improved through some lifestyle changes such as stopping smoking, controlling diabetes mellitus, eating a low-fat diet, controlling hypertension and hypercholesterolemia, and increasing the level of physical activity.[47]

Medical Intervention. Amputation (surgical resection) of the necrotic tissue is often required, particularly for cases of gangrene. Angioplasty may be performed and a stent inserted to keep the involved artery open. In other cases, a bypass surgery may be used, if the artery is severely damaged. Some of the medications that can be used include cholesterol-lowering medications such as statins and antiplatelet drugs to reduce the possibility of thrombus formation (clotting) in the arteries.

Physical Therapy Intervention. Physical therapy intervention is mainly related to the complications resulting from atherosclerosis. A major complication of PVD is the development of arterial insufficiency ulcers on the lower leg (refer to Chapter 8). The PTA will be required to treat these ulcers in the clinic as part of the wound-care team. These ulcers are nearly always located on the lower extremity over the lateral malleolus, over the bony prominence of the anterior aspect of the tibia, on the lateral border of the foot, and in the toe joints. The differences in treatment for arterial and venous ulcers must be understood and are described in Chapter 8. The symptoms that accompany such arterial ulcers include intermittent claudication, pain at rest, pain when legs are elevated, loss or reduction of dorsalis pedis pulse, and atrophy of the gastrocnemius and/or tibialis anterior muscle.

MAJOR ASPECTS OF PVD FOR THE PTA

1. Arterial disease results in lack of oxygen to the tissue involved. In complete occlusion of the arteries, gangrene can develop quickly.
2. Intermittent claudication in the lower leg is a general symptom of reduced blood supply to the muscles. Patients will be able to walk short distances, but if climbing stairs, walking rapidly, or running they will experience pain, particularly in the posterior lower leg muscles because the popliteal artery is most often affected. PTAs must know their anatomy, including the blood supply to the major muscle groups.
3. Because the area of tissue involved lacks oxygen supply, it is important that the area *not* be heated. The arteries are unable to cope with the normal circulation, and if heated, the tissue would become overheated and further damaged. Under normal circumstances, the circulation increases to disperse the effects of heat on tissues, but these arteries are damaged and unable to respond to extra demands placed on them.
4. Massage is contraindicated because it places too much demand on the arteries.
5. Advice to the patient should include ways to minimize the effects of the arterial insufficiency, such as raising the head end of the bed when sleeping. This places the patient in a position in which gravity assists the arterial flow to the extremities. If the feet were elevated, gravity would increase the difficulty of blood flow for the arteries to the lower extremities. Other advice is to stop smoking and keep blood pressure under control with a sensible diet and take any prescribed medications regularly as ordered by the physician.
6. Buerger-Allen exercises (previously described) can be taught to encourage the development of collateral circulation.

7. A progressive exercise routine can be taught to the patient, encouraging short bouts of exercise increasing in time as the level of tolerance to exercise improves. Rest must be included in the program.

8. Skin inspection techniques should be taught to the patient, including the use of a mirror for those patients unable to check the soles of the feet by any other means. Regular skin inspection is important for the distal lower extremities to identify the early warning signs of skin breakdown. The patient needs to see a doctor at the first sign of problems. Patients should be warned not to place the feet or lower legs too near a heat source such as an electric heating radiator, a fire, a bath that is too hot, or a heating pad, because they may sustain a burn. Shoes should be checked carefully before putting them on to make sure there is nothing sharp in them that could damage the skin. Feet must be dried carefully after washing.

9. Atherosclerosis problems are made worse by constrictive garments. The damaged arteries are unable to cope with the extra pressure from compression so it is important *not* to use compression stockings or have tight clothing such as knee-high socks that are tight round the area immediately distal to the knee

10. Treatment of arterial ulcers should be performed with caution. Normal average skin temperature is approximately 93° Fahrenheit or 34° Celsius. Whirlpool temperatures should be cool, 80° to 92° Fahrenheit or 27° to 33.5° Celsius, or neutral, 92° to 96° Fahrenheit or 33.5° to 35.5° Celsius to avoid overload to the arterially insufficient tissue (Sussman, 2001, p. 627).[48] When using cooler temperatures for a whirlpool treatment, the PTA should make sure that the surrounding air temperature is warm enough to prevent hypothermia and only treat the local area such as the lower leg for about 5 minutes. The use of neutral water temperatures allow for a longer period of immersion.[49] Any débridement of necrotic tissue should be performed with care taken that the area has sufficient arterial supply to allow the wound to heal. Many of these wounds will not heal unless the arterial blood supply is restored through arterial bypass surgery. A general rule is that sharp débridement for arterial ulcers should be performed by the physician or the PT.

Polyarteritis Nodosa

This disease is an inflammation with nodule formation of the small and medium-sized arteries. The condition mainly affects adults.

Etiology. No known cause of polyarteritis exists; however, it has been linked with hepatitis B and is thought to be autoimmune in nature.

Signs and Symptoms. Polyarteritis nodosa can cause aneurysm of the blood vessel and can occur anywhere in the body except the lungs. The disease can cause extensive organ damage. The main symptoms include abdominal pain, fatigue, possible fever, tachycardia, muscle and joint aches and tenderness on palpation, weakness, and weight loss.

Prognosis. With adequate treatment the prognosis is often good, but without treatment the condition becomes serious and can affect the kidneys and intestines. Major complications of the condition include stroke, renal failure, MI, and necrosis of the intestines.

Medical Intervention. The diagnosis of this condition is often difficult. Diagnostic tests performed may include blood tests to check the erythrocyte sedimentation rate (ESR) and the white blood cell count (WBCC), both of which are raised above normal levels in this condition, as well as a possible tissue biopsy of the arteries to detect inflammation. Medical management is through the use of immune system suppressants such as corticosteroids.[43]

Physical Therapy Intervention. Physical therapy is not indicated in this condition.

Raynaud's Disease or Syndrome

Raynaud's disease and phenomenon affects women more than men and is common in women between ages 20 and 49. Raynaud's can be classified as a peripheral vascular disease because it affects the blood vessels; however, there is also a neurological control component to the condition.

Etiology. Raynaud's is particularly common in people with connective tissue diseases such as scleroderma, rheumatoid arthritis, and systemic sclerosis, but in many cases, there is no known etiology. A genetic component to the disease may exist, and it has been found that Raynaud's is often a precursor to the development of connective tissue disease.[44]

Signs and Symptoms. People with Raynaud's disease or syndrome are acutely sensitive to cold. Onset of symptoms can also be brought on by emotional stress, smoking, and "working with vibrating machinery."[45] Symptoms are paleness of the skin, especially of the hands, and reduction of skin temperature (see Fig. 3-11).

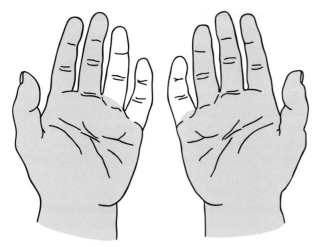

FIGURE 3.11 Hands of a patient affected by Raynaud's disease.

Prognosis. Raynaud's disease and Raynaud's phenomenon are not usually serious, but the patient cannot tolerate exposure to the cold.

Medical Intervention. Medical intervention is aimed at reducing the number of attacks of the condition, and preventing vascular damage and ulceration of the fingers, which may occur with vascular damage. Calcium channel blockers may be prescribed for improved vascular health.

Physical Therapy Intervention. The PT and PTA should not apply cold packs to patients with either the disease or the phenomenon because of the severe reaction to cold. In addition, aquatic therapy may not be possible unless the pool is heated to at least body temperature. The use of whirlpool treatments with the water at nonthermal temperatures should also be avoided.

Thromboangiitis Obliterans (Buerger's Disease)

Thromboangiitis obliterans is inflammation with thrombosis that affects the arteries and veins of the upper and lower extremities especially of the hands and feet.

Etiology. A high incidence of the disease exists in men aged 20 to 40 who smoke or chew tobacco.

Signs and Symptoms. Signs and symptoms include alterations in skin sensation, insensitivity to heat and cold, decreased or absent distal extremity pulses, and possible areas of gangrenous tissue. Acute, burning, tingling pain

may be experienced in the hands and feet at rest, and there is pain in the legs, ankles, and feet on ambulation with intermittent claudication. In addition, the hands and feet may be pale in color or red and cold, and there may be ulcerations of the hands and feet.

Prognosis. The disease can lead to permanent damage of the small vessels of the hands and feet, and severe cases can result in the need for amputation of the distal extremities. The symptoms of the disease may however resolve if the person stops smoking and the damage to the blood vessels is not too great. Complications of the disease include gangrene, and more extensive loss of the circulation other than in the affected limb.

Medical Treatment. Medical diagnostic tests include angiography or arteriography of the affected limb, Doppler ultrasound of the limb, and biopsy of the affected blood vessels. The main way to prevent the progression of the disease is to stop smoking. Because there is no cure, patients have to avoid cold temperatures. In some cases, surgery to cut the sympathetic nerve to the affected limb may reduce pain. In severe cases, amputation of the limb is performed.[46]

Physical Therapy Intervention. Although physical therapy is not directly indicated for this condition, there may be involvement with wound care if ulcerations form on the extremities. Gentle exercise programs to increase distal extremity circulation may be prescribed by the physician. See Chapter 8 for treatment of arterial insufficiency ulcers.

NOTE: *Diabetic ulcers are a combination of arterial and neuropathic problems. The patient with diabetes may have a peripheral neuropathy, creating loss of sensation in the affected limb. This means that diabetic ulcers will not be painful, but they are difficult to treat because the circulation to the area is impaired and healing is slow. A typical diabetic ulcer is located on the plantar surface of the foot. Diabetes is discussed at greater length in Chapter 9.*

Why Does the Physical Therapist Assistant Need to Know About Venous Diseases?

Many people with diseases of the venous system are treated with physical therapy interventions. Some of the more common interventions are related to venous insufficiency ulcers described in

Chapter 8. Other people with venous system diseases may attend physical therapy for other conditions. Physical therapy intervention is often affected by the presence of venous problems that may restrict the amount of exercise performed or the potential for functional recovery. An understanding of the mechanisms of the disease process in venous conditions provides the PTA with a greater ability to recognize potential problems and adjust intervention approaches as necessary for patient participation.

Venous Diseases

The venous diseases described in this section are characterized by pathology of the actual vessels of the venous system. These diseases can lead to systemic symptoms, as is the case for the arterial diseases. Refer to Chapter 8 for information regarding venous insufficiency ulcers.

Thrombophlebitis and Deep Venous Thrombosis

Thrombophlebitis means inflammation and clotting of veins. The condition usually affects either the deep or superficial veins of the lower extremities.

Etiology. Several causes of thrombophlebitis exist such as infection, trauma, surgery to the area involved, or a long period of immobility due to illness or prolonged hospitalization, which causes reduced circulation.

Signs and Symptoms. The signs and symptoms may include generalized fever, tenderness, and erythema (redness) over the area of the vein, induration (hardening of the tissue), and possible pain and tightness of the area. Signs of deep venous thrombosis (DVT) in the popliteal vessels of the lower leg can include pain in the central posterior calf, sometimes with swelling, acute tenderness to touch, and possible fever. Homan's sign is characterized by pain in the calf when the foot is passively or actively dorsiflexed, but it is not a reliable test for DVT.

Prognosis. The prognosis for thrombophlebitis depends on the extent of the condition and whether there is thrombus formation. Thrombus formation can result in death if the thrombus blocks a vessel in the heart, lungs, or brain. A cerebrovascular accident may occur if a thrombus travels to the brain. In many cases, the condition will be resolved successfully with medical intervention.

Medical Intervention. Diagnosis of the condition is performed through use of the Homan's test as described in the signs and symptoms section, and Doppler ultrasound studies of the vessels to detect potential blockages. The presence of typical signs and symptoms is indicative of the condition. Because of the danger of loosening the thrombus in the vein and creating an embolus, the patient is required to have bed rest. A compression bandage may be used and the patient placed on anticoagulant medications. Complications of a DVT are an embolus that could lodge in the lungs and cause death. Some individuals appear to be prone to the condition and are advised to wear elastic stockings and do exercises and activity after prolonged periods of rest. The use of compression pumps during periods of immobility is helpful in reducing the risks of DVT.

Physical Therapy Intervention. The PT and PTA are involved with ambulating and exercising patients early after surgery to reduce the risk of developing DVT. The PTA should be careful to note any lower extremity pain, particularly in postsurgical patients, that seems unusual, and immediately advise the supervising PT and physician as needed. In some cases, the emergency medical system may need to be initiated, and, at the least, the patient needs to be instructed to rest until a determination of the cause of pain is made. In some cases, there will not be any warning signs until the patient has a pulmonary embolus with chest pain. Occasionally, there may be sudden onset of extreme pain in the area of the hip. Any unusual sign noted by the PTA should be taken seriously. Wavering on the side of caution is always better than taking the risk of ignoring the problem.

Varicose Veins

Varicose veins are most often associated with the legs, but when present in the anus, they are called hemorrhoids. In the esophagus, varicose veins are called esophageal varices and may be caused by cirrhosis of the liver, which increases pressure in the portal vein. Esophageal varices can cause bleeding and death.

Etiology. Causes of varicose veins in the legs vary from a venous disease to a job that requires a lot of standing or heavy lifting. PTs, PTAs, nurses, and other health care workers are at risk for varicose veins because of the necessity for heavy lifting and standing. Pregnancy also increases risk of the problem.

Signs and Symptoms. In the lower extremities, varicose veins can be seen on the skin as superficial, twisted, darkened veins and usually involve the greater saphenous vein on the medial aspect of the leg. The valves in varicose veins do not work well. Pain and aching often occur particularly when standing still, and edema is often a problem.

Prognosis. Many people with varicose veins manage without having surgery. The amount of pain experienced in the area of the varicosity usually determines whether a person seeks medical help. However, varicose veins are sometimes a precursor to thrombus formation because of the static nature of the blood within the varicose vessels.

Medical Intervention. People with varicose veins should wear elastic support hose and avoid prolonged standing. PTs and PTAs should consider wearing support stockings to avoid the risk of developing the problem and shift weight regularly when standing. Regular exercise also helps to reduce the risk and to alleviate symptoms once the problem is present. Varicose veins may require surgical removal by stripping or injection with a sclerosing (hardening) agent to collapse the vein. Individuals with this condition should be warned of the possible harmful effects and seek medical advice if pain is experienced more than usual.

Physical Therapy Intervention. Physical therapy is not generally required for varicose veins, but the PT and PTA can give advice to health care workers for the prevention of the problem, such as regular exercise, not standing in one position too long, and the use of support hose.

Why Does the Physical Therapist Assistant Need to Know About Blood Disorders?

Although physical therapy intervention is not provided for specific blood disorders, the side effects of these conditions such as extreme fatigue, muscle weakness, debilitation and loss of mobility often indicate the need for physical therapy. PTAs are frequently involved in physical therapy interventions for people with these conditions. A knowledge of the pathological mechanisms involved in blood disorders assists when providing appropriate levels of exercise and activity for these patients and in recognizing potentially detrimental effects of the interventions.

Blood Disorders

Blood disorders are characterized by abnormalities of the cellular components of the blood. This section focuses mainly on the different types of anemia and leukemia. Some general terminology and descriptions regarding disorders of the blood are important for the PTA to be aware of. These include leukocytosis, leukopenia, polycythemia, and thrombocytopenia.

Leukocytosis is an increase in white cell count often related to an infection. Acute bacterial infections cause polymorphonuclear leukocytosis, chronic infections cause monocytosis, allergic reactions cause eosinophilia, and viral infections cause lymphocytosis. Certain neoplasms also cause leukocytosis.

Leukopenia is the reduction of white cells in the blood below normal levels. Leukopenia is mainly due to a lowered number of neutrophils (neutropenia) or, more rarely, lymphocytes (lymphopenia). The reduced white cell count to below 1,000 per microliter of blood results in reduction of the ability of the immune system to fight off infections.

Polycythemia is an increase in red blood cells (RBCs) and occurs in certain types of lung disease and heart disease, when living at high altitude, or when dehydrated after vomiting or diarrhea. Polycythemia increases the viscosity of the blood and can lead to a higher incidence of thrombosis and embolism, as well as to the development of leukemia.

Thrombocytopenia is a reduced number of platelets in the blood. Antibodies to the platelets in an autoimmune response in which the body destroys its own cells can cause thrombocytopenia.

Anemias and Other Disorders of Red Blood Cells

Many types of anemia exist, all of which are disorders of red blood cells. Anemias all cause a reduction of oxygen transportation by the blood. Anemia can be detected by doing a hematocrit count and hemoglobin levels from a blood sample, as previously described. Anemia can cause various changes to the red blood cells, including changes of size and shape and reduction in number. Hemolytic anemias are those in which the red blood cells do not live as long as usual. When the red cells are broken down, they release iron, which is used for formation of new red blood cells. Iron-deficient anemias are more common in developing countries, where it is estimated that up to 50% of the population suffers from the disorder. In industrialized countries, approximately 10% of people are affected by iron-deficient anemia.

Etiology. Causes of iron-deficient anemia include low iron in the diet, especially in vegetarians; malabsorption of iron by the body; high demands for iron during pregnancy and in infancy; or loss of blood as part of a disease process. Some serious diseases such as infections, rheumatoid arthritis, and neoplastic diseases such as Hodgkin's disease may also cause anemia. Immunohemolytic anemias are rare and are caused by patients developing antibodies to their own red blood cells. Red blood cells can also be destroyed by stress from cardiac disorders. Megaloblastic anemias are caused by poor nutrition, either through lack of folic acid or vitamin B_{12}, and cause a reduction of DNA synthesis. Folic acid–deficient anemia is found in pregnancy and in undernourished people such as the elderly. When vegetables are overcooked it destroys folic acid. Celiac disease and some drugs such as Dilantin and methotrexate restrict the absorption of folic acid, leading to anemia. Pernicious anemia is another type of megaloblastic anemia also caused by B_{12} deficiency and produces a demyelination of the peripheral nerves and spinal cord. Aplastic anemia affects bone marrow red blood cell production by stem cells. This may follow a viral infection and has been associated with non-A and non-B hepatitis as well as human immunodeficiency virus. Exposure to chemicals and radiation can also damage bone marrow and affect red blood cell production. This type of anemia may require bone marrow transplant. Sickle cell disease was covered in Chapter 2. Thalassemia is a hereditary disease causing a shape defect of the red blood cells. Thalassemia is common in Mediterranean populations and causes anemia and splenomegaly (enlarged spleen). The splenomegaly occurs as a result of absorption of the abnormally shaped red blood cells.

Signs and Symptoms. Characteristic signs and symptoms of anemia include fatigue, chest pain, and dyspnea. Pernicious anemia causes loss of muscle control due to demyelination of spinal nerves.

Prognosis. The prognosis depends on the cause and type of anemia.

Medical Intervention. Medical intervention depends on the type and cause of the anemia and correction of the cause if possible. In some cases, a blood transfusion is required. Diagnostic tests for anemia include blood tests for red blood cell count and hemoglobin levels and a physical examination by the physician.[50]

Physical Therapy Intervention. No physical therapy is indicated for anemia. However, patients receiving physical therapy may have anemia, and the therapist needs to be aware of the diagnosis and watch for signs of fatigue.

Leukemias

Leukemias are malignant neoplasms of the blood cells or blood-forming organs. Several types of leukemia are divided into two main classifications of acute and chronic, all of which are malignant and named according to the cells most involved.

Etiology. In most cases of leukemia, there is no known cause; however, some chemotherapy and radiation treatments for malignancy can cause the disease. ⊛ Acute lymphocytic leukemia (ALL) affects mainly children, whereas acute myeloblastic leukemia (AML) affects adults. Chronic myeloid/myeloblastic leukemia affects adults aged 25 to 60 and is due to a chromosome abnormality, whereas chronic lymphocytic/lymphocystic leukemia affects the over-50 age group.

Signs and Symptoms. Anemia occurs because of a lack of red blood cells with the related symptoms of fatigue, fever, debility, bleeding of gums, bone pain caused by increase of bone marrow that stretches the periosteum, and central nervous system symptoms such as headache and peripheral nerve problems. In acute leukemias, the stem cells fail to become mature blood cells, so there are not enough red cells, white cells, or platelets. Instead, there is an accumulation of cells called leukemic blasts in the bone marrow that prevent the formation of normal cells.

Prognosis. ⊛ Acute lymphocytic leukemia cure rates in children are about 80%, whereas in adults, the remission rate is 80%, with between a 30% and 50% cure rate.[51] In chronic lymphocytic leukemia, more than half of those in the early stages of the disease survive more than 12 years.[52] Complications of the disease may be a result of the chemotherapy treatments and include anemia, fatigue, and an increased risk of secondary malignancy.

Medical Intervention. Medical treatment for leukemias includes chemotherapy and radiation therapy, both of which have a debilitating effect on the patient. Certain characteristics of the disease, such as fatigue and debility, are further increased by chemotherapy. Another treatment option is bone marrow transplant.

Physical Therapy Intervention. The PTA may have to treat the patient to increase exercise and activity tolerance as the patient recovers.

> ### Why Does the Physical Therapist Assistant Need to Know About Lymphatic Disorders?
>
> The involvement of physical therapy interventions for people with lymphatic disorders is variable. Although people with some conditions such as Hodgkin's disease may not require physical therapy, most people with lymphedema benefit from specialized interventions to reduce the effects of the condition. Knowledge of the pathological mechanisms of lymphatic disorders is essential to the use of effective applicable interventions.

Lymphatic Disorders

The lymphatic system is closely linked to the venous part of the circulatory system. Inclusion of this section regarding lymphatic disorders is thus the final piece of the puzzle when discussing pathology of the circulatory system.

Hodgkin's Disease and Hodgkin's Lymphoma

Hodgkin's disease is a malignant disease of the white cells, called a malignant lymphoma. Other non-Hodgkin's lymphomas are common in patients with AIDS.

Etiology. The cause of the disease is unknown, but a virus is suspected.

Signs and symptoms. All lymphomas are malignant and affect the immune system. Detailing the various non-Hodgkin's lymphomas is beyond the scope of this book. Hodgkin's disease affects the lymph system, including the lymph nodes, spleen, liver, and bone marrow, causing swelling of one or many nodes. Signs and symptoms of the disease include fever, weight loss, fatigue, loss of appetite, and the swelling of lymph nodes, which is usually painless. Less common symptoms include hair loss and neck pain.

Prognosis. Cases of the disease are classified as Stage I through IV. Stages I and II have a better prognosis and are more easily treated with chemotherapy and radiation therapy. The survival rate for Stage I is 80% of patients living more than 10 years, with 60% of those in the later stages living more than 5 years.[53]

Medical Intervention. Treatment with chemotherapy and radiation regimens is used to disable the malignant white blood cells. Some survivors of the disease tend to develop leukemia or other malignant diseases after extensive chemotherapy and radiation therapy.

Physical Therapy Intervention. Physical therapy intervention is not indicated for Hodgkin's disease.

Lymphangitis and Lymphadenitis

Lymphangitis is acute inflammation of the lymphatic vessels, and lymphadenitis is inflammation of the lymph nodes.

Etiology. Lymphangitis and lymphadenitis are caused by infection of the lymphatic system. Infections are usually associated with cellulitis or abscesses caused by staphylococcal and streptococcal bacteria.

Signs and Symptoms. Characteristic signs and symptoms include fever, pain, general malaise, headache, muscle aches, and swollen and tender lymph glands. In lymphangitis there may be a red line extending from the infection site to the lymph nodes in the axilla, inguinal, or cervical areas with enlargement of lymph nodes in these areas. In lymphadenitis, the lymph nodes are tender to the touch, enlarged, and may be red and inflamed.[54]

Prognosis. Complete recovery from these infections usually occurs with the use of antibiotics/antimicrobials; however, the swelling of the lymph nodes may take a few weeks to subside. Complications that may occur include sepsis (infection throughout the body), cellulitis, and further abscess formation.

Medical Intervention. Diagnostic tests for lymphangitis and lymphadenitis include blood tests to determine infection and possible biopsy of the affected lymph nodes. Medical management is with specific antibiotic drugs after the type of infection is identified.

Physical Therapy Intervention. No physical therapy intervention is indicated for lymphangitis or lymphadenitis. The therapist may, however, detect enlarged lymph nodes within the musculature of the neck in patients with cervical problems due to this condition.

Lymphedema

Lymphedema is a chronic edema resulting from an increase of lymphatic fluid. Lymphedema may occur in the upper and lower extremities. Alternative terminology is elephantiasis.

Etiology. Damage to the lymph nodes can occur as a result of neoplasms (tumors), infection such as cellulitis, trauma or postsurgery (e.g., radical mastectomy—removal of the breast and associated axillary lymph glands), after extensive full-thickness burns, or following radiation treatment. In tropical countries, there is a parasitic worm called filariasis that enters the lymphatic vessels causing blockage.

Signs and Symptoms. In lymphedema, the involved arm or leg swells, and the skin becomes thickened (see Fig. 3-12).

Prognosis. Lymphedema is a chronic condition that requires constant attention and management over a person's lifetime. In some cases, the swelling does diminish a little over time, but it never completely resolves. Approximately 10% to 15% of patients who undergo radical mastectomy are estimated to have lymphedema in the upper extremity of the same side as the surgery.[55]

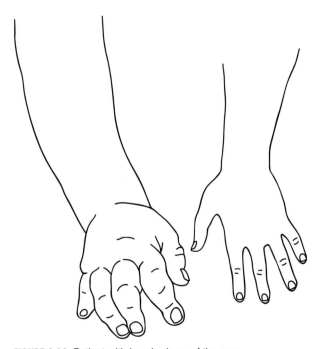

FIGURE 3.12 Patient with lymphedema of the arm.

Medical Intervention. Diagnostic tests performed include lymphangiography and magnetic resonance imaging. Medical management includes referral to a specialized center for lymphedema management where physical therapists and occupational therapist work together with the patient. Complications of the condition can include skin breakdown, chronic wounds, and ulcers, and therefore skin care and hygiene are emphasized.

Physical Therapy Intervention. Physical therapy intervention for lymphedema is a specialized field within physical therapy and involves clearing the proximal areas of the lymphatic system to stimulate the lymphatic system drainage. The PTA has the option of specialization in the management of lymphedema through further education and certification. Elevation of the limb; use of compressive, elastic garments; specific exercise programs; and special systems of massage techniques are all used in a total treatment regimen.

Why Does the Physical Therapist Assistant Need to Know About Cardiovascular System Failure?

PTAs may never observe people who are experiencing hypovolemic shock and organ failure unless they work in the intensive care unit or in an acute care facility. However, understanding the signs and symptoms in people who experience this condition may help to save a life.

Cardiovascular System Failure

When the cardiovascular system fails to function and there is a drop in blood pressure, the body goes into shock.

Hypovolemic Shock and Organ Failure

Hypovolemic shock is caused by the body's inability to supply oxygen to the body's tissues. If left untreated, it ultimately results in organ failure and death.

Etiology. The usual response of the body is to provide blood with essential oxygen to the brain for as long as possible, in which case other body organs may shut down before the brain. Shock can be due to an accident that severs an artery externally. Shock may also occur due to an internal loss of blood from an artery such as in a burst aneurysm or from an intestinal bleed. Cardiogenic shock occurs after a major MI or due to CHF when the heart is not able to pump enough oxygenated blood to the organs and tissues.

Signs and Symptoms. In cases of hypovolemic shock, there is a rise in heart rate with a rapid, weak, thready pulse rate; rapid breathing; a reduction in blood pressure; reduced urine output; confusion; anxiety; weakness; sweating; and possible loss of consciousness. If a person loses a lot of blood (i.e., more than one-fifth of the total blood volume), there is not enough total blood in the system to maintain blood pressure, and this is also termed hemorrhagic shock. In neurogenic shock, blood accumulates in the extremities, but not enough reaches the brain, and the neurons of the brain start to shut down.

Prognosis. Hypovolemic shock is a medical emergency, and the prognosis depends on the amount of blood lost, the speed of intravenous fluid therapy, and the age and medical status of the patient. Complications of hypovolemic shock are kidney and brain damage due to lack of oxygenation of the tissues.

Medical Intervention. Diagnostic tests are performed to identify the cause of the shock if these are not immediately evident. Such tests include a CBC, endoscopy, echocardiogram, and a Swan-Ganz (right heart) catheterization to rule out cardiogenic shock. Medical treatment includes the use of intravenous fluids to restore the fluid volume, medications to increase the blood pressure (e.g., epinephrine, norepinephrine, and dopamine), and prevention of hypothermia by keeping the person warm. Keeping the person flat or raising the legs above the level of head can help to reduce the symptoms of this condition. No fluids should be given by mouth.[56]

Physical Therapy Intervention. Physical therapy intervention is not indicated for organ failure and shock. Therapists may need to use basic first aid to stop external bleeding and severe blood loss in an emergency situation.

Physical Therapy Treatment and the Role of the PTA in Cardiac and Circulatory Conditions

PTAs need to remember that they will be part of a team approach to the treatment of the cardiac patient. The PT is ultimately responsible for the patient and delegation of a patient to a PTA will depend on several factors:

1. The condition of the patient: Is the patient fairly stable medically or is unstable and requiring constant reevaluation during treatment? The more stable patient will be a suitable candidate for the PTA to treat.
2. The PTA may treat the patient with a heart condition in the intensive care unit (ICU) or cardiac care unit (CCU) or may be more involved with the patient in the so-called step-down unit or in later stages of rehabilitation when the patient is more stable.

Other Considerations

1. Patients who are in ICU or CCU will be attached to cardiac monitors. When performing exercises, gait training, and bed mobility exercises, the leads may become loose, and there will be a loud bleeping noise to alert the nurse. Providing PT without causing a problem with the electrode connections is difficult, so it is important that the PTA inform the nurse in charge of the patient when PT intervention is being given. If electrode leads become loose during treatment, the PTA should inform the nurse so that they can be reattached. Patients with certain types of mobile heart monitors may have to receive PT on their floor because the monitors will not work in other areas of the hospital.
2. Try to coordinate treatment time with the schedule for pain medications, bathing activities, and other concerns. The patient should be as comfortable as possible when receiving PT. If pain medication makes the patient sleepy, it may be necessary to wait about 1 hour after medication is given to treat the patient. However, patients should be treated before the effects of the pain medication wear off.
3. Patients with cardiac conditions tend to fatigue rapidly. Remember that a few exercises and a short walk may be all they can tolerate during one visit in the early stages of recovery. Observe the patient carefully for signs of cyanosis, labored breathing, and trembling muscles, all of which can indicate fatigue. Check blood pressure and the perceived exertion level described by the patient regularly.
4. Keep the patient under close observation and monitor heart rate carefully before, during, and after treatment. Report any problems immediately to the PT and nurse. Be careful to document all findings in the patient chart.
5. Be sure to return patients to their room after treatment and leave the room as you found it. Make sure you put the bed rails up before leaving the room unless instructed otherwise by the nurse.

Home Health Physical Therapy

Many patients require home health management before attending an outpatient rehabilitation center for further treatment. The same points should be considered in the home setting. Careful monitoring of the patient must be performed by the PT or PTA before, during, and after treatment, including taking vital signs, monitoring the perceived rate of exertion (PRE), and closely observing the patient for signs of cyanosis, dyspnea, or respiratory distress. Exercise programs must follow a prescribed pattern developed by the physician and the PT. Overhead arm exercises are precluded in the first few weeks, and the patient should perform progressive ambulation exercises, building up gradually to stairs and slopes. Specific prescriptions for exercise may be given that detail the exercises to perform during each week after cardiac surgery or acute cardiac incident. The PTA must also closely observe and monitor the patient when administering these prescribed programs.

Outpatient Cardiac Rehabilitation

Cardiac rehabilitation is often divided into acute (Phase I), subacute (Phase II), intensive rehabilitation (Phase III), and ongoing rehabilitation (Phase IV). The outpatient phases of rehabilitation are those after discharge from the hospital in Phases II, III and IV. The Phase II rehabilitation may take place in an outpatient private PT office or in a hospital outpatient department. PT intervention starts within 1 or 2 days of hospital discharge and lasts up to 6 weeks, with a frequency of two to three visits per week. If patients are not well enough to attend an outpatient unit, they may have this treatment at home from the home health team. Patients are constantly monitored with ECG telemetry and taught how to monitor their own condition and vital signs. The PT individually designs the exercise program to the specific needs of the patient. The rehabilitation team may include a physician, physician assistant, nurse practitioner, social worker, a PT and PTA, an occupational therapist, a cardiac nurse, and a nutritionist. The Phase III program usually lasts for an additional 6 weeks with progressively more intense exercises, and treatment frequency is reduced to once or twice a week. In this phase, the patient performs much of the program at home and should be walking and performing weight-training exercises on a regular basis. The final phase of rehabilitation lasts for up to a year after onset of the program and is the period when the patient exercises regularly with weights, performs a walking program, and follows a heart-healthy lifestyle. As patients progress through the rehabilitation process, they should require less intensive monitoring, but observation should be continued to ensure there are no warning signs of cardiac symptoms. Patients are trained to detect warning signs for themselves and seek help if needed.

CASE STUDY 3.1

A 69-year-old male patient with a history of cardiac problems and mitral valve replacement 4 weeks earlier is coming to the rehabilitation unit for intervention. The PT has evaluated the patient, and the plan of care is for progressive ambulation and stair climbing; progressive exercises for strengthening of lower extremities, which are 3 out of 5 (3/5) on a scale of 1 to 5 strength overall; progressive exercises to increase exercise tolerance; and a home exercise and advice program. The patient is currently ambulating with a rolling walker and not doing stairs.

1. What kinds of monitoring would the PTA perform with this patient?

2. What symptoms would cause the PTA to alert the PT immediately?

3. Develop an exercise program to strengthen the lower extremities from a 3/5 to a 4/5 over the next 4 weeks.

4. Develop a home exercise program to include strengthening and increased exercise tolerance.

5. Give advice to the patient and family members on activities of daily living (ADLs), precautions to be aware of, and reasons to call the physician or PT.

CASE STUDY 3.2

An 80-year-old alert female patient is attending the outpatient department of the acute care hospital in which the PTA works for treatment of a venous stasis ulcer on the left lower leg over the area of the medial malleolus. Intervention is to include whirlpool for left leg, dressings, exercises, and ambulation training. The patient can only walk for 10 feet with a walker with maximal assistance of one person. Lower extremity general strength is 3/5. Upper extremity strength is 4+/5.

1. What are some warning signs the PTA needs to be aware of that would require alerting the PT?

2. Develop a progressive ambulation and lower extremity exercise program for the patient.

3. Develop a home program for the patient and instructions for the care provider.

4. Detail any specific instructions that may be appropriate for a patient with this particular diagnosis.

STUDY QUESTIONS

1. Take the dorsalis pedis pulse on yourself and two other people. Is the pulse easily detectable?

2. List the precautions that you would provide to a patient with peripheral vascular disease. Give the patient hints as to activities and positioning that would assist the patient in reducing symptoms.

3. Describe the symptoms of cardiac disease.

4. Explain to a patient what to expect when he or she goes for a stress test.

⦿ USEFUL WEBSITES

American Heart Association
http://www.americanheart.org

The Auscultation Assistant (Heart Sounds)
http://www.med.ucla.edu/wilkes/inex.htm

Centers for Disease Control and Prevention
http://www.cdc.gov

The Electrocardiogram (ECG) library
http://www.ecglibrary.com

HeartCenterOnline, Inc.
http://heart.healthcentersonline.com

University of Washington Department of Medicine

Heart sounds and murmurs
http://depts.washington.edu/physdx/heart/demo.html

Medline Plus, A.D.A.M., Inc.
http://www.nlm.nih.gov/medlineplus

Medscape
http://www.medscape.com

Normal Heart Sounds
http://www.medstudents.com.br/cardio/heartsounds/heartsou.htm

⦿ REFERENCES

[1] Synapse Publishing. (1996). *Normal heart sounds.* Retrieved 12.02.06 from http://www.medstudents.com.br/cardio/heartsounds/heartsou.htm.

[2] The Auscultation Assistant [heart sounds]. (n.d.). Retrieved from http://www.med.ucla.edu/wilkes/inex.htm

[3] Frownfelter, D., and Dean, E. (2006). *Cardiovascular and pulmonary physical therapy: evidence and practice,* 4th edition. St. Louis, MO: Mosby, Elsevier, p. 220.

[4] Ibid., p. 81.

[5] American Heart Association. (n.d.). Retrieved from http://www.heart.org/HEARTORG/Conditions/Arrhythmia/AboutArrhythmia/Tachycardia_UCM_302018_Article.jsp

[6] Gerred, S., & Jenkins, D. (2002). Retrieved 11.29.2006 from http://www.ecglibrary.com/stach.html

[7] Gerred, S., & Jenkins, D. (2002). ECG library available at http://www.ecglibrary.com

[8] American Heart Association. (n.d.). *Good vs. bad cholesterol.* Retrieved from http://www.americanheart.org/presenter.jhtml?identifier=180

[9] American Heart Association. (n.d.). *Good vs. bad cholesterol.* Idem

[10] Venes, D., Biderman, A., Fenton, B. G., Enright, A. D., Patwell, J., et al. (Editors) (2005). Blood urea nitrogen, *Taber's cyclopedic medical dictionary,* 20th edition. Philadelphia: F. A. Davis, p. 272.

[11] American Heart Association. (2006). *Heart disease and stroke statistics: 2006 update,* p. 13. Available at http://www.americanheart.org/downloadable/heart/1140534985281Statsupdate06book.pdf

[12] Medicinenet.com (n.d.). *Medications and drugs: nitroglycerin.* Retrieved from http://www.medicinenet.com/nitroglycerin/article.htm

[13] American Heart Association. (2006). *Heart disease and stroke statistics: 2006 update.* Retrieved from http://www.americanheart.org/downloadable/heart/1140534985281Statsupdate06book.pdf, p. 22.

[14] Frownfelter, D., & Dean, E. (2006). Ibid., p. 101.

[15] Austin, M. A., et al (2004). Familial hypercholesterolemia and coronary heart disease: a HuGe Association review. *Am J Epidemiol* 160:5, 421–441.

[16] Centers for Disease Control and Prevention. (2010). *High blood cholesterol prevention.* Retrieved from http://www.cdc.gov/cholesterol/prevention.htm

[17] National Institutes of Health and National Heart, Lung, and Blood Institute. (May 2001). *Third report of the National Cholesterol Education Program (NCEP), Expert panel on detection, evaluation, and treatment of high blood cholesterol in adults, Executive summary* (NIH Publication No. 01-3670), p. 5.

[18] American Heart Association. (n.d.). *Cardiac medications.* Retrieved 11.29.06 from http://www.americanheart.org/presenter.jhtml?identifier=4456

[19] American Heart Association. (2006). Heart disease and stroke statistics: 2006 update. Ibid., p. 10.

[20] American Heart Association. (2006). Ibid., p. 10.

[21] American Heart Association. (2006). Ibid., p. 11.

[22] American Heart Association. (2006). Ibid., p. 21.

[23] American Heart Association. (2010). *Congestive heart failure.* Retrieved from http://www.americanheart.org/presenter.jhtml?identifier=4585

[24] Gandhi, M. (2006). *Endocaritis. Medline Plus Medical Encyclopedia.* Retrieved 12.01.06 http://www.nlm.nih.gov/medlineplus/ency/article/001098.htm

[25] Frownfelter, D., and Dean, E. *(2006). Cardiovascular and pulmonary physical therapy: evidence and practice,* 4th edition. St. Louis, MO: Mosby, Elsevier.

[26] Centers for Disease Control and Prevention, U.S. Department of

Health and Human Services, National Center for Health Statistics. (2006). *Health, United States, 2006 with chartbook on trends in the health of Americans*. Retrieved 11.29.06 from http://www.cdc.gov/nchs/data/hus/hus06.pdf#executivesummary, p. 66.

[27] American Heart Association (n.d.). http://www.americanheart.org/presenter.jhtml?identifier=4720

[28] American Heart Association. (n.d.). *Silent ischemia and ischemic heart disease*. Retrieved from http://www.americanheart.org/presenter.jhtml?identifier=4720

[29] Gandelman, G. (2006). Myocarditis. *Medline Plus Medical Encyclopedia*. Retrieved 12.01.06 http://www.nlm.nih.gov/medlineplus/ency/article/000149.htm

[30] Ibid.

[31] Ibid.

[32] Vijayalakshmi, I. B., Mithravinda, J., Deva, A. N. (2005). The role of echocardiography in diagnosing carditis in the setting of acute rheumatic fever. *Cardiol Young* 15:583–588.

[33] Adis International Limited (2000). Rheumatic fever: a preventable and treatable public health problem. *Drugs Ther Perspect* 15:5–8. Retrieved 11.30.06 from http://www.medscape.com/viewpublication/89_toc?vol=15&iss=9

[34] Dressler, D. K. (2002). Heart transplantation. In *Organ transplantation: concepts, issues, practice, and outcomes* (chapter 13). Retrieved 11.30.06 from http://www.medscape.com/viewpublication/704_about

[35] Ibid.

[36] Leslie, M., Fitzgerald, D. C., & Mikanowicz, C. (2003). Musculoskeletal aching in the older adult: polymyalgia rheumatica and giant cell arteritis. *Topics Adv Pract Nurs eJournal* 3. Retrieved 11.30.06 from http://www.medscape.com/viewarticle/448336

[37] Eagle, K. A., & Armstrong, W. F. (2002). Diseases of the aorta: Takayasu arteritis and giant cell arteritis. *ACP Med Online*. Retrieved 11.30.06 from http://www.medscape.com/viewarticle/535386

[38] Ibid.

[39] Centers for Disease Control and Prevention, US Department of Health and Human Services, National Center for Health Statistics. (2010). Retrieved 1.3.11 from www.cdc.gov/stroke/facts.htm.

[40] Jauch, E. C., & Kissela, B. (2010). Acute stroke management: Frequency. *EMedicine from WebMD*. Available at http://emedicine.medscape.com/article/1159752-overview

[41] Jauch, E. C., & Kissela, B. (2010). Acute stroke management: Clinical history. *EMedicine from WebMD*. Available at http://emedicine.medscape.com/article/1159752-overview

[42] Thavendiranathan, P., et al. (2006). Primary prevention of cardiovascular diseases with statin therapy. *Arch Intern Med* 166:2307–2313.

[43] Christopher-Stine, L. (2006). Polyarteritis nodosa. *Medline Plus Medical Encyclopedia*. Retrieved 12.01.06 from http://www.nlm.nih.gov/medlineplus/ency/article/001438.htm

[44] Grader-Beck, T., & Wigley, F. M. (2005). Raynaud's phenomenon in mixed connective tissue disease. *Rheum Dis Clin North Am* 31:465–481. Retrieved 11.30.06 from http://www.medscape.com/medline/abstract/16084319?queryText=raynaud%20disease

[45] American Heart Association. (2006). *What is peripheral vascular disease?* Retrieved 12.1.06 from http://www.americanheart.org/presenter.jhtml?identifier=4692

[46] Hart, J. A. (2004). Thromboangiitis obliterans. *Medline Plus Medical Encyclopedia*. Retrieved 12.01.06 from http://www.nlm.nih.gov/medlineplus/ency/article/000172.htm

[47] American Heart Association. (2006). What is peripheral vascular disease? Retrieved 12.1.06 from http://www.americanheart.org/presenter.jhtml?identifier=4692

[48] Sussman, C., & Bates-Jensen, B. M. (2001). *Wound care: a collaborative manual for physical therapists and nurses*. Gaithersburg, MD: Aspen, p. 627.

[49] Sussman, C., & Bates-Jensen, B. M. (2001). Ibid.

[50] Brose, M. S. (2004). Anemia. *Medline Plus Medical Encyclopedia*. Retrieved 12.01.06 from http://www.nlm.nih.gov/medlineplus/ency/article/000560.htm

[51] Matsui, W. (2005). Acute lymphocytic leukemia. *Medline Plus Medical Encyclopedia*. Retrieved 12.01.06 from http://www.nlm.nih.gov/medlineplus/ency/article/000541.htm

[52] Brose, M. S. (2004). Chronic lymphocytic leukemia. *Medline Plus Medical Encyclopedia*. Retrieved 12.01.06 http://www.nlm.nih.gov/medlineplus/ency/article/000532.htm

[53] Matsui, W. (2006). Hodgkin's lymphoma. *Medline Plus Medical Encyclopedia*. Retrieved 12.01.06 http://www.nlm.nih.gov/medlineplus/ency/article/000580.htm

[54] Gandhi, M. (2005). Lymphadenitis and lymphangitis. *Medline Plus Medical Encyclopedia*. Retrieved 12.01.06 http://www.nlm.nih.gov/medlineplus/ency/article/001301.htm

[55] Lee, J. A. (2006). Lymphatic obstruction. *Medline Plus Medical Encyclopedia*. Retrieved 12.01.06 http://www.nlm.nih.gov/medlineplus/ency/article/001117.htm

[56] Perez, E. (2006). Hypovolemic shock. *Medline Plus Medical Encyclopedia*. Retrieved 12.01.06 http://www.nlm.nih.gov/medlineplus/ency/article/000167.htm

[57] O'Sullivan, S. B., & Schmitz, T. (2007). *Physical rehabilitation*, 5th edition. Philadelphia: F. A. Davis, p. 602.

[58] Ibid., p. 595.

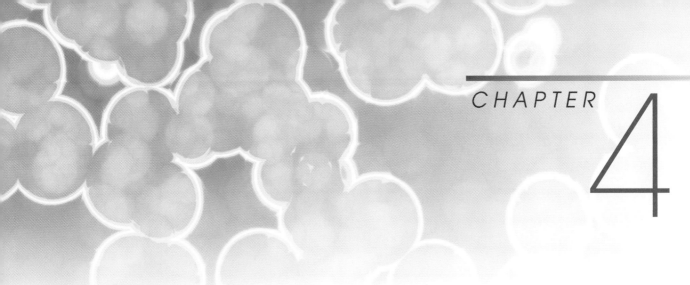

CHAPTER 4

Respiratory Diseases

LEARNING OBJECTIVES

After completion of this chapter, students should be able to:

- Review the anatomy and physiology of the respiratory system
- Describe the major functions of the lungs
- Describe common respiratory pathologies seen in physical therapy
- Recognize the general signs and symptoms of respiratory diseases
- Perform patient positioning for postural drainage of any given lung segment
- Analyze the appropriateness of exercise programs and treatment within the plan of care developed by the physical therapist for a patient with respiratory pathology
- Identify various tests that may be performed by the medical team for patients with respiratory diseases
- Discuss the types of surgery used for patients with severe respiratory pathologies
- Determine the contraindications and precautions for physical therapy intervention for patients with major respiratory conditions

CHAPTER OUTLINE

KEY TERMS

Atelectasis

Auscultation techniques

Bronchiectasis

Bronchopneumonia

Bronchopulmonary segments

Chest excursion

Controlled mechanical ventilation (CMV)

Empyema

Forced expiratory volume in 1 second (FEV1)

Graded exercise tolerance test (GXTT)

Hemoptysis

Metabolic equivalent (MET)

Nebulizer

Oxyhemoglobin dissociation curve

Pleural effusion

Pleural rub/friction rub

Positive expiratory pressure (PEP) therapy

Pyothorax

Surfactant

Ventilation-perfusion ratio (or quotient)

Introduction

This chapter reviews the anatomy and physiology of the respiratory system at both the cellular and organ levels. The most commonly used respiratory function tests are discussed. Diseases of the respiratory system are described, including the general signs and symptoms of all respiratory diseases and the etiology, prognosis, medical treatments, and physical therapy interventions for people with specific diseases. The chapter explains the role of the physical therapist assistant in working with people with respiratory pathologies, and details of appropriate physical therapy interventions are described.

Why Does the Physical Therapist Assistant Need to know About the Anatomy and Physiology of the Respiratory System?

Physical therapy interventions for people with respiratory pathologies are a vital part of physical therapy practice in many settings. The physical therapist assistant (PTA) sees patients with respiratory conditions within the acute care hospital, rehabilitation centers, and in certain outpatient settings. Whether the respiratory condition is the primary focus for the physical therapy management or a comorbid diagnosis for the physical therapy diagnosis, the PTA must have knowledge of the healthy lungs and respiratory system in order to provide the appropriate intervention as designated by the physical therapist (PT).

Anatomy and Physiology of the Respiratory System

This section provides a basic overview of the anatomy and physiology of the respiratory system, the respiratory contents of the thoracic cage, and the movements of the thorax and ribs. The muscles of respiration are described, and the mechanisms of ventilation and respiration at the cellular level are delineated, including normal and abnormal breathing patterns, ventilation control, lung capacity, gaseous exchange, and oxygen transport.

The Thoracic Cage and Its Contents

The heart and lungs are next to each other in the thoracic cavity, or thorax, and together with their associated blood vessels are jointly known as the cardiopulmonary system. The respiratory system is divided into the upper respiratory tract consisting of the nose, nasal passages, pharynx, and larynx (see Fig. 4-1), and the lower respiratory tract consisting of the trachea, bronchi, their branches of bronchioles, and the terminal alveoli within the lungs. The nose is divided by the nasal septum. The part of the nasal cavity closest to the nostrils has a lining of skin and hairs. These hairs help to trap particles that are inhaled, preventing them from entering the lower respiratory tract and potentially causing infection. The other areas of the nasal cavity and sinuses are lined with a mucous membrane, which possesses hairlike cilia to filter unwanted particles, and some mucous-producing glands. The pharynx extends superiorly from the upper end of the esophagus to the soft palate of the mouth and the posterior aspect of the nasal cavity. The larynx is a section of the pharynx that acts as a cartilaginous sphincter device situated in the lower part of the pharynx. The larynx is known in lay terms as the "Adam's apple." Actually the Adam's apple is only the thyroid cartilage part of the larynx. The larynx consists of

the hyoid bone and several cartilages including the cricoid, thyroid, epiglottic, corniculates, cuneiforms, and right and left arytenoids.[1] The vocal cords or vocal folds are structures of mucous membrane within the larynx that surround two vocal ligaments, which extend from the thyroid cartilage to the arytenoid cartilage. The vocal cords vibrate as air passes over them, causing sounds to be produced.[2] As a person swallows food, the epiglottis part of the larynx (a thin, fibrocartilaginous structure situated at the upper end of the larynx and at the base of the root of the tongue) closes over the trachea to prevent food from passing into the trachea.[3] The epiglottis also closes when the cough reflex is initiated so that pressure can be built up in the trachea to produce an effective cough. When the muscles that control the action of the larynx do not work, food or liquids can pass down the trachea, causing aspiration into the lungs. The larynx is innervated by a branch of the vagus nerve, which can become inactive after neurological events such as a cerebrovascular accident (CVA) or after general anaesthesia. Inactivity of the vagus nerve can increase the possibility of aspiration. To enable speech, air must pass over the vocal cords, and swallowing requires that the epiglottis be closed over the trachea to prevent aspiration. When trying to speak and eat at the same time, the epiglottis is not closed over the trachea, and thus fluids and food particles may pass into the trachea.

The trachea is the main airway from the nose and mouth cavity and bifurcates (divides into two) at the level of the suprasternal notch anteriorly and the level of the fifth thoracic vertebra posteriorly (see Fig. 4-2). This point is called the bifurcation of the trachea, and one of

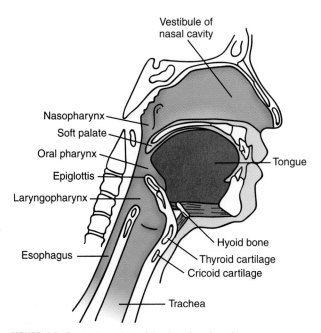

FIGURE 4.1 Sagittal section of the head and neck.

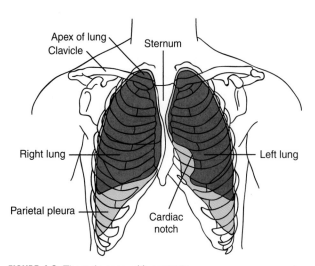

FIGURE 4.2 Thoracic cage with contents.

the cough reflex points is located here at the carina.[4] Other areas of possible stimulation of the cough reflex lie in the larynx, trachea, and lower bronchi.[5] The right bronchus runs distally as a continuation of the trachea, whereas the left bronchus deviates left at an angle. Most aspirated food and fluids pass down the trachea into the right lung because there is a straight line of access into the right lung via the right bronchus. In addition, the right bronchus is slightly larger in diameter than the left bronchus and thus allows food to pass through easily.[6] The trachea is composed of incomplete rings of cartilage, elastic and fibrous tissue, and some muscle. The structure of the trachea enables it to both move and stretch during breathing. The lining of the trachea is a mucous membrane with columnar epithelial cells. Each of these cells has more than 250 cilia, which are hairlike structures that beat toward the upper respiratory tract and attempt to take any foreign particles or mucus away from the lungs.[7]

The left and right bronchi enter the left and right lungs. These bronchi then branch many times, becoming progressively narrower from bronchi to bronchioles, to terminal bronchioles, to respiratory bronchioles, to alveolar ducts, and then to the alveolar sacs. The alveolar sacs, or alveoli, are small saclike structures that provide an increased surface area where gaseous exchange occurs. Oxygen is passed into the blood vessels from the lung, and carbon dioxide is passed from the tissues back into the bronchioles for disposal through the respiratory tract.

As described in Chapter 3, the pulmonary artery carries deoxygenated blood from the heart to the lungs, where it becomes oxygenated. The pulmonary vein carries oxygenated blood from the lungs to the left atrium of the heart where it is pumped to the rest of the body via the left ventricle. The heart and lungs are closely related in their functions so that when a problem arises with one, there is often a problem with the other. The thorax (rib cage) provides rigid, bony protection for the lungs and associated respiratory structures. The thorax consists of the 12 ribs, the 12 thoracic vertebrae posteriorly and the sternum and xiphoid process anteriorly. Ribs 1 through 7 are true ribs because they attach by joints to the vertebrae posteriorly and attach to the sternum anteriorly. The lower five ribs are called false ribs because they do not attach directly to the sternum. Ribs 8, 9, and 10 attach to the cartilage formed from the upper ribs, and ribs 11 and 12 are "floating" ribs because they do not attach to anything anteriorly. The longest rib is the seventh. Ribs 1 through 7 become progressively longer, and ribs 8 through 12 get progressively shorter. Each of the ribs has an articulation with two vertebrae and has a curve known as the "angle" of the rib.

The inferior border of each rib has a channel or groove that helps to protect the intercostal nerves and blood vessels. The intercostal muscles connect adjoining ribs, filling in the spaces between the ribs.

MOVEMENTS OF THE THORAX

Movements of the thorax are important to the function of the lungs. For inhalation, or intake of air from the atmosphere into the lungs, the thoracic cavity must increase in size. The reduction of size of the thoracic cavity, and thus the lungs, in exhalation enables expulsion of carbon dioxide from the body. Other names for the process of inhalation and exhalation from the lungs are ventilation or external respiration. Use of the terms ventilation, inhalation, and exhalation help to delineate between the process of external respiration and that of gaseous exchange at the cellular level of the alveoli, which is true respiration or internal respiration. For the purposes of this book, the intake of air into the lungs and the expulsion of air from the lungs are called inhalation and exhalation, respectively.

The thoracic spine does not have as much movement as the lumbar or cervical spines because the attachment of the ribs reduces the mobility of the thoracic spine to provide stability and protection of the thoracic contents. Two types of movement of the ribs exist known as "bucket handle" and "pump handle." The upper ribs move like a pump handle, causing the sternum to move forward and making the thorax larger in an anterior–posterior direction and also slightly in depth. The lower ribs tend to move out to the side in much the same way that a bucket handle moves and increase the lateral diameter of the thorax. Using these two types of movement, the thorax can increase in size during inhalation in all directions. In general, the ribs move up and out during inhalation, and down and in during exhalation, creating an increase and then a decrease, respectively, in the size of the thoracic cavity. The pleural cavity as a whole acts as a vacuum so that movement of the ribs creates a negative pressure during inhalation assisting expansion of the lungs and a positive pressure during exhalation that assists the compression of the lungs. The main increase in depth of the thorax is caused by contraction of the diaphragm muscle during inhalation; the muscles of ventilation are discussed later in the chapter.

THE LUNGS

People have two lungs, consisting of many cells that have the overall appearance of a sponge in texture. The left lung is narrower and smaller than the right because of the space occupied by the heart. However; the left lung is longer than the right because the liver pushes up beneath the diaphragm on the right side (see Table 4-1 for surface

Table 4.1 **Surface Marking for the Respiratory System**

STRUCTURE OF LUNG	SURFACE MARKING ON THE BODY
Apices (pleural of apex) of lung	2.5 cm superior to clavicles
Medial border right lung	Sternoclavicular joint to xiphisternum
Extent of inferior border right lung	Xiphisternum to sixth rib in midclavicular line, 8th rib in midaxillary line, and 10th rib from midscapular line (with arm at rest by the side)
Extent of medial border left lung	Sternoclavicular joint to mid sternum and then deviates for heart (cardiac notch) at level of 5 and 6 costal cartilages, then similar to right lung
Bifurcation of trachea	Sternal notch anteriorly/level 5th thoracic vertebra posteriorly

marking of the respiratory system). Each lung has an apex, or upper part, and a basal portion that lies adjacent to the diaphragm. Both lungs are divided into lobes separated by fissures (see Fig. 4-3). The right lung has upper, middle, and lower lobes. The left lung has only upper and lower lobes because of the space occupied by the heart. The lingular lobe of the left lung is sometimes considered to be the equivalent of the middle lobe but is really part of the upper lobe.[8,9] The three dimensional images from the National Institutes of Health (2004) Visible Human Project help to explain the relationships of the lobes of the lungs and the contents of the thoracic cavity.[10] Two layers of membranes called pleura cover the lungs. The inner layer of pleura is called the visceral pleura and is attached to the lung itself. The outer membrane is the parietal pleura, which lines the thorax and is actually an extension of the visceral pleura. The space between the

layers of pleura contains a small amount of fluid called **surfactant** to allow the two layers of pleura to glide over each other as the lungs expand during breathing. This potential space between the pleura serves to keep the parietal and visceral pleura together and also exerts a negative pressure that helps to draw the lung tissue to the walls of the thorax and prevents the lungs from collapsing.[11] The nerve supply of the lungs arises from the parasympathetic and sympathetic sections of the vagus nerve (10th cranial nerve).[12] The parasympathetic nervous system causes constriction (narrowing) of the bronchi, and the sympathetic nervous system causes dilation (bronchial relaxation).[13]

Each lung lobe is divided into **bronchopulmonary segments** (see Table 4-2) constituting the bronchial tree (see Figs. 4-4 and 4-5). The left lung consists of 9 bronchopulmonary segments, and the right lung consists of 10 segments. (Some sources say there are 8 segments in the left lung because they combine the apical and posterior segments of the left upper lobe.[14]) Some anatomical models may also combine the apical and posterior segments of the left upper lobe, which can be confusing for students. This discrepancy in description of the segments of the lungs does not change either the anatomy of the lungs or treatment aspects. The PTA should concentrate on understanding the position of the lung segments and the direction of the bronchioles entering these segments to facilitate airway clearance for patients with lung disease.

When placing patients into a position for postural drainage, the concept is to position them so that the lobar bronchi point upward against gravity. This position allows secretions collected in the lung lobes or segments to pass down into the bronchus with the help of gravity. After the secretions are in the bronchus, they can then pass to the

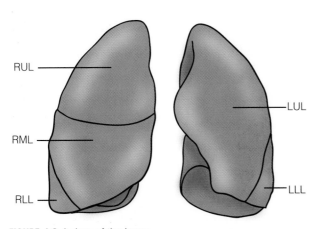

FIGURE 4.3 Lobes of the lungs.

Table 4.2 **Bronchopulmonary Segments of the Lungs**

RIGHT LUNG	SEGMENT	LEFT LUNG	SEGMENT
Upper lobe	Apical Posterior	Upper lobe	Apical Posterior (these two segments are combined in some sources)
	Anterior		Anterior
Middle lobe	Lateral Medial		Superior (lingular) Inferior (lingular)
Lower lobe	Superior (apical) Medial basal (cardiac) Anterior basal Lateral basal Posterior basal	Lower lobe	Superior (apical) (No medial basal because of position of heart)_____ Anterior basal Lateral basal Posterior basal

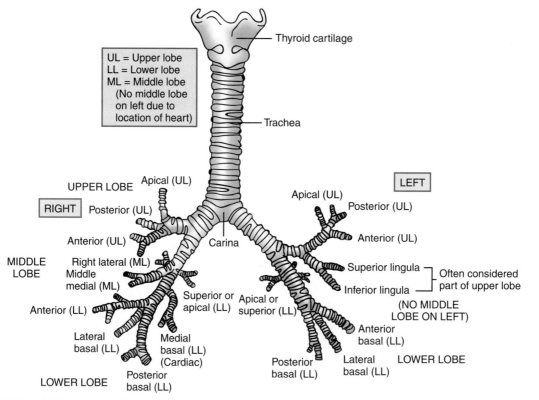

FIGURE 4.4 Bronchial tree showing bronchial branches to all segments of the lungs.

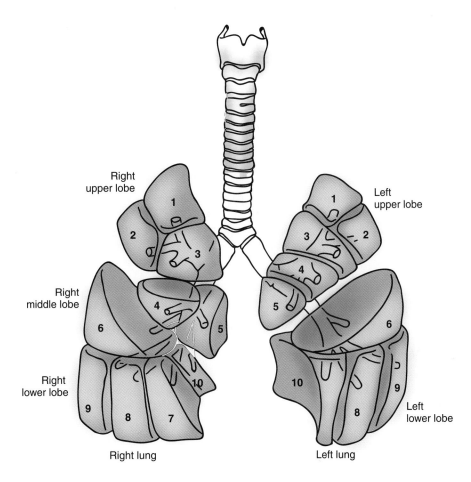

FIGURE 4.5 Bronchopulmonary segments of lungs: 1) apical (UL), 2) posterior (UL), 3) anterior (UL), 4) right lateral (ML), 4) left superior lingular (UL), 5) right medial (ML), 5) left inferior lingular (UL), 6) right and left superior or apical (LL), 7) right only medial basal (LL) (cardiac), 8) anterior basal (LL), 9) lateral basal (LL), and 10) posterior basal (LL).

major bronchi, where they can reach the carina and stimulate the cough reflex to remove the secretions. A three-dimensional model of the bronchi is helpful to understand the direction of the bronchi. Most anatomy departments have such models available for review (refer to Fig. 4-4).

Physiology of Ventilation and Respiration

The physiology of ventilation and respiration is controlled by neurological and muscular factors. The exchange of oxygen at the cellular level is affected by breathing patterns, voluntary and involuntary neurological control, lung capacity, and perfusion levels among various tissues of the respiratory system.

BREATHING PATTERNS

The normal resting rate of ventilations (inhalation and exhalation cycle) is between 12 and 20 breaths per minute (bpm) and is called eupnea. The terms used to describe abnormal breathing patterns are apnea for cessation of breathing, tachypnea for fast breathing, and bradypnea for slow breathing. The respiratory rate considered to be bradypnea is usually below 10 bpm and above 24 bpm to be considered tachypnea.[15] In the newborn, the respiratory rate is between 25 and 50 bpm and gradually reduces with age. The accepted values of respiratory rate for a 3-year-old child are 20 to 30 bpm, and at age 16 years, the rate is 15 to 20 bpm.[16]

Following are some of the more common breathing condition terms. *Sleep apnea* occurs when a person stops breathing, or has breathing that is too shallow to enable sufficient oxygen to perfuse in the lungs, when asleep, usually causing the person to awaken. This disturbed sleep pattern can lead to sleep deprivation and may affect mental functions and cause severe fatigue that can increase the likelihood of accidents.[17,18] *Hypopnea* is a symptom found in patients with respiratory disease in which there is reduced ventilation. Hypopnea, as well as sleep apnea, are more marked at night and may necessitate the use of nocturnal oxygen. A prolonged phase of exhalation may occur in patients with obstructive airways disease as a result of the smaller bronchioles closing down during exhalation, thus reducing the ability to expel air. If patients perform pursed-lip breathing, they may be able to control exhalation and prevent the collapse of the small bronchioles by maintaining a good pressure differential within the thoracic cage. A *Cheyne-Stokes breathing* pattern consists of irregular exhalation and inhalation with some deep breaths and some shallow. Cheyne-Stokes breathing is associated with severe medical problems such as heart failure and is often noted in patients who are dying. Patients with cerebellar dysfunction may experience *ataxic breathing,* which is characterized by irregular depth of breaths. Patients with brain damage may experience *apneustic breathing* in which there is a prolonged inhalation phase.

VENTILATION CONTROL

The control mechanisms of breathing are both involuntary and voluntary. Under normal circumstances, no thought has to be given to the act of breathing. A person can intentionally stop breathing for a few seconds during activities such as defecation, giving birth, or diving under water without any detrimental effects. Other activities that cause cessation of breathing for short periods of time are the involuntary responses such as yawning, laughing, and vomiting. When people speak, cough, or sing, they are using exhalation, and when sucking through a straw, they are using inhalation. The control centers for ventilation are centers in the brain and certain reflexes. Ventilation is so crucial to life that the involuntary control centers are in the more primitive areas of the brain in the reticular formation of the medulla and the pons.[19] Chemoreceptors in the medulla respond to changes in levels of carbon dioxide in the blood. If the partial pressure of carbon dioxide (pCO2) increases (the concentration of carbon dioxide in the blood), these chemoreceptors cause an increase in both the rate and depth of ventilation to bring more oxygen into the system.[20] Other chemoreceptors that cause an increased ventilation rate and depth of breathing are found in the carotid artery and the aorta. These receptors also respond to changes in the levels of carbon dioxide and oxygen in the blood.

Several reflexes affect ventilation. ⊛ The Hering-Breuer reflex is thought to have receptors in the smooth muscle walls of the trachea, bronchi, and bronchioles; however, research findings suggest that the reflex has more effect in the newborn than the adult.[21] The Hering-Breuer reflex is activated when the lungs are overinflated. In this situation, the Hering-Breuer reflex delays the start of the next inhalation; however, there must be a large increase in the lung volume to activate the reflex. The cough reflex is initiated when a stimulus affects the carina, or parts of the larynx, trachea, or lower bronchi. A stimulus could be a foreign particle such as food, dust, or mucus produced by the lungs. The cough reflex causes constriction of the bronchi and a high-speed exhalation that removes, or attempts to remove, any foreign particle in the trachea and propel it toward the mouth.[22] The stretch reflex may also play a part in the ventilatory control system.[23] Muscle spindles respond to elongation of the muscle where they are located. Muscle spindles are located both in the diaphragm and the intercostal muscles. When the muscle spindle is stimulated by stretch of the muscles, an impulse is sent to the spinal cord and the motor neurons of the anterior horn that initiates further contraction of the muscle.

The oxygen content of normal air is approximately 20% to 21%. When the muscles of inhalation enlarge the volume of the thoracic cage, the pressure in the alveoli is lowered. The pressure within the alveoli becomes lower than the atmospheric pressure of air, causing air to rush into the lungs from the atmosphere. The flow of air into the lungs during inhalation is called ventilation. A patient who cannot expand the chest enough to create negative pressure inside the lungs due to illness or paralysis of the respiratory muscles may need assistance with ventilation. Positive pressure ventilators are discussed later in this chapter and in Chapter 13 on intensive care. The muscles used for forced inhalation include the intercostals and diaphragm used in healthy breathing, plus the sternocleidomastoid, scalenes, serratus anterior, pectoralis major and minor, trapezius, and erector spinae. (See the section "Muscles of Ventilation" for further details.) The use of these additional accessory muscles of respiration accounts for the fact that many people with obstructive airways disease note muscle fatigue in these accessory muscles.

Exhalation occurs when the pressure inside the lung within the alveoli is greater than that of the atmosphere. During exhalation, the size of the thoracic cavity becomes smaller, which increases the alveolar pressure above that of the atmospheric air forcing air out of the lungs.[24] Exhalation is a result of the relaxation of the muscles that cause inhalation. Exhalation is thus a passive mechanism involving the relaxation of the muscles of inhalation, such as the diaphragm and intercostals, and the return of the ribs to their resting position. Forced expiration requires the use of the abdominal muscles as well as the internal intercostal muscles and the diaphragm.[25] Healthy lungs are easily inflated, which is known as compliance. Compliance is due both to the elastic nature of the lungs and to a fluid called pulmonary surfactant in the walls of the alveoli. The surfactant reduces surface tension in the alveoli and makes it easier for air to be taken into the alveoli.[26] If surfactant levels are low, the patient may need a ventilator to assist with breathing. The recoil of the thorax and the elasticity of the lungs contribute to keeping the lungs inflated inside the thorax. Healthy function of the lungs depends on both the elasticity of the lung tissue and the resistance of the chest wall, which causes a pulling motion on the lung tissue. These factors create a pressure gradient, which maintains lung inflation in the healthy individual. Full function of the lungs also depends on the ability of the airways to contract and relax. In individuals with respiratory diseases, the ability of the airways to contract and relax is impaired or altered. In persons with healthy lungs, resistance to the flow of air is reduced during inhalation because the airways dilate (enlargement in size of the internal diameter or lumen) and is increased during exhalation when the airways contract (reduction in size of the internal diameter or lumen of the airways).

LUNG CAPACITIES AND VOLUMES

Lung capacity (amount of air that can be inhaled into the lungs) values in Table 4-3 are for the average adult male; The lung capacities for an average adult female are approximately 25% less. Lung capacity for adults also varies according to height and age and tends to reduce with age. If the capacities are lower than usually expected, a lung function problem may be suspected.

The Vital Capacity (VC), sometimes called Forced Vital Capacity (FVC), and the **forced expiratory volume in 1 second (FEV1)** can both be measured using a spirometer. VC is the maximum amount of air exhaled after a maximal inhalation.[27] FEV1 is the volume of air forcibly expired after a maximal inspiration in one second. The FEV1 in a healthy individual young adult is normally approximately 80% of the VC. The percentage reduces with age even in a healthy adult to approximately

Table 4.3 **Lung Capacities in the Healthy Adult Male**

TYPE OF LUNG CAPACITY	DEFINITION	VOLUME OF AIR IN NORMAL ADULT MALE
Tidal volume (VT) or (TV)	Air inhaled/exhaled, each breath, in normal, quiet breathing	500 mL (0.5 L)
Inspiratory reserve volume (IRV)	Extra air that can be inhaled over tidal volume	2500 mL
Expiratory reserve volume (ERV)	Extra air that can be exhaled over tidal volume	1000 mL
Residual volume (RV)	Air that stays in lungs after forced expiration	1500 mL
Inspiratory capacity (IC)	Tidal volume + inspiratory reserve volume	3000 mL
Functional Residual Capacity (FRC)	Expiratory reserve volume + residual volume – air left in lungs after normal exhalation	2500 mL
Vital capacity (VC) or forced vital capacity (FVC)	Inspiratory reserve volume + tidal volume + expiratory Reserve volume – maximum amount of air exhaled after a maximal inhalation	4000 mL
Forced expiratory volume in 1 second (FEV1)	Volume of air that is forcibly expired after maximal inspiration in one second; usually 80% of VC	3200 mL
Total lung capacity (TLC)	All lung volumes added together	5500 mL
Minute ventilation (V)	Tidal Volume × Rate of Ventilation	500 × 15 = 7500

70% to 75%.[28] A change in the ratio of VC and FEV1 indicates lung pathology. The FEV1 reflects healthy, elastic, lung tissue because it shows that most of the air can be expelled from the lungs quickly. In obstructive airway diseases such as emphysema, asthma, and chronic bronchitis, the FEV1 is greatly reduced. In these patients the functional residual capacity (FRC), residual volume (RV), and total lung capacity (TLC) all are increased as a result of overinflation of the lungs. The combination of overinflation of the lungs and the reduced ability to exhale the air from the lungs creates a reduction of the ratio of FEV1/FVC. The ratio of FEV1/FVC can be as low as 70% and the FEV1 as low as 30% in persons with obstructive airways diseases.[29] If the airway disease is reversible, such as in asthma, the ratio will return to more normal values after the patient receives a bronchodilator medication (dilates the bronchi). In patients with restrictive airways diseases (inability of the lungs to fully expand) involving fibrosis (hardening) of the lung tissue or a collapsed lung, the ratio of FEV1/FVC may remain at 80%, but the VC, RV, and TLC all are reduced.[30]

GASEOUS EXCHANGE AND OXYGEN TRANSPORT

The process of transport of oxygen within the body includes the process of how oxygen is provided to all the tissues and also how deoxygenated blood is returned to the lungs for reoxygenation. PTAs need to be familiar with the basics of the oxygen transport system so that they can detect potential problems during physical therapy interventions for patients with cardiopulmonary conditions that require consultation by the PT. Air inhaled into the lungs (inhalation) and carbon dioxide exhaled (exhalation) from the lungs is called ventilation or external respiration. The exchange of oxygen and carbon dioxide within the cells is true respiration or internal respiration. Oxygen is required by the cells of the body to function, and carbon dioxide is the waste product of cellular activity.

Diffusion is the process by which oxygen is transported into the red blood cells from the alveoli of the lungs. Oxygen must pass through several layers of tissue and fluid on its journey from the atmosphere into the lungs including the surfactant, the alveolar membrane, and then through the capillary wall and into the red blood cell where it combines with hemoglobin. In some lung diseases such as chronic bronchitis and asthma, fluid builds up in the alveoli or the lung tissue becomes inflamed and thickened.[31-32] In such cases, oxygen cannot pass through the lung to the erythrocytes as readily, and levels of oxygen in the tissues are reduced.

Students should consult their physiology texts for a more detailed description of gaseous exchange. However, some important points to remember are the following:

- O_2 and CO_2 both are soluble in the cell membranes and thus easily pass through the alveolar membranes.
- O_2 does not dissolve in water as easily as CO_2. This becomes significant when there are secretions in the lungs that reduce the rate of diffusion of O_2 into the blood.
- CO_2 diffuses across the alveolar membranes much more quickly than O_2.
- Gaseous exchange is facilitated by the concentration of gases on either side of the membrane, both in a gaseous form and when dissolved in liquids. CO_2 will tend to move from an area of high concentration of CO_2 (within the tissues) toward an area of lower concentration (within the alveoli). The reverse is true for O_2.

In gases, diffusion is affected by the concentration of a particular gas such as O_2 within the area. This concentration is called the partial pressure of the gas. In simple terms, the concentration of a specific gas within a gaseous mixture is its partial pressure. Partial pressure of oxygen is noted as PO_2 and that of carbon dioxide PCO_2. When gases pass through the alveolar membrane they are affected by both gaseous and liquid physical principles as the result of the liquid surrounding the alveolar membrane and the gas within the alveolar sac.

The term "perfusion" relates to blood in the pulmonary vessels that supplies the lung tissue. The effect of gravity tends to make more blood available to supply the lower lobes of the lungs than the upper ones.[33,34] If perfusion is reduced in an area of the lung, there will also be a reduced ability for oxygen to diffuse from the lungs into the blood vessels for transport of oxygen to the tissues. This relationship is called the **ventilation-perfusion ratio or quotient**. In the healthy adult, the ventilation-perfusion ratio (V/Q ratio) is 0.8 (80%).[35,36] The values of the V/Q ratio enable the physician and PT to evaluate the need to administer oxygen to the patient. PTAs should follow the amount of oxygen dosage indicated by the physician and the PT when providing physical therapy intervention to the patient.

Oxygen combines with a protein in the blood called hemoglobin to form oxyhemoglobin, which is then transported to tissues that require oxygen. The oxygen in the hemoglobin is released when the level of oxygen in the tissues is lower than that in the blood. Because arterial blood is approximately 98% oxygen, any level of oxygen in the tissues below this level precipitates transfer of oxygen to these tissues. Hemoglobin has the ability to combine with large amounts of oxygen and is thus able to supply all the tissues in the body without ever losing all of its oxygen.[37] The lower the oxygen pressure in the tissues, the more oxygen is released from the hemoglobin. The relationship between the hemoglobin, and the release of oxygen from the hemoglobin, is called the **oxyhemoglobin dissociation curve.** The curve demonstrates the correlation between oxygen saturation levels of the hemoglobin and the partial pressure of oxygen in the blood.[38] Some diseases and pathological conditions, such as hypothermia and alkalemia, make it more difficult for oxygen to be released from the hemoglobin. Carbon dioxide is a by-product of cell metabolism and must be removed from the body. The venous blood carries CO_2 to the lungs where it is expelled. When the lungs do not function fully, the CO_2 is not removed, and because it is acid, it causes a drop in the normal pH of the lung causing acute respiratory acidosis.[39] If a patient hyperventilates, this can cause an increase in the pH level, leading to acute respiratory alkalosis.[40]

Oxygen is essential to all tissues of the body for life and energy. Adenosine triphosphate (ATP) is the substance at the basis of all energy production in the body. ATP fuels muscle contractions of all skeletal, heart, and internal organ muscles and stimulates nerve conduction. ATP is produced through complicated processes including the Krebs cycle and the electron transfer chain that occur in the mitochondria (refer to a physiology text for further details). Each of these processes requires the use of oxygen. The transport of oxygen to body tissues also relies on the heart and peripheral circulation. If the heart is malfunctioning, then oxygen delivery will be reduced, and respiratory function is compromised.

Muscles of Ventilation

Quiet or resting inhalation requires the muscle activity created mainly by the contraction of the diaphragm and the external intercostal muscles. The accessory muscles involved in inhalation are mainly used for increased expansion of the lungs, such as during exercise, or in the presence of respiratory or ventilation disease. These accessory muscles include the sternocleidomastoids, scalenes, serratus anterior, pectoralis major and minor, trapezius, and erector spinae. The muscles involved in quiet exhalation are the diaphragm and the internal intercostal muscles. During forced exhalation, the abdominal muscles are used to assist with the expulsion of air from the lungs by creating increased pressure in a superior direction on the diaphragm. Specific discussion of the muscles involved in respiration is provided in the following paragraphs.

DIAPHRAGM

The diaphragm is the main muscle of inhalation. The diaphragm is a dome-shaped muscle, with a central tendinous area, that separates the abdominal and thoracic cavities. The muscle attaches to the xiphoid process of the sternum, the internal aspects of the lower four ribs, and the bodies of lumbar vertebrae 1, 2, and 3. The esophagus, aorta, and superior vena cava all pass through the diaphragm. The phrenic nerve innervates the diaphragm. The phrenic nerve arises from cervical root levels 3, 4, and 5. The level of innervation of the diaphragm is significant to remember because in patients with spinal cord injuries affecting the cervical spine below the level of the phrenic nerve, the nerve supply to the diaphragm may still be intact to enable diaphragmatic breathing. Diaphragmatic breathing in patients with spinal cord injuries is when all lung expansion is achieved through movement of the diaphragm, and none through movement of the ribs.

When the diaphragm contracts, the dome shape of the muscle is flattened toward the abdomen, increasing the depth of the thoracic cavity. Up to two thirds of the vital capacity of the lungs is created by this flattening action of the diaphragm. In babies, the diaphragm is responsible for most of the ventilation. The diaphragm is also responsible for most of the resting ventilation in adults, particularly in a supine position. The parietal pleura of the lungs is attached to the diaphragm so that when the diaphragm contracts, it pulls the pleura with it and assists with the increased negative pressure between the pleura keeping the lungs adjacent to the thoracic walls.

EXTERNAL AND INTERNAL INTERCOSTAL MUSCLES

The external and internal intercostal muscles are the other main muscles involved in inhalation. The external intercostals are mainly involved with quiet ventilation, and the internal intercostals are involved more with forced ventilation. The muscles act to expand the ribs and provide tone to the intercostal spaces (spaces between the ribs), which prevents indrawing of these spaces when changes occur in the intrapleural pressure. The external intercostal muscles pass forward and downward from one rib to the adjacent rib immediately distal, whereas the internal intercostal muscles pass backward and downward from one rib to the adjacent rib immediately distal.

The accessory muscles of ventilation are mainly used during involuntary forced exhalation such as sneezing and coughing. The rectus abdominis plays a major role in forced exhalation by compressing the abdominal contents and pushing up on the diaphragm.[41] During forced inhalation, the accessory muscles include the sternocleidomastoids, which both work together to assist in lifting the rib cage up and out, the scalenes, the upper trapezius, serratus anterior, pectoralis major and minor, and the erector spinae muscles. These muscles also assist in elevation and stabilization of the upper ribs during forced exhalation. When a cough or sneeze occurs, the inhaled volume of air has to increase to allow for an explosive exhalation. These accessory muscles of ventilation enable the extra motion of the rib cage required to expand the thoracic cavity effectively.

Why Does the Physical Therapist Assistant Need to Know About Tests for Respiratory Function?

Some respiratory function tests are performed in the physical therapy department, and others are medical procedures administered by physicians or in the radiology department. People with respiratory conditions seen in the physical therapy department require monitoring during activities to ensure adequate oxygenation of tissues. The rate of respiration, breath sounds, and signs of shortness of breath and dyspnea must all be followed during physical therapy interventions. A knowledge of various lung function tests and their results is important so that the PTA can read the patient chart and determine the significance of test results for physical therapy interventions.

Tests for Respiratory Function

In this section, a variety of tests for determining respiratory function are described. Such tests include the subjective findings reported by patients such as shortness of breath and reduced tolerance to activity and the objective findings observed by the health care provider. Other tests encompass a variety of lung function tests for the measurement of lung capacity and determining the status of the respiratory system.

Subjective Findings
Subjective findings are those that the evaluating physical therapist and the treating PT or PTA learn directly from the patient, a care provider, or other person closely associated with the patient or client. The subjective history of the patient provides important insights into the life and health history of the patient that can be related to the appropriate and realistic physical therapy interventions for the patient. The symptoms expressed by the patient may provide good clues as to whether the disease process is resolving or worsening. PTAs do not diagnose or evaluate the patient, but they need to know whether the pulmonary condition is improving with physical therapy intervention. Patient reports of increased periods of shortness of breath, inability to walk up stairs without being very short of breath, and a reduction in the ability to perform activities of daily living may all indicate the need to refer the patient back to the PT for reevaluation and adjustment of the plan of care.

Objective Findings
Objective findings include those signs and symptoms associated with respiratory conditions that the PTA can observe. Objective findings include the measurement of excursion of the ribs (chest expansion), observation of abnormalities such as intercostal indrawing, and listening to breath sounds with auscultation techniques.

EXCURSION
The objective data gathered during the physical therapist evaluation and on a regular basis during physical therapy interventions include measurement of **chest excursion** (chest expansion) at full inhalation and full exhalation and the difference between the values is noted as the available excursion of the ribs. In a healthy "young adult between 20 and 30 years of age" the rib excursion is approximately 8.5 cm at the level of the xiphoid.[42] This measurement can be misleading in the patient with advanced stages of chronic obstructive pulmonary disease (COPD) because of the hyperinflated nature of the thoracic cavity. The PT will also use manual techniques during the evaluation process to assess the degree of rib excursion at apical, middle, and lower lung lobes looking for both the quality and quantity of motion.

INTERCOSTAL INDRAWING
Intercostal indrawing of the spaces between the ribs occurs in individuals with marked resistance to airflow during inhalation. The skin and intercostal muscle tissue between the ribs is drawn inward during inhalation as the result of an increased negative pressure in the thoracic cavity.[43] Intercostal indrawing can be seen more often in children than adults. A similar phenomenon can occur with paralysis of the intercostal muscles resulting from a cerebrovascular accident or spinal cord injury in which the intercostal spaces "collapse" during inhalation as a result of the negative pressure created within the chest.[44]

BREATH SOUNDS

Breath sounds are detected using **auscultation techniques.** Auscultation is the act of listening to sounds made by the body, particularly sounds of the heart and lungs. A stethoscope is used to listen to the sounds over the trachea and lung.[45] The exhalation (expiratory) tracheal breath sound is a little higher pitched and lasts slightly longer than the inhalation (inspiratory) tracheal breath sound.[46] Lung tissue sounds are termed vesicular sounds and are more difficult to detect than tracheal sounds. Inhalation breath sounds have a whooshing sound, and exhalation breath sounds are of short duration and barely detectable or have no sound at all. When auscultating over the lungs, no gap is detected between the inhalation and exhalation lung sounds. PTAs should familiarize themselves with normal breath sounds so that they are better able to alert the supervising PT if they suspect a change in the patient's status. The stethoscope is placed at different points over both lungs in a systematic pattern demonstrated in Figure 4-6.

Abnormal breath sounds include the following:

- Tracheal sounds heard over lung tissue areas that may be due to pneumonia when fluid is present in the lungs
- The absence of any sound may occur in cases of pleural effusion, collapsed lung, or pneumothorax (gas in the pleural cavity). In cases of asthma episodes, clinicians may not hear any breath sounds because of the obstruction of the bronchi and bronchioles.

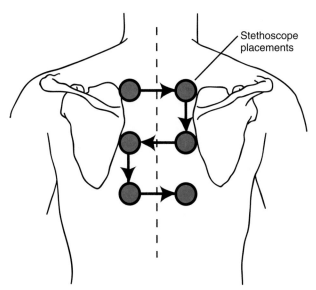

FIGURE 4.6 Pattern of stethoscope positions for listening to breath sounds.

- Unusual sounds over the lungs are called adventitious or extra sounds and include wheezing, rhonchi, crepitations, and crackles (rales).
- Wheezing and rhonchi indicate obstruction of the bronchi and bronchioles and may be either low-pitched or high-pitched sounds that increase in pitch as the airways become narrower.
- Crepitations and crackles are detected on inhalation and are short duration sounds resulting from the opening of closed airways.
- **Pleural rub** or **friction rub**[47] is heard as a squeak on both inhalation and exhalation. This sound is the result of either the rubbing together of inflamed pleura (pleurisy or pleuritis) or to the presence of a neoplasm in the pleura.
- Sometimes a patient is asked to whisper "one, two, three" while the clinician listens to the lungs through a stethoscope. If a disease process is active in the lung causing hardening or consolidation of the lung tissue, such as in pneumonia, the whisper will be heard quite clearly over the lung. Under normal circumstances, voice sounds cannot be heard clearly when listening to the lung.

Lung Function Tests

Lung function tests are procedures used to determine the physiological status of the lungs and include spirometry, peak expiratory flow measurement, arterial blood gases monitoring, acid and base balance of the blood, chest radiographs, computed tomography (CT), magnetic resonance imaging (MRI), pulmonary arteriography, bronchoscopy, exercise capacity and tolerance, hematological tests, and microbiology tests for infective agents.

SPIROMETRY

An incentive inspiratory spirometer is a device that encourages patients to inhale deeply after a pulmonary infection or thoracic surgery to prevent further complications. The incentive spirometer is widely used after surgery to prevent postoperative pulmonary complications such as **atelectasis** (collapse of a lung) by encouraging adequate inhalation to inflate all areas of the lungs.[48] One type of incentive spirometer is a simple machine with a ball that rises up a calibrated container in response to the amount of air exhaled into the machine. To use the spirometer, patients seal their lips round the tubing mouthpiece and slowly inhale. At the completion of inhalation, patients hold their breath for 2 seconds before exhaling again (see Fig. 4-7). The ball rises to a certain level in the container upon exhalation with patients aiming for a specific marker

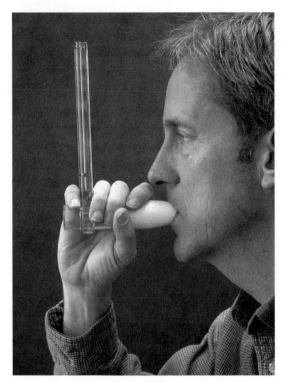

FIGURE 4.7 Incentive spirometer in use.

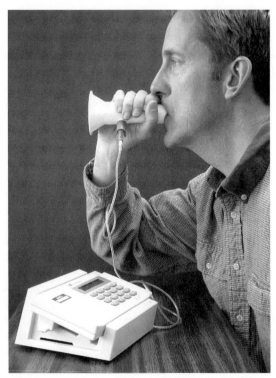

FIGURE 4.8 Electronic spirometer.

preset by the respiratory team. Use of the incentive spirometer should be accompanied by education in diaphragmatic and lateral costal breathing techniques. Breathing exercises are especially helpful for patients after abdominal surgery.

An electronic spirometer is used in the same way for incentive spirometry but can also be used to measure the expiratory values. The electronic spirometer provides more readings for analysis. Pathologies causing airways obstruction will reduce the FEV_1 value, but make little difference to the VC (see Fig. 4-8). Clinicians may attempt to record the FEV_1 and VC measurements at the same time. However, to obtain the FEV_1 patients have to expel air forcefully from the lungs as quickly as possible in the first second. Many patients with obstructive airways disease can increase the volume of air exhaled if they breathe out slowly, so a more accurate reading of the VC is obtained if the two measurements are taken separately. The FEV_1 is normally 80% of the VC.[49] According to the update on the Global Initiative for Chronic Obstructive Lung Disease, (2006)[50] COPD now includes four stages of classification related to spirometry values: Stage I: Mild; Stage II: Moderate; Stage III: Severe; and Stage IV: Very severe.[51] The diagnosis of the severity of the COPD relates to other findings as well as spirometry values (see Table 4-4).

A reduction in both the FEV_1 and the VC is called a "restrictive" pattern and indicates reduced lung volume. If the values of the FEV_1 and VC are more than two standard deviations from the normal for age, height, race, gender, and build, they are considered abnormal. Measurements of the FEV_1 and VC can be expressed in a flow/volume curve (see Fig. 4-9).

PEAK EXPIRATORY FLOW
Peak expiratory flow (PEF) is measured with a peak flow meter. PEF is reached at about 100 milliseconds into exhalation (expiration) and then starts to reduce as the air continues to be expelled from the lungs. The measurement of PEF is of most value in patients with asthma whose PEF fluctuates with the severity of the condition. A reduction in the PEF may indicate an impending asthmatic episode. Peak flow meters are issued to patients for home-monitoring purposes after they are taught how to use them effectively. The patient takes a deep breath in and then seals the lips round the mouthpiece of the meter and breathes out as quickly and fully as possible. Regular use of the PEF and tracking of outcomes and results can help the patient to predict the onset of asthmatic symptoms and enable the patient to take measures to avert an episode.

Table 4.4 Four Stages of Classification of Chronic Obstructive Pulmonary Disease (COPD) Related to Spirometry Values

STAGE OF COPD	LEVEL OF SERIOUSNESS OF CONDITION	FEV$_1$/FVC RATIO	FEV$_1$
Stage I	Mild	<0.70	50%–80% of predicted values
Stage II	Moderate	<0.70	50%–80% of predicted values
Stage III	Severe	<0.70	30%–50% of predicted values
Stage IV	Very severe	<0.70	30%–50% of predicted values plus chronic respiratory failure

FEV$_1$ = forced expiratory volume in 1 second.

(According to the 2006 update on the Global Initiative for Chronic Obstructive Lung Disease, Global Strategy for the Diagnosis, Management and Prevention of COPD, Global Initiative for Chronic Obstructive Lung Disease (GOLD) 2006. Available at: http://www.goldcopd.org.)

ARTERIAL BLOOD GASES

Arterial blood gas analysis provides values of the partial pressure of oxygen (PaO$_2$) in the blood. Hypoxemia is a reduction in the PaO$_2$ levels in the blood. Hypercapnia indicates a rise in the partial pressure of carbon dioxide (PaCO$_2$) in the blood. The normal values of PaO$_2$ are between 95 and 100 mm Hg, and normal levels for PaCO$_2$ are between 35 and 45 mm Hg (see Table 4-5). Hypercapnia refers to levels of PaCO$_2$ greater than 45 mm Hg.[52] To measure arterial blood gases during exercise testing, a catheter is inserted into the radial artery so that blood samples can be taken and analyzed at intervals of between 1 and 1.5 minutes. A pulse oximeter (see Fig. 4-10) can be used to provide an estimate of the levels of oxygen saturation in hemoglobin (SaO$_2$). A pulse oximeter is a small portable device with a sensor that attaches either to a finger, an ear, or the forehead. SaO$_2$ and PaO$_2$ levels correlate to some degree, and thus the pulse oximeter can be useful during physical therapy clinical intervention for monitoring patients with pulmonary pathology during ambulation and exercise.[53] During PT intervention, the SaO$_2$ level should be monitored closely. Accepted ranges of normal for pulse oximetry are between 96% and 100%. In patients with pulmonary disease, the usual range may be below this level but should be higher than 90%.[54] In cases in which the level drops below this level, the PTA should stop the intervention and consult the PT. The PT and PTA can observe the SaO$_2$ levels during intervention to ensure levels do not become too low. If SaO$_2$ levels fall below 90%, the patient may require oxygen therapy prescribed by the physician. The PTA should inform the supervising PT immediately if a reduction in the SaO$_2$ level below the level of 90% occurs during intervention. Even when using external oxygen, patients with pulmonary diseases should be monitored during PT intervention to ensure oxygen saturation levels remain within a safe limit.

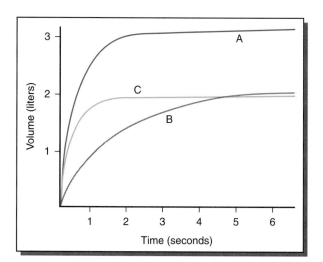

FIGURE 4.9 Spirometry flow/volume curves showing normal (A) and abnormal (B and C) forced expiratory volume in 1 second (FEV$_1$) and vital capacity (VC) value.

ACID/BASE BALANCE OF BLOOD

The normal acid/base (alkali) level of the blood is slightly basic (slightly alkaline) between 7.35 and 7.45 pH. The acid/alkali scale ranges from 0 (strongly acidic) to 14 (strongly basic; alkaline). The normal values for blood pH are therefore slightly basic but close to neutral.[55] A reduction in the pH level is called acidosis, and an increase is alkalosis. Respiratory acidosis results from a rise in the PaCO$_2$ and is present in patients with chronic bronchitis

Table 4.5 **Normal Levels in Arterial Blood Gas Samples**

NAME	ABBREVIATION	NORMAL VALUE IN ARTERIAL BLOOD
Partial pressure of oxygen	PaO_2	95–100 mm Hg
Partial pressure of carbon dioxide	$PaCO_2$	35–45 mm Hg
Acidity/alkalinity	pH	7.35–7.45

during episodes of exacerbations. Respiratory alkalosis occurs with a reduction in the $PaCO_2$ level and is present in persons with pneumonia.

CHEST RADIOGRAPHS

Chest radiographs are taken as part of a total approach to the diagnosis of lung pathology. They are valuable when taken at regular intervals to demonstrate changes in the condition of the lungs. Chest radiographs are taken in an anterior-posterior direction and from a lateral view, during maximum inhalation. In a radiographic (x-ray) image of healthy lungs, the trachea should be vertical and centrally placed in the chest cavity, and the heart should be approximately 50% of the total width of the chest at its widest part. The bones appear white on films, and air in the lungs appears dark. Lesions in the lungs may show up as gray or white areas called opacities or shadows. If these lesions are small and round, they may indicate the presence of such conditions as tuberculosis, carcinoma, or rheumatoid arthritis nodules. A shift from the midline position of the trachea, with a rise in the level of the diaphragm, may indicate a lung collapse. Opacity in a lung lobe may indicate a consolidation of that part of the lung tissue. The level of fluid may be seen as a straight line in the lung, possibly within a lung abscess or in a pleural effusion. The fluid appears as a dense opaque area with a straight edge.[56,57]

COMPUTED TOMOGRAPHY

CT is a sophisticated type of radiograph that takes a picture of an axial segment through the body. Patients lie on a bed that is passed through a chamber, which has x-ray tubes within it. The chamber rotates round patients to take views from various angles, and the computer then reconstructs these images into a radiograph. The images produced by computed tomography are detailed and enable the physician to make a more accurate diagnosis by localizing potential pathologies.[58] Chest CT scans are expensive to perform and thus are usually only used to confirm, or rule out, suspected pathologies noted on x-ray or as a first line of testing for people at high risk of lung disease.

MAGNETIC RESONANCE IMAGING

MRI is even more sophisticated than the CT scan. Patients lie on a table, which slides slowly through a tube surrounded by a large electromagnet. The machine produces radio and magnetic waves that "read" the protons in the body and formulate a computer image.[59] These computer images are clear and highly useful in diagnosis. No radiation is used, which is beneficial for patients. Some of the disadvantages of the MRI are that it is expensive to use, not always readily available, and sensitive to any motion of the body. Even breathing may interfere with the clarity of chest images. Metals that can be magnetized are unable to enter the room where an MRI machine is located including jewelry, watches, hair adornments, and metallic fasteners on underwear. In general, surgically implanted metals are made from titanium and are not magnetized by an MRI scan.[60] PTAs can help alleviate anxiety for patients going for an MRI by explaining the procedure. Patients should be warned that the MRI scan is very noisy and that they will wear earphones. The earphones have a

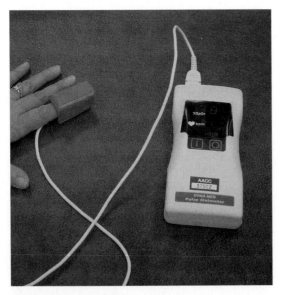

FIGURE 4.10 Pulse oximeter.

connection to the operator of the machine, who will speak to patients and tell them what is about to occur. Because the machine is rather claustrophobic, clinicians may suggest that patients close their eyes during the procedure. Soft music is often played through the headphones during the MRI to help patients relax. Patients need to stay as still as possible during the procedure to ensure good clarity of the images.

PULMONARY ARTERIOGRAPHY OR ANGIOGRAPHY

Pulmonary arteriography, also called pulmonary angiography, is a method of taking a visual image of the blood vessels of the lungs.[61] Pulmonary arteriography is an invasive procedure (one in which something enters the body) performed in a special laboratory or in the operating room. The procedure is used to detect pulmonary embolism and vascular irregularities.[62] A catheter is inserted into the femoral vein in the groin and guided up the vein into the heart using fluoroscopy (an opaque fluid injected into the veins so they will show up on x-ray via a viewing screen). The catheter tip is guided into the pulmonary artery, and a contrast medium is injected into the pulmonary artery through the catheter. Bronchial arteriography is performed by a similar method passing a catheter through the femoral artery into the aorta in the midthorax and then into the bronchial arteries. This procedure is performed when hemoptysis (bleeding) of the lung tissue is present in conditions such as bronchiectasis. Discovery of hemoptysis is immediately treated with a sclerosing or embolization agent to stop the bleeding. Superior vena cavography is performed for detection of abnormalities of the superior vena cava. If an obstruction is detected, a stent, a tube meshwork of metal, can be inserted to widen the lumen of the vessel.

BRONCHOSCOPY

Bronchoscopy is the examination of the trachea and bronchi by passing an endoscope or bronchoscope down the trachea. The bronchoscope has an optical viewer at the end of a flexible tube that enables the physician to see any abnormalities within the bronchi. Small surgical instruments can also be used through the bronchoscope for removal of tissue from the trachea or bronchi for a biopsy.

EXERCISE CAPACITY AND TOLERANCE

Exercise capacity and tolerance to activity is measured by tests performed during patient activity. These tests range from simple measurements, such as the distance ambulated by a patient within a specified time, for example, the 6-minute walk test,[63] to complex laboratory analyses of the physiological effects of exercise. The results of these tests provide objective findings regarding diagnosis and help the physician and PT to determine the possible level of disability and the interventions needed to assist patients. The presence of exercise-induced asthma can also be determined by such tests. Subjective information is also useful for developing realistic goals for patients such as their ability to climb stairs, talk while walking, speed of walking, and the ability to walk up slopes. The information gained from such questioning can indicate the need for more specific testing. In a simple timed walking test, patients are required to ambulate as quickly as possible for a specified time, and the distance is measured. Ambulation time may be 2, 6, or 12 minutes. The American College of Sports Medicine has established protocols, such as the Bruce protocol (performed on a treadmill with the heart monitored electronically), to test for exercise capacity and these protocols provide reliability and validity of test results.[64,65]

In the PT clinic, exercise capacity and tolerance tests are often performed on a treadmill to make the distance measurement and monitoring easier. However, if a treadmill is not available, the distances for ambulation can be measured along a corridor. Placing distance marks along the walls of a corridor close to the physical therapy department of a hospital, or within the physical therapy clinic can be helpful. During exercise capacity and tolerance testing, blood pressure, respiratory rate and pattern, heart rate, and O_2 saturation levels should be monitored carefully. In many cases, a simple timed walking test is sufficient to enable the PT to determine appropriate levels of exercise and activity for patients. If patients become short of breath after a few minutes, the simple solution may be to reduce the speed of ambulation to enable patients to ambulate a greater distance. If the uptake of O_2 is slow, reducing the speed of ambulation may considerably increase the functional ambulatory status of patients.

Higher level exercise capacity testing, or stress testing, is performed while patients use either a treadmill or a cycle ergometer. This stress test is also known as a monitored **graded exercise tolerance test (GXTT)** and can be used to determine both cardiac and pulmonary status.[66] Guidelines for exercise testing were reported in 1997 in a Report of the American College of Cardiology/American Heart Association Task Force on Practice Guidelines.[67] The data provided by a GXTT is in **metabolic equivalent (MET)**. One MET is the amount of oxygen required with the body at rest in a sitting position. Each MET is equal to about 3.5 mL/Kg of body weight per minute.[68] Basically, a 2 MET exercise activity takes twice the amount of energy required for sitting.[69]

Examples of 3 through 6 MET activities include

- walking at a moderate to brisk pace
- bicycling at 5 to 9 mph on level terrain

- playing a game of doubles tennis; recreational swimming
- horseback riding

To expend more than 6 METs, activities include

- race-walking (fast pace)
- bicycling more than 10 mph uphill
- playing a game of singles tennis
- playing most competitive sports such as soccer, football, basketball, and hockey

The readings of MET levels are different for healthy individuals as opposed to those with pulmonary pathologies. Charts are available from the Centers for Disease Control and Prevention web site at www.cdc.gov for the physician and PT to determine optimal levels of the METs when testing.

METs are a multiple of the resting amount of oxygen required (VO_2). Factors monitored during the GXTT include blood pressure, heart rate, respiratory rate, temperature prior to test, oxygen and carbon dioxide levels, oxygen saturation levels, and cardiac output. Generally patients who can achieve 65% to 75% of their predicted maximal heart rate without any symptoms of cardiopulmonary distress are candidates for exercise endurance and conditioning programs. However, aerobic conditioning exercises may be possible in patients who are deconditioned with as low as 50% to 60% of the predicted maximal heart rate.[70] Such patients should be monitored by the physical therapist as they require ongoing evaluation. During exercise, the level of exercise is dependent on keeping the heart rate within the 65% to 75% of predicted maximal heart rate parameters. The PTA must be aware of the test results before working with patients with pulmonary disease and monitor the blood pressure and heart rate to be sure each remains within the acceptable parameters set by the PT and physician for the specific patient.

The subjective report during physical therapy intervention developed by Borg called the Rating of Perceived Exertion scale (RPE) is a useful tool for assessing how patients perceive their level of energy and status during the therapeutic activity (refer to Chapter 3 for details). With many patients, the RPE is used in place of other monitoring when other techniques are not available or patients have so many cardiopulmonary complications that the RPE is the best tool.

HEMATOLOGICAL TESTS

A complete blood count (CBC) is often performed on patients with cardiopulmonary diseases. The PTA needs to be familiar with the terminology and abbreviations used and the normal values for these tests to read patients' charts effectively and understand when to refer patients back to the PT for reevaluation. Normal values for hematology tests vary according to the method used. Table 4-6 details various sections of the CBC and the normal value ranges. Table 4-7 details normal hematology values, and Table 4-8 details the description of the abbreviations of International System of Units (SI Units). The need to read a patient chart and determine hematological values for patients can be pertinent to physical therapy intervention. In patients with altered values on the CBC such as thrombocytopenia (low platelet count) the level of activity and exercise may need to be reduced depending on the degree of severity of the condition. If the white blood cell count (WBCC) is low (leukopenia), patients may be susceptible to complications and infections. Following standard precautions is extremely important when treating patients with a low WBCC, and the PTA should be scrupulous about hand washing and disinfection of equipment. Patients may need to wear a mask during contact with the public to reduce the risk of contracting infections.

Note: Occasionally there is confusion in the hospital when physical therapy is ordered. The PT needs to be careful that the order is truly for physical therapy and not for prothrombin time (also abbreviated PT) testing. The PTA also needs to be aware of this terminology when reading patient charts before each patient treatment.

MICROBIOLOGY

Microbiology is the study of micro-organisms such as bacteria, viruses, and molds as well as the study of cells. Samples such as blood, sputum, and the exudate from wounds are studied in the medical microbiology laboratory to determine the presence of infections. Tissue samples taken from a biopsy (removal of an area of tissue for testing), a culture swab (such as for Strep throat), or from surgery are analyzed for abnormalities such as cancer and infection. Patients with cardiac pathologies are at risk for infections, and microbiological analysis is frequently required to ensure patients are free from infection.

Microbiology analysis is performed on blood samples when infection is suspected. After the organism is identified in the blood, the site of the infection has to be determined and suitable drug therapy provided. In patients with pulmonary conditions, sputum cultures may be needed to identify the cause of pulmonary infections. Infected sputum may be yellow or green and, in some cases, foul smelling. The presence of a strong smell is often due to anaerobic bacteria in the sputum. The presence of bacteria in the sputum is not necessarily indicative of pulmonary infection because there can be contamination

Table 4.6 **Hematology Interpretation and Normal Values**

BLOOD FACTOR TESTED	COMMONLY USED ABBREVIATION	NORMAL RANGE IN SI UNITS	NORMAL RANGE IN CONVENTIONAL UNITS	SIGNIFICANCE
Hemoglobin	Hgb	Men: 8.1–11.2 mmol/L Women: 7.4–9.9 mmol/L	Men: 13–18 g/100 mL Women: 12–16 g/ 100 mL	Measures total red blood cell (RBCs) mass; low levels indicate anemia, and high levels indicate polycythemia or erythrocytosis (may indicate hypoxemic lung disease or cyanotic heart disease)
Hematocrit	Hct	Men: 0.45–0.52￼ Women: 0.37–0.48	Men: 45%–52% Women: 37%–48%	Erythrocytes as a percentage of total blood volume; normal level varies with age and elevation of habitat
Erythrocyte Count (Red Blood Cell count)	RBC	4.2–5.9 × 10 to power of 12/L	4.2–5.9 million/mm^3	Red cell count per specified volume of blood
Leukocyte count (White Blood Cell count)	WBCC	4.3–10.8 × 10 to power of 9/L	4,300–10,800/mm^3	High levels indicate presence of infection, parasites or allergic reactions
Platelet count	Plt	150–350 × 10 power of 9/L	150,000–350,000/mm^3	Thrombocytopenia (↓ platelet count) may indicate sepsis, or a drug reaction; often seen in critically sick patients, especially those on dialysis; thrombocytosis is an increase in platelet count
Mean corpuscular volume	MCV	86–98 fl	86–98 µm^3/cell	Measures size of RBCs; low levels are microcytosis and may indicate iron deficiency; high MCV is macrocytosis and may indicate vitamin B12 or folic acid deficiency
Mean corpuscular hemoglobin	MCH	1.7–2.0 pg/cell	27–32 pg/RBC	Hb divided by the total red cell count; provides the concentration of Hb in RBCs
Clotting profile 1. Prothrombin time 2. Partial thromboplastin time	PT PTT	Less than 2 sec deviation from control 25–38 sec	Less than 2 sec deviation from control 25–38 sec	Performed for those patients at high risk of developing bleeding or clotting problems; indicates clotting time
Erythrocyte sedimentation rate	ESR	Men: 1–13 mm/hr Women: 1–20 mm/hr	Men: 1–13 mm/hr Women: 1–20 mm/hr	Time taken for the RBCs to settle to the bottom of unclotted blood in the laboratory in 1 hour; if ESR is fast/higher, it indicates inflammation; inflammation causes RBCs to clump together, making them heavier

(Values based on *Taber's Cyclopedic Dictionary*, 20th edition, Appendix 3: Normal Reference Laboratory Values, pp. 2442–2445.)

Table 4.7 Hematology Electrolyte and Lipoprotein Interpretation and Normal Values

BLOOD FACTOR TESTED	COMMONLY USED ABBREVIATION	NORMAL RANGE IN SI UNITS	NORMAL RANGE IN CONVENTIONAL UNITS	SIGNIFICANCE
Proteins				
albumin		35–50g/L	3.5–5.0 g/100 mL	
globulin		23–35 g/L	2.3–3.5 g/100 mL	
Electrolytes				Balance of electrolytes is impor-tant for metabolic activity and transmission of electrical charges; alterations in elec-trolyte levels can affect the brain and nervous system, causing structures to swell or shrink, resulting in altered mental status
sodium	Na+	135–145 mmol/L	135–145 mEq/L	
potassium	K+	3.5–5.0 mmol/L	2.5–5.0 mEq/L	
calcium	Ca++	2.1–2.6 mmol/L	8.5–10.5 mg/100 mL	Na+ is crucial for nervous system function
chloride	Cl⁻	100–106 mmol/L	100–106 mEq/L	K+ is vital for neuromuscular function and alterations can effect the function of the heart
				Cl– levels fluctuate with dehydration
				If K+ levels fall below 3.2 or go higher than 5.1, physical ther-apy may be contraindicated due to possibility of arrhythmia/tetany
Cholesterol		<5.18 mmol/L	<200 mg/dL; over 240 mg/dL is high risk	Fatty compound found in bile; also found in plaque buildup in atherosclerosis
High density lipoproteins	HDL	Above 60 mg/dL = low risk[152] Men: below 37 mg/dL at risk Women: below 47 mg/dL at risk	Above 60 mg/dL = low risk[153] Men: below 37 mg/dL at risk Women: below 47 mg/dL at risk	"Good" cholesterol; vigorous exercise increases levels; estrogens thought to increase levels; higher levels of HDL are better
Low density lipoproteins	LDL	Optimal: <100 mg/dL[154] Near optimal: 100–129 mg/dL Borderline high: 130–159 mg/dL High: 160 – 189 mg/dL Very high: ≥190 mg/dL	Optimal: <100 mg/dL [155] Near optimal: 100–129 mg/dL Borderline high: 130–159 mg/dL High: 160–189 mg/dL Very high: ≥190 mg/dL	"Bad" cholesterol; increases during pregnancy, diabetes mellitus, chronic renal failure, hypothyroidism, and in those with genetic predisposition
LDL/HDL ratio	LDL/HDL	0.5–3.0 = low risk 3.0–6.0 = moder-ate risk >6.0–high risk	0.5–3.0 = low risk 3.0–6.0 = moderate risk >6.0–high risk	May indicate risk of coronary disease
Triglycerides		0.4–1.5 g/L	40–150 mg/100 mL	Fatty acids found in blood after food with high sugar or fat con-tent; decrease in response to exercise; may indicate increased risk of coronary disease

(Values based on *Taber's Cyclopedic Dictionary*, 20th edition, Appendix 3: Normal Reference Laboratory Values, pp. 2442–2445.)

Table 4.8 Explanation of the Abbreviations Used for the International System of Units (SI Units).

SI UNITS	INTERNATIONAL SYSTEM OF UNITS
g	gram
mmol	millimole
Mmol/L	Millimole per liter
pg	picogram
µL	microliter
mm^3	cubic millimeter
g/L	grams per liter
sec	second
mm/hr	millimeter per hour
dL	deciliter

from the mouth and trachea. If evidence of an increased white cell count in the blood, a fever, a reduction in PaO_2 levels, and chest x-ray abnormalities, combined with a bacterial colonization of sputum are present, then infection of the lungs is likely.

The rise in antibiotic resistant infections has increased the emphasis on standard precautions and infection control in the health care setting and is especially important for patients with cardiopulmonary conditions. See Chapter 2 for details of antimicrobial resistant infections.

Why Does the Physical Therapist Assistant Need to Know About Diseases of the Respiratory System?

People with respiratory conditions are treated in various physical therapy practice settings including the acute care hospital, rehabilitation centers, outpatient clinics, pediatric clinics, and home health care. In some instances, physical therapy interventions are provided for the actual pulmonary condition, and in others interventions are for strengthening, increasing exercise tolerance to activity, ambulation, and activities of daily living (ADL) training. The knowledge of respiratory diseases is essential for the PTA to understand the implications of the disease process on patient responses to interventions.

Diseases of the Respiratory System

In this section, the general signs and symptoms noted in most respiratory conditions are discussed and the respiratory diseases most commonly observed in physical therapy practice are described.

General Signs and Symptoms of Pulmonary Diseases

Pulmonary diseases present with a number of signs and symptoms. This section briefly describes some of the general signs and symptoms.

HINTS ON USE OF THE GUIDE TO PHYSICAL THERAPIST PRACTICE

The main Preferred Practice Pattern in the *Guide to Physical Therapist Practice* for pulmonary diseases is the "Cardiovascular/Pulmonary" Pattern 6.

- 6B, "impaired aerobic capacity/endurance associated with deconditioning" (p. 475): many pulmonary disorders cause decreased endurance and shortness of breath and patients with these symptoms may be placed in this pattern
- 6C, "impaired ventilation, respiration/gas exchange/endurance associated with airway clearance dysfunction" (p. 489): if there is dyspnea at rest and reduced gaseous exchange, which interferes with the ability to work or perform simple tasks, this is the most likely pattern
- 6E, "impaired ventilation and respiration/gas exchange associated with ventilatory pump dysfunction or failure" (p. 521): In cases of pulmonary fibrosis patients, may fall within this pattern; the use of oxygen may be required in such cases
- 6F, "impaired ventilation and respiration/gas exchange associated with respiratory failure" (p. 539): Patients with diagnoses such as asthma, adult respiratory distress syndrome, chronic obstructive pulmonary disease (COPD), and pneumonia, which cause dyspnea and increased respiratory rate at rest, impaired airway clearance, and impaired gaseous exchange fall under this pattern

(From the American Physical Therapy Association, 2003. *Guide to physical therapist practice*, revised 2nd edition. Alexandria, VA: APTA. Used with permission.)

COUGH

Cough is one of the most common indications of a respiratory problem. The cough is a basic protective system of explosive exhalation to attempt to rid the lungs and bronchial tree of foreign matter. In cases of respiratory disease, this foreign matter is sputum produced within the lungs in response to inflammation. A productive cough is one in which sputum is produced. The sputum may be either coughed up and spat out or swallowed. When performing chest physical therapy on a patient, a sputum sample is often required to send to the laboratory for diagnosis; therefore, patients should be encouraged to spit the sputum out into a sterile container. The nature of the sputum is indicative of the disease process and can determine whether infection exists (see Table 4-9). Abnormal breath sounds that accompany a cough may indicate the presence of secretions in the lungs, and can include wheezing, rhonchi, crepitations, and crackles (rales) as discussed earlier in this chapter.

DYSPNEA

Dyspnea is a state of breathlessness, shortness of breath, and varies in intensity. Dyspnea is a symptom of both pulmonary and cardiac conditions. Orthopnea is the type of dyspnea stimulated by a supine position. Paroxysmal nocturnal dyspnea (PND) is the type of dyspnea that causes patients to awaken in the night. PND can be a sign of congestive heart failure, and the symptoms can be increased with excessive exercise during the day. Platypnea is a form of dyspnea that occurs when sitting up from supine, and trepopnea is unilateral dyspnea that occurs when patients lie on their side and usually indicates unilateral lung pathology.

CYANOSIS

Cyanosis refers to a blue tinge of the skin and is termed central or peripheral. Central cyanosis can be seen mainly in the mucous membranes of the lips and tongue, when oxygen saturation levels reduce below 80% due to extensive lung disease. Peripheral cyanosis is seen more with cardiac pathologies when the heart is unable to maintain adequate peripheral circulation. Signs of peripheral cyanosis are seen in the fingers, nose, toes, and nail beds.

CHEST PAIN

Chest pain results from several factors as a consequence of pulmonary pathology. Pleuritic pain is caused by inflammation of the pleura. The pain arises from parietal pleura because pain nerve endings are not located in the visceral pleura or in lung tissue. Pleuritic pain is severe and sharp and is worse on inspiration, particularly when

Table 4.9 **Types of Sputum, Appearance, and Causes**

TYPE OF SPUTUM	TYPICAL CAUSES	OBSERVATION OF SPUTUM
Saliva	Normally present	Clear/watery
Frothy	Pulmonary edema	Bubbly either white or pink colored
Mucoid	Pulmonary conditions with no infection, e.g., asthma, chronic bronchitis	White and opaque
Mucopurulent	Cystic fibrosis, pneumonia, bronchiectasis	May have a slight yellow tinge and is slightly thicker than mucoid; may have a slight odor; cystic fibrosis sputum is often foul smelling due to infection
Purulent	Pulmonary infections, e.g., pseudomonas, pneumococcus bacteria	Thick, yellow or green; may be rust colored due to presence of old blood or red due to presence of fresh blood; often has a bad odor
Hemoptysis	Infections such as tuberculosis or bronchiectasis, pulmonary infarction, trauma causing damage to the lung, disorders of coagulation	Blood spots in sputum or a lot of blood; old blood appears brown and fresh blood red
Black sputum	Inhalation of smoke from cigarettes, fires, or heroin use; inhalation of coal dust	Spots of black in the sputum

coughing or deep breathing, due to stretching of the pleura. Occasionally pleuritic pain results from a pulmonary embolism, but it is more frequently a sign of pulmonary disease accompanied by fever and cough. Other causes of chest pain include a fractured rib and some lung tumors, which may cause a deep chest pain. Chest pain may also be caused by other pathologies that are beyond the scope of this book.

CHEST SHAPE AND REDUCED THORACIC MOBILITY

Chest shape and reduced thoracic mobility affect respiratory function. Several chest shapes are associated with pulmonary diseases. ⊛ Pectus carinatum (pigeon chest) is seen in children with asthma because the superior part of the sternum is in a permanently elevated position. A barrel chest is characterized by the thorax held in a permanently inspiratory position with large spaces between the ribs and a subsequent increase in the width and anterior-posterior diameter of the chest. A barrel chest may be seen in patients with emphysema. Kyphoscoliosis of the spine reduces the ability of the ribs to move and may restrict the function of one lung more than the other. An increased kyphosis of the thoracic spine with associated forward head position is typical of COPD and ankylosing spondylitis (AS). See Chapter 6 for information about AS.

Both pulmonary and cardiac diseases produce signs in the hands including clubbing of the fingers and toes (see Fig. 4-11). The tips of the toes and fingers become bulbous with a loss of the ridge between nail and finger.

PULMONARY EDEMA

Pulmonary edema is a build-up of fluid in the lungs with an accumulation of fluid in the alveoli and interstitial

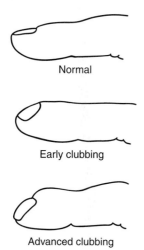

Normal

Early clubbing

Advanced clubbing

FIGURE 4.11 Clubbing of fingers.

spaces which prevents gaseous exchange, and usually occurs as a result of left ventricular failure with pulmonary hypertension. Pulmonary edema can also be a complication following thoracic surgery. Pulmonary edema causes many symptoms, including dyspnea, cough, excessive sweating, and possibly reduced cognition resulting from the lack of oxygen uptake.[71]

ATELECTASIS

Atelectasis is a condition in which either the whole or part of a lung collapses. ⊛ Atelectasis occurs in premature infants because of the lack of the production of surfactant by the immature lungs. If surfactant is not produced, the lungs collapse, and the infant can die if not placed on artificial ventilation. (See the sections "The Lungs," "Ventilation Control," and "Gaseous Exchange and Oxygen Transport" earlier in this chapter for details regarding surfactant.) In the adult, atelectasis can occur when fluid collects within the pleura as a result of pleural inflammation or heart failure, or air in the pleural cavity causing a pneumothorax. Localized atelectasis resulting from alveolar collapse can be due to a blockage in the bronchi. If no air enters an area of lung beyond the blockage, the existing air in the alveoli is absorbed, and the walls of the alveoli collapse.[72]

BRONCHIOLITIS

Bronchiolitis is an inflammation of the bronchi resulting in the production of secretions and inflammatory exudate in the lungs, causing a productive cough. Oxygen therapy is usually required for patients with bronchiolitis. Airway clearance techniques are helpful in loosening the secretions and helping the person to expectorate. Alveolitis is an inflammation of the alveoli. Alveolitis often occurs in response to an allergen and, if persistent, may develop into a chronic restrictive lung condition.

PNEUMOTHORAX AND PLEURAL EFFUSION

Pneumothorax is a life-threatening condition in which the lung collapses as a result of air entering the pleural cavity and changing the negative pressure that normally maintains the integrity of the lungs against the chest wall. Pneumothorax requires immediate medical intervention. Pneumothorax can be the result of trauma from a direct blow to the chest wall or a side effect of insertion of a central-line intravenous catheter, or it may be spontaneous in response to a lung condition such as asthma, cystic fibrosis, tuberculosis, COPD, or whooping cough.[73] In cases of certain pulmonary diseases, **pleural effusion** may result. Pleural effusion is the result of fluid filling the pleural cavity. Pleural effusion occurs most frequently in conditions such as congestive heart failure, pneumonia, tuberculosis, malignancy of the pleura, lung infections, asbestosis, and after thoracic surgery. [74]

> ### Why Does the Physical Therapist Assistant Need to Know About Pathological Conditions of the Respiratory Tract?
>
> The most common pathological conditions are those affecting the upper respiratory tract. These include viral and bacterial infections that result in inflammation of the upper respiratory tract. Examples of these conditions are sinusitis, pharyngitis, laryngitis, and acute rhinitis (the common cold). These conditions do not require physical therapy intervention unless they progress into lower respiratory tract infections. Patients with lower respiratory tract pathological conditions comprise the majority of people seen in physical therapy for respiratory intervention. Knowledge of these diseases and conditions, together with the possible medical and physical therapy interventions, is an essential part of the work of the PTA.

Pathological Conditions of the Respiratory Tract

The respiratory conditions discussed in this section comprise those affecting the lower respiratory tract of the trachea, lungs, and bronchi. Because conditions of the upper respiratory tract do not require physical therapy intervention, they are not included in this text.

Lung Abscess

A lung abscess is a localized cavity in the lung tissue, filled with pus and encapsulated by fibrous tissue. The incidence of lung abscess has reduced in recent years as a result of the use of antimicrobial medications but may be more prevalent in people with compromised immune systems.

Etiology. Lung abscess may occur as a result of carcinoma of the lung, as a complication of pneumonia, or in individuals with a compromised immune system.[75] Bacteria may also enter the lung secondary to stab or gunshot wounds and cause an abscess. Other cases of lung abscess may be caused by the aspiration of food or normal oral secretions. Most cases of aspiration occur in individuals who have swallowing difficulties after a cerebrovascular accident (CVA) or are under the influence of alcohol, illicit drugs, or prescribed medications such as sedatives.[76] In some cases, the abscess ruptures, resulting in **empyema** (pus in the space between the pleura) or septicemia (infection of the blood). If the abscess drains pus into the lung tissue, it can cause **bronchiectasis** (dilation of the bronchi with infection distal to the dilated portion). See Figure 4-12 for bronchiectasis.

Signs and Symptoms. The characteristics signs and symptoms of lung abscess can include fever, pain, dyspnea, cough, **hemoptysis** (blood in the sputum from the trachea or lungs), and halitosis (bad breath) due to pus-laden (infected) sputum.

Prognosis. Even though fairly uncommon, lung abscess and empyema are serious medical conditions that require immediate medical intervention. Severe infections left untreated can result in death.

Medical Intervention. A lung abscess is treated with antibiotics over a prolonged period of at least 6 to 8 weeks. The presence of empyema is often determined using diagnostic thoracentesis, which involves drawing fluid from the pleural space with a needle. This fluid is sent for laboratory analysis.[77] A surgical procedure used to drain infected fluid from the pleural space in cases of empyema is tube thoracotomy (or thoracoscopy) drainage.

Physical Therapy Intervention. The PT and PTA can facilitate drainage of the pus from the lungs through postural drainage positioning without deep inspiration. Deep breathing exercises to facilitate coughing are also

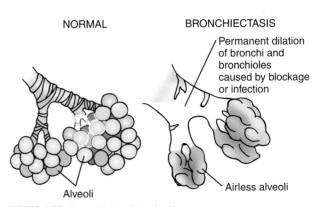

FIGURE 4.12 Bronchiectasis in the lung.

beneficial. All appropriate standard precautions should be followed, including the use of a mask and eye protection when treating a patient with a lung infection to prevent the occurrence of cross-infection.

Chronic Bronchitis and Emphysema

Chronic bronchitis and emphysema fall under the category of COPD. Chronic bronchitis and emphysema may actually occur in the same patient. Chronic bronchitis is a chronic inflammation of the bronchial tree, and emphysema is a disease of the alveoli. Prolonged chronic bronchitis may lead to emphysema, although emphysema may exist without marked chronic bronchitis. Two types of physical appearance are associated with COPD, the type A or "pink puffer" and the type B or "blue bloater." Although this terminology is becoming obsolete, it is a useful tool to help the PTA remember the characteristic appearance of patients with these diseases. Patients with predominant emphysema usually present as the "pink puffer" and ones with predominant chronic bronchitis present as a "blue bloater" (see Fig. 4-13).

Chronic Bronchitis

In clinical terms, chronic bronchitis is defined when a productive cough is present for at least 3 months of the year for 2 or more consecutive years. Bronchitis is an

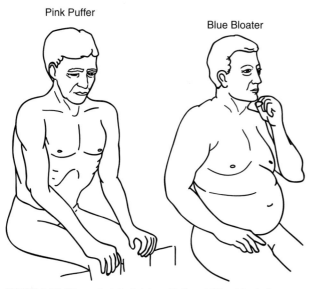

FIGURE 4.13 Characteristic "pink puffer" and "blue bloater" appearance in chronic obstructive pulmonary disease.

inflammation of the bronchi that produces excessive secretions that are expectorated (coughed up). In chronic bronchitis, the secretions are present for prolonged periods and lead to irreversible changes within the bronchi resulting in blockage with mucous plugs of the small bronchi and bronchioles. According to the 2010 American Lung Association Epidemiology and Statistics Unit Research and Program Services report based on the 2008 National Health Interview Survey approximately 9.8 million people in the United States have chronic bronchitis.[78]

Etiology. The main cause of chronic bronchitis is cigarette smoking. Other causative factors include environmental irritants such as secondhand smoke, air pollution, and occupational pollutants such as asbestos, chemicals, or types of dust.

Signs and Symptoms. The main signs and symptoms of chronic bronchitis are a productive cough during periods of exacerbation for at least 3 months of the year, dyspnea, and sensations of chest tightness.[79] Swelling of the lower extremities may occur as a result of right heart failure, and patients may use the accessory muscles of respiration excessively.[80]

Pathologically in chronic bronchitis, hypertrophy of the mucous membranes occurs with thickening of the submucosal glands in the trachea, bronchi, and bronchioles with eventual fibrosis of the mucous membranes. Also hyperplasia (increase in number) of the mucous producing glands, called goblet cells, in the walls of the bronchi results, causing an increase in the quantity of secretions. Ciliated epithelial cells in the linings of the airways lose many of their cilia as a result of the inflammatory response.[81]

Progression of the disease process in chronic bronchitis is gradual over a number of years, resulting in reduced pulmonary function and leading to progressive disability. A common complication of chronic bronchitis is bronchiectasis, which involves permanent dilation of the bronchi and bronchioles. Constant inflammation of the walls of the airways results in fibrosis of the walls of the bronchi and resultant dilation. In the presence of bronchiectasis, there is an increased risk of infection. Patients with this complication may develop fatigue, fever, and renal and hepatic failure. The appearance of patients with chronic bronchitis is usually that of the "blue bloater" (see Fig. 4-13).

The clinical picture of chronic bronchitis is detailed in Table 4-10. Diagnostically the FEV_1 is reduced in chronic bronchitis to 70% or less of the FVC. The FVC may be reduced overall, but it may take longer to expel all the air out of the lungs, making the exhalation (expiratory) phase of ventilation greater than normal.

Prognosis. People with chronic bronchitis are prone to contracting influenza and *Streptococcus pneumoniae* infections. Such infections can be life threatening if not treated effectively. Even though chronic bronchitis tends to become progressively worse, patients who stop smoking or avoid the substance causing the irritation to the bronchi will experience fewer acute exacerbations.

Medical Intervention. Medical intervention for patients with chronic bronchitis includes advice on smoking cessation, the use of bronchodilator inhalers, steroidal medications in inhaled or oral forms, and antimicrobial/antibiotic therapy for the management of infections. Some patients require oxygen therapy, especially if they have associated right heart failure. In addition, physicians recommend that patients with chronic bronchitis should receive an annual influenza vaccination and a pneumococcal vaccination every 5 to 6 years.[82,83] Physician referral may be provided for physical therapy, nutrition counseling, smoking cessation, and occupational therapy.

Physical Therapy Intervention. Specific interventions for patients with acute exacerbations of chronic bronchitis will include breathing exercises, airway clearance techniques, and pulmonary hygiene consisting of positioning for postural drainage with percussion, vibration, and shaking of the chest and cough facilitation. Home exercises and education to caregivers and patients are extremely important because patients need to learn how to position at home for postural drainage. Postural drainage positions are detailed later in this chapter. A progressive exercise rehabilitation program may be needed to increase exercise tolerance, aerobic capacity, and strength and mobility much the same as a cardiac rehabilitation plan.[84] In some cases, a progressive ambulatory training program with an appropriate assistive device may be required. In the initial stages of recovery, Stage I rehabilitation, patients use supplemental oxygen during the exercise program to ensure adequate perfusion of oxygen to the tissues. The PT and PTA need to ensure sufficient length of the oxygen tubing from the machine to patients to allow for ambulation. In the home-care setting, the PT will consult with the case manager, who may be a nurse, to ensure the necessary amount of tubing is provided.

Table 4.10   **Clinical Picture of COPD Conditions**

COPD CONDITION	CLINICAL PICTURE
Chronic bronchitis	Chronic productive cough
	Sputum clear/mucoid (purulent during infection)
	Chest infections recurrent
	Cyanosis of lips and nails
	Overweight
	"Blue bloater" or Type B COPD appearance (see Fig. 4-12)
	Associated with right heart failure and lower extremity edema
	Bronchiectasis
	Rhonchi and wheezing
	Expiration phase of breathing longer
Emphysema	No bronchial obstruction so no cough/sputum
	Chest enlarged in full inspiration position (barrel chest)
	Tachypnea—due to reduced alveolar surface area for gaseous exchange
	"Pink Puffer" or Type A COPD appearance (see Fig. 4-12)
	Hyperventilation to increase oxygen intake
	Regular use of accessory muscles of ventilation

It Happened in the Clinic

As a physiotherapy student in England in the last quarter of the 20th century, I was working on a male medical ward in the local teaching hospital. Many of the patients required chest physical therapy. At that time, the instructors in the physical therapy program also provided services at the hospital. Students in their final few months of education in those days worked almost independently; direct supervision was not required. I was performing postural drainage and chest percussion on a patient with chronic obstructive pulmonary disease when one of my instructors came to perform chest PT on the patient in the next bed. The instructor looked at the patient, who was smoking (it was allowed in hospitals at that time) and said if he wanted to kill himself, he could go ahead, but as a physical therapist, she was not going to treat him while he smoked; she then turned around and walked off the ward. As a young student,

I was in a state of shock at this abrupt refusal to treat the patient. However, the instructor went back later that afternoon and treated the patient. I saw the patient the next day, and he told me that it had been a real awakening for him to the dangers of smoking and that after the PT had left, he decided he had smoked his last cigarette. He had not touched a cigarette all day. I realized then that sometimes extreme conditions require unusual methods of treatment! This would perhaps be considered unethical and intrusive now, but because the PT returned and treated the patient later the same day, the intent of the "shock" tactics was effective and made the patient think about his health.

Emphysema

Emphysema is a COPD pulmonary condition. According to the 2010 American Lung Association Epidemiology and Statistics Unit Research and Program Services report based on the 2008 National Health Interview Survey, approximately 3.8 million people in the United States have emphysema.[85] Approximately 94% of people with emphysema are over age 45, and it has become more prevalent in females than males in the United States over the last few years, affecting 2 million women and 1.8 million men.[86]

Etiology. The main cause of emphysema is cigarette smoking, but it is not known why some people develop predominantly chronic bronchitis and others emphysema. Another contributing cause of emphysema is a congenital deficiency of a lung protecting protein called alpha 1-antitrypsin (AAT). The symptoms of AAT deficiency emphysema usually become apparent after age 32 and the symptoms are more severe if the person smokes.[87]

Signs and Symptoms. The clinical picture of patients with emphysema is detailed in Table 4-9. Most people with emphysema have the appearance of the "pink puffer" (refer to Fig. 4-13). Patients develop the typical barrel-shaped chest, exhibit hyperventilation and tachypnea in an attempt to increase oxygen uptake, and use the accessory muscles of ventilation to try and increase the volume of the chest. In the early stages of emphysema patients may be short of breath only on exertion, but eventually this condition progresses, and the person experiences dyspnea at rest. Patients with emphysema do not produce sputum or exhibit a cough because there is no bronchial obstruction or inflammation.

Pathologically in emphysema, the walls of the alveoli are destroyed by proteolytic enzymes released from leukocytes during the inflammatory process, thus reducing the surface area available for gaseous exchange (see Fig. 4-14). In addition, the walls of the alveoli lose their elasticity and thus their ability to expand and recoil. Air within the alveoli is not able to be exhaled, so it blocks fresh air from entering the alveoli, reducing the amount of oxygen available for gaseous exchange. Patients expand their chest wall using the accessory muscles in an attempt to inhale fresh air rich in oxygen. This upward and outward movement of the chest leads to the barrel chest typically noted in patients with emphysema. The FEV_1 and FVC are not affected in patients with emphysema unless there is associated chronic bronchitis.

Prognosis. Emphysema becomes a life-threatening condition as the alveolar destruction becomes more advanced. The possibility of infection increases the risks of serious complications.

Medical Intervention. Patients with advanced emphysema require oxygen therapy and may have to carry a portable oxygen tank at all times. In some cases, lung transplant may be an option for treatment. An alternative may be lung volume reduction surgery in which the most diseased areas of the lung are removed so that the other, uninvolved areas are able to work more effectively.[88] The most important advice from the physician and other health care providers is for the patient to stop smoking.

Physical Therapy Intervention. Physical therapy tests and measures for COPD include vital-sign monitoring, pulse oximetry, pulmonary function testing for FVC and

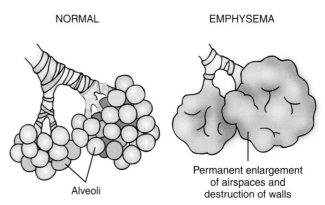

NORMAL EMPHYSEMA

Alveoli

Permanent enlargement of airspaces and destruction of walls

FIGURE 4.14 Emphysema in the lung.

FEV_1, measurement of chest excursion and breathing quality, assessment of cough, sputum and the ability to expectorate sputum, postural assessment, manual muscle testing, endurance assessment, and functional and home activity assessment. Following assessment by the PT, the plan of care is developed, and patients may be delegated to the PTA for intervention if they are sufficiently medically stable. Interventions provided by the PTA may include therapeutic exercise to increase endurance and strength, deep breathing exercises, and transfers and ambulation training with appropriate assistive devices.

The PTA may be required to monitor the use of the peak flow meter or spirometer with patients, and the pulse oximeter may be used during ambulation activities and exercise to monitor oxygen perfusion levels. Regular communication with the PT is essential during treatment of patients with COPD, especially if there are any changes in the status of patients. Many of these patients will be seen in the home setting and may use oxygen therapy. The PTA should be careful to follow the prescription for intensity of oxygen delivered to patients and not change the level of oxygen unless prescribed by the physician or the PT.

It Happened in the Clinic

Usually an oxygen saturation rate below 90% is a contraindication for performing physical therapy intervention. In a particular case in which a patient with severe emphysema was waiting for a lung transplant and receiving home PT, the physician had given permission for the PT to work with the patient carefully and allow an oxygen saturation level of anything above 75%! The patient was able to perform limited ambulation and exercises with close monitoring by the PT for signs of cyanosis, use of a pulse oximeter during activities, and use of oxygen at all times. This was an extreme case. Exercises and physical therapy should only be performed under such conditions by a PT and under strict adherence to the guidelines set by the treating physician. Because continuous evaluation of the patient's status is required, this would not be a patient scenario suitable for treatment by a PTA working alone. If the PTA were asked to do so, he or she should refer back to the supervising PT for advice and let the PT know that it is outside the scope of work of the PTA. The responsibility of designating patients to the PTA lies with the PT, but it is also the responsibility of the PTA to let the PT know if a patient is beyond the scope of work of the PTA.

Asthma

Asthma is an acute, reversible, inflammatory, obstructive pulmonary condition affecting both adults and children in which the bronchial system is acutely sensitive to external stimuli. Such stimuli can be extrinsic such as allergens or intrinsic as is the case with exercise-induced asthma. Asthma is common in the United States, and in 2008, 23.3 million Americans were estimated to have asthma. The percentage of the adult population with asthma ranges between 6.6% and 10.5% depending on the area of the country.[89] Asthma is estimated to cost the United States approximately $15.6 billion per year with $5.6 billion in prescription medications. In 2008, approximately 4.1 million children under age 18 were estimated to have asthma in the United States. The disease was estimated to be responsible for 14.2 million lost work days in 2008.[90]

Etiology. Extrinsic asthma cases present as Type 1 hypersensitivity; immune reactions; stimulated by allergens such as smoke, perfumes, or other strong smells; molds; animal dander; and insects such as cockroaches and dust mites.[91] Cases of intrinsic asthma are nonimmune in nature but are responses to environmental and internal factors, with the onset of symptoms affecting adults usually before age 40. Examples of intrinsic asthma include exercise-induced asthma, aspirin-induced asthma, a response to bronchial infection, psychological stress, and exposure to extremes of heat and cold.

Signs and Symptoms. The sensitivity of bronchi to certain stimuli is not fully understood. The mechanism of response is inflammation of the bronchial mucosa, with increased permeability of blood vessels in the linings of the bronchi and contraction and spasm of the smooth muscle walls of the bronchi. Mucous cells in the bronchi produce excess mucous as a result of the inflammatory process.

The characteristic signs and symptoms of asthma include wheezing, coughing, and dyspnea (see Table 4-10). During an asthmatic episode, patients may be in acute distress as a result of bronchospasm preventing the air exchange through the bronchi. During this phase, the cough is usually unproductive, but as the episode diminishes, plugs of sputum are expectorated. Respiratory patterns have a prolonged expiratory phase and the pulse is rapid. Both FEV_1 and FVC fall considerably both before and during an acute episode but return to normal values when the episode subsides.

Prognosis. Asthma is a reversible condition; however, deaths do occur because of uncontrolled asthmatic episodes of 24-hour duration called status asthmaticus, which do not respond to medication. An acute asthma episode of prolonged duration is considered to be a medical emergency.

Medical Intervention. Patients can be educated to predict an asthma event/episode by taking note of symptoms prior to an episode and by monitoring the FEV_1 and FVC regularly. Sometimes an occurrence can be avoided by taking medications at the first sign of problems. In most cases symptoms can be controlled by suitable medications. Medical treatment consists of bronchodilators such as salbutamol (also known as albuterol or Ventolin) and aminophylline administered through inhalers, nebulizers, or intravenously, and anti-inflammatory medications such as steroids. Antihistamine medications are prescribed for immune-mediated asthma, and oxygen therapy is required for severe cases.

Physical Therapy Intervention. Physical therapy tests and measures are the same as for COPD. Physical therapy interventions include postural awareness, breathing exercises to encourage chest excursion, relaxation training, and airway clearance techniques including postural drainage positioning, chest percussion, vibration, and shaking to facilitate removal of secretions. Discharge planning, home exercises, and education are important for these patients. ☺ The education of care providers is essential to enable use of postural drainage positioning and percussion techniques for children at home. Training of patients and care providers in the use of inhalers and nebulizer units is also important. The PTA may be involved with intervention for postural drainage and airways clearance techniques, breathing exercises, postural awareness education, home exercise and advice, relaxation techniques such as biofeedback for the upper chest and neck muscles, and discharge planning. ☺ Children with asthma become frightened at the onset of an incident, and physical therapy intervention can play a major role in helping them control breathing and relax muscles to minimize the effect of an episode or even prevent an episode from occurring.

Pneumonia

Pneumonia is a pulmonary disease involving inflammation of the alveoli and small bronchi. The disease affects mainly persons under 2 and those over age 65 years except for cases contracted by individuals who are immunosuppressed.

Etiology. Bacteria are responsible for 75% of pneumonia cases. Common bacterial causes of pneumonia are *Streptococcus pneumoniae*, *Haemophilus influenza*, *Staphylococcus*, *Escherichia coli*, and *Pseudomonas aeruginosa*, which are anaerobic bacteria. Legionnaires' disease is another form of pneumonia caused by the bacteria *Legionella pneumophila*. The name comes from cases in 1976 when members of the American Legion who were attending a convention were infected with the *Legionella* bacteria in a hotel via the air conditioning system. Viruses and fungi are also causative agents for pneumonia.[92] Viral pneumonia is transmitted by contact with an infected person. The causative virus or bacteria reaches the lung tissue through air droplets, aspiration from upper respiratory infections, aspiration of stomach contents or through sepsis of the blood. Patients susceptible to pneumonia include immunosuppressed individuals, those with serious infections, and those on life support or who are unconscious. Drug addicts contract bacterial pneumonia through contaminated intravenous needles.

Signs and Symptoms. Two basic types of pneumonia exist, alveolar pneumonia affecting the alveoli and bronchi and interstitial pneumonia affecting the alveolar septa.[93] Pneumonia can affect a lung segment, a whole lobe, or both lungs. If both lungs are involved the condition is termed **bronchopneumonia** and is usually the result of interstitial pneumonia of a viral cause. Bacteria commonly cause alveolar pneumonia, and when it affects a large portion of the lung, it is termed lobar pneumonia. Pneumonia is usually acute in nature, whether of viral or bacterial cause, but may be termed chronic if it recurs in people with conditions such as tuberculosis, cystic fibrosis, or fungal infections. Complications of pneumonia may include lung abscess, pleuritis (inflammation of the pleura; also called pleurisy), cardiac failure, pneumococcal meningitis, and chronic long-term lung disease or "honeycomb lung." Pleuritis is associated with severe, sharp pain caused by pleural effusion. If the pleural effusion is purulent, a **pyothorax** occurs (the whole pleural cavity is filled with pus). Abscess formation often occurs with *Staphylococcus* infections. The abscess destroys the wall of the bronchi and may lead to bronchiectasis. The clinical picture of pneumonia includes fever; chills; a productive cough with rusty, hemoptysis (blood), or mucopurulent (viscous and infected) sputum; dyspnea; tachypnea; and rales (see Table 4-11).

Table 4.11 **Clinical Picture of Some Pulmonary Conditions**

PULMONARY CONDITION	CLINICAL PICTURE
Asthma	Affects male:female in 2:1 ratio Extrinsic—Type 1 hypersensitivity response to allergens Intrinsic—stress, exercise, heat and cold, psychological stress, aspirin Inflammation bronchial mucosa and bronchospasm Wheezing, coughing, dyspnea Prolonged expiration phase Rapid pulse Reduced FEV_1 and FVC
Pneumonia	Affects mainly under 5 and over 70 age groups Bronchopneumonia (both lungs) 75% cases are due to bacterial pneumonia Fever, chills, cough productive of mucopurulent sputum, hemoptysis, dyspnea, tachypnea, rales May cause pleuritis with pleural pain
Cystic fibrosis	Hereditary disease of pancreas Intestinal malabsorption with fecal impaction, intestinal blockage, and foul-smelling feces Cough productive of purulent sputum Dyspnea, wheezing, failure to gain weight, sweat with high levels of sodium Hemoptysis, clubbing of fingers, delayed onset of puberty, male infertility Life expectancy varies with intensity of symptoms; early childhood up to thirties

FEV_1 = forced expiratory volume in 1 second; FVC = forced vital capacity.

Prognosis. Pneumonia is especially serious for people who have preexisting chronic lung conditions, heart disease, AIDS, have recently received transplant surgery, or have any form of chronic disease such as liver disease or sickle cell anemia. Individuals with any of these preexisting conditions are at a greater risk for developing pneumonia and of serious complications including death.[94] The disease is becoming more difficult to treat as a result of the development of strains of the bacteria resistant to antibiotics.[95]

Medical Intervention. The diagnosis of pneumonia is achieved through chest x-rays and laboratory studies to identify the bacteria in the sputum. Hematological tests may show high levels of lymphocytes and leukocytes and alteration in blood gases. Medical intervention consists of antimicrobial medications specific to the invading organism.

Physical Therapy Intervention. Physical therapy tests and measures are the same as described for asthma. Physical therapy intervention consists of airways clearance techniques, and postural drainage, much the same as for COPD. Exercises for strength and endurance after recovery are an important part of the rehabilitation.

GERIATRIC CONSIDERATIONS

Patients who are elderly are at particularly high risk of developing pneumonia during prolonged hospital stays for other medical reasons. Understanding the implications of immobility for any patient, particularly for the older population, is important for the PT and PTA. The sooner the patient is mobilized out of bed, the less the risk of pneumonia. The earlier the patient is transferred out of bed and ambulation commences, the sooner the patient can return home, the better the rate of recovery, and the less the likelihood of complications such as pneumonia.

Cystic Fibrosis

Cystic fibrosis (CF), also called fibrocystic disease of the pancreas, is a chronic, hereditary lung disorder. An estimated 10 million people are carriers of the disease in the United States.[96] The disease affects approximately 30,000 children in the United States and about 70,000 children throughout the world.[97] CF affects mainly Caucasian populations and rarely blacks or Asians. An estimated 5% of the white population of the United States are carriers of the gene for CF. The disease affects males and females equally and is the most common inherited genetic disease in the United States with an incidence of 1 in 2,000 births within the white population.[98]

Etiology. CF is a hereditary, autosomal recessive trait (defective gene and protein) located on chromosome 7.[99] This means that both parents must pass on the CF gene to the child for the child to have CF. If only one parent transmits the gene, the child becomes a carrier. The disease results in reduced pancreatic enzymes that cause malfunction of the mucous membranes and mucous-producing glands of the pancreas and lungs with resultant severe lung abnormalities. The disease affects the transport of chlorine ions within the body, mainly affecting the functions of the pancreas and lungs. The effects of this are seen mainly as intestinal malabsorption problems due to defects of the walls of the intestines and the production of excessive amounts of thick mucous in the bronchi.

Signs and Symptoms. High levels of sodium chloride are found in the sweat of patients with CF, which is significant for diagnosis. The main problems associated with CF are pancreatic insufficiency, resulting in nonabsorption of fats by the body causing malnutrition and chronic recurrent pulmonary infections with secretions that block the airways.[100] Mucus production in the lungs is excessive and viscid (thick), creating blockages within the bronchi. This buildup of mucus provides an ideal medium for the growth of bacteria, the secretions often become purulent (infected, yellow/green), and the bronchial walls become inflamed.

The clinical features of cystic fibrosis (see Table 4-10) include a highly productive cough with purulent (containing pus) sputum, dyspnea (shortness of breath), wheezing, failure to gain weight, diarrhea, fatigue, and high levels of sodium content in the sweat. A sweat chloride test is performed on infants as part of the diagnostic process.[101] During adolescence, the symptoms become worse with the development of COPD because of recurrent chest infections, hemoptysis (blood in the sputum) in the lungs, progressive breathlessness, wheezing, and cough, clubbing of the fingers, delayed onset of puberty, and frequently male infertility due to vas deferens blockage.

Pathologically patients with CF are born with normal lungs but abnormality of the pancreas. Deterioration of the lung tissue starts with mucus production, followed by bacterial growth in the mucus, which causes inflammation of the bronchial walls. The chronic inflammatory state of the bronchial walls causes bronchiectasis to develop. The airways become blocked with the viscous mucus, and the lung tissue fails to develop normally. Pancreatic abnormalities lead to malabsorption causing fecal impaction, intestinal obstruction, and foul-smelling feces. The stools of individuals with CF have a distinctive foul smell due to nonabsorption of fats. Patients tend to have distended abdomens and do not gain weight. Diabetes is common in persons with CF due to fibrosis of the pancreas. Intestinal obstruction is also common secondary to fecal impaction (hard stool blocking the intestine).

Prognosis. The life expectancy of patients with CF has improved over the past 60 years. Recent advances in

infection control have resulted in many patients living into adulthood, but the median life expectancy is 37 years.[102] Many children with CF still die in their teens and early 20s. The causes of death are usually pulmonary infections or intestinal malabsorption problems.

Medical Intervention. The medical intervention for families with a history of CF includes genetic counseling and genetic testing. Because the defective gene for CF is a recessive characteristic, which means that a defective gene is required from both parents to cause cystic fibrosis in a child, genetic testing can provide information regarding the possibility of having a child with CF.[103] Testing of the newborn can also help to provide early diagnosis of the condition and early medical intervention. The medical management for children with CF includes oxygen therapy, humidification, antibiotics, bronchodilators, and replacement of absent pancreatic enzymes. These children require close monitoring by the physician.[104]

One of the most common bacterial infections in patients with CF is *Pseudomonas aeruginosa,* and a drug of choice for this infection is inhaled tobramycin solution for inhalation (TOBI).[105] Mucolytic medications (inhaled mucus-thinning medications) such as Pulmozine are provided to help people expel the mucus more easily. Physicians provide advice regarding good nutrition and airway clearance techniques and refer the person for dietary counseling, respiratory therapy, and physical therapy.[106] One airway clearance technique is the use of **positive expiratory pressure (PEP) therapy.** The PEP therapy machine resists exhalation of air from the lungs and helps to keep the airways open.[107]

Physical Therapy Intervention. Physical therapy tests and measures follow the same pattern as other pulmonary diseases. Physical therapy intervention is vital for management of the disease. Patients need to follow an at least twice-daily postural drainage regime for the whole of their lives. Infection can be reduced to a minimum by maintaining clear airways. The PT and PTA teach postural drainage and airway clearance techniques[108] such as percussion, shaking, and vibrations, breathing exercises, and cough facilitation to the family and patient. The importance of pulmonary hygiene is emphasized. Mobility of the shoulder girdle and thorax are essential. A program of physical exercises and general fitness with endurance and aerobic activity is important, together with postural awareness and relaxation techniques. Physical therapy intervention is concentrated immediately after diagnosis of the disease to provide instruction in airway clearance procedures to care providers. A home program must be prescribed to include postural drainage, breathing exercises, and percussion techniques. During periods of infection, the PT and PTA may be involved with patients to assist with the treatment. Consultations by the PT may be needed for intermittent postural assessment and also in the terminal stages of the disease to improve quality-of-life issues and keep patients as comfortable as possible.

The psychological problems can be difficult to cope with for families affected by CF. ⊕ Children with CF require a lot of attention, so their siblings may become jealous and resentful. Parents often feel guilty because they have passed on the gene for the condition to the child and have to watch them suffer and ultimately die. The child is unable, in many cases, to participate in normal activities, especially as he or she grows older.

Tuberculosis

Tuberculosis (TB) is a type of bacterial lung disease, with similar effects to those of pneumonia. The incidence of TB is increasing particularly among immunosuppressed individuals such as those with HIV infection (see Chapter 10). A rise in cases of TB has also been noted in the homeless population and in prison inmates as a result of overcrowded conditions.

Etiology. TB is caused by the bacterium *Mycobacterium tuberculosis*. TB is an airborne infection transmitted via air droplets from one person to another through sneezing and coughing. Infection of individuals requires prolonged exposure to *Mycobacterium tuberculosis,* and thus the people more likely to become infected are those with compromised immune systems or who live in crowded conditions.

Signs and Symptoms. The main symptoms of tuberculosis are a productive cough and general body symptoms such as fatigue, weight loss, fever, chills, and night sweats.[109] The onset and progression of TB depends on the response of the individual patient. Lesions, or foci, develop in the lungs, which may become centrally necrosed. The necrosed areas then become enclosed by fibrous tissue creating granulomas, or the disease may progress to a more general pulmonary disease with widespread bodily symptoms, such as damage to kidneys, bone, joints, and the brain. When TB lesions become fibrosed, the disease is considered to be latent rather than

active. People with fibrosed lesions still have TB, but the disease process becomes inactive.

Prognosis. The prognosis for TB is generally good with the correct treatment including a healthy diet. Unfortunately, tuberculosis is one of the diseases developing drug-resistant strains that are becoming more difficult to treat. According to Gostin (2007), this drug resistance is turning into a "global crisis."[110] Tuberculosis is more prevalent among those individuals who are immunosuppressed and is a serious complication in patients with AIDS. Extensive lung damage with fibrosis can occur if the disease is not controlled. Fortunately, in many cases, the TB subsides into an inactive state with few residual effects.

Medical Intervention. Patients need to receive plenty of rest, fresh air, sunlight, good nutrition, and exercise to assist recovery from TB. Pharmacology management is more difficult as a result of the onset of drug resistant forms of the bacteria. Patients must take anti-TB medications for between 9 and 12 months, and compliance with the dosage and length of time is important to reduce the drug-resistant forms of the bacteria.

Physical Therapy Intervention. Physical therapy intervention is not usually required for patients with TB. However, PTAs need to be aware of the risks of TB transmission and be diligent in the use of standard universal precautions when treating patients with the disease. All health care workers are required to be tested annually for TB. On occasion, the PTA may see patients with chronic TB that has developed into joint and bone destruction of the spine and hips.

Lung Cancer, Benign Lung Tumors, and Malignant Lung Tumors

Tumors of the bronchi and lungs can be either benign or malignant. Approximately 1 million people die from lung cancer worldwide each year.[111] Lung cancer affects men slightly more than women. Benign lung tumors account for between 2% and 5% of all lung tumors. These benign tumors are not life-threatening but may predispose the person to becoming infected with pneumonia.[112]

Etiology. The relationship between smoking and lung cancer is widely accepted and places the smoker at much higher risk for cancer than the nonsmoker. Passive tobacco smoke inhalation, known as secondhand smoke, also raises the risk of lung cancer.[113]

Signs and Symptoms. Many tumors develop in the larger bronchi and spread to occlude the airways and cause atelectasis distal to the blockage. In some cases, tumors located in the lungs are secondary sites due to metastasis from a primary site somewhere else in the body, often from the brain or breast. The clinical picture of patients with lung cancer usually involves a dry cough, which often goes untreated because patients think it is caused by smoking. Other signs and symptoms include dyspnea, pain, hemoptysis (blood in the sputum), weight loss, and general feelings of fatigue.

Prognosis. The prognosis is varied depending on the type of tumor involved, the health of the individual, and the response to intervention. The general survival rate for patients with lung cancer was 15% over 5 years in 2002. According to the American Cancer Association the rates of death for this type of cancer have changed little since 2000 and are still significantly higher than for any of the other forms of more commonly diagnosed cancers such as breast, colon, and prostate cancers.[114] In 2010, the American Cancer Society predicted there would be 222,520 new cases of lung cancer in 2010 and that there would be 157,300 deaths from lung cancer accounting for 29% of all cancer deaths.[115] A reason for the higher death rate for persons with lung cancer may be the result of the highly vascular nature of the lung tissue, which facilitates metastasis to other areas of the body.

Medical Intervention. If the tumor is detected in an early stage, surgery can be performed to remove the section of involved lung followed by chemotherapy and radiation therapy. In cases of advanced-level tumors, the usual medical intervention will be with a combination of chemotherapy and radiation therapy.[116]

Physical Therapy Intervention. This may be required after surgery for postural drainage and vibrations to encourage removal of secretions. Percussion is contraindicated if there is a possibility of bone involvement in the ribs or hemoptysis. Postural drainage and vibrations may also be provided during the terminal phase of the condition to enhance the quality of life. Fatigue is common in people with cancer; therefore, aerobic activity and endurance exercises are also an important part of physical therapy intervention, with care being taken not to overfatigue patients. The wishes of patients should be followed, with the right to refuse treatment honored. The PTA needs to be aware of the grieving process taking place within the family to be able to provide optimal intervention. Home physical therapy may include instruction in the use of a mechanical lift to assist caregivers in the transfer of patients from chair to bed, some general mild exercises, and even ambulation and mobility exercises if appropriate. Instructions for lifting and transfer techniques for care providers are important to prevent injury to the care providers.

Pulmonary Infarction

Pulmonary infarction is a condition in which areas of the lung tissue are deprived of oxygen. Depending on the amount of time the tissue is deprived of oxygen, the lung tissue may recover or may become necrotic. Total infarction of the lungs is a comparatively rare occurrence. Infarction of areas of the lung is more common, and early diagnosis is the key to a good outcome for patients.

Etiology. A pulmonary infarction (death of cells in the lung) may develop secondary to a lower extremity pulmonary embolus (clot formation) that travels to the lungs. A large embolus can become lodged in the pulmonary artery and completely occlude the vessel, but this is fairly rare.[117] These so-called saddle emboli prevent blood from entering the lung, causing anoxia of lung tissue and death. Small emboli may occlude small bronchi and cause infarction of small areas of the lung supplied by that bronchus. Emboli may occasionally form after surgery and during physical therapy intervention. Other causes of blockage to the pulmonary artery are fat deposits, air (as in deep-sea diving), or pieces of bone or bone marrow as a result of major trauma.[118]

Signs and Symptoms. If infarcted areas in the lung are small, the person may experience pleural pain due to irritation of the pleura from the infarcted area. Pain associated with lower extremity emboli may be localized to the posterior lower leg or less commonly around the hip. The pain is usually intense and unlike the normal pain experienced after surgery or injury. Other symptoms of a pulmonary embolism may include dyspnea, seizures, or fever.

Prognosis. The prognosis for patients with saddle emboli is poor. Sudden complete occlusion of the pulmonary artery usually results in death. The prognosis for patients with small areas of pulmonary tissue infarction is generally good if the appropriate medical intervention is provided.

Medical Intervention. Diagnosis of a pulmonary embolism is dependent on chest radiographs, CT scans with radiocontrast, pulmonary angiography, MRI, echocardiography, and electrocardiograms.[119,120] The medical intervention is usually with anticoagulent medications such as warfarin and bed rest.

Physical Therapy Intervention. Physical therapy intervention is not indicated for patients with pulmonary infarction; however, an unexpected, unexplained increase in pain in the lower extremity during physical therapy intervention for other conditions should always be reported immediately to the supervising PT and the physician. A lower extremity embolus may travel to the lung and cause a pulmonary embolus. Some patients seem to be more predisposed to develop an embolus, and a history of emboli should be carefully noted when the PTA reads the patient charts prior to treatment.

Pneumoconioses

Pneumoconioses are a group of lung diseases caused by inhaling small particles from the air. Some of the more common forms of pneumoconioses include asbestosis, coal-worker's lung, and silicosis. People most susceptible to pneumoconioses are those who work in environments with a high level of dust or small organisms such as coal miners. According to the most recent Work-Related Lung Disease Surveillance Report 2002 (p. xxiii) published in 2005, 12.81 deaths per million of the population per year were attributed to all types of pneumoconioses in the United States in 1999 and 11.94 per million in 2002, demonstrating a slight decline in death rate from this condition.[121] The highest risk occupations for deaths due to pneumoconioses were insulation workers, boilermakers, and coal miners.

Etiology. Coal dust causes black lung disease or coal-worker's lung disease. The lungs actually turn black from inhalation of coal dust. This disease has been associated with a high level of tuberculosis in coal miners who worked for many years in the mines. Silicosis is caused by inhalation of crystals of silica in those who work as miners, cut stone, or do sandblasting. Asbestosis is caused by inhalation of small asbestos fibers, which become lodged in lung tissue. Smoking in patients with asbestosis greatly increases the risk of lung cancer.

Signs and Symptoms. All types of pneumoconioses can lead to fibrosis of the lungs with subsequent respiratory symptoms of dyspnea. The most dangerous pneumoconiosis

is considered to be asbestosis, which predisposes patients to developing lung cancers such as malignant mesothelioma.[122] Advanced levels of coal worker's pneumoconiosis can appear as diffuse areas of white patches on lung radiographs.[123]

Prognosis. According to the Centers for Disease Control and Prevention, the outcome for uncomplicated coal worker's pneumoconiosis is good. In the complicated form of the disease, the symptoms can get worse, causing cor pulmonale or tuberculosis. Death usually occurs as a result of complications from the disease rather than the disease itself.[124] The prognosis for people with asbestosis is not as good as for other forms of this condition and is especially poor for those who develop malignant mesothelioma. Seventy-five percent of people who develop malignant mesothelioma die within 1 year of diagnosis.[125]

Medical Intervention. Medical intervention for pneumoconiosis is similar to that for emphysema. In cases of pneumoconiosis, the fibrosis of the lungs prevents expansion of the lung tissue and oxygen therapy may be required. If lung secretions are a problem, inhalers will be prescribed. Referral to physical therapy may be initiated.

Physical Therapy Intervention. Physical therapy intervention may include postural drainage and percussion, general endurance exercises, and mobility training.

Sarcoidosis

Sarcoidosis is included in this section because of the affect the disease can have on the lungs. Sarcoidosis is an inflammatory condition with granuloma formation in various organs of the body including the lymphatic system and the lungs. Other areas of the body can be affected such as the skin, eyes, and liver.[126] The incidence of sarcoidosis is difficult to determine because many people with the condition are asymptomatic, but it may be more common than once thought. Estimates are that between 1 and 40 cases occur per 100,000 of the population in the United States.[127] Adults between the ages of 20 and 40 are most often affected. The black population in the United States is more at risk than others. People of Scandinavian and northern European origin are also at risk, and women are affected more often than men. Interestingly, those people most at risk of developing sarcoidosis include health care workers, teachers, and nonsmokers. [128]

Etiology. Sarcoidosis is thought to be an immune-mediated condition, but its cause is unknown. Granulation occurs in the lymph nodes throughout the body, but particularly in those within the thorax and lungs.

Signs and Symptoms. Many patients with sarcoidosis are asymptomatic (no symptoms). Others may develop symptoms such as dyspnea, fever, anorexia (inability to eat), skin ulcers, eye irritation, joint and muscle pain, headaches, lower extremity edema, cough, chest pain, and wheezing on ventilation.[129] Most patients with sarcoidosis develop symptoms in the lungs and thorax (95%).[130] Patients may have nodules in the lungs and enlarged lymph glands, often in the neck and chest. Sometimes the enlarged lymph nodes are painful.

Prognosis. Most patients recover spontaneously from sarcoidosis, but a small percentage of patients develop long-standing lung pathology or other organ pathology.

Medical Intervention. Diagnosis of sarcoidosis is made with the help of CT scans, MRI, chest x-rays, positron emission tomography scans, thallium and gallium scans (injection of radioactive substances into the body followed by a scan to track sites of inflammation), blood tests, and lung function tests. In such cases, medical treatment depends on the type of pathology experienced. In cases of lung pathology, medical treatment follows a similar pattern to those for lung conditions already described. Prednisone is often used to reduce the effects of inflammation depending on the severity of the condition.[131]

Physical Therapy Intervention. Physical therapy intervention is not indicated for patients with sarcoidosis.

Adult Respiratory Distress Syndrome

Adult respiratory distress syndrome (ARDS) is rapid lung failure as a result of many types of lung pathologies that lead to cardiopulmonary failure. In all cases, there is damage to the alveoli and anoxia occurs. About 150,000 people are affected by ARDS each year in the United States.[132]

Etiology. The causes of ARDS include pneumonia, other infections such as sepsis, cardiac failure, inhalation of toxic fumes or smoke, and near-drowning.

Signs and Symptoms. A typical clinical picture in ARDS starts with shortness of breath about 24 hours to 3 days after a precipitating event such as the onset of a critical disease or infection, near-drowning incident, or severe trauma. Symptoms can include tachycardia (fast heart rate), cyanosis of the skin, difficulty breathing, hyperventilation, and fatigue. The condition can progress to multiorgan failure and sepsis (acute total body inflammation in response to infection).[133]

Prognosis. The fatality rate for people with ARDS is reported to be between 40% and 70%.[134] Death is usually caused by general system failure as a result of multiple organ involvement and is associated with the lack of oxygenation of the tissues and sepsis. Most of the people who survive fully recover, but a few have long-term pulmonary problems associated with fibrosis of the affected lung tissue.[135,136]

Medical Intervention. Patients with ARDS require artificial ventilation and are usually treated in the intensive care unit or critical care unit in a hospital. Medications are usually administered for control of the causative bodily infection. Patients with ARDS are highly susceptible to additional infections.

Physical Therapy Intervention. Patients recovering from ARDS may require chest PT, exercise programs to gradually increase strength and endurance, and mobility for ambulation and functional activities of daily living. The precautions for the treatment of patients with ARDS are the same as for other severe pulmonary conditions. Vital signs should be taken before and after exercise, and the oxygen uptake should be monitored by a pulse oximeter to ensure adequate oxygenation of the tissues.

Bronchopulmonary Dysplasia in Pediatric Respiratory Distress Syndrome ⊛

The immature infant with respiratory distress syndrome (see atelectasis) who is placed on oxygen and a ventilator may develop bronchopulmonary dysplasia (BPD).

Etiology. BPD may be caused by pneumonia or meconium aspiration (aspiration of feces by the fetus in the womb). BPD is found frequently in immature or premature infants who have been placed on artificial ventilation for prolonged periods of time.

Signs and Symptoms. Bronchopulmonary dysplasia is characterized by respiratory distress and a dependency on oxygen. Signs and symptoms include cyanosis of the skin, tachypnea (rapid breathing), and dyspnea.

Prognosis. Chronic changes occur in the lungs of some of the infants who survive, including granulation of the bronchi and bronchioles, which sometimes close the airways, and cause emphysema, fibrosis, and atelectasis. In other milder cases, the child fully recovers after the first few years. The condition is also associated with right ventricular failure. Many infants require several months of ventilator treatment. BPD may predispose children to recurrent respiratory infections in childhood and later life.[137]

Medical Intervention. Even though one of the causes of BPD is the use of ventilators, infants with this condition require additional ventilator treatment to ensure oxygenation of the tissues. Anti-inflammatory medications such as prednisone to control edema, and diuretics to reduce the risk of fluid in the lungs may be used. Additional feeding through a nasogastric tube may also be necessary.[138]

Physical Therapy Intervention. Chest physical therapy with percussion and postural drainage positioning is helpful for the infant with BPD. Some children with BPD have neurodevelopmental delay and may require PT intervention during infancy and throughout the school years.[139]

Pulmonary Surgery

Two main types of thoracic surgical incisions are used for thoracic surgery for the heart or lungs. The posterolateral thoracotomy is an incision made in the intercostal space with patients in side-lying, affected side facing upward. Several muscles are cut during this surgery, including the serratus anterior, latissimus dorsi, intercostals, trapezius, rhomboids, and possibly the infraspinatus and teres major.[140] See Figure 4-15 for thoracotomy incision and the related incised muscles. An alternative method of a modified muscle sparing posterolateral thoracotomy is also used that does not cut through the muscles and thus reduces the rehabilitation time.[141]

An alternative incision is through a median sternotomy. In this procedure, the incision is straight through the sternum. This approach is mainly used for open heart surgery rather than pulmonary surgery. The addition of video-assisted surgery now allows the surgical team to be accurate during surgery through a smaller incision. The smaller incision reduces the healing time.

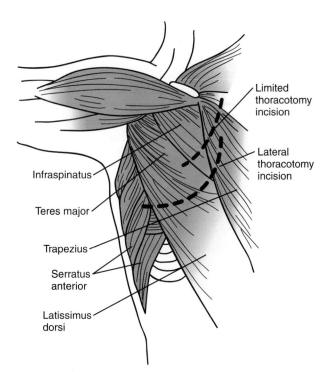

FIGURE 4.15 Thoracotomy incision with related muscles.

Pneumonectomy

Pneumonectomy is the surgical removal of a whole lung. Removal of the lung and the associated mediastinal lymph glands and parts of the chest wall is termed a radical pneumonectomy. An extrapleural pneumonectomy involving the removal of the lung plus part of the pericardium of the heart and sections of the diaphragm may be performed for severe forms of cancer such as malignant mesothelioma.[142] The indications for a pneumonectomy include carcinoma of the lung, severe tuberculosis, or bronchiectasis of the whole lung. The incision most often used for this surgery is a posterolateral thoracotomy.

The side effects of surgery can include damage to the phrenic nerve, causing reduced function of the diaphragm, and damage to the recurrent laryngeal nerve, which can result in loss of function of the vocal cords. Other complications can include empyema, pulmonary edema, pneumonia, and heart problems.[143] Patients may also have a reduction in the respiratory function and a reduced ability to cough immediately postsurgery.

Physical Therapy Intervention. Preoperatively the PT and PTA may be required to perform airway clearance techniques. Postoperatively, huffing can be taught rather than coughing because this technique is more suitable after thoracic surgery. Huffing causes less movement of the ribs and consequently is more comfortable for patients. See the section on "Coughing and Huffing" at the end of this chapter for further details about huffing techniques. Patients can also be instructed in how to support the surgical incision site during coughing by crossing the opposite arm across the chest and fixing it with the other arm for increased comfort during coughing postoperatively (see Fig. 4-16). Postsurgery, the space where the resected lung was removed becomes filled with fluid. A thoracic drain is used to obtain the optimum level of fluid in the surgical space. Eventually the space where the lung was removed will fibrose (tissues will organize into connective tissue that forms a scar). Physical therapy intervention is aimed at clearing secretions from the remaining lung without causing damage to the surgical site or risking injury to the severed ends of the bronchi within the thorax. Oxygen therapy or a ventilator may be required immediately after surgery. The use of an incentive spirometer helps patients to improve their ventilation. Upper extremity and spinal movements are encouraged to prevent loss of function, and breathing exercises are taught to keep the remaining lung functional. Postural reeducation is needed with a gradual return to strength, mobility, and endurance exercises. Placing patients in a Trendelenburg position (tipping patients with head down lower than the legs) is contraindicated when performing postural drainage for patients who have had a pneumonectomy. Placing patients in a head-down position may cause irritation of the surgical site and interfere with the consolidation of the lung space. If postural drainage is required to assist with removal of secretions, patients should be placed in a modified position in side lying. Patients should be encouraged to change position from side to side as often as possible.

Lobectomy

A lobectomy is the surgical removal of a lung lobe. The indications for the surgery are the same as for pneumonectomy, but the damage to the lung is not as extensive. A segmental resection is performed when the disease process affects only a lung segment.

Physical Therapy Intervention. Physical therapy intervention after segmental resection is to encourage expansion of the remaining area of lung on the surgical side. Intervention includes breathing exercises with huffing and support of the incision site for comfort. Vibrations can be performed on the unaffected lung from Day 1 postsurgery, progressing to the affected side if necessary after a few days, when patients are able to tolerate the procedure. Bed mobility exercises and progressive strengthening and endurance activities in the postoperative phase are essential to encourage patients to return to full function.

Hemothorax and Pneumothorax

Patients who have sustained chest trauma may have air or blood in their pleural cavity. Air in the pleural cavity

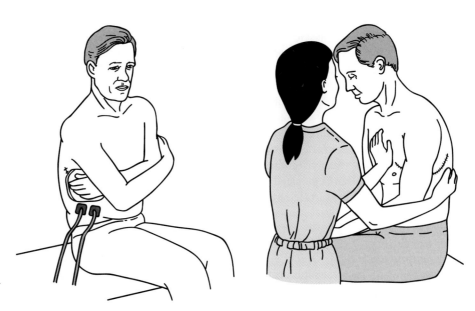

FIGURE 4.16 Hand and arm position to support incision after pneumonectomy.

is termed pneumothorax, and blood in the cavity is called a hemothorax. Removal of this air and blood is achieved by use of drainage tubes in the chest wall. Drainage tubes pass from patients into a container of water to prevent air passing back into the chest and causing a further pneumothorax.

Physical Therapy Intervention. If the PT and PTA treat patients with a chest tube in place, care must be taken to make sure the end of the tube stays in the water, that the tube remains free of external bends, and that the drainage container is lower than the thorax. Several types of drainage systems are available, including closed systems such as the Pleurovac (see Fig. 4-17). Many of these systems allow for patient mobility. The therapist can observe air draining from the chest cavity by noting air bubbles in the water of the container.

Note: The container with the tubes must always be kept on the floor or at least below the level of the thorax. If the container is raised above the level of the chest, water will drain backward into the chest from the drainage container. Any drainage of fluid back into the lungs will cause further lung congestion and possible infection.

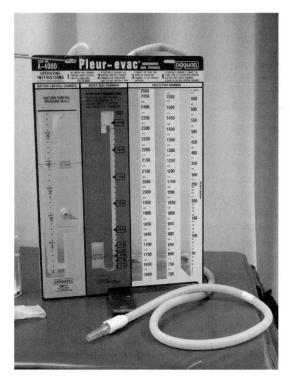

FIGURE 4.17 Photograph of Pleurovac unit.

Post–pulmonary Surgery Complications

Complications are possible after any surgery. Pulmonary surgery is major surgery, and complications can include lung infections, wound infection or adhesions, hemorrhage, pneumothorax, and collapse of the remaining lung tissue after a lobectomy or a segmental resection. Associated complications include deep venous thrombosis, restricted movement in the spine, shoulders and ribs, postural abnormalities, and muscle weakness from incised muscles during surgery. Muscle weakness is often found in the serratus anterior and latissimus dorsi because these muscles are cut most often during surgery. Other side effects of surgery may include atelectasis, muscle guarding, splinting (immobility from non-movement of patients), pulmonary embolism, pulmonary edema, and surgical emphysema. Surgical emphysema is caused by air in the subcutaneous tissues, usually surrounding a surgical site. Surgical emphysema can be palpated on the skin and feels like a bubbling under the surface of the skin.

Tracheotomy

In patients on mechanical ventilation resulting from serious disease or a life-threatening incident, a tracheotomy may be necessary. The trachea is divided, with patients under anesthesia, and a tracheal tube placed directly into the trachea from the anterior aspect of the neck. A tracheotomy makes it easier to provide ventilation to a patient who is either hypoxic or has ventilatory failure. The opening made during a tracheotomy surgery is termed a tracheostomy.

Lung Transplant

A lung transplant is performed usually as a last resort for people with severe lung disease. The surgery can involve the replacement of one lung or both. The suitable candidates for a lung transplant have to meet specific criteria set by the United Network for Organ Sharing (UNOS).[144] Individual hospital and medical systems may have their own criteria built on the basics from UNOS. The medical team determines whether people meet the criteria. Usually these criteria include people who are a maximum age of 60 or 65, who have the presence of a terminal lung condition, who are nonsmokers, and who are otherwise in fairly good health and with a good family support system after discharge.[145] A single lung transplant is usually performed through the posterolateral thoracotomy incision. The incision for a double lung transplant may be anterior and horizontal across the chest above the level of the diaphragm.

Physical Therapy Intervention. Patients will be on mechanical ventilation for the first 1 to 3 days after lung transplant surgery (see Chapter 13 for details of special considerations on intensive care unit and cardiac care unit). Constant monitoring of blood pressure, heart rate, and oxygen perfusion and saturation levels is required. Physical therapy intervention after lung transplant follows the format previously described for the thoracotomy procedure and includes encouraging upper extremity activity and bed mobility and assisting patients with getting out of bed. The goal is for gradual increase in exercise tolerance with an oxygen saturation level of over approximately 90%. A pulse oximeter is used during exercise and activity to monitor oxygen saturation levels. The PTA may be involved with treatment of these patients as part of the cardiopulmonary rehabilitation team. The PT must ensure that patients are sufficiently medically stable for the PTA to be involved in treatment.

Classes of Medications Used to Treat Respiratory Diseases

Antibiotics and antimicrobials may be indicated whenever an infection is present in the lower or upper respiratory tract as determined by the physician. A laboratory culture is performed using a sample of sputum or a swab of cells from the mouth or pharynx. An antibiotic is selected that is specific for the organism detected. Antibiotics should not be prescribed without determining the presence of infection because the infective organism can develop resistance to the antibiotic. Some examples of pulmonary diseases that require antibiotics are asthma with purulent sputum, bacterial pneumonia, empyema, and lung abscess.

Anti-inflammatory agents including corticosteroids may be used for the treatment of acute asthma exacerbations or episodes and other inflammatory conditions. Corticosteroids have an anti-inflammatory effect on the bronchi, reducing the edema of the bronchial linings. These medications can be administered either orally or through nebulizer inhalation.

Bronchodilators are used for the treatment of obstructive airways diseases including chronic bronchitis and asthma. They may also be used to treat bronchiectasis, emphysema, and bronchospasm. These medications act to relax muscle spasm in the bronchi, which results in dilation of the lumen of the bronchi. A common bronchodilator is salbutamol (Ventolin).

Humidification through a unit attached to oxygen, or purely a humidification unit, assists with the loosening and reduction of viscosity of secretions in the bronchi, making it easier for patients to expectorate the sputum. The oxygen is passed over a humidification unit, or **nebulizer**, that moistens the inhalant as it is inhaled by patients. Certain medications may be placed in the nebulizer unit for delivery with the oxygen. Medications include the bronchodilators previously mentioned and corticosteroids. Medications administered through a nebulizing unit take approximately 15 to 20 minutes to reach maximum effectiveness, and thus exercise programs should be performed after the medications have taken effect.

The Role of the PTA in Interventions for Patients With Respiratory Diseases

After patients have been evaluated and treated by the PT and have been determined to be medically stable, the PTA may treat patients with respiratory diseases. The PTA needs to remember that any changes in patient status must be immediately communicated to the PT and the physician. Oxygen saturation levels may need to be monitored with a pulse oximeter during treatment. Blood pressure and pulse must be taken before, during, and after treatment intervention, and peak flow or incentive spirometry measurements need to be taken to monitor patients' response to treatment. The PTA should be familiar with the particular dyspnea scale used in the facility. Such scales include the American Thoracic Society Dyspnea Scale, the Borg scale, and a simple visual analog scale. The perceived rate of exertion (PRE) can be used with patients familiar with their own symptoms. The PRE is a somewhat subjective procedure in which patients determine their own safe levels of exertion during exercise through their previous experience. However, the PRE is used widely during cardiac and pulmonary rehabilitation with patients demonstrating a high level of accuracy rating regarding their own exertion levels. Breathing exercises and postural drainage and percussion with vibration techniques may all be required. The PTA may also perform general pulmonary hygiene techniques and teach bed mobility exercises, progressive upper and lower extremity exercises, mobility programs, and use of oxygen therapy.

Specific Physical Therapy Treatment Interventions for Patients With Respiratory Pathologies

The goals of physical therapy intervention in the treatment of patients with pulmonary conditions include the following:

- Assist patients with removal of secretions from the lungs through airways clearance techniques
- Improve the quality of breathing and teach breathing control
- Teach mobilizing exercises for the thorax and upper extremities
- Reeducate in postural awareness and improve posture
- Teach relaxation techniques for all muscles of ventilation
- Increase exercise tolerance
- Teach use of assistive equipment when necessary

This text does not cover all physical therapy interventions for pulmonary pathological conditions, but postural drainage positions, coughing and huffing techniques, and some specific breathing exercises are described. A patient with secretions in the lungs resulting from any of the previously described pathologies will benefit from airways clearance techniques. The techniques may also be taught to patients and care providers for home management.

POSTURAL DRAINAGE AND AIRWAY CLEARANCE TECHNIQUES

Postural drainage is achieved by placing patients into a position such that the bronchial segment of the lung will drain, with the aid of gravity, into the larger bronchi where the lung secretions can stimulate a cough reflex and be expectorated. No special equipment is necessary for postural drainage. Many household furniture items can be adapted to provide good postural drainage positioning. Examples of patient positioning for chest percussion and vibration techniques are provided in Figure 4-18.

Remember to position patients so that the direction of the bronchi of the segment to be drained is facing up into the air against gravity. This positioning requires the PTA to have a good working knowledge of the bronchopulmonary segments and directions of the bronchi of the lungs. The illustrations in Figure 4-19 depict the positions used for drainage of several of the bronchopulmonary segments.

Many patients start coughing as soon as they are placed in a postural drainage position. Other patients require 10 to 15 minutes in a postural drainage position

Percussion

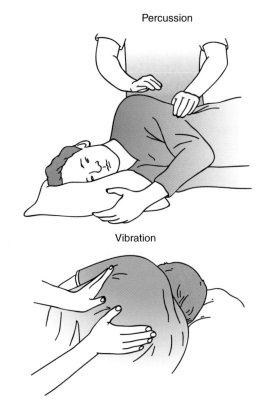

Vibration

FIGURE 4.18 Position for (A) chest clapping/percussion and (B) vibration of a patient for assisted airway clearance techniques.

followed by percussion and vibration techniques to facilitate expectoration of sputum. Postural drainage, percussion, and vibration techniques are performed by the physical therapist and the PTA. These techniques can be taught to family members for use at home. Other means of providing assistance for airway clearance is with the use of a mechanical device, such as a massage machine, that can be self-administered in some cases. (Consult a massage text for details of percussion and vibration techniques.) Some patients respond with positioning and immediate percussion. If the secretions are viscous, patients may benefit from a period of humidification to reduce the viscosity of the secretions prior to postural drainage. After patients start coughing, they should be encouraged to sit up and cough out the secretions into a receptacle. If a sputum sample is required for laboratory analysis, a sterile container should be used. Swallowing of secretions, especially those that are infected, can cause stomach irritation and should be discouraged. Patients with some pathological conditions and others who have had specific surgeries may not be suitable for postural drainage. See

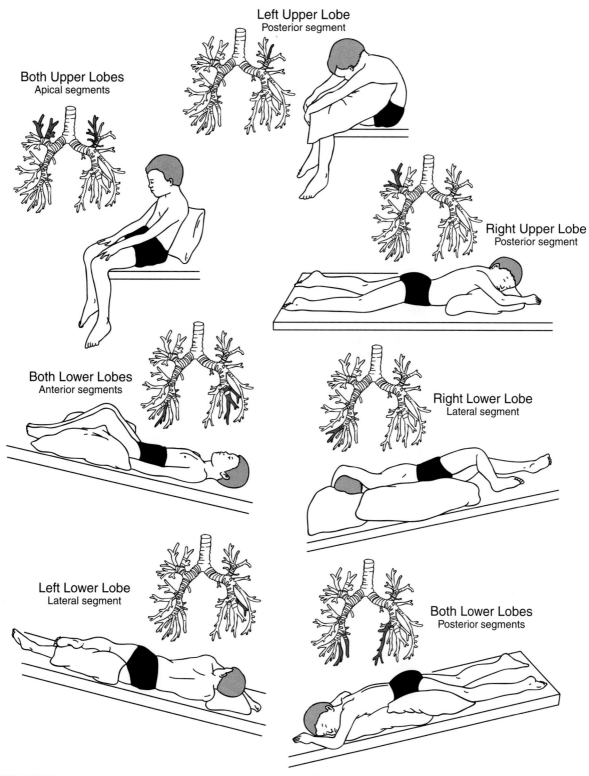

FIGURE 4.19 Various bronchopulmonary segment postural drainage positions.

Table 4-12 for details of these pathological conditions and surgical procedures, with the appropriate contraindications and precautions.

COUGHING AND HUFFING TECHNIQUES

An effective cough is elicited by instructing patients to take a deep inhalation breath and then tighten the abdominals before attempting a cough. Without a high volume of air in the lungs, patients may not be able to produce sufficient force in a cough to expel the secretions. Huffing is an alternative technique used especially when a forced cough may be uncomfortable or contraindicated, such as after thoracic surgery. Huffing, also called the forced expiration technique (FET) or the active cycle of breathing technique (ACBT),[146] can be taught rather than coughing because this technique is more suitable after

thoracic surgery. Huffing is performed by inhaling deeply and then exhaling forcefully either once or twice in a row, keeping the mouth open, without actually trying to cough.[147] Pryor and Webber (1998) stated that FET can also reduce the viscosity of the secretions within the lungs and make them easier to remove.[148] When combined with general deep-breathing exercises, including diaphragmatic breathing, this procedure helps to loosen secretions and enable expectoration (removal of lung secretions by coughing).

A combination of huffing and coughing may be required in some patients. When using huffing techniques, patients should rest after the technique is performed once or twice and use breathing exercises to reduce the possibility of bronchospasms. When bronchospasms occur, they reduce the amount of air exchange in the lungs and

Table 4.12   Contraindications and Precautions of Postural Drainage

TECHNIQUE	PATHOLOGICAL CONDITION	CONTRAINDICATED	PRECAUTIONS NEEDED
All postural drainage (PD)	Pulmonary edema with congestive heart failure	X	
	High intracranial pressure	X	
	Pulmonary embolism	X	
	Rib fractures	X	
	Empyema/hemoptysis/extensive pleural effusions	X	
	Recent head and neck trauma or spinal surgery or injury	X	
	Bronchopleural fistula after pneumonectomy	X	
	Patients with confusion		X (Use discretion; needs to be evaluated by PT)
Trendelenburg PD (head down)	Post-esophageal surgery	X	
	Lung carcinoma with hemoptysis	X	
	Any patient at risk for aspiration	X	
	Post-thoracotomy surgery	X	
Percussions/shaking	Osteoporosis/osteomyelitis of ribs/rib fractures	X	
	In presence of chest burns or skin grafts on chest	X	
	Surgical emphysema	X	
	Chest wall pain/lung contusions		
	Bronchospasms	X	
	In recent spinal anesthesia or pacemaker placement	X	
	In the very old or anxious		X (needs to be evaluated by PT)
Vibrations	May be performed in many of the above situations		

prevent the expectorant of secretions. Suctioning of secretions may be necessary to clear the airways of unconscious patients or those with reduced ability to cough. Suctioning is performed by the PT or the nurse. Suctioning is not a technique that a PTA is expected to perform. To perform suctioning, a catheter attached to a suction pump is passed down the trachea through the nasopharynx or pharynx, and secretions are removed. In many cases, once the suction tube reaches the carina at the bifurcation point of the trachea, the patient's cough reflex is stimulated, and the secretions can be easily removed.

BREATHING EXERCISES

Patients with respiratory disease experience fatigue and hypoxia due to poor breathing techniques. Instruction in lateral costal excursion exercises and diaphragmatic breathing assists patients in breathing more effectively. Relaxation plays an important part in effective breathing control. Many patients use accessory muscles of ventilation continuously, which contributes to the level of fatigue. Apical breathing is typically used by patients and is ineffective for ventilation of the lung bases. Most patients require assistance to inflate the basal area of the lungs. Observe carefully for patients who do a reversed abdominal breathing in which they tighten the abdominals during inhalation, which prevents the diaphragm from descending during inhalation. The PTA should instruct patients in effective diaphragmatic breathing (see Fig. 4-20). Patients are placed in a relaxed position and instructed to allow the abdomen to relax (go outwards) during inhalation/inspiration, and flatten during exhalation/expiration. Initial relaxed positions may include leaning against a wall, or sitting with the hands or elbows leaning on the knees to fix the upper chest and enable concentration on the abdomen. A gentle, relaxed breathing pattern is encouraged. Gradually patients can be taught to use this pattern during daily activities and progress to using it during specific exercise routines.

Lateral costal breathing to expand the basal segments of the lungs can be encouraged by using the hands. The principle of directional resistance is used to facilitate movement against the directional pressure of the force.

1. The PT/PTA places his or her hands on the lower lateral aspects of the thorax and allows patients to breathe, concentrating on using the lower part of the chest. As the patients take a deep breath, the therapist says, "Breathe in through your nose and out through your mouth and push your ribs out into my hands." When the inspiratory phase is completed, the therapist maintains pressure on the lower chest until patients have completed exhalation/expiration. At maximal exhalation/expiration the therapist applies overpressure to facilitate a deep breath and cause the chest to expand in the lateral costal area. Patients should not perform more than three maximal breaths at one time to avoid feelings of dizziness from hyperventilation. An increase in lateral costal excursion is usually elicited after the first cycle of ventilation.

2. Patients place their hands against their lateral costal area either with hands crossed over the chest or with elbows flexed and hands placed against the chest. The steps described in #1 are repeated. Both unilateral and bilateral expansion can be performed using this technique.

VENTILATORS, LIFE SUPPORT SYSTEMS, AND INTERMITTENT POSITIVE PRESSURE BREATHING

Management of patients using ventilatory and life support systems is discussed in greater detail in Chapter 13. Respiratory support systems are used for patients unable to breathe independently or who breathe insufficiently to provide adequate oxygenation. Mechanical ventilation machines include several types of machines. **Controlled mechanical ventilation (CMV)** is used when patients are paralyzed and unable to participate in breathing. An assist control (AC) unit completely controls breathing with the machine programmed at specific settings. Assisted mechanical ventilation provides specific delivery of oxygen, but patients can trigger the machine to work.[149] Patients have no control over intermittent mandatory ventilation (IMV). The machine delivers preset amounts of oxygen at intervals to supplement the breathing, while allowing patients to exhale.[150,151] Pressure support ventilation (PSV) provides patients with more control over the breathing, while ensuring a minimum level of inspiration. Another type of PSV is volume-assured pressure support (VAPS), which monitors the tidal volume of the lungs and assists in maintaining an adequate tidal volume. Intermittent positive pressure breathing (IPPB) machines are no longer being used for the most part.

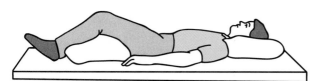

FIGURE 4.20 Initial relaxed position for diaphragmatic breathing exercises.

Some indications for using mechanical ventilation include the following:

- Pulmonary conditions when the PaO_2 falls below 60 mm Hg despite the use of oxygen therapy, as in patients with pneumonia or adult respiratory distress syndrome
- Pulmonary conditions when the $PaCO_2$ rises dramatically and patients become confused and exhausted, which may occur in asthma
- Severe muscle weakness or paralysis in which patients cannot breath independently (e.g., patients with high-level cervical quadriplegia)
- Severe thoracic trauma with impaired vital capacity, low PaO_2 of less than 60 mm Hg on oxygen, and inability to clear secretions
- Multiple trauma, septic shock, electrical burns

PEDIATRIC CONCERNS AND SPECIAL CONSIDERATIONS ⚘

In the infant, special considerations for pulmonary care need to be addressed:

1. The lumen of the bronchi in infants is much smaller than either in the child or the adult and as a result may become blocked much more easily by mucus.
2. The alveoli are immature and have a relatively smaller area for gaseous exchange to occur than the adult. The alveoli continue to multiply in number in the first few years of life.
3. Infant lungs have a low compliance, which requires more effort of breathing.
4. The diaphragm muscle is immature and fatigues rapidly.
5. The ribs are at a greater horizontal angle than in the adult and do not move as much to expand the chest. Most of the chest diameter expansion is from the diaphragm.
6. Postural drainage positioning can be performed while infants are in an incubator. Chest percussion can be performed using only a few fingers, and vibrations can be executed with the fingertips. Infants can be placed on the therapist's knee to elicit postural drainage positions. Patients usually tolerate this position well. As children get older, treatment has to be adapted to encourage them to be compliant.
7. Family involvement with the treatment for infants and children is essential.

CASE STUDY 4.1

A 75-year-old male patient with COPD is attending the outpatient physical therapy department in the local acute care hospital. No other significant pathologies or complications exist. The PT has evaluated the patient and determined that he requires breathing exercises, airways clearance techniques for the left lower lateral lobe, and monitoring with a pulse oximeter for oxygen saturation levels during a progressive exercise program to enhance strength and endurance.

1. Describe what particular precautions the PTA would take when working with this patient.

2. Using a model, perform the treatment program and include the following:
   - Teach the appropriate breathing exercises
   - Perform percussion techniques to facilitate airways clearance
   - Teach a family member (another student) how to perform percussion techniques and postural drainage positioning
   - Develop and teach a suitable progressive strengthening and endurance exercise program
   - Pay particular attention to the tests and measures used, as well as treatment and safety issues

CASE STUDY 4.2

An 8-year-old female with a history of cystic fibrosis is attending the physical therapy department for review of postural drainage positioning for home use. The PT has evaluated the patient and recommends postural drainage positions for all bronchopulmonary segments, including apical, with percussion and vibration techniques and facilitation of coughing.

1. Using a model, position the patient in all necessary postural drainage positions and perform percussion, vibration, and instruction in coughing techniques.

2. Teach another person to perform the same treatment, as you would instruct the child's parent.

3. Describe any precautions that might be taken.

4. Discuss a home program for the patient.

STUDY QUESTIONS

1. Teach basic breathing exercises, including lateral costal and diaphragmatic techniques, to a family member or friend with no medical knowledge. Concentrate on making the exercises easily understandable and effective. Teach huffing and coughing techniques.

2. The PTA is working with a patient with COPD for ambulation and endurance exercises. During ambulation with a walker, the oxygen saturation level falls to 75% as indicated by the pulse oximeter. What should the PTA do immediately? What subsequent steps should the PTA take to ensure the well-being of the patient?

3. What is the normal value for forced vital capacity (FVC) of the lungs in a healthy adult male?

4. What is the tidal volume of the lungs?

5. What is the normal relationship between the FVC and FEV_1? How does this ratio change in pulmonary pathology, and what significance does this have for the PTA? Give some examples of ratios for various pathologies.

6. Explain the concepts of the "blue bloater" and the "pink puffer."

7. List five of the typical signs and symptoms of pulmonary diseases.

8. Describe two pulmonary conditions that are considered to be COPD.

9. Describe how a patient can be assisted to cough after undergoing thoracic surgery.

10. Discuss with a fellow student the implications of antibiotic-resistant bacteria and name two such bacteria.

11. List three classifications of medications that can be used to treat pulmonary diseases.

12. Explain the mechanism of action for each classification type.

⊙ USEFUL WEB SITES

The U.S. National Library of Medicine's Visible Human Project
http://anatquest.nlm.nih.gov/

American Lung Association
http://www.lungusa.org

The Auscultation Assistant
http://www.med.ucla.edu/wilkes/inex.htm
Provides excellent audio of normal and abnormal breath and heart sounds

Radiological Society of North America
http://www.radiologyinfo.org
Provides excellent descriptions of all radiological procedures with graphics.

United Network for Organ Sharing
http://www.unos.org
Includes information regarding organ transplants

⊙ REFERENCES

1 The pharynx. (2000). *Gray's Anatomy of the Human Body.* Philadelphia: Lea & Febiger. New York: Bartleby.com. Retrieved 07.30.07 from http://education.yahoo.com/reference/gray/subjects/subject/244

2 The vocal folds. (2000). In ibid. Retrieved 07.30.07 from http://education.yahoo.com/reference/gray/subjects/subject/236

3 The epiglottis. (2000). In ibid. Retrieved 07.30.07 from http://education.yahoo.com/reference/gray/subjects/subject/236

4 The trachea and bronchi. (2000). In ibid. Retrieved 07.30.07 from http://education.yahoo.com/reference/gray/subjects/subject/237;_ylt=AopevdODIdCKzR3B.ESW2bIZvskF

5 Frownfelter, D., & Dean, E. (2006). *Cardiovascular and pulmonary physical therapy: evidence and practice,* 4th edition. St. Louis, MO: Mosby, p. 74.

6 The trachea and bronchi. (2000). *Gray's Anatomy of the Human Body.* In ibid. Retrieved 07.30.07 from http://education.yahoo.com/reference/gray/subjects/subject/237;_ylt=AopevdODIdCKzR3B.ESW2bIZvskF

7 Ibid.

8 Lister Hill National Center for Biomedical Communications, National Library of Medicine, National Institutes of Health. (2004). Visible human male images of the National Library of Medicine (NLM) right and left lungs. *Anatquest: anatomic Images On-line.* Retrieved

08.04.07 from http://anatquest.nlm.nih.gov/VisibleHuman/ImageData/Rendered/jpg/DSR110225739.jpg

9 Bergman, R., et al. (2006). *Anatomy atlases: a digital library of anatomy information*. Retrieved 08.04.07 from http://www.anatomyatlases.org

10 Lister Hill National Center for Biomedical Communications. Ibid.

11 Kaufman, D. (2006). Pleural effusion. *Medline Plus Medical Encyclopedia*. Retrieved 08.04.07 from http://www.nlm.nih.gov/medlineplus/ency/article/000086.htm#visualContent

12 Yale University School of Medicine (1998). *Cranial nerve X—vagus*. Retrieved 08.04.07 from http://www.med.yale.edu/caim/cnerves/cn10/cn10_1.html

13 University of the West of England, Bristol. (2005). *Respiratory tree: dilation and constriction of bronchioles*. Retrieved 08.04.07 from http://hsc.uwe.ac.uk/rcp/respiratory/treeDilation.asp

14 Frownfelter, D., & Dean, E. Ibid., p. 65.

15 O'Sullivan, S. B., & Schmitz, T. J. (2007). *Physical rehabilitation*, 5th edition. Philadelphia: F. A. Davis, p. 108.

16 Ibid., p. 82.

17 National Heart, Lung, and Blood Institute, U.S. National Library of Medicine, National Institutes of Health. (2007). *Sleep apnea*. Retrieved 08.04.07 from http://www.nlm.nih.gov/medlineplus/sleepapnea.html

18 Ibid. Retrieved 08.04.07 from http://www.nhlbi.nih.gov/health/dci/Diseases/SleepApnea/SleepApnea_WhatIs.html

19 Frownfelter, D., & Dean, E. Ibid., p. 73.

20 Ibid., p. 74.

21 Rabbette, P. S., et al. (1994). Hering-Breuer reflex and respiratory system compliance in the first year of life: a longitudinal study. *J Appl Physiol* 76:650–656.

22 Frownfelter, D., & Dean, E. Ibid., p. 74.

23 Ito, M., et al. (1999). Immediate effect of respiratory muscle stretch gymnastics and diaphragmatic breathing on respiratory pattern. Respiratory Muscle Conditioning Group. *Int Med* 38:126–132.

24 Frownfelter, D., & Dean, E. Ibid., p. 75.

25 Watchie, J. (1995). *Cardiopulmonary physical therapy: a clinical manual*. Philadelphia: W. B. Saunders, p. 36.

26 Clements, J. A., & Avery, M. E. (1998). Lung surfactant and neonatal respiratory distress syndrome. *Am J Respir Crit Care Med* 157:S59–S66.

27 Watchie, J. Ibid., p. 40.

28 Ibid., p. 49.

29 Frownfelter, D., & Dean, E. Ibid., p. 86.

30 Ibid., p. 96.

31 Ibid., pp. 91, 97.

32 American Lung Association (2010). *Asthma in adults fact sheet*. Retrieved 10.31.10 from http://www.lungusa.org/lung-disease/asthma/resources/facts-and-figures/asthma-in-adults.html

33 Frownfelter, D., & Dean, E. Ibid. p. 78.

34 West, J. B., & Dollery, C. T. (1960). Distribution of blood flow and ventilation-perfusion ratio in the lung, measured with radioactive CO_2. *J Appl Physiol* 15:405–410.

35 Ibid.

36 Treppo, S., Mijailovich, S. M., & Venegas, J. G. (1997). Contributions of pulmonary perfusion and ventilation to heterogeneity in Va/Q measured by PET. *J Appl Physiol* 82:1163–1176.

37 Hemoglobin test. (2002). *Healthline*. Retrieved 08.05.07 from http://www.healthline.com/galecontent/hemoglobin-test-1

38 Frownfelter, D., & Dean, E. Ibid., p. 82.

39 Hayes, J. A. (2005). Respiratory acidosis. *eMedicine from WebMD*. Retrieved 08.05.07 from http://www.emedicine.com/med/topic2008.htm

40 Ibid.

41 Watchie, J. Ibid., p. 36

42 Frownfelter, D., & Dean, E. Ibid., p. 223.

43 Pryor, J. A., & Webber, B. A. (1998). *Physiotherapy for respiratory and cardiac problems*, 2nd edition. Edinburgh, Scotland: Churchill Livingstone.

44 Frownfelter, D., & Dean, E. Ibid., p. 707.

45 Breath sounds. (n.d.). *The Auscultation Assistant*. Retrieved 08.05.07 from http://www.wilkes.med.ucla.edu/lungintro.htm

46 Kaufman, D. A. (2006). Breath sounds. *Medline Plus Medical Encyclopedia*. Retrieved 08.05.07 from http://www.nlm.nih.gov/medlineplus/ency/article/003323.htm

47 Friction rub. (n.d.). *The Auscultation Assistant*. Retrieved 08.05.07 from http://www.med.ucla.edu/wilkes/Rubintro.htm

48 Department of Patient education and Health Information, The Cleveland Clinic. (2005). *How to use an incentive spirometer*. Retrieved 08.05.07 from http://www.clevelandclinic.org/health/health-info/docs/0200/0239.asp?index=4302&src=news

49 Watchie, J. Ibid., p. 4.

50 Global Initiative for Chronic Obstructive Lung Disease. (2006). *Global strategy for the diagnosis, management and prevention of COPD*. Retrieved from http://www.goldcopd.org.

51 National Guideline Clearinghouse. (2007). http://www.guideline.gov/summary/summary.aspx?view_id=1&doc_id=10177

52 Hypercapnia. (2005). *Taber's cyclopedic medical dictionary*, 20th edition. (2005). Philadelphia: F. A. Davis, p. 1030.

53 Hill, E. & Stoneham, M. D. (2000). Practical applications of pulse oximetry. *Updates in Anaesthesia* 11:1–2. Retrieved 10.10.10 from http://www.nda.ox.ac.uk/wfsa/html/u11/u1104_01.htm

54 O'Sullivan, S. B., & Schmitz, T. J. (2007). *Physical rehabilitation*, 5th edition. Philadelphia: F. A. Davis, p. 102.

55 Disorders of nutrition and metabolism: acid/base balance. (2003). *Merck Manuals Online Medical Library for Healthcare Professionals*. Retrieved 10.10.10 from http://www.merck.com/mmhe/sec12/ch159/ch159a.html

56 Yale University School of Medicine. (2004). *Cardiothoracic imaging: pleural effusion*. Retrieved 08.06.07 from http://www.med.yale.edu/intmed/cardio/imaging/findings/pleural_effusion/index.html

57 Lababede, O. (2006). Pleural effusion. *eMedicine from WebMD*. Retrieved 08.06.07 from http://www.emedicine.com/radio/topic233.htm

58 Radiological Society of North America. (2007). Computed tomography (CT)—chest. *RadiologyInfo*. Retrieved 08.06.07 from http://www.radiologyinfo.org/en/info.cfm?pg=chestct

59 Radiological Society of North America. (2007). MRI of the chest. *RadiologyInfo*. Retrieved 08.06.07 from http://www.radiologyinfo.org/en/info.cfm?pg=chestmr

60 Ibid.

61 Hibbert-Bentley, S. (2007). Pulmonary angiography. *Medline Plus Medical Encyclopedia*. Retrieved 08.07.07 from http://www.nlm.nih.gov/medlineplus/ency/article/003813.htm

62 Nakano, T., et al. (1992). Pulmonary arteriography and bronchial arteriography in embolism [in Japanese]. *Nihon Kyobu Shikkan Gakkai Zasshi* 30 Suppl:254–263.

63 O'Sullivan, S. B., & Schmitz, T. J. Ibid., p. 338

64 Definition of Bruce protocol. (2006). *MedicineNet*. Retrieved 08.07.07 from http://www.medterms.com/script/main/art.asp?articlekey=30741

65 Irwin, S., & Tecklin, J. S. (2004). *Cardiopulmonary physical therapy: a guide to practice*. Philadelphia: Mosby, p. 259.

66 American Heart Association. (2007). *Exercise stress test*. Retrieved 08.07.07 from http://www.medterms.com/script/main/art.asp?articlekey=30741

67 Gibbons, R., et al. (1997). ACC/AHA guidelines for exercise testing: executive summary. A report of the American College of Cardiology/American Heart Association Task Force on Practice Guidelines (Committee on Exercise Testing). *Circulation* 96:345–354.

68 O'Sullivan, S. B., & Schmitz, T. J. Ibid., p. 605.

69 Centers for Disease Control and Prevention. (n.d.). *General physical activities defined by level of intensity*. Retrieved 09.30.07 from

http://www.cdc.gov/nccdphp/dnpa/physical/pdf/PA_Intensity_table_2_1.pdf

[70] O'Sullivan, S. B., & Schmitz, T. J. Ibid., p. 614.

[71] Gandelman, G. (2006). Pulmonary edema. *MedlinePlus Medical Encyclopedia.* Retrieved 08.07.07 from http://www.nlm.nih.gov/medlineplus/ency/article/000140.htm

[72] Kaufman, D. A. (2007). Atelectasis. *MedlinePlus Medical Encyclopedia.* Retrieved 08.07.07 from http://www.nlm.nih.gov/medlineplus/ency/article/000065.htm

[73] Kaufman, D. A. (2005). Pneumothorax. *Medline Plus Medical Encyclopedia.* Retrieved 08.08.07 from http://www.nlm.nih.gov/medlineplus/ency/article/000087.htm

[74] Kaufman, D. A. (2006). Pleural effusion. *Medline Plus Medical Encyclopedia.* Retrieved 08.08.07 from http://www.nlm.nih.gov/medlineplus/ency/article/000086.htm

[75] Mansharamani, N. G. (2003). Chronic lung sepsis: Lung abscess, bronchiectasis, and empyema. *Curr Opin Pulm Med* 9:181–185.

[76] Lung abscess. (2005). *Merck Manuals Online Medical Library for Healthcare Professionals* Retrieved 08.08.07 from http://www.merck.com/mmpe/sec05/ch053/ch053a.html

[77] Sahn, S. A. (2005). Diagnostic thoracentesis. *UpToDate.* Retrieved 08.08.07 from http://patients.uptodate.com/topic.asp?file=pleurdis/2076

[78] American Lung Association Epidemiology and Statistics Unit Research and Program Services January 2010. (2010). *Estimated prevalence and incidence of lung disease by lung association territory.* Retrieved 10.31.10 from http://www.lungusa.org/finding-cures/our-research/trend-reports/estimated-prevalence.pdf

[79] Bronchitis. (2007). *Medline Plus Medical Encyclopedia.* Retrieved 08.08.07 from http://www.nlm.nih.gov/medlineplus/bronchitis.html

[80] Frownfelter, D., & Dean, E. Ibid., p. 512.

[81] Ibid.

[82] American Academy of Family Physicians. (2005). Chronic bronchitis. *Familydoctor.org.* Retrieved 08.08.07 from http://familydoctor.org/online/famdocen/home/articles/280.html

[83] Heath, J. M., & Mongia, R. (1998). Chronic bronchitis. *Am Fam Physician* 57:2365–2372, 2376–2378.

[84] Frownfelter, D., & Dean, E. Ibid., p. 512.

[85] American Lung Association Epidemiology and Statistics Unit Research and Program Services January 2010. (2010). *Estimated prevalence and incidence of lung disease by lung association territory.* Retrieved 10.31.10 from http://www.lungusa.org/finding-cures/our-research/trend-reports/estimated-prevalence.pdf

[86] American Lung Association. (2010). Chronic obstructive pulmonary disease (COPD) fact sheet. Retrieved on 10.31.10 from http://www.lungusa.org/lung-disease/copd/resources/facts-figures/COPD-Fact-Sheet.html

[87] Ibid.

[88] Ibid.

[89] American Lung Association. (2010). Asthma in adults fact sheet. Retrieved on 10.31.10 from http://www.lungusa.org/lung-disease/asthma/resources/facts-and-figures/asthma-in-adults.html

[90] American Lung Association. (2010). *Asthma in adults fact sheet.* Ibid.

[91] National heart, Lung, and Blood Institute. (2008). *Asthma.* Retrieved 10.31.10 from http://www.nhlbi.nih.gov/health/dci/Diseases/Asthma/Asthma_WhatIs.html

[92] Blaivas, A. J. (2010). Pneumonia. *MedlinePlus Medical Encyclopedia.* Retrieved 10.31.10 from http://www.nlm.nih.gov/medlineplus/ency/article/000145.htm

[93] Saukkonen, J. J (2010). Lymphocytic interstitial pneumonia. *eMedicine from WebMD.* Retrieved 10.31.10 from http://emedicine.medscape.com/article/299643-overview

[94] National Institute of Allergy and Infectious Disease. (2006). Pneumococcal pneumonia. Retrieved 10.31.10 from http://www.niaid.nih.gov/topics/pneumonia/Pages/default.aspx

[95] National Institute of Allergy and Infectious Disease. (2009). *Pneumococcal disease.* Retrieved 10.31.10 from http://www.niaid.nih.gov/topics/pneumococal/Pages/PneumococcalDisease.aspx

[96] Cystic Fibrosis Foundation. (2007). *Testing for cystic fibrosis.* Retrieved 08.09.07 from http://www.cff.org/AboutCF/Testing

[97] *Cystic Fibrosis Foundation.* (2007). *What is cystic fibrosis?* Retrieved 08.09.07 from http://www.cff.org/AboutCF

[98] *Cystic Fibrosis Foundation.* (2007). *About cystic fibrosis.* Retrieved 04.21.07 from http://www.cff.org/AboutCF

[99] Umphred, D. A. (2001). *Neurological rehabilitation,* 4th edition. St. Louis, MO: Mosby, p. 294.

[100] Cystic Fibrosis Foundation. (2007). *About cystic fibrosis.* Ibid.

[101] Cystic Fibrosis Foundation. (2007). *Testing for cystic fibrosis.* Ibid.

[102] Cystic Fibrosis Foundation. *About cystic fibrosis.* Ibid.

[103] Cystic Fibrosis Foundation. (2007). Ibid.

[104] Lewis, R. A. (2007). Cystic fibrosis. *Medline Plus Medical Encyclopedia.* Retrieved 08.08.07 from http://www.nlm.nih.gov/medlineplus/ency/article/000107.htm

[105] Cystic fibrosis foundation. (2007). *Building strength: therapies for CF.* Retrieved 04.21.07 from http://www.cff.org/treatments/Therapies

[106] Ibid.

[107] Cystic fibrosis foundation. (2007). *Airway clearance techniques.* Retrieved 04.21.07 from http://www.cff.org/treatments/Therapies/Respiratory/AirwayClearance

[108] Ibid.

[109] Tuberculosis. (2007). *Medline Plus Medical Encyclopedia.* Retrieved 08.08.07 from http://www.nlm.nih.gov/medlineplus/tuberculosis.html

[110] Gostin, M. H. (2007, July). Extensively drug resistant tuberculosis: an isolation order, public health powers, and a global crisis. *JAMA* 298:83–86.

[111] Alberts, W. M. (2003). Lung cancer guidelines. *Chest* 123:1S–2S. Retrieved 08.08.07 from http://www.chestjournal.org/cgi/content/full/123/1_suppl/1S

[112] Mueller, D. K. (2007). Benign lung tumors. *eMedicine from WebMD.* Retrieved 08.08.07 from http://www.emedicine.com/med/topic2988.htm

[113] Alberg, A. J. (2003). Epidemiology of lung cancer. *Chest* 123:21S–49S. Retrieved 08.08.07 from http://www.chestjournal.org/cgi/content/full/123/1_suppl/21S

[114] Alberts, W. M. Ibid.

[115] American Cancer Society. (2010). *Cancer facts and figures 2010 tables and figures.* Retrieved 10.31.10 from http://www.cancer.org/Research/CancerFactsFigures/CancerFactsFigures/most-requested-tables-figures-2010

[116] Jett, J. R., et al. (2003). Guidelines on treatment of Stage IIIB non-small cell lung cancer. *Chest* 123:221S–225S. Retrieved 08.08.07 from http://www.chestjournal.org/cgi/content/abstract/123/1_suppl/221S

[117] Sharma, S. (2006). Pulmonary embolism. *eMedicine from WebMD.* Retrieved 08.08.07 from http://www.emedicine.com/med/topic1958.htm

[118] Kosmix Right Health. (2007). *Lung infarction.* Retrieved 08.09.07 from http://www.righthealth.com/Health/lung_infarction/-m-1-od-definition_Pulmonary__embolism-out-health—goog—sb-s

[119] Sharma, S. Ibid.

[120] Kosmix Right Health. Ibid.

[121] Centers for Disease Control and Prevention. (2005). *Work-related lung disease surveillance report 2002.* Division of Respiratory Disease Studies, National Institute for Occupational Safety and Health, U.S. Department of Health and Human Services, Public Health Service. Retrieved 10.31.10 from http://www2a.cdc.gov/drds/WorldReportData/csv/2005Figure06-01.csv

[122] Kaufman, D. A. (2007). Asbestosis. *MedlinePlus Medical Encyclopedia.* Retrieved 08.09.07 from http://www.nlm.nih.gov/medlineplus/ency/article/000118.htm

123 Taragin, B. (2006). Coal workers pneumoconiosis complicated # 2. *MedlinePlus Medical Encyclopedia*. Retrieved 08.09.07 from http://www.nlm.nih.gov/medlineplus/ency/imagepages/1604.htm

124 Kaufman, D. A. (2007). Coal workers pneumoconiosis. *Medline-Plus Medical Encyclopedia*. Retrieved 08.09.07 from http://www.nlm.nih.gov/medlineplus/ency/article/000130. htm#Expectations%20(prognosis)

125 Kaufman, D. A. Asbestosis. Ibid.

126 National Heart, Lung, and Blood Institute, U.S. Department of Health and Human Services. (2007). *What is sarcoidosis?* Retrieved 08.09.07 from http://www.nhlbi.nih.gov/health/dci/Diseases/sarc/sar_whatis.html

127 Gould, K. P., & Callen, J. P. (2009). Sarcoidosis: frequency. *eMedicine from WebMD*. Retrieved 10.31.10 from http://www.emedicine.com/DERM/topic381.htm

128 National Heart, Lung, and Blood Institute, U.S. Department of Health and Human Services. (2007). *Sarcoidosis: who is at risk?* Retrieved 08.09.07 from http://www.nhlbi.nih.gov/health/dci/Diseases/sarc/sar_whoisatrisk.html

129 National Heart, Lung, and Blood Institute, U.S. Department of Health and Human Services. (2007). *What are the signs and symptoms of sarcoidosis?* Retrieved 08.09.07 from http://www.nhlbi.nih.gov/health/dci/Diseases/sarc/sar_signsandsymptoms.html#chart

130 Baughman, R.P., et al. (2001). Clinical characteristics of patients in a case control study of sarcoidosis. *Am J Respir Crit Care Med* 164:1885–1889.

131 National Heart, Lung, and Blood Institute, U.S. Department of Health and Human Services. (2007). *How is sarcoidosis treated?* Retrieved 08.09.07 from http://www.nhlbi.nih.gov/health/dci/Diseases/sarc/sar_treatments.html

132 American Lung Association. (2006). *Adult (acute) respiratory distress syndrome (ARDS) fact sheet.* Retrieved 08.09.07 from http://www.lungusa.org/site/pp.asp?c=dvLUK9O0E&b=35012

133 Conrad, S. A. (2005). Respiratory distress syndrome: Adult. *eMedicine from WebMD*. Retrieved from http://www.emedicine.com/EMERG/topic503.htm

134 Ibid.

135 American Lung Association. (2006). *Adult (acute) respiratory distress syndrome (ARDS) fact sheet.* Ibid.

136 Ibid.

137 Kaufman, D. A. (2005). Brochopulmonary dysplasia. *MedlinePlus Medical Encyclopedia*. Retrieved 08.09.07 from http://www.nlm.nih.gov/medlineplus/ency/article/001088.htm

138 Ibid.

139 Frownfelter, D., & Dean, E. Ibid., p. 661.

140 Dürrleman, N., & Massard, G. (2006). Posterolateral thoracotomy. *Multimedia manual of cardiothoracic surgery.* European Association for Cardio-thoracic Surgery. Retrieved 08.09.07 from http://mmcts.ctsnetjournals.org/cgi/content/full/2006/0810/mmcts.2005.001453

141 Ashour, M. (1990). Modified muscle sparing posterolateral thoracotomy. *Thorax* 45:935–938. Retrieved 08.09.07 from http://thorax.bmj.com/cgi/content

142 Pneumonectomy. (2006). *Aetna InteliHealth.* Retrieved 08.09.07 from http://www.intelihealth.com/IH/ihtIH/WSIHW000/9339/23692.html

143 Ibid.

144 United Network for Organ Sharing. (2007). Retrieved from http://www.unos.org

145 Lung transplant. (2006). *Aetna InteliHealth.* Available from http://www.intelihealth.com/IH/ihtIH/WSIHW000/9339/31212.html

146 Frownfelter, D., & Dean, E. Ibid., p. 328.

147 Irwin, S., & Tecklin, J. S. (2004). *Cardiopulmonary physical therapy: a guide to practice,* 4th edition. St. Louis, MO: Mosby, p. 316.

148 Pryor, J. A., & Webber, B. A. (1998). Ibid., p. 144.

149 Nakayama, H. C., et al. (2003). Controlled versus assisted mechanical ventilation effects on respiratory motor output in sleeping humans. *Am J Respir Crit Care Med* 168:92–101.

150 Wylicil, P., Kardos, P., & Schladt, W. (1977). Intermittent mandatory ventilation—a new method in the treatment of severe respiratory insufficiency (German). *Med Klin* 72:166–170.

151 Valerón, L., et al. (2003). Intermittent mandatory ventilation. *An Pediatr* 59:86–92.

152 Zieve, D., Juhn, G., & Eltz, D. R. (2008). HDL test. *MedlinePlus Medical Encyclopedia*. Retrieved 10.31.10 from http://www.nlm.nih.gov/MEDLINEPLUS/ency/article/003496.htm

153 Ibid.

154 Zieve, D., Juhn, G., & Eltz, D. R. (2008). LDL test. *MedlinePlus Medical Encyclopedia*. Available from http://www.nlm.nih.gov/medlineplus/ency/article/003495.htm

155 Ibid.

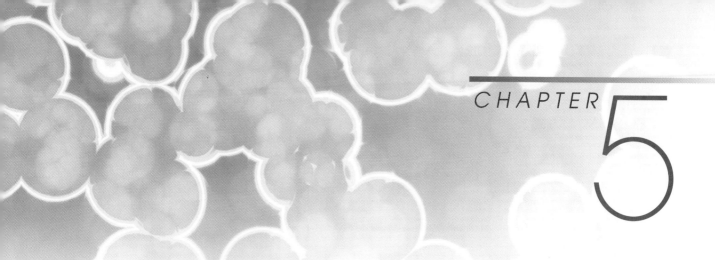

Degenerative Joint Diseases and Bone Pathologies

CHAPTER 5

LEARNING OBJECTIVES

After completion of this chapter, students should be able to:

- Describe the anatomy and physiology of bone and joints
- Describe the pathological mechanisms of osteoarthritis, osteoporosis, and other bone pathologies
- Describe the pathological mechanisms of tumors that affect bone and cartilage
- Discuss the physical therapy interventions for patients with osteoarthritis, osteoporosis, and other bone pathologies
- Determine the role of the physical therapist assistant in working with patients with osteoarthritis, osteoporosis, and other bone and joint pathologies
- Identify the contraindications and precautions for physical therapy intervention for patients with osteoarthritis, osteoporosis, and other bone and joint pathologies

CHAPTER OUTLINE

KEY TERMS

Avascular necrosis
Bouchard's nodes
Bursae
Crepitus
Eburnation
Fibrillation
Genu valgum
Genu varum
Hallux valgus
Hemarthrosis
Heberden's nodes
Hyperthyroidism
Hyperuricemia
Osteoarthrosis
Osteopenia
Osteophytes
Osteotomy
Pes planus
Radiculopathy
Retrolisthesis
Spondylolisthesis
Talipes equinovarus
Tophi
Trendelenburg gait pattern
Unicondylar knee resurfacing

CHAPTER OUTLINE (continued)

Introduction

This chapter begins with a review of the anatomy, physiology, and structure of normal joints and bone. Various degenerative joint diseases are then described with a focus on osteoarthrosis. An overview of the major surgical interventions applicable to people with degenerative joint diseases is included, and a description of the most commonly provided physical therapy interventions associated with these surgeries is discussed. A variety of diseases of the bone most commonly seen in physical therapy practice, including osteoporosis and tumors of the bone and cartilage, are described with their appropriate physical therapy interventions. Some of the most commonly acquired joint abnormalities and genetic bone abnormality conditions are also discussed.

Why Does the Physical Therapist Assistant Need to Know About Normal Joint Structure?

The anatomy of bones, joints, and muscles is the backbone of physical therapy practice. A basic understanding of the anatomy of a healthy joint is crucial to the understanding of the abnormalities that exist in joints for a variety of arthritic conditions and other pathologies and enables the physical therapist assistant (PTA) to be able to speak to other members of the rehabilitation team in a knowledgeable way. In addition, understanding how a joint is supposed to look, feel, and function in a healthy individual allows the PTA to determine when a person is having joint problems that require examination and evaluation by the physical therapist (PT).

The physical therapist assistant spends a great deal of time treating patients with degenerative joint diseases, and not always in an orthopedic setting. As many as 20 million people are affected by osteoarthritis, or osteoarthrosis, in the United States.[1] The incidence of osteoarthrosis increases with age, but people in their early 20s may have arthritic changes in their joints. An understanding of basic normal joint structure and bone physiology is required for the study of any form of arthritis. Bone, ligament, and tendon healing and the inflammatory response often associated with osteoarthrosis are detailed in Chapter 1.

Normal Joint Structure

The classification of joints falls into three general categories: 1) fibrous joints, which do not move and are called synarthroses; 2) slightly moveable joints with cartilage components; and 3) synovial joints (see Fig. 5-1), which are highly moveable and are called diarthroses (two components). Arthritic changes mainly occur in the synovial joints, and therefore these are discussed in detail.

Synovial joints have articular or hyaline cartilage covering their articular surfaces. The hyaline cartilage protects the bone ends and absorbs shock from the impact of weight bearing and activity. The cartilage is composed of approximately 80% water and provides a smooth surface that reduces the friction of the bone ends in the joints to a minimum. The cartilage consists of collagen fibers and proteoglycans formed by cartilage-producing cells called chondrocytes. The proteoglycans are responsible for the property of cartilage that allows it to absorb and expel water. When the cartilage is under pressure, it expels water and becomes thinner, and when the pressure is

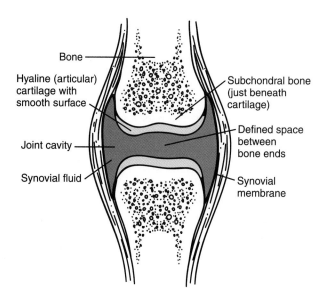

FIGURE 5.1 A synovial joint.

relieved, the cartilage absorbs water and swells. When the balance of proteoglycans is disturbed, the cartilage appears to lose some, or all, of the property to recover after pressure. Synovial fluid fills the joint space, providing lubrication and nutrition for the bone ends. The articular ends of the bones do not normally touch each other. A capsular ligament lined with a synovial membrane surrounds the joint. The synovial membrane produces the synovial fluid.

Ligaments, both external and internal to the joint, may be present, and some ligaments form an integral part of the capsule. If the ligaments are very strongly attached to the capsule they may reduce the available movement of the joint, as in the hip. In joints such as the shoulder, the ligaments are not as strong or integral with the capsule, and this allows more mobility of the joint. Many synovial joints have additional structures that increase stability, such as the menisci in the knee, the acetabular labrum in the hip, and the glenoid labrum in the shoulder. In the shoulder, joint stability is sacrificed to increase mobility, and in the hip mobility is sacrificed to provide the necessary stability.

Collagen is an important component of bone, cartilage, ligaments and tendons. (See Chapter 1 for further details of collagen). The hyaline cartilage is composed mainly of Type II collagen, while bone, ligament, and tendon are composed mainly of Type I. Collagen is organized into parallel fibers in tendons and ligaments to give strength to the structure. The capsule has both parallel fibers and a meshwork of connective tissue fibers that provide strength and a little flexibility.

Several other structures around the joint are impacted by the arthritic process. These structures include the bursae and periosteum. The **bursae** are sacs that are enclosed and have a small amount of lubricating fluid within them. They are located wherever a tendon passes over a bone or muscle, a muscle passes over a bone, or a ligament passes over another structure. The bursae act like a plastic bag when a hand is placed on either side of the outer surface and rubbed together. The double layer of slippery material provides a low friction medium so that structures can glide over each other. Periosteum covers the bones except within the articular surfaces. The periosteum is a connective tissue rich in blood vessels, nerve endings, and lymph vessels. Any damage to the periosteum results in pain because of the presence of many nerve endings within the periosteum.

Why Does the Physical Therapist Assistant Need to Know About the Normal Anatomy and Physiology of Bone?

Although the study of bone, bone injuries, and bone abnormalities is traditionally considered orthopedics, the PTA will work with people with these pathologies in a variety of practice settings. An understanding of the anatomical structure and physiology of bone is essential to the understanding of the diseased bone. In some instances, the PTA will work with people who have orthopedic conditions or mobility issues who have a comorbid diagnosis of a bone pathology, such as osteoporosis. The precautions and contraindications associated with these bone pathologies must be followed for patient safety when working with these people.

Normal Anatomy and Physiology of Bone

Bone serves as a support for the body and provides attachment for muscles so that movement can occur. The bones of the rib cage and spine also protect vital organs, such as the heart and lungs within the thoracic cavity. The normal function of bone depends on the health of the tissues within the bone and in the joints. Bone consists of collagen, elastin, and a large amount of ground substance. Proteoglycans, chondroitin sulphate, and glycoproteins comprise most of the ground substance, or osteoid, of bone, together with calcium phosphate in the form of hydroxyapatite. Long bones have Haversian canals, which run along the length of the bone carrying blood vessels for bone nutrition. Cross-channels called Volkmann's canals connect the Haversian canals (see Fig. 5-2 for the structure of a long bone). The osteocytes (bone cells) are contained in spaces called lacunae. The trabeculae, which are long, threadlike channels in the cancellous (spongy) bone provide strength to the bone. A good analogy for how the trabeculae give strength to the bone is that they act in the same way as several metal pipes placed together. One metal pipe is easy to bend, but if you place several pipes together, it is almost impossible to bend them. Bone generally has a high tensile strength and is able to withstand great forces placed on it. Osteoblasts are the cells that produce new bone, and osteoclasts resorb bone. The process of formation and resorption of bone is a constant activity that is normally in a state of homeostasis, maintaining the bone in a strong state. When the homeostasis of the bone is disturbed, as occurs in a fracture, the osteoblasts work overtime to heal it. If the osteoclasts are too active, the result can be osteoporosis.

The growth of bone occurs in both length and thickness. Growth in the length of bone is termed endochondral

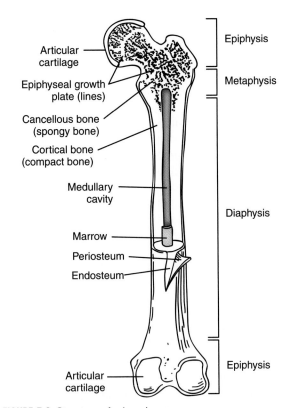

FIGURE 5.2 Structure of a long bone.

bone growth and occurs mainly in long bones. The growth in thickness of bone is called intramembranous growth and occurs to a greater extent in flat bones than in long bones. Endochondral bone growth occurs throughout childhood until the epiphysial plates (growth plates) ossify, sometime after puberty. Intramembranous ossification may continue throughout life under the influence of muscle stresses, which increase the strength and density of the bone, and through the actions of hormones such as parathyroid, cortisol, and growth hormone.

Why Does the Physical Therapist Assistant Need to Know About Degenerative Diseases of the Joints?

A major part of physical therapy practice comprises patients with arthritic conditions. Whether working in an outpatient orthopedic office or an inpatient acute care setting, the PTA will most likely be in daily contact with patients who have joint pathologies. Knowledge of joint pathology is essential for understanding the reasons for selected physical therapy interventions for patients with joint pathologies. Understanding the pathology also helps the PTA to remember the precautions and contraindications for selected physical therapy interventions when working with patients with joint problems.

Degenerative Diseases of Joints

The following degenerative joint conditions are those most commonly seen in physical therapy practice settings. The focus of this section is on the pathology of osteoarthrosis with its associated physical therapy interventions.

HINTS ON THE USE OF THE GUIDE TO PHYSICAL THERAPIST PRACTICE (OA, GOUT, AND INFECTIVE ARTHRITIS)

Several of the *Guide to Physical Therapist Practice* "Musculoskeletal" Practice Patterns may be appropriate for patients with osteoarthrosis (OA), gout, and infective arthritis.

- 4C, "impaired muscle performance" (p. 161): this pattern may be applicable in some cases of arthritis in which weakness is caused by muscle atrophy and pain inhibition

- 4E, "impaired joint mobility, motor function, muscle performance, and range of motion associated with localized inflammation" (p. 197): when the joint involved in the arthritis is in an active stage of inflammation, the preferred practice pattern is 4E; this pattern applies to OA, gout, infective arthritis, and any inflammatory response in a joint affecting the synovium, fascia, tendon, bursa, or ligament

- 4F, "impaired joint mobility, motor function, muscle performance, range of motion, and reflex integrity associated with spinal disorders" (p. 215): this pattern may be appropriate for patients with spondylolisthesis

- 4H, "impaired joint mobility, motor function, muscle performance, and range of motion associated with joint arthroplasty" (p. 251): This pattern applies to patients who have had a joint replacement arthroplasty; all the associated impairments and functional limitations such as reduced range of motion, functional limitations and muscle weakness are encompassed by this pattern

- 4I, "impaired joint mobility, motor function, muscle performance, and range of motion associated with bony or soft tissue surgery" (p. 269): this pattern is appropriate for those patients who have undergone other types of bone or soft tissue surgery such as bone grafting, muscle and ligament repairs, and open reduction and internal fixation of fractures

(From the American Physical Therapy Association, 2003. *Guide to physical therapist practice,* revised 2nd edition. Alexandria, VA: APTA. Used with permission.)

Osteoarthritis (Osteoarthrosis)

Osteoarthritis (OA) is a degenerative joint disease and as such does not fall into the same classification as rheumatoid arthritis, which is a true inflammatory arthritis. Patients with osteoarthritis undergo periods during which the osteoarthritic joint may become inflammatory in nature, but it is not specifically an inflammatory disease. This text therefore uses the term **"osteoarthrosis"** to delineate between degenerative arthritis and the inflammatory types of arthritis. OA can occur in any age group, although because it is largely a degenerative process due to wear and tear on the joints, most cases occur in people over 45 years old, and the incidence increases with age. Typically, under age 55, more men than women have OA, but this reverses after age 55.[2] According to the Arthritis Foundation, 21 million people in the United States have been diagnosed with osteoarthritis.[3] Statistics from the

Centers for Disease Control and Prevention (CDC) indicated that in 2005, there were 46.9 million people diagnosed with arthritis and associated conditions and that 22% of the total population had some sort of arthritis.[4]

Etiology. Two types of OA exist, primary and secondary. The etiology of primary OA is unknown. Secondary OA is the result of known factors such as previous injury to the joint, previous infection in the joint, a history of hypermobile joints, repetitive stress as a result of occupation or sports or hobbies, obesity, hemophilia with bleeding into the joint, or **hyperthyroidism**.[5] Repetitive stress injuries can occur from playing sports such as tennis, which may cause OA to develop in the shoulder, and soccer, which may cause knee injuries that predispose people to OA of the knee. Researchers are investigating whether there is some genetic predisposition to developing OA. The genetic tendency is thought to be especially associated with OA of the hands.[6] OA is usually unilateral in nature with perhaps one knee involved or one shoulder. OA is associated with loss of cartilage in the joint, resulting in reduced joint space between the bone ends of the joint. The loss of mobility of the affected joint results in long-term reduced function for patients.

Signs and Symptoms. Pathologically, OA is a largely noninflammatory condition with a course that is usually gradual, and progressively degenerative. The condition can ultimately interfere with functional activities depending on the location of the joint involved.

The characteristic signs and symptoms of OA include damage to the hyaline cartilage in the early stages. The mechanism of cartilage damage is through splitting of the collagen fibers and disorganization of the proteoglycans, causing the cartilage to absorb water. See Fig. 5-3 for the effects of OA in a synovial joint and Table 5-1 for the characteristics of specific joint structures in OA. The absorption of water by the cartilage causes cracks to develop in the surface of the cartilage, known as **fibrillation,** much as a chick emerging from an egg cracks the surface by pushing from within. These cracks join together, and pieces of cartilage flake off into the joint space. The pieces of loose cartilage can cause "locking" and discomfort if they become trapped in the joint line and may result in reduced range of motion of the joint. The synovial fluid will eventually absorb the cartilage pieces. The hyaline cartilage gradually becomes thinner and thinner until there is no cartilage remaining. The bone beneath the cartilage becomes shiny and smooth due to rubbing of bone against bone, causing **eburnation** (smooth and shiny

appearance) of the bone ends. The bone ends change shape as a result of the degenerative process with a flattening of the femoral head in the hip and flattening of the tibial condyles in the knee.[7] As a result of eburnation and

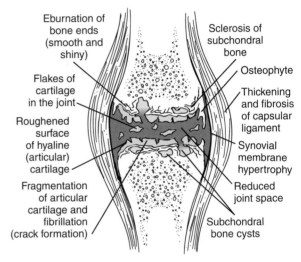

FIGURE 5.3 Effects of osteoarthrosis (OA) in a synovial joint.

Table 5.1 **Characteristics of Osteoarthritis (Osteoarthrosis)**

PART OF JOINT INVOLVED	CHARACTERISTIC
Articular cartilage	Fibrillation-softening, splitting, and fragmentation Splitting of collagen fibers Proteoglycan disorganized Cartilage absorbs water Fragments break off and cause "locking" of the joint
Bone	Eburnation of bone ends—shiny and smooth Cysts beneath bone end surface Osteophytes at joint margins Change in shape of bone ends—flattening
Synovial membrane	Hypertrophy Reduced synovial fluid production leads to reduced nutrition for the cartilage
Capsule	Fibrous degeneration Chronic inflammation
Ligaments	Contracted or stretched
Muscles	Disuse atrophy

other damage to the bone, cysts develop in the subchondral (just beneath the surface) bone. The stimulation of stresses to the exposed bone may produce osteophytic spurs. **Osteophytes** are bony spurs that develop at the margins of the arthritic joint. These osteophytes may interfere with joint motion and in some cases may break off and become lodged inside the joint. Irritation from bone fragments within the joint can cause synovitis (inflammation of the synovial membrane).

The synovial membrane becomes hypertrophied and starts to lose the ability to produce synovial fluid.[8] Because the synovial fluid provides nutrition for the hyaline cartilage, the loss of synovial fluid results in reduced nutrition for the hyaline cartilage. The capsular ligament and other ligaments closely associated with the joint, such as the anterior and posterior cruciate ligaments in the knee, consequently become inflamed, and start to degenerate. The muscles surrounding the affected joints atrophy due to the disuse caused both by the pain and the limited available motion of the joint.

Clinical Picture of OA

1. Pain on weight bearing, caused by synovial membrane nipping and hypertrophy, and bone pain as a result of the rubbing together of bone ends; night pain may also occur after extensive activity, as well as pain after exercise
2. Stiffness after inactivity that improves with movement
3. Reduced range of motion caused by muscle spasm, contractures, or bony blockage
4. Muscle atrophy, weakness, and spasm as a result of disuse and overstretching of the muscles
5. Joint deformity and enlargement
6. Joint **crepitus** (a grating noise within the joint) as a result of bone rubbing on bone or cartilage disintegration
7. Reduced function, or loss of function, as a result of pain and muscle weakness

The radiographic findings in a joint with OA include the loss of joint space, sclerosis of the bone ends, a flattened shape of the articular bone ends, and osteophyte formation at the margins of the joint.

OA can affect any joint in the body, but the main joints affected include the hip, knee, shoulder, and hands. Specific clinical features are associated with various joints.

OA of the Hip

In OA of the hip pain is often referred into the groin and distally along the anterior aspect of the upper leg as far as the knee. This pain referral pattern follows the dermatomes of the nerves that supply the hip joint. A dermatome is the area of skin supplied by a specific spinal nerve. The muscles involved include the hip flexors, adductors, and lateral rotators, all of which tend to spasm. The spasm results in deformity in the direction of the spasm. Muscle atrophy and weakness occur in all of the hip muscles but are most apparent in the hip extensors and abductors. The muscle weakness results in a lack of function, with patients having difficulty rising from a chair as a result of hip extensor weakness. Standing balance is also affected because of abductor weakness, causing the lack of pelvic stability. Patients develop a **Trendelenburg gait pattern** as a result of the inability of the hip abductors to maintain a level pelvis over a straight leg in the one-legged standing position. In this position, the hip abductors, particularly the gluteus medius, act in a closed kinetic chain (closed-chain) manner. In a Trendelenburg gait pattern, if the left hip abductors are weak, when patients place their weight on the left leg and raise the right leg off the ground, the pelvis drops away from the hip toward the right side. An alternative abnormal gait pattern is sometimes noted in patients with gluteus medius (hip abductor) weakness. In this gait pattern, also called a gluteus medius tilt, patients lean to the same side as the hip abductor weakness by side bending the lumbar spine so that the weight of the body is maintained over the affected hip to prevent a tilt of the pelvis in the opposite direction.

Closed kinetic chain

A closed chain action of muscles involves reversal of the usual mechanism of the muscle. The insertion point becomes the stationary part of the muscle, and the origin of the muscle is the part that moves. This can be considered a reversed origin/insertion of the muscle. In the open kinetic chain action of a muscle, the insertion of the muscle moves closer to the origin, but in a closed chain action, the origin moves toward the insertion.

OA of the Knee

In OA of the knee, muscle spasm frequently occurs in the hamstrings, causing a flexion deformity/contracture of the knee. The quadriceps muscles become atrophied and weak, and **genu valgus** deformity (knock-knee) occurs. The knee may appear very large as a result of the combination of atrophy of the quadriceps, especially the vastus medialis, and enlargement of the joint because of synovial hypertrophy. Pain is felt anteriorly, both toward the thigh and the ankle. Patients often limp as a result of both the pain and the lack of knee extension. Difficulty climbing stairs and walking on slopes is also experienced because of quadriceps weakness. A regular complaint from patients is the knee "giving way."

It Happened in the Clinic

A 70-year-old woman exhibiting bilateral arthritis symptoms in the knees was referred by her orthopedist for physical therapy for strengthening and mobility exercises. Because osteoarthrosis (OA) is almost invariably unilateral, this was unusual. On further questioning, it was learned that the client/patient had been a household servant and spent many hours on her knees, which accounted for the bilateral nature of her arthritis. Range of motion was severely limited in both flexion and extension, 10° to 60° on the right and 10° to 50° on the left, and the patient was experiencing considerable pain in the knees due to the 10° bilateral flexion deformity. Strength was 3+/5 in bilateral quadriceps muscles. Functionally, the patient had difficulty ascending and descending stairs and was unable to walk further than about 50 feet at a time due to pain. The patient increased her range of flexion with exercises to 10 to 70 on the right and 10 to 65 on the left but was unable to gain any further extension and the pain level remained high. Strength increased to 4/5 in bilateral quadriceps. Three months later, the patient had bilateral knee replacement surgery and after rehabilitation obtained 2° to 95° in the right knee and 0° to 90° on the left. She returned to full function on stairs and was able to walk up to 3 miles with a cane within 6 months.

OA of the Hands

OA of the hands (see Fig. 5-4) tends to develop slowly over many years and usually does not grossly impair function. OA in the hands has some unique characteristics. **Heberden's nodes** may be found on the distal interphalangeal joints (DIPs). These nodes are composed of cartilage or bone and sometimes become rather tender. Similar nodes may be found on the proximal interphalangeal joints (PIPs) called **Bouchard's nodes**. Radial or ulnar deviation of the distal phalanges may occur in advanced stages of OA. The hands may become quite deformed and be mistakenly identified as the hands of a person with rheumatoid arthritis unless the specific characteristics of OA are understood.

OA of the feet

OA of the feet mainly involves the first metatarsophalangeal joint (MTP) with a resulting **hallux valgus** deformity (bunions).

Prognosis. No current cure exists for OA. The progressive degeneration of the involved joints varies depending on the degree of activity, body weight, and other factors that are largely unknown.

Medical Intervention. Pharmacological intervention includes nonsteroidal anti-inflammatory drugs (NSAIDS), including COX-2 inhibitors for control of inflammation, and pain.[9] Although previous trials have been inconclusive, a recent study by the CDC, the Glucosamine/Chondroitin Arthritis Intervention Trial (GAIT) (2006), showed promising results for the use of a combination of chondroitin sulphate and glucosamine in patients with "moderate-to-severe knee OA pain."[10,11] The mechanism

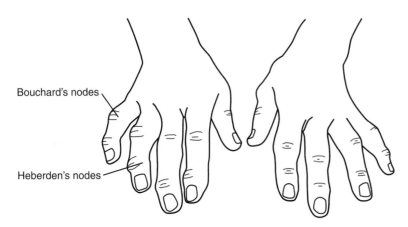

Bouchard's nodes

Heberden's nodes

FIGURE 5.4 Osteoarthrosis (OA) of the hands.

of effect of these drugs is not yet understood. A recent study from Denmark indicated the possibility of a calcitonin supplement reducing the risk of cartilage degradation in postmenopausal women.[12] According to the American College of Rheumatology (2007), this Danish study, performed on rats, has interesting implications for humans.[13]

In some cases of painful arthritic joints, injections of anti-inflammatory substances into the joint cavity by the physician can alleviate symptoms and allow patients to function more fully. In some cases of milder OA in which there is pain, arthroscopic surgery may be used to remove torn cartilage or small pieces of bone.

In severe cases of joint destruction, with loss of function of the joint and pain, patients may require joint replacement arthroplasty surgery.[14] A new surgery performed for OA in which only one side of the knee joint is affected by OA is called a **unicondylar knee resurfacing.** In this surgery a polyethylene tibial component and a metal femoral component are used to replace one side of the knee joint after removal of any diseased bone.[15] The advantage of this approach to surgery is that the range of motion of the knee after the surgery is usually greater than after a total joint replacement arthroplasty.

Physical Therapy Intervention. The physical therapy intervention for patients with OA is focused on improving the functional status of patients through exercise programs for strengthening weak muscle groups, endurance activities, and home exercise programs. The achievement of improved joint function also results in the reduction of pain. A change of diet with weight reduction is effective in patients who are overweight. The PT may request that the physician refer patients to a dietician for advice. Encouragement for any weight loss is beneficial. Even the loss of a few pounds will reduce the stress on joints during daily activities. The reduction in weight takes stress off the weight-bearing joints and decreases pain. Regular exercise is beneficial for patients, both aerobic exercise and specific exercises for weak muscle groups. Home exercise programs are essential for these patients, and compliance can be increased by providing patients with a logbook to check off each time that they perform their exercises. The exercises need to be kept to a manageable number of perhaps three to six exercises. If patients are given too many exercises to perform, it is more likely that they will not do any of them because of the time commitment.

Modalities used for the relief of pain include heat, ice, ultrasound, electrical stimulation, and massage. Paraffin wax baths may be effective for the hands. Passive motion of the patella may be helpful if structures around the knee are adherent. Stretching the hamstring muscles is performed if there is no bony blockage to movement at the knee. The advice given to patients by the PT or PTA should include the following:

1. Use a cane to prevent a limp. A limp could place stress on other joints.
2. Avoid keeping the joint in any one position for long periods. If forced to be in a sitting position, try to perform isometric exercises and gentle range of motion (ROM) exercises as frequently as possible.
3. Avoid prolonged standing in one position.
4. Exercise every day using the specific home exercise program provided by the PT/PTA.
5. Control weight by keeping to a low-fat diet. Even the loss of a few pounds can reduce stress on the joints.
6. Do *not* place a pillow beneath the knees. Using a pillow will encourage knee and hip flexion deformities.
7. Do *not* lift heavy weights that will place extra stress on joints.
8. Keep joints warm whenever possible. Cold weather can aggravate the pain of OA.
9. Use a moist heating pad at home for control of pain.
10. If knees swell, elevate the legs for 15 minutes, three times a day.
11. Try to walk as much as possible to maintain aerobic capacity, mobilize stiff joints, and strengthen muscles.
12. Try to pace activity to little and often, rather than too much at once.
13. Try to avoid sitting for prolonged periods, which encourages flexion deformity of the hip and knee.
14. Avoid crossing the legs, which will impair circulation.
15. Follow the physician's prescription for medications.

GERIATRIC CONSIDERATIONS

Osteoporosis is usually thought to be a disease of women, but the PTA should remember that in the elderly population, men have osteoporosis as well. When performing resisted exercises, always check for evidence of osteoporosis in the patient. Excessive pressure on bones can result in fractures. Osteoporosis is a "silent" disease, so no obvious signs and symptoms may be noted until a fracture occurs. Also remember: do *not* perform any spinal flexion exercises with a patient who has osteoporosis. Flexion of the spine increases the risk of compression fractures of the spine.

Spondylosis

Spondylosis is a degenerative disease affecting the intervertebral discs of the spine. Spondylosis frequently accompanies OA changes in the apophyseal joints (facet joints) of the spine. The term "spondylosis" is confusing and seems to be a catch-all word for a number of conditions involving arthritis of the spine. Most often the term applies to cervical spondylosis in which arthritic changes occur in the apophyseal joints (facet joints of the spine) along with a reduction in height of the intervertebral discs. Spondylosis occurs more often in people aged over 50 years, although younger people may also be affected.[16]

Etiology. Patients with spondylosis may have a history of poor posture due to lifestyles involving prolonged sitting or heavy lifting. A prior injury to the neck or spine can also predispose people to spondylosis. However, in most cases age seems to play a large part in the condition.

Signs and Symptoms. The pathology of spondylosis includes intervertebral disc deterioration with cracking of the annulus fibrosis and breakdown of the proteoglycans in the disc that enable the disc to absorb water and remain viable.[17] This deterioration results in loss of height of the disc. The characteristic signs and symptoms of spondylosis include "lipping" of the bodies of the vertebrae (extra growth of the bone in a lip formation at the margins of the vertebral bodies) seen on x-ray films. Loss of calcium in the vertebral bodies can also lead to crush or compression

---

Clinical picture and characteristics of spondylosis

1. Onset of symptoms after a period of worry or stress in a person's life
2. Headaches, neck ache, shoulder, and arm pain in patients with cervical spondylosis
3. Neck musculature weakness
4. Lipping of the vertebral bodies, reduced space between the vertebral bodies on X-ray films, and osteophytes around the margins of the apophyseal joints of the spine
5. Referred pain into the arm along a dermatome distribution as a result of nerve root pressure
6. Pain in the low back especially in the sacroiliac region, with pain into the buttocks and hips
7. Muscle spasms in the low back extensor muscles
8. Altered sensation and paresthesias along the dermatome distribution of the nerve root affected by the impingement
9. Limitation of motion in the spinal joints

---

fractures of the vertebrae.[18] Ligamentous thickening may occur, and the dura mater around the nerve root in the intervertebral canal can become inflamed, causing pain that may be both sharp and intense. Osteophytes may form at the apophyseal joints, which further reduces the lumen of the intervertebral canal causing impingement of the nerve root with an associated radiculopathy.

Prognosis. The prognosis for patients with spondylosis varies greatly with the individual. In many cases, people with spondylosis do not know they have the condition because they do not experience pain that interferes with function.

Medical Intervention. The medical management of spondylosis focuses on the reduction of pain and the relief of the neurological symptoms. If analgesics and anti-inflammatory medications do not work, decompressive surgery may be indicated to reduce the **radiculopathy** (pain due to compression on the nerve roots) or myelopathy (muscle weakness due to compression of the spinal cord).[19] Cortisone injections into specific areas of inflammation in the spine may be helpful.[20]

Physical Therapy Intervention. If the pain is great enough for patients to seek medical help physical therapy intervention may be provided. The goals of physical therapy intervention are to restore function through postural reeducation, muscle-strengthening exercises, flexibility exercises, mobilization of spinal joints, and the relief of pain. Postural reeducation plays a large role in the treatment of patients with spondylosis. Heat, relaxation exercises, relaxation techniques, and massage may all be used to reduce spasm and pain. Various modalities such as electrical stimulation, ultrasound, and traction may be used for the involved areas. Patients often respond well to hydrotherapy exercises, and the physical therapist may need to mobilize specific spinal segments. Advice provided to patients by the PT and PTA should include the following:

1. If you sleep supine (on your back) at night, use only one pillow to prevent a forward head posture (a position in which the head and neck are extended forward away from the body).
2. If you sleep on your side at night, place two pillows (or one thick pillow that keeps your head in line with your spine) under your head and one between your knees to prevent rotation of the low back and keep the hips and spine in alignment.
3. Perform regular stretching exercises throughout the day to help prevent stiffness in the spine.

4. Practice good sitting posture when at a desk or computer to prevent pain and stiffness. The computer monitor should be at a comfortable eye level, with the head looking straight forward. The keyboard should be at the level of the elbows when the arms are by the side, feet flat on the floor, back supported against a chair, and buttocks well back in the seat of the chair.
5. Move around regularly and do not sit, or remain in any one position, for long periods of time.

Spondylolysis

Spondylolysis is a disease process involving a defect in the pars interarticularis of the vertebrae of the lumbar spine. This condition should not be confused with spondylosis, which is an arthritic condition of the spine as described in the previous section. The pars interarticularis lies between the upper and lower articulating facets of the apophyseal joints of the vertebra (see Fig. 5-5).[21] Spondylolysis affects both children and adults. The incidence of spondylolysis in the United States is between 3% and 7% of the population. The incidence for certain types of athletes, particularly those involved with bodily contact sports and gymnastics, can be as great as 23% to 62%.[22]

Etiology. Spondylolysis is often caused by repeated microtrauma to the pars interarticularis that produces a stress fracture. This microtrauma may occur during participation in contact sports such as soccer, baseball, football, and wrestling, or in gymnastics and tennis. Another cause of spondylolysis is a genetic defect of the pars interarticularis. People with spina bifida occulta have an increased risk for development of the condition.[23]

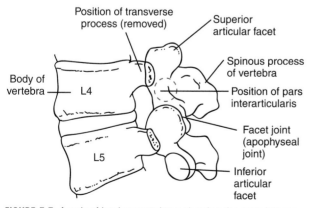

Position of transverse process (removed)
Superior articular facet
Spinous process of vertebra
Body of vertebra — L4
Position of pars interarticularis
Facet joint (apophyseal joint)
L5
Inferior articular facet

FIGURE 5.5 A pair of lumbar vertebrae showing the pars interarticularis and related structures.

Signs and Symptoms. Spondylolysis usually occurs in the lower lumbar spine at the level of L4/5 (lumbar 4/5) or L5/S1 (lumbar 5/Sacral 1). Clinically symptoms of spondylolysis may be absent, and the spinal defect may be discovered during an X-ray of the spine performed for other reasons.

Prognosis. In some cases, the defect starts to slip anteriorly. This condition is referred to as **spondylolisthesis.** If the condition is stable without slippage, the prognosis is good. People with diagnosed spondylolysis are checked periodically by a physician to ensure slippage has not occurred.

Medical Intervention. The diagnosis of spondylolysis is obtained through the use of computed tomography (CT) and magnetic resonance imaging (MRI) scans, x-rays, and bone-density tests. In some cases, a spinal fusion or an interbody fusion, in which the bodies of two vertebrae are fused together, may be required.[24] In athletes, a period of inactivity may be necessary to allow healing to take place and the associated pain to subside. Analgesic medications may be prescribed for the relief of pain associated with the condition.

Physical Therapy Intervention. Physical therapy intervention is provided for abdominal and extensor muscle strengthening exercises, postural reeducation, and lifestyle adaptations. Patients who are athletes may require intensive functional reeducation if the physician approves returning to the previous level of activity.

Spondylolisthesis

Spondylolisthesis occurs when a vertebral body slips anteriorly on the one immediately below it (see Figs. 5-5 and 5-6). If the vertebral body moves posteriorly, it is called **retrolisthesis.**[25]

As in spondylolysis, the usual sites of slippage in spondylolisthesis are L4/L5 and L5/S1. The slippage of the vertebra may cause a stenosis (narrowing) of the spinal canal, resulting in pressure on the spinal nerves. The usual age of onset of the condition is over 40, with females affected more than males. However, spondylolisthesis is also found in children with a birth defect of the spine.[26]

Etiology. Causes of spondylolisthesis include trauma involving a fracture of the pars interarticularis, which causes complete separation of the bone; subluxation of the apophyseal joints as a result of arthritic changes; or pathology of the bone, such as osteoporosis, or malignancy.[27]

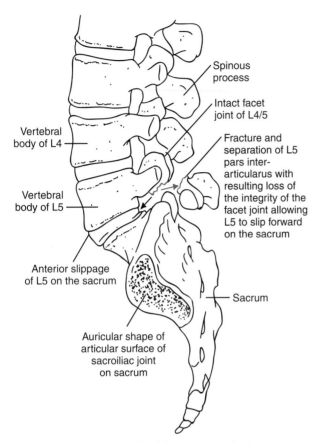

Labels on figure:
- Spinous process
- Intact facet joint of L4/5
- Vertebral body of L4
- Fracture and separation of L5 pars inter-articularus with resulting loss of the integrity of the facet joint allowing L5 to slip forward on the sacrum
- Vertebral body of L5
- Anterior slippage of L5 on the sacrum
- Sacrum
- Auricular shape of articular surface of sacroiliac joint on sacrum

FIGURE 5.6 Spondylolisthesis of the lumbosacral spine.

Signs and Symptoms. The characteristic signs and symptoms of spondylolisthesis include pain in the low back, which is often relieved when lying supine; muscle spasm in the lumbar paraspinal muscles; an increased lumbar lordosis; and referred pain into the lower extremities.

Prognosis. The symptoms of spondylolisthesis may be successfully treated in approximately 80% of patients through the use of therapeutic intervention, analgesics, and exercise. In severe cases when surgery is required, the success rate of the spinal fusion surgery is approximately 85% to 90%.[28]

Medical Intervention. In severe cases, a spinal fusion may be required, especially if there is evidence of nerve root symptoms or intractable pain (pain that cannot be relieved).

Physical Therapy Intervention. Physical therapy intervention for patients with spondylolisthesis may include progressive strengthening exercises for the abdominal muscles, postural reeducation, advice about avoidance of activities that cause extension of the spine, and the use of modalities including lumbar traction, when needed, for the relief of pain. An abdominal binder, or lumbosacral support, may be helpful in reducing symptoms.

Infective (Septic) Arthritis

Infective arthritis is most common in the very young or the very old, in people who are immunosuppressed, or those who abuse drugs. People with existing joint problems such as those with rheumatoid arthritis are more at risk for infective arthritis.[29] Sexually transmitted diseases, especially gonorrhea, are responsible for approximately 80% of infections of joints in younger, sexually active individuals.[30] Estimates are that approximately 20,000 people per year in the United States have some form of infective arthritis, but it is more common in the elderly and those who are immunosuppressed.[31]

Etiology. Several types of arthritis are caused by infections from viruses or bacteria or as a result of metabolic disorders. Bacterial infections may occur when a joint is directly infected after a puncture trauma involving the joint, through contamination from an infected wound such as a decubitus ulcer, or from septicemia (a systemic blood infection).[32] In some cases, the infection may occur after joint surgery. The most common causative organisms are *Staphylococcus aureus, Streptococci*, and *Pseudomonas*.[33] Other causes of joint infections are syphilis and gonorrhea (*Neisseria gonorrhoeae*), tuberculosis (TB), brucellosis, Lyme disease, and certain fungi and viruses.[34] TB and syphilis affect mainly the hips and spine, but other major joints, including the shoulder, may be affected. TB and syphilis were once thought to have been largely eradicated in the United States, but the emergence of the HIV infection and antibiotic-resistant bacteria has heralded an increase in the incidence of these diseases.[35]

Signs and Symptoms. Prolonged infection in a joint damages the articular cartilage. The characteristic signs and symptoms of infective arthritis are usually isolated to one joint and include a sudden onset of severe pain when resting, acute tenderness in the area of the joint and around the joint line, and all the other classic signs of inflammation, such as heat, swelling, erythema, and loss of function. The affected joint may become very stiff, and weight bearing may be impossible. The most commonly affected joint is the knee, but the hip and shoulder may also be involved.[36]

Prognosis. Some cases of infective arthritis can be life-threatening if they are caused by general septicemia caused by *Staphylococcus aureus*.[37] However, most cases are treated with antibiotics and resolve, leaving either no lasting damage or varying amounts of residual joint damage. This condition is a medical emergency requiring immediate intervention to prevent permanent damage to the joints. Often the PT or PTA is the one to recognize the signs and symptoms.

Medical Intervention. The diagnosis of infective arthritis may depend on the combination of results from a CT scan, MRI scan, x-rays, laboratory tests on aspirated (fluid removed with a needle) synovial fluid, and the past history and clinical signs. Medical treatment consists of rest and elevation of the limb, antibiotic therapy, and possible aspiration of the joint fluid by the physician. An external drain may be inserted to ensure that the infection does not intensify within the joint, and joint aspiration (joint tap) may be needed several times a day. A hospital stay is usually required until the infection is under control and may last for up to 11 days.[38]

Physical Therapy Intervention. Physical therapy intervention may be required after the infection has been fully treated by the physician. Joints may be stiff and muscles weak, resulting in functional problems. A progressive strengthening and stretching exercise program mixed with endurance activities is beneficial to patients. In cases in which there is damage to the joint, advice on resting positioning is helpful to prevent further joint deformity.

Hemophilic Arthritis

The arthritic effects of hemophilia have been noted for many years. A classic article by J. Albert Key in the *Annals of Medicine* in 1932 described the symptoms and provided many illustrations of x-rays and photographs of individuals severely affected with hemophilic arthritis.[39] Thanks to advances in medical science, it is now rare to see such severe deformities. Approximately 18,000 people in the United States have hemophilia.[40] (See Chapter 2 for other details about hemophilia.)

Etiology. Hemophilic arthritis is a specific type of arthritis present in patients with hemophilia that occurs when **hemarthrosis** (bleeding into the joint) is present. The presence of blood in the synovial fluid causes a deterioration of the articular cartilage that leads to arthritis in the affected joint.[41]

Signs and Symptoms. Approximately 75% to 90% of people with hemophilia have problems with hemarthrosis.[42] The characteristic symptom of hemarthrosis in people with

hemophilia is a sudden onset of pain in a joint, particularly following an injury of any kind or after prolonged unusual activity. Patients with hemophilia who develop pain in a joint should seek medical advice. Joint problems in patients with hemophilia start at an early age and tend to reoccur throughout life.[43] The prolonged presence of blood in a joint causes the cartilage to break down forming a type of arthritis. In addition, necrosis of the bone ends, cyst formation in the bone, and damage to the synovium may occur.

Prognosis. The long standing effects of hemarthrosis can be prevented by prompt treatment and removal of the blood from the joint. However, approximately 50% of patients with hemophilia have joint damage due to hemarthrosis. [44]

Medical Intervention. Diagnosis of hemarthrosis is performed using X-ray imaging, CT scan, ultrasonography, or MRI. Immediate aspiration of the blood from the joint is required to prevent damage to the internal surface of the joint.

Physical Therapy Intervention. The physical therapy intervention for people with hemophilic arthritis follows similar patterns for other forms of arthritis. Caution must be exercised to avoid causing additional bleeding into the joints in patients with hemophilia. Low-impact exercises are recommended.

Lyme disease

Lyme disease requires special attention because it is prevalent in the United States, particularly in the eastern states. The disease was first discovered in Lyme, Connecticut, in 1975. Although Lyme disease is an infection that causes problems in multiple body systems, it is associated with joint problems similar to those of arthritis. Approximately 20,000 cases of Lyme disease are reported each year in the United States.[45]

Etiology. Lyme disease is caused by the spirochete *Borrelia burgdorferi* and is transmitted to humans by two types of deer tick.[46]

Signs and Symptoms. Initial characteristics may include flulike symptoms, fever, chills, fatigue, and a skin rash. This skin rash may look like a "bull's-eye" with a central pale area including a small puncture surrounded by a red ring (see Fig. 5-7).

Prognosis. The long-term effects of Lyme disease can include arthritis in joints if the disease remains undetected

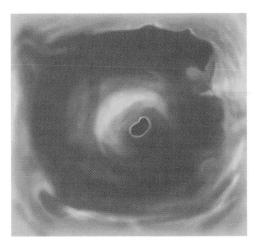

FIGURE 5.7 The bull's-eye rash of Lyme disease.

and untreated. The joint most affected is the knee. Other neurological symptoms can occur in rare cases.

Medical Intervention. A prolonged course of antibiotics is provided for treatment of the disease. New guidelines for the treatment of Lyme disease were published in 2007 by the CDC.[47] Blood tests are performed to determine the presence of antibodies to the *Borrelia burgdorferi* spirochete. However, these antibodies can take 3 to 6 weeks to develop in the system, and treatment usually takes place before the antibodies are detected if Lyme disease is suspected.[48,49]

Physical Therapy Intervention. The PT and PTA may see people with Lyme disease arthritis, which may be misdiagnosed or have gone undetected. Treatment usually focuses on muscle strengthening, joint mobility, and pain reduction to improve function.

Gout

Gout is commonly classified as a crystal arthritis. The term actually covers several types of arthritis-like conditions caused by crystals within the joints. Gout affects approximately 1% of the U.S. population, with males affected approximately twice as much as females.[50]

Etiology. The causes of gout are considered to be a mix of hereditary and environmental factors. Inherited gout involves a metabolic inability to process uric acid in the body.[51] The risk factors for gout include obesity, high blood pressure, taking certain medications such as aspirin or niacin, hypothyroidism (under active thyroid gland), recent surgery or trauma, overeating, starving, and heavy

alcohol intake.[52] Most patients have **hyperuricemia,** a high level of uric acid in the blood. ⊕ Another form of gout is due to a rare, X-linked recessive genetic condition called Lesch-Nyhan syndrome in which children lack an enzyme that assists with the metabolism of purines, resulting in high levels of uric acid in the blood.[53] Other types of gout are idiopathic, having no known cause. Normally uric acid is excreted in urine, but patients with gout have a reduced ability to excrete uric acid. After many years of buildup of this acid in the body, it collects in the joints as monosodium urate monohydrate crystals.[54,55] One form of pseudo-gout is associated with hyperparathyroidism (overactivity of the parathyroid gland), but in this form, the crystals in the joint are composed of calcium pyrophosphate and are not sharp.[56]

Signs and Symptoms. Most cases of gout start in the metatarsophalangeal joint of the great toe, but the condition can affect any joint in the body, especially the knee, ankle, and elbow. The uric acid crystals, which are elongated and sharp, stimulate an acute inflammatory reaction within the joint. Acute episodes of gout are extremely painful and may be associated with systemic symptoms including tachycardia, fever, and fatigue. Acute episodes last a few days, but further episodes tend to occur with progressively more regularity.[57,58] Chronic gout is less painful but is associated with bony deformity. Erosion of the bone ends occurs within the joints. Uric acid collects beneath the skin in lumps called **tophi** (see Fig. 5-8), which can be seen around the elbow, hands, ears, and sometimes the knee. The buildup of uric acid can also cause kidney dysfunction and kidney stones.

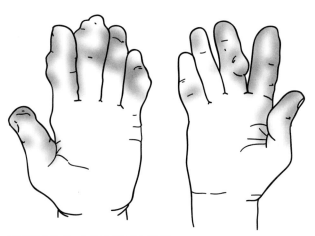

FIGURE 5.8 Gouty tophi in the hand.

Prognosis. Chronic gout can cause renal failure and hypertension. Gout can be controlled by a combination of medications and dietary adaptations, which reduce the intake of purines, and minimize the risk factors.

Medical Intervention. The diagnosis of gout is often determined by analyzing aspirated fluid from the joint and taking X-rays of the affected joint.[59] The treatment of gout is through lifestyle changes and medication. Reducing alcohol intake, losing weight, and maintaining adequate levels of hydration can be major factors in controlling acute episodes of gout.[60] Strong anti-inflammatory medications such as indomethacin or naproxen are used during acute flare-ups. During the latent phase (periods between attacks), medications such as allopurinol or probenecid may be prescribed to lower the uric acid levels in the blood and prevent an exacerbation.[61] These uric-acid-lowering medications are not effective during an acute gout episode.[62]

Physical Therapy Intervention. The PT and PTA do not play a major role in the management of gout but may assist with positioning for affected joints. Activity during an acute episode of gout is contraindicated because of the severe pain.

Surgical Intervention for Arthritis

Discussing surgery in detail for severe forms of arthritis is beyond the scope of this book; however, mention of the various types of surgery is essential when dealing with cases of arthritis. The PTA will be involved with the treatment and rehabilitation of patients after orthopedic surgeries associated with arthritis.

ARTHRODESIS

Arthrodesis of a joint is a surgery that fuses the joint and prevents motion. Arthrodesis is performed infrequently but may be indicated when the joint is severely damaged or patients are medically unsuitable for a total joint prosthesis. In cases of severe spinal pain or injury, arthrodesis may be performed on the spine.[63] The process of fusion of the joints is achieved with a combination of the use of pins, plates, screws, and wires and occasionally with the use of a bone graft. The most common sites for an arthrodesis are the ankle, knee, and hip. When a hip arthrodesis is performed on younger people, the body compensates by becoming hypermobile in the lumbosacral spine. A knee arthrodesis is limiting for patients because of the inability to flex the knee. Ankle arthrodesis is usually performed when there is extensive damage to the joints around the ankle to provide a pain-free

alternative for patients. The functional activity outcome must be considered before considering any surgical technique. In general, arthrodesis reduces the mobility of the joint but allows pain-free weight bearing.

HEMIARTHROPLASTY

Hemiarthroplasty is a one-sided replacement of a joint (see Fig. 5-9). In the hip, it would be the replacement of the femoral head, leaving the acetabulum intact.[64] Examples of this type of arthroplasty include the Thompson or Austin-Moore prostheses. The types of hemiarthroplasty include a monopolar prosthesis with a one-piece implant and a bipolar technique with two components consisting of a stem with a head and a separate cup that fit into, and articulate, with the acetabulum. In the bipolar type of prosthesis, the components move on each other to reduce the friction on the acetabulum.[65] The reasons for performing a hemiarthroplasty include a multiple fracture of the femoral neck of the femur, a tumor of the femoral neck or head, and OA with destruction of the femoral head but in which the acetabulum remains intact.

MENISCECTOMY

In some cases of OA involving damage to the meniscus of the knee, a meniscectomy may be sufficient. This surgery involves removal of any damaged areas of meniscus and

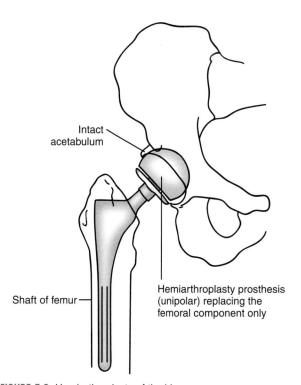

FIGURE 5.9 Hemiarthroplasty of the hip.

Intact acetabulum

Shaft of femur

Hemiarthroplasty prosthesis (unipolar) replacing the femoral component only any fragments of meniscus floating within the joint. A partial meniscectomy is removal of a piece of the damaged meniscus, whereas a total meniscectomy is removal of the entire meniscus. Usually the surgeon tries to preserve as much of the meniscus as possible to try to maintain the integrity and function of the knee joint. Repair of the meniscus may be possible if the damage is not too extensive. Meniscal surgeries are performed through the arthroscope. Small openings are made around the joint for passage of fiber-optic tubes into the joint allowing the surgeon to identify and excise the problem using small surgical instruments. Arthroscopic surgery reduces the recovery time for patients to a few days rather than several weeks because it is less invasive and has fewer side effects than surgery in which the joint is completely opened.

OSTEOTOMY

Osteotomy is a procedure in which a cut is made in the bone. A wedge osteotomy is a wedge-shaped cut in the bone. The osteotomy is usually performed to realign bones when there is a deformity such as genu varus. Osteotomy is performed more on the knee than the hip. A high tibial osteotomy is removal of a wedge of bone from the lateral aspect of the tibia to correct a varus deformity (bow legs) of the knee.[66] Osteotomy in the hip is usually performed to realign the hip joint and redistribute the stresses on the joint. Hip osteotomy is sometimes used as an alternative to total hip arthroplasty.[67]

RESECTION ARTHROPLASTY

Resection arthroplasty is the removal of a joint and can be performed for several joints in the body, including the sternoclavicular joint.[68] In some cases, the surgery may be performed on a site of a previously failed surgery. A resection arthroplasty of the hip, also known as a Girdlestone pseudoarthrosis, is an alternative surgery to joint replacement. A pseudo-joint forms where the joint is excised, the leg becomes shortened due to the removal of bone, and often there is no pain in the "joint." The procedure is sometimes used for patients who have a failed total hip arthroplasty or who have infection in the joint.[69] Girdlestone pseudoarthrosis is not often used because there is no actual joint replacement. Patients may require physical therapy intervention, focusing on an exercise program, and ambulation reeducation with an appropriate assistive device.

TOTAL JOINT ARTHROPLASTY

In many cases of arthritis, both the articulating surfaces of the joint are destroyed. In severe cases, the choice of surgery is usually a total joint arthroplasty in which both articulating surfaces of the joint are replaced. Examples of total joint replacements include total hip arthroplasty (THA; see Fig. 5-10), total knee arthroplasty (TKA; see Fig. 5-11), and total shoulder (see Fig. 5-12) and total elbow (see Fig. 5-13) arthroplasty. Contraindications for any total joint arthroplasty include the presence of infection in the joint, nerve damage, malignancy, and severe osteoporosis. A total knee arthroplasty may also be contraindicated in the presence of severe peripheral vascular disease. If patients are noncompliant, the results will not be as successful. If patients are very young, the durability of the prosthesis must be considered. The life of a total joint prosthesis is considered to be between 10 and 20 years, although some prostheses last longer. The life of the prosthesis depends on several factors, including the level of activity of the patient, body weight, and the general health condition of the bone and the body.[70]

TOTAL HIP ARTHROPLASTY

Total hip arthroplasty may be performed for patients with OA or rheumatoid arthritis who have extensive destruction of both the femoral and acetabular components of the joint, are in severe pain, and have limited functional abilities. Sir John Charnley, developed the first total hip prosthesis in the 1960s in England. The Charnley hip prosthesis consisted of a metal femoral head component with a small diameter femoral head, a squared-off stem, and a polyethylene (plastic) acetabular cup. The components

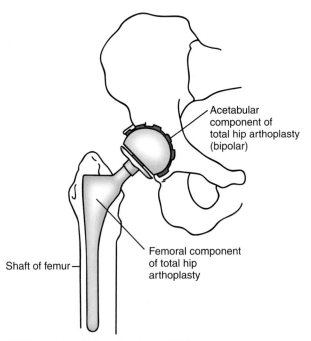

Acetabular component of total hip arthroplasty (bipolar)

Femoral component of total hip arthoplasty

Shaft of femur

FIGURE 5.10 Total hip arthroplasty (THA).

were fixed into place with acrylic cement after the original bone was removed. Recent innovations in total hip arthroplasty components have improved on the Charnley design by rounding off the femoral stem to make it stronger, although the basic concept remains the same.[71] Various sizes of femoral head and acetabular components are available to fit individual patients. Certain types of porous in-growth components allow the patient's own bone to grow into the device to provide fixation and may last longer than traditionally cemented types.[72] These prostheses are uncemented and require a postsurgical rehabilitation approach different from the traditional cemented prostheses. Uncemented prostheses work well with younger, more mobile patients because non-weight-bearing (NWB) is required for 6 to 8 weeks after surgery. Most hip replacements are performed through an incision in the posterolateral aspect of the hip.[73] Some hip replacements are performed using an anterolateral approach. The muscles cut during a posterolateral surgical approach include the gluteus maximus, tensor fascia lata, piriformis, the gemellus superior and inferior, obturator internus, and quadratus femoris.[74] These muscles are responsible for extension, lateral (external) rotation, and abduction of the femur. Cutting through these muscles during the surgery causes them to be weak. This approach to surgery makes patients susceptible to dislocating the arthroplasty if these muscles are put on stretch (placing the leg in internal rotation, adduction, and flexion). An alternative anterior approach to the surgery developed within the last few years avoids cutting of some of these muscles and may help to reduce both the rehabilitation time and the risk of dislocation of the prosthesis, although more experience over time is needed to evaluate the effectiveness of this technique.[75] The most likely position for dislocation of the prosthesis after an anterior surgical approach is with the hip in adduction, extension, and lateral (external) rotation.[76]

Physical Therapy Intervention for total hip arthroplasty.
Physical therapy intervention for THA must include patient education regarding the positions and actions that must be avoided after surgery. Instructions to patients after THA using a posterolateral approach should include:

1. Do not flex the hip beyond 90°.
2. Do not cross the affected leg beyond midline.
3. Do not cross your legs.
4. Do not lie on the unaffected side; this could produce flexion, adduction, and internal rotation of the hip and cause dislocation of the prosthesis.
5. Do not sit in a low chair or one that is soft.

6. Do not bend over to pick something up off the floor.
7. Do use an abduction wedge between the legs at night for the first few weeks after surgery.
8. Do sit in a firm, fairly high armchair so that you do not place the hip in more than 90° of hip flexion.
9. Do get in and out of bed either using an abduction wedge between the legs or keeping the legs together and straight, or making sure the affected leg does not pass beyond midline.
10. Do use a raised toilet seat over the existing toilet.
11. When standing up from a chair, scoot to the edge of the chair and lean more toward the unaffected hip to prevent flexion beyond 90° of the affected hip.
12. Do transfer from one surface to another leading with the "good" leg.
13. Do get up out of bed at least twice a day, on Day 1 or 2 after surgery as per physician's instructions.
14. Do ambulate with a walker or crutches for the first few weeks after surgery even if allowed to be full weight bearing (FWB). Progress to a cane in the opposite hand to the surgery for approximately 6 months to enable full healing and prevent a limp.
15. If a noncemented prosthesis is in place, use a walker with toe-touch weight bearing only for up to 8 weeks and then a cane as in Point 14 for 6 months.
16. Do perform your exercises at least twice a day, including quadriceps and gluteal sets, ankle pumps, hip abduction (isometric at first).
17. Do go up stairs with the "good" leg leading (Good up to heaven) and go down stairs with the involved leg leading (Bad down to hell).

If the surgery is performed through an anterolateral approach, the instructions are slightly different and involve avoiding a combination of hip adduction, extension, and lateral (external) rotation.[77] In this approach, the tensor fascia lata and gluteus medius and minimus are cut. The instructions to patients after the anterolateral approach surgery include prevention of adduction, extension, and lateral rotation of the hip.

Patients with a THA will be in the hospital for approximately 3 to 5 days and then will either return home or be transferred to a rehabilitation facility or nursing home for further treatment. PT intervention may continue at home or on an outpatient basis to assist patients with ambulation, strengthening exercises, and return to functional activity. In many cases, the PT will be the first person to get patients out of bed after a THA. To maintain safety precautions, more than one person is needed to assist patients out of bed for the first time after surgery.

The possible complications of total hip arthroplasty may include deep venous thrombosis (DVT), nerve or blood vessel damage, a fractured femoral shaft due to stresses placed on the rest of the bone from the prosthesis, dislocation of the prosthesis, leg-length discrepancy, and infection.

TOTAL KNEE ARTHROPLASTY

Total knee arthroplasty (TKA) is performed for patients with destruction of the knee joint due to severe arthritis or trauma (see Fig. 5-11). When considering patients for surgery, the surgeon looks at the loss of function, severity of pain, and inability to move the knee. The age and mobility of patients must also be taken into consideration. Total joint arthroplasty has a limited "life expectancy." However, in cases of severe arthritis, TKA may mean the difference between complete inactivity and a functional life for some younger patients. If the surgery is performed on a young patient, it is possible that a revision of the surgery will need to be performed after 10 to 20 years, depending on the level of activity of the person. The result, however, is that patients are able to live an active life for that period of time and may be willing to undergo another surgery if it means they can lead a comparatively pain-free, normal life in the interim. TKA has been performed since the 1960s, and recent developments have improved outcomes for patients. The articular surfaces of both the tibia and femur are replaced. Sometimes a patellar component is used, or the existing patella may be left intact. The surgical incision is usually at least 10 inches long on the anterior aspect of the knee. The surgery is very invasive, and there is a lot of swelling and bruising around the knee. Recovery from surgery is a painful process, and the PT and PTA need to provide encouragement and advice to patients. Ninety degrees of knee flexion must be achieved by patients after surgery to enable a return to normal function. In the United States and most of the Western world, everyday activities such as climbing stairs, sitting in a chair, stepping up a curb, and sitting down on the bed all require approximately 90° of knee flexion. In cultures where more knee flexion is required, such as in Japan where every day life requires sitting back on the heels to eat, a larger range of motion, up to 130° of flexion at the knee, may be required for return to full functional activity.

Unicondylar knee resurfacing is now offered as an alternative to total knee arthroplasty. In this surgery, one side of the joint is replaced by resurfacing the tibial and femoral articulating surfaces of the knee joint on the affected side. The recovery from this surgery is not as extensive as for a total knee arthroplasty, and the resulting range of motion is usually greater (see Fig. 5-11).[78]

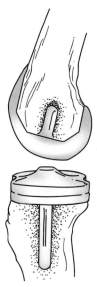

FIGURE 5.11 Total joint arthroplasty of the knee (TKA).

Physical Therapy Intervention for TKA. Physical therapy starts on Day 2 after surgery and, despite the presence of sutures or staples along the incision, knee flexion must be initiated immediately. Emphasize to patients the need to focus on mobilizing the knee to 90° within the first 2 weeks, otherwise adhesions may form and prevent the return of functional flexion. Return of flexion is a painful process and requires a lot of hard work and exercise. The return of full knee extension is also important. Many patients who receive a TKA have severe arthritis in the knee joint before surgery and already have a flexion deformity caused by mechanical problems in the joint or shortening of the hamstring muscle tendons. Weakness of the quadriceps muscles is also common before surgery, resulting in an extension lag (the inability to straighten the leg fully during a straight leg raise as a result of quadriceps muscle weakness). Physical therapy intervention for TKA includes active and passive knee extension exercises, active and passive knee flexion exercises, progressive strengthening exercises, wound care (if necessary), progressive ambulation training, and functional activities. The use of continuous passive motion machines is occasionally recommended by the orthopedic physician, although research studies have shown that the recovery rate is not affected after TKA with the use of adjunct machines.[79-80] The important emphasis for recovery of range of motion after surgery is an active and passive exercise program.

If the prosthesis is noncemented, patients will be non-weight-bearing (NWB) for the first 6 to 12 weeks, and the exercises must also be NWB. With a cemented TKA, patients can usually weight bear as tolerated (WBAT) immediately after surgery. The instructions regarding weight-bearing status provided by the surgeon must be followed. Patients need to be encouraged to remove the immobilizing knee brace to perform their exercises regularly and only use the brace for the first few days after surgery to provide comfort for ambulation. Functional outcomes for patients may be improved if the PT sees patients preoperatively to provide instruction and advice and emphasizes the need for early mobilization of the knee after surgery. Unfortunately, most insurance companies do not reimburse for presurgical education. Some joint replacement rehabilitation settings provide a total package that includes presurgical advice. If exercises are provided preoperatively, patients can start the program as soon as they are able to tolerate doing so after surgery. Most patients do well with TKA. The pain of recovery diminishes gradually, and patients can look forward to a pain-free, functional knee. A major complication that can occur after TKA is DVT, although recent studies have shown that the unicompartmental approach to surgery can reduce the incidence of this.[81,82] The PT and PTA need to be alert to the possible signs of a DVT, including an unusual increase in pain in the area of the knee, pain in the posterior central lower leg, acute tenderness on palpation over the central part of the gastrocnemius and soleus muscles, acute pain when dorsiflexing the ankle, or increased skin temperature or redness in the posterior lower leg. The PT refers patients to the physician immediately if a DVT is suspected.

TOTAL SHOULDER ARTHROPLASTY

The indications for a TSA are similar to those for the hip and knee (see Fig. 5-12). Approximately 23,000 shoulder replacements are performed in the United States annually.[83] Most of these surgeries are performed on arthritic shoulders, but some may be performed due to trauma. In most cases, pain is relieved after surgery, but there may be a reduction in motion of the joint. The reduction in motion is particularly noted in people with rheumatoid arthritis, although the range of motion is usually greater than before the surgery.[84] A surgery introduced into the United States in 2004 and developed in Europe in the 1980s is called a reversed shoulder arthroplasty. This surgery enables patients to obtain good range of motion even if the rotator cuff muscles are damaged. In this procedure, the ball is located at the site of the glenoid on the scapula and the concave articular surface is at the proximal end of the humeral component.[85,86] Many patients who need a shoulder arthroplasty have a combination of limited range of

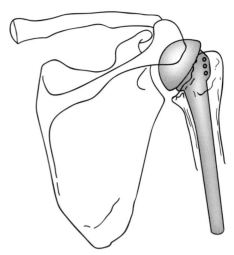

FIGURE 5.12 Total joint arthroplasty of the shoulder.

motion and severe pain before surgery. Because most patients do not usually return to full range of motion after surgery, the main reason for shoulder arthroplasty may be to relieve pain.

Physical Therapy Intervention for Total Shoulder Arthroplasty. Physical therapy is indicated for the rehabilitation of patients who have had a shoulder arthroplasty. The individual surgeon's protocol should be followed. Patients must keep the shoulder immobilized in a sling for the first two weeks in between sessions of passive stretching, and also at night, for approximately 1 month. Lifting restrictions apply for the first 6 weeks after surgery, including no driving.[87] Gradual, progressive, active exercises are instituted approximately 2 weeks after surgery, and full rehabilitation may take several months to restore functional motion and strength. In general, gentle passive and isometric exercises are performed several times a day, starting the day after surgery, to maintain the range of motion achieved during surgery and start to strengthen the muscles. In the second week after surgery, Codman's pendulum exercises are usually instituted, with a gradual progression to resisted exercises after the first 6 weeks.[88]

OTHER JOINT ARTHROPLASTY

The reasons for total elbow arthroplasty are different from the arthroplasties previously mentioned. This surgery is not commonly performed but may restore stability and function for an unstable elbow (see Fig. 5-13).[89] Total ankle arthroplasty is now performed, and arthroplasty for the wrist is in the early stages of development.[90,91] Arthroplasty for the

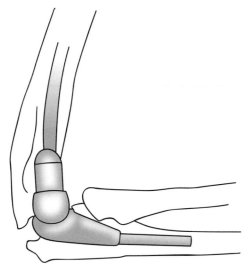

FIGURE 5.13 Total joint arthroplasty of the elbow.

metacarpophalangeal joints and interphalangeal joints of the hands is usually performed for people with severe, rheumatoid arthritis who have both deformity and loss of functional use of the hands.[92]

Why Does the Physical Therapist Assistant Need to Know About Diseases of the Bone?

Although physical therapy is not indicated for the treatment of many bone diseases other than osteoporosis, patients with bone diseases are seen for physical therapy intervention for other conditions. An awareness of the signs and symptoms of bone diseases is essential for the PT and PTA to recognize instances when physical therapy might be contraindicated. An understanding of the pathological processes of bone diseases enables appropriate development of exercise programs and other interventions that take into consideration comorbid (associated diagnoses that are not being treated directly) diagnoses for patients.

Diseases of Bone

The diseases of the bone included in this section reflect metabolic, infective, and neoplastic etiological pathologies. Probably the most significant pathology for the PTA is that of osteoporosis.

Osteoporosis

Osteoporosis is a disease of the bone in which the bone loses density and strength (see Fig. 5-14). An understanding of osteoporosis is of major importance to the practice of physical therapy because in many cases, the possibilities for physical therapy intervention are limited. Osteoporosis is a silent disease in the initial phases and may be discovered only when an x-ray for another problem reveals reduced bone density, or when a fracture occurs. Osteoporosis causes many thousands of fractures each year in the United States at a cost of about $10 billion per year. According to the Surgeon General's 2004 report, 1.5 million people a year experience a fracture due to osteoporosis. The condition affects 10 million people in the United States over 50 years of age, with an additional 34 million having osteopenia.[93] The report also indicated that the monetary cost directly related to fractures from osteoporosis is estimated to be between $12.2 and $17.9 billion annually. The greatest cost is in lives lost due to fractures. The reduction of independence in the elderly is incalculable. Osteoporosis affects women more than men until men reach the age of 70, and then the incidence is more equal. The disease affects Caucasians and Asians more than blacks, and particularly those with small bones.

Etiology. After age 30, women lose approximately 0.5% of their bone mass per year and after menopause this bone

Normal appearance of cancellous bone

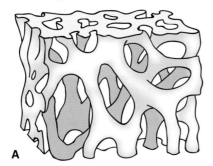

A

Cancellous bone affected by osteoporosis showing thinning and irregularities of bone matrix

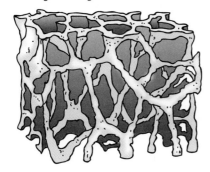

B

FIGURE 5.14 Osteoporotic bone.

loss increases to between 1% and 3% per year. Women are particularly susceptible to osteoporosis after the onset of menopause (cessation of menstruation) when calcium levels in the body become reduced due to the reduction of estrogen production. Prolonged use of corticosteroid drugs and cigarette smoking can cause osteoporosis. The primary form of osteoporosis occurs mainly in the elderly. Secondary osteoporosis may occur in any age group as a result of hormone imbalance, intestinal malabsorption problems causing reduced calcium intake, prolonged periods of immobility after trauma or severe illness, tumors, and certain types of drug therapy. Certain types of osteoporosis are hereditary with no known predisposing causative factors and are not well understood.

Signs and Symptoms. The main bones affected by osteoporosis are the spine, pelvis, and hip. Fractures of the femoral head and crush fractures of the vertebrae in elderly women are often the result of osteoporosis. Estimates are that up to 50% of all women over 50 will fracture a bone because of osteoporosis.[94] The characteristic signs and symptoms of osteoporosis include spinal changes such as an increased thoracic kyphosis with the classical

"Dowager's Hump" that result from crush fractures of the thoracic spine. A loss of height may occur, and this can cause breathing problems and difficulty eating because of compression of the thoracic and abdominal cavities. Fractures of the wrist and hip are also common. Patients often complain of low back and neck pain.

Prognosis. Osteoporosis is not usually life threatening, but it can cause significant pain. If the osteoporosis is severe, individuals may not be able to work if their job entails heavy manual labor or heavy lifting. The increased risk of fracture may also reduce activity levels for sports and other activities, resulting in necessary lifestyle changes.

Medical Intervention. Prevention of osteoporosis is the best course of action because the disease is not easily treated once the bone has lost density. Some studies have shown that estrogen replacement therapy for postmenopausal women and after total hysterectomy (removal of the uterus and ovaries) may reduce bone loss, but the use of replacement estrogen is not usually prescribed because of recent findings regarding the risks of estrogen therapy, including increased risks of breast cancer and heart disease.[95] Extra supplements of calcium and vitamin D, regular weight-bearing exercise, low levels of alcohol consumption, and smoking cessation are recommended for postmenopausal women to minimize the risks of developing osteoporosis.[96]

Physical Therapy Intervention. Patients with osteoporosis are often seen in the physical therapy clinic. Knowledge of osteoporosis, including the contraindications and precautions affecting these patients, is essential to prevent further injury and ensure effective physical therapy intervention. Spinal flexion exercises are contraindicated for patients with osteoporosis because they further increase the stress on the vertebral body and can cause crush fractures. Osteoporosis is also a contraindication for any form of mobilization techniques or traction. Measurements of joint range of motion and muscle strength are performed with care to avoid applying too much resistance.

Physical therapy intervention for osteoporosis takes place on several levels and is provided as part of a health care team approach. Female patients postmenopause with back pain should always be carefully screened by the evaluating PT for the presence of osteoporosis. If osteoporosis is suspected, the patient should be referred back to the physician for bone density tests.

The preventive intervention may consist of advice from the PT and PTA for an activity program involving low-impact, weight-bearing exercises; regular walking; postural advice; spinal extension exercises; and seating positioning. Advice from a dietician may be necessary for dietary adaptations to increase calcium and vitamin D intake. The physician will advise patients about reduction of alcohol intake, smoking cessation, and hormone replacement therapy (HRT). After people have osteoporosis, they may have low back or neck pain from loss of intervertebral space and compression fractures (crushing of vertebral bodies).

Heat and gentle extension exercises with massage may help to reduce symptoms. People with osteoporosis in the spine may also be helped by a spinal support, but the PTA should remember that these supports tend to cause further weakness of the back muscles because patients rely on the support. Appropriate back extension exercises are even more important for patients using spinal supports. Elderly patients with osteoporosis may require balance reeducation to help reduce the risk of falls.

GERIATRIC CONSIDERATIONS

It is important to remember that many people with osteoarthrosis (OA) are also often elderly. Because OA is caused by the wear and tear on joints as well as injury, the older the population, in general the more likely the signs of OA. If an elderly person with OA of the knee has a joint replacement, the main concern is to promote return of functional flexion up to 90°. However, often the person has waited a long time before seeking orthopedic assistance, the lower extremity muscles are weak, and the range of motion presurgery is very limited. A knee flexion deformity may be present, and the patient may be unable to extend the knee fully. Prolonged positioning with the knee in flexion causes the hamstrings to tighten and shorten and this will require attention after the surgery. Always remember that the patient's aerobic capacity may be compromised as well. Rehabilitation after joint replacement may include not only knee range of motion exercises including passive stretching into knee extension to stretch out the shortened knee flexors but may include endurance and aerobic capacity exercises to return the patient to a functional level. In the patient with Alzheimer's disease, the rehabilitation process may take some innovative thinking on the part of the PT and PTA to encourage return to functional status.

Rickets ⊕

Rickets is the result of vitamin D, calcium, or phosphate deficiency in childhood. Because the skin produces vitamin D in response to sunlight, a higher incidence of rickets is reported in areas without much sun and in people who spend most of their time indoors.[97,98] Fortunately, the incidence of rickets in the United States is rare.

Etiology. Insufficient absorption of calcium occurs during bone formation in children, which results in weak bones that tend to bend. This condition is considered to be a type of osteopenia (bone loss). Osteopenia is considered to be a precursor to osteoporosis. Dietary deficiencies coupled with a lack of sunlight further increase the risk of rickets.

Signs and Symptoms. Children with rickets often have bowed legs as a result of actual bowing of the long bones of the femur and tibia. This bowing is not caused by an abnormality of the knee. Children with rickets who are left untreated tend to be smaller than usual for their age and may have spinal and pelvic deformities, a pigeon chest (the chest is increased in anterior-posterior diameter), and delayed dental formation. These children often have a "pot belly," an increased thoracic kyphosis, swelling of the joints, and deformities of the chest and pelvis.[99]

Prognosis. If diagnosed in young children, the skeletal deformities can often be avoided, but if the condition remains undiagnosed until after bone growth has ended, permanent bony deformities are generally present.[100]

Medical Intervention. Medical intervention includes the use of vitamin D and calcium supplements and advice to parents and care providers on providing a balanced diet containing sufficient amounts of the vitamins and minerals to prevent further problems.

Physical Therapy Intervention. Physical therapy intervention is not usually indicated for this disease in childhood, but if skeletal deformities develop later in life as the result of undetected rickets, intervention may be necessary to assist with postural awareness, muscle strengthening, and general mobility.

Osteomalacia

Osteomalacia is a pathological, metabolic condition of bones caused by the lack of vitamin D, calcium, or phosphate absorption in adulthood. Osteomalacia causes softening and weakening of the bones. As a result, fractures are common in people who have the condition.

Etiology. The causes of osteomalacia include lack of calcium absorption in the intestine, loss of phosphates as a result of malfunctioning kidneys, hyperthyroidism, and hyperparathyroidism. A lack of vitamin D, or an inability to process the vitamin, can also lead to hypocalcemia (low levels of calcium in the body). Lack of vitamin D may be found in some people who are strict vegetarians or those who are on a very low fat diet.[101] Osteomalacia can also be a secondary complication of disorders of the small intestine, liver, pancreas, gallbladder, or bile duct. The elderly are more prone to this disease because of a higher incidence of intestinal problems. The use of certain medications such as phenobarbital and antacids as well as prolonged use of anticonvulsant drugs (seizure medications) may also deplete the levels of calcium and vitamin D in the body, which can lead to hypophosphatemia (low levels of phosphates in the body) and hypocalcemia.[102]

Signs and Symptoms. The characteristic signs and symptoms of osteomalacia include general body aches and pains, muscle weakness, bone pain, postural changes such as an increased thoracic kyphosis, and bowing of the long bones of the lower extremities, stress fractures, and weight loss. In some instances, patients may exhibit a Trendelenburg gait pattern (see the previous information on Trendelenburg gait).[103]

Prognosis. The prognosis of people with osteomalacia varies depending on the severity of the condition. The condition can cause long-standing deformities of the bones and joints if it remains untreated.

Medical Intervention. In some cases, supplements of vitamin D or phosphates may be prescribed by the physician. In other cases, parenteral feeding (intravenous or gastric tube feeding) may be needed to restore nutrition to the body. Surgery may be required to correct bone and joint deformities caused by long-standing osteomalacia.[104]

Physical Therapy Intervention. Physical therapy is not indicated for general cases of osteomalacia. However, if muscle weakness is an ongoing problem after medical intervention, physical therapy intervention may be required to rehabilitate patients for muscle strength and endurance.

Legg-Calvé-Perthes Disease ⊛

Legg-Calvé-Perthes is a pediatric disease.

Etiology. Legg-Calvé-Perthes disease is caused by **avascular necrosis** (loss of blood supply and disintegration of the bone) of the proximal femoral epiphysis (growth plate). The causes of the disease are not fully understood, but some theories include possible trauma to the hip or leg in which inflammation interferes with the blood supply to the head of the femur or a defect in the blood coagulation mechanism, which has the same effect.

Signs and Symptoms. The characteristic signs and symptoms of Legg-Calvé-Perthes are a flattening of the head of the femur or a collapse of the head of the femur. These problems with the femoral head can lead to arthritis in later life. The disease affects young males more than females in a 3-5:1 ratio, with 1 in 1,200 children younger than 15 years affected in the United States, usually between the ages of 3 and 12 years. In approximately 80% of cases, the condition occurs in only one leg.[105] The signs and symptoms include a gradually developing limp, pain and stiffness in the involved hip, groin pain, anterior thigh and knee pain, atrophy of leg muscles, tenderness to palpation over the hip, and reduced range of motion in hip abduction and medial rotation.[106]

Prognosis. Many cases of Legg-Calvé-Perthes disease do not require any treatment. In general, if the person is diagnosed after age 8, the prognosis for the long-term effects on the hip joint is not as favorable, often resulting in OA changes in the hip later in life. Girls appear to have more severe disease in the hip than boys.[107]

Medical Intervention. Medical diagnosis is achieved through a combination of x-rays, bone scans, MRI, arthrograms, and blood tests. Children are encouraged to ambulate with a brace that keeps the hip in abduction and medial rotation to reduce possible deformity and to rest as much as possible to relieve weight from the hip.[108] Leg traction combined with bed rest may be ordered, and in some cases, surgery may be required for fixation of the femoral head to the femoral shaft.[109] Some children are susceptible to the development of OA in the hip later in life, but most have no residual effects of the disorder if treatment is performed.

Physical Therapy Intervention. Physical therapy may be required for gait training, particularly if crutches are needed for non-weight-bearing on the affected leg. Exercise programs to strengthen the hip muscles and increase the range of motion at the hip, as well as parental advice for suitable activities for children with a brace, may be indicated. If both legs are affected by the condition, children may be confined to a wheelchair until the condition is stable enough to allow weight bearing.

Slipped Capital Femoral Epiphysis ☺

Slipped femoral epiphysis is a condition similar to Legg-Calvé-Perthes disease except that the femoral head slides on the femur at the epiphysis during growth of the bone and the femur becomes laterally rotated.[110] A slipped femoral epiphysis is more common in boys than in girls.[111]

Etiology. The condition is sometimes caused by a traumatic twisting injury and most often occurs in boys and girls between the ages of 11 and 16 years. Boys are affected about twice as often as girls. Children who are obese or who are growing rapidly are at a greater risk of developing the condition.[112,113]

Signs and Symptoms. The characteristic signs and symptoms of a slipped femoral epiphysis include pain and restriction of movement at the hip and knee pain as a result of referred pain from the hip and altered ambulation patterns.

Prognosis. The outcomes for children with slipped capital femoral epiphysis are generally good with return to full function. In severe cases involving destruction of the femoral head, there is an increased risk of hip arthritis later in life.

Medical Intervention. Surgical intervention with pins is usually necessary to fix the femoral head to the femoral shaft.[114] Children are expected to perform partial weight bearing for approximately 6 to 8 weeks after surgery.

Physical Therapy Intervention. Physical therapy intervention may be necessary for strengthening exercises, and gait reeducation with crutches for non-weight-bearing or partial weight-bearing as prescribed by the surgeon. Patients should be advised to avoid adducting the leg beyond midline.

Paget's Disease

Paget's disease, also called osteitis deformans, is a disease of bone in which the healthy structure of the bone is replaced by a more solid structure that reduces the strength of the bone (see Fig. 5-15). Paget's disease is a disease of the older adult affecting primarily people aged

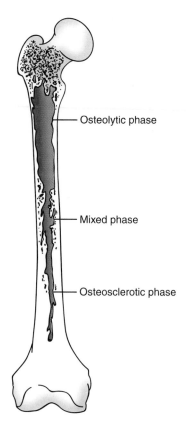

FIGURE 5.15 Paget's disease of bone.

over 70 years, but it can affect those over 40. The disease is most common in Europe, the United States, Australia, and Canada and least common in Asian countries.[115] The disease is thought to have originated in Britain and Europe and migrated to other colonial countries through emigration.

Etiology. The cause of Paget's disease is not known, but the most recent theory is that a slowly developing virus of the osteoclasts is responsible. A genetic tendency within families is also suspected.[116]

Signs and Symptoms. In the first phase of Paget's disease, increased activity of the osteoclasts that resorb bone tissue is present. The osteoblasts are unable to replace the bone tissue quickly enough, and so fibrous tissue is deposited. In the second phase, the osteoblasts work overtime and cause abnormal thickening and sclerosis of the bone. The bone is weakened through a change of structure, not loss of minerals. The disease mainly affects the spine, pelvis, femur, tibia, and skull. Many patients experience minimal signs and symptoms with this condition.

When the skull is affected, the signs and symptoms are enlargement of the skull, loss of hearing, headaches, and vertigo.[117] Other signs and symptoms noted in patients with severe or longstanding Paget's disease include fatigue, general joint stiffness, bone pain, increased thoracic kyphosis, gait disorders, frequent fractures, and occasionally heart disease. Bone tumors (sarcomas) occur in some patients with Paget's disease.[118]

Prognosis. Most people with Paget's disease have minimal symptoms. The prognosis for people with severe forms of the disease varies depending on the person's age when the disease begins.[119]

Medical Intervention. Medications to inhibit the resorption of bone are often used to treat Paget's disease including bisphosphonates and calcitonin. Analgesic medications may also be necessary to reduce pain.

Physical Therapy Intervention. Physical therapy intervention for patients with Paget's disease is directed toward prevention of falls, ambulation reeducation, and general strengthening and endurance exercises.

Osteomyelitis

Osteomyelitis, as its name suggests, is inflammation of bone caused by infection. The incidence of osteomyelitis is approximately 2 in 10,000 people in the United States.[120] The condition most commonly affects children, and boys more than girls. In older adults, the people most susceptible to osteomyelitis are those who are intravenous drug users and those with sickle cell anemia, AIDS, recent surgery involving prosthetic insertion such as a joint arthroplasty, recent trauma, or chronic joint diseases. Immunosuppressed adults such as those with diabetes or alcoholism or those on corticosteroid or immunosuppressive medications may also be susceptible to osteomyelitis.[121]

Etiology. The causes of osteomyelitis are infectious agents such as bacteria, fungi, viruses, or parasites. One of the main bacteria responsible is *Staphylococcus aureus*. In children, the inflammation usually occurs via the circulatory system in highly vascular areas such as the metaphysis of the long bones of the leg and arm. Osteomyelitis often causes infection into the joint close to the infected bone such as the knee or elbow if left untreated. In adults, the infective organism is usually spread from direct puncture wounds into the bone or from respiratory or urinary tract infections.[122]

Signs and Symptoms. The characteristic signs and symptoms of osteomyelitis may include fever associated with the sudden onset of pain in the affected bone, tenderness on palpation over the area, fatigue, and the symptoms associated with inflammation such as pain, edema, warmth, and an inability to bear weight on the affected limb. Pus develops in the area of infected bone leading to necrosis of bone tissue. Adults with chronic osteomyelitis may develop a pathological fracture. In some cases of osteomyelitis, the body temperature is within normal limits indicating an absence of fever.[123] Undetected infections may lead to necrosis of the bone, destruction of the joint cartilage, and joint deformity in children.

Medical Intervention. Medical diagnosis is achieved through a combination of bone scans, MRI, CT scans, x-rays, and ultrasonography. Medical treatment is usually with intravenous (IV) antibiotics and aspiration of the infected material from the affected bone.[124] Surgical débridement of the bone may be necessary if the infection does not respond to IV antibiotics.

Prognosis. If the infection is diagnosed early, the prognosis is usually good.

Physical Therapy Intervention. Physical therapy intervention is not indicated for patients with osteomyelitis in the infectious stage, but knowledge of the signs and symptoms may enable the PT to determine a need for referral back to the physician. In some cases, a patient treated for suspected arthritis in a joint may have a fever and be unresponsive to therapy. Such symptoms alert the PT to refer patients back to the physician. Physical therapy may be involved with exercise programs and gait reeducation after resolution of the infection. In addition, whirlpool therapy with débridement may be indicated after surgical débridement of the affected bone.

Bone Diseases Associated With Hyperparathyroidism and Hypoparathyroidism

The function of the parathyroid hormone (PTH) is to maintain optimum calcium levels in the body. The parathyroid hormone affects the absorption rate of calcium from the intestine by increasing vitamin D production by the kidneys and also activates osteoclasts in the bone to increase resorption of bone. In either over- or underproduction of PTH, problems occur as the result of abnormal levels of calcium in bones. With hyperparathyroidism (overproduction of PTH), the osteoclasts become more active and bone density is reduced.[125,126] Hypoparathyroidism (reduction of PTH) can also cause bone problems. If the parathyroid glands are underactive or removed by surgery, the level of calcium in the serum is decreased. Calcium and vitamin D are required to restore the calcium balance.[127] The bony effects of hypo- and hyperparathyroidism may cause secondary osteoporosis.

Tuberculosis in the Bone

Tuberculosis (TB) is primarily a condition affecting the lungs (see Chapter 4), but in severe cases that are left untreated, the disease becomes extrapulmonary (spreads beyond the lungs). Bone infection in extrapulmonary TB can occur via the circulatory system from the infected lungs. The bony areas most affected by TB are the spine and the long bones, particularly at the knee and hip.[128] The problem of TB in bone is most prevalent in developing countries but is becoming a problem in immunodeficient individuals in the Western world, such as those with acquired immunodeficiency syndrome (AIDS). The TB organism is developing a resistance to antibiotic drugs and is becoming more difficult to treat.

Etiology. Infection with the *Mycobacterium* tuberculosis is spread to the bones via the vascular system or from the adjacent infected lymph nodes.

Signs and Symptoms. The TB bacillus thrives in places with high oxygen content and is thus attracted to the synovial membrane of the joints. The infection then spreads to the bone, where it stimulates an inflammatory response causing caseous necrosis and destruction of bone. **Pott's disease** refers to TB infection of the vertebral bodies and causes the collapse of vertebrae and neurological symptoms

Prognosis. People with TB of the bone are usually in an advanced stage of the TB infection, in some cases, many years after initial infection with the bacteria. Patients with Pott's disease (TB of the spine) may sustain multiple collapsed vertebrae and even atlantoaxial subluxation resulting in paraplegia.[129]

Medical Intervention. The medications used to treat TB are antitubercular drugs, otherwise known as antimycobacterial drugs. These drugs are specific antibiotic/antimicrobial drugs used to treat mycobacteria and include rifampin (Rifadin), ethambutol, pyrazinamide, and ciprofloxacin. Surgical intervention may be necessary

for bone disease that has destroyed the hip or knee joints.

Physical Therapy Intervention. Physical therapy intervention consists of a program designed to strengthen muscles, improve endurance to activity, and restore functional independence. In the acute active phase of TB joint disease, positioning and bed mobility exercises are needed to minimize stress on the involved joint. A team approach to treatment is advisable to provide psychosocial support for patients due to the chronic disease process. The PT and PTA must use standard precautions when treating patients with active TB in order to prevent the spread of infection to other patients and to the therapist.

Syphilis

Syphilis is a sexually transmitted disease, which if untreated can invade the bone and nervous system. It is covered in detail in Chapter 10.

Gonococcal Arthritis (Disseminated Gonococcal Infection)

Gonococcal infections are transmitted by sexual contact.

Etiology. Gonococcal arthritis is an acute infectious type of arthritis caused by the sexually transmitted *Neisseria gonorrhoeae* organism. The condition is found more in females than males and most frequently in pregnant or menstruating women. This type of arthritis is also more common in the male homosexual population.[130]

Signs and Symptoms. The characteristic signs and symptoms of gonococcal arthritis appear soon after infection with the *Neisseria gonorrhoeae* organism. The signs and symptoms include pain in the distal joints such as the wrists, ankles, feet, knees, and elbows, a skin rash, often on the soles of the feet or palms of the hands, tenosynovitis, and a fever.[131] Patients may not have any genital or urinary symptoms and thus may not be aware they have been exposed to a sexually transmitted infection.

Prognosis. Most patients with gonococcal arthritis symptoms recover after treatment with the appropriate antibiotics. In rare cases, destruction of joints result from the infection.[132]

Medical Intervention. Antibiotic resistant strains of *Neisseria gonorrhoeae* are developing from the overuse and improper use of antibiotics requiring most patients with the disease to be treated in a hospital with intravenous antibiotics. The 2007 guidelines from the CDC recommend the use of cephalosporin (Ceftriaxone) for the treatment of disseminated gonococcal arthritis.[133,134] The treatment is effective within 48 hours.

Physical Therapy Intervention. Physical therapy is not indicated unless joint arthritis is involved. Physical therapy treatment would follow the same principles as for other forms of joint arthritis.

HIV/AIDS-Related Arthritic Symptoms

Many patients with human immunodeficiency virus (HIV) and autoimmune deficiency syndrome (AIDS) develop arthritic symptoms, which may resemble Reiter's syndrome, osteoarthrosis, or psoriatic arthritis (see Chapter 6). The joint problems may be noted before the diagnosis of HIV is confirmed. The joints commonly involved are the knees and ankles. HIV and AIDS are detailed in Chapter 10.

Bone Tumors

Bone tumors are abnormal growths within bone and may be either benign or malignant. Some tumors of bone result from the metastasis of tumors in other parts of the body.

Osteosarcoma

One of the more common bone tumors is malignant osteosarcoma, also known as osteogenic sarcoma. Osteosarcomas are slightly more common in males than females under 30 years of age and are found in adolescent boys who are going through rapid phases of bone growth. These tumors tend to develop in long bones, especially those involving the knee such as the distal femur and the proximal tibia, although they can occur in the humerus and other bones.[135]

Etiology. The etiology of osteosarcoma is largely unknown, although other conditions already described such as Paget's disease and chronic osteomyelitis can predispose patients to develop an osteosarcoma. Most tumors develop spontaneously.

Signs and Symptoms. The main characteristic symptom of an osteosarcoma is pain in the affected bony area. Associated edema of the affected limb at the site of the tumor with erythema and stiffness of the joint closest to the lesion may also occur.[136] In some cases, a pathological fracture may be the first sign of a problem.[137]

Prognosis. Osteosarcomas are serious forms of cancer, can be life threatening, and require aggressive treatment. These tumors tend to metastasize to the lungs.[138] As with most malignant tumors, the prognosis depends on the stage of the tumor when diagnosed.

Medical Intervention. Diagnostic tests for osteosarcoma involve MRI, CT scan, x-rays, and tissue biopsy. Medical treatment may consist of chemotherapy, radiation therapy, and surgery to remove the affected bone. Both an orthopedist and an oncologist are involved with the extensive surgery for removal of osteosarcomas. In many cases, a joint such as the knee has to be replaced with a prosthesis as a result of the tumor location at the ends of the bones near the joint.[139] In some severe cases, amputation may be necessary.

Physical Therapy Intervention. Physical therapy intervention is required to assist patients to return to functional activity after surgery. Patients are likely to spend time in a rehabilitation facility and may require home PT after discharge.

Osteoma, Osteoid Osteoma, and Osteoblastoma

Osteomas, osteoid osteomas, and osteoblastomas are all rare benign tumors of bone. Osteomas are more common in the older age group and are usually located on the head or neck.[140] Osteoid osteomas are small tumors found mainly in the long bones of the lower extremity in males between the ages of 20 and 30. Osteoblastomas are larger than osteoid sarcomas and are often located in the spine of both males and females between the ages of 20 and 30.[141] Osteoblastomas are rare, accounting for only 1% of all bone tumors.[142]

Etiology. The cause of these tumors is unknown.

Signs and Symptoms. Osteomas are benign tumors of a bony consistency attached to the bone surface and often occur in the head and neck. Osteomas may cause limitation of range of motion if they are close to a joint and may cause hearing problems, vertigo, or sensation loss if located near the inner ear or close to a cranial nerve.[143] Osteoid osteomas occur mainly in the cortex of the femur or tibia. Osteoid osteomas are less than 2 cm in diameter but can cause joint pain. Osteoblastomas are usually found in the spine and are larger than osteoid osteomas. These tumors affect males more than females and are more likely to cause pain due to their location in the spinal column.

Prognosis. The prognosis for patients with these benign bone tumors is good. Occasionally a benign tumor may turn into a malignant osteosarcoma.[144]

Medical Intervention. Medical treatment depends on the location of the tumor and whether it causes restricted range of motion or pain. Tumors that cause pain may be treated symptomatically with analgesic medications or may require surgical excision (removal).[145] In most cases with no functional impairments, the tumor is not treated surgically. A medical diagnosis is advised to rule out malignancy.

Physical Therapy Intervention. Physical therapy intervention is more likely to be indicated for patients with osteoblastomas because excision of the tumor often causes extensive bone loss with a need for partial or non-weight-bearing gait reeducation. Patients with vertigo may also benefit from physical therapy intervention for balance reeducation.

Osteochondroma ☻

Osteochondromas, also called exostoses, are the most common benign tumors of bone that are composed of bone with a covering of cartilage. These tumors, or extra bone growths, occur in children and are most commonly located in the distal femur, proximal tibia, and proximal humerus close to the epiphysis (growth plate).[146]

Etiology. Osteochondromas are formed from the metaphysis of the bone near the epiphysis. The cause of the extra bone growth is unknown.

Signs and Symptoms. Most osteochondromas are painless. In some cases, inflammation of the area surrounding the exostosis is noted. Fractures of the affected bone may occur, occasional irritation of the nerve causing altered sensation of the skin. Osteochondromas may also interfere with the growth plate of the bone, resulting in a limb length discrepancy.[147,148]

Prognosis. After children stop growing, these tumors also tend to stop growing as well. If surgical intervention has been necessary, long-term effects on mobility may be present as a result of uneven limb length.

Medical Intervention. Medical diagnosis is determined with the use of MRI, CT scan, X-ray, bone scan, and blood tests. Medical intervention with surgical excision is only indicated if the growth limits motion or function or is cosmetically unsightly.

Physical Therapy Intervention. Physical therapy intervention is rarely needed for children with osteochondromas unless surgical intervention is necessary. If physical therapy intervention is required, it focuses on restoration of functional mobility, strength, and endurance.

Giant cell tumor of bone

Giant cell tumors of bone, otherwise called osteoclastomas, are usually benign and composed of mononuclear cells and giant cells, which resemble osteoclasts. However, in 5% to 10% of patients, the tumors are malignant.[149] The tumors occur in both males and females and are most common between the ages of 20 to 40.[150] The usual sites of the tumors are at the proximal end of the tibia, the distal end of the femur, the distal radius, and the proximal humerus. The tumors may also develop in the vertebrae, particularly the sacrum.[151]

Etiology. The cause of giant cell tumors is unknown. Patients with Paget's disease of the bone are more at risk for developing giant cell tumors.[152]

Signs and Symptoms. Pain arises at the site of the tumor and is usually mild at first, progressively increasing with the size of the tumor. Pain may also be felt with movement of the joint adjacent to the tumor and increase with the level of activity. A swollen mass may be palpated at the site of the tumor, and a fracture may occur as a result of the growth of the tumor in the bone.[153]

Prognosis. The benign giant cell tumors are not life threatening, although they can affect joint function. Malignant giant cell tumors may metastasize to the lungs and follow the same prognosis as other malignant tumors depending on the staging of the growth at diagnosis.

Medical Intervention. The physician may keep a patient with a giant cell tumor under observation to ensure malignancy is not likely. If the tumor becomes large, surgical removal (curettage) is performed, and the resulting hole is filled with either a bone graft or cement. In cases of malignancy with metastases to the lungs, the affected part of the lung is excised.[154]

Physical Therapy Intervention. Of particular note to the PT and PTA is that these tumors often develop close to joints and may mimic arthritis. If patients do not respond to arthritis treatment, it is advisable to refer them back to the physician for further studies.

Ewing's sarcoma ⊛

Ewing's sarcoma, also called peripheral primitive neuroectodermal tumor (PNET), is a rapidly progressing malignant tumor of the bone, which frequently affects the soft tissue surrounding the bone as well as the bone itself. The tumors are most commonly located in the long bones, the pelvis, and the chest, although they can occur in any bone. Ewing's sarcoma mainly occurs in children, adolescents, and young adults between the ages of 5 and 20. The tumor is one of the more commonly occurring bone tumors in children.[155]

Etiology. The cause of Ewing's sarcoma is not known, but the tumor usually develops in the bones of children experiencing a rapid phase of growth, often during puberty.

Signs and Symptoms. Signs and symptoms of Ewing's sarcoma vary. In some cases, no symptoms are reported; in other cases, the tumor development is accompanied by fever, pain, and swelling. Pathological fractures of the bone may also occur. The tumor may metastasize to the lungs and other bones.[156]

Prognosis. Early detection and intervention is necessary for a good survival rate.

Medical Intervention. Medical treatment consists of surgical excision of the tumor, radiation therapy, and chemotherapy.

Physical Therapy Intervention. Physical therapy intervention focuses on the return of individuals to functional ambulation and activities of daily living after surgery or chemotherapy.

Fibrous Dysplasia ⊛

Although not strictly a tumor, fibrous dysplasia resembles a tumor. In cases of fibrous dysplasia, the structure of the trabecular bone is replaced by fibrous tissue. The condition can affect one bone, or many bones, and results in weakening of the bones leading to fractures.

Etiology. The cause of fibrous dysplasia is unknown. A genetic mutation occurs in the developing fetus that causes a bone development anomaly.[157] The onset of fibrous dysplasia may also be associated with endocrine problems.[158]

Signs and Symptoms. When only one bone is involved, the disease most often affects the growing bones of the jaw, long bones of the leg, or the ribs. Fractures of these bones may alert the physician, but often the problem remains undiagnosed. If the disease affects many bones, the cranium, pelvis, femur, and shoulder girdle are most often affected, and deformities occur that can limit function, including the ability to walk.[159,160] Fibrous dysplasia accompanied by endocrine problems associated with the pituitary, or thyroid gland, are fairly rare and affect mainly females. In this combination type of the disease, also known as McCune-Albright Syndrome, the bone abnormalities are associated with café-au-lait spots on the skin and the early onset of puberty.[161,162]A similar disease called osteitis fibrosa cystica (Von Recklinghausen's disease) can be associated with Cushing's syndrome and hyperthyroidism. In this disease, the bones become softened as a result of the release of too much parathyroid hormone.[163]

Prognosis. Mild cases of fibrous dysplasia cause relatively few problems. Severe cases of the condition can lead to bone deformities, including scoliosis, fractures, abnormalities of the cranium that result in vision or hearing loss, and the development of arthritis in adjacent joints.[164]

Medical Intervention. The medications used to prevent the breakdown of bone include the same ones used to treat osteoporosis, which are bisphosphonates such as alendronate (Fosamax).[165] Patients with severe cases of fibrous dysplasia may require surgery for removal of the affected bone, fixation of a fracture, or reduction of nerve pressure.[166]

Physical Therapy Intervention. Physical therapy intervention is focused on the return to functional activity after surgery for patients. In most cases, PT is not indicated for patients with mild cases of fibrous dysplasia.

Multiple Myeloma

Multiple myeloma is a type of myeloma and is a malignant tumor of plasma cells in bone marrow that is also known as plasma cell myeloma. Depending on the type of multiple myeloma, the spread of the disease to many bones within the body may be fast or slow. The usual onset of the disease is after the age of 65, although younger people may be affected, with approximately 50% greater incidence in black males than white males.[167] The frequency of the condition is estimated to be approximately 5 to 6 cases per year per 100,000 people.[168] Males are affected more often than females. The incidence of multiple myeloma is a significant problem in those patients with acquired immunodeficiency syndrome (AIDS).[169,170]

Etiology. The etiology of multiple myeloma is unknown. The risk of developing the disease seems to be higher when people are exposed to external factors such as petroleum products, heavy metals, asbestos, and agricultural dust that contains herbicides and insecticides.[171]

Signs and Symptoms. Signs and symptoms are often nonexistent in the early stages of the condition. The characteristic signs and symptoms of multiple myeloma include bacterial infections as a result of damage to the immunoglobulins that normally help to fight disease, bone pain, fatigue, pathological fractures, renal disease, anemia due to destruction of the bone marrow, and osteoporosis.[172] Multiple myeloma affects mainly the skull, pelvis, and spine. If the spine is involved, extensive nerve damage may be present, with back pain, bowel and bladder problems, and paraplegia in the later stages of the disease. Amyloidosis may occur in association with the myeloma. Amyloidosis is a condition characterized by protein fragments building up in tissues of the body, causing stiffness.[173] The stiffness can affect muscles and nerves and is particularly a problem in the carpal tunnel, where it causes classic carpal tunnel symptoms of pain, tingling at the wrist and hand, and numbness in the hand.

Prognosis. The prognosis for people with multiple myeloma varies according to the stage of the disease at diagnosis. In people with Stage III disease the prognosis is not as good, with a higher mortality rate. According to the American Cancer Society, approximately 19,900 new cases of multiple myeloma will be diagnosed in 2007.[174] The 5-year survival rate after diagnosis for people with multiple myeloma is approximately 33%, with slightly higher survival rates in younger people.[175]

Medical Intervention. The diagnosis of multiple myeloma involves bone biopsy, x-rays, CT scans, MRI, blood tests for a complete blood count (CBC), and serum protein electrophoresis to measure the protein levels in the blood.[176] An increase in the number of plasma cells in the bone marrow and an increased level of proteins in the blood and urine are indications for the presence of multiple myeloma.[177] Medical treatment of multiple myeloma includes chemotherapy, radiation therapy, and stem cell transplantation.[178] Medical trials are in place to monitor the use of thalidomide for the treatment of multiple

myeloma. Thalidomide is thought to boost the immune system and inhibit angiogenesis (the formation of new blood vessels to supply the tumor with nutrients).[179] Other medications for the treatment of multiple myeloma include bisphosphonates to increase bone density[180,181] and bone-reducing drugs or radiopharmaceuticals such as Quadramet.[182] These drugs are also effective in reducing bone pain in many cases.

Physical Therapy Intervention. Physical therapy is not usually indicated for people with multiple myeloma.

Bone Metastases

Several carcinomas in the body have a tendency to metastasize to bone, including those in the breast, lung, kidney, and prostate.[183] The flat bones such as the skull and ribs are usually affected most, as well as the vertebrae.

Etiology. Bone metastases are usually secondary sites of a primary tumor located elsewhere in the body. Cells from the primary site seed to the secondary location and develop into new tumors. In the case of bone metastases, the primary sites are most often located in the breast or lung.[184]

Signs and Symptoms. Although metastases may cause pain, they are not usually detected until a minor injury causes a bone to fracture. X-ray imaging of the affected bones reveals the condition. In many instances, the ribs are affected by bone metastases.

Prognosis. Bone metastases usually indicate a serious spread of the primary cancer due to diffuse progression of the carcinoma. In some cases, this metastasis indicates a terminal phase of the cancer. However, recent advances in medical treatment for carcinomas is increasing the life expectancy for people with bone metastases.

Medical Intervention. The diagnosis of bone metastases is performed with the assistance of x-rays, CT scans, bone scans, MRI scans, and positron emission tomography scans. The initial medical treatment for bone metastases is usually directed against the location of the primary cancer, with the use of chemotherapy and radiation therapy. Radiopharmaceutical medications may be prescribed, such as strontium-89 (Metastron) and samarium-153 (Quadramet).[185] In addition, bisphosphonate medications may be prescribed to strengthen the affected bone. In some cases, surgery may be needed to insert a metal rod or plate to prevent the bone from fracturing.[186]

Physical Therapy Intervention. Physical therapy is not directly indicated for bone metastases. However, patients with bone metastasis may receive physical therapy to reduce the symptoms of fatigue and debilitation, and for postsurgical rehabilitation. Physical therapy may include transfer training, gait training, advice regarding bed and chair positioning, and education of the caregivers. In some cases, instructions on the use of a mechanical lift, such as a Hoyer lift, may be indicated.

Cartilage Tumors

Cartilage tumors are characterized by abnormal growths of tissue within the cartilaginous structures of the body. Some of these tumors are benign (nonspreading), whereas others are malignant and spread to other parts of the body.

Chondroma

Chondromas are benign, usually encapsulated tumors, of cartilage consisting of hyaline cartilage, seen most frequently in the bones of the feet and hands.[187] These tumors develop either in the medullary cavity of the bone or on its surface and in all age groups. Chondromas may occur singly or in multiple groups. If many chondromas are present, the risk of developing malignancy increases. Two syndromes associated with chondromas are Ollier's disease,[188] in which one side of the body is affected by multiple chondromas, and Maffucci's syndrome,[189] in which multiple chondromas and vascular tumors, called angiomas, are present in the associated soft tissues.

Etiology. The etiology of chondromas is unknown, although Maffucci's syndrome is thought to be hereditary.

Signs and Symptoms. When chondromas are located in the periosteum, or in the tendon sheaths, pain is the most likely symptom. The majority have no signs or symptoms.

Prognosis. In rare cases, a chondroma can turn into a malignant tumor, but usually the chondroma causes no problem.

Medical Intervention. If the chondroma is causing pain due to pressure on the periosteum of the bone or as a result of its location within a tendon sheath, the tumor will be excised. In most cases, no treatment is required.[190]

Physical Therapy Intervention. PT intervention is not indicated for patients with chondromas unless restricted ROM, weakness, or some other impairment results from the location of the tumor or the excision of the tumor.

Chondrosarcoma

Chondrosarcomas are malignant tumors found within bone originating from cartilage tissue. Chondrosarcomas are usually diagnosed in people over 40 years of age, with most cases occurring in people over 80 years old; however, younger people may be affected.[191,192] The overall incidence of chondrosarcomas is approximately 8 in 1 million people.[193] Chondrosarcomas can occur in any bone, but they are more common in the shoulder, pelvis, ribs, and femur.

Etiology. The cause of these tumors is unknown.

Signs and Symptoms. The most common symptom is pain, often worse at night. Localized edema may be present. If the tumor is located near a joint, joint effusion and restricted joint motion may be present.

Prognosis. This tumor may develop rapidly and often metastasizes to the lungs hematogenously (through the circulatory system). The 5-year survival rate for people with a Grade I tumor that does not metastasize is approximately 90%. The 5-year survival rate for people with a Grade III tumor that grows aggressively and metastasizes is approximately 23%.[194]

The American Joint Committee on Cancer developed a staging mechanism for malignant tumors called TNM that is used by physicians to describe the stage, or progression, of a tumor. The "T" designates the site of the primary tumor, the "N" describes whether the cancer has spread to the lymph nodes, and the "M" indicates the state of metastasis of the tumor to distant areas of the body.[195] The TNM system of tumor grading also designates numbers after each letter to describe the size of the tumor. After this system has been followed, a numeric grade for the tumor is established by the physician that ranges from Stage I through Stage IV. The seriousness and invasive nature of the tumor becomes progressively greater from Stage I to Stage IV, with Stage I being the least serious.[196]

Medical Intervention. Diagnosis of chondrosarcoma is achieved with the help of X-rays, CT scans, and MRI. The typical choice of treatment is surgical excision (removal) of the tumor.

Physical Therapy Intervention. Physical therapy is not usually indicated for treatment of patients with chondrosarcoma unless there is reduced mobility as a result of the surgery or the disease.

Joint Abnormalities

The joint abnormalities included in this section are limited to genu valgum and genu varus of the knees, which can usually result from diseases of the knee joint.

Genu valgum (Knock-Knee) ⊛

Genu valgum is a condition in which the child or adult has knock-knees in a standing position and is unable to put the feet close together (see Fig. 5-16). Genu valgum is the most common cause of anterior knee pain in adolescents.[197] During the first year of development, most infants have genu valgum, but this usually resolves by the age of 5 or 6.

Etiology. A genu valgum deformity usually occurs as a result of a disease that affects the knee joint (see Chapter 7 for rheumatoid arthritis). In children the condition is often caused by a developmental abnormality, which may resolve on its own. These children also tend to have a **pes planus** (flat foot). Other causes of genu valgum include malnutrition, and hereditary or genetic conditions such as Down syndrome, skeletal dysplasia, or osteogenesis imperfecta. Other causative diseases include rheumatological conditions, hemophilia, and rickets. In some cases, the deformity may develop as a result of uneven growth at the physis and epiphysis during adolescence.[198]

Signs and Symptoms. Children and adolescents with genu valgum tend to develop a circumduction gait pattern in which they throw the leg laterally to avoid hitting the other leg during walking. Anterior and medial knee pain is common as a result of the stress placed on the patellofemoral ligaments and the medial collateral ligament of the knee.

Prognosis. The prognosis for adolescents with this condition is good if the deformity is corrected before maturation of the bones. If the condition remains untreated, there can be damage to the menisci, and underdevelopment of the lateral condyle of the femur, resulting in lateral compartment problems in the knee.[199]

Medical Intervention. A variety of medical interventions may be used to correct genu valgum. In some cases, progressive bracing is used, but the results are not always successful. A tibial osteotomy (a wedge of bone surgically removed from the proximal end of the tibia) on the medial aspect of the tibia may be used to correct the deformity in people who have completed bone growth. An alternative surgery is a guided growth procedure, in which a plate and

screws are inserted on either side of the epiphysis (growth plate of the bone) to slow the growth of the tibia and femur on the medial aspect of the knee (Stevens & Holmstrom, 2007).[200] The guided growth procedure is a minimally invasive surgical technique that requires follow-up every few months to make sure the deformity is not overcorrected.

Physical Therapy Intervention. Physical therapy intervention for patients with genu valgum deformity focuses on strengthening of the muscles of the lower extremity and encouraging a more normal gait pattern. Physical therapy intervention is rarely the only treatment provided for this condition. After surgery to correct the deformity, physical therapy techniques for strengthening, gait reeducation, and activities to encourage return to normal function are provided.

Genu Varum (Bow Legs) ⊛

Genu varum is a condition in which the legs are bowed laterally. The condition can occur in childhood and continue into adulthood or can be the result of other pathologies.

Etiology. Genu varum may be due to a deformity at the knee caused by osteoarthrosis or rheumatoid arthritis, or it may result from general bowing of the long bones in the lower extremities such as that found in rickets (see Fig. 5-16). Some cases of childhood genu varum are caused by skeletal dysplasia.[201] Other causes of genu varum include trauma,

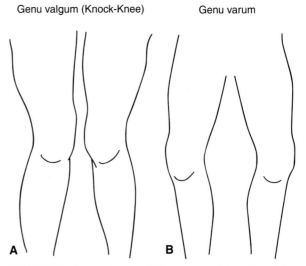

FIGURE 5.16 Genu valgum and Genu varum deformities of the knees.

osteochondroma, rickets, osteogenesis imperfecta,[202] and Blount's disease (a disorder that affects the growth of the medial aspect of the proximal tibial physis).[203]

Signs and Symptoms. Normal alignment of the tibia and femur are usually noted when infants are approximately 14 to 16 months old. If the normal alignment of the tibia and femur are not seen by the time the child is 16 months old, genu varum may be suspected.

Prognosis. Most cases of genu varum in young infants correct themselves.[204] In cases of pathological genu varum, the cause of the problem is corrected. Some less severe cases of correct themselves by age 9 years without intervention. In more severe cases, the bowing of the tibia and femur may persist into adolescence and cause gait abnormalities.

Medical Intervention. Infants are checked regularly by a physician to monitor their development and ensure that genu varum corrects itself before age 2 to 3 years. In cases of continued genu varum, the physician may recommend corrective surgery such as a lateral wedge tibial osteotomy or progressive bracing to encourage the bones into a more normal growth pattern.[205]

Physical Therapy Intervention. Physical therapy intervention for children with genu varum may be necessary after surgical correction to ensure gait reeducation, muscle strengthening, and correct application of any bracing or orthoses.

Genetic Bone Abnormalities

The bone abnormalities described in this section are characterized by genetically inherited conditions. Some of these resolve in infancy with appropriate medical intervention, whereas others persist throughout life.

Talipes Equinovarus (Clubfoot) 🔊

Talipes equinovarus, or clubfoot, is a genetic condition affecting 1 in 1,000 live births. The condition affects males more than females in a 2:1 ratio.[206,207]

Etiology. Most cases of talipes equinovarus are of unknown etiology. Talipes equinovarus can result from a genetic trait, especially in those with a family history of the condition, and is also present in children with cerebral palsy and spina bifida.[208]

Signs and Symptoms. The foot and ankle are held in a position of plantarflexion and inversion. The condition may be bilateral or unilateral (see Fig. 5-17). The ankle is plantar flexed, and the subtaloid and mid-tarsal joints are both adducted and inverted.[209]

Prognosis. Many cases of talipes equinovarus are corrected by serial splinting, but some severe cases may not be fully corrected. The outcome for children with talipes equinovarus who have received treatment is usually good.

Medical Intervention. The condition may be merely positional or postural, in which case no treatment is necessary. Treatment of the condition usually consists of serial splinting over many months. The foot is placed in a series of casts with gradually more and more of a normal position achieved by applying a continuous passive stretch to the soft tissues and joints. In cases in which the talipes equinovarus is fixed or rigid, surgical correction may be necessary if the condition is resistant to serial splinting.[210]

Physical Therapy Intervention. Physical therapy intervention may involve assisting with positioning and stretching of the child's foot to facilitate casting. Passive stretching of the ankle and lower extremity may be performed if the condition is diagnosed at birth and treatment is initiated early. After completion of the serial casting and achievement of a better foot and ankle position, the PT and PTA may be intermittently involved with facilitating weight-bearing activities as the child develops.

Developmental Dysplasia of the Hip 🔊

Development dysplasia of the hip (DDH), or developmental dislocation of the hip, was formerly called congenital dislocation of the hip (CDH). DDH is a genetic condition

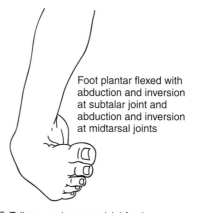

Foot plantar flexed with abduction and inversion at subtalar joint and abduction and inversion at midtarsal joints

FIGURE 5.17 Talipes equinovarus (clubfoot).

in which the head of the femur dislocates from the acetab-ulum of the pelvis. DDH may affect one or both hips, occurs in approximately 1 in 1,000 births, and affects girls more than boys in a 6:1 ratio.[211]

Etiology. DDH is often hereditary and can be due to hip ligament laxity or a shallow shape of the acetabulum. Infants born by breach delivery and first babies are more at risk for the condition. Children with Down syn-drome are prone to DDH as a result of the associated ligamentous laxity.[212]

Signs and Symptoms. If DDH is not diagnosed, shorten-ing of the affected leg may occur as a result of hip disloca-tion, and the gait pattern will be affected. Infants with DDH may not move the affected leg as much, and the leg may be externally rotated compared with the other leg.[213] Patients will often develop a Trendelenburg gait pattern as a result of weakness of the hip abductors (dropping of the pelvis away from the affected hip). Spinal scoliosis and increased lumbar lordosis are commonly associated with DDH, and arthritis in the hip and spine may develop in later life.

Prognosis. The key to a good outcome with DDH is early diagnosis and intervention. People with arthritis second-ary to DDH are candidates for arthroplastic replacement of joints in later life.

Medical Intervention. Infants are checked for DDH at birth, but the condition may go undetected. Early detec-tion is important to avoid arthritis in the hip and gait irreg-ularities later in life. If the hips are placed in a double hip spica cast or splint such as a Pavlik harness with the lower extremities maintained in an abducted position for several months after birth, complications can be avoided, and the femoral head may remain in the acetabulum (see Fig. 5-18). Surgery to reduce a hip dislocation is rarely used unless the condition is severe.[214]

Physical Therapy Intervention. Physical therapy inter-vention for infants may be needed to teach parents how to manage the hip spica brace for home use. In adults who develop arthritis as a result of undiagnosed DDH, the physical therapy intervention follows the same course as for other forms of osteoarthrosis.

Torticollis ☻

Torticollis, also called wryneck or cervical dystonia, is the name given to a condition in children with the head and neck held in a side-flexed and rotated position. The term

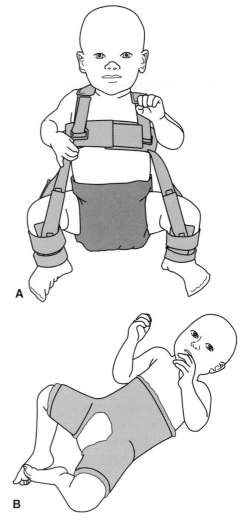

FIGURE 5.18 Hip spica devices for developmental dysplasia of the hip. (A) Pavlik harness. (B) Hip spica cast.

also refers to acquired cases of torticollis in adulthood. The condition in adults is more common in females in a ratio of 2:1 with males.[215]

Etiology. In many cases of infant torticollis, the cause is unknown. In other cases the cause can be a result of injury of the sternocleidomastoid (SCM) muscle or injury of the blood or nerve supply to the muscle before or during birth, a genetically inherited trait, the result of an ear or throat infection, or the position of the fetus in the uterus before birth. In rare cases, the condition may be caused by a spinal cord tumor or a brain abnormality, usually located in the basal ganglia.[216,217] In both children and adults, the condition can also develop as a result of injury to the mus-cle tissue, nerves, or blood vessels of the SCM muscle.[218]

Signs and Symptoms. Torticollis is not usually immediately apparent after birth but develops over a period of a few months when contraction of the SCM muscle occurs. Infants born with this condition tend to develop asymmetry of the face as a result of lying with one side of the head rotated against the pillow or mattress.[219] The shoulder on the affected side may be elevated as a result of the pull of the shortened SCM muscle and the associated tightening of the upper trapezius muscle. As a result of the shortening of the SCM muscle, the head is side flexed to the same side as the affected muscle and rotated away from the affected side. The range of motion of the cervical spine is limited, all the cervical muscles tend to be stiff, and cervical pain is often a problem.

Prognosis. The prognosis for infants with torticollis is good with appropriate treatment. The prognosis in adults with the condition depends on the resolution of the cause. In chronic cases that do not respond to stretching, nerve root compression may occur resulting in numbness and tingling in the dermatome and myotome areas of the nerve root.[220]

Medical Intervention. The condition in infants is usually diagnosed during regular visits to the physician. Treatment includes stretching and positioning to encourage lengthening of the affected SCM muscle. In cases that do not respond to this conservative treatment, surgical release of the affected SCM muscle may be required.[221]

Physical Therapy Intervention. Physical therapy is often required for soft tissue stretching of the SCM muscle. The stretching is performed by a combination of rotating the head toward the affected side and side flexing away from the affected side. A sustained, gentle but firm, passive stretch is needed to facilitate lengthening of the muscle. The care providers must be taught to perform the passive stretching safely and effectively and position the infant correctly to encourage stretching of the SCM.

Achondroplasia ☉

Achondroplasia or dwarfism is a condition affecting the stature of individuals, resulting in a reduction in growth of the long bones and a normal-sized head and torso.

Etiology. Achondroplasia can result from an autosomal dominant genetic disorder that affects the growth of the cartilage in the epiphyseal plate and prevents normal growth of the long bones. However, in approximately 80% of cases, a spontaneous mutation of the gene occurs without a prior history of the condition in the family.

Prognosis. Most people with achondroplasia live a normal life span.

Signs and Symptoms. Individuals with achondroplasia have short arms and legs; a relatively normal-sized head, although the jaw may be small and the forehead slightly bulged; and normal-sized body, hands, and feet.[222] The mental status of children with achondroplasia is usually normal. Other signs and symptoms may include an increased thoracic kyphosis and lumbar lordosis, bowing of the legs, hypotonia (low tone), a waddling gait pattern, an anomaly of the hand called "trident hand" resulting in increased space between the index and ring finger, and spinal stenosis (narrowing of the spinal canal resulting in spinal cord compression).[223]

Medical Intervention. Medical intervention is not needed at birth for people with achondroplasia. If spinal stenosis or hypotonia cause neurological problems, these are treated as necessary. In rare cases, children with achondroplasia are born with hydrocephalus or clubfoot, and these conditions require immediate medical intervention.[224]

Physical Therapy Intervention. Physical therapy generally is not needed for children with achondroplasia. Physical therapy intervention is indicated for children with hypotonia to facilitate muscular development. Children born with hydrocephalus may have a resultant developmental delay that requires physical therapy intervention.

Osteogenesis Imperfecta ☉

Osteogenesis imperfecta (OI) is also known as "brittle bone disease" and affects 6 to 7 in approximately 100,000 births all over the world.[225] OI is a disorder of bones and connective tissue that results in extremely fragile bones. Eight types of osteogenesis imperfecta have been identified. Unlike other forms of staging, the types of OI cannot be assumed as progressively worse from Type I to Type VIII. Type I OI is the least severe and most common, and type II is the most severe. All the other types of OI fall somewhere between Types I and II as far as the severity of the disorder are concerned.[226]

Etiology. OI is a rare condition resulting from an autosomal dominant or recessive inherited factor resulting in a genetic defect on the COL1A1 or COL1A2 genes. These genes are responsible for Type I collagen synthesis. The interference with collagen synthesis results in brittle bones.[227]

Signs and Symptoms. Children with this condition sustain fractures easily. Many infants have fractures when still in the uterus. Other symptoms may include brittle teeth, weak muscles, hearing problems, and scoliosis.[228] The characteristic signs and symptoms of OI range from a triangular-shaped head flattened across the top of the skull, fragile bones, osteoporosis, thin skin, reduced enamel on the teeth, spinal scoliosis, and a small stature with bone deformities where fractures have healed. The condition may be complicated further by weak heart valves, including mitral valve insufficiency.[229] The lack of growth of long bones causes a decrease in height. Many children also bruise easily and have lax ligaments.

Prognosis. Many children survive into adulthood, particularly in less severe cases, but some with severe disease have a limited life expectancy. Children with Type II OI are often stillborn or die within a short time after birth.[230]

Medical Intervention. The medical diagnosis of OI is often difficult. The first signs of problems may occur when children fracture a bone for the first time.[231] Physicians avoid performing surgery as much as possible for children with OI, but in some cases, a fracture may require internal fixation. Casting, bracing, and splinting are used to immobilize fractured limbs with early mobility whenever possible.[232] Pharmacological intervention includes the use of oral or intravenous bisphosphonates to increase bone strength.[233]

Physical Therapy Intervention. Physical therapy may be required in the home and school to provide advice for seating and activity and to encourage gross motor skills such as ambulation, transfers, and appropriate exercise. Many of these children need a power wheelchair with specially molded inserts for mobility. Assistive devices may be needed for ambulation, such as a wheeled walker for safety. Severely affected children need constant supervision when ambulating, use of a gait belt for all activities, and restriction of play activities with other children. When handling children with OI, extreme care must be taken to avoid causing a fracture. Despite careful handling, fractures do occur. Resisted and passive exercises are contraindicated for these children, and family and teachers should be taught how to handle the child effectively to reduce the risk of fractures. Aquatherapy is useful for these children and enables strengthening exercises without stress to the bones. Occupational and physical therapy involvement also includes the use of splints and braces for some children to improve function.

Osteopetrosis ☺

Osteopetrosis, also called marble bone disease or Albers-Schonberg disease, is a rare genetically transmitted disease affecting the development of osteoclasts (bone absorption cells). The incidence of the disease is 1:100,000 to 500,000 people.[234]

Etiology. A genetic defect in the formation of osteoclasts causes bone to become dense in the medulla of the bone, thus reducing the ability of the bone to resist stress.[235] The disease takes various forms including an early onset disease in infancy and a late onset after the age of 40.[236]

Signs and Symptoms. The bones are thick and prone to fracture in much the same way as the bones in persons with Paget's disease. Pain due to pressure on the nerves is also common. The defect in the osteoclast function inhibits the production of red blood cells and causes anemia. In some cases, particularly in infants, osteopetrosis can cause deafness and blindness.[237]

Prognosis. The prognosis depends on the severity of the disease. The condition in infants has a poor prognosis if the symptoms are severe and include neurological problems.[238] Without bone marrow transplant, the prognosis is poor, and death usually occurs before age 10.[239]

Medical Intervention. Infantile osteopetrosis is treatable with bone marrow transplantation. Treatment for adult-onset osteopetrosis is generally symptomatic for fractures.

Physical Therapy Intervention. Physical therapy is not indicated for osteopetrosis unless patients with fractures require intervention for gait training and strengthening.

Marfan's Syndrome ☺

Marfan's syndrome affects the growth of the skeleton. The incidence of Marfan's syndrome is 1 in 5,000 births in the United States among all ethnic backgrounds and affects males and females equally.[240] Marfan's syndrome has an incidence of only 1 in 10,000 births in parents without the gene mutation. President Lincoln was thought to have had Marfan's syndrome.

Etiology. Marfan's syndrome is usually an autosomal dominant hereditary condition of connective tissue (see also Chapter 2). However, in 25% of the cases of Marfan's syndrome, the disorder is due to a spontaneous mutation of the gene at conception. The hereditary form of Marfan's syndrome is autosomal dominant. This means that if one parent has the defective gene, there is a 50% likelihood of the child inheriting the gene. The defective gene in individuals with Marfan's syndrome affects the structure of the protein fibrillin that is one of the constituents of connective tissue. Children have the genetic defect at birth, but the effects of the disease may not be apparent until adulthood.

Signs and Symptoms. Marfan's syndrome can affect any structure in the body that has connective tissue. Typically the bones and blood vessels are affected, and defects of the aorta are common. The condition often remains undiagnosed. Individuals with Marfan's syndrome tend to be tall and thin with arachnodactyly (long fingers and toes) and have an asymmetry of the face and head. They may also have thoracic deformities, lax joint ligaments, and heart mitral valve incompetence. Serious complications may include dislocation of the lens of the eye, detached retina, aortic rupture, and spontaneous pneumothorax (see Chapter 4).[241]

Prognosis. If the condition is untreated, life expectancy is usually about 60 years. However, if the condition is diagnosed early, the more severe side effects such as heart disease and aortic dilatation can be minimized, and people can live a normal life span.[242]

Medical Intervention. Diagnosis of Marfan's syndrome is difficult. Much of the diagnosis depends on observation of the child and the family, although genetic testing for the presence of the defective gene may be performed. Some of the more typical signs and symptoms of Marfan's syndrome may enable the physician to determine the presence of the condition. Surgeries for heart and blood vessel abnormalities may be necessary. In some cases, surgery may also be required for the eye, especially in instances of a detached retina or cataracts.

Physical Therapy Intervention. Any physical therapy intervention would be related to specific manifestations of the syndrome, such as heart disease or musculoskeletal problems. Intervention would be specific to the functional limitations.

CASE STUDY 5.1

A 50-year-old white male with diagnosis of osteoarthrosis (OA) in the left knee secondary to severe trauma at age 20 is attending the physical therapy clinic. The PT has evaluated the patient. Manual muscle testing reveals a 4+/5 strength in

the right lower extremity overall, and ⅗ in the left quadriceps, hamstrings, and anterior tibialis. Range of motion of right knee flexion is 0° to 130° and left is 10° to 90°. Girth measurements reveal a 2-inch reduction of girth of the left leg compared with the right, at a level 3 inches superior to the base of the patella, and an increase of 1 inch girth of the left knee compared with the right at the level of the base of the patella. A marked limp is noted during ambulation, and the patient has great difficulty rising from a low chair and climbing and descending stairs. He complains of severe pain and "cracking" in the left knee during ambulation, which is aggravated when climbing stairs or walking up or down slopes. He is restricted in his normal activities, which include taking a one-mile walk on level surfaces and slopes around his neighborhood every day and playing 18 holes of golf twice a week. The plan of care developed by the PT includes short-term goals for the patient to strengthen the quadriceps, hamstrings, and anterior tibialis to 4/5 in 4 weeks; ambulate 100 feet without severe pain in two weeks; and increase range of motion to 5° to 95° in two weeks. Long-term goals are for the patient to strengthen the weak muscles and to improve muscle endurance to enable ambulation of one mile and tour of the golf course in two months and to increase range of motion of left knee to 0° to 100° to enable functional stair climbing and slope walking in two months. The plan of care developed by the physical therapist includes moist heat and electrical stimulation to the left knee; progressive resistive exercises for quadriceps, hamstrings, and anterior tibialis, increasing to a maximum of 6-pound weights; range of motion exercises to increase range of flexion and extension of the left knee; and progressive ambulation on level and uneven surfaces and on stairs with an appropriate assistive device to alleviate pain and reduce gait abnormalities. Treatment will occur twice per week for 1 week and once per week for another 6 weeks, for a total of 8 treatments (the patient's HMO will only sanction 8 treatments). The PT asks the PTA to take over the treatment of this patient.

1. Develop a progressive resistive exercise (PRE) program for the patient in the clinic within the guidelines of the PT plan of care. Provide the patient with a home exercise program with clear instructions and diagrams.

(Continued)

2. Develop a range of motion exercise program for the patient that he can continue at home without purchasing expensive equipment.

3. Describe the assistive device of your choice for this patient and explain the progression of ambulation to the patient. What will your advice be to the patient?

4. How will you determine the progress of the patient with only one session per week after the first week, and how will you encourage him to do his exercises?

STUDY QUESTIONS

1. Name three characteristics of osteoarthrosis (osteoarthritis).

2. Describe the changes in the bone ends within a joint affected with osteoarthrosis.

3. Describe a gait pattern caused by weak hip abductor muscles and demonstrate the gait abnormality to another person.

4. Describe two types of hip arthroplasty.

5. What is the etiology of osteoarthritis?

6. Explain why the author prefers to call osteoarthritis "osteoarthrosis."

7. Describe five items of advice the PTA should provide to the patient with osteoarthrosis.

8. Describe five aspects of the clinical picture of a patient with spondylosis.

9. Explain the difference between osteoporosis and osteopenia.

10. Develop an exercise program for a patient with moderate osteoporosis in the spine. Consider carefully the contraindications when developing this program.

11. What precautions would you take when treating a child with osteogenesis imperfecta?

12. Name four precautions you would give to a patient who has just had a total hip arthroplasty (THA).

13. Describe one malignant and one benign tumor of bone with the likely age of onset and prognosis.

14. Why do you think it is important to know about tuberculosis and its effects on bone?

15. Syphilis and gonorrhea are both sexually transmitted diseases. Why is it helpful for the PT and PTA to understand the signs and symptoms of these diseases?

16. Explain the differences among spondylosis, spondylolysis, and spondylolisthesis.

● USEFUL WEB SITES

Arthritis Foundation
http://www.arthritis.org
Go to the Surgery Center on this Web site to view an animation of several joint surgeries, including total knee arthroplasty and unicondylar knee resurfacing.

National Osteoporosis Foundation
http://www.nof.org/professionals/index.htm
University of Washington Department of Medicine
Susan Ott, MD

Osteoporosis and bone physiology
http://courses.washington.edu/bonephys/index.html
This site includes x-rays, slide shows, video clips, and information regarding osteomalacia and osteoporosis.

American Cancer Society
http://www.cancer.org

American Joint Committee on Cancer
http://www.cancerstaging.org

● REFERENCES

[1] Osteoarthritis (degenerative arthritis). (2007). *MedicineNet.* Retrieved 08.19.07 from http://www.medicinenet.com/osteoarthritis/article.htm

[2] Arthritis Foundation. (2007). *Osteoarthritis. Who is at risk?* Retrieved 08.17.07 from http://www.arthritis.org/disease-center.php?disease_id=32&df=whos_at_risk

[3] Ibid.

[4] National Center for Health Statistics, Centers for Disease Control and Prevention. (2006). *Arthritis morbidity.* Retrieved 8.17.07 from http://www.cdc.gov/nchs/fastats/arthrits.htm

[5] Arthritis Foundation. (2007). *Osteoarthritis. What causes it?* Retrieved 08.17.07 from http://www.arthritis.org/disease-center.php?disease_id=32&df=causes

[6] Ibid.

[7] Shiel, W. C. (2007). Osteoarthritis (degenerative arthritis). *Medicine Net*. Retrieved 08.17.07 from http://www.medicinenet.com/osteoarthritis/page2.htm

[8] Stitik, T. P., & Foye, P. M. (2006). Osteoarthritis. *eMedicine from WebMD*. Retrieved 08.19.07 from http://www.emedicine.com/pmr/topic93.htm

[9] Arthritis Foundation. (2007). *2007 Drug guide.* Retrieved 08.17.07 from http://www.arthritis.org/types-of-drugs.php?dt_id=1

[10] Arthritis Foundation. (2006). *Top ten arthritis advances of 2006. The Glucosamine/chondroitin Arthritis Intervention Trial (GAIT).* Retrieved 08.17.07 from http://www.arthritis.org/top-10-2006.php

[11] National Center for Complementary and Alternative Medicine (NCCAM), National Institutes of Health, Department of Health and Human Services. (2007). *Questions and answers: NIH Glucosamine/Chondroitin Arthritis Intervention Trial (GAIT).* Retrieved 08.17.07 from http://nccam.nih.gov/research/results/gait/qa.htm

[12] Sondergaard, B. C., et al. (2007). The effect of oral calcitonin on cartilage turnover and surface erosion in an ovariectomized rat model. *Arthritis Rheum* 56:2674–2678.

[13] American College of Rheumatology. (2007). *A potential new disease modifying drug for osteoarthritis.* Retrieved 08.17.07 from http://www.rheumatology.org/press/2007/0730drugosteo.asp

[14] Arthritis Foundation. (n.d.). *Total knee surgery animation.* Retrieved 08.17.07 from http://ww2.arthritis.org/conditions/surgerycenter/surgerycenterflash/totalknee.html

[15] Arthritis Foundation. (n.d.). *Unicondylar knee resurfacing.* Retrieved 08.17.07 from http://ww2.arthritis.org/conditions/surgerycenter/surgerycenterflash/uni.html

[16] Freedman, K. B. (2006). Cervical spondylosis. *MedlinePlus Medical Encyclopedia.* Retrieved 08.18.07 from http://www.nlm.nih.gov/medlineplus/ency/article/000436.htm

[17] Johannessen, W., et al. (2006). Assessment of human disc degeneration and proteoglycan content using T1 (rho) weighted magnetic resonance imaging. *Spine* 31:1253–1257.

[18] Freedman, K. B. Ibid.

[19] Kalfas, I. H. (2002). Role of corpectomy in cervical spondylosis [review]. *Neurosurgery Focus* 12(1):E11.

[20] Freedman, K. B. Ibid.

[21] Weinberg, E. P. (2005). Spondylolysis. *eMedicine from WebMD.* Retrieved 08.18.07 from http://www.nlm.nih.gov/medlineplus/ency/article/001260.htm

[22] Ibid.

[23] Ibid.

[24] Ibid.

[25] Shen, M., et al. (2007). Retrolisthesis and lumbar disc herniation: A pre-operative assessment of patient function. *Spine J.* 7(4):406-413.

[26] Chen, A. L. (2006). Spondylolisthesis. *MedlinePlus Medical Encyclopedia.* Retrieved 08.18.07 from http://www.nlm.nih.gov/medlineplus/ency/article/001260.htm

[27] Ibid.

[28] Ibid.

[29] Infective arthritis. (2003). *The Merck Manuals On-line Medical Library.* Retrieved 08.18.07 from http://www.merck.com/mmhe/sec05/ch065/ch065c.html

[30] Brusch, J. L. (2005). Septic arthritis. *eMedicine from WebMD.* Retrieved 08.18.07 from http://www.emedicine.com/med/topic3394.htm

[31] Ibid.

[32] Lee, S. (2007). Septic arthritis. *MedlinePlus Medical Encyclopedia.* Retrieved 08.18.07 from http://www.nlm.nih.gov/medlineplus/ency/article/000430.htm

[33] Ibid.

[34] Ibid.

[35] Ibid.

[36] Ibid.

[37] Ibid.

[38] Ibid.

[39] Key, J. A. (1932). Hemophilic arthritis. *Ann Surg* 95:198–225. Retrieved 08.18.07 from http://www.pubmedcentral.nih.gov/articlerender.fcgi?artid=1391531

[40] National Heart, Lung, and Blood Institute. (2007). Hemophilia. *MedlinePlus Medical Encyclopedia.* Retrieved 08.18.07 from http://www.nlm.nih.gov/medlineplus/hemophilia.html

[41] Key, J. A. Ibid.

[42] Kilcoyne, R. F. (2004). Hemophilia, musculoskeletal complications. *eMedicine from WebMD.* Retrieved 08.18.07 from http://www.emedicine.com/radio/topic909.htm

[43] Ibid.

[44] Ibid.

[45] Centers for Disease Control and Prevention, Department of Health and Human Services. (2007). CDC reports high Lyme disease rates in 10 states. Retrieved 08.18.07 from http://www.cdc.gov/od/oc/media/pressrel/2007/r070614.htm

[46] Lyme disease. (2007). *MedlinePlus Medical Encyclopedia.* Retrieved 08.18.07 from http://www.nlm.nih.gov/medlineplus/lymedisease.html

[47] Clinicians clash over new Lyme disease guidelines. (2007). *MedlinePlus Medical Encyclopedia.* Retrieved 08.18.07 from http://www.nlm.nih.gov/medlineplus/news/fullstory_52188.html

[48] Lyme disease: anti–*Borrelia burgdorferi* IgM/IgG. (2006). *Lab Tests On-line.* Retrieved 08.18.07 from http://www.labtestsonline.org/understanding/analytes/lyme/test.html

[49] National Institute of Allergy and Infectious Diseases, National Institute of Arthritis and Musculoskeletal and Skin Diseases, National Institutes of Health. (2003). *Lyme disease: the facts, the challenge.* Retrieved 08.18.07 from http://www.niaid.nih.gov/publications/lyme/niaid%20lymedisbookf2.pdf

[50] Francis, M. L. (2006). Gout. *eMedicine from WebMD.* Retrieved 10.05.07 from http://www.emedicine.com/med/topic924.htm

[51] Shiel, W. C. (2007). Gout and hyperuricemia. What are gout and hyperuricemia? *MedicineNet*.com. Retrieved 08.19.07 from http://www.medicinenet.com/gout/article.htm

[52] Shiel, W. C. (2007). Gout and hyperuricemia. What are the risk factors for gouty arthritis? *MedicineNet.* Retrieved 08.19.07 from http://www.medicinenet.com/gout/page2.htm

[53] National Institute of Neurological Disorders and Stroke. (2007). *NINDS Lesch-Nyhan syndrome information page.* Available at http://www.ninds.nih.gov/disorders/lesch_nyhan/lesch_nyhan.htm

[54] Laurent, R., & Gleeson, R. (2000). Synovial fluid analysis in the investigation of arthritis. *Palms Info Link.* Retrieved 08.19.07 from https://portal.nsccahs.health.nsw.gov.au/palmstst/Education/Pubs/Infolink/issue9.shtml

[55] Akahoshi, T., Murakami, Y., & Kitasato, H. (2007). Recent advances in crystal-induced acute inflammation. *Curr Opin Rheumatol* 19:146–150. Available at http://www.medscape.com/viewarticle/551887

[56] Schumacher, R. H. (2006). *Pseudogout.* Retrieved 08.19.07 from http://www.rheumatology.org/public/factsheets/pseudogout_new.asp?aud=pat

[57] Shiel, W. C. (2007). Gout and hyperuricemia. What are symptoms of gout? *MedicineNet.* Retrieved 08.19.07 from http://www.medicinenet.com/gout/page2.htm

[58] Gout. (2007). *MedlinePlus Medical Encyclopedia.* Retrieved 08.19.07 from http://www.nlm.nih.gov/medlineplus/gout.html

[59] Shiel, W. C. (2007). Gout and hyperuricemia. How is gouty arthritis diagnosed? *MedicineNet.* Retrieved 08.19.07 from http://www.medicinenet.com/gout/page3.htm

[60] Shiel, W. C. (2007). Gout and hyperuricemia. How is gout treated? *MedicineNet*. Retrieved 08.19.07 from http://www.medicinenet.com/gout/page4.htm

[61] The Cleveland Clinic. (2003). *Allopurinol*. Retrieved 08.19.07 from http://www.clevelandclinic.org/health/health-info/docs/0600/0654.asp?index=4771

[62] Shiel, W. C. (2007). Gout and hyperuricemia. How is gout treated? Ibid.

[63] Levesque, M. C., editor. (2007). Arthritis: joint fusion surgery (arthrodesis) to treat arthritis. *WebMD*. Retrieved 08.19.07 from http://www.webmd.com/osteoarthritis/guide/joint-fusion-surgery

[64] Internet Society of Orthopaedic Surgery and Trauma. (2006). Hemiarthroplasty of the hip. *Orthogate*. Retrieved from http://www.orthogate.org/patient-education/hip/hemiarthroplasty-of-the-hip.html

[65] Ibid.

[66] Brouwer, R. W., et al. (2006). Osteotomy for medial compartment arthritis of the knee using a closing wedge or an opening wedge controlled by a Puddu plate: a one year, randomized, controlled study. *J Bone Joint Surg* 88:1454–1459. Retrieved 08.19.07 from http://findarticles.com/p/articles/mi_qa3767/is_200611/ai_n16888159/pg_1

[67] Erstad, S., & Rodgers, E. (2005). Osteotomy for osteoarthritis. *WebMD*. Retrieved 08.19.07 from http://www.webmd.com/osteoarthritis/Osteotomy-for-osteoarthritis

[68] Rockwood, C. A., Wirth, M. A. & Grassi, F. A. (1997). Resection arthroplasty of the sternoclavicular joint. *J Bone Joint Surg* 79:387–393. Available at http://www.ejbjs.org/cgi/content/abstract/79/3/387

[69] Huddleston, H. D. (2007). *Arthritis of the hip joint: other surgical treatment alternatives*. Retrieved 08.19.07 from http://www.hipsandknees.com/hip/hiptreatment.htm

[70] Surgical challenges in revision total knee replacement. *Medscape*. Retrieved 09.07.07 from http://www.medscape.com/viewarticle/413058_3

[71] Delauney, C. (n.d.). The Charnley total hip replacement: the gold standard of primary hip replacement, 36 years on. *Maitrise Orhtopédique, The French Orthopaedic Web Journal*. Retrieved 08.19.07 from http://www.maitrise-orthop.com/corpusmaitri/orthopaedic/mo83_delaunay/delaunay_us.shtml

[72] Jana, A. K., et al. (2001). Total hip arthroplasty using porous-coated femoral components in patients with rheumatoid arthritis. *J Bone Joint Surg* 83:686–690. Retrieved 08.19.07 from http://findarticles.com/p/articles/mi_qa3767/is_200107/ai_n8995888

[73] Freedman, K. B. (2006). Hip joint replacement. *MedlinePlus Medical Encyclopedia*. Retrieved 08.19.07 from http://www.nlm.nih.gov/medlineplus/ency/article/002975.htm

[74] Rohd, B. (2007). THR: posterolateral approach. Duke Orthopaedics presents *Wheeless' Textbook of Orthopaedics*. Retrieved 09.07.07 from http://www.wheelessonline.com/ortho/thr_posterolateral_approach_1

[75] Matta, J. M. (n.d.). *The anterior approach for total hip arthroplasty: background and operative technique*. Anterior Total Hip Arthroplasty Collaborative. Retrieved 08.19.07 from http://hipandpelvis.com/physicians_corner/AAsurg-tech.pdf

[76] Donatelli, R. A., & Wooden, M. J. (2001). *Orthopaedic physical therapy,* 3rd edition. New York: Churchill Livingstone, p. 444.

[77] Ibid.

[78] Arthritis Foundation. (2001). *Unicondylar knee resurfacing*. Retrieved 08.19.07 from http://ww2.arthritis.org/conditions/SurgeryCenter/surgerycenterflash/unikneeop.swf

[79] Beaupré, L. A., et al. (2001). Exercise combined with continuous passive motion or slider board therapy compared with exercise only: a randomized controlled trial of patients following total knee arthroplasty. *Phys Ther* 81:1029–1037.

[80] Denis, M., et al. (2006). Effectiveness of continuous passive motion and conventional physical therapy after total knee arthroplasty: a randomized clinical trial. *Phys Ther* 86:174–185

[81] Chotanaphuti, T., et al. (2006). The prevalence of thrombophilia and venous thromboembolism in total knee arthroplasty. *J Med Assoc Thailand* 90:1342–1347.

[82] Hitos, K., & Fletcher, J. P. (2006). Venous thromboembolism following primary total knee arthroplasty. *Int Angiol* 25:343–351.

[83] American Academy of Orthopaedic Surgeons. (2005). *Shoulder joint replacement*. Retrieved 08.19.07 from http://orthoinfo.aaos.org/fact/thr_report.cfm?Thread_ID=291&topcategory=Shoulder

[84] Laberge, M. (2004). Shoulder resection arthroplasty. *HealthLine*. Retrieved 08.19.07 from http://www.healthline.com/galecontent/shoulder-resection-arthroplasty/2

[85] Shoulder replacement surgery. (n.d.). *ShoulderSurgeon*. Retrieved 08.19.07 from http://www.shouldersurgeon.com/shoulder_replacement_surgery/index.htm

[86] American Academy of Orthopaedic Surgeons. (2005). Ibid.

[87] Ibid.

[88] Shankman, G. A. (2004). *Fundamental orthopedic management for the physical therapist assistant*. St. Louis, MO: Mosby.

[89] Matsen, F. A., III. (2006). *Total elbow joint replacement for elbow arthritis: surgery with a dependable, time-tested prosthesis can lessen pain and improve function in elbows, especially those with rheumatoid arthritis*. University of Washington, Orthopaedics and Sports Medicine. Retrieved 08.19.07 from http://www.orthop.washington.edu/uw/elbowreplacement/tabID__3376/ItemID__61/Articles/Default.aspx

[90] Getting an ankle replacement. (n.d.). *JointReplacement.com*. Retrieved 08.19.07 from http://www.jointreplacement.com/xq/ASP.default/mn.local/pg.cat/joint_id.7/cat_id.3/joint_nm.Ankle/local_id.38/qx/default.htm

[91] Haddad, S. L. (2003). Total ankle arthroplasty: case report. *Orthoped Technol Rev* 5(2). Retrieved 08.19.07 from http://www.orthopedictechreview.com/issues/marapr03/case.htm

[92] The British Society of Surgery of the Hand. (n.d.). *Rheumatoid arthritis*. Retrieved 08.19.07 from http://www.bssh.ac.uk/documents/Rheumatoid_arthritis.pdf

[93] U.S. Department of Health and Human Services. (2004). *Bone health and osteoporosis. A report of the surgeon general*, pp. 3–4. Retrieved 08.19.07 from http://www.surgeongeneral.gov/library/bonehealth/docs/exec_summ.pdf

[94] Osteoporosis. (2007). *MedlinePlus Medical Encyclopedia*. Retrieved 08.19.07 from http://www.nlm.nih.gov/medlineplus/osteoporosis.html

[95] Haines, C. (2005). Understanding osteoporosis prevention. *WebMD*. Retrieved 09.07.07 from http://www.webmd.com/solutions/hs/osteoporosis/prevention

[96] Ibid.

[97] VanVoorhees, B. W. (2006). Rickets. *MedlinePlus Medical Encyclopedia*. Retrieved 09.07.07 from http://www.nlm.nih.gov/medlineplus/ency/article/000344.htm

[98] Finberg, L. (2006). Rickets. *eMedicine from WebMD*. Retrieved 09.07.07 from http://www.emedicine.com/ped/topic2014.htm

[99] VanVoorhees, B. W. (2006). Ibid.

[100] Ibid.

[101] Rohd, B. (2007). Osteomalacia. Duke Orthopaedics presents *Wheeless' Textbook of Orthopaedics*. Retrieved 09.09.07 from http://www.wheelessonline.com/ortho/osteomalacia

[102] Ibid.

[103] Ibid.

[104] Ott, S. (2007). *Osteoporosis and bone physiology*. University of Washington Department of Medicine. Retrieved 09.09.07 from http://courses.washington.edu/bonephys/index.html

[105] Khan, A. N. (2007). Legg-Calvé-Perthes disease. *eMedicine from WebMD*. Retrieved 10.06.07 from http://www.emedicine.com/radio/topic387.htm

[106] Ibid.

[107] Ibid.

[108] University of Virginia Health System. (2004). *Legg-Calvé-Perthes disease: what is Legg-Calvé-Perthes disease?* Retrieved 10.06.07

from http://www.healthsystem.virginia.edu/uvahealth/peds_orthopaedics/lcpd.cfm

[109] Ibid.

[110] Joseph, T. N. (2006). Slipped capital femoral epiphysis. *MedlinePlus Medical Encyclopedia*. Retrieved 10.06.07 from http://www.nlm.nih.gov/medlineplus/ency/article/000972.htm

[111] Ibid.

[112] Ibid.

[113] Marano, H. (2006). Slipped capital femoral epiphysis. *eMedicine from WebMD*. Retrieved 10.06.07 from http://www.emedicine.com/sports/topic122.htm

[114] Ibid.

[115] Hurd, R. (2006). Paget's disease. *eMedicine from WebMD*. Retrieved 10.06.07 from http://www.nlm.nih.gov/medlineplus/ency/article/000414.htm

[116] Paget's disease of bone. (2007). *MedlinePlus Medical Encyclopedia*. Retrieved 10.06.07 from http://www.nlm.nih.gov/medlineplus/pagetsdiseaseofbone.html

[117] Hurd, R. (2006). Ibid.

[118] Paget's disease of bone. (2007). Ibid.

[119] Paget's disease. (2006). *MedicineNet*. Retrieved 10.06.07 from http://www.medicinenet.com/pagets_disease/article.htm

[120] Babcock, H. M. (2006). Osteomyelitis. *MedlinePlus Medical Encyclopedia*. Retrieved 10.06.07 from http://www.nlm.nih.gov/medlineplus/ency/article/000437.htm

[121] Ibid.

[122] King, R. W. (2006). Osteomyelitis. *eMedicine from WebMD*. Retrieved 10.07.07 from http://www.emedicine.com/emerg/topic349.htm

[123] Ibid.

[124] Ibid.

[125] Mayo Clinic. (2007). *Diseases and conditions: hyperparathyroidism*. Retrieved 10.07.07 from http://www.mayoclinic.com/health/hyperparathyroidism/DS00396/DSECTION=2

[126] The Endocrine and Metabolic Diseases Information Service, National Institute of Diabetes, and Digestive and Kidney Diseases, National Institutes of Health. (2006). *Hyperparathyroidism*. Retrieved 10.07.07 from http://endocrine.niddk.nih.gov/pubs/hyper/hyper.htm

[127] Halpern, J. (2005). Hypoparathyroidism. *eMedicine from WebMD*. Retrieved 10.07.07 from http://www.emedicine.com/emerg/topic276.htm

[128] Batra, V. (2006). Tuberculosis. *eMedicine from WebMD*. Retrieved 10.07.07 from http://www.emedicine.com/ped/topic2321.htm

[129] Ibid.

[130] Keith, M. P. (2007). Gonococcal arthritis. *eMedicine by WebMD*. Retrieved 10.07.07. from http://www.emedicine.com/med/topic2928.htm

[131] Koopman, W. J. (1997). *Arthritis and allied conditions: a textbook of rheumatology*, Volume 2, 13th edition. Baltimore: Williams & Wilkins.

[132] Keith, M. P. Ibid.

[133] Ibid.

[134] Centers for Disease Control and Prevention. (2007). *Updated recommended treatment regimens for gonococcal infections and associated conditions— United States, April 2007*, p. 2. Retrieved 10.07.07 from http://www.cdc.gov/std/treatment/2006/GonUpdateApril2007.pdf

[135] Mehlman, C. T. (2005). Osteosarcoma. *eMedicine by WebMD*. Retrieved 10.16.07 from http://www.emedicine.com/orthoped/topic531.htm

[136] Patton, D. (2005). Childhood cancer: osteosarcoma. *Kidshealth*, Nemours Foundation. Retrieved 10.16.07 from http://www.kidshealth.org/parent/medical/cancer/cancer_osteosarcoma.html

[137] Levy, A. S. (2006). Osteosarcoma. *MedlinePlus Medical Encyclopedia*. Retrieved 10.16.07 from http://www.nlm.nih.gov/medlineplus/ency/article/001650.htm

[138] Ibid.

[139] Mehlman, C. T. (2005). Osteosarcoma. *eMedicine by WebMD*. Retrieved 10.16.07 from http://www.emedicine.com/orthoped/topic531.htm

[140] DeGroot, H., III. (2004). Osteoma. *Bonetumor.org*. Retrieved 10.17.07 from http://www.bonetumor.org/tumors/pages/page12.html

[141] Zileli, M., et al. (2004). Osteoid osteomas and osteoblastomas of the spine. Neurological Focus, *Medscape from WebMD*. Retrieved 10.17.07 from http://www.medscape.com/viewarticle/465365

[142] Papavassiliou, E., & Jichici, D. (2007). Benign skull tumors. *eMedicine from WebMD*. Retrieved 10.17.07 from http://www.emedicine.com/NEURO/topic33.htm

[143] Ibid.

[144] Ibid.

[145] Ibid.

[146] Children's Hospital Boston. (n.d.). *Osteochondroma (exostosis)*. Retrieved 10. 17. 07 from http://www.childrenshospital.org/az/Site1079/mainpageS1079P0.html

[147] Ibid.

[148] Brooks, D., Jelinek, J., & Kumar, D. (2002). *Benign, malignant and metastatic bone tumors*. Washington Cancer Institute at Washington Hospital Center, Washington Musculoskeletal Tumor Center. Retrieved 10.24.07 from http://www.sarcoma.org//main.php-page=review.htm

[149] Goh, L. A., & Peh, W. C. G. (2007). Giant cell tumor. *eMedicine from WebMD*. Retrieved 10.17.07 from http://www.emedicine.com/radio/topic307.htm

[150] American Academy of Orthopaedic Surgeons. (2007). *Giant cell tumor of bone*. Retrieved 10.21.07 from http://orthoinfo.aaos.org/topic.cfm?topic=A00080&return_link=0

[151] Goh, L. A., & Peh, W. C. G. (2007). Giant cell tumor. *eMedicine from WebMD*. Retrieved 10.17.07 from http://www.emedicine.com/radio/topic307.htm

[152] Ibid.

[153] American Academy of Orthopaedic Surgeons. (2007). Ibid.

[154] American Academy of Orthopaedic Surgeons. (2007). Ibid.

[155] Brooks, D., Jelinek, J., & Kumar, D. Ibid.

[156] Nanda, R. (2006). Ewing's sarcoma. *MedlinePlus Medical Encyclopedia*. Retrieved 10.24.07 from http://www.nlm.nih.gov/medlineplus/ency/article/001302.htm

[157] Mayo Foundation for Medical Education and Research. (2007). *Fibrous dysplasia*. Retrieved 10.24.07 from http://www.mayoclinic.com/health/fibrous-dysplasia/DS00991/UPDATEAPP=0

[158] Ibid.

[159] Ibid.

[160] Ballas, C. (2005). Fibrous dysplasia. *MedlinePlus Medical Encyclopedia*. Retrieved 10.24.07 from http://www.nlm.nih.gov/medlineplus/ency/article/001234.htm

[161] Mayo Foundation for Medical Education and Research. (2007). Ibid.

[162] Anand, M. K. N. (2007). Fibrous dysplasia. *eMedicine from WebMD*. Retrieved 10.24.07 from http://www.emedicine.com/radio/topic284.htm

[163] Hurd, R. (2006). Osteitis fibrosa. *MedlinePlus Medical Encyclopedia*. Retrieved 10.24.07 from http://www.nlm.nih.gov/medlineplus/ency/article/001252.htm

[164] Mayo Foundation for Medical Education and Research. (2007). Ibid.

[165] Ibid.

[166] Ibid.

[167] American Cancer Society. (2006). *Detailed guide: multiple myeloma. What are the risk factors for multiple myeloma?* Retrieved 10.24.07 from http://www.cancer.org/docroot/cri/content/cri_2_4_2x_what_are_the_risk_factors_for_multiple_myeloma_30.asp

[168] Lonial, S. (2005). *Intro to myeloma*. Multiple Myeloma Research Foundation. Retrieved 10.24.07 from http://www.multiplemyeloma.org/about_myeloma/index.php

[169] Saif, M. W., & Shannon, K. (2005). Multiple myeloma and HIV infection: an association or a coincidence? *J Appl Res* 5: 318–324.

[170] Pantanowitz, L., & Dezube, B. J. (2003). Multiple myeloma and HIV infection—causal or casual coincidence? *AIDS Read* 13:383–324. Retrieved 10.24.07 from http://www.medscape.com/viewarticle/460735_side1

[171] Lonial, S. (2005). *Intro to myeloma.* Ibid.

[172] Lonial, S. (2005). Multiple myeloma: symptoms. Retrieved 10.24.07 from http://www.multiplemyeloma.org/about_myeloma/index.php

[173] Mayo Clinic. (2007). *Amyloidosis.* Retrieved 10.24.07 from http://www.mayoclinic.com/print/amyloidosis/DS00431/DSECTION=all&METHOD=print

[174] American Cancer Society. (2006). *Detailed guide: multiple myeloma. What are the key statistics about multiple myeloma?* Retrieved 10.24.07 from http://www.cancer.org/docroot/CRI/content/CRI_2_4_1X_What_are_the_key_statistics_for_multiple_myeloma_30.asp?rnav=cri

[175] Ibid.

[176] Lonial, S. *Diagnosis and staging.* Multiple Myeloma Research Foundation. Retrieved 10.24.07 from http://www.multiplemyeloma.org/about_myeloma/2.05.php

[177] Lonial, S. Intro to myeloma. Ibid.

[178] Multiple myeloma. (2007). *MedlinePlus Medical Encyclopedia.* Retrieved 10.24.07 from http://www.nlm.nih.gov/medlineplus/multiplemyeloma.html

[179] International Myeloma Foundation. (2006). *Understanding thalidomide therapy.* Retrieved 10.24.07 from http://myeloma.org/pdfs/Understanding_Thalidomide.pdf

[180] International Myeloma Foundation. (2006). *Understanding bisphosphonate therapy.* Retrieved 10.24.07 from http://myeloma.org/pdfs/UnderstandingBisphos_b3.2.pdf

[181] American Cancer Society. (2006). *Detailed guide: multiple myeloma. Treatment options by stage.* Retrieved 10.24.07 from http://www.cancer.org/docroot/CRI/content/CRI_2_4_4X_Treatment_Options_by_Stage_30.asp?sitearea=

[182] International Myeloma Foundation. (2006). *Understanding Quadramet.* Retrieved 10.24.07 from http://myeloma.org/pdfs/Understanding_Quadramet.pdf

[183] Coleman, R. E. (December, 2000). Management of bone metastases. *The Oncologist* 5:463–470.

[184] Ibid.

[185] American Cancer Society. (2007). *Detailed guide: bone metastasis. How is bone metastasis treated?* Retrieved 10.24.07 from http://www.cancer.org/docroot/CRI/content/CRI_2_4_4X_How_Is_Bone_Metastasis_Treated_66.asp

[186] Ibid.

[187] Danciu, M., & Mihailovici, M. S. (2004). Chondroma. *Atlas of Pathology.* Retrieved 10.24.07 from http://www.pathologyatlas.ro/Chondroma.html

[188] Cluett, J. (2007). Ollier's disease. *About.com: Orthopedics.* Retrieved 10.24.07 from http://orthopedics.about.com/cs/tumors/g/olliers.htm

[189] American Association of Enchondroma Diseases. (2005). *Maffucci's syndrome.* Retrieved 10.24.07 from http://www.aamed.net/modules.php?name=Content&pa=showpage&pid=5

[190] Vanni, R. (2003). Bone: chondroma. *Atlas of Genetics and Cytogenetics in Oncology and Haematology.* Retrieved 10.24.07 from http://atlasgeneticsoncology.org/Tumors/ChondromaID5147.html

[191] Hide, G. (2005). Chondrosarcoma. *eMedicine from WebMD.* Retrieved 10.24.07 from http://www.emedicine.com/radio/topic168.htm

[192] American Cancer Society. (2006). *Detailed guide: bone cancer. Types of bone cancer. Primary bone tumors: chondrosarcoma.* Retrieved 10.24.07 from http://www.cancer.org/docroot/CRI/content/CRI_2_4_1X_What_Is_bone_cancer_2.asp

[193] Hide, G. (2005). Ibid.

[194] Ibid.

[195] American Joint Committee on Cancer. (n.d.). *What is cancer staging?* Retrieved 1.30.07 from http://www.cancerstaging.org/mission/whatis.html

[196] American Cancer Society. (2007). *Detailed guide: cancer. What is staging?* Retrieved 11.30.07 from http://www.cancer.org/docroot/CRI/content/CRI_2_4_3X_What_is_staging.asp?sitearea=

[197] Stevens, P. M., & Holmstrom, M. C. (2007). Genu valgum, pediatrics. *eMedicine from WebMD.* Retrieved 10.25.07 from http://www.emedicine.com/orthoped/topic495.htm

[198] Ibid.

[199] Ibid.

[200] Ibid.

[201] Duke Orthopaedics. (n.d.). Pediatric genu varum. *Wheeless' Textbook of Orthopaedics.* Retrieved 10.25.07 from http://www.wheelessonline.com/ortho/pediatric_genu_varum

[202] Ibid.

[203] Duke Orthopaedics. (n.d.). Blount's disease. *Wheeless' Textbook of Orthopaedics.* Retrieved 10.25.07 from http://www.wheelessonline.com/ortho/blounts_disease

[204] Marshall, I. (2006). Bowlegs. *MedlinePlus Medical Encyclopedia.* Retrieved 10.25.07 from http://www.nlm.nih.gov/medlineplus/ency/article/001585.htm

[205] Connecticut Children's Medical Center. (2007). *Orthopaedics: bowlegs and knock knees.* Retrieved 10.25.07 from http://www.ccmckids.org/services/orthopaedics_bowlegs2.asp

[206] Patel, M., & Herzenberg, J. (2005). Clubfoot. *eMedicine from WebMD.* Retrieved 10.25.07 from http://www.emedicine.com/orthoped/topic598.htm

[207] Thomas, J. N. (2006). Clubfoot. *MedlinePlus Medical Encyclopedia.* Retrieved 10.25.07 from http://www.nlm.nih.gov/medlineplus/ency/article/001228.htm

[208] Patel, M., & Herzenberg, J. Ibid.

[209] Ibid.

[210] Ibid.

[211] Rauch, D. (2006). Developmental dysplasia of the hip. *MedlinePlus Medical Encyclopedia.* Retrieved 10.25.07 from http://www.nlm.nih.gov/medlineplus/ency/article/000971.htm

[212] Duke Orthopaedics. (n.d.). Developmental dislocation of the hip. *Wheeless' Textbook of Orthopaedics.* Retrieved 10.25.07 from http://www.wheelessonline.com/ortho/developmental_dislocation_of_the_hip

[213] Rauch, D. Ibid.

[214] McCarthy, J. (2005). Developmental dysplasia of the hip. *eMedicine from WebMD.* Retrieved 10.25.07 from http://www.emedicine.com/orthoped/topic456.htm

[215] Reynolds, N. C., Jr., & Ma, J. (2006). Torticollis. *eMedicine from WebMD.* Retrieved 10.26.07 from http://www.emedicine.com/neuro/topic377.htm

[216] Children's Hospital & Regional Medical Center, Seattle, Washington. (n.d.). *Orthopedics: torticollis.* Retrieved 10.26.07 from http://orthopedics.seattlechildrens.org/conditions_treated/torticollis.asp

[217] Reynolds, N. C., Jr., & Ma, J. Ibid.

[218] Greene, A. (2006). Torticollis. *MedlinePlus Medical Encyclopedia.* US National Library of Medicine, *National Institutes of Health.* Retrieved 10.26.07 from http://www.nlm.nih.gov/medlineplus/ency/article/000749.htm

[219] Ibid.

[220] Ibid.

[221] Ibid.

[222] Rauch, D. (2006). Achondroplasia. *MedlinePlus.* US National Library of Medicine, *National Institutes of Health.* Retrieved 10.26.07 from http://www.nlm.nih.gov/medlineplus/ency/article/001577.htm

[223] Rauch, D. (2006). Achondroplasia. *MedlinePlus Medical Encyclopedia.* Retrieved 10.26.07 from http://www.nlm.nih.gov/medlineplus/ency/article/001577.htm

[224] Ibid.

[225] Genetics Home Reference, US National Library of Medicine, National Institutes of Health. (2007). *Osteogenesis imperfecta.* Retrieved 10.26.07 from http://ghr.nlm.nih.gov/condition=osteogenesisimperfecta

[226] Ibid.

[227] Ibid.

[228] National Institute of Arthritis and Musculoskeletal and Skin Diseases. (2007). Osteogenesis imperfecta. *MedlinePlus Medical Encyclopedia*. Retrieved 10.26.07 from http://www.nlm.nih.gov/medlineplus/osteogenesisimperfecta.html

[229] American Academy of Orthopaedic Surgeons. (2007). *Osteogenesis imperfecta*. Retrieved 10.26.07 from http://orthoinfo.aaos.org/topic.cfm?topic=A00051&return_link=0

[230] Ibid.

[231] Osteogenesis Imperfecta Foundation. (n.d.). *Diagnosis and testing*. Retrieved 10.26.07 from http://www.oif.org/site/PageServer?pagename=DiagTest

[232] American Academy of Orthopaedic Surgeons. (2007). Ibid.

[233] Ibid.

[234] Bhargava, A. (2007). Osteopetrosis. *eMedicine from WebMD*. Retrieved 10. 26.07 from http://www.emedicine.com/med/topic1692.htm

[235] McKusick, V. A., Tiller, G. E., & O'Neill, M. J. F. (2007). *Osteopetrosis, Autosomal recessive1; OPTB1*. Online Mendelian Inheritance in Man # 259700. Retrieved 10.26.07 from http://www.ncbi.nlm.nih.gov/entrez/dispomim.cgi?id=259700

[236] Bhargava, A. Ibid.

[237] Osteopetrosis.org. (2002). *Osteopetrosis*. Retrieved 10.26.07 from http://www.osteopetrosis.org/

[238] Carolino, J., Perez, J. A., & Popa, A. (1998). *Osteopetrosis*. American Academy of Family Physicians. Retrieved 10.26.07 from http://www.aafp.org/afp/980315ap/carolino.html

[239] Bhargava, A. Ibid.

[240] National Institute of Arthritis and Musculoskeletal and Skin Diseases. (2001). *Questions and answers about Marfan syndrome*. Retrieved 08.17.07 from http://www.niams.nih.gov/hi/topics/marfan/marfan.pdf

[241] Ibid.

[242] National Institute of Arthritis and Musculoskeletal and Skin Diseases. (2001). *Questions and answers about Marfan syndrome*. National Institutes of Health. Retrieved 08.17.07 from http://www.niams.nih.gov/hi/topics/marfan/marfan.pdf

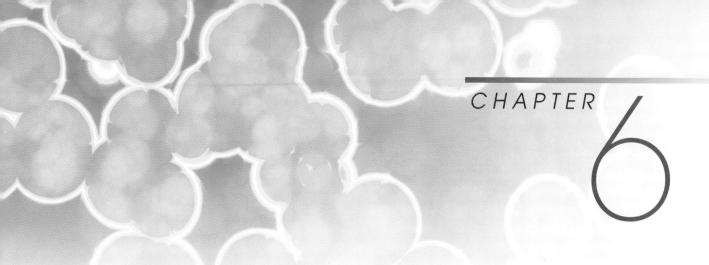

Rheumatoid Arthritis and Related Conditions

LEARNING OBJECTIVES

After completion of this chapter students should be able to:

- Describe the pathological mechanisms of rheumatoid arthritis, juvenile rheumatoid arthritis, and Still's disease
- Describe the pathological mechanisms of ankylosing spondylitis, psoriatic arthritis, systemic lupus erythematosus, scleroderma, Sjögren's syndrome, and several of the more common forms of rheumatoid-related inflammatory joint pathologies and connective tissue diseases
- Discuss the pathological mechanisms of muscular dystrophy, myasthenia gravis, and other muscular diseases
- Identify the differences between inflammatory arthritis and systemic connective tissue diseases
- Determine the physical therapy intervention for patients with the described rheumatoid conditions and muscular diseases
- Analyze the role of the physical therapist assistant in working with patients with the described rheumatoid conditions and muscular diseases
- Determine the contraindications, precautions, and special considerations for PT/PTA intervention for patients with rheumatoid arthritis, juvenile rheumatoid arthritis, and Still's disease, ankylosing spondylitis, psoriatic arthritis, systemic lupus erythematosus, scleroderma, and several of the more common forms of rheumatoid related inflammatory joint pathologies and connective tissue diseases

KEY TERMS

Ankylosis
Arthritis mutilans
Bamboo spine
Boutonnière's deformity
Enthesitis
Felty's syndrome
Fusiform-shaped fingers/spindle fingers
Hallux valgus
Hammer toes
Malar rash/butterfly rash
Myofascial pain syndrome
Pannus
Pencil-in-cup deformity
Raynaud's phenomenon
Rheumatoid factor
Sacroiliitis
Sjögren's syndrome
Swan-neck deformity
Ulnar drift

CHAPTER OUTLINE

Introduction

This chapter covers information regarding the inflammatory and systemic arthropathies such as rheumatoid arthritis (RA), rheumatoid-related inflammatory pathologies, connective tissue diseases, and muscle diseases. People with RA and other related pathologies described in this chapter are frequently seen in physical therapy practice.

Why Does the Physical Therapist Assistant Need to Know About Rheumatoid Arthritis?

Rheumatoid arthritis (RA) is one of the more common arthritic conditions seen by the physical therapist (PT) and the physical therapist assistant (PTA) in clinical practice. As a result of the systemic nature of RA, the approach to intervention is different from that of individuals with osteoarthritis. Understanding the pathological processes involved in RA assists the physical

therapist in developing an individualized plan of care and enables the physical therapist assistant to follow that plan of care, keeping in mind the various precautions and contraindications of the disease process.

Rheumatoid Arthritis

HINTS ON USE OF THE GUIDE TO PHYSICAL THERAPIST PRACTICE

Rheumatoid arthritis (RA), juvenile rheumatoid arthritis, and Still's disease are classified in the *Guide to Physical Therapist Practice*, Musculoskeletal Preferred Practice Pattern 4.

- 4C, "impaired muscle performance" (p. 161): This pattern is appropriate in some cases
- 4D, "impaired joint mobility, motor function, muscle performance, and range of motion associated with connective tissue dysfunction" (p. 179): This pattern

is the more likely one to use for these conditions due to the extensive nature of the symptoms of this group of diseases; associated impairments and functional limitations in these conditions include muscle weakness, pain, swelling and/or joint effusion and reduced range of motion

- 4G, "impaired joint mobility, muscle performance, and range of motion associated with fracture" (p. 233): Because many patients with RA are placed on steroid medications and prolonged use of these increases the risk of fractures, this pattern may be appropriate in specific cases

- 4H, "impaired joint mobility, motor function, muscle performance, and range of motion associated with joint arthroplasty" (p. 251): Joint replacement for severely affected joints is an option for patients with RA and after these procedures the patient may be placed in pattern 4H

- 4I, "impaired joint mobility, motor function, muscle performance and range of motion associated with bony or soft tissue surgery" (p. 269): If soft tissue or bone surgery other than an arthroplasty is performed the appropriate pattern will then be 4I

NOTE: RA is a systemic disease that affects the internal organs as well as the joints; therefore, patients may have symptoms that require classification into a cardiovascular/pulmonary pattern. The physical therapist must decide which pattern is appropriate depending on the focus of the rehabilitation at any given time.

(From the American Physical Therapy Association, 2003. *Guide to physical therapist practice,* revised 2nd edition. Alexandria, VA: APTA. Used with permission.)

Rheumatoid arthritis is an inflammatory, systemic (total body), connective tissue, and autoimmune disease characterized by bilateral, symmetrical arthritis. RA is a true inflammatory polyarthritis affecting many joints in the body.[1] The condition affects many body organs, including the heart, liver, eye, skin, bones, and lungs. The symptoms of the disease range from mild to severe with varying degrees of joint deformity, and soft tissue, and organ involvement. See Table 6-1 for a comparison of the characteristics of osteoarthritis (OA) and RA. In the *Guide to Physical Therapist Practice,* RA falls within several patterns of the Musculoskeletal section depending on the structures involved. Individuals with RA may experience impaired posture, gait, joint mobility, motor function, and muscle performance, noted in several of the

musculoskeletal patterns (see Hints on Use of the Guide to Physical Therapist Practice, Box 6-1). The PT and PTA must consider the involvement of the individual to determine which section of the *Guide to Physical Therapist Practice* is most appropriate to determine preferred practice patterns.

RA predominantly affects females, with an incidence of a 3:1 female to male ratio.[2] The age of onset varies from the teenage years to the 60s, with some cases occurring in children. Most instances involve people between the ages of 25 and 55.[3] Childhood rheumatoid conditions are described separately later in the chapter.

Etiology. The etiology of RA is largely unknown. However, in 60% of people with RA in the United States, a genetic trait called HLA-DR4 is present that may predispose people to develop the disease. Hormones, especially the sex hormones, are considered a factor in some people. In some cases, the autoimmune nature of the disease, in which the cells of the immune system attack the individual's own body structures, could be initiated by a virus. The rubella and Epstein-Barr viruses are suspected to play a role in the onset of RA, but the evidence is as yet inconclusive.[4] The autoimmune response leads to the formation of immune complexes that further increase the inflammation.

Signs and Symptoms. The signs and symptoms of RA can be divided into articular (joint) changes, and nonarticular changes. The following sections detail both the articular and nonarticular changes that occur in RA.

Articular (Joint) Pathological Changes

The joint pathology of RA involves synovitis with deposition of immune complexes that leads to hypertrophy and thickening of the synovium and an excessive production of synovial fluid. When the inflammation becomes chronic, villi (finger-like projections) form on the internal surface of the synovial membrane and grow along the joint margins forming a covering called **pannus.** The pannus is an abnormally invasive layer of tissue that consists of macrophages, synoviocytes, lymphocytes, plasma cells, and mast cells. Cytokines, such as interlukin-1, within the pannus stimulate the "synoviocytes to produce cartilage-degrading enzymes" (Tsou, 2007, p. 1)[5], which destroy the hyaline cartilage and the bone beneath. The destruction of the hyaline cartilage results in a reduced joint space and rubbing of the bone ends on each other within the joint. Some joints may become ankylosed (fixed) by fibrous tissue or bone. Inflammation in the joint

Table 6.1 **Comparison of Osteoarthritis and Rheumatoid arthritis**

	OSTEOARTHRITIS	RHEUMATOID ARTHRITIS
Etiology	Wear and tear Prior trauma to joint Onset gradual	Largely unknown Heredity/environment/autoimmune (?) Viral trigger Onset gradual or sudden and may start with general malaise or joint pains
Characteristics	Asymmetrical (one joint involved); knees and hips most commonly affected; hands in women Fibrillation and fragmentation of articular cartilage, eburnation of bone ends, cysts beneath bone end surface, osteophytes at joint margins and change in shape (flattening) of bone ends, with hypertrophy of synovial membrane Ligaments contracted or stretched Disuse atrophy of muscles Fibrous degeneration of capsule and reduced joint space	Symmetrical involvement with inflammation in peripheral joints; joints of hands and feet most commonly affected initially; progresses to proximal peripheral joints Rheumatoid factor in blood Hypertrophy of synovium with synovitis and deposition of immune complexes; villi formation on synovium leading to pannus that destroys articular cartilage and bone Osteoporosis or osteopenia of bones adjacent to affected joints, reduced joint space Muscle atrophy, ruptured tendons and ligaments, skin nodules Severe fatigue, anemia, weight loss, vitamin B deficiency, leucopenia, Felty's syndrome, scleritis, Sjögren's syndrome
Deformities	Heberden's nodes (DIP) Bouchard's nodes (PIP) Genu varus (bow legs) more common	Boutonnière's deformity (ext DIP/flex PIP/hyperextension MCPs) Swan-neck deformity (flex DIP/ext PIP) Trigger finger (flexor tenosynovitis) Ulnar drift Genu valgum (knock knees) more common Atlantoaxial subluxation
Clinical picture/characteristics	Pain on weight bearing in affected joint(s); asymmetrical joint involvement Stiffness after inactivity that reduces with movement Reduced range of motion with or without pain Muscle atrophy, weakness, and spasm Joint deformity and enlargement Joint crepitus Reduced function or loss of function in the affected joint(s)	Pain at rest and on weight bearing; night pain common; multiple symmetrical joints involved Early-morning stiffness that lasts >1 hour Reduced range of motion with pain Involvement of PIPs and MCPs hands and feet Severe fatigue General body symptoms including lung and heart complications, vasculitis with skin ulcers, Raynaud's phenomenon Increased incidence of fracture due to osteoporosis Severe reduction or loss of function Inflammation
Medications	NSAIDs in the stage of inflammation {osteoarthritis is not an inflammatory condition; however, inflammation can be present} Aspirin, other analgesics	NSAIDs, aspirin (salicylic acid), acetaminophen Corticosteroids, Gold, Methotrexate, Penicillamine DMARDs or SAARDs
Prognosis	No cure Symptoms helped by weight loss Severe cases may require joint replacement to improve function Regular exercise beneficial	No cure Varied; depends on onset Severe cases may require joint replacement to improve function Specific exercise and treatment protocols are often beneficial Joint protection is paramount

DIP = distal interphalangeal joint; DMARD = disease-modifying antirheumatic drugs; MCP = metacarpophalangeal joint; NSAID = nonsteroidal anti-inflammatory drug; PIP = proximal interphalangeal; SAARD = slow-acting antirheumatic drugs.

can cause breakdown of adjacent ligamentous tissues resulting in subluxation of the joints. Pressure on the muscle tendons may lead to rupture of the tendons. Osteoporosis may develop in the distal ends of the bones adjacent to joints with RA changes (see Fig. 6-1).

The onset of RA usually begins as symmetrical arthritis in the distal joints of the upper and lower extremities, especially the hands and feet.[6] General body illness can, however, be the first sign of the disease. Some individuals experience an acute onset characterized by sudden, unexplained, severe pain and stiffness, whereas others have a more gradual onset over a matter of several months.

The early stages of RA are mainly inflammatory, and therefore the cardinal signs of inflammation are apparent. Joints are swollen with joint effusion, soft tissue edema around the joint, or both. The involved joints are acutely painful, hot to the touch, and the skin around the joint may have an erythema. **Rheumatoid factor** (RF), an antibody to immunoglobulin G (IgG), is present in the blood and synovial fluid of many people with RA. Individuals with RF are classified as seropositive, and those without RF as seronegative. Loss of function of the joints is also noted. The joints most affected in the early stages are the proximal interphalangeal joints (PIPs) and metacarpophalangeal joints (MCPs) of the hands, the wrists, and the PIPs and metatarsophalangeal joints (MTPs) of the feet. Later manifestations of the disease may include involvement of the hips, knees, shoulders, elbows, cervical spine, and temporomandibular joint.

The pain experienced by people with RA can be both acute and severe. One of the identifying features of RA is pain experienced at rest, at night, and in the early morning. Tenderness on palpation is apparent around the involved joints together with edema of the soft tissues and joint effusion. The joint effusion contributes to one of the signs of RA known as **spindle fingers, or a fusiform-shaped finger,** in which the finger takes on the shape of a spindle due to swelling of the PIP joint (see Fig. 6-2).[7] Early-morning stiffness is another distinctive feature of RA. Unlike stiffness in individuals with OA, this stiffness may last several hours after awakening in the morning. According to a research study performed by Yazici and coworkers in 2004, a direct link exists between the level of early morning stiffness and the degree of functional problems in individuals with RA than can be noted just by observing joint swelling or the results of blood tests.[8] Functionally, individuals with severe RA require considerable amounts of time to dress and get moving in the morning and may need to get up very early to be able to go to work.

Muscle atrophy can be extensive in RA and may result from disuse. Painful and stiff joints make the individual less likely to exercise, and thus the muscles become atrophied. The already edematous joints appear even more edematous as a result of the lack of muscle mass around the joint. The loss of motion in RA joints can be attributed to many factors. The restricted motion may be a result of pain on movement causing the individual to keep the joints in one position or due to damage of the tendons, ligaments, or the joint itself.

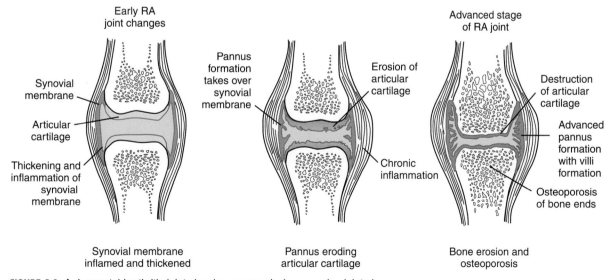

FIGURE 6.1 A rheumatoid arthritis joint showing progressively worsening joint changes.

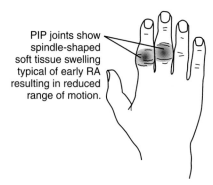

PIP joints show spindle-shaped soft tissue swelling typical of early RA resulting in reduced range of motion.

FIGURE 6.2 One of the signs of rheumatoid arthritis is "spindle finger," also known as a fusiform-shaped finger, in the proximal interphalangeal joints.

Several specific joint deformities are associated with RA such as trigger finger, **Boutonnière's deformity, Swan-neck deformity, and ulnar drift,** also called Z deformity. Trigger finger is a painful condition caused by finger flexor tenosynovitis (inflammation of the tendon sheath). Trigger finger results in a snapping type motion when attempting to flex and extend the finger. Trigger finger may be caused by rheumatoid nodules situated close to the flexor tendons or result from flexor tendon ruptures. The flexor tendon ruptures are usually caused by the tendons passing over roughened areas of bone in the area over which the tendon passes.

Boutonnière's deformity of the finger involves hyperextension of the distal interphalangeal joint (DIP) joint, flexion of the PIP and hyperextension of the MCP joint (see Fig. 6-3) Three stages of severity are considered in Boutonnière's associated with RA. Stage I is characterized by mild PIP joint synovitis, a normal MCP joint, and a DIP joint that may or may not be hyperextended. At this stage, any extensor lag of the PIP joint can be corrected manually. In Stage II, the PIP joint demonstrates a moderate flexion contracture of 30° to 40°, hyperextension is noted at the MCP joint, and although passive extension of

the PIP joint may still be possible some loss of function of the finger is noted. Stage III Boutonnière's is characterized by destruction of the PIP joint that is apparent on radiograph.[9] In Stage III, the most severe form, surgery may be performed. The DIP joint is usually fused as it does not provide a lot of bony area for insertion of a joint arthroplasty. The PIP joint may be fused, but a more functional option is a joint arthroplasty. See the section "Surgical Intervention" later in this chapter for details regarding the PIP and MCP joint arthroplasties.

Swan-neck deformity of the finger involves flexion of the DIP joint and hyperextension of the PIP joint (see Fig. 6-4). This deformity can also be found in other orthopedic and neurological conditions. Swan-neck deformity resulting from RA is usually caused by adhesions and the associated shortening of the finger extensor tendons and the joint capsule (Koopman, p. 1044).[10] In the later stages of swan-neck deformity when hand function is limited, PIP arthroplasty is considered. During the earlier stages of the deformity, a splint may be used to maintain the joint in a functional position.

Ulnar drift deformities in the hand are the result of disruption of the collateral ligaments of the MCP joints.[11] The fingers "drift" toward the ulnar side of the hand (see Fig. 6-5). This is sometimes called a Z deformity because of the shape the hand adopts. An MCP arthroplasty may be performed to correct these deformities. An arthroplasty usually improves the range of motion (ROM) of the joint, but functionally the grip may not be improved.

The radioulnar joint is often affected in RA. A synovitis occurs, which results in limited and painful motion during pronation and supination of the forearm. The ligaments surrounding the wrist become damaged as a result of constant stretching, resulting in subluxation of the head of the ulna. In severe cases, the ulnar head is excised, and a wrist arthroplasty is performed. Total wrist arthroplasty is performed only rarely, in severe cases of RA. A Biaxial prosthesis for the wrist has shown more promising results.[12,13] One of the problems in wrist prosthetics is there

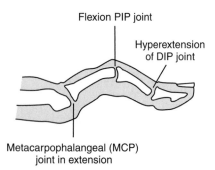

Flexion PIP joint

Hyperextension of DIP joint

Metacarpophalangeal (MCP) joint in extension

FIGURE 6.3 Boutonnière's deformity in a hand with rheumatoid arthritis.

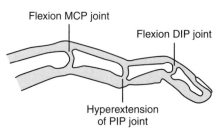

Flexion MCP joint

Flexion DIP joint

Hyperextension of PIP joint

FIGURE 6.4 Swan-neck deformity in a hand with rheumatoid arthritis.

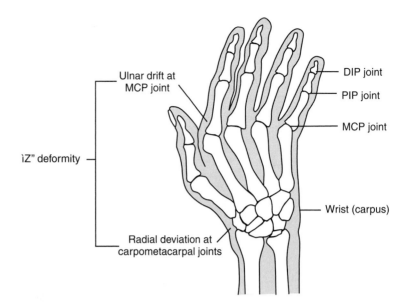

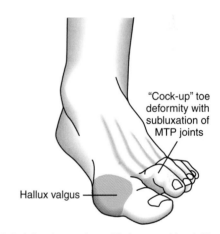

FIGURE 6.5 Ulnar drift in a hand with rheumatoid arthritis (Z deformity).

is little bone to attach the parts of the prosthesis.[14] Another complication of the wrist replacement surgery is loosening of the prosthesis.[15]

Carpal tunnel syndrome is common in RA. Inflammation of tendons and tendon sheaths at the wrist, and swelling within the carpal tunnel causes pressure on the median nerve. The most observable sign is usually atrophy of the muscles of the thenar eminence in the hand, which is associated with lack of sensation on the palmar surface of the thumb, index, and middle fingers and the radial half of the ring finger. The lack of sensation coincides with the dermatome distribution of the median nerve. Depending on the severity of the nerve compression, the individual will have reduced function of the thumb because the ability to oppose the thumb is affected.

Changes in the rheumatoid foot occur mainly at the level of the midfoot and forefoot as a result of synovitis and tendonitis of the posterior tibialis tendon, often resulting in loss of the longitudinal arch of the foot.[16] RA in the feet can cause severe subcalcaneal pain. The deformities of the foot in RA include subluxation of the metatarsal heads causing "cock-up" toes. Deviation of the toes toward the fibula and inflammation of the tibiotalar joint with associated reduction of motion contribute to changes of posture and pressure on the calcaneum, which stimulate bursitis around the calcaneum. The change in weight bearing on the metatarsal heads results in calluses and pain on weight bearing.[17] Claw toes, **Hallux valgus** (bunion), **hammer toes,** and mallet toes are also common. The problems are usually bilateral (see Figs. 6-6 and 6-7).

FIGURE 6.6 A foot in a patient with rheumatoid arthritis.

The knees and hips are also affected in RA. The knees in people with RA tend to assume a position of genu valgus (knock-knees) as opposed to the genu varus (bowlegs) exhibited in people with OA (refer to Chapter 5). However, either genu varus or valgus may be seen as well as flexion deformity at the knees[18] (see Fig. 6-8). Symptoms of pain in the hips and knees may be the result of acute synovitis in the joints. Because such soft tissue signs and symptoms are not revealed on radiographs, severe pain is not necessarily correlated with severe bony changes on radiographic findings.

Cervical spine involvement in RA is perhaps the most dangerous aspect of the articular disease process. Although RA affects all of the synovial joints of the cervical spine,

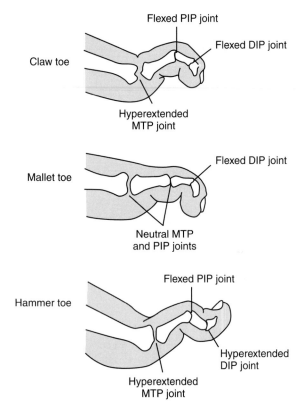

FIGURE 6.7 Toe deformities in RA: claw toe, mallet toe, hammer toe.

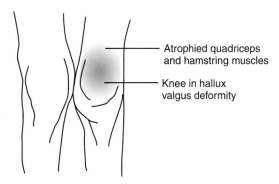

FIGURE 6.8 Rheumatoid knees.

the most commonly affected joint is the atlantoaxial joint. According to Calleja and Hide (2006) approximately 83% of people with RA have an anterior atlantoaxial subluxation only two years after onset of the disease.[19] In addition, the use of corticosteroid medications increases the risk of atlantoaxial joint inflammation and instability. The involvement at the atlantoaxial joint may include synovitis, ligamentous subluxation, and vertebral body fractures as well as osteopenia in the bones.[20] If the ligaments of the

cervical spine are affected by the disease process, an increased risk of the odontoid process of the axis vertebra becoming detached may exist, which can lead to compression of the spinal cord. In severe cases, this can result in quadriparesis (altered sensation in all four limbs), quadriplegia or tetraplegia (weakness in all four limbs), and even death. In less severe cases, pressure on the cervical nerves can result in headaches and radicular pain in the dermatome (area of skin supplied by a spinal nerve) or myotome (muscle supplied by a spinal nerve) distribution of the spinal nerve involved.[21] Pressure on the blood vessels in the cervical area may result, which can cause transient ischemic attacks (TIA). A TIA causes disruption in the blood supply of the affected blood vessel, which can cause symptoms of ischemia (lack of blood) to the area supplied by the particular blood vessel. TIAs may cause changes in blood pressure. Cervical spine involvement may also cause vertebral artery insufficiency, also known as vertebral basilar insufficiency. Vertebral artery insufficiency is caused by restriction of blood flow in the vertebral and basilar arteries in the posterior aspect of the skull and upper cervical spine. The reduced blood flow may result in insufficient blood flow to the posterior aspect of the brain and onset of symptoms, such as ataxia, dizziness, motor and sensory changes, vertigo, and visual deficits.[22,23]

Nonarticular (Nonjoint) Pathological Changes
The nonarticular (nonjoint) signs and symptoms of RA include severe fatigue, which may be related to anemia, anorexia, **Felty's syndrome,** or weight loss.[24] Fatigue is a symptom of RA that cannot always be easily explained. Approximately 30% to 70% of people with RA have anemia of chronic disease.[25] This type of anemia is thought to be caused by the release of cytokines as a result of the inflammatory process that decreases the production of red blood cells by the bone marrow.[26] Other causes of anemia in people with RA may include iron deficiency as a result of poor nutrition or the loss of blood caused by intestinal bleeding resulting from taking large quantities of nonsteroidal anti-inflammatory medications (NSAIDS).[27]

Felty's syndrome is a serious side effect of RA and usually occurs in people with severe or long-standing RA. Felty's syndrome causes splenomegaly (enlargement of the spleen), liver enlargement in some cases, swollen lymph nodes, and leukopenia (reduction of white cell count).[28] People with Felty's syndrome are prone to infections, vasculitis, and skin lesions, and the syndrome may be the cause of death in individuals with severe RA.[29] Skin nodules affect approximately 20% to 25% of people with RA. Skin nodules are usually associated with seropositive

RA and can indicate a more severe disease process.[30,31] Rheumatoid skin nodules are mainly found on the forearms, scapulae, sacrum, ischial tuberosities, and Achilles tendons (see Fig. 6-9). The nodules consist of fibrous necrotic tissue and chronic inflammatory cells. These nodules are usually painless but may become problematic if they open and become infected. Nodules of a similar nature develop in the heart and lungs. In the heart, the nodules may cause problems with the heart valves. In the lungs, the nodules can lead to coughing and dyspnea.

Eye problems in people with RA include scleritis and nodule formation within the sclera, which can lead to reduced vision and blindness in severe cases. In some severe cases of scleritis, glaucoma may develop as a result of corneal inflammation.[32] Cataracts are also fairly common, and the formation may be exacerbated by the use of corticosteroid medications to control the RA disease process.[33] **Sjögren's syndrome** is another side effect of RA that includes symptoms of dry eyes and photophobia (sensitivity to light).[34] Pulmonary complications are some of the more common nonarticular complications in people with RA.[35] The types of lung pathologies seen in individuals with RA include pleural effusion and lung nodules, interstitial lung disease, bronchiolitis, bronchiectasis, and respiratory infections.[36] Osteoporosis is also a common finding in RA largely due to steroid medications but also due to the disease process itself. Osteoporosis is seen mainly in the ends of the bones involved in the RA-affected joints. Vasculitis (inflammation of the blood vessels) is common in those with seropositive RA and may lead to skin ulcers, gangrene, or "glove" or "stocking" neuropathies due to loss of blood supply to the peripheral nerves.[37] **Raynaud's phenomenon** is also often seen in people with RA. Raynaud's phenomenon is a vasospasm (closing down of the superficial blood vessels) of the hands in which the skin becomes white or blue in response to cold or emotion, and then turns red and painful when the circulation returns to the fingers.[38] Amyloidosis, a progressive metabolic disease in which amyloid protein deposits accumulate in internal organs, occurs in rare cases of RA.[39] The protein crystals deposited in the heart, kidneys, and other internal organs as a result of this complication can cause severe malfunction of these organs and even death.[40]

Prognosis. When diagnosis and treatment are provided in the early onset of the condition, the signs and symptoms of RA can be better controlled. Some people with RA have a severe disease process that causes considerable joint deformity and reduced mobility. The nonarticular signs and symptoms of RA such as lung and heart disease can cause complications that result in early mortality.

Medical Intervention. The first step in medical intervention for RA is determining the diagnosis. The American Rheumatism Association developed revised criteria for the diagnosis of RA in 1987 with an update in 2003.[41] An earlier set of criteria were developed by the same association in 1958 and Bennett and Burch also developed criteria in 1967 known as the New York criteria. The American Rheumatism Association criteria include morning stiffness of 1 hour or more duration, symmetrical arthritis of at least three joints associated with soft tissue swelling of more than six weeks' duration, arthritis of hands, rheumatoid skin nodules, and positive results on tests for rheumatoid factor. For a person to be diagnosed with RA, at least four of the separate criteria must be met.[42]

"It Happened in the Clinic"

A man in his 50s was referred for physical therapy. His diagnosis was rheumatoid arthritis (RA). The PT examination revealed weakness in bilateral upper extremities and lower extremities. Of particular note was the 2/5 manual muscle test (MMT) for shoulder abduction bilaterally. Functionally, the patient was able to ambulate up to 1 mile and climb stairs without difficulty. Upper-extremity function was limited resulting from reduced range of motion bilaterally, 120° elevation through flexion on the left, and 115° on the right. Observation of the patient without a shirt, from both posterior and anterior views, identified that the contour of both shoulders was altered. Closer examination revealed that bilateral deltoid muscles were completely atrophied with a flattened area where the rounded shape of the deltoid muscle

(Continued)

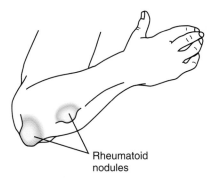

Rheumatoid nodules

FIGURE 6.9 Rheumatoid nodule in the forearm.

should have been. After referral back to the physician, an electromyogram test revealed the nerve supply (Axillary Nerve, C5, 6) was damaged, and thus the muscle was no longer innervated. The physician determined that the RA disease process was the cause of the nerve damage and that it was irreversible.

Radiological Testing. Radiographs show joint abnormalities including reduced joint space and bony changes in people with RA (see Fig. 6-10). They may also show a slightly dense area when profuse soft tissue swelling is present. Osteoporosis may also be evident on radiographs with the areas of least bone density observed at the bone ends located close to the joints affected with RA. Radiographs of the cervical spine are taken to determine whether a subluxation of the atlantoaxial joint exists. People with RA are susceptible to atlantoaxial subluxation, which is a life-threatening condition.

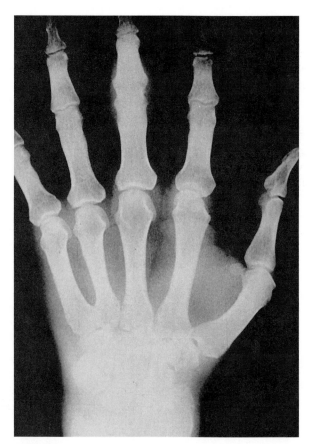

FIGURE 6.10 X-ray showing severe RA of hand. (From Koopman, W.J. (1997). *Arthritis and Allied Conditions. A Textbook of Rheumatology,* 13th edition, Vol. 1, p. 883, fig. 44.12A. Used with permission.)

Laboratory Testing. Laboratory tests are performed to verify the diagnosis of RA and also to monitor the progression of the disease. Rheumatoid factor (RF) is an antibody present in approximately 80% of people with RA. The RF antibody combines with IgG to form an immune complex, which creates an inflammatory process within the tissues of the body. [43] High levels of RF in people with RA seem to be associated with severe forms of RA and the development of nonarticular symptoms, such as rheumatoid nodules and lung disease.[44] Rheumatoid factor is also found in the blood of individuals with certain infective conditions such as infectious mononucleosis, hepatitis, and tuberculosis, and in people with the connective tissue disease systemic lupus erythematosus.[45] Elevated erythrocyte sedimentation rates (ESR) are also noted in people with RA as a result of the inflammatory process. As noted earlier, individuals with RA may develop anemia of chronic disease, or iron-deficient anemia may be present from the loss of blood into the intestines caused by the use of NSAIDS. Regular blood and urine tests are performed on individuals who take NSAIDS to make sure they are not developing anemia.

Surgical Intervention. People with RA have varying levels of disability and loss of function. Deformity of the joints is not sufficient for performing surgery. The most common reasons for doing surgery are to reduce severe pain and to improve function. Because the peripheral joints are the ones most commonly involved in RA, these joints are the candidates for arthroplasty. In some cases of severe functional loss in the hands, a Silastic prosthesis total joint replacement is performed for joints of the fingers. The PIP arthroplasties may be a hinged type such as the Swanson Silastic replacement and the Neuflex Silastic replacement, or have two separate components—for example, the pyrolytic carbon MCP replacement by Ascension.[46,47] Silicone joint replacements for the MCP joints have been performed since the early 1960s with good long-term results.[48] Details of surgical procedures for the hand are beyond the scope of this book. For interested readers, Koopman's *Arthritis and Allied Conditions* provides the details of specific surgical procedures. Other types of surgeries performed include tendon repairs, as well as **osteotomies** in which deformities are reduced by removal of a section of bone. Osteotomies are most commonly performed at the knee with removal of a section of the tibia. An arthrodesis may be performed to permanently fix an extensively damaged joint in a functional position. This procedure is used most often in the spine and the ankle, usually relieving pain. In many cases, the synovium becomes inflamed causing severe joint pain and edema. In such cases, a synovectomy may be performed to remove the synovium. Total joint arthroplasty is performed on the shoulder and elbow in severe cases. In OA, hip and knee arthroplasty is performed when necessary to improve function and to reduce pain.

In cases of joint deformities of the hand, when conservative methods of intervention fail to improve function, surgery is the final option to restore function. Surgery is performed only if the function of the hands is reduced to the point of disability. Many people with RA may have deformed hands that remain functional. The decision to perform surgery must be carefully weighed because the surgery may not be successful, resulting in less function than before surgery. Recent advances in finger joint arthroplasty have increased the chance for good functional outcomes.

Pharmacology. Pharmacological therapy is essential in the treatment of RA to attempt to control the inflammatory process and to prevent severe complications and deformities that lead to loss of function and disability. Individuals may require different types of medications at various stages of the disease process. People may become sensitized to certain medications, resulting in a decreased ability to control symptoms. In some cases, people accommodate to a medication resulting in less effective control of symptoms. Physicians may have a difficult time finding an appropriate level of long-term drug therapy for patients. Several classifications of medications are used to treat RA, each having its own mode of action on the inflammatory process. The classification of the medications used to treat RA and some of the brand names are provided here to familiarize the PTA with the general concept that a variety of medications are needed to treat symptoms of RA. Salicylates (aspirin) or NSAIDs such as Celebrex and Cox-2 inhibitors are frequently used as the medications of choice for the person with RA. Disease-modifying antirheumatic medications (DMARDs) include a wide variety of medications that work in different ways to reduce inflammation. Medications classified as DMARDs include cyclosporine, gold salts, hydroxychloroquine, penicillamine, and sulfasalazine. Corticosteroids such as prednisolone, prednisone, betamethasone, cortisone, dexamethasone, and triamcinolone all suppress the immune response to control inflammation and also may be used to treat RA. More recent pharmacological agents have been developed classified as "biologic drugs." This new classification of medications includes abatacept (Orencia), etanercept (Enbrel), adalimumab (Humira), and anakinra (Kineret).[49] In many instances, people with RA may require a combination of several medications for effective management of the disease.[50]

The possible side effects of any of these medications may include damage to the liver, kidneys, skin, intestines, and heart (see Table 6-2).[51] Close monitoring of blood chemistry is required when a person is placed on many of these drug regimens. Intra-articular injections are frequently used for RA joints that are very symptomatic. Steroid injections are performed into the joint and sometimes give pain relief for many months. Most physicians do not inject any one joint more than four or five times because the steroid can cause joint damage if concentrations are too high.

Splinting. The preservation of joint integrity is essential for function. Splinting of joints is used to prevent, or minimize, joint deformity and to protect the involved joint in people with RA. Splints may be dynamic or passive and worn during the day or at night. A simple resting splint to keep the knee in extension at night to prevent flexion deformity may be required (see Fig. 6-11). Splints can be custom made by an orthotist or can be made in the PT or OT department. In some cases, an off-the-shelf knee-immobilizing splint may be used. Splints must be well padded to prevent skin abrasions, because people with RA have sensitive skin that is prone to breakdown.

Finger splints to correct swan-neck and Boutonnière's deformities may be worn to improve function of the hand. Simple "ring" type splints may be used to keep either the PIP or the DIP joints in a functional position (see Fig. 6-12). Ring splints are now made in a variety of materials including silver so that they look like jewelry.[52] Several types of wrist splints may be used. A thumb spica splint may be necessary at night to protect the thumb and keep the thumb in a functional slightly abducted position. A general "cock-up" splint for the wrist, that keeps the wrist in a functional extended position may help during daily activities (see Fig. 6-13). Splints often need to be modified to assist the person with RA.

Physical Therapy Intervention. Physical therapy evaluation and intervention for clients with RA requires a full systems approach. PT management is directed toward improvement in functional activity, minimization of joint deformity and joint preservation, increasing joint ROM, reduction of pain, strengthening of muscles, client education, and adaptations to activities of daily living (ADLs) necessary to promote independence.[53,54] When using the

Table 6.2 **Some Medications Used to Treat Rheumatoid Arthritis With Effects and Side Effects**

MEDICATION/MEDICATION CLASSIFICATION	EFFECTS OF MEDICATION	POSSIBLE ADVERSE SIDE EFFECTS
Aspirin (salicylic acid)	Anti-inflammatory Analgesic Reduces fever Reduces clotting thus increasing bleeding time	GI: nausea, heartburn, indigestion, ulceration Central nervous system: vertigo, hearing problems, dizziness (reversible) Liver toxicity (rare) Kidney damage (variable)
Acetaminophen	Analgesic Reduces fever	Liver toxicity in large amounts (rare)
NSAIDs (e.g., Celebrex, Cox-2 inhibitors)	Anti-inflammatory Analgesic Reduce the production of prostaglandins and reduce inflammation	GI irritation CNS: dizziness, headaches Liver toxicity Renal toxicity
Corticosteroids (e.g., prednisone, prednisolone, betamethasone, cortisone, dexamethasone, triamcinolone)	Anti-inflammatory Immunosuppressive	GI: nausea, stomach ulcers, weight gain CNS: vertigo, headaches, neuritis Dermatological: thin skin, edema, poor healing Musculoskeletal: muscle weakness, osteoporosis Cardiac: hypertension, atherosclerosis Endocrine: Cushing's syndrome Ophthalmic: glaucoma, cataracts
DMARDs (also called SAARDs; e.g., azathioprine, cyclosporine, gold salts, hydroxychloroquine, methotrexate, penicillamine, sulfasalazine)	Anti-inflammatory Immunosuppressive	<u>General</u> GI: nausea, vomiting, diarrhea CNS: headaches, depression, fatigue, peripheral neuritis, neuropathy, myopathy Ophthalmic: retinopathy with night blindness, blurred vision <u>Gold Salts</u> GI: diarrhea, nausea Dermatological: sensitivity to sun Liver toxicity Renal toxicity Bone marrow damage <u>Penicillamine</u> GI: diarrhea, nausea, vomiting, pain Hematological: thrombocytopenia, leukopenia Skin: rash, mouth ulcers Renal: proteinuria <u>Sulfasalazine</u> Hematological: neutropenia, thrombocytopenia, hemolysis

CNS = central nervous system; GI = Gastrointestinal; NSAID = nonsteroidal anti-inflammatory drug; SAARD = slow-acting antirheumatic drugs.

Guide to Physical Therapist Practice, note that the preferred practice pattern used depend on the level of involvement of the individual patient. Some people will fall completely within the musculoskeletal practice patterns, whereas others may have additional problems that fall within the realm of the neuromuscular practice patterns. Still others may have some areas that need to be addressed within the integumentary practice patterns. The complexity of symptoms for the people with RA and JRA cross many areas of expertise for the PT and PTA. When possible, the physical therapy interventions should begin soon after diagnosis of RA.[55] A team approach for intervention is most beneficial for people with RA involving the services of the occupational therapist, nutritionist, and social worker as well as the PT and PTA.[56] When working with clients with RA, the evaluation must be comprehensive. A more

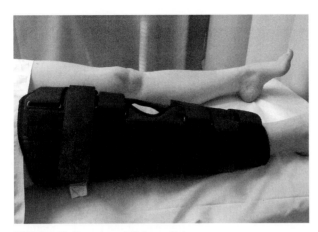

FIGURE 6.11 Knee immobilizing splint.

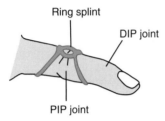

Ring splint

DIP joint

PIP joint

FIGURE 6.12 "Ring" splint for swan-neck and Boutonnière's deformity.

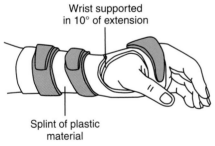

Wrist supported
in 10° of extension

Splint of plastic
material

FIGURE 6.13 Modified "cock-up" splint for rheumatoid arthritis.

holistic approach is required than with many other patients. Approach to the treatment of people with RA is a team concept that includes the physician, physical therapist, occupational therapist, social worker, psychiatrist, nutritionist, and possibly the recreational therapist. The PTA must be aware of the total body involvement of the condition and not focus on one specific problem to the detriment of other areas. Because the person with RA has multiple joint and internal organ involvement, treating one area of the body may cause an adverse effect on another area and result in serious side effects. The PT and PTA need to listen carefully to everything the client relates to them and adapt the treatment as necessary. Endurance and tolerance to treatment and activities are likely to be

dramatically reduced in people with RA as a result of the systemic nature of the disease.

Gait patterns and assistive devices require particular attention (see Fig. 6-14). When in an acute exacerbation, patients may require a wheelchair. Because severe weakness may be an issue, a power chair may be necessary. The choice of assistive device(s) depends on the functional level of the individual. Lofstrand (elbow) crutches are helpful if more stability is required. The adult with severe RA may require a walker. A wheeled walker reduces the amount of lifting required, and a wheeled walker with forearm supports may be necessary for patients with hand involvement, poor grip, and minimal strength. Wheeled walkers with a built-in seat can be helpful to allow the person to rest as necessary. Special canes with a molding to the contours of the hand are available for patients unable to grip a regular cane (see Fig. 6-15). Other canes have a wide grip, which facilitates use. If funding is an issue, foam tubing may be placed over the handle of a curved handle straight cane to facilitate the grip. All handle adaptations help to reduce additional stress on the already deformed joints of the hand and wrist and preserve joint integrity.

GERIATRIC CONSIDERATIONS

Many patients diagnosed with rheumatoid arthritis (RA) are on steroidal anti-inflammatory medications. Prolonged usage of the medication as well as the aging process increases the risk of the skin becoming delicate and susceptible to damage. Extreme care should be taken to avoid damage to the skin. A slight abrasion can become an open wound. Suggestions for protection of the skin are as follows:

- Encourage patients to wear long pants to cushion the shin area from damage. An occupational therapist in England made "protective splints" out of a soft splinting material for patients with RA to wear around the lower leg to protect the shins. These fastened with Velcro and were easily removable and highly effective in protecting the shins from damage.
- Ensure the patient does not have sharp-edged corners in the home on coffee tables or other obstacles that might cause injury to the legs.
- If a walker is required, patients may bump their legs on the walker. A wheeled walker may help to reduce the risk of injury.
- When using electrical stimulation modalities do not use tape to attach the electrodes. Use soft straps to apply the electrodes.

Hydrotherapy. Hydrotherapy is a wonderful medium for people with RA. Recommendations for hydrotherapy range from a series of six sessions to daily use within the home for some people.[57] The water should be at approximately body temperature or slightly higher, between 98° and 100° Fahrenheit, although some people use a temperature of 85° to 95°.[58] Cold water may cause cramping and discomfort for people with RA and is not recommended, although some people with RA may benefit from ice baths. Patients should be warned to limit exercise in the water when first starting a program. Movement is likely to feel easier in the water as a result of the effect of buoyancy leading to overexertion without the person realizing. The PT and PTA need to ensure that the client increases the amount of exercise and time in the water gradually. A good initial trial in the pool is between 10 and 15 minutes working gently to determine the person's reaction to the treatment. The exercise program should be increased gradually ensuring good body mechanics and correct exercise technique. Patients should be encouraged to rest after pool therapy. Pool therapy is contraindicated in an acute exacerbation of RA when the joints are acutely inflamed. Gait reeducation may be started in the water, and both stretching and strengthening exercises performed using the properties of buoyancy and resistance of the water. PTs and PTAs should refer to an aquatic exercise book for further details of pool therapy.

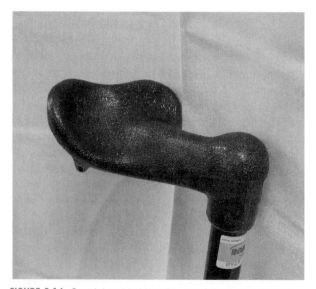

FIGURE 6.14 Special molded handle cane for use with persons with reduced grip.

Passive Stretching. Passive stretching for people with RA needs to be approached with caution. Gentle passive stretching for muscles may be beneficial, but the PT should examine clients for any contraindications and consult with the physician regarding this treatment. Passive stretching of joints is best performed through gentle, restricted exercise, positioning, and splinting. Resting splints to maintain good joint position are an integral part of the treatment approach. Reducing the risk of joint deformity in patients with RA is essential. The patient and caregiver should be given clear instructions regarding positioning at night and during rest periods. Pillows should not be used beneath the knees because this encourages flexion deformities. A large part of the PT/PTA treatment will be spent teaching positioning techniques to reduce the risk of joint deformity. Any forced joint maneuvers are contraindicated in RA. The disease process results in the loss of integrity of ligaments and joint capsule and increased susceptibility to rupture, thus cervical traction, or cervical mobilization techniques are *contraindicated for patients with later stage RA* because of the possibility of cervical instability. In the early stages of the disease process extreme caution should be used in the application of cervical traction or mobilization techniques. In some cases, serial casting may be necessary to assist with joint stretching in the lower limbs. Serial casting requires a cast or splint to be applied with some stretch placed on the joint and then reapplied with a slightly more stretching angle after one to two weeks. In this way, a joint can be stretched gradually. In the knee joint, the splint may be applied at an angle of 20° of flexion and then later at 15° until progressive stretching and splinting reduces the flexion deformity to zero or a functionally acceptable position. Care must be taken to avoid pressure on the skin during serial casting by providing adequate padding within the cast. Such splinting techniques should ideally be performed by a person experienced in the application of splints for this patient population. Health care providers fabricating serial casts include orthotists, physical therapists, occupational therapists, and orthopedic nurses.

Active Exercise. Active exercise is an essential part of the physical therapy program for patients with RA. Innovative approaches by the PT and PTA are often needed to enable these people to be able to perform their exercises. Exercise programs should be developed concentrating on strengthening the weak muscle groups, improving cardiovascular conditioning, and assisting patients to achieve a maximal functional level. This often involves a program that addresses multiple systems because of the extensive nature of the condition. All exercises should be performed within client tolerance and without exacerbating pain levels or producing excessive fatigue, because ligaments are vulnerable to damage. Gentle and progressive knee exercises should emphasize quadriceps activity in a closed chain and open chain manner without the use of excessive weights. Hip mobility exercises and upper extremity ROM and strengthening are usually required. Wand exercises are helpful for the upper extremities. Exercises that appear easy for people with orthopedic diagnoses may be extremely difficult for patients with RA. Home instructions should be practical and the number of exercises kept within a manageable level. People with RA tend to have a low exercise tolerance as a result of general body symptoms. The emphasis should be placed on the quality of performance of the exercises rather than on the quantity. Often a few specific exercises concentrated on the most problematic areas will meet client needs. Patients should be warned to discontinue the exercises if they experience increased pain or unexpected side effects. Exercises also need to be discontinued if the RA symptoms exacerbate.

Electrical Modalities and Thermal Agents. The use of electrical modalities such as neuromuscular electrical stimulation may be combined with active exercises to help build muscle mass and strength.[59] Neuromuscular electrical stimulation is contraindicated in the acute stage of the disease process. The use of interferential therapy may be helpful for the relief of pain and can be used during acute exacerbation phases of the disease. When using interferential therapy, the suction cup electrodes must be avoided because they may damage the fragile skin of many people with RA. Ultrasound can be helpful for the reduction of pain and edema and to assist with increasing joint mobility during the nonacute stage of the disease process. Recent studies on rats confirm that the use of transcutaneous electrical nerve stimulations (TENS) may prove useful for the treatment of painfully inflamed joints in either the acute or chronic stages.[60] Thermal (hot and cold) modalities have been used for many years for the symptomatic relief of pain and inflammation. Recent innovations such as laser-light therapy (LLT) continue to be evaluated for effectiveness. Both the use of electrical and thermal agents continue to be studied to provide evidence of the effectiveness of the interventions.[61]

Orthotics. Other considerations for treatment of people with rheumatoid arthritis include the use of various orthotics, such as a firm cervical collar to address instability of the cervical spine. Some patients with severe instability of the cervical spine may have to wear a rigid collar at all times including when sleeping. Other people with cervical symptoms may be helped with a soft collar to assist in relaxing the cervical muscles. The decision to utilize supports is at the discretion of the physician and the PT. The PTA should be aware of cervical manifestations in patients and report any change in symptoms to the supervising PT immediately. Shoe orthotics may be helpful in relieving foot pain in some clients. Frequently a custom-fitted shoe with increased toe depth will alleviate foot discomfort. An apparent, or an actual, leg length discrepancy may be caused by a scoliosis, or a fixed flexion deformity of the hip or knee. Leg length discrepancies may be addressed by inserting a heel lift into the shoe or fitting clients with an elevated shoe. Prone-lying may assist with reducing the risk of or addressing hip flexion contractures.

Pain Reduction. Analgesics and anti-inflammatory medications may reduce the pain associated with RA. Physical therapy intervention can help reduce pain with the use of modalities in the nonactive phases of the disease. People with RA usually respond well to warmth. Many patients with RA have Raynaud's phenomenon and react adversely to extremes of temperature, especially cold. Skin sensitivity in these people requires extra precautions when applying heat. The skin tends to become red and blistered quickly, so the clinician must check the skin regularly during treatment and caution the patient about the risk of a burn. Home programs may include use of heat modalities, but again the patient must be cautioned regarding the risk of burns. The goal of PT is to return the person to maximal functional level to provide as much independence as possible through provision of a home program that will help the patient to maintain independence. In today's managed care environment, clinicians may not be able to treat patients long-term. More beneficial effects may be obtained by seeing individuals once a week for several weeks to progress and monitor their home program of exercises and activities. Caregivers, teachers, and parents also need to be educated about treatment and management.

Psychosocial Aspects. The psychological aspects of RA can be detrimental to patients. Occasionally, people with RA exhibit euphoria, a false sense of elation. As with many conditions associated with chronic pain, people with RA may have difficulty accepting their limitations and dealing with chronic pain and become depressed and even suicidal. If the PT or PTA suspects any of these symptoms, the physician and social worker should be contacted immediately.

Nutrition. Nutritional concerns stem from many factors for people with RA. A side effect of some of the medications for RA is loss of appetite, and therefore reduced nutritional status, and even malnutrition, may be an issue. Weight loss has been linked to the production of cytokines in people with RA as a result of the chronic inflammation, and folic acid deficiency is linked with the use of methotrexate.[62] The gastric side effects of some medications used to treat RA may also cause appetite suppression. In many cases, individuals with RA may be unable to prepare meals and shop for food. All of these factors increase the risk of nutritional deficits in people with RA.[63] Steroid medications also cause retention of fluid, which can lead to obesity. People with RA may require nutritional supplements.

PRECAUTIONS, CONTRAINDICATIONS, AND SPECIAL CONSIDERATIONS FOR PT INTERVENTION FOR PATIENTS WITH RA

1. No cervical traction for RA in the later stages; may use with caution in the early phase.
2. No spinal flexion exercises in the presence of osteoporosis.
3. No forced stretching of RA joints.
4. No mobilization/manipulation of rheumatoid joints.
5. No use of pillows or rolls beneath the knees during treatment or when resting at home (unless true fixed flexion deformity prevents full extension).
6. Care when using heat to prevent burning the patient; the skin is very sensitive. Use extra towels and padding when using moist heat packs in the clinic and adequately instruct patients regarding home hot pack use.
7. When using electrodes for electrical stimulation, do not use tape or suction cups that could easily damage sensitive skin. Always use flexible straps to keep electrodes in place and make sure the straps are not too tight.
8. Caution patients to stop exercises if pain increases or unusual symptoms develop.
9. Instruct patients to check the safety of ambulatory assistive devices. Patients often keep these pieces of equipment for many years. Suggest regular replacement of rubber cane/walker tips. Check bolts on walkers.
10. Skin care
    - Skin is delicate from both medications and the RA disease process itself. Warn patients to be extra careful to avoid walking into objects. Recommend wearing pants to provide some degree of protection for the legs. Take extra care when using a wheelchair to prevent hitting the legs with the foot rests.
    - Do not wear any type of jewelry that could scratch the patient and cause a wound.
    - Warn patients to avoid wearing jewelry that could scratch their skin and cause a wound.
    - Keep fingernails manicured and short to prevent scratching the patient and causing a wound.
    - Educate patients how to use a mirror on a long handle to inspect skin that they are unable to see, such as on the back of their legs or under their feet.
11. Refer the patient to occupational therapy for adaptive equipment to use in the bathroom, kitchen, and so on. If unavailable, refer patients to a catalog with samples of adaptations. Make certain patients are safe in the bathroom with the use of a tub transfer seat if needed. Suggest reasonable ways of adapting eating utensils with foam tubing that will fit over existing cutlery.
12. Suggest patients sit in a firm, elevated chair to facilitate rising from sitting.
13. Remember that patients with RA will fatigue easily, and you may need to adapt their treatment protocols accordingly.

Why Does the Physical Therapist Assistant Need to Know About Juvenile Rheumatoid Arthritis and Still's Disease?

Children with juvenile rheumatoid arthritis and Still's disease are seen in a variety of physical therapy practice settings. In the school system, children may need adaptations and interventions to enable them to participate in the education process. These children may also be seen by PTAs in private practice, acute care hospital, and rehabilitation settings. The systemic nature of these diseases means that children are often debilitated and easily fatigued. Physical therapy interventions must be adapted to suit the specific needs of these children according to the signs and symptoms of their disease process.

Juvenile Rheumatoid Arthritis and Still's Disease

Juvenile rheumatoid arthritis (JRA) is otherwise known as juvenile chronic arthritis (JCA), juvenile idiopathic arthritis, or Still's disease. Still's disease was named for George Frederick Still, who identified systemic manifestations in association with joint problems in children in 1897. Still's disease is usually the term used for JRA with systemic manifestations and accounts for approximately 10% to 20% of all cases of JRA.[64] A type of adult-onset systemic arthritis, not discussed here, is also classified as Still's disease and has similar signs and symptoms to those of the juvenile form. The incidence of JRA in the United States is approximately 50 to 100 per 100,000 children, and the disease is thought to affect between 25,000 and 50,000 children.[65,66]

Etiology. The etiology of JRA and Still's disease is unknown. The disease is thought to be autoimmune, similar to that of RA. In some cases, the disease is considered to be precipitated by infection.

Signs and Symptoms. The onset of juvenile forms of RA is usually more acute in nature than the adult type. Although JRA follows the pattern of adult RA, in many ways it is also different as a result of growth factors in the child. JRA is identified in children aged under 16 years.[67,68] JRA is a connective tissue, autoimmune disorder affecting multiple areas of the body and is usually seronegative for rheumatoid factor (RF). One main difference from adult RA is that JRA tends to affect the larger peripheral joints such as the knees and hips, rather than the smaller joints of the hands and feet, although the wrists are often affected in Still's disease.[69] A general classification of arthritis in children is recognized for those having symptoms that last from 6 weeks to 6 months or more. Several subcategories of JRA have been identified, including pauciarticular (affecting four or less joints), polyarticular (affecting five or more joints), and systemic (affecting multiple body systems) with a persistent fever 39° Centigrade or higher for more than 2 weeks.[70] The characteristic signs and symptoms of JRA include pain and stiffness in the affected joints with joint contractures present in severe cases. Bone growth retardation may occur, particularly in the long bones and the mandible, systemic symptoms such as a skin rash may appear, and heart pathologies such as pericarditis are often evident. (See Table 6-3 for a comparison of the characteristics of JRA and Still's disease.) Children with JRA experience fatigue and loss of aerobic capacity conditioning, with muscle spasms, atrophy, and osteoporosis caused by both the disease process and the medications used to treat the disease. As a general rule, children with systemic symptoms of JRA have a rapid progression of the disease process. Children with systemic symptoms also have a worse prognosis than those without any systemic symptoms. In addition to the previously mentioned signs and symptoms, children with Still's disease have a fluctuating high fever, arthritis in several joints, a skin rash, enlargement of the spleen and liver, a sore throat, swollen lymph glands, and may have lung and

Table 6.3 **Characteristics of Still's Disease and Juvenile Rheumatoid Arthritis (JRA)**

CHARACTERISTICS OF STILL'S DISEASE	CHARACTERISTICS OF JRA
Systemic inflammatory disease affecting body organs and multiple joints	Chronic and inflammatory disease of joints
Etiology: unknown	Etiology: unknown
Fever of 39°C or more lasting more than 2 weeks	Pauciarticular: involves four or fewer joints
Skin rash on body and limbs	Polyarticular: involves five or more joints
Pericarditis/hepatitis	Symptoms last from 6 weeks to ≥6 months
Anemia	Growth retardation of bones
Growth retardation of bones	

heart problems such as pericarditis, pleuritis, and pleural effusion.[71]

Prognosis. The more joints that are involved in the disease process, the more severe the problems experienced and the greater the likelihood of joint problems persisting into adulthood. However, approximately 75% of all children with JRA have a remission of the disease by the time they are adolescent with minimal loss of function.[72] The remaining 25% of children will continue to have arthritis associated disease throughout their adult life. Children who have Still's disease may also have lasting damage to the heart and lungs. Many children with JRA have joint damage and problems with joint mobility that affect their functional abilities. Joint replacement surgery is usually an option only after the child has stopped growing.

Medical Intervention. The medications prescribed for JRA are similar to those used for RA. NSAIDs are used whenever possible to avoid the long-term side effects of steroidal anti-inflammatory medications. Celebrex was approved for the treatment of nonsystemic JRA in 2006 by the U.S. Food and Drug Administration.[73] The medications required for the treatment of the systemic symptoms of Still's disease may include the use of corticosteroids and some of the DMARDs described under the section on RA. Steroid medications may make children hungry, causing them to overeat. However, in other cases, children with JRA fail to grow. In all cases, both children and adults may require nutritional supplements. Frequently the intervention of an orthotist is necessary to provide a custom-fitted shoe with increased toe depth which will alleviate foot discomfort. Footwear for children with JRA is particularly important to provide sufficient room for growth and reduce the risk of foot deformities. Children with JRA often become depressed because they cannot participate fully in school activities and are often in pain. The disease may affect children's appearance, creating joint deformities that make them self-conscious. A financial burden often exists for people with JRA and their families as a result of the high cost of medications and therapeutic interventions. Expensive adaptations may be necessary to the home to accommodate wheelchairs and other assistive devices. The involvement of a social worker is usually essential for these patients to coordinate the support services needed to enhance functional independence.

Physical Therapy Intervention. The PTA should remember that the family members must be an integral part of the treatment program for children with JRA. Treatment is directed toward reduction of pain, with control and reduction of the development of contractures and the preservation and promotion of functional activity. As in adults, splinting to prevent joint deformities is important. Children often do not understand why physical therapy treatment is uncomfortable, therefore the cooperation and understanding of the family is essential to treat the child effectively. As with RA, active joint pathology with acute inflammation is a contraindication for any exercise, mobilizing technique, or electrical modality. Children with JRA have varying degrees of joint pathology with exacerbations that require considerable time off school. Teachers and other school personnel must be aware of the child's limitations and medical condition. Children may have mornings when they are so stiff that they require several hours to prepare for school, or they may not be able to go to school at all. Educating other children in the class about JRA is also important. Physical education (PE) activities will most likely be limited, and the PE teacher may need to develop innovative ways to include the child in the regular classroom setting. The PT/PTA may be able to assist with developing techniques within the classroom to enable participation by the child as fully as possible.

Exercise programs should include group work in physical therapy programs and inclusion in physical education programs wherever possible. Active exercise is an essential part of the physical therapy program for patients with JRA. Passive stretching for children with JRA needs to be approached with caution. As with adults with RA, gentle passive stretching for muscles may be beneficial, but the PT should examine clients for any contraindications and consult with the physician regarding this treatment. Positioning of joints while at rest and the use of resting splints to maintain good joint position is essential. Reducing the risk of joint deformity in children with JRA is important to ensure growing bones and joints are protected. Recent studies suggest that children with JRA demonstrate increased aerobic function with any exercise program and that the program does not need to be intensive and difficult for the child.[74] Because severe weakness may be an issue with children with JRA, a power chair may be necessary. Children with JRA may require a power chair for use at school to enable them to function and to participate in the education setting. A light-weight sports wheelchair may be a good alternative for some children. Children with RA may have days when they do not need the power chair if they can ambulate for some part of the day. The understanding of the teacher is essential to enable children with RA to adapt to individual situations. Assistive ambulatory devices such as walkers, canes, or Lofstrand (elbow) crutches may be needed. Lofstrand crutches are often more acceptable to a child than a walker, because they provide greater mobility. Aquatherapy in a warm pool is a beneficial treatment for children with JRA. Some children with JRA may benefit from ice baths, but caution must be used as some children will react adversely to cold therapy.

Why Does the Physical Therapist Assistant Need to Know About The Rheumatoid-Related Inflammatory Joint Pathologies?

Multiple varieties of rheumatoid and arthritis related conditions exist. This book is not intended to describe all such conditions but only the more commonly known ones. The PT and PTA are frequently faced with people with these conditions during everyday practice. The PT or PTA may encounter patients with these conditions and be asked to treat people with the signs and symptoms of the condition, or the condition may be an added complicating factor to another injury or illness. In either case, the PTA must have knowledge of the pathology of the condition and its potential impact on the proposed PT intervention.

Rheumatoid-Related Inflammatory Joint Pathologies

Rheumatoid-related inflammatory joint pathologies include the seronegative spondyloarthropathies and polyarticular arthropathies, such as ankylosing spondylitis, psoriatic arthritis, and reactive arthritis, also called Reiter's syndrome.

HINTS ON USE OF THE GUIDE TO PHYSICAL THERAPIST PRACTICE

Ankylosing spondylitis is classified in the *Guide to Physical Therapist Practice*, Musculoskeletal Preferred Practice Pattern 4.

- 4E, "Impaired joint mobility, motor function, muscle performance, and range of motion associated with localized inflammation" (p. 197): Patients with ankylosing spondylitis (AS) are classified in this "Musculoskeletal" Practice Pattern because the inflammation is usually around the joints of the spine and the sacroiliac joints. If the AS becomes a more general condition affecting the body organs, then the practice pattern would perhaps be altered according to the evaluation findings of the physical therapist.
- 4H, "Impaired joint mobility, motor function, muscle performance, and range of motion associated with joint arthroplasty" (p. 251): If a patient has had a joint replacement performed, this would become the most appropriate classification.

(From the American Physical Therapy Association, 2003. *Guide to physical therapist practice*, revised 2nd edition. Alexandria, VA: APTA. Used with permission.)

Ankylosing Spondylitis

Ankylosing spondylitis (AS), also called Marie-Strümpell disease, is a progressive, inflammatory, rheumatoid-related disease, affecting the joints and ligaments of the spine and occasionally peripheral joints as well as internal organs.[75,76] AS is classified as one of a group of diseases called seronegative spondyloarthropathies.[77] AS is more common in Caucasians, especially those of northern European descent and has a very high incidence in some Native American populations. The disease is rare in Asian populations, particularly the Japanese, and in the black and African populations.[78] AS is approximately 3 times more common in men than in women and onset occurs mainly between ages 15 and 40

years.[79] The incidence of AS in the general population is approximately between 0.1% and 0.2%.[80] A separate form of AS, known as juvenile ankylosing spondylitis, which falls under the general classification of juvenile spondyloarthropathies, occurs before age 16.[81,82]

Etiology. One theory about the cause of AS is an immunological component based on the high incidence of the presence of the HLA B27 antigen in people with the disease. Recent research has determined the presence of two other genes associated with AS, ARTS1, and IL23R.[83] In families with AS, a higher incidence of the disease exists, suggesting a genetic tendency to develop the disease likely, especially if the associated genes are present in the individual.[84] The presence of the genes associated with AS does not, however, mean that the person will develop the disease, as demonstrated by the fact that approximately 7% of the U.S. population have the genes associated with AS, but only 1% of those with the genes actually develop the disease.[85]

Signs and Symptoms. The characteristic signs and symptoms of AS include **ankylosis** (fusion/stiffening of the joints), which affects mainly the spine and sacroiliac joints but can also involve the shoulders, hips, and knees. The disease is seronegative for rheumatoid factor in the blood. Approximately 90% to 95% of people with AS have a tissue type genetic marker known as human leukocyte antigen (HLA B27), which is also found in certain other inflammatory diseases such as inflammatory bowel disease, psoriatic arthritis, Reiter's syndrome and some inflammatory eye conditions.[86]

Symptomatically, AS often starts with pain and stiffness in the low back as a result of inflammation in the sacroiliac joints and the joints of the lumbar spine. Fatigue is apparent in the early stages of the disease. Sometimes the low back pain is severe and acute, and in other cases, the pain is gradual and more of an ache. Sciatic nerve pain is often noted, with radiation down the posterior aspect of the thigh, which may be accompanied by severe spasm in the lumbar paraspinal muscles. In the early stages of the disease, the symptoms of stiffness and pain are often greater in the early morning and may be alleviated during the day with movement and exercise.

Pathologically, inflammation may affect the synovial joints of the spine or may be in the junction of the ligaments and the bone **(enthesitis)**. The areas affected by enthesitis include the junction of the annulus fibrosus of the intervertebral disk at the margins of the vertebral bodies, the symphysis pubis, and the sternal joints. Occasionally, enthesitis is present in the Achilles tendon junction at the calcaneum and in the feet.[87] All joints of the spine are involved with the ligaments of the spine first becoming fibrosed and then converting to bone causing the typical **"bamboo spine"** effect noted on X-ray films (see Fig. 6-15). The process of ankylosis starts in the lumbar spine and the sacroiliac region as **sacroiliitis** and progresses up the spine to include the costovertebral and manubriosternal joints.[88] After ankylosis occurs, the part of the spine involved becomes fused and immobile, creating mobility problems for the person. The pain is reduced after ankylosis has occurred, but during the active inflammatory phases of the disease the pain can be severe.

Other characteristics of the disease include loss of chest expansion as a result of ankylosis of the costovertebral and manubriosternal joints. Individuals must rely on use of the diaphragm to breathe due to the lack of thoracic mobility, and therefore, the vital capacity is reduced. In later stages of the disease, deformities can include forward flexion of the spine with increased thoracic kyphosis, flattening of the lumbar lordosis, and a forward head position (see Fig. 6-16). Pain, stiffness, and even ankylosis can progress to the shoulders, hips, and knees. People may complain of "hip pain" due to referred pain from the sacroiliac joint. Complications can include aortic incompetence, iritis (inflammation of the iris of the eye), uveitis (general inflammation of structures of the eye), heart abnormalities, and osteoporosis.[89] In severe and rare cases, subluxation of the atlanto-occipital or atlantoaxial joints similar to that of RA may occur. A pseudoarthrosis can also form in the spine if a "fracture" of the ankylosed area is present, causing a false joint. This pseudoarthrosis can be dangerous because it can cause instability of the spine. Given the possibility of the formation of a pseudoarthrosis, patients should be advised to avoid participation in contact sports. Ankylosis of the spinal column reduces the shock-absorbing qualities of the spine,

increasing the susceptibility to fracture. People with AS may experience fractures of the spine with minimal trauma. The muscles of the body become generally atrophied and individuals become weak and easily fatigued.

Prognosis. The progression of AS in most people includes periods of exacerbations (worsening of the condition) and remissions (symptoms subside). After each remission phase, individuals usually do not return to their prior level of function. AS is not curable, but persons with AS can be helped with medications and physical therapy intervention. Some people become very immobile, whereas others maintain some limited mobility of the spine depending on the severity of the condition. The condition does not reduce life expectancy. In most people, the reduction of functional mobility progresses slowly over a period of years. However, in 10% to 20% of those with AS, the loss of mobility and function occur fairly rapidly.[90] The presence of peripheral joint involvement and early onset of the disease seem to indicate an increased possibility of rapid progression of the disease with reduced functional capacity.[91]

Medical Intervention. The medical diagnosis of AS is often determined by the physician ruling out other related conditions because AS has similar symptoms to other disease processes. The most recent diagnostic criteria for AS were developed in New York and Rome in the 1960s and

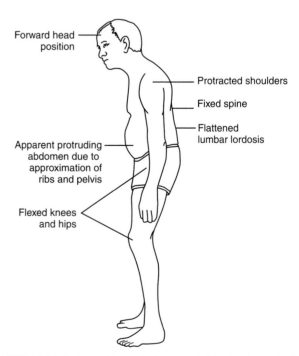

FIGURE 6.16 Patient with ankylosing spondylitis showing typical posture.

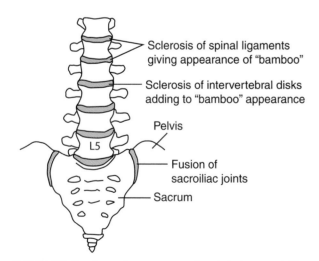

FIGURE 6.15 Bamboo spine appearance in ankylosing spondylitis.

were modified in the 1980s.[92] The criteria used for the diagnosis of AS include unilateral or bilateral sacroiliitis (inflammation of the sacroiliac joint), low back pain experienced for at least 3 months that is relieved by exercise, limitation of spinal motion in more than one plane, and reduction of chest expansion compared to age and gender equivalent healthy individuals[93,94] The use of MRI and CAT scans, as well as X-rays assist in the diagnosis of AS.

The pharmacological intervention for people with AS includes a variety of medications. Often-prescribed medications include NSAIDs such as ibuprofen, indomethacin, naproxen, and Celebrex. Analgesics and muscle relaxants may also be prescribed. The more recent biologics or tumor necrosis factor alpha (TNFa) blockers such as Enbrel (etanercept), Remicade (infliximab), Humira (adalimimub), and Simponi (golimumab) are effective in slowing down the progression of the joint disease process.[95] Sulfasalazine is used for its effects of reducing both pain and inflammation. Other medications sometimes prescribed are methotrexate in smaller doses than those given for patients with rheumatoid arthritis and corticosteroids.[96] The use of pharmacological agents allows the client to remain functional during periods of pain and stiffness. Sometimes a physician will inject areas affected by enthesitis (inflammation of the junction between bone and tendon) with corticosteroids, and radiation therapy may also be used for these local areas of problem. The use of radiation therapy has largely declined in recent years due to the side effects. The side effects from radiation therapy vary according to the area of the body irradiated. These side effects include, but are not limited to, skin reactions, nausea and vomiting, digestive, bladder and fertility problems, a low white blood cell count, fatigue, and hair loss.[97] In people with severe AS, especially those in which the ankylosis has affected the spine as well as other joints such as the hips, knees, and shoulders, surgical intervention may be necessary to improve functional mobility. If the spine and the hips are rigid as a result of ankylosis, performing bilateral hip arthroplasty surgery may allow the person to be functional.[98]

"It Happened in the Clinic"

A male patient in his 20s was referred to PT with a diagnosis of ankylosing spondylitis. The PT examination revealed minimal motion in his spine; range of motion (ROM) of bilateral hips was severely limited, 0 to 40° flexion right hip and 0 to 45° flexion left hip. ROM of bilateral knees was within normal limits. Strength of lower extremity muscles ranged from 2+/5 to 3+/5. Upper extremity ROM and strength were grossly within normal limits. His postural deficits included an increased kyphosis in the thoracic spine, forward head position, and flexed position at the hips with bilateral knees hyperextended. His mobility was severely compromised because he was unable to flex either his spine or hips. He could not bend down, and had difficulty getting up out of a chair. Ambulation was reduced to half a mile. The patient rated his pain in the lumbar spine and sacroiliac joints as 8/10. The patient was unable to participate in any of his usual leisure activities, including playing baseball. As a teacher, he was no longer able to write on the blackboard or stand for the prolonged periods needed to lecture. After extensive PT to increase ROM and strength, the patient was still unable to gain sufficient ROM in spine and hips to be functional in activities of daily living. The rheumatologist suggested bilateral total hip replacements, but the patient was young and undecided about the procedure. After discharge, the patient returned home, and 6 months later decided to have the bilateral hip replacements. His recovery postsurgery was rapid and dramatic. He gained functional range of motion in his bilateral hips and was able to return to work and resumed playing recreational baseball 1 year postsurgery.

Physical Therapy Intervention. Physical therapy intervention can provide essential education to patients with AS to maintain mobility of the spine and the proximal peripheral joints as long as possible.[99] Emphasis should be placed on extension of the spine for as long as possible, particularly prior to the ankylosis of the spine. Acute exacerbations of the condition, which include severe pain, can be treated with modalities and postural awareness training. Exercise can assist in reducing deformity and improving the functional outcomes for patients including increased chest expansion and spinal mobility.[100] The use of aquatherapy is also extremely beneficial for people with AS.[101] The effects of water buoyancy can improve the ability to move by supporting the limbs and the spine when performing range of motion exercises. Aquatherapy exercises should include lower extremity mobility including ambulation forward, backward, and sideways in different depths of water, cycling exercises with the person resting on a back rest, general swimming motions for upper extremity (UE) and spinal mobility, and strengthening exercises with the use of paddles and flotation devices.

Specific PT interventions may include the following:

1. Measurements of spinal movements during the PT evaluation process and testing of lung vital capacity. Use of special measurement devices such as a spondylometer

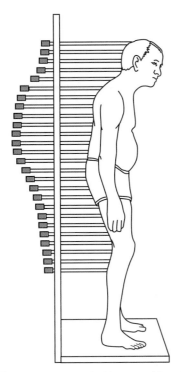

FIGURE 6.17 Patient measured with a spondylometer.

(see Fig. 6-17) and flexible measuring devices that can be translated to a drawing on paper for comparison at a later date. Photographs of the patient may also be helpful.

2. PT evaluation of levels of fatigue can be performed by using an analog scale or a numerical rating scale, similar to that of a pain numerical rating scale. The PTA may repeat this measurement periodically to gauge a patient's progress. This is an attempt to make a subjective assessment of pain and fatigue as objective and reproducible as possible.

3. Pain relief and reduction of muscle spasm through use of modalities. Caution should be used with modalities if individuals have received radiation therapy.

4. Improvement and/or maintenance of spinal mobility through exercise programs:
   a. Use of hydrotherapy/aquatherapy to increase mobility of spine and peripheral joints
   b. Breathing exercises to improve thoracic expansion
   c. Spinal mobility exercises including a home program to be performed every day (Keep the exercise program as short as possible to encourage the patient to actually do the exercises. Patients benefit from performing at least some exercise rather than none at all.)
   d. Patient education on positioning at home to include lying prone to stretch the hips and spine
   e. Stretching exercises for spine and extremities
   f. Relaxation exercises

g. Reduction of deformity through postural awareness training in sitting, standing, and walking
   h. Improvement and maintenance of lung vital capacity through breathing exercises and postural training
   i. Strengthening, endurance, and aerobic exercises for general health and fitness
   j. Group activities to benefit the patient psychologically and physically, including group exercise and referral to support groups

5. Advice on ADL, use of appropriate assistive devices, and possible referral to other health care providers such as occupational therapy for help with adaptations to the daily routine and environment.

6. Advice to desist participation in contact sports due to the danger of pseudoarthrosis and fracture of the spine.

7. Referral to the social worker, rheumatologist, pastoral counselor, or other health care provider as appropriate.

"It Happened in the Clinic"

A 40-year-old woman was admitted to the hospital with severe pain in both hands, swelling of the fingers, reduced motion of the distal interphalangeal (DIP) joints, minimal pitting of the finger nails, and the inability to pick up even the lightest of weights, including the towel to dry the dishes. She complained of difficulty walking and climbing stairs, pain in both feet, and severe stiffness and pain in her lumbar spine that made her unable to get moving in the morning to go to work. She was examined by the rheumatologist and his team of physicians and medical students, and a diagnosis of rheumatoid arthritis was suspected. The rheumatologist recognized that the case was not typical of someone with RA and looked under the hairline of the head at the base of the occiput. In this area was a small area of psoriasis that had been hidden by the hair. Psoriatic arthritis was now the suspected diagnosis, and x-rays and blood tests were ordered. The presence of HLA-B27 was confirmed in the blood, no rheumatoid factor was present, and x-rays and CT scan of her hands and spine revealed arthritis of the DIP joints of the hands and some changes in the sacroiliac joints indicating inflammation. Anti-inflammatory medications and physical therapy were prescribed. Physical therapy consisted of modalities for the hands, feet, and spine to reduce inflammation and pain and an exercise program for increasing mobility of the spine and strengthening hands, feet, and spinal muscles. After 6 weeks, the patient had improved in all areas in range of movement and strength and was discharged with an appropriate home exercise program and advice on modifications for activities of daily living.

Psoriatic Arthritis

Psoriatic arthritis is another of the group of seronegative spondyloarthropathy diseases and is characterized by inflammation of the joints, skin psoriasis, and occasional systemic symptoms. According to the National Psoriasis Foundation (2005), five types of psoriatic arthritis exist: symmetric, asymmetric, distal interphalangeal predominant, spondylitis, and arthritis mutilans. Of these five types, the distal interphalangeal predominant and the arthritis mutilans are the most rare, each affecting only 5% of the people who have psoriatic arthritis.[102] Conflicting figures exist for the incidence of psoriatic arthritis as a result of the difficulty experienced in accurate diagnosis of the condition. Psoriasis affects between 2% and 5% of the white population of North America (United States and Canada), and approximately 1 million people in the United States.[103] The National Psoriasis Foundation estimates that between 10% and 30% of people with psoriasis also have psoriatic arthritis,[104] whereas other sources estimate that between 5% and 8% of people with psoriasis develop psoriatic arthritis.[105,106] Psoriatic arthritis particularly affects people of North European descent and North American Caucasians, with males and females equally affected. ⊛ A juvenile form of the disease exists with the age of onset between 9 and 12 years; however, the usual age range of onset for psoriatic arthritis is between 35 and 55 years.[107]

Etiology. The exact etiology of psoriatic arthritis is unknown, but evidence points to a combination of factors including an autoimmune factor, a genetic tendency for development of the disease, and environmental factors.[108] Some sources also note that physical or psychological trauma, or infection, may precipitate psoriatic arthritis in people who have psoriasis.[109] This autoimmune disease is now known to be mediated by the T cells (part of the immune system), which produce cytokines such as tumor necrosis factor-alpha and interferon-gamma and damage the joints.[110]

Signs and Symptoms. Psoriatic arthritis affects mainly the distal joints of the hands and feet, but can involve sacroiliitis and spondylitis. The symptoms of psoriatic arthritis tend to go through phases of exacerbation and remission.[111] The sacroiliitis is usually unilateral, unlike that of AS except in the symmetrical type of the disease. See Table 6.4 for a comparison of the five types of psoriatic arthritis. No rheumatoid factor is present in the blood of people with psoriatic arthritis. Other characteristic signs and symptoms of the disease include iritis, aortic valve disease, colitis, urethritis, and mouth ulcers.[112] The presence of psoriasis may be difficult to determine but may be noted at the base of the skull under the hairline in the occipital region. Many cases of arthritis may be associated with psoriasis but remain undiagnosed as psoriatic arthritis. Approximately 50% of people with psoriatic arthritis have the HLA-B27 antigen in their blood. The severest form of psoriatic arthritis is called **arthritis mutilans**.[113]

Pathologically, in psoriatic arthritis, inflammation of the synovium of the affected joints is present similar to

Table 6.4 Types of Psoriatic Arthritis

TYPE	PERCENTAGE OF TOTAL PSORIATIC ARTHRITIS POPULATION	CHARACTERISTICS
Type 1: distal interphalangeal predominant	8%–16%	Mainly DIP joint involvement and may be associated with pitting of finger nails of affected digits
Type 2: arthritis mutilans	Less than 5%	Disabling form of psoriatic arthritis with severe involvement of joints of hands and feet; sacroiliitis may be present
Type 3: symmetrical	5%	Symmetrical polyarthritis similar to that of rheumatoid arthritis; DIPs more involved than PIPs; seronegative for rheumatoid factor
Type 4: asymmetrical	15%–70%	Asymmetrical oligoarticular arthritis; affects one joint of the hands, feet or larger joints such as knee
Type 5: spondylitis	Less than 5%	Affects axial skeleton with sacroiliitis and/or spondylitis; usually unilateral sacroiliac involvement; tends to be found more in males

DIP = distal interphalangeal joint; PIP = proximal interphalangeal.

that seen in RA. The synovial membrane then becomes thickened, and cartilage and bone erosion occurs. The main joints involved are the distal interphalangeal joints (DIP joints). Inflammation of the synovium of the affected joints leads to destruction of the joint and eventually destruction and deformity of the ends of the bones (see Fig. 6-18). A typical deformity noted on x-ray in DIP predominant psoriatic arthritis and in arthritis mutilans is the **pencil-in-cup deformity** (see Fig. 6-19). Pitting of the fingernails may also be noted in cases of psoriatic arthritis (see Fig. 6-20) and a thickening of the fingers often called "sausage fingers."

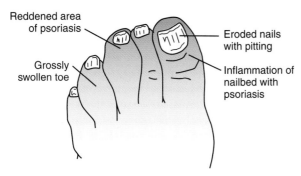

FIGURE 6.18 Foot in a patient with psoriatic arthritis.

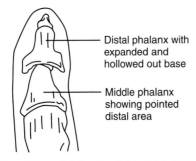

FIGURE 6.19 "Pencil-in-cup" deformity of the distal phalanx.

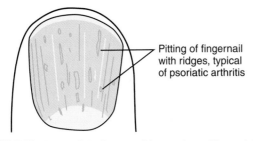

FIGURE 6.20 Pitting of the finger nail in a patient with psoriatic arthritis.

Prognosis. The prognosis for people with psoriatic arthritis is generally good. No cure exists for the condition, but it usually progresses slowly with only approximately 11% of cases involving severe functional deficits. The most disabling form of the disease is the arthritis mutilans.[114] Some of the indications for more severe forms of the disease include a strong family history of the disease, extensive and severe psoriasis, female gender, and the presence of HLA-B27 in the blood.[115]

Medical Intervention. The diagnosis of psoriatic arthritis is achieved through the use of x-rays, computed tomography (CT) scans, magnetic resonance imaging (MRI) scans, and laboratory tests. People with psoriatic arthritis have a raised ESR and are negative for rheumatoid factor. Pharmacological intervention is usually through the use of NSAIDs. Other medications used are slow-acting antirheumatic medications (SAARDs) and methotrexate to control the psoriatic skin lesions and nail pitting. The use of antitumor necrosis factor therapy medications has also shown some promising results.[116] In people with severe joint involvement, intra-articular injections with corticosteroids may be used.[117]

Physical Therapy Intervention. Physical therapy intervention for persons with psoriatic arthritis is aimed at reducing symptoms through use of modalities such as paraffin hand baths, moist hot packs, and cold packs. Exercise programs to improve hand and spinal function and improve and maintain ROM are helpful. In individuals with low back pain and sacroiliitis, modalities and exercises can be effective in reducing symptoms. Hydrotherapy can be beneficial for these patients in providing increased mobility for joints.[118] People with psoriatic arthritis can also be encouraged to perform hand exercises in warm water hand baths at home. Sufficient rest for patients with psoriatic arthritis is necessary to prevent undue fatigue.[119]

Reactive Arthritis (Reiter's Syndrome)

Reactive arthritis, Reiter's syndrome, and Reiter's disease are all terms for the same disease. Reactive arthritis is another of the group of diseases classified as seronegative polyarticular spondyloarthropathies[120](see Table 6.5). No rheumatoid factor (RF) is present in people with reactive arthritis. The disease affects men approximately 25 times more than women with the usual onset of the disease between the ages of 30 and 40.[121] The incidence of reactive arthritis in the United States is approximately 3.5 per 100,000 and is more common in the white population.[122]

Table 6.5 Comparison of Several Seronegative Polyarticular Arthropathies

CONDITION/DISEASE	SIGNS AND SYMPTOMS
Ankylosing spondylitis	Ankylosis of spine/hips Sacroiliitis Bamboo spine Enthesitis Low back pain (LBP) Increased thoracic kyphosis/ 　forward head position Difficulty breathing/reduced 　vital capacity Fatigue
Psoriatic arthritis	Psoriasis Peripheral arthritis in hands 　and feet Sacroiliitis Iritis Swelling of digits Urethritis Mouth ulcers
Reiter's syndrome	Arthritis, usually polyarthritis Urethritis/uveitis Conjunctivitis Fever and weight loss after 　infection Plantar fasciitis Sacroiliitis/low back pain Skin lesions on feet, hands, 　and genitalia

Etiology. The actual etiology of reactive arthritis is unknown, but symptoms usually occur about 1 to 4 weeks after an intestinal or venereal infection. Some of the infections thought to be responsible for the onset of reactive arthritis include gonococcus, HIV, shigella, salmonella, streptococcus, and chlamydia.[123,124] The presence of the genetic marker HLA-B27 in the blood is thought to be a genetically predisposing factor for people to develop the disease after an infection.[125]

Signs and Symptoms. The classic diagnostic criteria for reactive arthritis consist of a triad of symptoms including arthritis, urethritis, and conjunctivitis, although all three symptoms may not occur in some individuals.[126] The characteristic signs and symptoms of reactive arthritis include inflammation of the synovium of the knees, ankles, feet; of the Achilles tendon; and of the plantar fascia. People usually complain of low back pain and have swelling of the fingers and toes; a skin rash on the feet, hands, or genitalia; and mouth ulcers, urethritis, uveitis, conjunctivitis,

and sacroiliitis.[127] The HLA-B27 antigen is present in the blood of approximately 65% of all people with reactive arthritis.[128] The disease is characterized by both acute and chronic stages. In the acute phase of the disease, fever and weight loss may be noted. In an acute episode, there is considerable pain and swelling in the affected joints. Acute episodes may occur frequently, and occasionally the symptoms mimic those of ankylosing spondylitis.

Prognosis. The prognosis for people with reactive arthritis is varied. The disease can be severe or mild. Some individuals have reoccurrence of the symptoms, especially joint problems, over many years, but others do not.

Medical Intervention. The diagnosis of reactive arthritis may be difficult. Laboratory tests may reveal anemia and a raised ESR, but these results are not specific for reactive arthritis. Pharmacological intervention usually involves the use of the stronger NSAIDs, such as indomethacin.[129] Some evidence suggests that the use of antibiotics may be beneficial in preventing reoccurrence of the disease or in prevention of continued symptoms beyond the initial stages of infection.[130] In the later stages of the disease, joint abnormalities may be noticed on x-ray, but such tests reveal nothing significant in the early stages of the condition. In severe cases, joint replacement surgery may be an option.

Physical Therapy Intervention. The goals of physical therapy intervention in the acute phase are to reduce pain and inflammation with ice packs and reduce or minimize possible deformities through positioning and splinting.[131] In the subacute phase, the goals are to reduce pain and inflammation with the application of modalities, improve joint mobility, strengthen muscles and provide advice to the patient for improvement of functional activities. Ultrasound and electrical stimulation may be helpful to reduce plantar fasciitis and Achilles tendonitis. The use of foot and heel orthotics may also help to reduce heel pain, which is a common symptom in this condition.

GERIATRIC CONSIDERATIONS

Many patients with rheumatoid-related conditions have normal life expectancy. These patients will have more problems as they age compared with the general population as a result of the arthritic condition and the associated reduction in joint ROM and muscle strength. In some cases, the PTA will treat a patient for a specific condition not related to the arthritis such as a muscle strain or ligamentous sprain. In all

(Continued)

cases, the PTA should read the PT evaluation carefully to determine the comorbid diagnoses. If a patient has a rheumatoid-related condition, both the rate of recovery from injury and the extent of recovery may be affected. Exercise protocols must be adapted to the level of ability of the patient. Listen carefully to the patient regarding the level of usual physical function and plan and adapt the treatment session accordingly.

HINTS ON USE OF THE GUIDE TO PHYSICAL THERAPIST PRACTICE

Scleroderma and systemic lupus erythematosus are classified in the *Guide to Physical Therapist Practice*, Musculoskeletal Preferred Practice Pattern 4.

- 4D, "Impaired joint mobility, motor function, muscle performance, and range of motion associated with connective tissue dysfunction" (p. 179): Patients with scleroderma, systemic lupus erythematosus (SLE), and psoriatic arthritis have connective tissue diseases associated with rheumatoid arthritis (RA) and as such tend to be included in this Practice Pattern.

(From the American Physical Therapy Association, 2003. *Guide to physical therapist practice*, revised 2nd edition. Alexandria, VA: APTA. Used with permission.)

Why Does the Physical Therapist Assistant Need to Know About Connective Tissue Diseases?

Connective tissue diseases are generally systemic diseases affecting all areas of the body. The focus of the signs, symptoms and effects of these diseases in areas of joints, muscles, ligaments, and tendons means that physical therapy interventions are frequently indicated. General mobility is often an issue for people with these diseases and PT interventions include ADL and functional ambulation and mobility. Most of the connective tissue diseases are rare, but some, including systemic lupus erythematosus, fibromyalgia, and myofascial pain syndrome, are frequently seen in people attending physical therapy clinics. An understanding of the pathology of the connective tissue diseases is thus essential when working with people with these conditions.

Connective Tissue Diseases

Connective tissue diseases are those conditions that affect any area of the body with connective tissue. These diseases tend to be systemic (involve the whole body) and include scleroderma, systemic lupus erythematosus (SLE), fibromyalgia, giant cell arteritis, polymyalgia rheumatic, myofascial pain syndrome, and polyarteritis nodosa.

Scleroderma

Scleroderma, also known as systemic sclerosis, circumscribed scleroderma, dermatosclerosis, and morphea, is a systemic, autoimmune, connective tissue disease. [132] Because the disease is systemic in nature, affecting multiple organ systems, the effects of the disease are more severe than those of the nonsystemic arthritis-related diseases. The two main forms of the disease are the diffuse form and the limited form. The incidence of scleroderma is approximately 20 per million annually in the United States. The disease affects all ethnic groups, and it affects women more than men in a 3:1 ratio or more.[133,134]

Etiology. The etiology of scleroderma is unknown. One theory is that the disease is partly hereditary, although family members sometimes have associated conditions such as SLE, rather than scleroderma. Exposure to solvents and radiation are also thought to play a part in development of the disease.[135] A drug-induced form of SLE can be caused by certain antihypertensive, antiseizure, and antituberculosis medications, as well as penicillamine. Once the medications are discontinued, the symptoms usually disappear.[136]

Signs and Symptoms. Scleroderma is inflammatory in nature in the initial stages and progresses to a chronic condition of thickening and loss of elasticity of the skin with progressive fibrosis involving body organ systems. Thickening of the skin of the face, trunk, and limbs and sclerosis (scarring) of body organs, including the heart, lungs, kidneys, and esophagus, are found in the diffuse form of the disease.[137] Involvement of the body organs can cause hypertension and result in headaches and fatigue. The limited form of scleroderma tends to affect mainly the skin of the face and hands. The milder, limited form of the disease is characterized by CREST. CREST is an acronym for:

Calcinosis (deposition of calcium in the superficial layers of the skin)
Raynaud's phenomenon (see later in this chapter)
Esophageal hypomotility (reduced ability of the esophagus to propel food due to weakness of esophageal muscles)

Sclerodactyly (thickening and tightness of skin of fingers and/or toes)

Telangiectases (areas of dilated superficial capillary blood vessels apparent on the skin).

Other characteristic signs and symptoms of the disease include edema of the fingers; thickening and tightening of the skin of hands (see Fig. 6-21), feet, and face, which may cause a pursed lip appearance or a pulling back of the lips; and loss of skin creases (see Fig. 6-22). In severe cases of scleroderma, joint contractures may be present as a result of tightening of the skin over joints. Occasionally gangrene of the distal fingers occurs with loss of the distal part of the digits. Joint stiffness of the fingers, wrists, knees, and ankles is common. Weakness and atrophy of muscle occurs, especially over the contracted joints. Joint involvement can include the

temporomandibular joint (TMJ), making eating difficult. The esophagus is affected in most cases, increasing swallowing difficulties. Effects on the gastrointestinal tract cause bowel problems of constipation and diarrhea, with the associated loss of control of the bowel sphincters.[138] Other organs that may be affected by the disease are the liver, pancreas, and thyroid gland. Sjögren's syndrome (dry mouth and eyes) is another side effect of the condition. See Table 6.6 for signs and symptoms of scleroderma and SLE. The symptoms of early morning stiffness and multiple joint pains can lead to misdiagnosis as RA.

Prognosis. Recent studies indicate that most organ damage occurs during the first 3 years of skin symptoms; however, damage does not occur in all people.[139] Approximately 70% of people with scleroderma have lung complications and these are responsible for many deaths in this condition. The effects of scleroderma on

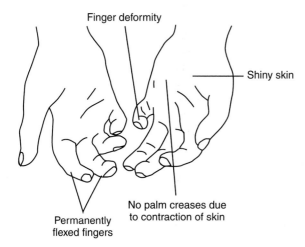

FIGURE 6.21 Hands of a patient with scleroderma.

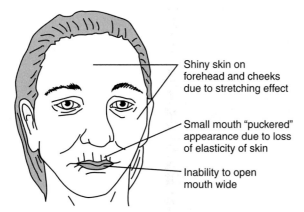

FIGURE 6.22 The typical facial appearance of a woman with scleroderma.

Table 6.6 **Signs and Symptoms of Scleroderma and Systemic Lupus Erythematosus**

CONNECTIVE TISSUE DISEASE	CHARACTERISTICS, SIGNS, AND SYMPTOMS
Scleroderma	Edema of fingers/thickening and tightening of skin/weakness and atrophy of muscles/joint contractures due to tight skin over joints
	Pursed lip appearance/swallowing difficulties due to esophageal hypomobility
	Urethritis
	Conjunctivitis
	Scleroderma/sclerosis
	CREST
	Lung complications
	Gastrointestinal problems
	Renal disease
	Sjögren's syndrome
	Liver, pancreas and thyroid disease
Systemic lupus erythematosus	Butterfly (malar) rash across nose and cheeks
	Arthritis of hands
	Raynaud's phenomenon
	Photosensitivity
	Raised erythrocyte sedimentation rates
	Cardiopulmonary problems
	Neurological problems
	Renal disease
	Gastrointestinal symptoms

the heart can include left ventricular congestive failure, pericarditis, hypertensive heart disease, and atherosclerosis. The effects on the kidney known as "scleroderma renal crisis," and pulmonary symptoms are frequently the cause of death for people with renal involvement.[140]

Medical Intervention. The diagnosis of the disease is through a combination of blood tests for the presence of antinuclear antibodies (ANA); which are suggestive of an autoimmune response; chest x-rays; electrocardiogram; and an extensive history of signs and symptoms.[141] Because corticosteroids affect the kidneys and the disease also affects the kidneys, this is not a drug of choice. Some medication trials have been performed with the use of angiotensin-converting enzyme inhibitors, which appear to show mixed but promising results.[142,143] The use of medications is focused on the prevention of thrombosis (blood clots) with the use of low doses of aspirin; the prevention of acid reflux with medications such as omeprazole (Prilosec), esomeprazole (Nexium), or lansoprazole (Prevacid); and the suppression of the immune system with medications such as penicillamine, azathioprine, and methotrexate.[144] The immune system suppressive medications do not reverse any fibrosis that has occurred in the skin or internal organs.[145] Skin lotions may also be used. Advice should be provided about practicing good skin care, reducing the intake of caffeine, smoking cessation, avoiding exposure of the skin to the cold, avoiding skin trauma, and avoiding large doses of vitamin C that stimulate collagen production.[146]

"It Happened in the Clinic"

A 35-year-old white woman was seen in the rheumatology clinic. Her main complaints were pain and stiffness in her fingers, difficulty swallowing food, extreme early morning stiffness, pain in multiple joints throughout her body, dry eyes and mouth, and feeling weak. The rheumatologist's team noted that her hands were in a "clawlike" position, and she seemed unable to extend her fingers fully. She complained of pain in the temporomandibular joint area and demonstrated limited mandibular depression. The symptoms had been progressing for approximately 3 months, and the patient eventually decided to visit the physician. The patient was diagnosed with scleroderma after confirmation from blood tests. Anti-inflammatory medications and a program of physical and occupational therapy were initiated. The physical therapy consisted of paraffin baths for the hands, gentle stretching exercises for the fingers, exercises for opening of the mouth, ambulation training, and general aerobic and strengthening exercises including the stationary bike. She was advised to use hand lotion several times a day and to use rubber gloves when her hands were in water. The occupational therapist worked with the patient on dressing skills and cooking to help with assistive devices for the kitchen. In approximately 4 weeks, the patient was beginning to have less early-morning stiffness and had increased mobility in her hands. She returned to work as a secretary part-time for the first few months and was able to resume full-time work within 6 months.

Physical Therapy Intervention. Physical therapy intervention is directed toward maintaining gentle stretching of joints to minimize contractures, providing soft tissue mobilizing and massage techniques, and improving general aerobic fitness. Active exercise programs are important for patients. A 6-minute walk test is useful to determine the general physical capacity of patients and the PT may be involved in lung function testing.[147] The correlation between hand function and the ability to perform ADL is still under investigation, but the stiffness and loss of dexterity experienced by people with scleroderma is a major problem for performing ADL.[148] The use of exercise in combination with paraffin baths for the hands appears to improve hand function more than exercise alone.[149] Care must be taken to avoid overstretching the joints, which could produce skin breakdown. Advice should be given for use of lotions on the skin to help keep the skin moist and avoiding exposing the skin to water for prolonged periods. Use of rubber gloves when using cleaning materials is recommended to reduce irritation of the skin. A daily hand exercise program assists in reducing the loss of joint range of motion. Referral to the occupational therapist, speech and language pathologist, and dentist is usually required. Stretching of the mouth is needed to enable patients to open the mouths to eat. These exercises may be taught by the speech and language pathologist or may be initiated by the PT and followed up with the PTA. A team approach to patient management is essential for people with scleroderma.

Systemic Lupus Erythematosus

Systemic lupus erythematosus is, as its name suggests, a systemic disease that affects multiple body organs. SLE is classified as a rheumatoid-related, systemic, chronic, autoimmune, inflammatory, connective tissue, and collagen disorder. The average annual incidence of SLE in the United States is approximately 1 in 10,000, with a higher incidence in some European countries. Approximately 1 in 2,000 people in the United States has SLE. ⊛ The general age of onset of the disease is from 14 to 64, mainly during the childbearing years.[150] The disease is more prevalent in females than males in a 9:1 ratio, and is more common in black women than white women.

Etiology. The etiology of SLE is unknown; however, research suggests genetic, hormonal, and external environmental factors involvement. The disease is rarely found in African countries, which has led to the hypothesis that environmental factors may be a main cause of the disease because African American women have a higher incidence than white women. Another aspect of the disease is an alteration in apoptosis (normal programmed death of cells) that increases the rate of cell death in the body.[151] Several genetic markers have been isolated for SLE indicating a predisposition to develop the disease. These include HLA-DR2, HLA-DR3, and ANA.[152]

Signs and Symptoms. The signs and symptoms of SLE vary widely and range from slowly developing to rapidly progressing. The characteristic signs and symptoms of SLE include a rash on the face known as a **malar rash** or "butterfly" rash because of the shape of the marking across the bridge of the nose and on either side of the face onto the cheeks, which resembles a butterfly (see Fig. 6-23). Some people have a discoid (small oval plaques) rash on various parts of the body that may mimic other types of skin conditions. Individuals who exhibit discoid rashes and do not have general organ involvement

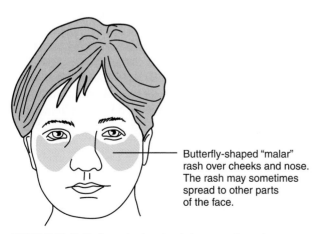

Butterfly-shaped "malar" rash over cheeks and nose. The rash may sometimes spread to other parts of the face.

FIGURE 6.23 Butterfly rash of systemic lupus erythematosus.

are classified as having discoid lupus.[153] People with all types of SLE may experience fatigue, general feelings of malaise or fever, weight loss or gain, alopecia (loss of hair), and Raynaud's phenomenon.[154] Arthritis-like symptoms are noted, especially in the fingers, feet, knees and wrists, that resemble those of RA. Body organ involvement includes arterial necrosis; anemia; renal disease; cardiopulmonary disease, including pleurisy and pleural effusions; central nervous system problems, such as anxiety, depression, seizures, Parkinsonism, and myelopathy; and gastrointestinal symptoms.[155,156] Conjunctivitis and blurred vision are also common symptoms of SLE. The disease process involves exacerbations and remissions of the symptoms with progressively greater involvement of the internal organs. People with SLE have a raised ESR and the presence of ANA and anti-deoxyribonucleic acid antibodies.[157] Their presence is the result of the body developing antibodies to its own tissues in an autoimmune response. See Table 6.6 for the signs and symptoms of scleroderma and SLE.

Prognosis. The prognosis for people with SLE has greatly improved in recent years because of advances in drug therapy. However, the greater the internal organ involvement, the worse the prognosis tends to be. In people with severe cardiovascular, renal, or neurological involvement, death can occur within 5 years. The survival rate for 10 years beyond diagnosis of the condition is now at 90%, which is much improved from the 1950s, when the rate was 50%.[158]

Medical Intervention. The diagnosis for SLE involves multiple testing using laboratory blood tests to detect whether someone has the genetic markers, check the ESR for the presence of inflammation, creatinine kinase tests to monitor kidney function, and urine tests to check for proteinuria (protein in the urine). Other diagnostic tools include MRI, chest x-rays to detect pulmonary symptoms, and echocardiograms to determine heart problems. The pharmacological intervention for SLE includes anti-inflammatory medications such as corticosteroids and NSAIDs such as aspirin and ibuprofen.[159] Antimalarial medications are also sometimes helpful in controlling symptoms.[160] The physician will provide advice to patients regarding the avoidance of sunlight and ultraviolet light exposure as a result of the photosensitivity experienced by people with SLE. The use of hats, sunscreen, and protective clothing is recommended. Patients must be aware of additional symptoms that might indicate an infection and alerted to visit the physician with any unusual symptoms; they must also be monitored for blood pressure and cholesterol regularly.

A study published in December 2007 raised some excitement about the treatment of SLE. Greg Lemke, a professor of molecular neurobiology at the Salk Institute, and his associates have discovered a "TAM" amino acid tyrosine protein kinase receptor, akin to the cytokines, that inhibits inflammation.[161] The TAM receptor is normally activated by a factor in the blood to shut down the inflammation after an initial period. This TAM receptor does not work in people with autoimmune diseases. A possibility exists for giving a blood factor called protein S to persons with autoimmune diseases to prompt the shutdown of the overactive immune system that destroys the body's tissues.[162]

Physical Therapy Intervention. The physical therapy intervention for clients with SLE is much the same as that for persons with RA. The therapeutic positioning of joints during acute exacerbations to prevent deformity and active exercise in the subacute and more chronic phases is essential. Fatigue is a limiting factor for people with SLE; therefore, patients need to be directed to work within their tolerance to exercise. Individuals with SLE should avoid exercising at times of the day when they feel tired in order to conserve energy. At the same time, exercises to increase endurance and aerobic activity are helpful. As in all arthritis-related conditions, physical therapy intervention should include ROM, stretching, and strengthening exercises, and posture reeducation. Teaching patients skin care is important. The PTA needs to be aware of any changes in the signs and symptoms of people with SLE during treatment sessions and refer to the supervising PT if changes are noted. Because these people are susceptible to renal problems, they should be monitored for changes in blood pressure during treatment and observed for signs of edema. Edema and hypertension result from the inability of the kidneys to secrete fluids, causing a buildup of fluids, particularly in the lower extremities, and an increased resistance to blood flow, resulting in a rise in blood pressure. If in doubt, the PTA should immediately refer the patient to the PT for reexamination.

Fibromyalgia

Fibromyalgia, also known as fibromyalgia syndrome, or FMS, is a chronic pain syndrome characterized by multiple areas of muscle tenderness and frequently joint pain, although the condition does not directly affect the joints.[163] The incidence of fibromyalgia is higher in women than men, especially those between the ages of the early teens to mid-60s. Fibromyalgia is more commonly diagnosed in middle-aged women and in people with rheumatoid arthritis or other autoimmune diseases such as SLE and ankylosing spondylitis.[164] Fibromyalgia occurs in 2% to 4% of the U.S. population.[165]

Etiology. Onset of the characteristic signs and symptoms of fibromyalgia may be associated with trauma, especially to the cervical spine, stress, hyperthyroidism, or possibly after an infection. A link with sleep disorders, dietary factors, psychosocial, and environmental factors may be noted. A genetic predisposition to develop the condition is thought to exist, because fibromyalgia tends to occur in families. Another possible cause is the dysfunction of the hormonal linkage system of the hypothalamus, pituitary, and adrenal glands.[166] People with fibromyalgia have high levels of substance P in their spinal fluid. This chemical is responsible for the transmission of pain nerve impulses to and from the brain and is thought to increase the pain signals, resulting in the heightened sensation of pain in those with fibromyalgia.[167,168] In addition to the high levels of substance P, serotonin levels are often decreased in people with fibromyalgia, and the combination of the two factors may be responsible for the increased pain perception.[169] Serotonin is a hormone present in blood platelets, the digestive tract, and the brain that acts as a chemical mediator for the transmission of nerve impulses and is known to alter mood, emotion, sleep, and appetite. High serotonin levels are responsible for some cases of depression, and low levels may increase the perception of painful stimuli.[170]

Signs and Symptoms. The signs and symptoms of fibromyalgia include many specific sites of tenderness on palpation in the muscles. A positive diagnosis exists when 11 out of a possible 18 points on the body are hypersensitive to palpation (see Fig. 6-24). People with fibromyalgia may also experience headaches or migraines, fatigue, chest pain, profuse sweating, cognitive deficits such as poor memory, and inability to concentrate, early morning stiffness, swelling, low back pain, neck pain, urinary and bowel symptoms such as irritable bowel syndrome, restless leg syndrome, anxiety, depression, dizziness, Raynaud's phenomenon, and sleep disorders.[171] A heightened sensitivity to external stimuli such as sound, smell, temperature extremes, taste, and light may be present.[172] The symptoms of fibromyalgia seem to be aggravated by cold and damp and relieved in warm and dry weather. Lack of sleep and physical or emotional stress may also increase the symptoms. The main areas of tenderness in persons with fibromyalgia are located in the cervical and shoulder areas with some in the low back and hips. The major muscles involved include the trapezius, supraspinatus, gluteals, and the suboccipital insertion of the cervical muscles. Other areas of tenderness may include the lateral epicondyles, greater trochanters, costochondral junctions of the second rib and the medial joint line of the knees (see Fig. 6-24). The most important symptom according to patients is that of considerable pain, which interferes with daily functional activities.

Prognosis. Fibromyalgia is not a life-threatening condition, although it can cause severe debility and reduced functional capacity.

Medical Intervention. The diagnosis of fibromyalgia is complex and entails the elimination of other possible diagnoses before fibromyalgia is identified, therefore this is a diagnosis of exclusion. According to the American College of Rheumatology Criteria for the Classification of Fibromyalgia, a positive diagnosis is made when there are at least 11 tender points present out of a possible 18, with

9 on each side of the body.[173] The medical management of people with fibromyalgia involves a team approach. Medications prescribed by the physician may include antidepressants such as amitriptyline (Endep), fluoxetine (Prozac), paroxetine (Paxil), or duloxetine (Cymbalta), which also help to improve sleep patterns; muscle relaxants such as cycloflex and flexeril; analgesics such as acetaminophen (Tylenol) and tramadol (Ultram); and pain medications such as NSAIDs including aspirin, ibuprofen and naproxen sodium.[174] The extent and strength of the medications depends on the individual's needs. In 2007, pregabalin (Lyrica) became the first specific drug for the treatment of fibromyalgia in adults to be approved by the Food and Drug Administration (FDA). Pregabalin was already approved to treat seizures and some types of nerve pain, and in randomized, placebo-controlled trials, it was found to benefit people with fibromyalgia.[175] Injections of analgesics and/or cortisone into the tender muscle areas may help to reduce pain, although inflammation is not associated with fibromyalgia.[176] In addition, cognitive behavioral therapy with a psychologist, psychiatrist, or behavioral scientist is often helpful, combined with a

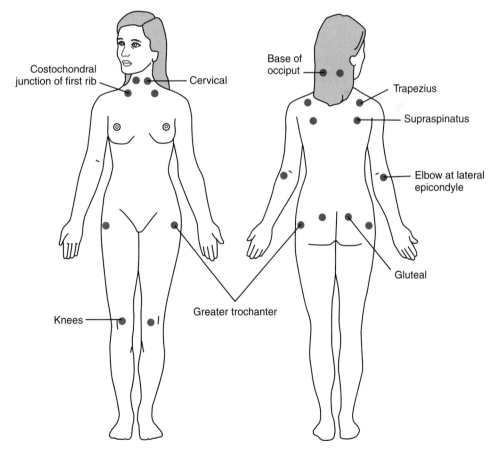

FIGURE 6.24 Location of tender points in fibromyalgia.

regular exercise program and physical therapy and occupational therapy as needed.[177]

Physical Therapy Intervention. Interventions for people with fibromyalgia include stress reduction, adaptation of the workplace environment, aerobic exercises, and other moderate exercise routines. People with fibromyalgia appear to have increased symptoms when they either do not exercise at all or exercise too much.[178] Physical therapy intervention must strike a balance in moderation of activity and exercise to help in the management of symptoms. Pain management strategies, teaching self-management, and home exercise programs are all helpful in reducing symptoms and essential for these patients because the symptoms may last for many months and even several years.[179] Modalities to reduce pain such as biofeedback have been shown to be effective in reducing both the number and severity of tender points and the overall pain level in people with fibromyalgia.[180] Some studies have shown that low-level laser therapy (LLLT) improved morning stiffness and reduced the number of tender points.[181] Because fatigue is often a major symptom in fibromyalgia, patients should be advised to take frequent rest periods when performing aerobic exercise routines. A study of patients in Scandinavia found that physical therapy had a positive impact on patients' well-being over the long term, which helped them to cope with pain and maintain functional activity for longer than without the physical therapy intervention.[182]

Giant Cell Arteritis

Giant cell arteritis, also called temporal arteritis, is a multiple system and multiple symptom condition that affects older adults, usually over age 50 and is more common in women than men in a 2:1 ratio. The incidence of the disease increases with age and a higher incidence is noted in the white population.[183] The annual incidence of the disease in both the United States and the United Kingdom is between 188 and 220 cases per million of the population.[184] According to estimates, 40% to 60% of people with giant cell arteritis also have polymyalgia rheumatica. (See the section on polymyalgia rheumatica for details.)[185]

Etiology. The actual cause of the disease is unknown. Giant cell arteritis is usually classified with rheumatology as a result of the inflammatory nature of the disease. Several cytokines are thought to be involved in the development of the disease including tumor necrosis factor (TNF) and interleukin-6.[186] The diagnosis of giant cell arteritis is

considered an emergency because the complications of the disease can be life-threatening.

Signs and Symptoms. Giant cell arteritis is a condition that involves chronic inflammation of the major arteries of the body including the carotid arteries, aorta, femoral, and subclavian arteries in 50% of patients.[187] Giant cells are present in the walls of the arteries in most people with the condition. The characteristic signs and symptoms of giant cell arteritis are many, but the main indication of the disease may be severe temporal or occipital headaches that occur suddenly or sudden blindness or vision impairment in one or both eyes.[188] Some of the signs and symptoms of giant cell arteritis include sensitivity to touch over the temporal arteries, located in the temporal area of the head, and temporal or occipital headaches. The general, systemic symptoms may include weight loss, feelings of malaise, ulcerations in the mouth, scalp pain, necrosis of the scalp, depression, neck pain, head and neck swelling, a low-grade fever, muscle aching, and vertigo. The more severe symptoms of giant cell arteritis include loss of vision as a result of inflammation of the optical arteries, transient ischemic attacks (TIA), myocardial infarction (MI), and cerebrovascular accident (CVA/stroke).[189,190]

Prognosis. Giant cell arteritis is considered a medical emergency as a result of the extreme side effects of blindness, MI (heart attack), and CVA, which can occur in some people.[191] Although these side effects are comparatively rare, they can be fatal.

Medical Intervention. The diagnosis of giant cell arteritis is extremely important as a result of the possible severe side effects of the disease. The diagnostic tools used include the use of positron emission tomography (PET) scans, MRI, and CT scans. These scans can detect the inflammation in the major arteries, including the temporal artery, and may also be used to detect infarcts in the brain.[192,193] Laboratory blood tests may also reveal a raised erythrocyte sedimentation rate (ESR) in most people. The pharmacological management of giant cell arteritis is usually with the administration of oral or intravenous corticosteroids.[194] An attempt has been made to try to reduce the dosage of corticosteroids prescribed as a result of side effects of the medication. A recent study by Mahr and coworkers (2007) suggested that the use of methotrexate at the same time as corticosteroids may allow lower dosages of corticosteroids to be effective in reducing the inflammation of the arteries.[195]

Physical Therapy Intervention. No physical therapy intervention is indicated for individuals with giant cell arteritis; however, the PT/PTA should be aware of the disease in case a patient develops severe headaches in the temporal area that are previously undiagnosed by the physician. An immediate referral to the physician may prevent complications for the patient.

Polymyalgia Rheumatica

Polymyalgia rheumatica (PMR) is a chronic and systemic condition often associated with giant cell arteritis. Approximately 10% to 15% of people with PMR develop, or already have, temporal arteritis (giant cell arteritis). The onset of PMR is usually in the 60-plus age group, and it is rarely diagnosed under age 50. The annual incidence of PMR is approximately 20 to 50 per 100,000 people worldwide.[196] The incidence in women is twice that of men.[197]

Etiology. The etiology of polymyalgia rheumatica is not fully known. Some of the theories regarding the cause of PMR include the possibility of both environmental and genetic predisposition factors. Infection with chlamydia and certain viruses are thought to cause onset of the disease.[198]

Signs and Symptoms. The characteristic signs and symptoms of PMR include aching, stiffness, and pain in multiple areas of the body including the neck, low back, shoulders and legs, with most joint stiffness focused in the proximal joints of the shoulder and pelvic girdles.[199] Onset of aching and stiffness may be sudden, which is worse after periods of inactivity and in the early morning or the pain and stiffness may progress gradually. Night pain is common, making it difficult for people to get out of bed in the morning as a result of the morning stiffness that lasts up to an hour. People with PMR often require a considerable amount of time to get moving in the morning, thus they have to awaken early to get ready for work. The associated symptoms of PMR may include fever, depression, fatigue, night sweats, edema of the hands and feet, weight loss, and inflammation of the synovial membranes causing joint pain.[200] A raised ESR is commonly present, the red blood cell count may be lower than normal, and no RF is apparent.[201]

Prognosis. PMR is not life threatening unless associated symptoms of giant cell arteritis are present that may result in the onset of a MI or a CVA.

Medical Intervention. The diagnosis of PMR is performed by the physician following a set of criteria that includes morning stiffness, depression, weight loss, and bilateral upper extremity tenderness. To meet the criteria for PMR,

patients must have at least three of the defined symptoms.[202] The pharmacological intervention for PMR is corticosteroids such as prednisone, which frequently provides immediate or rapid relief of the symptoms.[203] Other pharmacological interventions may include methotrexate to attempt to reduce the dosage of corticosteroids required, aspirin to reduce blood clotting, and the use of anti-osteoporosis medications to offset the effects of the corticosteroids.[204] Corticosteroid injections into the affected joints may also be performed.[205,206]

Physical Therapy Intervention. Physical therapy intervention is focused on the maximization of functional activity. A combination of modalities to reduce pain and stiffness, mobilizing exercises within pain tolerance, aerobic conditioning exercises, a home management program, and adaptive strategies for the work and home environments may be used. Severe muscle weakness is rarely associated with the condition, so muscle strengthening exercises may not be the main focus of the treatment.

Myofascial Pain Syndrome

Myofascial pain syndrome, also called myofascial pain dysfunction or fibrositis syndrome, is often confused with polymyalgia rheumatica and fibromyalgia. The identification of trigger points in myofascial pain syndrome is credited to Janet Travell, M.D.

Etiology. An association between myofascial pain syndrome and repetitive stress syndromes has been identified. Other causes of myofascial pain syndrome are thought to be infection and stress.

Signs and Symptoms. Clinically the most significant finding in myofascial pain syndrome is the presence of trigger points in the muscles involved. Pressure on the trigger point areas results in pain referred to another site in the body. Myofascial pain is usually localized to one or just a few areas, whereas fibromyalgia is more profuse in nature. The tender points associated with fibromyalgia do not trigger referred pain. Janet G. Travell, M.D., and her coauthor David G. Simons, M.D., are generally regarded as the people who developed the concept of the trigger point as a recognized physiological and pathological entity. Travell describes a trigger point as "a hyperirritable locus within a taut band of skeletal muscle, located in the muscular tissue and/or its associated fascia."[207] Trigger points are "active" when they give pain to the person. Trigger points are called "latent" when they do not cause pain but are activated easily into a pain mode when the muscle is stressed as a result of a muscle pull or other minimal trauma. New theories on trigger points reveal an abnormal depolarization of the motor endplates that cause excess amounts of acetylcholine to be transmitted across the synapse. This excess of acetylcholine causes hypersensitivity of the muscle tissue, resulting in the formation of trigger points.[208]

Prognosis. Myofascial pain syndrome can cause severe amounts of muscular pain and can be difficult to treat effectively. A chronic pain syndrome can result from this condition.

Medical Intervention. The use of Travell's press and stretch technique to trigger points can be effective. In some cases, a physician may inject the trigger point with an analgesic and/or muscle relaxant, such as lidocaine or bupivacaine.[209,210] Some studies have shown that "dry needling" used in acupuncture can also be effective in reducing the trigger points.[211]

Physical Therapy Intervention. The physical therapist needs to identify the trigger points before the use of intervention techniques. Trigger points are detected by palpation and can be felt as tight bands or tight points within the muscle. In a true trigger point, pressure over the area causes referral of pain to a distant site in a specific pattern. For example, pressure over the infraspinatus muscle belly trigger point elicits referred pain down into the arm. Because interpretation of palpation findings is outside the scope of work of the PTA, PTAs should recognize the existence of trigger points and become familiar with the feel of a trigger point

in case the PT requests acupressure or other interventions over the trigger point area. Physical therapy intervention may consist of desensitization of a trigger point with specific manual pressure over the area, electrical stimulation, ultrasound, and stretching techniques to the involved muscle, including spray and stretch techniques with fluoromethane spray (see Fig. 6-25). A recent study by Srbely and Dickey (2007) showed that ultrasound and stretching to trigger point areas can reduce the pain and increase the pain threshold over these areas.[212] Another study by Esenyel and coworkers (2007) demonstrated the effectiveness of using lidocaine and Botox injections combined with stretching exercises and the use of ultrasound, at both conventional doses and high power doses, for the relief of trigger points.[213] More general intervention for people with myofascial pain syndrome should also include postural reeducation and exercises for aerobic conditioning.[214] More important, a study by Dommerholt, Bron, and Franssen (2006) explained the importance of a multidisciplinary approach to the treatment of people with myofascial pain syndrome to maximize the effectiveness of any intervention.[215]

Polyarteritis Nodosa

Polyarteritis nodosa is included in this chapter because it is a systemic vasculitis, autoimmune disease affecting the collagen and connective tissue of the skin and throughout the body. An alternative term for the disease is "systemic necrotizing vasculitis." Polyarteritis is a rare disease. The incidence of polyarteritis nodosa in the United States is between

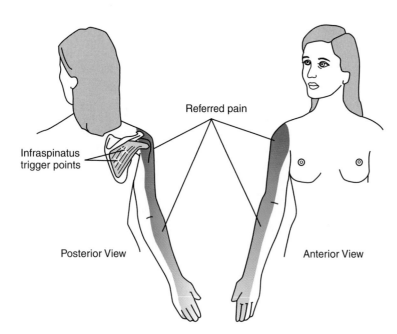

FIGURE 6.25 Infraspinatus trigger point location showing area of referred pain down the arm.

3 and 4.5 cases in 100,000 per year. The condition is mainly diagnosed between ages 40 and 60. ⊛ However, polyarteritis nodosa may also occur in children and teenagers.[216] The disease is more common in males than in females with a 6:1 ratio.[217] The incidence is higher in countries where hepatitis B is common. In 33% to 52% of cases of polyarteritis nodosa, the digestive system is affected.[218]

Etiology. Although no known cause for the disease has been identified, the etiology of polyarteritis nodosa is closely linked with hepatitis B and results in the formation of immune complexes in the walls of the involved arteries. As many as 10% to 30% of people with polyarteritis nodosa may also have hepatitis B.[219,220] Other infectious diseases such as the Epstein-Barr virus are also known to precede the disease.[221]

Signs and Symptoms. Pathologically, polyarteritis nodosa involves inflammation of the small and medium arteries in the body resulting in nodule formation in the walls of the arteries as a result of aneurysms. These aneurysms produce scar tissue, which can cause a reduction in the size of the lumen of the vessel or complete closing of the lumen. The most common sites for the involvement are in the arteries of the joints, muscles, kidneys, gastrointestinal tract, reproductive organs, and the skin.[222] People with polyarteritis nodosa often have associated involvement of the nerves lying close to the blood vessels, which increases the level of pain involved with the condition. The characteristic signs and symptoms of polyarteritis nodosa can include skin lesions, especially of the fingertips and thighs, where the appearance of the nodules can be like blood blisters. Other characteristics of the condition include vasculitis, skin mottling, fever, sweating, anorexia, polyarthralgia (pain in several or many joints), hypertension, a raised ESR rate, edema of the lower extremities, and abdominal pain.[223,224] Nodules may also occur within the central nervous system and in the lungs, kidneys, and gastrointestinal tract.[225] Peripheral neuropathy symptoms are present in approximately 60% of people with polyarteritis nodosa.[226]

Prognosis. The prognosis for individuals with polyarteritis nodosa is poor if no treatment is provided. A generalized vasculitis can occur if the condition is untreated, which can cause death.[227]

Medical Intervention. Diagnosis of the condition is often confirmed with a biopsy of the nodules in the skin or other organs affected by the disease.[228] Other diagnostic procedures include angiograms and arteriograms in which a dye is injected into the circulatory system, and x-rays are taken of the appropriate areas of the body. An MRI may be used, and laboratory tests for blood may show a raised ESR. The pharmacological intervention is usually with the use of corticosteroids.[229] Immunosuppressive medications may also be used, such as cyclophosphamide or azathioprine. People who have hepatitis B may also be given an antiviral medication such as interferon-alpha.[230]

Physical Therapy Intervention. Physical therapy intervention is not indicated for persons with this condition, but the PT and PTA should have some awareness of the signs and symptoms. Because the condition may occur in the muscles and joints, people may be misdiagnosed and referred to physical therapy for pain control/management.

HINTS ON USE OF THE GUIDE TO PHYSICAL THERAPIST PRACTICE

Reflex sympathetic dystrophy is classified in the *Guide to Physical Therapist Practice*, Musculoskeletal Preferred Practice Pattern 6.

- 6H, "Impaired circulation and anthropometric dimensions associated with lymphatic system disorders" (p. 569); Patients with reflex sympathetic dystrophy have altered skin reactions and sensation; pain and edema and are classified under this Practice Pattern.

(From the American Physical Therapy Association, 2003. *Guide to physical therapist practice*, revised 2nd edition. Alexandria, VA: APTA. Used with permission.)

Why Does the Physical Therapist Assistant Need to Know About Other Rheumatoid and Connective Tissue-Associated Diseases?

People with some of the rheumatoid-associated diseases that do not fit strictly under the classification of either rheumatoid or connective tissue disease are seen in physical therapy practice either as stand-alone diagnoses or as signs and symptoms of other rheumatoid or connective tissue diseases. The PTA needs to be familiar with the pathology of these diseases to understand the complexity of the rheumatoid related diseases and the implications of this pathology for physical therapy interventions.

Other Rheumatoid- and Connective Tissue–Associated Diseases

The other rheumatoid- and connective tissue-associated diseases are those conditions and diseases that do not directly fit into the categories of either rheumatoid-related inflammatory pathologies or connective tissue diseases. The diseases described in this section include complex regional pain syndrome (CRPS), also called reflex sympathetic dystrophy (RSD), rheumatic fever, sarcoidosis, and Sjögren's syndrome.

Complex Regional Pain Syndrome

Complex regional pain syndrome (CRPS), also known as reflex sympathetic dystrophy (RSD), reflex sympathetic dystrophy syndrome, shoulder-hand syndrome, and causalgia, is a chronic pain syndrome involving a disturbance of the vasomotor control of the affected limb. The condition can occur in either the upper or the lower extremities, although it is more common in the upper.[231] Women are affected 3 times more often than men, and the age of onset is usually in adults between ages 25 and 55, although people of any age can be affected. An estimated 3 to 6 million people are affected by CRPS in the United States.

Etiology. The cause of CRPS is unknown, but it is most common in people with coronary artery disease, hemiplegia, peripheral nerve injury, and Colles' fracture and following trauma.[232] As many as 90% of people with CRPS may have had some form of trauma before the onset of CRPS.[233] Why some people with these conditions develop the condition and others do not is unknown. The development of CRPS is not directly proportional to the severity of the injury. A relatively minor injury may result in CRPS. Pathologically, theories differ as to the cause of CRPS. An alteration in the autonomic nervous system is thought to occur that alters the pain signals after injury, but the exact nature of the problem is not understood.

Signs and Symptoms. The characteristic signs and symptoms of a limb affected by CRPS include severe pain, edema, and skin changes including thinning, shininess, sweating, acute sensitivity, loss of wrinkles, and excessive hair growth.[234] Contractures of the digits may occur in the later stages of the condition. The PT/PTA should become suspicious of the presence of the condition if patients are progressing well with intervention after trauma and then suddenly develop severe pain in the

hand or foot for no apparent reason. The extremity may be acutely sensitive to touch, and pain in both the hand and shoulder is common.

Prognosis. No cure exists for CRPS. The prognosis is varied. In some cases, CRPS resolves spontaneously, whereas in other cases, the pain becomes more severe and the condition results in loss of function of the limb and deformity.[235] As many as 30% of people with CRPS may not respond to therapeutic intervention of any kind.[236]

Medical Intervention. Several medications may be used for the management of persons with CRPS to reduce the pain. Corticosteroids or opiates may be necessary and many people are placed on antidepressants. Topical analgesics may be helpful in reducing some of the pain and sensitivity of the limb.[237] In severe cases, a sympathetic nerve block may have to be performed by a neurosurgeon, or an intrathecal drug pump may be surgically inserted for the delivery of pain medications.[238]

Physical Therapy Intervention. Physical therapy intervention for CRPS is controversial. Early mobilization of the limb after injury may reduce the risk for the development of CRPS. The intervention often involves both physical therapy and occupational therapy. Intervention may include the use of thermal modalities, exercise, and desensitization of the limb using textures of fabric starting with soft and progressing to rougher materials. Other interventions may include contrast baths, fluidotherapy, or electrical stimulation under water with the charges reversed to attempt to reduce both the pain and the hypersensitivity to heat and cold. Advice regarding the reduction of guarding of the affected limb is also provided.[239] The physical therapy management and intervention for CRPS is difficult and the outcome is not always successful.

Rheumatic Fever ⊛

Rheumatic fever is a systemic, inflammatory disease of childhood that affects mainly the heart and joints. Refer to Chapter 3 of this text for more information on this disease.

Sarcoidosis

Sarcoidosis is a systemic, sometimes chronic disease, possibly autoimmune in nature, that can affect any body organ. The disease could equally well be included as part of the pulmonary diseases, but speculation surrounds the autoimmune nature of the disease, and patients have arthritic manifestations; therefore, it is included in this chapter.

Sarcoidosis occurs mainly between ages 20 and 40.[240] The occurrence of sarcoidosis is worldwide. In the United States, the estimated incidence in Caucasians is 5 in 100,000, but it is 40 in 100,000 in African Americans. The incidence of the disease in Scandinavia is 64 in 100,000 people.[241]

Etiology. The cause of sarcoidosis is unknown; however, some evidence indicates that cytomegalovirus (CMV), hepatitis C, rubella, and other viruses or environmental factors, such as types of dust and metals, may play a role in its development.[242,243] The disease is complex in nature and causes an abnormal response of the immune system.

Signs and Symptoms. Sarcoidosis affects the lymph nodes, lungs, liver, eyes, skin, joints, muscles, and the nervous system. Granulomas (lumps of tissue) develop in the body spontaneously for no apparent reason. The granulomas can manifest themselves as swollen lymph glands, which may or may not be evident to the person. The common signs and symptoms of sarcoidosis include fatigue, chest pain, shortness of breath, skin lesions, and joint pains.

Prognosis. The outcome for people with sarcoidosis can vary from being asymptomatic to death in approximately 1% to 6% of cases.[244] Between 60% and 70% of people with sarcoidosis experience spontaneous healing within a period of 24 to 36 months, whereas 20% to 30% of patients have some permanent lung damage.[245]

Medical Intervention. The diagnosis of sarcoidosis is a diagnosis of exclusion. That is, diagnostic testing rules out other causes of illness, such as tuberculosis, rheumatoid arthritis, rheumatic fever, and cancer.[246] None of the tests for sarcoidosis are conclusive except for the tissue biopsy. The possible tests for diagnosis include the following:

- Blood tests for the detection of high levels of angiotensin converting enzyme secreted by the granulomas
- Chest x-rays
- Pulmonary function tests
- Biopsy of the lungs or other tissues such as the lymph glands
- Bronchioalveolar lavage, in which the lungs are rinsed and the fluid is examined for different types of cells that may indicate inflammation (e.g., white blood cells)
- Fiberoptic bronchoscopy, in which a flexible, narrow tube with a light at the end and a tiny camera is passed into the lungs
- Thallium or gallium scanning in which radioactive gallium-67 or thallium is injected into the venous system, and a body scan is performed to see where the gallium is concentrated in the areas of inflammation
- CT or MRI scans
- PET scan, which also uses radioactive dye injections and may be more helpful in locating the areas of inflammation

Most people with sarcoidosis do not require any treatment. In these individuals, the condition resolves over a period of 24 to 36 months with the physician monitoring patients for any signs of organ damage.[247] When the symptoms of sarcoidosis become more chronic and internal body organs are at risk of damage, the medications prescribed by the physician are usually corticosteroids. The corticosteroids reduce both the inflammation and the production of granulomas.[248] Other medications may include methotrexate, azathioprine, hydroxychloroquine, the biologic tumor necrosis factor inhibitors such as adalimumab (Humira) and infliximab, and immunomodulatory agents such as thalidomide.[249]

Physical Therapy Intervention. Physical therapy intervention is only indicated for patients with lung damage or joint problems. Treatment intervention for the joint problems associated with sarcoidosis follow the same pattern as for other arthritic conditions. Pulmonary hygiene techniques may be implemented for people with long-term pulmonary effects.

Sjögren's Syndrome

Sjögren's syndrome can either be a primary diagnosis with no other disease process or a secondary group of signs and symptoms found as part of a diagnosis for many pathological conditions, especially those of connective tissue, and autoimmune diseases such as rheumatoid arthritis, systemic lupus erythematosus, scleroderma, polyarthritis, polymyositis and dermatomyositis, and autoimmune thyroiditis (Hashimoto's thyroiditis).[250,251,252] Approximately 50% of the 4 million people in the United States with the syndrome have primary Sjögren's syndrome and 50 percent have secondary.[253] The incidence of Sjögren's syndrome is largely in women, with a 9:1 female to male ratio. The age of onset is primarily between the ages of 40 and 60.[254]

Etiology. Sjögren's syndrome is a systemic and autoimmune disease. Although the exact cause is unknown, research indicates a strong genetic tendency is involved.[255]

Signs and Symptoms. The signs and symptoms of the syndrome include dry eyes and mouth as a result of dysfunction of the mucous membranes and inflammation of the lacrimal (tear) and salivary glands, caused by an autoimmune response.[256] Dental and gum problems can occur as a result of the mouth dryness. The symptoms of primary Sjögren's syndrome also include severe fatigue, depression, arthralgia (joint pain), and fibromyalgia.[257,258]

Prognosis. Currently, no cure has been discovered for Sjögren's syndrome. The symptoms of fatigue, joint pain, and vision problems can cause impairment of the quality of life.[259] In rare cases, damage can occur to vital body organs such as the lungs, kidneys, and lymph nodes, resulting in pneumonia, kidney failure, or lymphoma, all of which can be life threatening.[260]

Medical Intervention. The diagnosis of Sjögren's syndrome may be made by the family physician and confirmed by an ophthalmologist. Blood tests often reveal the presence of antinuclear antibodies (ANA) and RF in some patients.[261] The pharmacological interventions for people with this disease are aimed at relieving the symptoms rather than curing the disease. Artificial tears and artificial salivary substances may be used. People with severe manifestation of the disease causing internal organ involvement may be prescribed corticosteroids and other immune suppressive medications such as azathioprine (Imuran) or cyclophosphamide (Cytoxan). Frequent dental care is recommended to prevent oral complications.[262] When musculoskeletal problems occur the medications of choice are often NSAIDs.[263]

Physical Therapy Intervention. The PTA is not involved with specific treatment for persons with the condition, unless patients have musculoskeletal symptoms. However, the PTA may be treating someone with a related pathological condition who happens to have this condition. Therefore, the PTA should be aware of the implications of this condition on patients' rehabilitation.

Why Does the Physical Therapist Assistant Need to Know About Muscle Diseases?

In physical therapy practice, the PTA will provide interventions for many people with muscle diseases as well as musculoskeletal and orthopedic conditions. Patients with muscular dystrophy are seen frequently in the pediatric physical therapy setting. Knowledge of the pathology of muscular dystrophy and other muscle diseases is essential to provide people with the necessary therapeutic interventions to encourage as much functional independence as possible and to teach self-management techniques.

Muscle Diseases

The muscle diseases described in this section include those most frequently seen in physical therapy practice including muscular dystrophy, myasthenia gravis, and the inflammatory myopathies.

HINTS ON USE OF THE GUIDE TO PHYSICAL THERAPIST PRACTICE

Although muscular dystrophy (MD), myasthenia gravis, and myopathies are not listed in all the following practice patterns, they may be classified in the *Guide to Physical Therapist Practice*, Musculoskeletal Preferred Practice Patterns 4 through 7.

- 4A, "Primary prevention/Risk reduction for skeletal demineralization" (p. 133): Patients with muscular dystrophy are at risk for bone demineralization in the later stages of the disease as a result of lack of weight bearing on the lower extremities.
- 4D, "Impaired joint mobility, motor function, muscle performance, and range of motion associated with connective tissue dysfunction" (p. 179): The lack of dystrophin in the muscles makes this pattern the most appropriate for MD.
- 5G, "Impaired motor function and sensory integrity associated with acute or chronic polyneuropathies" (p. 411): Although MD results from lack of dystrophin in the muscles this practice pattern most closely resembles the needs of patients with MD; This pattern is also appropriate for patients with myasthenia gravis and myopathies.
- 6B – "Impaired aerobic capacity/endurance associated with deconditioning" (p. 475): This pattern is appropriate for several of the muscular diseases including MD and myasthenia gravis.
- 7B, "Impaired integumentary integrity associated with superficial skin involvement" (p. 601): Patients with MD are at risk for skin break-down as a result of poor mobility.

(From the American Physical Therapy Association, 2003. *Guide to physical therapist practice*, revised 2nd edition. Alexandria, VA: APTA. Used with permission.)

Muscular Dystrophy ⊛

Muscular dystrophy (MD) occurs in many forms. Multiple types of MD exist, but only those most commonly observed in physical therapy practice are described here.

Duchenne MD (DMD) and Becker's MD (BMD) are the two most common forms. Both DMD and BMD are diagnosed in childhood and result in progressive weakness and atrophy of muscles. Of the two, DMD is the more severe and more rapidly progressing form.[264] Other types of MD include fascioscapulohumeral MD, which is diagnosed during the teenage years; limb-girdle MD, which can have an onset between the teenage years and adulthood; and myotonic MD, which has an adult onset.[265] Both DMD and BMD occur almost exclusively in males, with females in affected families becoming carriers of the disease. Fascioscapulohumeral, myotonic, and limb-girdle MD occur in both males and females, with males affected more frequently.[266,267] The incidence of DMD in the United States is 1:3500 to 5,000 male births, with 400 to 600 reported new cases each year.[268] The other forms of MD are much more rare.

Etiology. DMD and BMD are x-linked, recessive, inherited, genetic diseases that cause progressive weakness and atrophy of muscles.[269] In both DMD and BMD, the genetic defect lies on the X chromosome. In DMD, the genetic defect causes a lack of dystrophin in the muscle. In BMD, the dystrophin is present but altered so that it does not function normally.[270] A study by Cyrulnik and coworkers (2008)[271] hypothesized that the lack of dystrophin in DMD may also affect the development of the pathways between the cerebellum and cerebrum in the brain, causing cognitive deficits in some people with DMD. The genetic defect in limb-girdle MD can be either autosomal dominant (affecting females and males) or autosomal recessive (affecting males only). Facioscapulohumeral MD is caused by an autosomal dominant genetic trait and affects both females and males.[272]

Signs and Symptoms. The onset of DMD is usually diagnosed between ages 2 and 6, whereas the onset of BMD is more often from 5 to 25 years. The characteristic signs and symptoms of MD include many that may not immediately cause concern. The first signs that something may not be right with muscle development are when children do not walk as expected at age 1 or start to walk and do not progress as expected with their balance and running. In addition, children may be toe walkers, exhibit a waddling gait pattern as a result of hip abductor and extensor weakness (gluteus maximus and gluteus medius), have frequent falls, have problems getting up from a sitting or lying position, and have the appearance of enlarged or hypertrophied lower leg muscles, especially the gastrocsoleus complex.[273,274] Often children with DMD or BMD

are labeled as clumsy before they are diagnosed with the condition. The muscles of the posterior lower leg tend to look hypertrophied, resulting from an accumulation of connective tissue in the muscles. If children push up to standing by walking the hands up the legs, this is known as "Gower's sign" and usually indicates a peripheral weakness, that requires further diagnostic testing.[275]

In DMD and BMD the progressive muscle weakness starts in the proximal muscle groups of the pelvic and shoulder girdles and progresses to the distal extremities and the respiratory muscles. Children with DMD are usually unable to walk by age 12 and have to rely on the use of a wheelchair for mobility.[276] Many, but not all, children with DMD demonstrate mental retardation. The signs and symptoms of BMD progress more slowly than DMD and affect mainly the pelvic and shoulder girdles. Other signs and symptoms of DMD include seizures; scoliosis, which may be severe; and susceptibility to respiratory infections, particularly in the later stages of the disease, as a result of the lowered forced vital capacity (FVC) of the lungs.[277] The lowered FVC often occurs as a direct result of the scoliosis, which compresses the thoracic cavity and reduces the volume of the lungs.

Various other types of MD affect localized muscle groups. Facioscapulohumeral MD may start in the teens through adulthood and slowly progress to affect the face, neck, and shoulder musculature. Limb-girdle MD also affects people in the teens and into adulthood and is focused on the pelvic and shoulder girdles. Limb-girdle MD tends to progress slowly. Myotonic MD may either be present from birth in the congenital form or start in adulthood. People with myotonic adult onset MD have symptoms including muscle spasms, cataracts, and cardiac and endocrine disorders.[278] In ocular MD, the onset is from 5 to 30 years, and the effects are on the ocular (eye) muscles, with some weakness in the facial, neck, and upper extremity muscles.

Prognosis. Currently, no cure exists for MD. Most children with DMD do not survive more than 15 to 20 years from onset, although life expectancy is steadily increasing, and some people live into their 30s.[279] The life span for people with BMD, fascioscapulohumeral MD, myotonic adult onset MD, and limb-girdle MD life is usually normal.

Medical Intervention. The diagnosis of MD may take some time because the family may not recognize the motor deficits, and referral to a physician may be delayed for some time. Blood tests for the diagnosis of DMD include the detection of increased levels of serum creatine phosphokinase (CPK) in the blood. The CPK is detectable before the symptoms of the disease become apparent as a result of breakdown of the muscle tissue but is not present in all persons with the disease and is not a definitive test for MD.[280] A multiplex polymerase chain reaction (PCR) genetic test or a single condition amplification/internal primer sequencing test of the blood can be performed to detect genetic deletions of the dystrophin gene.[281,282] Recent research is promising for the use of stem-cell therapy for the treatment of muscular dystrophy. Most research has been performed on mice, and some studies have demonstrated that muscle tissue with dystrophin has been successfully stimulated to grow in the animal models.[283,284] The techniques have yet to be tested on humans with DMD. Other techniques used for the diagnosis of MD include ultrasonography of the muscles, which demonstrates an increased echo effect as a result of the deposition of connective tissue (scar tissue) in the muscle, and muscle biopsy. Monitoring of people with MD includes the use of electrocardiograms (ECGs) to check for cardiac problems and pulmonary function tests (PFTs) to check the status of the lungs.

In patients with severe scoliosis, surgery may be required to provide improved lung expansion and reduce the problems that occur with appropriate seating. Spinal fusion is often the surgery of choice for people with MD. The pharmacological interventions may include the use of anticonvulsants to prevent seizures in susceptible persons, the use of immunosuppressants thought to perhaps delay muscle damage, and antibiotics for respiratory infections as needed.[285] Referrals from the physician are common for physical therapy, occupational therapy, respiratory therapy, and speech therapy. The recommendation for involvement with support groups for families with a child with MD and other resources are also beneficial.

Physical Therapy Intervention. Physical therapy intervention may be needed for any type of MD. The role of PT for individuals with MD is to provide home exercise programs to maintain strength and function as long as possible, without overtiring the patient. Advice on home adaptations, wheelchair measurement and ordering, power-chair choices to provide optimal mobility, and instruction to the family for management of the child are essential. A team approach with the physical therapist, PTA, occupational therapist, certified occupational therapy assistant (COTA), social worker, speech and language pathologist (if needed), respiratory therapist, physician, teacher, and family is important. Families with a child with MD require numerous home and transport adaptations. In the later stages of the disease process, hoists may be needed for patient transfers. Therapeutic positioning of patients is crucial to minimize deformities and contractures. In many cases, special molded inserts for the wheelchair will be required to provide comfort and pressure relief for people with MD.

Myasthenia Gravis

Myasthenia gravis (MG) is a chronic autoimmune disease in which the body produces antibodies that destroy the acetylcholine receptors at the synapse in the neuromuscular junctions resulting in muscle weakness.[286] The incidence of the disease in the United States is between 1:10,000 and 3:10,000 of the population.[287] The onset of the disease may be either sudden or gradual. In women, the onset of the disease occurs mainly in the adult years before age 40, and in adult men over age 60.[288]

Etiology. The pathology of the disease is partly related to the thymus. Antibodies mediated by T and B cells block or destroy the acetylcholine receptors in the muscle at the myoneural (neuromuscular) junction preventing the transmission of nervous impulses to the muscle fibers.[289] The actual cause of the thymus dysfunction, which results in myasthenia gravis, is unknown.

Signs and Symptoms. The characteristic signs and symptoms of MG include weakness of the eye, skeletal, and respiratory muscles, which is most evident later in the day because fatigue of muscles is the main symptom of MG. The most frequent first signs of the disease are weakness of the eye and face muscles causing ptosis (eyelid drooping), diplopia (double vision), swallowing and chewing difficulties, speech abnormalities such as slurring, and problems holding the head in an upright position.[290] The muscles of inspiration and expiration are often involved causing breathing difficulties, which may lead to respiratory failure in untreated cases.

Prognosis. The prognosis for MG varies greatly. Some people live comparatively normal lives, whereas others with severe symptoms may only live a few years. Infectious disease, especially of the respiratory system, creates risks for these people as a result of the level of muscle fatigue. A study by Romi and coworkers demonstrated that patients with seropositive MG were more likely to have a severe disease progression than those who were seronegative.[291]

Medical Intervention. MG is diagnosed by the physician using the Quantitative Myasthenia Gravis (QMG)

Score for Disease Severity. The system has 13 separate assessments for diagnosis of the condition.[292] Some of the tests performed include blood tests to detect the presence of acetylcholine receptor antibodies, an edrophonium test in which edrophonium chloride is administered intravenously to temporarily reduce the muscle weakness, and a CT scan of the thymus.[293] The medical treatments for MG vary and continue to be adjusted in light of evolving research findings. The pharmacological intervention usually involves a combination of immunosuppressive corticosteroid medications such as prednisone, azathioprine, or cyclosporine, and cholinesterase inhibitors to improve the neuromuscular transmission of acetylcholine.[294,295] Other treatments may include thymectomy (removal of the thymus), plasmapheresis (removal of blood and separation of the red cells and plasma to remove the antibodies to acetylcholine, and then return of blood to the body), or a complete blood plasma exchange to remove the abnormal antibodies that attack the acetylcholine receptors.[296,297] A study by Romi and coworkers indicated that an early thymectomy may increase the chances of a better outcome for patients with myasthenia gravis.[298]

Physical Therapy Intervention. Physical therapy intervention may include providing assistive devices for ambulation and ADL, and teaching the patient and care providers techniques to assist with transfers and ambulation. Generally, people with MG benefit from intervention early in the day, when their fatigue levels are lower. Individuals with MG require regular rest periods during their treatment routine. Exercise programs, if used, should consist of minimal repetitions to reduce the effects of fatigue on the muscles. Functional activities that include breathing exercises should be the emphasis of any intervention. The level of severity of the disease varies greatly with some people demonstrating minimal weakness and others exhibiting severe weakness. Most likely, only the individuals with severe skeletal muscle weakness will be seen by the PTA in the PT department or office.

Inflammatory Myopathies

Several types of inflammatory myopathies exist, including polymyositis and dermatomyositis. This group of diseases cause weakness of skeletal muscles and are considered rheumatoid related diseases.[299] Polymyositis occurs most frequently in people between the ages of 31 and 60.[300]

Etiology. The exact cause of this group of diseases is not known. Pathologically an autoimmune response mediated by the T-cells attacks the muscle fibers. Possible theories of triggering factors for myositis include injury, infection, or a virus, or other autoimmune disease processes such as RA, SLE, scleroderma, or Sjögren's syndrome.[301] A separate group of infectious myositis diseases, which is not described in detail here, are caused by bacteria, viruses, and parasites.

Signs and Symptoms. The characteristic signs and symptoms of this group of diseases mainly consist of weakness of the proximal shoulder, shoulder girdle, and neck muscles. The specific characteristics of polymyositis include gradual or sudden onset of symmetrical, proximal muscle weakness, cardiac problems including congestive heart failure and pericarditis, and weight loss.[302] People with dermatomyositis have a facial skin rash associated with the symptoms of weakness, which may progress to the upper body, mainly on the extensor aspects of the limbs.[303] In rare and severe cases of myositis, the muscle fibers are replaced with fatty deposits resulting in fibrosis.

Prognosis. No cure exists for myositis, but the symptoms can be controlled with medications and physical therapy.[304] In rare cases, respiratory and cardiac problems may cause serious health problems and even death.

Medical Intervention. The diagnosis of myositis is often complicated. Some of the tests used include the following: blood tests such as creatine phosphokinase (CPK) and aldolase, both of which are present in larger quantities in the presence of muscle damage; blood tests for antinuclear antibodies (ANA) and specific myositis antibodies; ESR for detection of inflammation; a muscle or skin biopsy; an MRI; and an electromyogram (EMG) to detect possible changes in the electrical conductivity of the muscles.[305] The pharmacological intervention for myositis includes corticosteroids or other immunosuppressive medications such as azathioprine or methotrexate.[306]

Physical Therapy Intervention. Physical therapy intervention consists of exercise programs, manual muscle testing, aquatic therapy, assistance with ADL, and advice regarding home exercise programs and energy conservation. When the person requires bed rest, the PT and PTA may be involved with positioning and prevention of contractures. The PTA needs to proceed carefully with these patients, referring to the supervising PT regularly to protect the person. Damage to muscle fibers can be irreversible if the patient is pushed too hard in an exercise program or is not stable before PT intervention. Both the physician's and PT's instructions must be followed carefully.

CASE STUDY 6.1

A 26-year-old woman with rheumatoid arthritis (RA) attends the clinic where you are working. She has been diagnosed with RA for 5 years and has been referred by her rheumatologist for functional activities and strengthening and mobilizing exercises. The physical therapist examines and evaluates the patient and determines that the patient has an overall strength of 3/5 in the lower extremities. Genu valgum is present at the knees. AROM of the knees is limited with the patient lacking 20° of extension in the left knee and lacking 25° of extension in the right knee. The shoulders have gross weakness of 3/5 in all shoulder muscles. Shoulder AROM is limited as follows: left shoulder elevation through flexion is 0 to 90°, right shoulder elevation through flexion is 0 to 100°. She is not in an acute stage and has minimal pain at this time. The patient has difficulty rising from a chair, great difficulty climbing stairs due to weakness in the lower extremities, and is not sleeping well as a result of discomfort at night. The hands show signs of the beginning stages of swan-neck deformity in the right index and middle fingers and Boutonniere's deformity of the left index finger and right ring finger. In addition, grip strength is 10 pounds on left and 15 pounds on right. The patient is right-handed. The PT plan of care includes strengthening exercises for the quadriceps and hamstrings, shoulder mobility exercises, hand exercises for increasing strength, functional activities to include sit-to-stand-to-sit and stair climbing, and gait training on level and uneven surfaces with an appropriate assistive device. A home exercise and activity program is also prescribed.

1. Develop an exercise program to strengthen the quadriceps and hamstrings. Consider all precautions and contraindications when deciding on the exercise program and decide what specific instructions you will provide to the patient. Create the exercise program in a numerical list with subcategories beneath each item.

2. Develop three activities that the patient can perform to encourage knee extension. Provide advice for home management to increase knee extension.

3. Provide four exercises for the hands to help develop grip strength without damaging tendons or joints.

4. Develop an exercise program for mobilizing the shoulders.

5. Develop a home exercise program for the patient with four exercises for the shoulders and four for the lower extremities.

6. What advice will you give the patient to assist her with functional and day-to-day activities?

7. What type of assistive device would you recommend for this patient? Describe any specific instructions you would give her when using the device at home considering her diagnosis.

CASE STUDY 6.2

An 8-year-old boy is attending the outpatient clinic where you work. He was diagnosed with juvenile rheumatoid arthritis (JRA) 1 year ago. He attends school and manages well, ambulating with Lofstrand crutches most of the time. Occasionally, he can manage with a straight cane. The supervising physical therapist has been working with the child for several weeks and has decided to delegate the treatment program to you. He has 3/5 strength in bilateral quadriceps and hamstrings, and his grip strength is very poor. She requests that you develop some activities to incorporate quadriceps strengthening exercises and hand grip strength exercises into games that will hold his attention. He likes to read and work on the computer and can at times ride an adaptive bike with small wheel stabilizers when he is not in too much pain. He has missed a significant amount of school this year due to severe pain in the knees. At the moment, he is not in severe pain.

1. Think of three games you could play with this little boy that will encourage strengthening of the quadriceps and hamstring muscles without putting too much stress on the knee joints.

2. Think of two activities for the hands to increase hand grip strength.

3. Develop a home program for the child.

4. Consider a plan of action for speaking to the mother regarding home activities to continue his improvement.

CASE STUDY 6.3

A 23-year-old male patient with a diagnosis of anky-losing spondylitis is attending the outpatient clinic where you work. He is reporting significant pain in the spinal region and is having difficulty dressing himself in the morning as a result of the stiffness of his whole spine. The PT has evaluated the patient and deter-mined that he has almost no motion available in the lumbar spine, strength of lower extremities is 4/5 over-all, and upper extremities are 4+/5. The range of mo-tion of the upper and lower extremities is within nor-mal limits. The patient is starting to develop a forward head position. The PT has asked you to work in the warm rehabilitation pool with the patient to encour-age increased range of motion of the spine and in-crease the strength and mobility of the lower extremi-ties to improve overall functional abilities. Additionally, you are requested to provide heat packs for the spine to reduce pain, followed by active exercises on land for strengthening of the upper and lower extrem-ities, extension exercises for the spine, and postural reeducation to address the forward head position.

1. Describe the ambulatory exercises you could have the patient perform in the pool to encourage in-creased range of motion of the lower extremities.

2. What exercises for the spine could be performed and what motion of the spine will you try to encourage as much as possible?

3. What position will you place the patient in to apply the hot packs for the spine?

4. Develop three exercises for lower extremity strengthening and three for the upper extremities that the patient can perform at home.

5. Discuss the postural training you will provide for the patient to address the forward head position.

STUDY QUESTIONS

1. What is the etiology of rheumatoid arthritis (RA)?

2. Name the type of juvenile arthritis that is character-ized by systemic disease.

3. Name three deformities of the hand that can occur in RA.

4. Name three deformities of the foot that can occur in RA.

5. Describe a deformity that often occurs at the knees in RA. How does this differ from the more common deformity found in osteoarthritis (OA)?

6. Describe three contraindications or precautions to consider when treating patients with RA.

7. What medications would be prescribed for a patient with RA? Name three types.

8. What types of splinting devices might be used by the patient with RA? Discuss any special precautions that need to be taken when advising the patient about wearing prescribed splinting devices.

9. How would management of a patient with RA differ from that of a patient with OA? What are some of the things that would need to be taken into consider-ation? Compare and contrast OA and RA.

10. A 22-year-old patient with ankylosing spondylitis (AS) attends the outpatient clinic where you work. He pres-ents with severe ankylosis of the whole spine, sacroil-iac joints, and bilateral hips. He can move his knees through full range. He is awaiting bilateral hip arthro-plasties. Provide the patient with some strategies to use to increase function prior to surgery, such as how to put on his shoes, get in and out of bed, and rise from a chair. You cannot improve range of motion of the spine or hips, so your strategies cannot be exercise-related for these areas. (Try to imagine the difficulties involved if you were unable to move your spine or your hips.)

11. Develop a progressive home exercise program within the plan of care developed by the PT to span a period of 3 weeks, for a 34-year-old female patient diag-nosed with fibromyalgia, bearing in mind that fatigue is a common symptom for persons with this disease.

12. A 3-year-old boy diagnosed with Duchenne muscular dystrophy has been evaluated by the PT. The child needs a home exercise program to help with independent transfers from floor to chair and floor to bed. He is able to walk short distances up to 50 feet, but his balance is insufficient to enable him to run. He falls frequently because of balance problems. He can climb steps when able to touch the wall for balance. Develop a home pro-gram so the family can encourage the patient to be as in-dependent as possible. What play activities can you de-velop to help with transfers? What advice will you give the caregivers and parents regarding transfers and play? What are your impressions about a motorized wheel-chair versus an ordinary light-weight wheelchair?

USEFUL WEB SITES

American College of Rheumatology
http://www.rheumatology.org

American Rheumatism Association
http://www.rxed.org

Association of Rheumatology Health Professionals
www.rheumatology.org/arhp

Centers for Disease Control and Prevention
http://www.cdc.gov

Lupus Research Institute
http://www.lupusresearchinstitute.org

Muscular Dystrophy Association
http://www.mdausa.org

The Myositis Association
http://www.myositis.org

National Institute of Arthritis and Musculoskeletal and Skin Diseases
http://www.niams.nih.gov

National Institute of Neurological Disorders and Stroke (NINDS)
http://www.nlm.nih.gov

National Psoriasis Foundation
http://www.psoriasis.org

Scleroderma Foundation
http://www.scleroderma.org

The Sjögren's Syndrome Foundation
http://www.sjogrens.org/syndrome/

SLE Lupus Foundation
http://www.lupusny.org

Spondylitis Association of America
http://www.spondylitis.org

REFERENCES

[1] Shiel, W. C. (2007). Rheumatoid arthritis. *MedicineNet.com.* Retrieved 11.08.10 from http://www.medicinenet.com/rheumatoid_arthritis/article.htm

[2] Matsumoto, A. K. (2007). *Rheumatoid arthritis: Clinical presentation.* The Johns Hopkins Arthritis Center. Retrieved 11.08.10 from http://www.hopkins-arthritis.org/arthritis-info/rheumatoid-arthritis/rheum_clin_pres.html

[3] Rheumatoid arthritis. (2010). *MedlinePlus Medical Encyclopedia.* Retrieved 11.08.10 from http://www.nlm.nih.gov/medlineplus/rheumatoidarthritis.html

[4] Smith, H. R. (2010). Rheumatoid arthritis: Causes. *eMedicine from WebMD.* Retrieved 11.08.10 from http://emedicine.medscape.com/article/331715-overview

[5] Tsou, I. Y. Y., Peh, W. C. G., & Bruno, M. A. (2010). Rheumatoid arthritis, hand. *eMedicine from WebMD.* Retrieved 11.08.10 from http://www.emedicine.com/radio/topic877.htm

[6] Ibid.

[7] Koopman, W. J. (1997). *Arthritis and allied conditions: A textbook of rheumatology*, 13th edition, Volume I. Baltimore: Williams and Wilkins, p. 1043.

[8] Yazici, Y., et al. (2004). Morning stiffness in patients with early rheumatoid arthritis is associated more strongly with functional disability than with joint swelling and erythrocyte sedimentation rates. *J Rheumatol* 9:1723–1726.

[9] Likes, R. L. (2010). Boutonnière deformity. *eMedicine from WebMD.* Retrieved 11.08.10 from http://www.emedicine.com/orthoped/topic24.htm

[10] Koopman, W. J. Ibid., p. 1044.

[11] Koopman, W. J. Ibid., p. 1046.

[12] Neumeister, M., Nguyen, M-D., & Wilhlmi, B. J. (2008). Hand, rheumatoid hand. *eMedicine from WebMD.* Retrieved 11.08.10 from http://www.medscape.com/viewarticle/420502

[13] Lakshmanan, P., & Sher, L. (2008). Wrist arthritis. *eMedicine from WebMD.* Retrieved 11.08.10 from http://emedicine.medscape.com/article/1245097-overview

[14] Neumeister, M., et al. Ibid.

[15] Ibid.

[16] Koopman, W. J. Ibid., p. 1047.

[17] Ibid., p. 1048.

[18] Ibid., p. 1048.

[19] Calleja, M., & Hide, G. (2008). Rheumatoid arthritis, spine. *eMedicine from WebMD.* Retrieved 11.08.10 from http://www.emedicine.com/RADIO/topic836.htm

[20] Ibid.

[21] Koopman, W. J. Ibid., p. 1049.

[22] Ibid., p. 1050.

[23] The Nebraska Medical Center. (2008). *Neurosurgery: vertebral basilar insufficiency.* Retrieved 11.08.10 from http://www.nebraskamed.com/services/neuro/neurosurgery/vertebral_basilar_insufficiency.aspx

[24] Shiel, W. C. (2007). Felty's syndrome. *MedicineNet.com.* Retrieved 11.08.10 from http://www.medicinenet.com/feltys_syndrome/article.htm

[25] Swaak, A. (2006, August). Anemia of chronic disease in patients with rheumatoid arthritis: aspects of prevalence, outcome, diagnosis, and the effect of treatment on disease activity. *J Rheumatol.* Retrieved 11.08.10 from http://www.jrheum.com/subscribers/06/08/1467.html

[26] Ibid.

[27] Golding, A. (2006). *Anemia of inflammation: The missing link.* The John Hopkins Arthritis Center. Retrieved 11.08.10 from http://www.hopkins-arthritis.org/physician-corner/cme/rheumatology-rounds/anemia_inflammation_rheumrounds5.html

[28] Borigini, M. J. (2009). Felty's syndrome. *MedlinePlus Medical Encyclopedia.* Retrieved 11.08.10 from http://www.nlm.nih.gov/medlineplus/ency/article/000445.htm

[29] Shiel, W. C. (2007). Felty's syndrome. *MedicineNet.com.* Retrieved 11.08.10 from http://www.medicinenet.com/feltys_syndrome/article.htm

[30] Rheumatoid nodules. (n.d.). Duke Orthopaedics presents *Wheeless' Textbook of Orthopaedics.* Retrieved 11.08.10 from http://www.wheelessonline.com/ortho/rheumatoid_nodules

[31] King, R. W. (2006). Arthritis, rheumatoid. *eMedicine from WebMD.* Retrieved 11.08.10 from http://www.emedicine.com/EMERG/topic48.htm

[32] Maksimowicz-McKinnon, K., & Wilke, W. S. (2004). *Rheumatoid arthritis.* The Cleveland Clinic Foundation, Department of Rheumatic and Immunological Disease. Retrieved 11.08.10 from http://www.clevelandclinicmeded.com/medicalpubs/diseasemanagement/rheumatology/rheumarth/rheumarth.htm

[33] Ibid.

[34] Ibid.

[35] Marx, A. (1998–2007). *Case rounds—Case round #6.* The Johns Hopkins Arthritis Center. Retrieved 11.08.10 from http://www

.hopkins-arthritis.org/physician-corner/case-rounds/case6/6_case. html#overview

[36] Ibid.

[37] Shiel, W. C., & Stöppler, M. C. (2006). Vasculitis (Angiitis). *MedicineNet.com*. Retrieved 11.08.10 from http://www .medicinenet.com/vasculitis/article.htm

[38] Borigini, M. J. (2007). Raynaud's phenomenon. *MedlinePlus Medical Encyclopedia*. Retrieved 11.08.10 from http://www.nlm. nih.gov/medlineplus/ency/article/000412.htm

[39] Husby, G. (1985). Amyloidosis and rheumatoid arthritis. *Clin Exp Rheumatol* 3:173–180.

[40] Haggerty, M. (2002). Amyloidosis. *Healthline*. Retrieved 11.08.10 from http://www.healthline.com/galecontent/amyloidosis

[41] Arnett, F. C., et al. (1988, March). The American Rheumatism Association 1987 revised criteria for the classification of rheumatoid arthritis. *Arthritis Rheum* 31:315–324.

[42] American Rheumatism Association. (2003). *Diagnostic criteria for RA (2003 update)*. Retrieved 11.08.10 from http://www.rxed.org/ umce/TNFtable1.htm

[43] Borigini, M. J. (2007). Rheumatoid factor. *MedlinePlus Medical Encyclopedia*. Retrieved 11.08.10 from http://www.nlm.nih.gov/ medlineplus/ency/article/003548.htm

[44] Shiel, W. C. (2008). Rheumatoid factor. *MedicineNet.com*. Retrieved 11.08.10 from http://www.medicinenet.com/rheumatoid_factor/ article.htm

[45] Ibid.

[46] Morris, J. (2008). Joint replacement surgery of the hand. *MedicineNet.com*. Retrieved 11.08.10 from http://www.medicinenet.com/ joint_replacement_surgery_of_the_hand/page4.htm

[47] Neumeister, M., Nguyen, M-D., & Wilhlmi, B. J. (2008). Hand, rheumatoid hand. *eMedicine from WebMD*. Retrieved 11.08.10 from http://www.medscape.com/viewarticle/420502

[48] Morris, J. (2008). Ibid.

[49] Understanding rheumatoid arthritis medications. (2006). *eMedicine from WebMD*. Retrieved 11.08.10 from http://www.emedicinehealth. com/understanding_rheumatoid_arthritis_medications/article_em. htm

[50] Donahue, K. E., et al. (2008, Jan). Systemic review: comparative effectiveness and harms of disease-modifying medications for rheumatoid arthritis. *Ann Int Med* 148(2):124-134.

[51] Understanding rheumatoid arthritis medications. (2006). Ibid.

[52] Murphy ring splints. *North Coast Medical*. Retrieved 11.08.10 from http://www.ncmedical.com/item_1082.html

[53] Ahlman, A. (2004). Pathway to independence: physical therapy for patients with rheumatoid arthritis. *Medscape Today from WebMD*. Retrieved 11.08.10 from http://www.medscape.com/viewarticle/ 474935

[54] Iverson, M. D. (2007). Rehabilitation interventions are most effective when started early—physical therapy for the management of rheumatoid arthritis. *J Musculoskel Med* 24:269–276.

[55] Ibid.

[56] Clark, B. M. (2000). Rheumatology, 9. Physical and occupational therapy in the management of arthritis. *Can Med Assoc J* 163:999-1105.

[57] Houghton, S. (2006). Hydrotherapy for rheumatoid arthritis. Retrieved 11.08.10 from http://www.bestbets.org/cgi-bin/bets. pl?record=01041

[58] *Endless Pools. Rheumatoid arthritis aquatic therapy*. Retrieved 01.24.08 from http://www.endlesspools.com/why/therapy/ ther_alldredge.html

[59] Piva, S. R., et al. (2007, Aug). Neuromuscular electrical stimulation and volitional exercise for individuals with rheumatoid arthritis: a multiple-patient case report. *Phys Ther* 87:1064–1076.

[60] Vance, C. G. T., et al. (2007). Transcutaneous electrical nerve stimulation at both high and low frequencies reduces primary hyperalgesia in rats with joint inflammation in a time-dependent manner. *Phys Ther* 87:44–51.

[61] Ottawa Panel. (2004). Ottawa panel evidence-based clinical practice guidelines for electrotherapy and thermotherapy interventions in the management of rheumatoid arthritis in adults. *Phys Ther* 84:1016–1043.

[62] Koch, C. (n.d.). *Arthritis management: nutrition and rheumatoid arthritis*. The Johns Hopkins Arthritis Center. Retrieved 1.24.08 from http://www.hopkins-arthritis.org/patient-corner/disease-management/nutinra.html

[63] Ibid.

[64] Still's disease: systemic onset juvenile rheumatoid arthritis. (2007). *MedicineNet.com* Retrieved 11.08.10 from http://www.medicinenet. com/stills_disease/article.htm

[65] Ibid.

[66] Lee, S. (2007). Juvenile rheumatoid arthritis. *MedlinePlus Medical Encyclopedia*. Retrieved 1.24.08 from http://www.nlm.nih.gov/ medlineplus/ency/article/000451.htm

[67] Ibid.

[68] Juvenile rheumatoid arthritis. (2008). *MedlinePlus Medical Encyclopedia*. Retrieved 11.08.10 from http://www.nlm.nih.gov/medlineplus/ juvenilerheumatoidarthritis.html

[69] Still's disease: systemic onset juvenile rheumatoid arthritis. (2007). Ibid.

[70] Brewer, et al. (1973). Criteria for the classification of juvenile rheumatoid arthritis. *Bulletin Rheumatic Diseases* 1973:23:712–719

[71] Ibid.

[72] Lee, S. (2007). Ibid.

[73] U.S. Food & Drug Administration. (2006). *Celebrex approved to treat juvenile rheumatoid arthritis*. Retrieved 1.24.08 from http://www.fda.gov/bbs/topics/NEWS/2006/NEW01530.html

[74] Singh-Grewal, D., et al. (2007). The effects of vigorous exercise training on physical function in children with arthritis: a randomized, controlled, single-blinded trial. *Arthritis Rheum* 57:1202–1210.

[75] American College of Rheumatology. (n.d.). Ankylosing spondylitis. Retrieved 1.24.08 from http://www.rheumatology.org/public/ factsheets/as.asp?aud=pat

[76] Genetics Home Reference. (2008). *Genetic conditions: ankylosing spondylitis: what is ankylosing spondylitis?* Retrieved 3.30.08 from http://ghr.nlm.nih.gov/condition=ankylosingspondylitis

[77] American College of Rheumatology. (n.d.). Ibid.

[78] Brent, L. H., & Kalagate, R. (2010). Ankylosing spondylitis and undifferentiated spondyloarthropathy. *eMedicine from WebMD*. Retrieved 11.08.10 from http://emedicine.medscape.com/article/ 332945-overview

[79] Shiel, W. C. (2010). Ankylosing spondylitis. *MedicineNet.com*. Retrieved 11.08.10 from http://www.medicinenet.com/ankylosing_ spondylitis/article.htm

[80] Peh, W. C. G. (2009). Ankylosing spondylitis. *eMedicine from WebMD*. Retrieved 11.08.10 from http://www.emedicine.com/ RADIO/topic41.htm

[81] Arthritis Foundation. (2010). *Juvenile spondyloarthropathy*. Retrieved 11.08.10 from http://www.arthritis.org/disease-center.php?disease_ id=39

[82] Spondylitis Association of America. (2009). *Juvenile spondyloarthritis*. Retrieved 11.08.10 from http://www.spondylitis.org/about/ juvenile.aspx

[83] Shiel, W. C. (2008). Ankylosing spondylitis. Ibid.

[84] Ibid.

[85] Ibid.

[86] Di Lorenzo, A. L. (2006). HLA-B27 syndromes. *eMedicine from WebMD*. Retrieved 1.24.08 from http://www.emedicine.com/oph/ topic721.htm

[87] Brent, L. H., & Kalagate, R. (2010). Ankylosing spondylitis and undifferentiated spondyloarthropathy. *eMedicine from WebMD*. Retrieved 11.08.10 from http://www.emedicine.com/MED/ topic2700.htm

[88] Ibid.

[89] Ibid.

90 Peh, W. C. G. Ibid.

91 Brent, L. H. Ibid.

92 Van der Linden, S., Valkenburg, H. A., & Cats, A. (1984). Evaluation of diagnostic criteria for ankylosing spondylitis. a proposal for modification of the New York criteria. *Arthritis Rheum* 27:361–368.

93 Koopman, W. J. Ibid., p. 1198.

94 Peh, W. C. G. Ibid.

95 Spondylitis Association of America. (2009). *Medications used to treat ankylosing spondylitis and related diseases.* Retrieved 11.08.10 from http://www.spondylitis.org/about/medications.aspx

96 Ibid.

97 American Cancer Society. (2008). *Radiation therapy effects.* Retrieved 3.30.08 from http://www.cancer.org/docroot/MBC/MBC_2x_RadiationEffects.asp

98 Spondylitis Association of America. (2009). *Ankylosing spondylitis: Treatment.* Retrieved 11.08.10 from http://www.spondylitis.org/about/as_treat.aspx

99 Mayo Clinic. (2009). *Ankylosing spondylitis: treatments and drugs.* Retrieved 11.08.10 from http://www.mayoclinic.com/health/ankylosing-spondylitis/DS00483/DSECTION=treatments-and-drugs

100 Gonca, I., et al. (2006). Effects of a multimodal exercise program for people with ankylosing spondylitis. *Phys Ther* 86:924–935.

101 Arthritis: ankylosing spondylitis. (2008). *WebMD.* Retrieved 3.30.08 from http://www.webmd.com/back-pain/guide/ankylosing-spondylitis

102 National Psoriasis Foundation. (2005). *Psoriatic arthritis.* Retrieved 3.30.08 from http://www.psoriasis.org/about/psa/types.php

103 Hammadi, A. A., & Badsha, H. (2010). Psoriatic arthritis. *eMedicine from WebMD.* Retrieved 11.08.10 from http://emedicine.medscape.com/article/331037-overview

104 Levine, N. (2009). Psoriatic arthritis. *WebMD.* Retrieved 11.08.10 from http://arthritis.webmd.com/psoriatic-arthritis/psoriatic-arthritis-overview

105 Lohr, K. M. (2005). Psoriatic arthritis. *eMedicineHealth.* Retrieved 1.24.08 from http://www.emedicinehealth.com/psoriatic_arthritis/article_em.htm

106 Martin, D. (n.d.). *Psoriatic arthritis.* The Johns Hopkins Arthritis Center. Retrieved 02.03.08 from http://www.hopkins-arthritis.org/arthritis-info/psoriatic-arthritis/

107 Hammadi, A. A., & Badsha, H. Ibid.

108 National Psoriasis Foundation. Ibid.

109 Fearon, U., & Veale, D. J. (2001). Pathogenesis of psoriatic arthritis. *Clin Exp Dermatol* 26:333–337.

110 Myers, W., Opeola, M., & Gottlieb, A. B. (2004). Common clinical features and diseases mechanisms of psoriasis and psoriatic arthritis. *Curr Rheumatol Rep* 6:306–313.

111 Hammadi, A. A., & Badsha, H. Ibid.

112 Ibid.

113 National Psoriasis Foundation. Ibid.

114 Hammadi, A. A., & Badsha, H. Ibid.

115 Martin, D. Ibid.

116 Fearon, U., & Veale, D. J. Ibid.

117 Hammadi, A. A., & Badsha, H. Ibid.

118 Emery, P. (2004). *Psoriatic arthritis.* American College of Rheumatology. Retrieved from http://www.rheumatology.org/public/factsheets/psoriatic_new.asp

119 Hammadi, A. A., & Badsha, H. Ibid.

120 Burns, B., & Soliman. C. E. (2010). Reactive arthritis. *eMedicine from WebMD.* Retrieved from http://emedicine.medscape.com/article/808833-overview

121 Borigini, M. J. (2010). Reactive arthritis. *MedlinePlus Medical Encyclopedia.* Retrieved 11.08.10 from http://www.nlm.nih.gov/medlineplus/ency/article/000440.htm

122 Burns, B., & Soliman. C. E. Ibid.

123 Barth, W. F., & Segal, K. (1999). Reactive arthritis (Reiter's syndrome). *Am Fam Physician* 60:499–503.

124 Burns, B., & Soliman. C. E. Ibid.

125 Barth, W. F., & Segal, K. Ibid.

126 Ibid.

127 Borigini, M. J. Ibid.

128 Barth, W. F., & Segal, K. Ibid.

129 Ibid.

130 Borigini, M. J. Ibid.

131 University of Washington School of Medicine. (2005). *Reiter's syndrome: management and treatment.* Retrieved 1.24.08 from http://www.orthop.washington.edu/uw/tabID__3376/ItemID__52/mid__0/PageID__7/Articles/Default.aspx

132 Scleroderma. (2007). *MedlinePlus Medical Encyclopedia.* Retrieved 1.24.08 from http://www.nlm.nih.gov/medlineplus/scleroderma.html

133 Shiel, W. C., & Davis, C. (2010). Scleroderma. *MedicineNet.com.* Retrieved from http://www.medicinenet.com/scleroderma/page4.htm

134 Jiminez, S. A., et al. (2010). Scleroderma. *eMedicine from WebMD.* Retrieved 11.08.10 from http://www.emedicine.com/MED/topic2076.htm

135 Ibid.

136 Shiel, W. C. (2010). Systemic lupus erythematosus. *MedicineNet.com.* Retrieved 11.08.10 from http://www.medicinenet.com/systemic_lupus/article.htm

137 Shiel, W. C. (2007). Scleroderma. Ibid.

138 Ibid.

139 Ibid.

140 Jiminez, S. A., et al. Ibid.

141 Scleroderma. (2007). Ibid.

142 Koopman, W. J. (1997). Ibid., p. 1452

143 Steen, V. D. (2001). Treatment of systemic sclerosis. *Am J Clin Dermatol* 2:315–325.

144 Shiel, W. C. (2007). Scleroderma. Ibid.

145 Varga, J., & Abraham, D. (2007). Systemic sclerosis: a prototypic multisystem fibrotic disorder. *J Clin Invest* 117:557–567.

146 Jiminez, S. A., et al. Ibid.

147 Van Laar, J. M., Stolk, J., & Tyndall, A. (2007). Scleroderma lung: pathogenesis, evaluation and current therapy. *Drugs* 67:985–996.

148 Snadqvist, G., Eklund, M., Akesson, A., & Nordenskiöld, U. (2004). Daily activities and hand function in women with scleroderma. *Scand J Rheumatol* 33:102–107.

149 Sandqvist, G., Akesson, A., & Eklund, M. (2004). Evaluation of paraffin bath treatment in patients with systemic sclerosis. *Disabil Rehabil* 26:981–987.

150 Borigini, M. J. (2010). Systemic lupus erythematosus. *MedlinePlus Medical Encyclopedia.* Retrieved 11.08.10 from http://www.nlm.nih.gov/medlineplus/ency/article/000435.htm

151 Bartel, C. M., & Muller, D. (2010). Systemic lupus erythematosus. *Emedicine from WebMD.* Retrieved 11.08.10 from http://www.emedicine.com/MED/topic2228.htm

152 Ibid.

153 Ibid.

154 Ibid.

155 Ibid.

156 Borigini, M. J. (2010). Systemic lupus erythematosus. Ibid.

157 Bartel, C. M., & Muller, D. Ibid.

158 Ibid.

159 Borigini, M. J. (2010). Systemic lupus erythematosus. Ibid.

160 Bartel, C. M., & Muller, D. Ibid.

161 Rothlin, C. V., et al. (2007). TAM receptors are pleiotropic inhibitors of the innate immune response. *Cell* 131:1124–1136.

162 Lupus Research Institute. (2008). *Profound immune system discovery opens door to halting destruction of lupus.* Retrieved 3.30.08 from http://www.lupusresearchinstitute.org/press_article.php?2007_profound_discovery

163 Chakrabarty, S., & Zoorab, R. (2007). Fibromyalgia. *Am Fam Physician* 76:247–254.

164 *Fibromyalgia.* (2008). *MedlinePlus Medical Encyclopedia.* Retrieved 3.30.08 from http://www.nlm.nih.gov/medlineplus/fibromyalgia.html#cat5

165 American College of Rheumatology. (2010). *Fibromyalgia*. Retrieved 11.08.10 from http://www.rheumatology.org/practice/clinical/patients/diseases_and_conditions/fibromyalgia.asp

166 Chakrabarty, S., & Zoorab, R. Ibid.

167 U.S. Food and Drug Administration. (2007). *Living with fibromyalgia, first drug approved*. Retrieved 3.30.08 from http://www.fda.gov/consumer/updates/fibromyalgia062107.html

168 American College of Rheumatology. (2010). Ibid.

169 Shiel, W. C., Jr. (2007). Fibromyalgia (fibrositis). *MedicineNet.com*. Retrieved 1.24.08 from http://www.medicinenet.com/fibromyalgia/page2.htm

170 Schloss, P. W. (1998). The serotonin transporter: a primary target for antidepressant drugs. *J Psychopharmacol* 12:115–121.

171 Shiel, W. C., Jr. Ibid.

172 American College of Rheumatology. (2010). Ibid.

173 Chakrabarty, S., & Zoorab, R. Ibid.

174 Arthritis Foundation. (2010). *Fibromyalgic treatment options*. Retrieved 11.08.10 from http://www.arthritis.org/disease-center.php?disease_id=10&df=treatments

175 U.S. Food and Drug Administration. (2007). Ibid.

176 Shiel, W. C., Jr. Ibid.

177 Chakrabarty, S., & Zoorab, R. Ibid.

178 Mannerkorpi, K., et al. (2008). Experience of physical activity in patients with fibromyalgia and chronic widespread pain. *Disabil Rehabil* 30:213–221.

179 Rooks, D. S., et al. (2007). Group exercise, education, and combination self-management in women with fibromyalgia: a randomized trial. *Arch Int Med* 167:2192–2200.

180 Babu, A. S., et al. (2007). Management of patients with fibromyalgia using biofeedback: a randomized control trial. *Indian J Med Sci* 61:455–461.

181 Armagan, O., et al. (2006). Long-term efficacy of low level laser therapy in women with fibromyalgia: a placebo-controlled study. *J Back Musculoskel Rehabil* 19:135–140.

182 Hävermark, A-M., & Langius-Eklöf, A. (2006). Long-term follow-up of a physical therapy programme for patients with fibromyalgia syndrome. *Scand J Caring Sci* 20:315–322.

183 Giant cell arteritis [editorial]. (2007). *Rev Optom* 144(suppl):56A–58A.

184 Treatment of polymyalgia rheumatica and giant cell arteritis: are we any further forward [editorial]? (2007). *Ann Int Med* 146:674–676.

185 Alger, B. S., & Meskimen, S. (2006, October). Polymyalgia rheumatica (PMR). *Cortlandt Forum*, pp. 72–78.

186 Treatment of polymyalgia rheumatica and giant cell arteritis: are we any further forward [editorial]? Ibid.

187 Ibid.

188 Ibid.

189 Ibid.

190 Sowka, J. W., & Kabat, A. G. (2007). Which way to treat GCA? *Rev Optom* 144:90–91.

191 Kumar, A., & Costa, D. D. (2007). Insidious posterior circulation stroke with rapid deterioration due to vertebral giant cell arteritis. *Age Ageing* 36:695–697.

192 Szmodis, M. L., Reba, R. C., & Earl-Graef, D. (2007). Positron emission tomography in the diagnosis and management of giant cell arteritis. *J Head Face Pain* 47:1216–1219.

193 Bley, T. A., et al. (2007). Influence of corticosteroid treatment on MRI findings in giant cell arteritis. *Clin Rheumatol* 26:1541–1543.

194 Bley, T. A., et al. (2008). Mural inflammatory hyperenhancement in MRI of giant cell (temporal) arteritis resolves under corticosteroid treatment. *Rheumatology* 47:65–67.

195 Mahr, A. D., et al. (2007). Methotrexate to reduce corticosteroid doses. *Arthritis Rheum* 56:2789–2797.

196 Nothnagl, T., & Leeb, B. F. (2006). Diagnosis, differential diagnosis and treatment of polymyalgia rheumatica. *Drugs Aging* 23:391–402.

197 Munson, B. L. (2006). Myths and facts about polymyalgia rheumatica. *Nursing* 36:28–28.

198 Nothnagl, T., & Leeb, B. F. Ibid.

199 Alger, B. S., & Meskimen, S. (2006, October). Polymyalgia rheumatica (PMR). *Cortlandt Forum*, pp. 72–78.

200 Ibid.

201 Nothnagl, T., & Leeb, B. F. Ibid.

202 Ibid.

203 Ibid.

204 Alger, B. S., & Meskimen, S. Ibid.

205 Ibid.

206 Waxman, J. Ibid.

207 Travell, J. G., & Simons, D. G. (1983). *Myofascial pain and dysfunction: the trigger point manual*. Baltimore: Williams & Wilkins, p. 12.

208 McPortland, J. M., & Simons, D. G. (2006). Myofascial trigger points: translating molecular theory into manual therapy. *J Manual Manipulative Ther* 14:232–239.

209 Ibid.

210 Minty, R., Kelly, L., & Minty, A. (2007). The occasional trigger point injection. *Can J Rural Med* 12:241–244.

211 Ga, H., et al. (2007). Dry needling of trigger points with and without paraspinal needling in myofascial pain syndromes in elderly patients. *J Altern Complement Med* 13:617–623.

212 Srbely, J. Z., & Dickey, J. P. (2007). Randomized controlled study of the antinociceptive effect of ultrasound on trigger point sensitivity: novel applications in myofascial therapy? *Clin Rehabil* 21:411–417.

213 Esenyel, M., et al. (2007). Myofascial pain syndrome: efficacy of different therapies. *J Back Musculoskel Rehabil* 20:43–47.

214 McPortland, J. M., & Simons, D. G. Ibid.

215 Dommerholt, J., Bron, C., & Franssen, J. (2006). Myofascial trigger points: an evidence-informed review. *J Manual Manipulative Ther* 14:203–221.

216 Klusmann, A., et al. (2006). Painful rash and swelling of the limbs after recurrent infections in a teenager: polyarteritis nodosa. *Acta Paediatr* 95:1317–1320.

217 Chung, S. (2006). Polyarteritis nodosa. *eMedicine from WebMD*. Retrieved from http://www.emedicine.com/NEURO/topic314.htm

218 Hervé, F., et al. (2006), April). Ascites as the first manifestation of polyarteritis nodosa. *Scand J Gastroenterol* 41:493–495.

219 Shiel, W. C. (2007). Polyarteritis nodosa. *Medicinenet.com*. Retrieved 3.30.08 from http://www.medicinenet.com/polyarteritis_nodosa/page2.htm

220 Chung, S. Ibid.

221 Caldeira, T., et al. (2007). Systemic polyarteritis nodosa associated with acute Epstein-Barr virus infection. *Clin Rheumatol* 26(10):1733-1735.

222 Hervé, F., et al. Ibid.

223 Kato, T., et al. (2006, June). A case of cutaneous polyarteritis nodosa manifested by spiking high fever, arthralgia and macular eruption like adult-onset Still's disease. *Clin Rheumatol* 25:419-421.

224 The Johns Hopkins Vasculitis Center. (n.d.). *Polyarteritis nodosa*. Retrieved from http://vasculitis.med.jhu.edu/typesof/polyarteritis.html

225 Levine, N. (2007). Ulceration of left ankle and swelling of both legs. *Geriatrics* 62:32–32.

226 Chung, S. Ibid.

227 Shiel, W. C. Polyarteritis nodosa. Ibid.

228 Klusmann, A., et al. Ibid.

229 Hervé, F., et al. Ibid.

230 Shiel, W. C. Polyarteritis nodosa. Ibid.

231 National Institutes of Neurological Disorders and Stroke, National Institutes of Health. (2010). *NINDS complex regional pain syndrome information page*. Retrieved 11.08.10 from http://www.ninds.nih.gov/disorders/reflex_sympathetic_dystrophy/reflex_sympathetic_dystrophy.htm

232 National Institutes of Neurological Disorders and Stroke, National Institutes of Health. (2008). Ibid.

233 Duman, I., et al. (2007, September). Reflex sympathetic dystrophy: a retrospective epidemiological study of 168 patients. *Clin Rheumatol* 26(9):1433-1437.

234 National Institutes of Neurological Disorders and Stroke, National Institutes of Health. (2008). Ibid.

235 Ibid.

236 Duman, I., et al. (2007, September). Ibid.

237 National Institutes of Neurological Disorders and Stroke, National Institutes of Health. (2008). Ibid.

238 Ibid.

239 Swan, M. E. (2004). *Treating complex regional pain syndrome: a guide for therapy.* Reflex Sympathetic Dystrophy Syndrome Association. Retrieved 3.30.08 from http://www.rsds.org/pdf/ptotbrochure_604.pdf

240 National Heart Lung and Blood Institute. (2007). *Sarcoidosis.* Retrieved 3.30.08 from http://www.nhlbi.nih.gov/health/dci/Diseases/sarc/sar_whoisatrisk.html

241 Shiel, W. C. (2008). Sarcoidosis. *MedicineNet.com.* Retrieved 3.30.08 from http://www.medicinenet.com/sarcoidosis/page8.htm

242 Ibid.

243 Gould, K. P., & Callen, J. (2009). Sarcoidosis. *eMedicine from WebMD.* Retrieved 11.08.10 from http://emedicine.medscape.com/article/1123970-overview

244 Ibid.

245 Shiel, W. C. Sarcoidosis. Ibid.

246 Turchin, I., Nguyen, K., & Ménard, H. A. (2008). Cough, fever, joint pain, and tender nodules: what is your call? *Can Med Assoc J* 178:151–152.

247 Shiel, W. C. Sarcoidosis. Ibid.

248 Ibid.

249 Gould, K. P. Ibid.

250 Lwin, C. T-T., et al. (2003). The assessment of fatigue in primary Sjögren's syndrome. *Scand J Rheumatol* 32:33–37.

251 Shiel, W. C. (2010). Sjögren's syndrome. *MedicineNet.com.* Retrieved 11.08.10 from http://www.medicinenet.com/sjogrens_syndrome/page4.htm

252 The Sjögren's Syndrome Foundation. (2008). *About Sjögren's syndrome* Retrieved 11.08.10 from http://www.sjogrens.org/home/about-sjogrens-syndrome

253 Ibid.

254 Shiel, W. C. (2010). Sjögren's syndrome. Ibid.

255 Ibid.

256 Ibid.

257 Lwin, C. T-T., et al. Ibid.

258 Ostuni, P., et al (2002). Fibromyalgia in Italian patients with primary Sjögren's syndrome. *Revue du Rheumatisme* 69:56–63.

259 National Institutes of Neurological Disorders and Stroke, National Institutes of Health. (2008). NINDS Sjögren's syndrome information page. Retrieved 11.08.10 from http://www.ninds.nih.gov/disorders/sjogrens/sjogrens.htm

260 Sjögren's syndrome. (2003). *Merck Manuals Online Medical Library for Healthcare Professionals.* Retrieved 3.30.08 from http://www.merck.com/mmhe/sec05/ch068/ch068d.html

261 Shiel, W. C. (2007). Sjögrens syndrome. Ibid.

262 Ibid.

263 National Institute of Neurological Disorders and Stroke, National Institute of Health. (2007). Ibid.

264 Muscular Dystrophy Association. (2007). *Duchenne muscular dystrophy.* Retrieved 3.30.08 from http://www.mdausa.org/disease/dmd.html

265 Muscular Dystrophy Association. (2007). *Limb-girdle muscular dystrophy (LGMD).* Retrieved 3.30.08 from http://www.mdausa.org/disease/lgmd.html

266 National Institutes of Neurological Disorders and Stroke, National Institutes of Health. (2010). *NINDS muscular dystrophy information page.* Retrieved 11.08.10 from http://www.ninds.nih.gov/disorders/md/md.htm

267 Fascioscapulohumeral muscular dystrophy. (2009). *PatientUK.* Retrieved 11.08.10 from http://www.patient.co.uk/showdoc/40001404/

268 Centers for Disease Control and Prevention. (2008). *Duchenne/Becker muscular dystrophy.* Retrieved 4.21.08 from http://www.cdc.gov/Features/MuscularDystrophy/

269 Twee, D. (2007). Muscular dystrophy. *eMedicine from WebMD.* Retrieved 3.24.08 from http://www.emedicine.com/orthoped/topic418.htm

270 Muscular Dystrophy Association. (2007). Duchenne muscular dystrophy. Ibid.

271 Cyrulnik, S. E., et al. (2008). Duchenne muscular dystrophy: a cerebellar disorder? *Neurosci Behav Rev* 32:486–496.

272 Muscular Dystrophy Association. (2007). Duchenne muscular dystrophy. Ibid.

273 Ibid.

274 Twee, D. Ibid.

275 Ibid.

276 National Institutes of Neurological Disorders and Stroke, National Institutes of Health. NINDS muscular dystrophy information page. Ibid.

277 Twee, D. (2007). Ibid.

278 National Institutes of Neurological Disorders and Stroke, National Institutes of Health. NINDS muscular dystrophy information page. Ibid.

279 Centers for Disease Control and Prevention. Ibid.

280 Twee, D. Ibid.

281 Ibid.

282 Zeigler, T. (2003). Accurate and affordable diagnosis of Duchenne muscular dystrophy. National Institutes of Neurological Disorders and Stroke, National Institutes of Health. Retrieved 1.24.08 from http://www.ninds.nih.gov/news_and_events/news_articles/news_article_dmd_test.htm

283 Liu, Y., et al. (2007). Flk-1 adipose-derived mesenchymal stem cells differentiate into skeletal muscle satellite cells and ameliorate muscular dystrophy in MDX mice. *Stem Cells Dev* 16:695–706.

284 Ozasa, S., et al. (2007). Efficient conversion of ES cells into myogenic lineage using the gene-inducible system. *Biochem Biophys Res Commun* 357:957–963.

285 National Institutes of Neurological Disorders and Stroke, National Institutes of Health. (2008). NINDS muscular dystrophy information page. Ibid.

286 National Institutes of Neurological Disorders and Stroke, National Institutes of Health. (2007). *Myasthenia gravis fact sheet.* Retrieved 1.24.08 from http://www.ninds.nih.gov/disorders/myasthenia_gravis/detail_myasthenia_gravis.htm

287 Kantor, D. (2006). *Myasthenia gravis.* University of Maryland Medical Center. Retrieved 1.24.08 from http://www.umm.edu/ency/article/000712.htm

288 National Institutes of Neurological Disorders and Stroke, National Institutes of Health. *Myasthenia gravis fact sheet.* Ibid.

289 Ibid.

290 Hampton, T. (2007). Trials assess myasthenia gravis therapies. *JAMA* 298:29–30.

291 Romi, F., et al. (2006). Myasthenia gravis: disease severity and prognosis. *Acta Neurolog Scand* 183:24–25.

292 Hampton, T. Ibid.

293 National Institutes of Neurological Disorders and Stroke, National Institutes of Health. (2007). *Myasthenia gravis fact sheet.* Ibid.

294 Ibid.

295 Options for immunomodulatory therapy. (2001). *Drug Ther Perspect* 17(21).

296 Hampton, T. Ibid.

297 Options for immunomodulatory therapy. Ibid.

298 Romi, F. et al. Ibid.

299 Myositis. (2008). *MedlinePlus Medical Encyclopedia*. Retrieved 7.21.09 from http://www.nlm.nih.gov/medlineplus/myositis.html#cat42

300 National Institutes of Neurological Disorders and Stroke, National Institutes of Health. (2007). NINDS polymyositis information page. Retrieved 7.21.09 from http://www.nlm.nih.gov/medlineplus/myositis.html#cat42

301 Myositis. Ibid.

302 National Institutes of Neurological Disorders and Stroke, National Institutes of Health. Ibid.

303 National Institutes of Neurological Disorders and Stroke, National Institutes of Health. (2007). NINDS dermatomyositis information page. Retrieved 1.24.08 from http://www.ninds.nih.gov/disorders/dermatomyositis/dermatomyositis.htm

304 Ibid.

305 The Myositis Association. (2007). *Diagnosis of myositis*. Retrieved 3.30.08 from http://www.myositis.org/template/page.cfm?id=8

306 National Institutes of Neurological Disorders and Stroke, National Institutes of Health. Ibid.

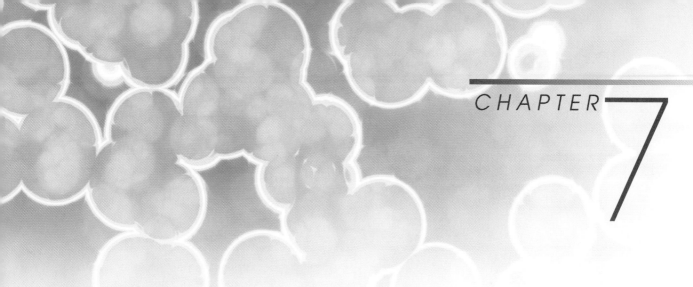

CHAPTER 7

Neurological Disorders

LEARNING OBJECTIVES

After completion of this chapter, students should be able to:

- Review the anatomy and physiology of the central nervous system
- Review the anatomy and physiology of the peripheral nervous system
- Describe central nervous system and peripheral nervous system diseases and conditions
- Identify specific medical tests used for people with neurological conditions
- Determine specific physical therapy interventions used for people with neurological conditions
- Analyze the use of the *Guide to Physical Therapist Practice* when treating people with neurological conditions

CHAPTER OUTLINE

KEY TERMS

Absolute refractory period

All-or-none response

Ascending and descending spinal tracts

Athetosis

Autogenic inhibition reflex

Axonotmesis

Blood-brain barrier

Brodmann's area of the brain

Choreiform movements

Clasp-knife effect

Clonus

Corticospinal tract and pyramidal decussation

Hemiballismus

Hydrocephalus

Meningocele and myelomeningocele

Motor unit

Myoclonus

Neurodevelopmental therapy/ training

Neuropraxia

Neurotmesis

Radiculopathy

Reciprocal inhibition reflex

Referred pain

Introduction

This chapter begins with a review of the anatomy and physiology of the neurological system at both the cellular and structural levels. The development of the nervous system in the fetus is explained and the motor development of the infant outlined. The various areas of the brain and central nervous system are described, as are the vestibular, limbic, autonomic, and peripheral nervous systems. Peripheral nerve lesions are explained, and a variety of medical and physical therapy tests performed on people with neurological disorders are described. Some of the more commonly used physical therapy interventions for people with neurological disorders are detailed. Finally, the neurological disorders, including those resulting from developmental abnormalities, are fully described to provide the pathological basis on which physical therapy interventions are predicated.

Why Does the Physical Therapist Assistant Need to Know About the Anatomy and Physiology of the Neurological System?

Physical therapy intervention can make a huge difference for people with neurological conditions, helping them to be more independent. The field of neurological medicine is fascinating and well worth the effort of learning how the neurological system works. Knowledge of the nervous system is crucial to an understanding of neuropathology. The complex central and peripheral nervous systems, the cellular structure of the neurons, and neural transmission need to be understood to unravel the complexity of neurological conditions. Many people, of all ages, with neurological conditions receive physical therapy intervention. Whether working in an acute care hospital, rehabilitation center, outpatient, home health, nursing home, or pediatrics setting, PTAs most likely will treat people with neurological conditions.

The Anatomy and Physiology of the Neurological System

The human nervous system is extremely complex. This section attempts to simplify the information as much as possible while still conveying an understanding of how this system works. The content of this chapter is not intended to be a definitive explanation of the human nervous system but rather to highlight its important aspects for gaining an understanding sufficient for the physical therapist assistant (PTA).

The nervous system consists of the central nervous system, including the brain and spinal cord and the peripheral nervous system, which consists of the spinal and cranial nerves. The main sections of the brain are the cerebrum; cerebellum; the brainstem, consisting of the pons, medulla, and midbrain; and the diencephalon, consisting of the epithalamus, subthalamus, hypothalamus, and the thalamus (see Fig. 7-1). The brain as a whole is the body's sophisticated computer system, processing all information received through the senses of hearing, smell, vision, taste, and touch. The brain also controls movement; enables speech, memory, cognition, and abstract thinking; controls the endocrine system; and regulates all the essential autonomic, nonvolitional (not consciously controlled by the mind) functions of life, such as heart rate, blood pressure, breathing, bladder and intestinal control, and temperature regulation. In addition to all these functions, the brain controls the emotions. This complex system regulated by the brain enables people to carry out the multiple functions a human being is capable of performing.

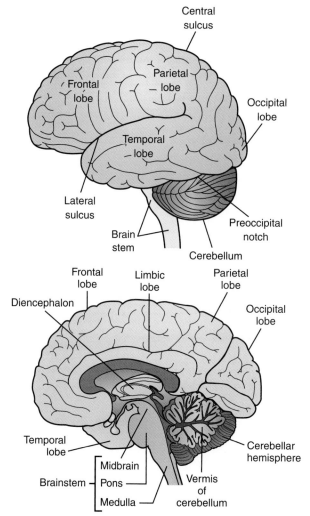

Central sulcus

Parietal lobe

Frontal lobe

Occipital lobe

Temporal lobe

Lateral sulcus

Preoccipital notch

Brain stem

Cerebellum

Frontal lobe

Limbic lobe

Parietal lobe

Diencephalon

Occipital lobe

Temporal lobe

Cerebellar hemisphere

Midbrain

Brainstem — Pons

Medulla

Vermis of cerebellum

FIGURE 7.1 The brain. (A) Showing lateral view (external surface). B. Showing medial view of one side of the brain.

Development of the Nervous System in the Fetus

The development of the nervous system begins during the first few weeks of gestation (development of the fetus within the uterus) and continues beyond birth. The myelination of the neurons begins about Week 8 of gestation and is not completed until approximately the age of 3 to 4 years in the child. After fertilization of the ovum by the sperm, a blastocyst of cells develops with the inner layers of cells, becoming the embryo. The early embryo has three layers: the ectoderm and endoderm, with the mesoderm in between. The ectoderm develops into the epidermis, the nervous system, and the sensory organs. The mesoderm becomes the dermis, skeleton, muscles, and

circulatory system. The endoderm becomes the digestive tract, liver, pancreas, and respiratory system. A neural tube of tissue starts to form out of the ectoderm at approximately 18 days of gestation of the embryo. This neural tube is the basis for the development of the whole nervous system. The neural tube starts as an open-ended structure, but once the tube closes at approximately 28 days of gestation, the brain starts to develop. The neural tube enlarges to form the rhombencephalon (hindbrain), mesencephalon (midbrain), and the prosencephalon (forebrain). The rhombencephalon becomes the pons, medulla, and cerebellum. The mesencephalon remains the midbrain, and the forebrain develops into the diencephalon consisting of the thalamus and hypothalamus, and the telencephalon consisting of the lateral ventricles and the cerebral hemispheres. At the same time the neural tube is developing, the mesoderm of the embryo starts developing into the vertebrae and skull from the part of the mesoderm called the sclerotome. Another section of the mesoderm, called the myotome, develops into skeletal muscle, and the dermatome develops into the dermis. The epithelial cells of the neural tube develop into neurons. As the neural tube develops further, axons from neurons associate with a group of muscles forming a myotome innervated by one spinal nerve, and an area of skin called a dermatome also supplied by one spinal nerve. The neural tube cavity becomes the spinal canal, through which the spinal cord passes and by which it is protected.

PRIMITIVE REFLEXES

Primitive reflexes, also called postural reactions or abnormal postural reflexes, are reflexes present in the child or adult which are no longer a normal response to stimuli after a certain age. In most instances, the presence of these reflexes indicates a central nervous system (CNS) problem. Each of the specific reflexes is characterized by a pattern of movement typical for that reflex.

One of the first people to describe these reflexes and their effect on movement disorders in CNS conditions was the physical therapist Berta Bobath (1985) in her book *Abnormal Postural Reflex Activity Caused by Brain Lesions* first published in 1965.[1] The presence of these reflexes is important to recognize when working with people who have CNS conditions. The knowledge is used in a system of physical therapy interventions known as **neurodevelopmental therapy (NDT),** based on the principles developed by Berta Bobath and her husband Karel Bobath. The following descriptions of the primitive reflexes are based on the concepts noted by Berta Bobath. The primitive reflexes can be subdivided into supporting reactions, and tonic neck and labyrinthine reflexes stimulated by the movement of the head on the body. In addition to these primitive reflexes, normal postural reactions, such as righting reactions and equilibrium reactions, start to develop after birth. In general, righting reactions start to develop immediately after birth and the equilibrium reactions at about age 7 months. These righting and equilibrium reactions continue throughout life unless a neurological problem arises. Some other responses and reflexes are associated with childhood development and maturity of the nervous system. Each of these is outlined in Tables 7-1 and 7-2.

Table 7.1 **Primitive Reflexes and Reactions**

NAME OF REFLEX OR RESPONSE	STIMULUS THAT PROMOTES REFLEX OR RESPONSE	EFFECT OF REFLEX OR RESPONSE
Positive supporting reaction	Passive dorsiflexion of the ankle/foot	Lower extremity (LE) extensor muscles contract
Negative supporting reaction	Return to plantar grade (90°) position of foot after dorsiflexion	Relaxation of the extensors of the lower extremity (in people with LE spasticity, full relaxation does not occur)
Crossed extension reflex	Weight bearing on foot	Increased extensor tone in weight-bearing leg and reduced extensor tone in opposite leg, allowing flexion to occur
Asymmetrical tonic neck reflex	Rotation of head on the body	Extension of the limbs on side toward which head is rotated with flexion on the opposite side
Symmetrical tonic neck reflex	Extension of the head	Increased extensor tone in upper extremities and increased flexor tone in lower extremities
	Flexion of the head	Increased flexor tone in upper extremities and increased extension tone in LEs
Tonic labyrinthine reflexes (often occurs with symmetrical tonic neck reflexes and difficult to separate the effects of each)	Supine position	Overall extension of spine and neck with shoulder retraction and extension and adduction of legs

Table 7.2 **Normal Postural Reactions and Other Associated Responses**

NAME OF POSTURAL REACTION OR ASSOCIATED RESPONSE	STIMULUS THAT PROMOTES REACTION OR RESPONSE	EFFECT OF REACTION OR RESPONSE
Labyrinthine righting reactions acting on the head	Stimulated by the effects of the position of the head on the inner ear	Keep the head in a normal position in space relative to gravity
Body righting reactions acting on the head	Stimulated by contact of the body with the ground or other surface through the tactile sensory receptors	Keep the head in a normal position in space relative to gravity and orient the person in space
Neck righting reflexes	Movement of the head causes the body to follow; proprioceptors in the neck muscles are stimulated	Keeps the body and head in alignment
Body righting reflexes acting on the body	Stimulation of tactile sensory receptors in the skin	Keeps the body in a normal position even when the head is not in the correct position

Table 7.2   **Normal Postural Reactions and Other Associated Responses** (continued)

NAME OF POSTURAL REACTION OR ASSOCIATED RESPONSE	STIMULUS THAT PROMOTES REACTION OR RESPONSE	EFFECT OF REACTION OR RESPONSE
Optical righting reflexes	Input to the optical centers in the occipital lobes of the cerebrum from the eyes	Keeps the eyes in a level orientation at all times
Parachute reaction	Response to a fall	Arms extend at the elbows and the fingers extend and abduct to protect the head during the fall; develops at 6 months of age in a forward direction, 8 months for sideways, and between 10 and 12 months in a posterior direction
Landau reflex	Extension of the head in prone	Extension of head is followed by extension of the whole body; this reaction usually disappears after 2 years of age.
Head righting response	Newborn placed in a vertical position with head balanced on the body	Newborn can maintain the head upright on the body in a vertical position for a few seconds
Primary standing	Newborn held vertically with feet on ground	Newborn can keep feet on ground once placed and extend the legs
Automatic walking	Newborn held vertically with feet on ground and moved forward	Infant starts taking steps
Moro reflex/response	Infant held in supine	If head goes into extension, the upper and lower limbs extend and adduct immediately followed by opening of the hands and flexion of the limbs to the midline. This response disappears at about 6 months of age.
Placing response	Infant held upright with dorsum of foot against the edge of a table	Infant steps with the leg and places the foot on the table; reaction occurs after about 10 days of age
Galant's reflex	Touching the skin of the infant between the 12th rib and the iliac crest	Lateral flexion of trunk toward the side of the stimulation
Crossed extension	Infant held with one leg in extension and the sole of the foot is rubbed	Opposite leg flexes and then extends and adducts with the toes in extension and abduction; this reaction disappears before 1 month of age
Grasp reflex/tonic reaction of finger flexors	Light pressure on palm of infant hand	Flexion of fingers and thumb of the hand; reaction disappears at 4 or 5 months of age
Toe grasp reflex/tonic reaction of toe flexors	Strong pressure applied to the sole of the infant foot	Flexion of toes; reaction disappears between 9 and 12 months of age
Rolling response	Infant placed in supine and the head is turned to one side	The hips and legs start to roll followed by the shoulders and thorax; this start of disassociated movement occurs at 4 months of age; before this, the infant rolls like a log in one piece when the head is turned
Balancing reactions	Child tilted to one side in sitting	The spine curves to keep the head in a position with the eyes level; occurs at the age of 5 months; newborns tilt their head to keep the eyes level

MOTOR DEVELOPMENT

Motor development of the infant and young child generally progresses at an accepted rate. The ability to evaluate the developmental level of a child relies on this sequence of progressively developing motor skills at an age-appropriate time. Some children do not go through the developmental process in exactly the prescribed sequence and may skip some of the stages. The age for performing a certain motor activity varies within a "normal" range. Several of the major milestones of motor development are listed in Table 7-3 as a guide to

Table 7.3 **Some Major Milestones of Motor Development**

AGE	MOTOR ABILITIES
1–3 months	Head lag during pull to a sitting position Rising on forearms Prone creeping
3–6 months	Vertical head control Rolls from prone to supine Sits with trunk support Prone resting on forearms or hands with head control
6–9 months	Rolls supine to prone and back Sits without support Reaches to play with feet Maintains an all fours position Takes weight through feet and steps if held upright
9–12 months	Moves from lying to sitting Crawls Stands supported Pulls up to stand Cruises in standing holding on to furniture Walks with hand held or alone at 12 months
12–18 months	Walks alone—wide base of support Kneels upright Squats when playing Stoops from standing to pick up toys Crawls up stairs, down on buttocks Starts to walk up stairs by 18 months Starts to run stiffly by 18 months
18 months to 2 years	Runs, changes direction, and stops Walks upstairs and downstairs holding on, one step at a time Walks backwards with toys Throws ball and attempts to kick a ball
2–2 ½ years	Climbs stairs without holding on, may alternate feet Descends stairs holding on, one foot at a time Runs Climbs simple apparatus Jumps both feet at once Stands on tiptoe Kicks large ball Walks with mature gait pattern Starts to ride a tricycle
2.5–3 years	Climbs stairs alternating feet Descends stairs alternating feet by 3 years Climbs more complex apparatus Able to walk in all directions and avoid obstacles Runs and walks on tiptoe Stands on one leg for a few seconds Walks on narrow board with assistance
3–4 years	Climbs ladders and trees Hops on one leg Throws and catches a ball Uses a bat
4–5 years	Dances Skips Hops for several yards on either foot Walks along a narrow line

the developmental sequence. This list only details some of the major gross motor activities of interest to physical therapist assistants; other developmental sequences include fine motor skills and cognitive functions, which develop along with the gross motor skills. This list is purely a guide and not intended to be part of an evaluative process performed by the physical therapist (PT).

The Neuron

The functional cells of the nervous system are neurons (refer to Fig. 7-2). Approximately 100 billion neurons are contained within the brain, all of which are present at birth. As a general rule, neurons do not regenerate, so once a neuron dies, it is gone permanently. These cells include a cell body, containing a nucleus, mitochondria, and Golgi apparatus; an axon that can be up to several feet long to extend the length of the spinal cord from the brain and transmits information to other parts of the body; and dendrites, attached to the cell body through which the

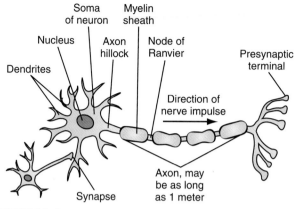

Soma of neuron
Myelin sheath
Nucleus
Axon hillock
Node of Ranvier
Dendrites
Presynaptic terminal
Direction of nerve impulse
Axon, may be as long as 1 meter
Synapse

FIGURE 7.2 A neuron.

neuron receives information from surrounding neurons or other cells. Some neurons are unipolar, having one axon, and others are bipolar with two axons.[2] Some axons are covered with a myelin sheath that insulates the axon and allows nerve impulses to travel faster along the length of the axon. Other neurons do not have a myelin sheath. Each neuron has a specific function. The sensory neurons detect stimuli from the senses such as touch, temperature, sharp and dull sensation, and the motor neurons supply the muscles with stimuli from the brain.

The myelin sheath wraps around the axon of the neuron in segments called internodes (areas of myelin between the nodes of Ranvier) with gaps between the segments called nodes of Ranvier. The internodes of axons in the peripheral nervous system are formed by an individual Schwann cell, whereas within the central nervous system the myelin is formed by other glial cells (nervous system cells) called oligodendrocytes. Yet other glial cells called astrocytes provide a network of support for the neuron cell bodies within the gray matter of the brain and spinal cord and for the bundled axons throughout the white matter.[3] Some other glial cells are macrophages that destroy any pathogens such as bacteria and viruses and the resultant debris that is produced when damage occurs to the neurons.

NERVE TRANSMISSION

The network of neurons only allows a one-way flow of information along the nervous system. If the information were to flow in both directions, the messages would be scrambled. Afferent neurons transmit information from the sensory nerve endings to the brain and efferent (think E for exit) neurons relay information from the CNS to the muscles. Interneurons make connections between neurons within the nervous system.

The mechanism of nervous transmission consists of both electrical energy (ions) and chemical transmitters. Neurons are able to change their electrical energy across the cell membrane rapidly. This electrical change is termed the electrical potential. These changes in electrical potential across the neuron cell membranes are responsible for the transmission of impulses along the neuron with passage of Na+ (sodium), K+ (potassium), and Cl– (chlorine) ions across the cell membrane. Under normal circumstances when the neuron is not transmitting any impulses, the concentration of NA+ and Cl- ions is higher on the outside than the inside of the cell, and the concentration of K+ ions is higher on the inside of the neuron. The actual potential within the neuron during the resting phase is more negative than that outside the cell. This is called the resting potential of the neuron with a value of approximately –70 mV (microvolts).[4] An electrical charge across the cell membrane ensures that the neuron is ready to receive electrical charges created by impulses within the brain or from sensory nerve endings within the tissues of the body. During the resting potential phase, ions pass freely in and out of the semipermeable neuron cell membrane. The active exchange of Na+ and K+ ions requires assistance from the adenosine triphosphate pump, which causes sodium ions to leave the neuron and potassium ions to enter the cell. When the membrane potential becomes less negative than the resting potential of the cell (e.g., changes from –70 mV to –55 mV), depolarization of the neuron occurs, creating an excitatory state during which an electrical impulse can be transmitted along the neuron. During depolarization Na+ ions pass into the neuron attracted by both the negative charge inside the cell and pushed by the high Na+ concentration outside the cell. Immediately after, depolarization a state of hyperpolarization occurs, during which the membrane potential becomes more negative than the resting potential of the neuron as K+ ions pass out of the neuron. During this hyperpolarized state, the neuron is less likely to transmit an electrical signal. Immediately after the hyperpolarization period repolarization of the neuron occurs with the neuron returning to its resting potential. After the neuron has transmitted an electrical impulse, a rest is needed to prevent impulses being transmitted in the opposite direction and to allow the neuron to return to its resting potential and become ready to receive further electrical impulses. This rest is called the refractory period. The refractory period is divided into the **absolute refractory period,** during which no stimulus can be transmitted, and the relative refractory period, when a stimulus must be extremely strong to create any effect on the neuron.

Several factors are responsible for changing the resting potential of the neuron. For an impulse to be transmitted along the neuron an action potential must be initiated. This action potential is a large depolarization of the neuron cell membrane sufficient to cause an electrical impulse to be transmitted. Cell membrane potentials are constantly changing, causing local changes in electrical potential. However, in order to activate a stimulus and thus an action potential the strength of the electrical impulse must exceed the threshold level for that particular neuron. Each type of neuron has a different threshold level specific to the purpose of the neuron. This initiation of the action potential is **all-or-none,** meaning that the stimulus is either large enough to exceed the threshold and stimulate an action potential, or it is not. The stimulus to create an action potential may be caused by either one large input or an accumulation of smaller impulses called a summation of impulses. Action potentials travel along the axon of the neuron from one node of Ranvier to another. The myelin sheath around the axons helps to reduce the leakage of voltage from the axon during the transmission of the impulse and speeds up the rate of transmission of the impulse. Each node of Ranvier has many voltage gated channels that increase the electrical potential as it travels along the neuron. In addition, electrical potentials exist at the synapses (junctions) between the axons of neurons and other cells or neurons at the synapse (see Fig. 7-3).

Each neuronal axon has between one and thousands of synapse connections with other neurons or cells. The synapse is a connecting gap between the end of the axon and the dendrites of other neurons or the cell body of another type of cell such as a muscle receptor. This gap is miniscule with a distance between 10 nm and 20 nm separating the two cells.[5] The synapse consists of the presynaptic and postsynaptic elements. The presynaptic element is the end of the axon of one neuron, and the postsynaptic element is the surface of the dendrites and part of a cell body of another type of cell. The presynaptic element releases neurotransmitter amine, amino acid, or peptide chemical substances into the synapse which enhance the transmission of the impulses across the synapse by changing the permeability of the receiving cell to accept the impulse. Several different neurotransmitters exist, some of which are listed in Table 7-4. Acetylcholine is the neurotransmitter produced at the neuromuscular junctions. The transmission of impulses across the synapse may be either fast or slow depending on the chemical makeup of the neurotransmitter. Acetylcholine causes a rapid transmission of impulses at the neuromuscular junctions. Other neurotransmitters, such as dopamine, serotonin, and norepinephrine, tend to mediate slower rates of transmission across the synapse. Depolarization occurs at the synapse much the same as in the axon of the neuron, except it is not called an action potential. The postsynaptic element of the synapse depolarizes in an excitatory postsynaptic potential (EPSP) similar to the action potential that serves as a reservoir for the electrical potential to reach a threshold necessary for the electrical impulse to be transmitted across the synapse. This is followed by an inhibitory postsynaptic potential (IPSP), which is a reversal or reduction of the threshold. Unlike the neuron

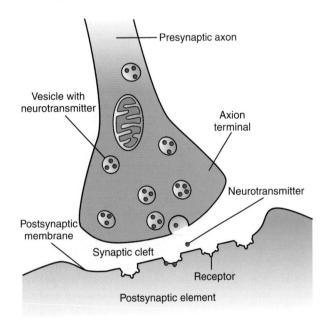

FIGURE 7.3 A synapse.

Labels: Presynaptic axon; Vesicle with neurotransmitter; Axon terminal; Neurotransmitter; Postsynaptic membrane; Synaptic cleft; Receptor; Postsynaptic element

Table 7.4 **Some of the Neurotransmitters Produced at Synapses**

TYPE OF NEUROTRANSMITTER	NAME OF NEUROTRANSMITTER
Amines	Acetylcholine
	Serotonin
	Dopamine
	Norepinephrine
Amino acids	Glycine
	Glutamate
Neuropeptides	Angiotensin II
	Endorphin
	Enkephalin
	Neurotensin
	Substance P

transmission, once a synapse has been activated, it becomes sensitized to additional impulses and may remain in a state of long-term potentiation, which allows the rapid transmission of impulses across that synapse for days or weeks. One of the theories for the development of memory and learning is that this long-term potentiation at the synapse opens up new pathways within the brain.[6] These new pathways enable the expansion of the network of neurons and increase the number of synaptic connections enhancing memory and learning.

Clinically, the refractory period for neurons is significant because in people with neurological conditions, the refractory period may become lengthened, and a longer rest period may be necessary between exercises to allow the neuron to return to its resting potential. The knowledge regarding electrical transmission along neurons is relevant when using electrical stimulation modalities. A number of medications can alter the rate of transmission of impulses across the synapse. Some of the medications that can enhance or depress synaptic transmission can be seen in Table 7-5.

MOTOR NEURONS

Approximately 1 million motor neurons exist in the human body.[7] The lower motor neurons lie in the spinal cord and the brainstem, and the primary motor cortex (upper motor neurons) lies in the cerebrum immediately anterior to the central sulcus of the cerebrum (see Fig. 7-4). Each motor neuron innervates an individual neuromuscular junction of a set of nerve fibers. The motor neuron and the muscle fibers innervated by that motor neuron are called **a motor unit.** The size of each motor unit varies. When a large degree of fine motor control is needed, such as in the muscles of the hand, the size of the motor unit is smaller. In such cases each neuron innervates fewer muscle fibers to control the muscle better. Larger motor units exist in larger muscles such as the quadriceps or hamstrings, because each neuron supplies many muscle fibers. Each muscle contains three types of muscle fiber—red, white, and intermediate fibers. The red fibers contain many mitochondria and are capable of sustaining a weak muscle contraction for a prolonged period of time. The white fibers have few mitochondria and are responsible

Table 7.5   **More Commonly Known Substances That Either Enhance or Depress Synaptic Transmission**

MEDICATIONS AND SUBSTANCES THAT ENHANCE SYNAPTIC TRANSMISSION	EFFECT
L-dopa	Converts into dopamine in the brain, able to cross the blood-brain barrier, used in the treatment of Parkinson's disease and other basal ganglia disorders
Benzodiazepine tranquilizers (e.g., diazepam, Valium)	Open channels in the axons
Barbiturate sedatives	Increase the opening time of gated channels in axons
Morphine mimics (e.g., opioid peptides)	Bind to receptors causing analgesia
Fluoxetine (i.e., Prozac)	Antidepressant that blocks serotonin reuptake
Cocaine	Blocks monoamine reuptake
Medications and Substances That Depress Synaptic Transmission	**Effect of substance**
Botulinum toxin	Blocks release of acetylcholine causing paralysis of the muscles
Strychnine	A poison that blocks gated channels within the axons causing convulsions
Curare	Arrow tip poison that blocks the nicotine acetylcholine receptors, causing paralysis
Haloperidol (Haldol)	Antipsychotic that blocks dopamine receptors

for more powerful, short, twitch contractions. The characteristics of the contraction of the intermediate fibers is somewhere between those of the red and white fibers. Even though three types of muscle fiber exist, each individual motor unit only consists of one type of muscle fiber. Because three types of muscle fiber exist and each motor unit includes only one type of muscle fiber, it should come as no surprise that there are three types of motor unit. The motor units are as follows:

- Type S = slow twitch (low force for a prolonged period of time)
- Type FF = fast twitch, easily fatigued (large force for a short period of time)
- Type FR = fast twitch, resistant to fatigue (moderate force for moderate period of time)

The control over the motor neurons is achieved through the primary motor cortex in the cerebrum (see Fig. 7-4). Areas of the body such as the feet, hands, and lips have a comparatively larger area of motor areas in the motor cortex than other areas of the body because they require a lot of fine motor control and therefore a greater number of motor units and neurons. An area of the cerebrum of the brain on either side of the central sulcus is called the sensorimotor cortex. This area includes the motor cortex, the premotor cortex, and the supplementary motor area (see Fig. 7-4). All three areas work together to control motor function. This extremely large area of the brain indicates the importance of muscle control for the body. When the upper motor neurons (UMN) are affected

by conditions such as a cerebrovascular accident, the effects can be divided into two separate responses. The immediate result of injury is a flaccid paralysis of the affected limbs due to spinal shock when the control over the lower motor neurons by the brain is lost. This flaccid paralysis is followed in a matter of days by spasticity in the affected limbs as the lower motor neurons (LMN) take over control of the muscles. This loss of control by the motor cortex has clinical implications because it results in increased stretch reflexes causing muscle tone to increase when muscles are quickly and suddenly stretched. If a slow stretch is applied to the muscles, less resistance is noted. Other manifestations of loss of UMN control include a **clasp-knife effect** in which there is a sudden release of spasticity and resistance during stretching of a muscle when Golgi tendon organs inhibit the motor neurons as part of the autogenic inhibition reflex; **clonus** or a rapid, intermittent contraction in response to a sudden stretch of the muscle; and the return of some primitive reflexes such as the Babinski reflex. A positive Babinski reflex is demonstrated when plantar stimulation is applied to the foot and the foot is withdrawn. This reflex usually is overridden by the motor cortex in the first few weeks of life; therefore, the presence of this reflex is indicative of damage to the CNS.

Central Nervous System

The CNS is generally divided into the cerebrum with its two hemispheres; the cerebellum; the diencephalon consisting of the epithalamus, subthalamus, hypothalamus,

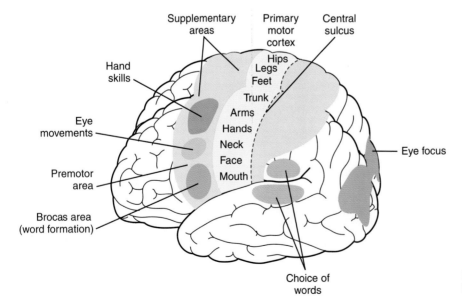

FIGURE 7.4 Location of motor areas in the cortex of the brain.

and the thalamus; the medulla, pons, and midbrain of the brainstem; the basal ganglia; and the spinal cord. For ease of understanding, the following section starts with descriptions of the blood supply to the brain and the cerebrospinal fluid (CSF), and then of the brain and the spinal cord. The cranial nerves, autonomic, parasympathetic and sympathetic nervous systems, and vestibular and limbic systems are also included in this section. No simple approach exists for the description of the CNS because all parts of the system are closely interrelated both anatomically and functionally. At times it may seem as if the description of one area does not make sense until the whole section has been read. Indeed, without a description of each part of the CNS, the whole cannot be understood, and it is impossible to describe the whole system at the same time.

The meninges are the protective coverings of the CNS. The outer layer of meninges is the dura mater, which attaches to the inner surface of the skull. This outer layer is thicker and consists of more collagen than the other two layers, has a blood supply from the meningeal arteries, has a nerve supply from the trigeminal nerve, and is sensitive to pain. The dura mater also provides a means of separating areas of the brain in the dural septa (singular septum). The septa between the two cerebral hemispheres is called the falx cerebri, and between the cerebrum and the cerebellum is the tentorium cerebella. The middle layer of meninges is the arachnoid mater. The pia mater covers the surface of the CNS and attaches to the brain. No real spaces exist between the layers of the meninges. The so-called epidural space lies between the skull and the dura mater, and the subdural space lies between the dura mater and the arachnoid mater. The CSF and the cerebral arteries and veins pass between the pia mater and the arachnoid mater in the subarachnoid space. The meninges continue down the spinal cord.

BLOOD SUPPLY TO THE BRAIN

The blood supply to the brain tissue is served by a network of arteries and both deep and superficial veins. The tissue of the brain is supplied by branches of the internal carotid artery and the vertebral arteries. The internal carotid artery divides into the middle cerebral and anterior cerebral arteries which supply most of the cerebral cortex and the diencephalon. The vertebral arteries supply blood to the brainstem, cerebellum, spinal cord, and the occipital and temporal lobes of the cerebral cortex. Two of the vertebral arteries join together near the medulla and form the basilar artery, which gives rise to the two posterior cerebral arteries and the anterior inferior cerebellar and superior cerebellar arteries. A unique system of arterial

supply to the brain through the circle of Willis ensures that the brain has alternative ways of receiving blood supply if one artery becomes blocked. This circle of Willis is formed at the base of the brain by connections between the anterior cerebral, internal carotid, and posterior cerebral arteries (see Fig. 7-5 for details). Some people who have a cerebrovascular accident have blockage of one of the arteries within the circle of Willis. Another unique feature of the blood supply to the brain is that the arterial vessels supplying the brain tissue form a **blood-brain barrier**. This barrier is formed by a combination of the arachnoid mater layer of the meningeal covering of the brain, the blood and CSF, and the endothelial cell layers of the cerebral capillaries. The capillaries have specialized selectively permeable membranes which allow glucose and lipid (fat) soluble substances to pass through but prevent transmission of bacteria into the brain tissue. One problem with this system is that it also prevents the passage of medications such as antimicrobials from reaching the tissue in the event of a bacterial infection resulting from direct trauma. The venous system of the brain is a network of superficial and deep veins of the cerebrum that ultimately drain into the jugular veins. The deep cerebral veins are different from other veins in that they have no valves since they drain downward. Within the brain itself the superficial veins empty into the superior sagittal sinus and the deep veins empty into the straight sinus, both of which are major collecting drainage vessels for the veins.

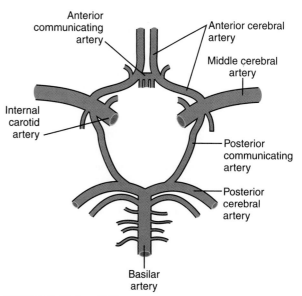

FIGURE 7.5 Circle of Willis.

CEREBROSPINAL FLUID

The CSF is a fluid that surrounds the brain and spinal cord. The cerebrospinal fluid is formed within the four ventricles of the brain. These ventricles are the lateral ventricle in each cerebral hemisphere, the third ventricle of the diencephalon, and the fourth ventricle within the pons and medulla of the brainstem between the lobes of the cerebellum. The two lateral ventricles communicate with the third ventricle via the interventricular foramina also known as the foramina of Monro, and the third and fourth ventricles communicate via the cerebral aqueduct (aqueduct of Sylvius). Thus all four ventricles are interconnected. The CSF is formed by the choroid plexus membrane within each ventricle. A total of approximately 150 mL of CSF is present within the brain and around the spinal cord, and only 25 mL of this lies within the ventricles.[8] New CSF is formed at a rate of approximately 0.5 L each day. This means that the total amount of CSF is renewed and replaced several times each day. The CSF circulates throughout the brain and spinal cord and is recycled through absorption into the venous system. The CSF serves several functions. This fluid acts as a shock absorber and buffer between the soft tissue of the brain and the skull, effectively creating a fluid bath in which the brain floats. The CSF also bathes the neurons of the CNS and assists the transport of hormones activated by the nervous system. When the drainage system for the CSF is compromised in any way, the amount of CSF within the ventricles builds up, expanding the ventricles and increasing the pressure on the brain tissue. This buildup of pressure is called **hydrocephalus.** The occurrence of hydrocephalus is a medical emergency that requires reduction of the pressure of fluid to prevent damage to brain tissue. A surgical procedure is performed to reroute the CSF away from the brain via a shunt and tubing draining into the abdominal cavity.

BRAINSTEM

The brainstem consists of the medulla, pons, and midbrain. The brainstem is the most primitive part of the brain, which is present in all the lower animals as well as humans and other mammals. Functionally this structure serves like a major highway system throughway for ascending sensory tracts to reach the thalamus and the cerebellum and descending motor tracts to reach the muscles via the spinal cord. The brainstem is a junction box for many of the cranial nerves and acts like a network computer for integrating control over the nonvolitional functions such as the respiratory and cardiac systems and level of consciousness. In addition, the brainstem integrates some of the more complex motor patterns of activity, such as walking, through its reticular formation.

The central canal of the medulla is a continuation of the spinal cord. At the junction of the medulla lies the pyramidal decussation where the spinal tracts cross over to the other side of the brain. Several cranial nerves emerge from the medulla, including the glossopharyngeal (IX), vagus (X), and hypoglossal (XII) nerves. See Table 7-6 for more information about the cranial nerves. Part of the vestibular network is housed in the medulla as the vestibular nuclei, and bulges of neuron cell bodies called trigones for the hypoglossal and vagus nerves are located here. Structurally the pons looks as if it is a bridge to the cerebellar hemispheres. This structure connecting the medulla and midbrain consists of the basal pons, the middle cerebellar peduncles, and part of the fourth ventricle. Other cranial nerves exit from the pons, including trochlear (IV), trigeminal (V), abducens (VI), facial (VII), and the vestibulocochlear (VIII) nerves. The third section of the brainstem is the midbrain, which consists of four mounds called the superior and inferior colliculi, two cerebral peduncles, the substantia nigra, and the reticular formation. The oculomotor nerve (cranial nerve III) emerges from the midbrain (see Table 7-5).

The midbrain is the center of the brain responsible for control of breathing, heart rate, blood pressure, and levels of arousal and consciousness. Different areas of the midbrain are under the control of various neurotransmitters, including norepinephrine, dopamine, serotonin, and acetylcholine (refer to Table 7-4). The reticular formation is a specialized area of the midbrain, which serves as a relay station for the sensory nervous system. In addition, the reticular formation modulates pain sensation through the pain-control pathways. Parts of the reticular formation also provide connections with the cerebellum. This area of the brain gives rise to the reticulospinal tracts, which control spinal motor neurons and regulate spinal reflex arcs to prevent unnecessary triggering of the deep tendon reflexes. These tracts carry descending motor tracts for some of the more basic, but complex, movements such as running and walking.

The substantia nigra releases the neurotransmitter dopamine and controls functions of movement including initiation of movement and normal resting muscle tone. Damage to the substantia nigra results in Parkinson-type problems, such as inability to initiate movements, muscle rigidity, and tremors.

Most of the 12 cranial nerves emerge from the brainstem. Exceptions to the rule include: the olfactory nerve (I) that arises as bundles of nerve axons in the olfactory

Table 7.6 **Cranial Nerves**

NO. OF CRANIAL NERVE	NAME	ORIGIN	FUNCTION	MUSCLES SUPPLIED	EFFECT OF DAMAGE TO NERVE
I	Olfactory	Olfactory bulb attached to cerebrum	Smell	None	Loss of smell
II	Optic	Diencephalon	Vision	None	Loss or partial loss of sight
III	Oculomotor	Midbrain	Eye movements	Eye: Inferior rectus Inferior oblique Medial rectus Superior rectus Levator palpebrae superioris	Ptosis of upper eyelid (drooping) Dilation of pupil Unable to move eyeball medially Lateral strabismus (eyeball moves laterally)
IV	Trochlear	Pons	Eye movements	Eye: Superior oblique Superior rectus	Vertical double vision—difficult to walk down stairs
V	Trigeminal	Pons	Sensory for skin of head Motor for muscles of mastication (chewing)	Mastication: Masseter Temporalis Lateral pterygoid Medial pterygoid	Inability to chew Trigeminal neuralgia or tic douloureux—severe pain in nerve distribution
VI	Abducens	Pons	Eye movements	Eye: Lateral rectus	Medial squint
VII	Facial	Pons	Sensory: taste buds, external ear Parasympathetic—salivary and lacrimal glands Motor—muscles of facial expression	Facial expression: Platysma Stylohyoid Digastric Stapedius of middle ear	Facial palsy of one side of the face—Bell's palsy
VIII	Vestibulo-cochlear (Cochlear nerve and vestibular nerve)	Pons and medulla	Auditory (cochlear) and balance (vestibular) Impulses from vestibular nerve are transmitted to the cerebellum	Vestibular nucleus complex acts as a relay station for impulses to the cerebellum; act on muscles of the eyes, neck and trunk Cochlear nerve	Balance disorders, loss of equilibrium Deafness—may be temporary or permanent

(table continues on page 276)

Table 7.6 **Cranial Nerves** (continued)

NO. OF CRANIAL NERVE	NAME	ORIGIN	FUNCTION	MUSCLES SUPPLIED	EFFECT OF DAMAGE TO NERVE
IX	Glossopharyngeal (tympanic nerve, carotid branch, pharyngeal branch, tonsillar branch, lingual branches)	Medulla	Sensory: taste, pain, temperature, touch for tongue; Visceral for control of blood pressure; Motor: pharynx, larynx, esophagus	Stylopharyngeus Salpingopharyngeus (sensory fibers to pharynx, tonsil, and posterior tongue)	Alteration of taste; Swallowing problems
X	Vagus	Medulla	Sensory: taste, pain, temperature, touch for tongue, pain for dura of brain; Visceral for thorax and abdomen to control cardiovascular respiratory, and alimentary functions; Motor: muscles of pharynx, larynx, and esophagus	Striated muscle of esophagus; Muscles of larynx and soft palate	Paralysis of soft palate and larynx; Difficulty breathing, swallowing
XI	Accessory	Medulla and ventral horn spinal cord	Motor to trapezius and sternocleidomastoid	Trapezius Sternocleidomastoid (SCM)	Paralysis or weakness of trapezius and SCM
XII	Hypoglossal	Medulla	Intrinsic and extrinsic muscles of tongue	Extrinsic tongue: genioglossus styloglossus hyoglossus	Deviation of tongue toward the weak side

bulb, which is attached to the interior part of the cerebrum close to the brainstem; the optic nerve (II) forms the optic chiasm where half of the nerves cross over to supply the opposite eye and is closely related to the diencephalon (thalamus); and the accessory nerve (XI), which arises both from the medulla and the ventral horn of the upper spinal cord.

BASAL GANGLIA

The basal ganglia lie within the brainstem enfolded by the cerebral cortex. This collection of neuronal motor cell bodies consists of the caudate nucleus, putamen, nucleus accumbens, globus pallidus, substantia nigra, and the subthalamic nucleus. The function of the basal ganglia is control of body movement by inhibiting the thalamus. The basal ganglia also produce neurotransmitter substances, of which dopamine is the most prevalent. The two areas of

the basal ganglia most commonly heard about are the globus pallidus and substantia nigra since damage or dysfunction of these areas is responsible for most of the movement disorders associated with the basal ganglia. The caudate and putamen receive input from the cerebral cortex, with the output going to the globus pallidus and substantia nigra. Both the substantia nigra and globus pallidus receive input from the caudate and putamen and send information to the thalamus.

Damage to the basal ganglia may result in a variety of movement disorders depending on the area affected. Some of these include the increased muscle tone resulting in lead-pipe rigidity and cogwheel rigidity associated with Parkinson's disease; resting tremors also associated with Parkinson's disease; involuntary **choreiform movements** associated with Huntington's disease; the slow, involuntary, writhing movements of limbs known as **athetosis**;

and **hemiballismus,** the flailing movements of one arm or leg associated with damage to the subthalamic nucleus.

Diencephalon

The diencephalon lies deep within the brain and consists of the epithalamus, subthalamus, hypothalamus, and the thalamus. The main areas of interest for the physical therapist assistant are the hypothalamus and the thalamus. The thalamus accounts for approximately 80% of the diencephalon.[9] The thalamus acts as a relay station for the sensory pathways from peripheral sensory receptors to the cerebellum, basal ganglia, and limbic system and also receives input from the cerebral cortex. The thalamus is functionally like the main sorting area of a post office, which decides which mail is sent priority and which is considered junk mail. The thalamus selects which impulses will be transmitted to the cerebral cortex. The difference in the thalamus is that not all the incoming impulses "mail" will reach other areas of the brain. The epithalamus contains the pineal gland, which secretes the neurotransmitter melatonin and is thought to be associated with circadian rhythms (the sleeping and waking cycles) and sexual behavioral urges. The subthalamus contains part of the substantia nigra and acts as a channel for the sensory pathways on route toward the thalamus, cerebellum, and basal ganglia. The hypothalamus functions like a major electrical connection box for neuronal pathways to the limbic system, the motor and sensory centers of the brain, and the pituitary gland. The hypothalamus is discussed further in the section on the limbic system.

Cerebellum

The cerebellum partially surrounds the brainstem and is sometimes called the little brain. The cerebellum receives inputs from the vestibular, spinal, and cerebral cortical tracts and from the visual and auditory centers of the brain. The outgoing information is relayed to the brainstem and the thalamus through the Purkinje cells within several nuclei of the cerebellum. The main function of the cerebellum involves postural control of muscles, balance, and coordination. The use of functional magnetic resonance imaging (fMRI) scanning has shown that the cerebellum also works with the cerebrum for motor planning activities, motor learning, and cognitive functions (activities of the brain that require reasoning). Much of the function of the cerebellum has been discovered through people with disorders affecting this part of the brain. Damage to the cerebellum causes motor deficits which result in loss of coordination of voluntary movement, such as a staggering gait with a broad base of support with the feet set wide apart, ataxia (an uncoordinated movement of the body), changes in muscle tone including hypotonia (increased muscle tone), dysmetria (over- or underestimating distance when performing an activity such as picking up a glass), dysdiadochokinesia (inability to perform rapidly alternating movements), and a scanning speech resulting from problems using the muscles of the mouth characterized by words spoken deliberately, and slowly, with pauses between each word.

Cerebrum

The cerebrum consists of two cerebral hemispheres, the right and left, covered by a layer of cerebral cortex containing approximately 25 billion neurons, the outer part of which is the neocortex. The two cerebral hemispheres are connected by the corpus callosum and the anterior commissure. Each hemisphere is divided into several lobes. Different areas of the cerebral cortex are associated with different functions. The functions of the cerebrum include language, abstract thought, perception, movement, and adaptation to the environment. Some of the neurons of the cerebrum are called pyramidal cells, and those specific to the motor cortex are Betz cells. The pyramidal cells have long axons that connect with other parts of the brain. Other neurons within the cerebral cortex are nonpyramidal and have shorter axons. The pyramidal cells have dendritic spines, which are thought to be associated with learning. The primary sensory areas receive input from the nuclei of the thalamus. The primary motor area or primary motor cortex, known as **Brodmann's area,** is the origin of the corticospinal tract. Together with the premotor and supplementary motor area, this motor cortex controls all muscle movement (refer to Fig. 7-4). The association areas of the cerebrum are related to auditory, visual, and higher mental functions. The visual area lies in the occipital region (posterior part of the head) and the auditory area in the temporal lobe of the cerebrum (area beneath the temporal bones of the skull). The cerebrum also connects with the limbic system, which is described separately. Many areas of the cerebrum still have unknown functions.[10]

As a general rule, the left cerebral hemisphere is the dominant one (the opposite hemisphere) in 95% of people who are right-handed. Left-handed people often have the left hemisphere as dominant but more likely have the right side of the brain as the dominant hemisphere. The dominant cerebral hemisphere is responsible for the production and comprehension of language. In left-handed people, the language centers may be in the right hemisphere or partially in both hemispheres. The language centers of the left hemisphere are known as Broca's area and Wernicke's area. Functionally the left hemisphere is known to control language, mathematical ability, and logical problem solving abilities. The right hemisphere is responsible for spatial orientation, the ability to produce tonal differences and understand tonal changes in other people's language, the ability to recognize faces, and musical ability. These are generalizations when discussing the functions of the cerebrum because the connecting network still is not understood fully. Some of the deficits caused by loss of function in areas of the cerebrum are described in Table 7-7. The cerebrum also is involved in the regulation of the sleep cycle together with parts of the midbrain, pons, medulla, and hypothalamus. During paradoxical sleep, sometimes called desynchronized sleep or rapid eye movement (REM) sleep, the cerebral cortex may be in an active state, although the sensory pathways usually are inhibited so that no actual muscular movement occurs. During this phase of sleep, there is little muscle tone, the blood pressure is reduced, the heart rate and breathing rate become rather erratic, and REM occurs. During the synchronized/slow-wave sleep often called deep sleep, the muscle tone is reduced significantly, and both the heart rate and blood pressure are reduced.[11]

SPINAL CORD

The spinal cord is part of the CNS extending approximately 42 to 45 cm in length from the base of the brain to the level of the junction between the first and second lumbar vertebrae (L1/L2). At its widest point, the spinal cord is approximately 1 cm in diameter. The spinal cord runs through the spinal canal formed by the vertebrae. The cord is divided into 31 segments by the spinal nerve roots, 8 cervical, 12 thoracic, 5 lumbar, 5 sacral, and 1 coccygeal. The nerve roots from cervical 1 (C1) to cervical 7 (C7) exit superior to (above) the vertebra of the same number, whereas cervical 8 (C8) exits distal to (below) the seventh cervical vertebra and the rest of the nerve roots exit distal to each vertebra of the same number. The nerve roots from the dorsal and ventral sides of the cord join together to form a dorsal root ganglion, which contains sensory neuron cell bodies that supply that particular

Table 7.7 **Some Deficits Resulting From Damage to Areas of the Brain**

AFFECTED AREA	NAME (IF APPROPRIATE)	DESCRIPTION
Left cerebral hemisphere	Aphasia	Loss of ability to use language
Broca's area	Broca's aphasia	Loss of ability to speak and write language (may still comprehend language)
Wernicke's area	Wernicke's aphasia	Unable to understand language and sequencing is incorrect; still able to produce words
	Paraphasia	Substitution of words or phrases with incorrect words or phrases
	Neologisms	The use of meaningless words
	Jargon aphasia	Use of words and phrases that do not make any sense
Right cerebral hemisphere	"Neglect" of one side of the body	Loss of spatial orientation as a result of damage to the right cerebral hemisphere; often appears as left-sided neglect for people who have had a right cerebrovascular accident
	Agnosia	Inability to recognize objects which may be visual, tactile, or both
	Apraxia	Inability to perform movements on command
	Motor aprosodia	Inability to put any tone or emotion in speech
	Sensory aprosodia	Inability to be able to understand the tone or emotion in other people's speech
Dorsal and lateral prefrontal cortex of cerebrum	Loss of working memory	Inability to plan any activities, solve problems, or concentrate and be attentive
Amygdala	Short-term and working memory loss	Impulsivity, inappropriate actions

spinal nerve root. Each spinal nerve segment (except C1) innervates an area of skin called a dermatome and an area of muscle called a myotome. Two enlargements are situated along the spinal cord. The cervical enlargement gives rise to the nerve roots of C5 through T1, which supply the upper extremities, and the lumbosacral enlargement gives rise to the L2 through S3 nerve roots that supply the lower extremities. The distal tip of the spinal cord is called the conus medullaris, and it is anchored to the coccyx by the filum terminale. The dural sheath that surrounds the spinal cord is a continuation of the meninges surrounding the brain and ends at the level of the second sacral vertebra (S2). Between the end of the spinal cord at the level of L1/L2 and the end of the dural sheath at S2 lies the lumbar cistern. Within the lumbar cistern lie the dorsal and ventral nerve roots of the cauda equina, so named because it looks like a horse's tail.[12] These nerve roots are bathed in CSF, which lies within the subarachnoid space. The lumbar cistern is an ideal location to draw samples of CSF because it contains no spinal cord, and there is less possibility of causing nerve damage with a needle. Unlike the epidural space of the brain, the epidural space of the spine is an actual space that contains connective tissue and the vertebral veins.

On cross-section the spinal cord appears fairly round with an H-shaped area of gray matter and the surrounding areas of white matter (see Fig. 7-6). In general, the gray matter is composed of neuronal cells, giving it a more dense appearance and the white matter consists of the axons of neurons. The white matter consists of the spinal tracts of ascending sensory neuron axons and the descending motor neuron axons. **Ascending tracts** (sensory) go from the sensory receptors of the skin and viscera to the brain and the **descending tracts** (motor) go from the brain to the muscles. See Table 7-7 for details of ascending and descending tracts. A small area called the anterior white commissure connects the two uprights of the "H." The motor neuron cell bodies to skeletal muscles lie in the anterior horn (ventral horn) of the spinal cord. The anterior horn is larger in the cervical and lumbar areas of the cervical and lumbosacral enlargements of the spinal cord as a result of the vast number of motor neurons for supply to the upper and lower extremities respectively. The cell bodies of these large motor neurons also are known as lower motor neurons because they lie within the spinal cord rather than the brain. Two other parts of the anterior horn include the spinal accessory nucleus in the upper cervical area where the accessory nerve forms and the phrenic nucleus between C3 and C5 where the phrenic nerve exits to supply the diaphragm. The posterior horn

(dorsal horn) of gray matter mainly contains sensory neurons to the viscera. The tip or cap of the posterior horn is the substantia gelatinosa and contains sensory fibers for pain and temperature. The area of gray matter between the anterior and posterior horns called the intermediate area contains the neurons of the autonomic nervous system. A specialized area of autonomic neurons called the Clarke's nucleus or nucleus dorsalis lies in this area between the levels of T1 and L2. Clarke's nucleus is of special interest to physical therapists because the neurons located here are specialized for communicating with the cerebellum for balance and coordination and also transmit proprioceptive information to the thalamus.

As previously described, the white matter of the spinal cord contains the ascending sensory and descending motor tracts. The ascending tracts transmit neuronal fibers (axons) to the thalamus, cerebellum, and the brainstem. The descending fibers (axons) pass from the cerebral cortex and brainstem to the motor neurons of the spinal gray matter of the anterior horn. An extensive number of tracts exist, but some specific tracts are relevant to the physical therapist assistant and are detailed in Table 7-8 and highlighted in Figure 7-6. The ascending tracts start with the prefix "spino" for spinal and end with the name of the destination. The descending tracts start with the prefix according to the area of the brain they arise from and end with the suffix "spinal." The most important descending pathway is the **corticospinal tract** responsible for carrying information from the cerebral cortex, through the pons and medulla, and to the anterior horn of the spinal cord, where it goes to the muscles responsible for voluntary movement. Most of the fibers in this tract cross over to the opposite side of the spinal cord at the **pyramidal decussation** immediately distal to the medulla. This crossing over of the fibers in the tracts accounts for damage to the motor cortex of the brain resulting in weakness or paralysis of muscles on the opposite side of the body from the brain damage. Of note is that damage to the upper motor neurons in the motor cortex of the brain results in spastic weakness and paralysis of muscles whereas damage to the lower motor neurons in the anterior horn of the spinal cord usually results in flaccid (floppy) paralysis and the loss of deep tendon reflexes.

Several reflex arcs are formed within the spinal cord. These reflex arcs mainly are concerned with protection because feedback from the brain is not required to elicit a response. The main four spinal reflex arcs of significance for the physical therapist assistant are: the **stretch reflex** (see Fig. 7-7 for details) also called the **deep tendon reflexes** or the tonic stretch reflex; the **withdrawal reflex**,

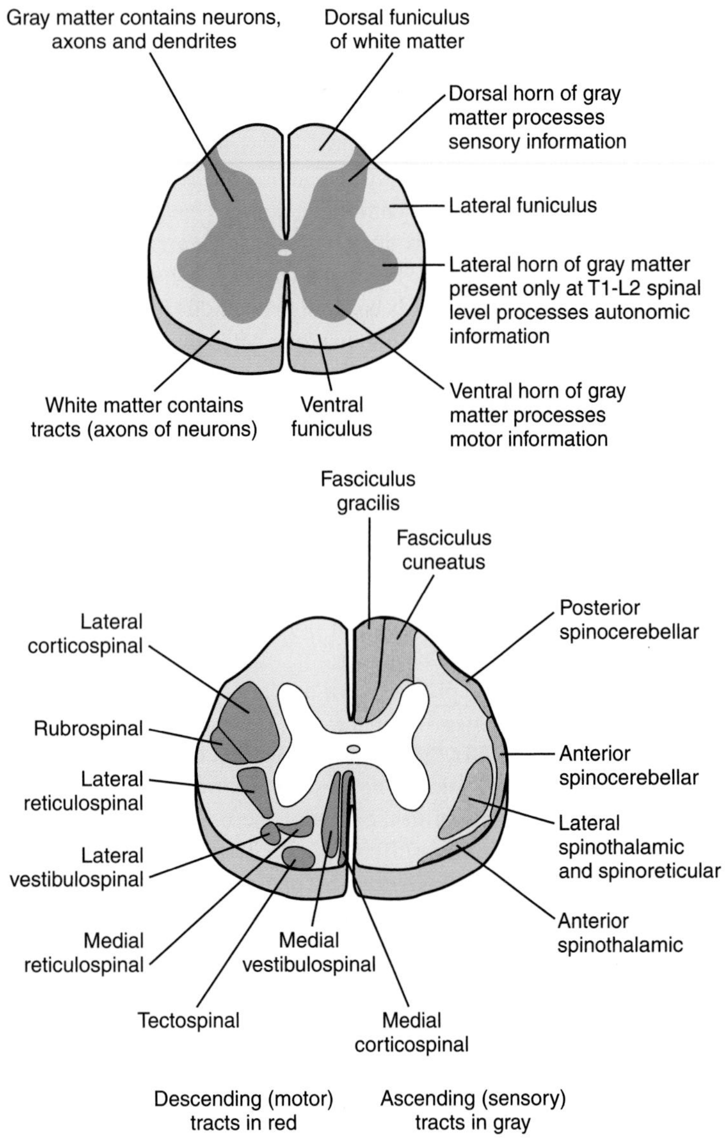

Gray matter contains neurons, axons and dendrites

Dorsal funiculus of white matter

Dorsal horn of gray matter processes sensory information

Lateral funiculus

Lateral horn of gray matter present only at T1-L2 spinal level processes autonomic information

Ventral horn of gray matter processes motor information

White matter contains tracts (axons of neurons)

Ventral funiculus

Fasciculus gracilis

Fasciculus cuneatus

Posterior spinocerebellar

Lateral corticospinal

Rubrospinal

Lateral reticulospinal

Lateral vestibulospinal

Anterior spinocerebellar

Lateral spinothalamic and spinoreticular

Anterior spinothalamic

Medial reticulospinal

Medial vestibulospinal

Tectospinal

Medial corticospinal

Descending (motor) tracts in red

Ascending (sensory) tracts in gray

FIGURE 7.6 Cross section of the spinal cord. (A) Main areas of gray and white matter. (B) Ascending (sensory) tracts and descending (motor) tracts. (The descending and ascending tracts travel on both sides of the spinal cord. The figure shows them separately for clarity.)

Table 7.8 **Some of the Main Spinal Tracts of the White Matter of the Spinal Cord With Their Functions**

TRACT	TYPE OF FIBERS TRANSMITTED
Ascending tracts Anterior spinocerebellar	Coordination, complex tactile information, reflex information (tract crosses to opposite side of the brain in the spinal cord)
Posterior spinocerebellar	Proprioception, pressure, tactile sensation (tract does not cross over)
Spinocervical	Tactile information
Spinothalamic	Pain and temperature
Descending tracts Lateral corticospinal (Pyramidal)	Voluntary muscles mainly of the limbs (this tract crosses within the decussate pyramid)
Anterior corticospinal	Voluntary muscles mainly of the trunk (fibers do not cross)

reciprocal inhibition reflex, and **autogenic inhibition** reflex. These simple feedback loops are contained within the spinal cord and consist of two neurons and one synapse. When stretch is applied to a tendon, such as the patella tendon with a reflex hammer, an afferent fiber from the muscle spindle transmits the information to an alpha motor neuron in the anterior horn of the spinal cord which then loops back to the muscle causing it to contract. This particular stretch reflex is the knee-jerk reflex. The withdrawal reflex is elicited when skin receptors detect a sharp or hot stimulus that is potentially dangerous. The feedback loop of the spinal reflex causes the affected part to be withdrawn away from the stimulus. This reflex also has a crossover response. If the foot or hand is withdrawn from a stimulus in a flexor response, the opposite limb responds by going into extension to counteract the unbalancing effect of the movement response. The reciprocal inhibition effect occurs in all of the spinal reflexes causing a simultaneous relaxation through inhibition of the neurons of the antagonist muscles at the same time as the synergist muscle is stimulated to contract. In effect the reciprocal inhibition prevents the antagonists from interfering with the action of the agonist muscles during contraction. An autogenic inhibition occurs when specific Ib neuron fibers from the Golgi tendon organ are stimulated and actually inhibit the muscle from contracting through a system of inhibitory interneurons within the spinal cord between the incoming afferent and outgoing efferent neurons for the reflex. In a person with an intact nervous system, the autogenic inhibition serves to prevent overstretching to a muscle by reducing the contraction of the muscle, and may prevent tendon and muscle tears.[13] This autogenic inhibition effect is sometimes noted in neurological conditions in which the descending motor neurons are damaged. The spasticity of the muscles resists movement of the joints. When manual force is applied to the limb, a sudden release of spasticity is noted, thought to be the result of the autogenic inhibition. The sudden release of the spasticity of muscles during such a movement is termed the clasp-knife effect because the sudden release of the muscle is similar to a folded knife clicking back into place when closed.

VESTIBULAR SYSTEM

The vestibular system is concerned with the position of the body in relation to gravity and the position of the eyes in relation to the environment to keep the body in a stable position. The system comprises the semicircular canals, utricle, and saccule of the labyrinth and the cochlear of the inner ear (the vestibular part of the inner ear is described in Chapter 14); the vestibular nerve (cranial VIII) with its neuron cell body located in the vestibular ganglion of the spinal cord; the eyes; and the four vestibular nuclei, lateral, medial, superior, and inferior of the medulla. Some input from the vestibular nerve goes from the inner ear directly to the cerebellum, thalamus, and cerebral cortex. The spinal tracts associated with the vestibular system are the ascending vestibulo-ocular to the eyes, and the descending motor medial and lateral vestibulospinal tracts. The descending vestibulospinal tracts terminate in the postural muscles of the upper and lower extremities, the trunk, and cervical spine. Information from the semicircular canals indicates movement of the head. This is transmitted to the muscles, which then respond to keep the body in a stable position according to gravity.[14] During static posture, the utricle and saccule relay information to the muscles so that the body can determine where the head is in space. This function plays a part in maintenance of normal postural alignment.[15] The sensory input to the vestibular system is provided by proprioceptors in the joints and muscles and pressure and tactile skin receptors. Disorders of the vestibular system can result in a variety of symptoms, including loss of balance, anxiety and fatigue, dizziness, vertigo (spinning sensation), and inability to concentrate.[16]

LIMBIC SYSTEM

The limbic system is the name for a collection of structures within the brain associated with emotions, especially fear and anger, mood, and social behavior, including sexual activity and appetite for food, recognition of emotions in others, and long-term memory. These areas of the brain

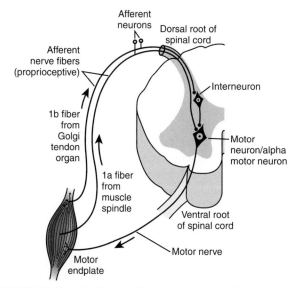

FIGURE 7.7 Spinal reflex arc showing the stretch reflex.

comprise the amygdala, hippocampus, hypothalamus (including the parahippocampal gyrus and cingulate gyrus), and the olfactory cortex (smell) located on the medial surface of the temporal lobe of the cerebral cortex.[17,18] The hypothalamus connects with all parts of the limbic system and acts as a central station for the neural pathways of the functions of emotions, as well as for the endocrine system and autonomic functions. The hippocampus is largely associated with the storage of declarative memory (long-term memory). The amygdala is associated with the response to learned stimuli and emotional responses to events. The sensation of fear is connected with the amygdala and results in the flight or fight response. The amygdala receives input from the visual and auditory centers and the somatosensory cortex. Outputs from the amygdala go to the hypothalamus, the autonomic centers of the brainstem, sympathetic neurons, and the frontal cortex of the cerebrum.[19] This extensive network of the limbic system explains how the sense of smell can elicit strong emotions, and also how emotions can be tied to the learning process for long-term memory storage. Recent studies using fMRI scans have demonstrated the extensive connections within the brain associated with learning and emotions. Events associated with strong emotions seem to be remembered more readily.[20]

AUTONOMIC NERVOUS SYSTEM

The autonomic nervous system is a network of neurons that control the nonvolitional muscles (not under voluntary control), basic body functions, and helps to keep the body in a state of homeostasis (a state conducive to normal function). Thus, this system controls the internal organs such as the smooth muscle of the heart, the smooth muscles of the bronchi, and the muscles of the intestines. The branch of the nervous system that controls voluntary muscles is known as the **somatic motor system.** The functions under the control of the autonomic nervous system include the urinary system; the gastrointestinal tract; blood pressure and heart rate regulation; body temperature; respiration; sweat, saliva, and tear secretion; the control of the pupil and lens of the eyes; and male sexual function. The autonomic nervous system is largely a motor system of efferent neurons but also contains sensory neurons that provide feedback from the organs to the CNS. The autonomic system is divided into the sympathetic (SNS) and parasympathetic (PNS) nervous systems. The PNS also is called the craniosacral system. The SNS is responsible for the "fight-or-flight" response and tends to be in a high state of excitement during stress and exercise. The PNS is active during rest when the body is replenishing its resources. In general, the two systems supply their effectors through two neurons, a preganglionic and postganglionic neuron to the organs they supply. The originating cell bodies (preganglionic) of the two systems lie in the brain or spinal cord. The postganglionic cell bodies lie in ganglia. The ganglia of the SNS are located either in paravertebral ganglia close to the spinal cord or in other areas distant from the organ they supply. The ganglia of the PNS lie close or within the organ they supply. The preganglionic axons of both systems are myelinated, whereas the postganglionic neurons of both systems are unmyelinated. Because the neurons of the PNS are close or within the organ they supply, their postganglionic axons are short. Those of the SNS are long as a result of being situated far from the organ supplied. The preganglionic neurons of both systems release the neurotransmitter acetylcholine. The postganglionic neurons of the SNS release norepinephrine and those of the PNS release acetylcholine. The effects of the SNS can be either specific or more widespread. The PNS tends to have a specific effect on the organs it supplies.

The autonomic nervous system has a number of reflexes associated with it. These reflexes are essential for the functioning of the parts of the body not under volitional control. Examples of these reflexes include the baroreceptor reflex and the micturition and defecation reflexes. Each reflex consists of sensory receptors, a control section, and motor fibers to the muscles of the organ. The baroreceptor reflex controls blood pressure. The baroreceptors are located in the junction of the internal and external carotid arteries at the carotid sinus. Impulses from the baroreceptors join with the glossopharyngeal (cranial nerve IX) and vagus nerves (cranial nerve X) and go to the medulla.[21] The efferent fibers from the medulla transmit to the sympathetic preganglionic neurons, which innervate the smooth muscle of the walls of the blood vessels, causing them to dilate or constrict to alter the blood pressure. The other autonomic reflexes work in a similar manner. The micturition reflex is triggered when the bladder is full but can be overridden by conscious control. The PNS causes the bladder to contract, and the SNS causes the internal urethral sphincter to contract. The external urethral sphincter is under voluntary control.

Peripheral Nervous System

The peripheral nervous system comprises the spinal nerves and peripheral nerves to the trunk and limbs and the sensory receptors within the organs of the body. Basically, any nerve component that is not part of the CNS is classified as belonging to the peripheral nervous system. Some authors consider the autonomic nervous system to be part of the peripheral system. The peripheral nerves have meningeal coverings similar to those of the CNS. These coverings are named the epineurium for the outer layer, the inner endoneurium, and the perineurium lying between the two. The perineurium functions like the arachnoid barrier in the brain, creating a blood-nerve barrier similar to the blood-brain barrier of the CNS. Three types of nerve fibers exist in the peripheral system. The myelinated "A" fibers are both sensory and motor and are the largest diameter and fastest conducting nerves. The "B" fibers are smaller in diameter and myelinated, and the "C" fibers are small in diameter, unmyelinated, and conduct impulses more slowly.

Sensory nerve receptors are numerous throughout the body. Many types of receptors exist for a variety of functions. Interoceptors monitor the internal organs of the body. Proprioceptors monitor body position and change of position. Exteroreceptors consist of teloreceptors that monitor the external environment for sound and vision and contact receptors that monitor the environment and perceive pain and tactile stimulation. Other types of receptors include chemoreceptors for the detection of metabolic changes, chemical balance, smell, and taste; photoreceptors for vision; thermoreceptors for heat and cold; mechanoreceptors for touch, muscle length, and audio and vestibular functions; nociceptors for pain; and cutaneous receptors of the skin that monitor the immediate environment for pain, pressure, touch, and vibration. The

cutaneous receptors are described in Table 7-9, and further details can be found in Chapter 8. Some specialized receptors that deserve to be mentioned are the muscle spindles, which monitor muscle length and proprioception, and the Golgi tendon organs, which monitor muscle tension and joint position. The nociceptors are free nerve endings for the detection of mechanical painful stimuli and are myelinated to allow the rapid transmission of impulses so the body can respond by withdrawing from the noxious stimulus. Polymodal nociceptors have no myelin and provide the slower response to painful stimuli for safety.

Throughout the body, the spinal nerves exit from the spinal cord and supply joints, ligaments, muscles, skin, and tendons. This network of peripheral nerves supplies the body in a sequence. The upper cervical nerves largely supply the muscles of the neck and the skin of the head and neck. The upper extremities are supplied by nerves that exit high in the spinal cord in the cervical and upper thoracic areas, the trunk by nerves below those of the upper extremities mainly from the thoracic area, and the lower extremities are supplied by nerves from the lumbar and sacral areas of the spine. Two major networks of peripheral nerves are identified. The brachial plexus comprises the nerves that supply the upper extremities and the lumbar and sacral plexus for the nerves supplying the lower extremities. The first four cervical nerves form a small cervical plexus. The brachial plexus is formed by

Table 7.9 **Cutaneous Sensory Receptors**

NAME	LOCATION	TYPE OF RECEPTOR	CUTANEOUS FUNCTION
Free nerve endings	Subcutaneous tissue, dermis, and epidermis	Nonencapsulated free nerve ending Myelinated C fibers and nonmyelinated A fibers	Pain sensation
Merkel endings	Stratum basale of epidermis	Non-encapsulated	Respond to mechanical and tactile stimuli
Peritrichial nerve endings	Surround hair follicles	Non-encapsulated	Mechanical/tactile for light touch on the hairs
Meissner's corpuscles	Dermis especially in ridges of fingertips	Encapsulated Myelinated axon	Mechanical/tactile for touch and texture of any object or surface
Pacinian corpuscles	Dermis and subcutaneous tissue	Encapsulated Non-myelinated axon	Vibration
Ruffini endings	Dermis and subcutaneous tissue	Encapsulated Myelinated axon	Pressure and stretch of skin

the branches of cervical 5, 6, 7, 8, and thoracic 1. The 5th and 6th cervical nerve roots join to form the upper trunk of the brachial plexus, the 7th cervical forms the middle trunk, and the 8th cervical and 1st thoracic form the lower trunk. These trunks divide into lateral, medial, and posterior cords. See Figure 7-8 for the cervical plexus, Figure 7-9 for the brachial plexus, Figure 7-10 for the lumbar plexus, and Figure 7-11 for the sacral plexus. The cervical nerves, the thoracic nerves, and the peripheral nerves arising from the brachial plexus with their nerve root innervations and muscles and other structures they supply are detailed in Table 7-10. The distribution of the peripheral nerves from spinal nerve roots to muscles, joints, blood vessels, skin, and underlying structures is a complex system. Because these nerve roots supply internal organs as well as skin and muscle, any pain detected in the internal organs or muscles may be referred to areas of the skin supplied by the same nerve roots. This is termed **referred pain.** A generalized description of myotomes is contained in the section on neurological testing later in this chapter.

PERIPHERAL NERVE LESIONS

Damage to a peripheral nerve may be reversible or irreversible. The nature of the damage depends on the length of time the damage is sustained and the intensity of the damaging event. Three main classifications of axonal damage to the nerves can be described: **neurapraxia,** **axonotmesis,** and **neurotmesis.** Neurapraxia is temporary damage to a nerve caused by pressure on the axon that does not cause any structural changes. Neurapraxia does not cause muscle atrophy but may result in temporary paralysis of the muscles supplied by the damaged nerve as a result of the inability of the axon to transmit impulses and create action potentials. In most cases, people with

(text continues on page 288)

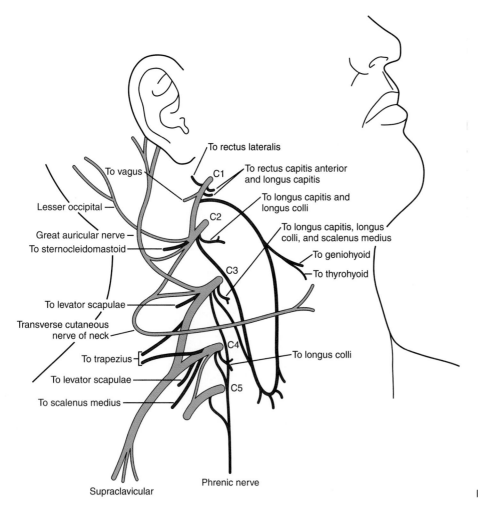

FIGURE 7.8 Cervical plexus.

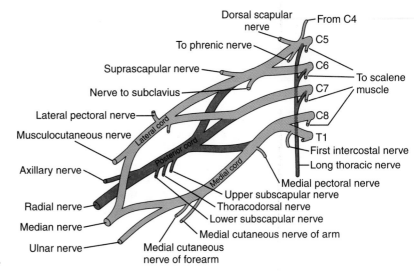

FIGURE 7.9 Brachial plexus.

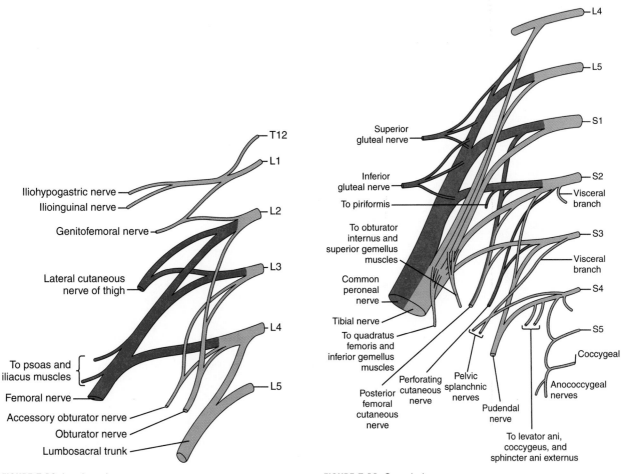

FIGURE 7.10 Lumbar plexus.

FIGURE 7.11 Sacral plexus.

Table 7.10   **Cervical and Thoracic Peripheral Nerves, Nerve Root Derivation, and Muscle and Other Innervations**

NERVE	NERVE ROOTS	MUSCLES SUPPLIED	OTHER STRUCTURES SUPPLIED BY NERVE
Cervical 1	C1	Obliquus capitis inferior Obliquus capitis superior Semispinalis capitis Rectus capitis lateralis Rectus capitis anterior (C1, C2) Longus capitis (C1–3) Hyoid muscles	Branch joins with vagus nerve
Cervical 2	C2	Longus colli (C2–4)	
Accessory nerve	C2 and 3	Sternocleidomastoid	
Supraclavicular nerves	C3, C4	None	Sternoclavicular joint Skin over pectoralis major and deltoid Skin of upper and posterior shoulder
Phrenic nerve	C3–5	Diaphragm	Branches supply parts of lower lungs, and abdominal viscera
Cervical C4–8	Nerve roots C4–6 close to exit from intervertebral foramen	Scalenus anterior Scalenus medius Scalenus posterior Longus colli	
Axillary nerve	C5, C6	Deltoid Teres minor	Skin overlying deltoid and long head of triceps
Dorsal scapular nerve	C5	Levator scapulae Rhomboids	
Long thoracic nerve	C5–7	Serratus anterior	
Median nerve	C5–8, T1 (lateral and medial cord of brachial plexus)	Pronator teres Flexor carpi radialis Palmaris longus Flexor digitorum superficialis Flexor pollicis longus Flexor digitorum profundus Pronator quadrates Flexor pollicis brevis Abductor pollicis brevis Opponens pollicis Lumbricals 1–3 1st dorsal interosseus	Elbow joint Proximal and distal radioulnar joints Wrist joint Intercarpal, carpometacarpal, and intermetacarpal joints Skin over thenar eminence, lateral thumb, anterior and lateral digits, terminal digits, and posterior aspect of middle and distal phalanges Sheaths of long flexor tendons Digital arteries, sweat glands of hand, and nail beds Vascular to brachial artery

Table 7.10 Cervical and Thoracic Peripheral Nerves, Nerve Root Derivation, and Muscle and Other Innervations (continued)

NERVE	NERVE ROOTS	MUSCLES SUPPLIED	OTHER STRUCTURES SUPPLIED BY NERVE
Musculocutaneous nerve	C5–7	Coracobrachialis Biceps, long and short heads Brachialis	Elbow joint Humerus Skin anterior forearm
Nerve to subclavius	C5, C6	Subclavius	
Pectoral nerves	C5–8, T1	Pectoralis major and minor	
Radial nerve	C5–8, T1	Triceps Anconeus Brachioradialis Extensor carpi radialis longus Brachialis Extensor carpi radialis brevis Supinator Extensor digitorum Extensor digiti minimi Extensor carpi ulnaris Extensor pollicis longus Extensor indicis Abductor pollicis longus Extensor pollicis brevis	Elbow joint Distal radioulnar joint Intercarpal and intermetacarpal joints Metacarpophalangeal and proximal interphalangeal joints Skin on posterior aspect upper arm Skin lateral aspect of lower half of upper arm Skin on lateral and posterior aspect of forearm to the wrist
Subscapular nerves	C5, C6	Subscapularis Teres major	
Suprascapular nerve	C5, C6	Supraspinatus Infraspinatus	Glenohumeral joint Acromioclavicular joint Scapula
Thoracodorsal nerve	C6–8	Latissimus dorsi	
Medial cutaneous nerve of forearm	C8, T1		Skin over biceps Skin of parts of medial aspect of forearm
Medial cutaneous nerve of arm	C8, T1		Skin on medial aspect of lower part of upper arm
Ulnar nerve	C (7), 8, T1	Flexor carpi ulnaris Flexor digitorum profundus Palmaris brevis Abductor digiti minimi Flexor digiti minimi Opponens digiti minimi Interossei Lumbricals 3 and 4 Adductor pollicis Flexor pollicis brevis	Elbow joint Wrist joint Intercarpal, carpometacarpal, and intermetacarpal joints Vascular to ulnar artery, and palmar arteries Skin medial side little finger, adjacent sides of little and ring fingers, adjacent sides of ring and middle fingers, medial side of palm of hand

(table continues on page 288)

Table 7.10   Cervical and Thoracic Peripheral Nerves, Nerve Root Derivation, and Muscle and Other Innervations (continued)

NERVE	NERVE ROOTS	MUSCLES SUPPLIED	OTHER STRUCTURES SUPPLIED BY NERVE
Thoracic nerves	T1–12	External and internal intercostals muscles (supplied by nerve at same level) Serratus posterior (T9–12) External oblique abdominal muscles (lower six thoracic nerves) Internal oblique abdominal muscles (lower six thoracic and L1) Transversus abdominis (lower six thoracic and L1) Rectus abdominis (lower six or seven thoracic)	Sensory to diaphragm (lower six thoracic nerves)

neurapraxia fully recover from the injury. Axonotmesis occurs from a more serious injury to the nerve axon.[22] This injury is often caused by prolonged pressure on the nerve and results in atrophy of the muscles supplied by the nerve and degeneration of the neuronal axon. The neural sheath of the nerve remains intact in axonotmesis. In some cases, the axon of the nerve may grow back along the length of the sheath, and in others the nerve axon never fully returns to its previous length resulting in permanent atrophy or paralysis of the affected muscles. The axon grows back at a slow rate of approximately 1 mm per day. The most serious nerve injury is neurotmesis in which both the axon and the axon sheath are damaged. Recovery from neurotmesis is more problematic because the regrowing axon does not have a path to follow. Surgical suturing of the nerve may be performed to facilitate the regrowth and direction of the axon. The process of damage to the axon after axonotmesis and neurotmesis is called Wallerian degeneration. The myelin sheath of the axon deteriorates back to the previous node of Ranvier in the Schwann cells, and debris builds up that can impair the regrowth of the axon.[23]

Specific peripheral nerve lesions involve compression, or external trauma to the nerve axon. Compression may be the result of chronic inflammation, a tumor, or some other space occupying lesion that compresses the nerve. When compression of the nerve occurs where the nerve root exits the intervertebral foraminae of the spine the condition is called a **radiculopathy.** Whether the damage is to a peripheral nerve or a spinal nerve root, the effects of the compression or damage result in a loss or reduction of the nerve supply to muscles, joints, and skin beyond the level of the injury and pain. Because blood vessels usually follow the path of the peripheral nerves, compression injuries may also cause ischemia to the associated tissues. The median nerve may be compressed by inflammation caused by repetitive stress, or pregnancy, or as a result of an anatomically narrow carpel tunnel, as it passes through the wrist at the carpal tunnel. This compression results in weakness and atrophy of the intrinsic muscles (small muscles with both origin and insertion within the hand) of the thenar eminence of the hand supplied by the median nerve. Compression of the radial nerve as it winds around the head of the humerus may occur if constant pressure is placed on the nerve by leaning against a wall or other hard object. This condition is often termed "Saturday night palsy" as a result of the compression occurring when people are under the influence of alcohol or drugs. Radial nerve compression causes permanent or temporary weakness of all the muscles of the upper extremity supplied by the radial nerve distal to the site of injury. Another radial nerve compression injury known as "crutch palsy" may occur in people using axillary crutches incorrectly by placing weight through the axilla onto the crutch when resting. Also, a fractured humerus may compress the radial nerve.[24] Thoracic outlet syndrome is another peripheral nerve compression disorder. This syndrome is caused by compression of the nerves of the brachial plexus and subclavian blood vessels as they pass from the cervical spine to the axilla through the space between the clavicle and the first rib. Occasionally the presence of a cervical rib (a fairly common anatomical anomaly) increases the risk of compression by further reducing the size of the space.[25] Trauma to the shoulder may cause inflammation, which reduces the size of the space. Compression of the subclavian blood vessels results in pallor of the skin of the upper extremity, reduced temperature of the skin, and weak or absent pulses. Compression of the nerves results in weakness of the muscles supplied by the nerves and when severe the weakness is termed Gilliat-Sumner hand. Numbness and pain occur in the associated dermatomes of the upper extremity.[26] (See Fig. 7-12 for dermatomes and Table 7-10 for muscles supplied by the peripheral nerves of the upper extremity arising from the brachial plexus). Another, more common lower extremity compression nerve injury concerns the common peroneal nerve as it winds around the head of the fibula in the lower extremity. People who have a below-knee cast in place may experience compression of the common peroneal nerve with associated symptoms in the muscles supplied by the nerve. See Table 7-11 for the muscles

(text continues on page 292)

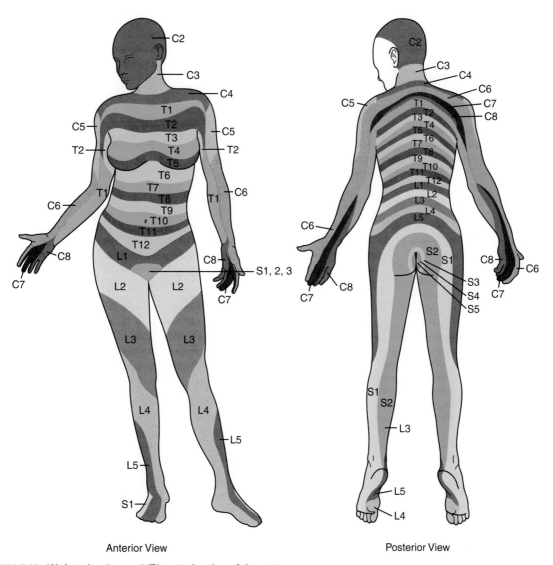

Anterior View

Posterior View

FIGURE 7.12 (A) Anterior view and (B) posterior view of dermatomes.

Table 7.11 **Lumbar and Sacral Peripheral Nerves, Nerve Root Derivation, and Muscle and Other Innervations**

NERVE	NERVE ROOTS	MUSCLES SUPPLIED	OTHER STRUCTURES SUPPLIED BY NERVE
Iliohypogastric	L1	None	Cutaneous—skin of anterolateral buttock, and skin of abdomen near pubis
Ilioinguinal	L1	Internal oblique abdominals	Cutaneous—skin upper and medial thigh, skin over male genitalia, skin over mons pubis and labia majora in females
Genitofemoral	L1, L2	Cremaster	Cutaneous—Skin of scrotum in male, skin of mons pubis and labia majora in female and skin over the femoral triangle Femoral artery
Nerve to psoas major	L1–3 (branches of ventral rami)	Psoas major Psoas minor (L1)	
Lateral cutaneous nerve of thigh	L2, L3 (dorsal branches of ventral rami)	None	Peritoneum of the iliac fossa Cutaneous—skin of anterior and lateral thigh to the knee
Femoral	L2–4 (dorsal branches of ventral rami)	Pectineus Sartorius Iliacus Rectus femoris Vastus lateralis Vastus medialis Vastus intermedius	Articular to hip and knee joints Femoral artery
Intermediate cutaneous nerve of thigh	L2–4 (anterior division of femoral nerve)	Sartorius	Cutaneous—skin of anterior thigh
Medial cutaneous nerve of thigh	L2–4 (anterior division of femoral nerve)	None	Cutaneous—skin of medial thigh and lower leg
Saphenous nerve	L2–4 (cutaneous branch of femoral nerve)	Rectus femoris Vastus lateralis Vastus medialis Vastus intermedius	Articular to knee joint Skin over patella and lateral knee Cutaneous—skin medial side of foot
Obturator	L2–4 (ventral branches of ventral rami)	Adductor longus Adductor brevis Adductor magnus Gracilis Obturator externus Pectineus	Articular branch to hip joint Cutaneous—Skin of medial thigh Femoral artery, popliteal artery Articular to knee joint and capsule
Accessory obturator	L3, 4 (Ventral rami)	Pectineus	Articular to hip joint
Nerve to quadriceps and Gemellus inferior	L4, L5, S1 (Ventral branches ventral rami)	Gemellus inferior Rectus femoris Vastus lateralis Vastus medialis Vastus intermedius	Articular to hip joint

Table 7.11 **Lumbar and Sacral Peripheral Nerves, Nerve Root Derivation, and Muscle and Other Innervations** (continued)

NERVE	NERVE ROOTS	MUSCLES SUPPLIED	OTHER STRUCTURES SUPPLIED BY NERVE
Nerve to Obturator internus and Gemellus superior	L5, S1, S2 (ventral branches, ventral rami)	Obturator internus Gemellus superior	None
Nerve to piriformis	S1, S2 (dorsal branches ventral rami)	Piriformis	None
Superior gluteal	L4, L5, S1 (dorsal branches ventral rami)	Gluteus medius Gluteus minimus Tensor fascia lata	None
Inferior gluteal	L5, S1, S2 (dorsal branches ventral rami)	Gluteus maximus	None
Posterior femoral cutaneous	S2, S3 (ventral branches ventral rami) S1, S2 (dorsal branches ventral rami)	None	Cutaneous—skin of gluteal region over the gluteus maximus muscle, perineum, posterior thigh and lower leg including popliteal fossa, upper medial thigh, and genitalia
Sciatic	L4, L5, S1–3 (ventral divisions sacral plexus)	Biceps femoris Semitendinosus Semimembranosus Adductor magnus (ischial head)	Articular to hip joint
Tibial (terminal branch of sciatic nerve that divides into sural, and medial and lateral plantar nerves)	L4, L5 S1–3	Gastrocnemius Plantaris Popliteus Soleus Tibialis posterior Flexor digitorum longus Flexor hallucis longus Abductor hallucis (medial plantar) Flexor digitorum brevis (medial plantar) Flexor hallucis brevis (medial plantar) First lumbrical (medial plantar) Flexor digitorum accessories (lateral plantar) Abductor digiti minimi (lateral plantar) Flexor digiti minimi brevis (lateral plantar) Interossei (medial and lateral plantar) Adductor hallucis (lateral plantar) Second, third, and fourth lumbricals (lateral plantar)	Articular to knee and ankle joints, superior and inferior tibiofibular joints, and tarsal and metatarsal joints Cutaneous to lateral and posterior lower one-third of the lower leg and lateral foot and heel (sural), medial plantar surface of foot (medial plantar nerve). Skin of toes, nail beds, lateral plantar surface of foot (lateral plantar nerve)

(table continues on page 292)

Table 7.11 **Lumbar and Sacral Peripheral Nerves, Nerve Root Derivation, and Muscle and Other Innervations** (continued)

NERVE	NERVE ROOTS	MUSCLES SUPPLIED	OTHER STRUCTURES SUPPLIED BY NERVE
Common peroneal (terminal branch of sciatic nerve which divides into the deep peroneal or anterior tibial nerve, and the superficial peroneal nerve also called the musculocutaneous nerve)	L4, L5, S1, S2 (dorsal branches ventral rami)	(See anterior tibial and superficial peroneal)	Articular to anterior knee joint, superior tibiofibular joint Cutaneous—skin of proximal lower leg
Anterior tibial/ deep peroneal (terminal branch of common peroneal nerve)	L4, L5, S1, S2	Tibialis anterior Extensor hallucis longus Extensor digitorum longus Peroneus tertius Extensor digitorum brevis First and second dorsal interossei	Articular to ankle joint, and tarsal and metatarsophalangeal joints of second, third, and fourth toes
Superficial peroneal/ musculocutaneous (terminal branch of common peroneal nerve)	L4, L5, S1, S2	Peroneus longus Peroneus brevis	Cutaneous—skin of toes, lateral ankle, and distal lower leg
Perforating cutaneous	S2, 3 (dorsal divisions sacral plexus)	None	Cutaneous—medial and lower parts of skin overlying the gluteus maximus
Pudendal—nerve to levator ani, coccygeus, and sphincter ani	S2–4 (ventral divisions sacral plexus)	Sphincter ani externus Pelvic floor muscles Levator ani Coccygeus Muscles of penis and clitoris	Cutaneous—skin of perineum, rectum, anal canal, penis and scrotum in males and labia in females Sensory to vagina Pelvic viscera

supplied by the peripheral nerves to the lower extremity arising from the sacral plexus.

Testing for the Neurological System

A variety of tests are used to check the integrity of the nervous system. Some of these tests require the use of machines while others can be completed by the examiner. The following tests are commonly used for neurological testing.

CT SCAN

The computed tomography (CT) scan is used to scan the brain for areas of damage, bleeding, and changes to the brain tissue. The cross-sectional nature of the radiographs obtained from CT is useful in determining the location of brain damage and the position changes of brain structures such as the ventricles associated with hydrocephalus

(buildup of fluid in the ventricles causing pressure on the brain tissue). Brain tumors can also be identified using a CT scan. The use of CT scan is general procedure when people are suspected of having a CVA. Use of the CT scan can help to determine whether the CVA is caused by a hemorrhagic or ischemic event. Determining the cause of the CVA helps physicians to determine the appropriate treatment intervention as well as the prognosis.

DERMATOMES

A dermatome is an area of skin supplied by one particular nerve root. Dermatomes can provide a method of checking the integrity (working function) of the nerve roots. Because a specific area of skin is supplied by each nerve root, testing the sensation in this area of skin can help to determine whether the nerve root is functional. Refer to Figure 7-12 for skin supplied by nerve roots.

Deep Tendon Reflexes

The deep tendon reflexes (DTRs) are spinal cord reflexes as previously described. Each deep tendon reflex is innervated by a discreet nerve root or nerve roots. Testing these reflexes can provide information regarding the integrity of the nerve roots responsible for each of these reflexes. These reflexes are tested by striking the tendon with a tendon hammer, also called a reflex hammer, to stretch the tendon eliciting contraction of the muscle. The biceps DTR measures cervical (C) 5/6; triceps and brachioradialis DTR measures C7; patellar quadriceps DTR measures lumbar (L)3/4; and the ankle jerk DTR measures sacral (S)1. The measurement of the quality of DTRs is designated by the following scale:

– or 0 = absent
– or 1 = diminished
+ or 2 = average
++ or 3 = exaggerated
+++ or 4 = clonus[27]

Electrodiagnostic Testing: Electromyography and Nerve Conduction Studies

Electromyography tests the electrical activity present in muscles. All functioning muscles have electrical energy. In this procedure, needles are inserted into the muscle to be tested and the electrical activity of the muscle is recorded at rest and during contraction.

Nerve conduction studies usually are performed in conjunction with an EMG. Surface electrodes are placed along the length of the nerve to be tested at various intervals. The nerve is electrically stimulated and the rate of transmission of the nerve impulse is recorded. A slower than usual nerve conduction indicates damage to the nerve. The specific site of the injury can be determined with this test. Nerve conduction studies are used to diagnose nerve compression conditions such as carpal tunnel syndrome (median nerve), thoracic outlet syndrome (brachial plexus compression), ulnar nerve entrapment at the elbow, and cervical radiculopathy (nerve root compression in the cervical spine). The studies are repeated to determine the recovery of the nerves.[28]

Glasgow Coma Scale

The Glasgow Coma Scale (GCS) was developed by Teasdale and Jennett in 1974[29] and revised in 1976.[30] The purpose of the GCS is to facilitate more accurate measurement of the level of consciousness of patients admitted to the hospital and assess progress once in the hospital. The scale consists of a three-part assessment of the level of consciousness/coma: eye opening response, verbal response, and motor response. In each section, several types of responses are given points. At the completion of the assessment, the number of points given for each of the three sections is added and the total score provides an assessment for the level of consciousness. The points given in each section of the assessment are as follows:

Eye-opening response
- Spontaneous—open with blinking = 4 points
- To verbal stimuli, command, speech = 3 points
- To pain only = 2 points
- No response = 1 point

Verbal response
- Oriented = 5 points
- Confused conversation, able to answer questions = 5 points
- Inappropriate words = 3 points
- Incomprehensible speech = 2 points
- No response = 1 point

Motor response
- Obeys commands for movement = 6 points
- Purposeful movement to painful stimuli = 5 points
- Withdraws in response to pain = 4 points
- Flexion in response to pain (decorticate posturing) = 3 points
- Extension response to pain (decerebrate posturing) = 2 points
- No response = 1 point

According to the American College of Surgeons (1993) as noted by the Centers for Disease Control and Prevention (CDC),[31] the range of total scores reflects the following:

- Coma score = 3 to 8, no response to all categories
- Severe head injury = GCS score of 8 or less
- Moderate head injury = GCS score of 9 to 12
- Mild head injury = GCS of 13 to 15

The GCS is not a definitive assessment scale because it does not provide accurate predictions regarding the recovery of people after coma or head injury. However, the scale allows assessment of people who are unconscious to be performed in a systematic way.

Magnetic Resonance Imaging (MRI)

MRI of the brain is used when a neurological insult such as a cerebrovascular accident is suspected that is not exhibited on the CT scan. A CT scan is faster in an emergency situation. However, an MRI is preferred if time allows because it provides a better image. Use of the MRI is more expensive than the CT scan, and thus the choice of using the machine is dependent on the physician. The detail of the radiographs obtained through the MRI is greater than that of the CT scan and may provide valuable information for the diagnosis and appropriate treatment of people with neurological problems. People with pacemakers and metal implants may not be able to undergo MRI as a result of the high magnetic field generated by the machine.

MUSCLE STRENGTH TESTING

Muscle strength testing may be combined with the testing of the myotomes. The muscle testing may be manually performed by the therapist or a dynamometer may be used. Dynamometers may be handheld devices or large computerized machines called isokinetic dynamometers. Testing grip strength with a hand dynamometer is performed regularly in physical therapy practice. Examples of isokinetic dynamometers include the Cybex machine and the Biodex System. The use of a dynamometer improves the reliability of the test results but is more time-consuming to perform. The isokinetic dynamometer controls the velocity of movement against the patient's maximal force through range of motion. Accurate positioning of patients on the isokinetic dynamometer is essential for reliable measurements. The axis of the joint must be directly aligned with the axis of the arm of the machine, and the rest periods, patient position, and all settings on the machine must be the same each time a test is performed to ensure the greatest accuracy of the test results. The validity of the test results depends on all these criteria being met. The tests on one patient may be compared with subsequent tests of the same patient to monitor progress in muscle strengthening. The greatest validity of results is achieved if the same therapist performs the test each time (intrarater or intratester reliability).[32] If different people perform the test each time on individual patients (interrater or intertester), the reliability is greatly reduced.[33]

Manual muscle testing (MMT) is the most frequently used method of measuring the strength of muscles by the physical therapist and physical therapist assistant. Several measurement scales are used in the clinic to record the strength of muscles. Each of these scales measures the strength of either individual muscles or groups of muscles in relation to gravity and manually applied resistance. The three most frequently used MMT scales are as follows:

1. 0–10 (Kendall, 1993)[34]
2. N (normal), G (good), F (fair), P (poor), Trace, and zero
3. 0–5

The Kendall 0–10 scale is based on static resistance to the muscle or muscle group whereas the other two scales require resistance to be applied throughout the muscle's range. A comparison can be made between measurements on each of the scales, but the same scale should be used when testing patients. Controversy exists about what constitutes "normal" for MMT. Normal muscle strength generally means that the joint can move through range of motion against gravity with strong manual resistance applied.[35] Some clinicians add the provision that a normal strength muscle must also be able to fully function in everyday activities. The intrarater/intratester reliability for MMT is considered quite valid,[36] but the interrater/intertester reliability is not as valid. In general the same person should perform the MMT on individual patients each time of testing. See Table 7-11 for a comparison of the different manual muscle testing grading systems.

MYOTOMES

Myotomes can be a useful tool in evaluating the level of spinal nerve damage in neurological disorders such as peripheral nerve injuries. As previously described, a myotome consists of muscles supplied by a particular nerve root. The distribution of the spinal nerves allows the physical therapist to test the muscles supplied by that nerve root to determine if the nerve supply to the muscles is intact. The nerve roots supply groups of muscles and so testing individual muscles is usually not necessary.[37] Table 7-13 indicates the spinal nerve root supply to groups of muscles.

NEURAL TENSION TESTING/NERVE STRETCHING

The process of testing for tension of the nerves has been incorporated into evaluations by physical therapists for many years. All neuromuscular structures need to be free to move to allow for functional activity. Several authors and proponents of neuromuscular mobilization, such as David Butler, James Cyriax, and David Maitland, have used the concept of testing the mobility of the nervous system before performing mobilizations and manipulations.[38] More recently, the concept of neural tension testing has become part of general orthopedic and neurology practice. The concept of neural tension testing is to place the whole of the nervous system on stretch to determine whether there is any tethering, damage, or inflammation along the length of the nerve. Because the nervous system is all connected, positioning of the spine and extremities can affect the perception of pain in a nerve of the peripheral nervous system. The specific tests and positions used for testing the nervous system are also incorporated into treatment techniques. A few of the neural tension tests are outlined in this section to familiarize the physical therapist assistant with the concept.

Table 7.12   Manual Muscle Testing Grades

GRADES	ABBREVIATION	0–5 SCALE	0–10 SCALE	CRITERIA
Normal	N	5	10	Full available ROM, against gravity, strong manual resistance
Good plus	G+	4+	9	Full available ROM, against gravity, nearly strong manual resistance
Good	G	4	8	Full available ROM, against gravity, moderate manual resistance
Good minus	G-	4-	7	Full available ROM, against gravity, nearly moderate manual resistance
Fair plus	F+	3+	6	Full available ROM, against gravity, slight manual resistance
Fair	F	3	5	Full available ROM, against gravity, no resistance
Fair minus	F–	3-	4	At least 50% of ROM, against gravity, no resistance
Poor plus	P+	2+	3	Full available ROM, gravity minimized, slight manual resistance
Poor	P	2	2	Full available ROM, gravity minimized, no resistance
Poor minus	P-	2-	1	At least 50% of ROM, gravity minimized, no resistance
Trace plus	T+	1+		Minimal observable motion (less than 50% ROM), gravity minimized, no resistance
Trace	T	1	T	No observable motion, palpable muscle contraction, no resistance
Zero	0	0	0	No observable or palpable muscle contraction

ROM = range of movement.

(From O'Sullivan, S. B., & Schmitz, T. J. 2007. *Physical rehabilitation,* 5th edition. Philadelphia: F. A. Davis, p. 181. Used with permission)

Passive Neck Flexion Test. The passive neck flexion test can be one of the first tests used for neural tension testing. The neck is flexed passively by the examiner. People without any underlying problems would not have any pain on flexing of the neck. A positive test for neural tension would elicit pain somewhere along the length of the nerve such as in the spine or lower extremity. If the straight leg raising test is added to the neck flexion, some symptoms of pain may also occur in people positive for neural tension.[39] The passive neck flexion test is also part of the slump test.[40]

Slump Test. The slump test is an extension of the straight-leg raise test for detection of tightness or impingement of the sciatic nerve. The slump test is performed with patients in a sitting position with hands behind their backs to keep the hands out of the way and prevent them putting pressure through the hands. The test has several levels and the pain perception is noted after each of these levels. Patients are instructed to "slump" forward at the spine keeping the head upright. Next the slump is maintained and the neck is flexed. Extension of the knee is added to the mix keeping the ankle relaxed. The final phase is dorsiflexion of the ankle maintaining all other positioning. The examiner may add passive overpressure to people by gently pressing on the head and neck or by extending the knee and flexing the ankle more fully. The interpretation of test results is in the realm of the physical therapist, not the

Table 7.13 **The Spinal Nerve Root Supply to Groups of Muscles**

LEVEL OF NERVE	MUSCLE GROUP
Cervical Nerve Roots	
C1–2	Upper cervical flexion
C2	Upper cervical extension
C3	Cervical lateral flexion
C4	Shoulder girdle elevation
C5	Shoulder abduction
C7	Elbow extension
C8	Thumb extension, finger extension
Thoracic Nerve Roots	
T1	Finger adduction and abduction
T2–L1	None
Lumbar Nerve Roots	
L2	Hip flexion
L3	Knee extension
L4	Dorsiflexion and inversion of ankle
L5	Extension of great toe
Sacral Nerve Roots	
SI	Eversion of foot, buttock contractions, knee flexion
S2	Knee flexion, standing on toes
S3–4	Pelvic floor muscles, bladder and genital function (saddle)

PTA. In approximately half of the general population, the full slump position will cause some pain in the midthoracic region, and most people will not be able to extend the knee fully. However, the lack of knee extension may be the result of tightness in the hamstring muscles as well as neural tightness.[41]

Straight Leg Raise Test. The most appropriate use of the straight leg test is for assessment of the spine. The test should be performed passively by the examiner. With patients in supine one leg is raised by the examiner keeping the knee fully extended and preventing the limb from rotating to either side. A wide variability exists of the angle of flexion achieved at the hip without pain in the posterior part of the limb. Again, the issue is that hamstring tightness may affect the results of the test. Additional stress can be placed on the nerves by dorsiflexing the ankle or having patients flex the neck. Any pain experienced by patients should be noted as to location and description.[42]

Upper Limb Tension/Nerve Tests. A series of upper limb nerve tension tests (ULTT/ULNT) have been described by Butler (1991)[43] for testing of the medial, radial, and ulnar nerves in the upper extremities. These tests are also classified as neurodynamic tests. These tests usually are performed passively by the examiner after allowing patients to actively place the limb in the position of testing to relieve anxiety. The concept of the tests is to place the nerve to be tested in a position of progressively more stretch to determine where the tightness of the nerve is located as noted by the pain perception and location by patients.

The median nerve is tested using the ULNT1 passive test. This test is performed with patients in supine. The arm is placed in a progressively stretched position of shoulder abduction, wrist and finger flexion, supination of forearm, shoulder lateral rotation, elbow extension, and cervical lateral flexion away from the side tested.[44] Many people cannot tolerate the full stretch but with intervention for stretching of the nerve may achieve more mobility without pain. Even in people with normal neural tension, some tightness, discomfort, and tingling sensation may be noted.

The radial nerve is tested using the ULNT2. The sequence of positioning of the upper extremity for this test is as follows: patients in supine, shoulder girdle depression, elbow extension, internal rotation of the arm, and wrist flexion.[45]

The ulnar nerve test is the ULNT3. The sequence for this test is performed with patients in supine starting with passive wrist extension and followed by forearm pronation, elbow flexion, lateral rotation of the shoulder, depression of the shoulder girdle, and shoulder abduction. This test also may be performed in reverse with the proximal part of the upper limb placed in position first followed by the progressively more distal positions.[46]

PALPATION

Palpation is the process of feeling with the hands, particularly with the fingers. The procedure is useful in detecting abnormal muscle tightness or tissue density changes, the temperature of the area, joint effusion, and edema. Palpation is used extensively by physical therapists to detect abnormalities of soft tissue structures such as muscles, as well as joints and spinal structures. Palpation techniques can be improved with practice and are a valuable tool for evaluation and ongoing assessment of people with all types of medical conditions including neurological disorders.

POSTTRAUMATIC AMNESIA SCALES

The length of time people experience posttraumatic amnesia can be used to determine the severity of the head injury and the possible prognosis. In addition to the Glasgow Coma Scale, other tests performed to determine the level of posttraumatic amnesia of people with head injuries include the Galveston Orientation and Amnesia Test (GOAT),[47] the Modified Oxford Posttraumatic Amnesia Scale (MOPTAS), and the Westmead Posttraumatic Amnesia Scale (WPTAS).[48] Each of these scales is based on 12 items considering the age of the patient, the time of day the test is administered, the first memory after injury, the last memory before injury, and recall of faces, names, and selected pictures of objects. Additional cognitive tests also may be performed such as the Mini-Mental State Examination (MMSE),[49] the Visual Naming Language Test,[50] the Verbal Selective Reminding Test (VerbalSR),[51] and the Visual Selective Reminding Test (VisualSR).[52] These tests usually are performed by the speech and language pathologist or the psychiatrist/psychologist. The physical therapist assistant only needs to be aware that these tests exist so they can be recognized in the patient chart.

RANCHO LOS AMIGOS LEVELS OF COGNITIVE FUNCTIONING

The Ranchos Los Amigos was developed at the Rancho Los Amigos National Rehabilitation Center in 1972 as an assessment tool for the people with brain injuries.[53] The levels of functioning are based on the levels of consciousness and the ability to problem solve, concentrate, behave appropriately for the social situation, have judgment, and memory. The levels of cognitive function are:

Level I—**No response**
Level II—**Generalized response:** Body response to any stimuli. May be blinking, body movement, slow to respond
Level III—**Localized response:** Inconsistent specific responses to stimuli
Level IV—**Confused/agitated:** Bizarre behavior, unable to process information, minimal concentration
Level V—**Confused, inappropriate, nonagitated:** Responds to simple commands but confused by complex commands, easily distracted
Level VI—**Confused, appropriate:** Consistently follows simple instructions, poor memory for tasks, poor concentration

Level VII—**Automatic, appropriate:** Seems appropriate in familiar surroundings, reduced insight, judgment and problem-solving abilities, unable to plan future events
Level VIII—**Purposeful, appropriate:** Alert and oriented, functional in society, but may still lack judgment and problem-solving abilities

RANGE OF MOTION

Range of motion measurement is central to physical therapy interventions. Although some physical therapists visually estimate range of motion, this is not an accurate way to record measurement. The preferred method for measurement of joints is performed using a goniometer.[54] The most commonly used are universal goniometers, which are protractors that have a measurement range between 180° and 360° (see Fig. 7-13). These goniometers are available in plastic and metal and are of different sizes for the measurement of different joints. A specialized universal goniometer called a cervical range of motion instrument (CROM) may be used to measure motion of the cervical spine. A large universal goniometer is used for the measurement of joints such as the hip and knee. The large goniometers have longer arms and provide more accurate measurements. The axis of the goniometer must be placed over the anatomical axis of the joint to be measured. One arm is fixed (fixed arm of the goniometer) in place by the hands of the operator along the length of the proximal bone of the joint to be measured, and the other arm is moved (moveable arm of goniometer) with the distal bone of the joint. The measurement of joints using a goniometer has a fairly high intrarater (intratester, same person) reliability, with a less reliable interrater (intertester, different operator) value.[55] Smaller goniometers are useful for the measurement of smaller joints.[56] The same type of goniometer should be

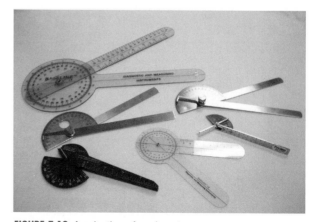

FIGURE 7.13 A selection of goniometers.

used each time a joint is measured to ensure the best re-liability of results. Small finger goniometers are available for measuring the interphalangeal joints. Another type of goniometer is like a compass combined with a spirit level, called an inclinometer. The instrument may have either a digital or analogue recording device. The inclinometer can be used to measure any joint but is used most often when measuring the range of motion of the spine (see Fig. 7-14).

Other methods for measuring range of motion include a tape measure and a wire shaped around the flexed joint. The tape measure is often used to determine the range of motion of the spine. The tape measure is placed with the "0" at the spinous process of an identified verte-bra and a measurement taken in standing to the next de-fined vertebra. The measurement is taken again after the person moves through full flexion or extension of the spine, the two measurements are compared, and the difference between the two is noted. This difference can be used as a comparison for the next time the measurement is taken to determine an increase in the range of motion of the spine. A wire shaped around the joints of the fingers is frequently used when measuring the small joints of the hands. The wire is molded to the shape of the flexed finger, and a tracing of the shape is made on paper for comparison at the next measurement. The use of a flexible wire has been determined to be less reliable than a goniometer.[57]

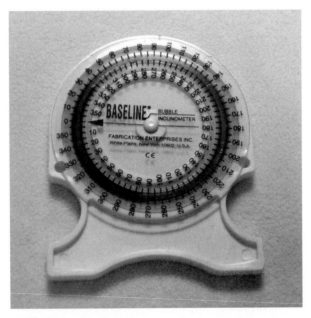

FIGURE 7.14 An inclinometer.

SOME SPECIFIC PERIPHERAL NERVE TESTS

The peripheral nerve tests described in this section are used to diagnose a variety of neurological conditions. These tests are used by the physical therapist, physicians, and other rehabilitation providers.

Phalen's Wrist Flexion Test for the Median Nerve. Phalen's wrist flexion test is specific for median nerve in-jury at the carpal tunnel. In this test, the nerve is further compressed by allowing the wrists to flex with gravity and then pressing the backs of the hands together to increase the flexion. A positive test causes tingling and/or paresthe-sia in the dermatome distribution of the median nerve of the hand over the thumb, index and middle fingers, and lat-eral palm. The tingling takes in excess of 60 seconds to oc-cur.[58] A reverse Phalen's test also tests the integrity of the median nerve. In the reverse Phalen's, a fist is made with the wrist placed into extension. Pressure is applied over the carpal tunnel for 60 seconds. A positive test is a paresthe-sia in the distribution of the median nerve in the hand.

Tinel's Sign (Any Nerve). Tinel's sign is a test used to detect irritation of a nerve by compression or other injury. This test is often referred to as a "distal tingling on per-cussion" test or DTP. The test involves percussing (tap-ping) lightly over the nerve. A positive sign is tingling or "pins and needles" in the dermatome distribution of the nerve. The response of tingling is thought to occur as a re-sult of hypersensitivity of the nerve due to the injury and inflammation. Tinel's sign may be used to detect any in-jured nerve but is frequently used in the diagnosis of carpal tunnel syndrome caused by compression of the me-dian nerve at the wrist.[59]

Thoracic Outlet Tests. Thoracic outlet syndrome is caused by compression of nerves and blood vessels as they pass between the clavicle and the first rib on their way to the upper extremity. The compression may be the result of tightness of the anterior scalene or pectoralis mi-nor muscles, the presence of a cervical rib, or a reduced space between the first rib and the clavicle. This fairly rare condition may result in any or all of the following symp-toms: edema of the upper extremity, neck and shoulder pain, pallor (paleness) of the skin of the upper extremity, weakness and atrophy of hand muscles, tingling of the hand and forearm, and poor circulation to the forearm and hand resulting in cyanosis.[60] Many different tests may be performed to diagnose thoracic outlet syndrome. Some of the more commonly used tests include the Allen test, Adson's maneuver, and a provocative elevation test.

The Allen test is performed with patients in a sitting position. The shoulder is abducted to 90°, and the examiner performs horizontal extension and lateral rotation of the arm with the elbow flexed. A positive Allen test for thoracic outlet syndrome is demonstrated by disappearance of the radial pulse when the patient rotates the head to the opposite side from the tested arm while the position of the arm is maintained by the examiner.[61] Adson's maneuver involves the patient rotating the head to the side to be tested. The examiner extends and laterally rotates the shoulder with the arm in full extension and the patient extends the head in the rotated position. A positive test is demonstrated by disappearance of the radial pulse when the patient takes a deep breath. However, this test is not definitive for thoracic outlet syndrome because many people have a positive response to the test even though they do not have the condition.[62] Some sources do not describe placing the arm in lateral rotation and extension but merely having the patient extend and rotate the head.[63] The provocative elevation test for thoracic outlet syndrome is performed by the patient. Both arms are elevated above the head, and the patient is asked to make a fist and then open the hand for 15 repetitions. A positive test is indicated by symptoms of cramping, fatigue, and tingling in the forearms and hands.[64]

TWO-POINT DISCRIMINATION
The two-point discrimination test is frequently used to determine skin sensation changes resulting from neurological conditions including diabetic neuropathy.[65] The tester uses an instrument with two sharp points that can be moved to varying distances from each other. The two points are touched to the skin at the same time, and subjects state whether they can feel two points or one. The perception of sensation by people is recorded, together with the distance apart the points are when the sensation is felt. In some areas of the body, two points will be detected as close together as 5 mm, whereas in other areas, 20 mm will be the smallest space when two points are discerned. The test relies on the skin receptors for pain and pressure in the skin. Certain areas of the body such as the hands are more sensitive to stimulation. People can usually detect the two points closer together in the hand than elsewhere on the body. The problem with this test is that the closer the two points become, the less reliable the response.[66] Several recent research studies have suggested that the two-point discrimination test should not be the only test performed for tactile responses of the skin.[67]

VERTEBRAL ARTERY TEST FOR CERVICAL SPINE
The use of the vertebral artery test for the detection of vertebrobasilar insufficiency (VBI) has become rather controversial. The test is a combination of passive neck extension and rotation to elicit compression of the vertebral arteries in the cervical spine. The test is supposed to indicate the presence of ischemia to the brainstem resulting from atherosclerosis of the basilar, subclavian, or vertebral arteries or compression of these arteries in cervical spondylosis. The signs and symptoms of VBI are varied and can include dizziness, lightheadedness, vision, speech and swallowing problems, nausea, and syncope. According to an extensive literature search performed in 2005 by Richter and Reinking, there is little evidence to support the reliability of vertebral artery testing. False negative results can occur, and the test itself can in some cases result in the onset of VBI.[68] In view of these findings it is suggested that the physical therapist and PTA students do not practice this test on each other in the classroom setting. Using the test selectively in the clinical setting is also recommended.

Physical Therapy Treatment for People With Neurological Conditions

A variety of physical therapy treatment approaches may be used when working with people with neurological conditions. The following section describes some of them.

Adverse Mechanical/Neural Tension
Treatment of the nervous system with the concept of adverse mechanical/neural tension is based on the principles of neural tension testing described in the section on "testing of the nervous system." Adverse mechanical or neural tension treatment is attributed to David Butler, an Australian physiotherapist, in his 1991 book *Mobilization of the Nervous System*.[69] The principle of adverse neural tension is that when there is a dysfunction in the musculoskeletal system, many structures are involved in addition to joints and muscles. Butler advocates a "multifactorial approach to patient examination and management" (1991, p. xiii) of patients with musculoskeletal disorders that includes assessment of the mobility of the nervous system.[70] The nervous system is considered as a total entity with the peripheral nerves an extension of the CNS. This system is continuous through the electrical impulses, chemical neurotransmitters, and the structure of the connective tissue of the nerves themselves. This connectedness means that if a part of the nervous system is not fully mobile, the rest of the system is affected. Nerves can be restricted from movement as a result of arthritic

changes, joint inflammation, scar tissue, or fibrosis of the neural tissue or may be compressed by muscle hypertension or inflamed tendons and ligaments. The ability of the nerves to stretch is necessary for full joint mobility and muscle function.[71] The elasticity of the nervous system is tested through a series of movements designed to identify both abnormalities in the ability of the nerves to stretch and the possible location of the problem. The principle tests used for the nervous system are not specific to individual peripheral nerves but to areas of the body. These tests are described in the section on "nervous system testing" and include passive neck flexion, straight leg raise (SLR), slump test, prone knee bend (PKB), and upper limb tension tests (ULTT) 1, 2, and 3. Once the physical therapist has interpreted the neural tension tests, similar positions of stretch used in the testing procedures can be used for mobilization treatment of the affected area. The mobilizations are graded according to the degree of severity of the injury and require constant reevaluation. The use of these techniques is beyond the scope of the physical therapist assistant. However, some positions of gentle stretch for the affected nerves can be provided as a home exercise program. These exercises should be combined with any appropriate strengthening exercises and postural advice.[72]

Alexander Technique

The Alexander technique is a complementary and alternative medicine treatment that reeducates the mind and body through a series of movements and exercises. The technique involves unlearning poor movement habits developed throughout the lifetime of clients using movement, postural awareness, and reduction of tension.[73] Although many people are trained in Alexander methods for the reduction of back pain and postural problems, the technique is sometimes used for people with other movement disorders resulting from neurological disorders.

Brunnstrom Approach

Signe Brunnstrom was a Swedish physical therapist and educator who developed a system of treatments for people with neurological conditions, particularly cerebrovascular accident (CVA). Her theories were based on the reduction of return of primitive reflex patterns of movement after CVA. This technique involves movement patterns used to stimulate the return of normal tone and posture. Stimulation of the skin overlying the agonistic muscles creates a contraction of the agonist muscles and a relaxation of the antagonist muscles (muscles in spasticity). This technique of "brushing" the skin is still used in practice, particularly during the early rehabilitation of people after a CVA to elicit contraction of affected muscles and inhibit the onset of spasticity.[74]

Constraint-Induced Movement Therapy

Constraint-induced movement therapy (CIMT) is a technique that involves restricting the use of the unaffected upper extremity in people who have experienced a CVA. The general practice of this technique is to restrict the use of the unaffected arm for a period of 2 weeks with the use of a sling or constraint-induced mitten for approximately 90% of the waking hours. At the same time, an intensive physical rehabilitation program for repetitive use of the affected upper extremity is performed. This combination of immobilization of the unaffected arm and intensive use of the affected arm has been shown to "produce a massive use-dependent cortical reorganization that increases the area of cortex involved in the innervation of movement of the more-affected limb" (Taub et al.)[75] as shown on neural imaging and functional MRI studies. ⊛ The CIMT method has proved useful in improving both the quality and quantity of movement in the affected upper extremity for people who are in either the acute, subacute, or chronic stages of rehabilitation after a CVA[76,77] and for children.[78] In addition, the positive effects of the intervention seem to continue over the long term.[79] Other variations of the technique include CIMT for the lower extremity involving constant use of the affected lower extremity during walking, and functional activities such as going from sit to stand, step climbing, and other exercises with the use of a weight supporting harness if necessary.[80] The CIMT also is used for people who have experienced traumatic brain injury, spinal cord injury, multiple sclerosis,[81] and phantom limb pain after amputation. When used to reduce phantom limb pain patients are provided with a temporary prosthesis early in the rehabilitation phase.[82] A derivative of the CIMT concept is "forced use" of the affected extremity involving immobilization of the unaffected upper limb without the intensive, repetitive rehabilitation for the affected limb. This "forced use" usually is intended for self-exercise of patients at home in conjunction with outpatient rehabilitation. Mixed results are attributed to this type of "forced use" therapy in the subacute phase of recovery from a CVA.[83]

Craniosacral Therapy

Craniosacral therapy is a form of complementary and alternative medicine that uses gentle manual, light-touch, small-range movement techniques to facilitate increased movement, function, and reduced pain. This technique facilitates the body's own healing mechanisms by focusing on the skull, face, and sacrum during treatment. The concepts of the craniosacral system were proposed by osteopathic physician William Sutherland in the early 20th century. The osteopath John Upledger developed the treatment techniques associated with the craniosacral concept in the 1980s after observing the rhythmic movement of the dura mater during a surgical procedure.[84] The principles of the technique are not fully understood but are based on the craniosacral rhythm created by the circulation of cerebro-spinal fluid (CSF). The effectiveness of the technique has yet to be verified by valid research data. Current studies performed regarding craniosacral therapy do not verify the effectiveness of the treatment technique, although anecdotal results are often positive.[85,86]

Feldenkrais Method

The Feldenkrais method is another form of complementary and alternative medicine that evolved out of the lifelong work of Moshe Feldenkrais and his book *Body and Mind,* published in 1980. Dr. Moshe Feldenkrais (1904–1984) was a physicist, engineer, and martial arts expert.[87] The Feldenkrais concept is "based on principles of physics, biomechanics, and an empirical understanding of learning and human development" (Standards of Practice of the Feldenkrais Method as adopted by the International Feldenkrais Federation (IFF) General Assembly in May 1994). Two general methods are used in Feldenkrais: Awareness Through Movement and Functional Integration. The Functional Integration method is a gentle hands-on approach by the practitioner, whereas the Awareness Through Movement is a system of specific exercises. The method involves the use of the somatic senses to increase awareness of the posture, balance, position in space, and kinesthetic awareness leading to improved balance and movement. Research studies are starting to demonstrate the effectiveness of this technique of treatment.[88] One recent study by Vrantsidis et al. (2009) demonstrated a statistically significant improvement in older people in balance after completion of an 8-week program of Getting Grounded Gracefully based on the Awareness Through Movement lessons of the Feldenkrais method.[89] A 2006 study by Stephens et al. demonstrated positive results for hamstring stretching using the Feldenkrais Awareness Through Movement program compared with traditional stretching techniques.[90] Another study by Batson and Deutsch (2005) demonstrated positive improvements in balance for a small group of people who had experienced neurological deficits as a result of CVA.[91] Anecdotally, people treated with this method indicate positive results.

Myofascial Release

The development of the concept of treatment using myofascial release (MFR) in physical therapy is attributed to the physical therapist John F. Barnes. The concept of MFR was originally developed by osteopathic physicians, but Barnes developed the treatment approach. This treatment format is a complementary and alternative medicine approach to musculoskeletal deficiencies that uses hands-on techniques to reduce myofascial restrictions and thus reduce pain and restore functional movement. The concept is based on the principle that fascia is a complete network of connective tissue within the body and restriction of one area of fascia affects the rest of the body. Scarring of the fascia as a result of injury, trauma, chronic poor posture, or inflammation all reduce the extensibility of the fascia and result in pain and reduced mobility and function.[92] Two of the main forms of treatment technique include myofascial mobilization and myofascial unwinding.[93] Both techniques use light touch by the practitioner. Unwinding involves working on the extremities or head and neck to release restrictions of movement using the person's own inherent movement patterns. According to Remvig et al. (2008), research studies to date have not provided statistical evidence of the effectiveness of the myofascial release technique.[94] However, many people who have obtained positive results from undergoing myofascial release therapy would take issue with this fact. No doubt exists that more research needs to be performed to prove the efficacy of MFR.

Neurodevelopmental Therapy/Bobath Techniques

Neurodevelopmental therapy or treatment (NDT) is based on the work of physical therapist Berta Bobath (1907–1991) and her physician husband Karel Bobath. The Bobaths wrote several books including *A Neurophysiological Basis for the Treatment of Cerebral Palsy, Abnormal Postural Reflex Activity Caused by Brain Lesions, Motor Development in the Different Types of Cerebral Palsy*, and *Adult Hemiplegia: Evaluation and Treatment*. The Bobaths worked with many children with cerebral palsy and developed a treatment approach for CNS upper motor neuron (UMN) problems based on restoring as normal movement as possible to the affected areas of the body.[95] The evaluation and observation of the primitive reflexes and responses seen in people with these neurological deficits, the suppression of inappropriate movement patterns, and the stimulation of normal developmental sequence movement patterns is central to the Bobath treatment. The Bobath method has been adapted over several decades to include treatment for people of all ages with CNS dysfunction. Restoration of control of the hip and shoulder girdle muscles and the reduction of spasticity in the typical lower extremity synergy and upper extremity flexor synergy patterns assist with the return of more normal movement patterns during walking and functional activities. The treatment method continues to evolve as new evidence related to neuromuscular disorders is discovered.[96]

Proprioceptive Neuromuscular Facilitation

The concept of proprioceptive neuromuscular facilitation (PNF) was developed by Dr. Herman Kabat in the 1940s in response to the outbreak of poliomyelitis. Margaret Knott and Dorothy Voss were instrumental in writing the first book about the concept and developing treatment techniques in conjunction with Dr. Kabat and Dr. Sedgwick Mead. These techniques were found to be applicable for people with many musculoskeletal and neurological diagnoses.[97] The patterns of motion used in PNF are based on the normal, functional, combined movements of rotation and diagonals performed by the upper and lower extremities. The purpose of PNF exercises is to increase strength, range of motion, coordination, balance, stability, and proprioceptive and kinesthetic awareness. A system of directional graded resistance through full available range of motion, verbal commands, visual observance by the patient, and overstretch at the beginning of movements is applied by the therapist administering the treatment. Each diagonal motion is followed with a reversal of the direction of motion. Variations can be added to the diagonal motions by flexing the intermediate joint of the elbow or knee and by increasing the amount of resistance applied during specific parts of the range of motion. Several specific patterns of PNF movement exist for the upper and lower extremities. Some of the terms used to describe the different techniques applied during PNF include the following:

- *contract-relax*—resisted contraction of the antagonist muscles, which are restricting range of motion or contraction of the agonist muscles if the antagonist muscles are too weak or painful
- *dynamic reversals*—reversal of the diagonal of movement
- *hold-relax*—resisted contraction of the antagonist muscles followed by relaxation of the same muscles
- *overflow*—the principle of overflow of a resisted contraction from adjacent muscles to those which are weak
- *repeated stretch and contractions of muscles*—the stretch reflex is stimulated by the overstretch of the muscle by the therapist

- *rhythmic initiation*—movement of the limb through range at a set speed and pace
- *rhythmic stabilizations*—isometric contractions against resistance for opposing muscle groups often used to stimulate the muscles for balance in standing or sitting
- *stabilizing reversals*—therapist pushes against the force of the muscles and prevents movement

Although the main patterns of movement are for the upper and lower extremities, PNF is used for total body movements during progressive treatment sessions called chopping and lifting. PNF also may be used during mat activities and ambulation training.[98] Patterns may be performed unilaterally or bilaterally. The main upper and lower extremity patterns of motion are as follows:

Upper extremity diagonal 1—D1 flexion—flexion, adduction, external rotation
Upper extremity diagonal 1—D1 extension—extension, abduction, internal rotation
Upper extremity diagonal 2—D2 flexion—flexion, abduction, external rotation
Upper extremity diagonal 2—D2 extension—extension, adduction, internal rotation
Lower extremity diagonal 1—D1 flexion—flexion, adduction, external rotation
Lower extremity diagonal 1—D1 extension—extension, adduction, internal rotation
Lower extremity diagonal 2—D2 flexion—flexion, abduction, internal rotation
Lower extremity diagonal 2—D2 extension—extension, adduction, external rotation

Sensory Integration

A. Jean Ayres, PhD, (1920–1988) developed the concept of sensory integration (SI) therapy in the 1970s. Dr. Ayres was an occupational therapist, psychologist, and educator who also developed several standardized test instruments including the Southern California Sensory Information Tests, the Southern California Postrotatory Nystagmus Test, and the Sensory Integration and Praxis Tests.[99] The concepts developed by Dr. Ayres are used extensively in occupational and physical therapy and speech and language pathology interventions with children who have sensory integration dysfunction. SI therapy is often combined with neurodevelopmental therapy when working with children with developmental delay. The theory of SI is based on postural and balance problems stemming from vestibular dysfunctions, poor visual perception, tactile deficits, and lack of kinesthetic and proprioceptive awareness. All of these factors are considered essential for the normal development of behavior, eye-hand coordination, motor planning, perception, motor learning, and cognitive learning. Sensory integration therapy focuses on addressing these sensory processing deficits.[100] The intervention using sensory integration involves using tactile stimulation and a system of stimulating balance and postural reactions using a variety of equipment such as therapy balls, platform swings, bolsters and bolster swings, and balance boards.

Tai Chi Chuan in Rehabilitation

Tai Chi Chuan is an ancient Chinese martial art, movement, and self-defense system dating back to the 13th century. The prescribed movements are slow, controlled, and consistent. The movements promote relaxation, concentration, muscle control, balance, muscle endurance, core abdominal strength and postural stability, and general muscle strength and flexibility. In recent years, Tai Chi has been used effectively in many aspects of physical therapy. As part of an exercise program for cardiac rehabilitation Tai Chi improves cardiovascular function while reducing stress. Perhaps as important is that the practice of Tai Chi encourages daily exercise, which is beneficial to the cardiovascular system.[101] Tai Chi has been shown to improve balance, strength, flexibility, and functional mobility and reduce the number of falls as well as the fear of falling.[102] Tai Chi is thus a natural choice for rehabilitation for people with many types of dysfunction including neurological conditions. ☯ The exercise is particularly appropriate for the elderly but offers a dynamic yet comparatively gentle form of exercise for all age groups, including children.

Why Does the Physical Therapist Assistant Need to Know About Neurological Disorders?

People with neurological disorders often seek physical therapy intervention, and the treatment of people with these conditions comprises a large portion of the physical therapy clientele. Many types of practice settings are available for the treatment of people with these disorders, including acute care hospitals, neurological units in hospitals, rehabilitation centers, pediatric settings such as school systems and neonatal intensive care units (NICU), outpatient practices, and home health physical therapy. All PTAs are likely to treat people with neurological conditions and need to be aware of the pathology leading to these disorders. Physical therapy intervention makes a positive difference for people with neurological conditions.

Neurological Disorders

HINTS ON USE OF THE GUIDE TO PHYSICAL THERAPIST PRACTICE

Neurological disorders are classified in the *Guide to Physical Therapist Practice*, Neuromuscular Preferred Practice Pattern 5.

- 5A "Primary prevention/risk reduction for loss of balance and falling" (p. 307): This pattern is appropriate when working with people with balance dysfunctions resulting from vestibular or cerebellar lesions resulting from neurological disorders.
- 5B "Impaired neuromotor development" (p. 319): Most physical therapy intervention with the pediatric neurological population involves this pattern.
- 5C "Impaired motor function and sensory integrity associated with nonprogressive disorders of the central nervous system—Congenital origin or acquired in infancy or childhood" (p. 339): Cerebral palsy, hydrocephalus, infectious diseases affecting the nervous system, spinal bifida, traumatic brain injury, and prematurity are all included in this pattern.
- 5D "Impaired motor function and sensory integrity associated with nonprogressive disorders of the central nervous system—Acquired in adolescence or adulthood" (p. 357): This pattern encompasses a wide range of neurological disorders resulting from traumatic head injury, cerebrovascular accident, seizures, near-drowning, and infectious diseases of the CNS.
- 5E "Impaired motor function and sensory integrity associated with progressive disorders of the CNS" (p. 375): The management of people with Alzheimer's disease, amyotrophic lateral sclerosis, Huntington disease, multiple sclerosis, Parkinson disease, and seizures would fall within this practice pattern.
- 5F "Impaired peripheral nerve integrity and muscle performance associated with peripheral nerve injury" (p. 393): Any peripheral nerve lesion would be included in this pattern; the more common ones of note are carpal tunnel syndrome, Erb's palsy, and traumatic peripheral nerve lesions.

(Continued)

- 5G "Impaired motor function and sensory integrity associated with acute or chronic neuropathies" (p. 411): People with neuropathies would fall under this practice pattern. These would include alcoholic or diabetic neuropathies, Guillain-Barré syndrome, and post-polio syndrome.
- 5H "Impaired motor function, peripheral nerve integrity, and sensory integrity associated with non-progressive disorders of the spinal cord" (p. 429): The conditions associated with this practice pattern include complete and incomplete spinal cord injury, infectious diseases involving the spinal cord, spondylosis and other degenerative joint disease of the spine, herniated intervertebral disk, and osteomyelitis.
- 5I "Impaired arousal, range of motion, and motor control associated with coma, near coma, or vegetative state" (p. 447): Any person in a low state of awareness is included in this pattern; causes of the coma state could include cerebrovascular accident, traumatic brain injury, infections of the CNS, and neoplasia.

(From the American Physical Therapy Association, 2003. *Guide to physical therapist practice,* revised 2nd edition. Alexandria, VA: APTA. Used with permission.)

For ease of description, the neurological disorders are divided into two sections. These sections are the conditions resulting from deficits in the development of the nervous system or birth injury and neurological disorders listed in alphabetical order. Spina bifida is described in Chapter 2.

Neurological Conditions Resulting From Deficits in the Development of the Nervous System or Birth Injury

The following neurological conditions result from damage to the fetus during the developmental stage of the fetal growth or through injury sustained during the birthing process.

Anencephaly ⊛

Anencephaly is a neural tube defect of the nervous system associated with the disturbance of development of the fetus within the uterus. The condition results in lack of development of the brain. The incidence of anencephaly varies between 1 in 1,000 and 1 in 20,000 infants.[103]

Etiology. The actual cause of anencephaly is unknown. Some known factors contributing to the cause are genetic, dietary, and chemical.[104] Exposure of women during early pregnancy to certain pesticides such as methyl parathion has been demonstrated to increase the risk of having a child with anencephaly.[105] The risk factors for mothers of having a child with anencephaly include low levels of education and poor socioeconomic status.[106] The risk for having a child with anencephaly also is linked closely with other neural tube defects such as spina bifida and congenital hydrocephalus.[107]

Signs and Symptoms. Infants with anencephaly may have a rudimentary brainstem but lack the cerebral hemispheres and other parts of the brain. The vault of the skull may be absent altogether or incomplete. These infants are usually blind, deaf, unconscious, and lack the ability to respond to external stimulation.[108]

Prognosis. The prognosis of infants born with anencephaly is poor. An infant cannot survive long without a brain. Of the infants born with anencephaly, only 40% survive more than 24 hours, and 5% of those may live for up to 7 days. The diagnosis of this condition within the first or second trimester of pregnancy is paramount, and genetic counseling is provided for parents. Many fetuses with anencephaly spontaneously abort during the first trimester of pregnancy.[109]

Medical Intervention. The diagnosis of anencephaly can be determined through the detection of high levels of maternal serum alpha-fetoprotein and low levels of estriol, both of which are predictive of neural tube defects and particularly of anencephaly.[110] Transabdominal and transvaginal ultrasonography can detect the abnormality during the first trimester (first 3 months) of pregnancy.[111] A 2004 CDC report indicated a dosage of 400 µg per day of folic acid would reduce the incidence of neural tube defects by between 50% and 70%. In 1998, a mandate from the CDC was put in place for folic acid supplements before and during pregnancy.[112]

Physical Therapy Intervention. No physical therapy intervention is indicated for infants with anencephaly.

Arnold-Chiari Malformation/ Chiari Malformation ⊛

Chiari malformation is a rare developmental deficit of the fetus resulting in a structural defect of the cerebellum and the skull. The defect causes a blockage of the circulation of CSF within the skull and spinal cord. Parts of the cerebellum may protrude downward into the spinal canal through the foramen magnum (the exit foramen for the spinal cord from the skull), creating pressure on the spinal cord. Pressure also may be reflected upward into the cerebrum. The prevalence of Chiari I is approximately 0.1% to 0.5% with slightly more females affected than males.[113]

Etiology. The causes of the defects of the cerebellum and skull are largely unknown. Genetic tendencies within certain families seem to be the most likely etiology. Recent research has indicated a linkage with the condition and chromosomes 9 and 15. However, some people with the malformation do not have a family history of the condition.[114]

Signs and Symptoms. The characteristic signs and symptoms of Chiari malformation range from none to severe neurological deficits. The more common symptoms are dizziness, muscle weakness or paralysis, lack of skin sensation, vision deficits, headaches, and poor balance and coordination. Three types of Chiari malformation are identified. People with Type I may have no visible signs or symptoms or in some cases may have sleep apnea.[115] Other common symptoms of people with Type I include neck pain, myelopathy (muscle weakness), and dysarthria and dysphagia associated with brainstem lesions.[116] Type II known as Arnold-Chiari malformation is accompanied by myelomeningocele (defect of spinal column) and partial or complete paralysis below the level of the spinal lesion. Other symptoms of Type II may include swallowing and feeding problems, nystagmus (involuntary oscillation of the eyes), and a weak cry. Type III is the most severe and is often accompanied by hydrocephalus (accumulation of CSF in the ventricles of the brain), syringomyelia (disease of spinal cord with cyst and cavity development on cord), and scoliosis (abnormal lateral and rotational curvature of the spine).[117] Some sources describe a Type IV level of the condition as the most severe.

Prognosis. People with Type I Chiari malformation may have no problems, whereas those with Type III may be permanently paralyzed below the level of the myelomeningocele.

Medical Intervention. Type I Chiari malformation is usually diagnosed in adults or older children, whereas Chiari Type II is diagnosed in infants and young children. No cure exists for the condition. The defect of the cerebellum and skull may need to be corrected surgically with a decompression of the cervicomedullary junction (junction of the cervical region and the medulla) to restore the flow of CSF.[118] People with a myelomeningocele defect of the spine (spina bifida) must have the defect closed immediately after birth or in utero.

Physical Therapy Intervention. Physical therapy intervention may be indicated for balance and coordination disorders. The outcomes of therapy will depend on the extent of the neural damage. Early-childhood intervention for infants may be helpful in teaching the family management of the condition.

Autism Spectrum Disorder ☺

The term autism, or autism spectrum disorder (ASD), encompasses a wide range of neurodevelopmental disorders including classical autism, Asperger syndrome, Rett syndrome, childhood disintegrative disorders, and pervasive developmental disorders not otherwise specified (PDD-NOS). The CDC 2007 figures for the incidence of autism in the United States indicate that 1 in 150 is affected by the disorder and as many as 1 in 94 boys. Males are 4 times more likely to be affected than females.[119]

Etiology. The cause of autism is not fully understood. A combination of genetic and environmental factors are thought to be responsible. Environmental factors under investigation include heavy metals such as mercury and lead, viral infections, and exposure to toxic chemicals.[120] Abnormal levels of serotonin in the brain have been identified in many children with the condition leading to the theory that the disruption of neurotransmission results from a defect in normal brain development in the fetus.[121]

Signs and Symptoms. The signs and symptoms of autism spectrum disorder vary. Children with all types of the disorder exhibit impairment of social interaction. They are largely unresponsive to people, do not make eye contact, have a short attention span, and are unable to focus on facial expressions or interpret the facial and nonverbal expressions of others. They respond well to a strict routine and become agitated when the routine is altered. Children do not interact with other children well in a play situation, often preferring to play alone. They may be aggressive. Some children are passive, whereas others are overactive. Speech development is often delayed. Typical repetitive behaviors include rocking, rotating, self-biting, head banging, hand flapping, rubbing surfaces and toys, and twirling objects in the hands.[122] Extreme sensitivity to light, touch, sound, and visual media also may be noted.[123] Children with Asperger syndrome exhibit autistic behaviors but have well-developed language skills. In children with childhood disintegrative disorder, development is normal up to the age of between 3 and 10 years, then autistic behaviors start to occur and previously learned skills are lost. A specific type of autism called Rett syndrome affects females. This is a sex-linked genetic disorder causing social withdrawal, impaired language skills, and a characteristic hand-wringing motion.[124] Autism is often accompanied by other conditions such as tuberous sclerosis (brain tumors), seizures, Tourette syndrome, learning disabilities, and attention-deficit disorder. Between 20% and 30% of children with autism develop epilepsy seizures.[125]

Prognosis. No cure exists for autism. Therapeutic and behavioral interventions can reduce the symptoms and help children to become more functional.

Medical Intervention. The diagnosis of autism is determined through a multidisciplinary team of neurologists, psychiatrists, psychologists, speech and language pathologists, occupational therapists, and physical therapists. Neurological, cognitive, and language tests are performed. Hearing tests are completed to rule out hearing deficits, which can result in behaviors similar to those of autism. Once a specific diagnosis of the type of autism spectrum disorders is established, educational and behavioral interventions using applied behavioral analysis and family counseling are initiated. Medications may be helpful to reduce depression, anxiety, and obsessive-compulsive behaviors. Antipsychotic medications are prescribed for severe behavioral issues and anticonvulsants for seizures. Medications used for attention-deficit disorder also may be prescribed.[126]

Physical Therapy Intervention. Children with ASD exhibit a range of developmental delays in gross and fine motor development. Both the physical and occupational therapist may be involved with interventions to stimulate more normal movement patterns. In general, the younger the child is when the intervention begins, the better the outcome.[127] A wide variety of treatment options are used with children with ASD including neurodevelopmental therapy (NDT/Bobarth), PNF, balance and coordination training, and relaxation exercises. The PT, occupational therapist, and speech and language pathologist can work together as a team to provide intervention for children with autism. Many children with ASD have problems with motor planning, and reeducating this type of planning is helpful. Difficulties with motor planning make sudden changes in anticipated activity difficult for people with this condition.[128] Although many people with autism will have symptoms their whole life, the effects of the symptoms can be greatly reduced with the help of therapeutic interventions. Some studies suggest that regular exercise program interventions can help to reduce the stereotypical behaviors of children with ASD.[129]

Cerebral Palsy

A discussion of cerebral palsy is contained in Chapter 2. Many of the physical therapy interventions described in this chapter are appropriate for individuals with cerebral palsy. The choice of physical therapy interventions is related to the presentation of motor deficits in individuals affected by this wide range of nonprogressive neurological disorders.

Fetal Alcohol Spectrum Disorders ⊛

The broad category of fetal alcohol spectrum disorders encompasses fetal alcohol syndrome (FAS), alcohol-related neurodevelopmental disorder (ARND), and alcohol-related birth defects (ARBD). This is a group of disorders related to alcohol consumption in pregnancy that result in a wide array of physical, behavioral, cognitive, and musculoskeletal disorders. FAS, ARND, and ARBD affect between 2 and 6 in every 1,000 live births in the United States, with the highest incidence in the Native American population.[130]

Etiology. The cause of this group of disorders is alcohol consumption by the mother during pregnancy. Although higher intake of alcohol seems to result in greater severity of abnormalities in the infant, no "safe" level of alcohol consumption is known.

Signs and Symptoms. A variety of physical, behavioral, musculoskeletal, and cognitive signs and symptoms are characteristic of children with FAS and other alcohol-related disorders. Physical appearance is often marked by facial characteristics such as small eyes, wide and flat nasal bridge, a small jaw, a cleft palate and lip, and eye and ear abnormalities. Cardiac defects are common. Growth retardation occurs during gestation and after birth, and microcephaly (small brain) is common. Mental retardation is usually present with an IQ of below 79 noted in most children. Cognitive deficits may include poor attention span, low levels of concentration, memory deficits, impaired judgment, poor comprehension, and abstract reasoning, and learning disabilities. Behavioral manifestations include hyperactivity and impulsivity, mood swings, poor social skills, inappropriate sexual behavior, and aggressive tendencies. Approximately 50% of children with FAS have poor coordination, hypotonia (low muscle tone), and attention-deficit/hyperactivity disorder (ADHD).[131]

Prognosis. No cure exists for children with FAS, ARND, and ARBD. The mental retardation, cognitive and behavioral deficits continue throughout life. People with severe FAS also are prone to chemical dependency as adults. However, therapeutic and behavioral interventions can improve function and modify behaviors.

Medical Intervention. Medical management is focused on the prevention of the condition. Women who are pregnant or wish to become pregnant are counseled to stop consuming alcohol and educated about the possible effects on the fetus of drinking alcohol during pregnancy. The diagnosis of infants is important to enable early intervention of the necessary physical, psychological, and behavioral therapies.[132]

Physical Therapy Intervention. Early physical therapy intervention is preferred for infants and children with fetal alcohol spectrum disorders. The motor development levels of these children correlates more closely with mental equivalent age than the chronological age. A thorough evaluation is performed by the physical therapist of range of motion, muscle tone, and developmental gross motor levels of development. One of the standardized assessment tools may be used, such as the Bayley Scales of Infant Development, the Peabody Developmental Motor Scales, the Denver Developmental Screening Test, or the Bruininks-Oseretsky Test of Motor Proficiency. The type of intervention will depend on the manifestations of the disorder and is individualized. Neurodevelopmental physical therapy is commonly used, and other treatment may focus on balance and coordination. Other physical problems noted in children with fetal alcohol spectrum disorders include ataxia, dysdiadochokinesis (inability to perform rapidly alternating movements), tremors, postural problems, and gait deficits, all of which need to be addressed.[133] Screening by the physical therapist includes looking for accompanying problems such as congenital hip dislocation, talipes equinovarus (club foot), and scoliosis.[134] After the evaluation is completed, the physical therapist assistant will be involved with the ongoing intervention for these children.

"It Happened in the Clinic"

Jane was evaluated in the outpatient department of a specialized pediatric hospital after referral from the Early Childhood Intervention program. She was 1 year old and had only recently been noted to have developmental delay problems because her mother had not been taking her for her postnatal checkups at the baby clinic. Her mother was 15 years old with a history of drug and alcohol abuse. Jane had been placed in a day-care center during the past month, and the child care workers noticed that Jane did not seem to be developing at the usual rate for her gross motor skills for her age. She still was not sitting independently nor was she interacting with the other children. At times she appeared to be aggressive to the other children if they approached her. In the pediatric hospital, it was noted that Jane had some of the typical signs and symptoms of fetal alcohol syndrome (FAS). She had a cleft palate that had been surgically repaired soon after birth, a small jaw, and small eyes. She exhibited a poor attention span and was unable to concentrate on playing with a soft toy for longer than a few seconds. Her limbs and trunk were hypotonic (low tone), which interfered with her ability to sit independently on the floor. She was able to roll from supine to prone but showed no inclination to crawl. After evaluation from the physician, physical therapist, occupational therapist, and psychologist, it was determined that Jane had FAS as a result of her young mother drinking alcohol during her pregnancy. Jane was immediately admitted to the hospital to initiate further evaluation and initiation of physical therapy and occupational therapy services to assist with her gross and fine motor development. She continued to be monitored by Early Childhood Intervention services on her discharge and received continuing PT and OT services.

Holoprosencephaly

Holoprosencephaly is a neurological development defect in the forebrain of the embryo or fetus. The prosencephalon (forebrain of the embryo) fails to divide into two cerebral hemispheres. The incidence in the United States is 1 in 5,000 to 20,000 live births. This statistic is misleading because most fetuses with the condition die in utero.[135] The actual incidence of holoprosencephaly may be as high as 1 in 250.[136]

Etiology. The cause of holoprosencephaly is largely unknown. Genetic factors are responsible in some families, and most infants with the condition have identified genetic abnormalities with the trisomy of chromosomes 13 and 18 the most common.[137] Risk factors for having a child with holoprosencephaly include maternal diabetes, and maternal infections such as syphilis, rubella, herpes, and cytomegalovirus during pregnancy. The use of alcohol, over-the-counter and prescription medications, and illicit drugs also increase the risk of having a child with this condition.[138]

Signs and Symptoms. The signs and symptoms depend on the level of severity of the condition. Three classifications exist. Alobar is the most severe form of the condition in which the cerebrum is not divided and severe facial deformities occur. In semilobar holoprosencephaly there is partial separation of the cerebrum into lobes. The least severe form is lobar in which two cerebral hemispheres are formed and the brain may function normally. The most common facial deformity is premaxillary agenesis (cleft lip). In more severe cases, the nose may be either missing altogether, or there may be a tubular proboscis above the single eye. Some infants may have cyclopia, a single eye located in the middle of the forehead. A less common deformity is ethmocephaly, a proboscis located between two closely set eyes.[139] Other facial characteristics are cebocephaly (a single nostril nose), hypotelorism (close-set eyes), and a single upper middle tooth. Associated signs and symptoms may include mental retardation, hydrocephalus (buildup of CSF in ventricles of the brain), microcephaly (small brain), epilepsy, and abnormalities of the internal organs and musculoskeletal system.[140] Children may also have a short stature or exhibit failure to thrive.[141]

Prognosis. Only 3% of fetuses with holoprosencephaly develop to full term and delivery.[142] In some infants born with less severe forms of the condition, the brain may be functionally normal, and the child may live a normal life span. Infants with severe forms of the condition may survive from a few days to a few years.

Medical Intervention. No specific treatment is suitable for all infants with this condition. The intervention will depend on the severity of the malformation. Facial reconstruction surgery may be provided for infants with mild facial abnormalities such as cleft palate and cleft lip. Some infants with mild forms of the condition do not require any medical intervention. Some of the medical interventions may include hormone replacement therapy for pituitary dysfunction, medications for epilepsy, shunt placement for hydrocephalus, gastrostomy tube placement for feeding difficulties, and genetic counseling for parents.[143]

Physical Therapy Intervention. Infants with mild to moderate holoprosencephaly can benefit from neurodevelopmental physical therapy to stimulate the developmental sequence. Children with the mildest forms of the condition may not require any physical therapy intervention.

Common Neurological Disorders

This section presents some of the most common neurological disorders observed in physical therapy practice in alphabetical order.

Alzheimer's Disease (Also See Dementia—Non-Alzheimer's)

Alzheimer's disease is recognized as a progressive degenerative, organic brain syndrome that destroys the neurons of the cerebral cortex causing dementia. Over 5.2 million people in the United States have been diagnosed with Alzheimer's disease. Each year, half a million people are diagnosed with the disease.[144] The incidence rises with age. Approximately 6% of those older than 65 years have Alzheimer's, rising to 20% in those over 80. Although it is generally a disease of the older population, Alzheimer's can start much earlier.

Etiology. The etiology of Alzheimer's is not yet known. Some factors that may increase the risk of developing Alzheimer's are the presence of cerebrovascular disease, especially atherosclerosis, and a genetic tendency in families with a history of Alzheimer's. The brains of people with Alzheimer's disease have tangles of neurofibrils, which are normal to some degree in the aging brain but are present in large numbers in Alzheimer's. Plaques and amyloid tissue accumulate in the nerve tissue. Amyloid is a protein substance of abnormal consistency that builds up in tissues and is thought to be a by-product of abnormal physiological function in cells and organs. One theory states that the amyloid has an effect on the neurofibrils causing them to break down and become tangled. The effect is to prevent the transmission of nerve impulses along the neural axons and thus destroy the function of sections of the cerebral cortex. New studies indicate that the presence of difficulty performing activities of daily living (ADLs) is a major factor in predicting the onset of dementia.[145]

Signs and Symptoms. The characteristic signs and symptoms of Alzheimer's disease include a variety of memory and behavioral deficits. Unlike other types of dementia, people with Alzheimer's forget both recent and distant events so that their memories are destroyed. In other types of dementia patients mainly lose memory of recent events but retain distant ones. Other signs and symptoms include loss of the ability to learn new things, problems with word retrieval, loss of recognition of family and friends, personality changes, alteration of sleep patterns, loss of functional abilities, and changes in mood. In many cases individuals become quite the opposite in personality from their normal. Some people who were quiet become loud and in some cases may become violent.[146] The symptoms of Alzheimer's disease may progress very slowly or more rapidly. A staging of the patient with Alzheimer's is divided into seven stages by the Alzheimer's Association with the first stage exhibiting no impairments and the final stage resulting in loss of mobility, inability to speak or eat, and coma.[147] The seven stages are described in Table 7-14.

In addition to the signs and symptoms experienced by people with Alzheimer's, the family or caregivers often experience anxiety, depression and emotional and physical stress. This stress may lead to an increase in elder abuse if the person with dementia is cared for at home. In the nursing home setting stress can take its toll on caregivers and result in less than optimal care.[148]

Prognosis. The length of time from the onset of symptoms of Alzheimer's disease to death varies from patient to patient, but usually is between 7 and 11 years, with a possibility of between 3 and 20 years.[149] In patients who

have severe symptoms in the later stages of the disease many die from pneumonia or other infections. Some patients lapse into a coma state before death.

Medical Intervention. The diagnosis of Alzheimer's disease is difficult because the neurofibrillary tangles within the brain are only detectable at autopsy. Recent findings suggest that a combination of brain scans with MRI and CT scan, memory tests, detection of specific proteins called p-tau181 and beta-amyloid in the body fluids, and presence of the risk genotype ApoE-e4 for Alzheimer's may help to predict the onset of Alzheimer's disease.[150] The effective diagnosis of Alzheimer's disease as opposed to other forms of dementia such as vascular dementia is important for the early management of the disease.[151] Medical intervention is now focusing on prevention of Alzheimer's disease as well as research for a cure. Maintaining a healthy diet of fruits, vegetables, and fish seems to reduce the risk of developing Alzheimer's. People who have higher levels of education also seem to be at less risk.[152] Although there is currently no cure for Alzheimer's disease, some medications that increase the levels of acetylcholine in the body have been shown to have an effect of slowing down the regression for a few months. Other medications and substances thought to be effective in delaying the disease process are large doses of vitamin E

Table 7.14 **The Stages of Alzheimer's Disease**

NAME OF STAGE	SIGNS AND SYMPTOMS OF THE STAGE
No impairment	No impairment
Very mild cognitive decline	Forgetfulness marked by loss of familiar objects such as keys and inability to remember the names of people who are friends and family
Mild cognitive decline	Word retrieval problems; friends and family notice changes; reduced ability to organize or plan; reduced concentration; reduced comprehension of written material; performance changes at work
Moderate cognitive decline	Loss of memory of recent events; impaired ability to perform mathematical tasks; inability to plan and organize daily activities such as preparing meals and handling finances; may become socially withdrawn and uncomfortable in socially challenging situations
Moderately severe cognitive decline	Unable to recall phone numbers and personal history details; confused as to day, time, season; difficulty with simple arithmetic; know the names of close family members
Severe cognitive decline	Inability to perform daily tasks; need help with activities of daily living; experience sleep disruption and changes in sleep-wake cycle; urinary and fecal incontinence may be present; personality changes that can lead to delusions; may wander and become lost
Very severe cognitive decline	Final stage of the disease; inability to walk without assistance ; need help with feeding and toileting; inability to speak coherently; generally incontinent

(Adapted from Alzheimer's Association information.)

and estrogen hormone replacement therapy. Some physicians recommend regular use of anti-inflammatory drugs to slow the plaque formation in the brain by theoretically reducing the inflammatory response involved in the development of the plaques. Recent research using stem cells is showing some promising results for the return of memory in animal models and may have implications for use in humans.[153] Another new treatment from researchers at Mount Sinai School of Medicine is a compound in the second stage of human research trials called NIC5-15, which is thought to slow the progression of Alzheimer's disease dementia by preventing the formation of beta-amyloid plaques.[154] Many patients with Alzheimer's have to be placed in a long-term care setting due to behavioral and safety issues. Massage has been shown to have a positive effect on people who have agitation associated with Alzheimer's. The main improvements are noted in wandering, physical and verbal aggression, and being resistive to care within the nursing home setting.[155]

Physical Therapy Intervention. Physical therapy treatment concentrates on encouraging functional independence as long as possible. Exercise programs can be helpful in keeping people active.[156] Although Alzheimer's disease causes mainly cognitive problems the resultant inactivity of the patient leads to muscle weakness and loss of functional abilities. Physical therapy may entail working with patients to encourage activity levels, work on balance reeducation, strengthening and mobility exercises, and modalities as necessary for pain management. If the cognitive impairment is too great, the PT or PTA may work with patients in a group setting with general exercises. Some patients do a lot of aimless walking and are likely to fall. This presents several problems such as fatigue due to too much walking and falls resulting from balance problems. Whether patients are in a long-term facility or at home, minimizing clutter in the environment can reduce the risk of falls. This may be accomplished by simply taking up loose rugs or may require reducing or rearranging the amount of furniture in the rooms the patient uses most. Preventing patients from walking around is not the answer, unless they are at severe risk of falls, because it reduces overall mobility levels and may cause anger. When speaking to anyone with dementia, the PT or PTA should use simple short commands and be sure to use the patient's name. Advice and education of caregivers is extremely important so that consistency of approach to patients is achieved. Patients may require assistance with transfers and ambulation and must be supervised when performing exercise programs. Involving patients with group activities in the long-term care facility often is helpful.

"It Happened in the Clinic"

Mrs. Cowen was 90 years old and diagnosed with Alzheimer's disease just over 2 years ago. She was experiencing an increase of arthritis symptoms in her right knee with pain and loss of the ability to go up and down stairs. Her reduced mobility was creating a problem at the sheltered home where she lived because she was unable to negotiate the stairs or ambulate for more than 50 feet without a rest. The dining room where she ate all her meals was 150 feet from her room, and she now required a wheelchair to get to the dining room. Physical therapy intervention in the home was provided to help her increase the range of motion and strength in her right knee and to increase the distance of ambulation. The cognitive impairment resulting from Alzheimer's disease affected her ability to retain new information, and it proved difficult to ensure she performed her exercises or increased her ambulation distance. With the permission of the sheltered home staff, the physical therapist placed a photograph of Mrs. Cowan's family members at 25-feet intervals along the corridor from her room to the dining room. She was instructed to go and see her son, daughter, or grandson rather than specifying a distance. This worked as a motivational goal to increase the distance of ambulation over a period of 2 weeks, and she was able to return to the dining room for her meals without using a wheelchair.

Amyotrophic Lateral Sclerosis

Amyotrophic lateral sclerosis (ALS) is also known as Lou Gehrig's disease after the baseball player who developed the disease. ALS is a progressive, degenerative disease of the nervous system affecting both upper and lower motor neurons. The sensory system remains intact.[157] ALS mainly occurs in people between the ages of 40 and 60 with men affected more than women. People from all ethnic and racial backgrounds are affected by the disease. The incidence of ALS in the United States is approximately 1 in 100,000 people.[158] Approximately 20,000 Americans are living with ALS, and 5,000 people are diagnosed with the disease each year. The disease occurs worldwide.[159]

Etiology. The cause of ALS is largely unknown. The disease is similar to poliomyelitis, but no specific pathogen (virus or bacteria) has been identified associated with ALS. Approximately 5% to 10% of cases are attributed to inherited genetic factors. For the other 90% to 95% of people with ALS, the disease occurs randomly with no known cause. Several etiology theories include a virus, toxic levels of certain metals or minerals, and even an autoimmune disease triggered by the aging process. Of the people with familial ALS, approximately 20% carry a genetic defect causing mutation of the neurotransmitter enzyme superoxide dismutase 1 (SOD1). Another neurotransmitter, glutamate, may also be responsible for the disease. High concentrations of glutamate in the cerebrospinal fluid (CSF) destroy neurons and most people with ALS have high levels of this substance.[160]

Signs and Symptoms. Early symptoms of the disease usually involve muscle weakness, involuntary movements, spasticity, twitching and cramping in the distal extremities. The symptoms progress to include atrophy and paralysis of all the muscles in the limbs, trunk and face. Sensory systems are not affected. Fatigue is a progressive symptom regardless of the age of onset of the condition.[161] Dysarthria (speech problems associated with speaking and forming words) and dysphagia (swallowing and chewing difficulties) may exist as a result of paralysis or weakness of the facial muscles.[162] Hyperreflexia occurs (heightened responses to reflexes) including a more sensitive gag reflex, and a positive Babinski sign.[163] Respiration and feeding are affected by the muscle weakness. Psychological problems may include depression and suicidal thoughts.[164] Cognitive impairments include dementia in some people, changes in behavior, alterations in personality, and loss of the ability to plan. The memory usually remains intact.[165]

Prognosis. People with ALS progressively become weaker and weaker over a 3- to 10-year period and usually die from respiratory failure or complications from malnutrition and dehydration.[166]

Medical Intervention. The diagnosis of ALS consists of ruling out other diseases that can cause muscle weakness. The initial diagnosis relies on the medical history and physician observations. An electromyogram can help to determine whether the weakness is caused by peripheral neuropathy, and MRI and blood and urine tests can rule out other causative factors.[167] Medical intervention is with medications such as diazepam to control muscle spasms. Many people with ALS are candidates for the use of intermittent positive pressure ventilation (IPPV) machines in the later stages of the disease. Patients and their families must make hard decisions about whether to use ventilator assistance. A tracheostomy will be inserted if the decision is made to use IPPV. Advances in gene therapy

are showing promise for the treatment and delay of symptoms associated with ALS.[168] The only medication approved by the Food and Drug Administration to specifically treat ALS is riluzole (Rilutek), which slows the progression of the disease by decreasing the release of glutamate.[169,170] A speech and language pathologist and occupational therapist may be recommended to assist with swallowing and eating problems. The team approach to management of people with ALS is vitally important. Those involved with the management of people with ALS include the home care and hospice nurses, physical therapist, physician, psychologist, nutritionist, occupational therapist, respiratory therapist, social worker, and speech and language pathologist.[171]

Physical Therapy Intervention. Physical therapy interventions are directed at assisting patients to maintain as much independence and functional movement for as long as possible including ADL. Reduction of pain, education of patients and families, assistive equipment, home modifications advice, and exercise programs all play a part in the overall interventions.[172] Regular reevaluation by the PT is necessary as a result of the progressive nature of the disease. The PTA may work on functional mobility including measurement for a wheelchair and instruction in its use, balance, strengthening, stretching, and mobility exercises, low-impact aerobic exercises in the initial stages of the disease, breathing exercises, postural drainage, and chest PT.[173]

Cerebrovascular Accident and Transient Ischemic Attack

People experiencing a cerebrovascular accident (CVA), also known as a stroke or, more recently, a brain attack, may require a period of time in the intensive care unit (ICU) after onset of the condition. A CVA is considered to be a medical emergency. CVAs are the third leading cause of death in the United States. Approximately 600,000 to 800,000 people per year experience a CVA in the United States with a 30% per year fatality rate.[174] A CVA is generally diagnosed if the symptoms last more than 24 hours. If symptoms of a CVA last only a few minutes or a few hours, the diagnosis is usually a transient ischemic attack (TIA). However, a TIA can be a predictor of a future CVA.[175]

Etiology. A CVA can be precipitated by a ruptured aneurism in a blood vessel within the brain. In such cases, the blood from the aneurism seeps into the tissue and creates pressure on the brain tissue, resulting in various symptoms depending on the location of the injury. This is called a hemorrhagic CVA. In other cases, the CVA is caused by an embolus (a blood clot) developed from an area of atherosclerosis of the large blood vessels. The embolus travels along the blood vessels until it blocks a smaller blood vessel in the brain, resulting in anoxia of the brain tissue supplied by the vessel. This can result in brain tissue necrosis due to lack of oxygen. This type of CVA is known as an ischemic CVA. One of the leading causes of CVA and other cardiovascular diseases is smoking.[176] In addition, the Surgeon General's report in 2006 reported that secondhand smoke is estimated to account for a further 46,000 deaths of people from coronary heart disease and CVA each year.[177]

Signs and Symptoms. A variety of symptoms may be related to a TIA. Weakness of one side of the face may cause a lop-sided tilt to the mouth as the mouth is pulled toward the strong side. This causes difficulty with smiling. People may experience headaches, transient difficulties with blurred vision, speech, or swallowing, and a weakness or tingling of one side of the body. A short period of confusion is common with a TIA.[178] These problems may resolve in a matter of minutes or hours, but people should go to the emergency room for assessment because TIAs have been noted to precede a CVA in many cases. People with CVA may have hemiplegia with weakness or loss of function of one side of the body that includes the upper and lower extremities. Because the spinal tracts cross over within the spinal cord, a CVA on the right side of the brain affects the limbs on the opposite side of the body. Therefore, a right-sided CVA will cause weakness on the left side of the body. Some people have swallowing problems (dysphagia) after a CVA and require a semiliquid diet. Others may have speech difficulties (dysphasia). If the location of the neurological insult is in the cerebellum, the effects may be loss of balance. Severe symptoms can occur if the CVA affects the brainstem. The brainstem is a primitive part of the brain that controls major body functions such as breathing. Patients who experience a brainstem CVA are likely to be managed in the ICU. Some patients may be confused or mentally disoriented. Some patients fail to recognize relatives and may not be able to recognize familiar objects such as a spoon or fork. This may last a few hours or many days or may be permanent. Patients may be unaware of the existence of the affected side of the body and "neglect" that side. Perception of the position of the body in space may be lost (loss of proprioception and lack of kinesthetic awareness). In many instances, patients with a CVA spend the initial few days after onset of the problem in the ICU where vital signs and general condition can be monitored closely.

Prognosis. Various factors affect the prognosis of people with a CVA such as the location and extent of the brain damage and the general health of the patient. The prognosis for patients with a brainstem CVA is poor. Seeking medical help immediately can make a difference. In cases in which the problem is due to an embolus, medications can be administered to dissolve the clot and reduce the overall brain damage. People who experience TIAs have a 9% risk of having another TIA or a CVA.[179]

Medical Intervention. A quick diagnosis of people experiencing the symptoms of either a TIA or CVA is essential for a good outcome. An MRI scan is useful for diagnosing the cause of the CVA.[180] The recommendation is for intervention within the first 90 minutes after the onset of CVA or TIA symptoms.[181] An ischemic CVA is treated with anticoagulants, whereas treatment of a hemorrhagic CVA is focused on controlling the hypertension and bleeding within the brain. The risk of CVA after a TIA is high, especially in the days and weeks immediately after the TIA.[182] The immediate interventions include reducing hypertension, lowering blood cholesterol using statin medications, and the use of antiplatelet treatments or anticoagulant therapy with warfarin (Coumadin). Long-term interventions include smoking cessation, reduction of alcohol consumption, increased amounts of exercise, weight loss or control, the use of a low-dose daily aspirin (81 mg), precautionary measures such as an annual flu shot and a pneumonia vaccination, and stroke rehabilitation if necessary. CVA caused by atherosclerosis may require surgery to prevent further instances.[183] Such surgery is often a carotid endarterectomy, in which the carotid artery is replaced by a blood vessel taken from the person's leg such as the saphenous vein. Alternatively, a stent (mesh device to keep the artery open) may be surgically inserted into the carotid artery.

Physical Therapy Intervention. Physical therapy intervention for the patient post-CVA in the ICU may include bed mobility exercises, range of motion of the affected limbs, active assisted exercises for the affected limbs, and active exercises for the unaffected limbs. Good results for increased range of motion and the ability to reach have been noted with exercises involving weights and weight-bearing for abduction of the weak upper extremity (Ellis, 2009).[184] The PT and PTA are involved with assisted transfers from bed to chair and ambulation as possible and as allowed by the physician. Encouragement may be needed to help patients turn to the affected side if they have a neglect problem. Demonstrate exercises to family members and caregivers and allow them to watch the treatment. However, if the patient is distracted and unable to concentrate, ask the family to leave the room during the treatment. The PT and PTA should decide the best course to follow with this matter. In the later stages of rehabilitation, the PT and PTA may want the family present during treatment. Patients may be on oxygen, be attached to the electrocardiogram monitor, have an indwelling catheter, and may have a nasogastric feeding tube if they have problems with swallowing resulting from the CVA. Patients may be mentally disoriented or confused and unable to understand or concentrate on instructions.

PRECAUTIONS AND CONSIDERATIONS FOR PHYSICAL THERAPY INTERVENTION

Several general precautions and considerations are required when working with patients with CVA in the ICU:

1. Read patient charts carefully before treatment.
2. Check with the nurse before treatment.
3. Check vital signs before treatment.
4. Follow all specified recommendations regarding patient position change to prevent pressure ulcers.
5. Observe patients closely during treatment for signs of changes in vital signs and discoloration of lips, or ears for signs of cyanosis.
6. Observe patients closely for signs of fatigue.
7. Observe patients closely for any signs of increased weakness or changes in speech such as slurred speech, which might indicate a further CVA. If in any doubt call the nurse and contact the supervising PT.
8. Lock the bed in place or push it up against a wall if moving patients out of bed.
9. Document the volume of any fluids given to patients during treatment because fluid intake and output is monitored on the ICU.
10. If patients are on a thickened liquids diet due to swallowing problems be sure *not* to give them water to drink. They might aspirate a thin liquid.
11. Encourage patients to turn their head toward the affected side by standing on the side of the bed of the affected side.
12. Speak to patients and explain exactly who you are and what you are going to do.
13. Be encouraging but make patients do as much as possible for themselves.
14. Keep instructions to simple one word commands or short sentences.
15. Keep treatments fairly short to prevent undue patient fatigue.
16. When getting patients into a sitting position or transferring them out of bed into a chair, ensure that the catheter bag is on the side of the bed the patient is exiting. Keep the catheter bag below the level of the pelvis to prevent flow back of urine into the bladder.
17. Remember that it may not be possible to do more than a few exercises with patients for the first few days. Getting patients into a chair may be the most they can tolerate in one session.
18. Move all intravenous and feeding hookups to the side of the bed patients will exit.
19. Ask for assistance to perform transfers, particularly for the first attempt.
20. If there is a major difference between the description of the PT's prior treatment and what you observe during treatment be sure to talk to the supervising PT and defer treatment if necessary.
21. Make patients comfortable on completion of the PT session ensuring they are in a good position, have an alarm close to hand, and can reach their essentials such as the telephone.
22. Inform the nurse upon completion of the treatment session and verify any change in patient positioning.
23. If family members were requested to leave the room during PT, remember to inform them that they may return to the room. Remind them that the patient may be fatigued after the PT session.
24. Try not to get drawn into discussions with the family regarding prognosis. This is the role for the physician and the PT. Keep discussion to current treatment issues and how the family can help the patient during recovery.

GERIATRIC CONSIDERATIONS

When working with older people who have sustained a cerebrovascular accident (CVA, or stroke), particular consideration must be given to the prior functional abilities of the person. Because rehabilitation of people with a CVA involves complex activities, this prior function must include the non-involved side of the body. The medical chart must be carefully read to determine the past medical history. Often family members may be able to fill in gaps in the medical chart. If the range of motion of the lower or upper extremity of the involved side is not within full range, the problem may be the result of a prior arthritic condition. Trying to return the person to a level of range of

(Continued)

motion in the affected joint more than previously available may not be realistic. Conversely, there may be limitation of motion in joints of the unaffected side resulting from previous injury or arthritis. This makes it difficult to make a comparison between one side of the body and the other as is usually required when taking range of motion measurements. Other factors complicating the rehabilitation may include prior medical conditions such as diabetes mellitus, congestive heart failure, respiratory conditions, and peripheral vascular disease. All these diagnoses will affect the amount and intensity of the rehabilitation tolerated by the patient.

Creutzfeldt-Jacob Disease

Creutzfeldt-Jakob disease (CJD) is actually a group of rare, prion, degenerative neurological disorders. Various types of the disease exist including sporadic, hereditary, acquired, and variant. The age of onset of CJD in humans usually is after 60 years of age.[185] A form of CJD found in cattle is bovine spongiform encephalopathy (BSE) or "mad cow disease." The prevalence of BSE in the United States is low. The worldwide prevalence of CJD and other prion diseases is 1 per 1 million people, with between 200 and 300 cases occurring in the United States annually.[186] Approximately 85% of people with CJD have the sporadic form, 5% to 10% have the hereditary type, and the remaining 5% to 10% have acquired CJD.[187]

Etiology. The sporadic form of CJD accounts for approximately 85% of all cases of the disease and is of unknown cause. Some people with the sporadic form are infected through direct contact with infected transplant materials such as corneal transplants and dura mater grafts. However, all blood and body tissues are now specially treated in the United States to prevent transmission in this way. Another method of transmission is through direct contact with infected brain tissue and CSF during brain surgery or autopsy.[188]

The hereditary/genetic form of CJD is either transmitted from one parent through an autosomal dominant gene or develops as a spontaneous mutation of the PRNP gene. The PRNP gene is responsible for making prion protein (PrP). This protein plays a part in the transport of copper in the body and may protect the neurons of the brain from damage. A mutation of the PRNP gene causes abnormalities to occur in the development of the prion proteins. The abnormal prions build up in the brain tissue, destroying neurons resulting in extensive brain damage.[189]

A relationship between the BSE in cattle and the variant form of Creutzfeldt-Jakob disease (vCJD) in humans is suspected. BSE is caused by alterations in the normal proteins called prions, which then infect the animal. The infection is thought to be transmitted by animal feed that contains infected materials from other animals. Outbreaks of BSE in Britain in the 1970s and 1980s were correlated with a few cases of vCJD in humans after an incubation period of approximately 10 years.[190]

Signs and Symptoms. The characteristic signs and symptoms of CJD include multiple mental and neurological symptoms such as a rapid and progressive dementia accompanied by severe mental impairment with changes in personality, reduced judgment, and an inability to think clearly. Depression and insomnia (inability to sleep) are common. Motor deficits include loss of coordination of movement, severe muscle weakness, **myoclonus** (involuntary muscle movements), loss of the ability to speak, and eventual immobility. During the end stages of the disease, blindness may occur, and people often lapse into a coma.[191]

Prognosis. CJD is a fatal disease; no cure currently exists for it. Approximately 90% of people die within 1 year of diagnosis.[192]

Medical Intervention. The diagnosis of CJD is one of ruling out other possible causes for the neurological symptoms such as dementia, encephalitis, or meningitis. Diagnostic procedures include a spinal tap for testing of CSF, an electroencephalogram (EEG), and CT scan to rule out CVA or brain tumors. More specific tests include MRI, which can detect degeneration of the brain tissue typical of CJD,[193] and a brain biopsy. However, a brain biopsy is rarely used because the risks are greater than the benefits. An autopsy of the brain after death can confirm the diagnosis, but precautions must be taken so that the people involved do not have direct contact with the brain tissue or the CSF. The main treatment for people with CJD is to alleviate any symptoms. Opiate medications may be prescribed to reduce pain, and muscle relaxants such as clonazepam and sodium valproate may be used to reduce myoclonus. In the final stages of the disease, people must be repositioned frequently to prevent decubitus ulcers.[194]

Physical Therapy Intervention. Physical therapy intervention is indicated to help people maintain mobility for as long as possible. A combination of strengthening and mobility exercises is used within patients' tolerance and assistive devices for ambulation provided as needed.

Dementia—Non-Alzheimer's (Lewy Body, Senile Dementia, Vascular Dementia)

Although Alzheimer's disease has gained a lot of publicity as a result of the prevalence of the condition, other types of dementia exist. Such dementias include Lewy body dementia, senile dementia, vascular dementia, and dementias precipitated by other diseases. These types of dementia affect people in a wide age range and often under age 65.[195]

Etiology. Lewy body dementia is one of the leading causes of dementia next to Alzheimer's disease and vascular dementia. The dementia is caused by a buildup of Lewy body proteins in the brain.[196] The Lewy bodies disrupt the production of neurotransmitters in the brain. Dopamine production by the basal ganglia and the production of acetylcholine are both reduced.[197] Vascular dementia is caused by vascular disease of the vessels to the brain resulting in ischemia. Dementia may be precipitated by many other diseases such as Creutzfeldt-Jakob disease, depression, Down syndrome, HIV, Huntington's disease, numerous inherited metabolic and neurological conditions, multiple sclerosis, parkinsonism, substance abuse, and traumatic brain injury. Temporary conditions such as infections, thyroid dysfunction, and vitamin B_{12} deficiency may cause reversible dementia. Other factors that cause dementia-like conditions include toxic substances and some pharmacological medications. Some of the medications that may cause symptoms of dementia include psychotropic medications such as lithium and tricyclic antidepressants, antihypertensive (blood pressure lowering) medications including diuretics, anticancer medications, antibiotics such as penicillin, and even aspirin, digitalis, and amphetamines. Exposure to heavy metals such as aluminum, gold, lead, mercury, nickel, thallium, and tin may cause dementia symptoms.[198] Exposure to smoking and secondhand smoke is also thought to be linked to the development of a variety of types of dementia.

Signs and Symptoms. Lewy body dementia is a progressive dementia resulting in rapid problems with cognitive functions, Parkinson-like motor deficits, functional deficits, and hallucinations.[199] Other types of dementia result in various levels of cognitive and motor dysfunction, memory loss, word retrieval problems, poor judgment, aggression, depression, anxiety, and aimless wandering.[200]

Prognosis. The prognosis for people with dementia depends on the causative factors. Treatment of the underlying cause of the dementia may resolve or reduce the symptoms. Some types of dementia are largely untreatable such as those caused by Creutzfeldt-Jakob disease and AIDS related dementia.

Medical Intervention. The diagnosis of specific types of dementia is often difficult. The early onset of dementia often indicates a cause other than Alzheimer's disease, although early-onset Alzheimer's exists. A medical history is performed to determine whether some of the diseases that can be associated with dementia can be identified. The medical treatment of dementia symptoms will depend on the causative factors. The use of antidepressants may be the first intervention to make sure that depression is not the causative factor. Other diagnostic tools include a cognitive screening test such as the Mini-Mental State Examination, and radiological imaging with a CT scan or MRI to detect any changes in brain anatomy. Blood tests are performed for thyroid function tests and levels of vitamin B_{12}. People with suspected alcohol or other substance abuse are advised to stop taking the substance to see if that is causing the dementia.[201] People with Lewy body dementia are treated with cholinesterase inhibitors, which seem to reduce the symptoms of the dementia and hallucinations.[202] The treatment of other types of dementia is specific to the causative disease. Group discussions, support groups for both patients and families, and the use of reminiscence therapy may be helpful. Reminiscence therapy uses photographs and familiar objects to stimulate recall for people with dementia.

Physical Therapy Intervention. Physical therapy intervention is directed not toward treatment of dementia but of the neurological and musculoskeletal manifestations of the disease process that may be causing the dementia. Ambulation, strengthening, stretching, and endurance exercises, balance and coordination activities, and functional training may be needed. Strategies for interventions have to be adjusted to accommodate the altered cognitive state of people with these conditions. Short, simple instructions and a firm, calm voice, help to maximize the rehabilitation potential of interventions. Providing intervention within a familiar location such as the home can alleviate the stress of unfamiliar surroundings that may often cause further confusion. Ensuring that people have ready access to a large calendar and clock in their room also can help to reduce levels of confusion by orienting them to time and place. Some research is currently being conducted for the use of robots to assist people with dementia to be more interactive and able to remain in their own home longer. The participation in activities such as music therapy and arts and crafts has been demonstrated to keep people with dementia more active, and interaction with people is beneficial.[203]

Epilepsy, Seizure Disorder, and Epileptic Syndromes

Epilepsy is a condition in which numerous neurons in the brain are fired simultaneously leading to a large burst of electrical energy that triggers seizures involving multiple involuntary contractions of muscles in the body. Worldwide more than 50 million people are affected by epileptic seizures.[204] In the United States, 1 in 100 people experience a seizure during their lifetime, but to be diagnosed with epilepsy, at least two seizures have to occur with no known cause.[205] Many types of epileptic syndrome exist. Some of the more well known include West syndrome, Lennox-Gastaut syndrome, juvenile myoclonic epilepsy, Rolandic epilepsy, Landau-Kleffner syndrome, Rasmussen's encephalitis, progressive myoclonic epilepsy, temporal lobe epilepsy, frontal lobe epilepsy, and childhood absence epilepsy. [206]

Etiology. Many types of seizure disorders are of unknown cause. Some are the result of genetic traits that seem to run in families. Other types are the result of other disease processes such as meningitis, viral encephalitis, AIDS, dementia, CVA, or myocardial infarction (heart attack). Brain damage resulting from a head injury or developmental disorders may precipitate seizure disorders. Men are affected slightly more than women, and young children and people over the age of 65 are at greater risk of developing the condition.[207] The pathological cause of the seizures are the result of abnormalities within the neurons of the brain or of the balance of neurotransmitters, which cause multiple neurons to be triggered at once and result in abnormal muscle contractions and sensory changes.

Signs and Symptoms. The onset of seizure disorders often is during early childhood including Lennox-Gastaut syndrome, Rolandic epilepsy, Landau-Kleffner syndrome, juvenile myoclonic epilepsy, and childhood absence epilepsy. The general signs and symptoms of seizure disorders are uncontrolled, involuntary muscular contractions of various intensities, and convulsions. These contractions may be absence seizures, atonic, myoclonic/myotonic, or tonic-clonic. Absence seizures are often called "petit mal" seizures and are characterized by brief periods of loss of consciousness, staring, and minimal changes in body movements. People with atonic seizures experience a temporary loss of muscle tone resulting in collapse and falls. Myoclonic or myotonic seizures are characterized by jerking and twitching movements. Tonic-clonic seizures also known as "grand mal" are more serious with loss of consciousness, stiffness and shaking, and loss of bladder control. Some seizures affect a smaller area of the brain and are known as simple partial seizures or complex partial seizures. People who experience simple partial seizures do not lose consciousness but have temporary changes in emotions and sensations such as tingling, flashing lights, changes in taste and smell, and muscle jerks or twitches. Complex partial seizures cause altered levels of consciousness, staring, twitching, and unusual movements such as hand rubbing.[208]

Prognosis. No cure exists for seizures, but approximately 80% of people with epilepsy have their seizures under control with antiepileptic medications. In some people, seizures resolve with age. In most cases, seizures do not cause brain damage. ☻ Children who experience seizures tend to have behavior and emotional problems resulting from the disruption to social activities. The normal life span usually is not affected by seizures unless a life-threatening status epilepticus seizure occurs that lasts for more than 5 minutes and can lead to brain damage or death. A rare complication of epilepsy is sudden unexplained death in epilepsy (SUDEP). Driving accidents during a seizure and drowning incidents in the bathtub or when swimming are more likely in people with epilepsy.[209,210]

Medical Intervention. The diagnosis of seizure disorders is achieved through a detailed medical history, EEG studies of the brain and brain scans with CT or MRI. The diagnosis of seizures in children with developmental or learning disabilities can be challenging.[211] Antiepileptic medications include diazepam (Valium), carbamazepine (Tegretol), clobazam, felbamate, topiramate, valproic acid (Depakene), valproate, and zonisamide.[212,213] More recently approved medications include carisbamate, lacosamide, retigabine, rufinamide, and stiripentol. All of these antiepileptic medications act on the synaptic neurotransmitters to either inhibit or stimulate specific chemical transmitters.[214] Vagus nerve stimulation helps some people whose seizures are not adequately controlled with medications. A small electrical stimulation unit is implanted under the skin of the anterior chest wall, which sends electrical impulses to the vagus nerve every few minutes. The unit can be triggered by the person if a seizure is imminent. Vagus nerve stimulation reduces the number of seizures for many people.[215,216] When all other medical interventions are unsuccessful in controlling seizures, brain surgery to remove the area of the brain causing the focal seizures may be performed.[217] In people with multiple daily seizures that are not controlled, a hemispherectomy may be performed.[218] Another possible intervention is placing people on a ketogenic diet consisting of a high fat content and no sugars. This ketogenic diet reduces the number of seizures experienced by some people. People with epileptic seizures are advised to stop drinking alcohol because this can interfere with the effectiveness of the antiepileptic medications. Advances in gene therapy and stem cell research provide hope for people with epilepsy.[219]

Physical Therapy Intervention. Physical therapy is indicated for the treatment of people with epilepsy who have sustained a fracture. ☺ Some children with specific types of epilepsy associated with developmental delay may attend physical therapy for intervention with NDT, ambulation, and exercises for balance, coordination, strengthening, stretching, and endurance. When working with people who have experienced a CVA or a head injury, PTAs need to be aware of the possibility for seizures.

Guillain Barré Syndrome and Acute Inflammatory Demyelinating Neuropathy

Guillain Barré syndrome (GBS) is an autoimmune, neurological disease triggered by a previous infection or traumatic event that causes the immune system to attack the neural tissue. This syndrome can affect people in any age group and occurs in 1 in 100,000 of the population.[220]

Etiology. Guillain Barré syndrome usually occurs after an infection. Respiratory and gastrointestinal infections are most likely to cause the syndrome. Occasionally surgery may trigger the symptoms. Vaccinations are not proven to cause the syndrome.[221] A rare cause of Guillain Barré is a medication called pegylated interferon alpha 2a prescribed for chronic hepatitis C infection and other viral infections.[222] The reason why some people develop this syndrome is unknown. The theory is that the immune system is somehow misled into thinking the body's own neural tissue is foreign and starts attacking the myelin sheath and axons of the peripheral nerves causing disruption of the electrical signals to the muscles.

Signs and Symptoms. The signs and symptoms of Guillain Barré syndrome evolve rapidly over a period of days, weeks, or hours. People tend to be at their weakest approximately 3 weeks from the onset of symptoms. The initial symptoms include weakness of muscles and tingling sensations in the skin of the lower extremities that spreads to the upper body and upper extremities. The syndrome can result in almost total paralysis of the muscles. The muscle weakness is usually bilateral, the deep tendon reflexes are absent, and the CSF contains an abnormally high level of protein biomarkers such as neurofilament, tan, and glial proteins. People with severe forms of the syndrome may have paralysis of the respiratory muscles and even the heart.[223]

Prognosis. The general prognosis for people with Guillain Barré syndrome is fairly good. Most people will recover even after severe symptoms. Total paralysis may be life-threatening as a result of the effect on respiration and heart rate, and patients may require a ventilator. Some people may experience continued residual muscle weakness. The recovery may take weeks to years.[224] A correlation exists between high levels of protein biomarkers in the CSF and a less favorable outcome for people with the syndrome.[225] Higher levels of cortisol in the plasma also seem to correlate with an increased risk of respiratory failure during the acute phase of the disease.[226] Older people with the syndrome who need to be placed on a mechanical ventilator have a higher risk of mortality.[227]

Medical Intervention. No known cure exists for this disease. The diagnosis can be difficult as the symptoms are similar to other demyelinating neurological diseases. However, the sudden onset of the signs and symptoms is indicative of Guillain Barré syndrome. A spinal tap may be performed because the CSF of people with the condition contains high levels of protein biomarkers such as neurofilament, tan, and glial resulting from the breakdown of the myelin and neuronal axons.[228] Blood tests for levels of cortisol in the plasma will reveal higher than normal levels.[229] Nerve conduction velocity tests indicate a slowing of nerve transmission to the muscles resulting from the demyelination of the nerves and the destruction of neuronal axons. CT scans and MRIs of the brain may be performed to rule out other neurological diseases. Most people with the signs and symptoms of the disease are admitted to the hospital and monitored in the ICU. People with severe paralysis may require a respirator. The medical intervention may include plasmapheresis (plasma exchange). During this procedure, the blood is removed from the body, and the plasma is separated from the blood cells. Only the blood cells are returned to the body, and the plasma volume is restored by the body. This procedure is sometimes effective in reducing the intensity of the autoimmune response and is thought to remove some of the toxic immune system components within the blood plasma. Intravenous injections of high doses of immunoglobulin may help to reduce the progression of the disease by restoring some of the body's immune defenses.[230] Other medical interventions are aimed at ensuring adequate hydration when people are unable to swallow, preventing skin breakdown during paralysis by regular turning and repositioning, and support of essential body systems affected by the disease. During the recovery phase, the neurologist, nursing, physical therapy, occupational therapy, speech and language therapy, respiratory therapy, social work, and psychological counseling are all indicated. Psychological support for the family is important. People with this condition are often admitted to an inpatient rehabilitation unit before they return home. Ongoing interventions after discharge home usually are required as in-home or outpatient care. The need for a hospital-type adjustable bed and adaptations to the home are assessed by the intervention team before discharge from the hospital.

Physical Therapy Intervention. During the initial phases of the disease process, the physical therapy intervention may include instruction to nursing and families regarding passive or active assisted range of motion exercises to all of the affected limbs to reduce the risk of joint and muscle contractures. Physical therapy is paced according to the recovery of the peripheral nerves. People fatigue rapidly during recovery and should not be overfatigued in therapy. Interventions may include analysis of gait patterns using a digital computerized gait analysis machine;[231] functional mobility training in a wheelchair and progressive ambulation with appropriate assistive devices, such as walkers and ankle-foot orthoses;[232] ADL training; progressive resistive exercises for all extremities and trunk muscles; breathing exercises and pulmonary hygiene interventions, such as percussion and vibrations; neurodevelopmental therapy;[233] and balance and coordination reeducation.[234] Combining treatment sessions with other rehabilitation disciplines and psychology can be beneficial for maximizing patient outcomes and goals. Biofeedback has proven effective in reducing pain perception and encouraging muscle strengthening.[235]

Huntington's Disease

Huntington's disease is a progressive, hereditary, degenerative neurological disease. The disease affects approximately 1 in 20,000 people in the United States and 1 in 10,000 worldwide.[236]

Etiology. This hereditary disease is autosomal dominant (only one parent has to have the defective gene), caused by a single defective gene. The genetic mutation is located on the fourth chromosome and called the CAG trinucleotide repeat expansion of the HTT gene. This abnormality leads to a long version of the HTT gene responsible for the production of huntingtin protein.[237] The resultant abnormally long protein breaks into segments that coagulate and build up in the neurons of the brain. The longer the protein, the more likely it is to cause early onset of the disease. The normal huntingtin protein is thought to protect neurons of the brain from self-destruction, and the abnormal protein removes this protection causing break down of the neurons within the brain.[238]

Signs and Symptoms. The signs and symptoms of Huntington's disease usually start people in their 30s and 40s, although younger people may develop the symptoms. Symptoms usually progress slowly. When the disease affects younger people, the onset may be similar to Parkinson's disease with muscle rigidity, tremors, and slow movements.[239] The more characteristic signs and symptoms of Huntington's disease involve several movement disorders. Chorea (involuntary, jerky, uncoordinated movements), dystonia (increased muscle tone accompanied by involuntary movements with rotation that last for prolonged periods of time), myoclonus (involuntary twitching and spasm of muscles), movement tics (brief, repetitive, muscular spasms usually involving the face), and Parkinson-like movements are common. People with the disease also exhibit hallucinations; sleep changes; slurred speech and difficulty swallowing; behavioral changes, such as aggression, agitation, anger, and poor concentration and attention; dementia; severe mood swings; psychiatric disorders; seizures; and progressive cognitive deficits.[240,241]

Prognosis. Huntington's disease cannot be cured and results in death approximately 10 to 30 years after the onset of the signs and symptoms.[242,243] Medical management can reduce the symptoms of the disease to increase the length of time people can remain functional.

Medical Intervention. The diagnosis of Huntington's is achieved through a detailed family medical history, with possible psychiatric evaluation and genetic testing for the faulty gene associated with the disease. CT and MRI of the brain may indicate any changes in the brain tissue and rule out other diseases.[244] No medications exist to cure or prevent the disease. The medical management is aimed at controlling the symptoms of the disease to allow people to function better. Because the symptoms are a combination of motor deficits and behavioral and psychiatric disorders, a variety of different medications may be used. The first medication approved by the CDC specifically to control the movement disorders of people with Huntington's disease was tetrabenazine (Xenazine).[245] Other types of medications include antiepileptics to control seizures; antidepressants such as fluoxetine (Prozac) or nortriptyline (Pamelor) to control both depression and obsessive-compulsive disorder; acetylcholinesterase inhibitors, such as rivastigmine[246] to reduce synaptic transmission and minimize the muscle disorders and dementia; and botulinum toxin injections to affected muscles. Antipsychotic medications such as haloperidol and clozapine help to control hallucinations and violent outbursts, and lithium is used for the control of severe mood swings.[247] Surgical interventions such as deep brain stimulation (implantation of an electrode in the brain) and stem-cell transplants are undergoing medical trials for effectiveness.[248,249] People with Huntington's disease benefit from speech and language pathology to help with speech and feeding problems, occupational therapy for adaptations to the home for safety and ADL, and physical therapy interventions. The psychological and physical burdens on the caregivers of people with HD is considerable.[250,251] Care givers are provided with resources for support groups and respite care, and admission to a skilled nursing facility may become necessary for people in the later stages of the disease.[252]

Physical Therapy Intervention. Physical therapy intervention is indicated for people with Huntington's disease. A study by Bosse and coworkers in 2008 indicated a need for further research regarding the appropriate provision of physical therapy services related to the stage of the disease process. Many physical therapists do not see people diagnosed with early HD, and by the time a referral is made, the disease is advanced, which may have an impact on the effectiveness of physical therapy intervention.[253] The focus of PT is to keep people independent for as long as possible. Strategies include strength, flexibility, and endurance exercise programs; balance exercises and fall prevention strategies; ambulation and transfers training; advice on energy conservation techniques; home exercise programs; and instruction for care providers and family members. In the later stages of the disease, instruction on the use of a mechanical lift may be provided.

Multiple Sclerosis

Multiple sclerosis (MS) is an autoimmune, chronic, degenerative, demyelinating neurological disorder of the CNS. Two general types of the disease are recognized: primary progressive multiple sclerosis and relapsing, remitting multiple sclerosis.[254] In the United States, the prevalence of MS is higher in Caucasians than other groups. MS affects approximately 400,000 people in the United States, with people between the teenage years and age 50 at the highest risk for the disease. Women are affected 2 to 3 times as often as men.[255]

Etiology. The exact cause of multiple sclerosis has not been clearly identified. The causative factors are thought to be both genetic and environmental. Recent genetic studies in people with MS have identified a defect in the interleukin 2 and 7 receptor alpha genes that reduces the ability of the T-cells to switch off the immune response causing an autoimmune attack on the myelin surrounding the CNS nerves.[256] The prevalence of MS is higher in countries further away from the equator in both the Northern and Southern hemispheres in the more temperate climates, which leads to the theory that environment is a causative factor. Other factors that may cause triggering of the disease in genetically susceptible individuals are viruses such as measles, herpes, and influenza and the concentration of sex hormones. Scar tissue from sclerosis of the demyelinated nerves causes plaques to build up on the nerves. These plaques build up in the spinal cord and brain, disrupting brain function and neural transmission of electrical impulses.[257]

Signs and Symptoms. The signs and symptoms of multiple sclerosis vary from person to person. The onset of symptoms may occur gradually or very quickly between the ages of 20 and 40 years in both males and females. Demyelination of the nerves causes the primary symptoms, such as changes in skin sensation of tingling, numbness, burning, and pricking and sensitivity to heat; vision disturbances of blurred vision, double vision, and optic neuritis, which develops in approximately 55% of all people with MS; muscle weakness resulting in speech and swallowing problems, gait deficits, tremors, fatigue, dizziness and loss of balance, and poor coordination of movements; cognitive problems including memory and concentration deficits; and bowel and bladder incontinence. The secondary symptoms occur as a result of the primary symptoms such as pressure sores that develop in people who are inactive and frequent urinary tract infections due to incontinence. Other tertiary symptoms that cannot be overlooked are those that affect social, psychological, and vocational functioning. Depression has a major impact on these areas of life.[258]

Prognosis. No cure exists for multiple sclerosis, but people with the disease can be helped with medications that slow down its progression. Some people have mild effects from the disease, and others become completely debilitated.

Medical Intervention. A team approach to the treatment of people with MS is required. The team may comprise the physician, neurologist, psychologist/psychiatrist, social worker, nurse, physical therapist, occupational therapist, and speech and language pathologist. The diagnosis of multiple sclerosis is a difficult process. Other disease processes such as idiopathic inflammatory demyelinating disorders (IIDD) have to be eliminated before the diagnosis is made. Physicians use the McDonald Criteria consisting of data from an MRI, the presence of some myelopathy, and a unilateral optic neuritis during the diagnostic process.[259] Some of the rehabilitation assessment instruments are described under the physical therapy intervention. Physicians, psychologists, and therapists may administer the Minimal Assessment of Cognitive Function in MS (MACFIMS) test to determine the level of cognitive deficits present in people with suspected MS.[260] Several medications are approved for the treatment of multiple sclerosis. The majority of the medications reduce the autoimmune mechanism that destroys the myelin. These medications reduce the development of new brain lesions and slow down the progression of the disease in people with relapsing-remitting MS and include interferon (Avonex, Betaseron, Rebif); glatiramer acetate (Copaxone); mitoxantrone (Novantrone); and natalizumab (Tysabri).[261]

Physical Therapy Intervention. The physical therapy intervention for people with MS is extensive. Several studies have demonstrated the efficacy of strengthening, stretching, and aerobic exercises for people with MS on levels of mobility, quality of life, and reduction of the effects of fatigue both in the short term and long term. Exercise programs may involve several weeks of physical therapy group or individual exercise programs interspersed with home exercises.[262,263] Although fatigue should be avoided, new evidence suggests that resistance training is appropriate for people with mild to moderate symptoms of MS.[264] Balance and fall prevention should also be incorporated into the rehabilitation program.

Functional electrical stimulation may be used to improve ambulation abilities in people with gait deviations resulting from the weakness of MS.[265] Some success has been noted using constraint-induced movement therapy for people with hemiparetic (one-sided) weakness symptoms of MS,[266] and pool exercises in water below body temperature as a result of heat sensitivity can be beneficial.[267] Many standardized assessment tools exist for use by the physical therapist to evaluate and monitor the musculoskeletal and neurological effects of the disease. Probably the most commonly used are the range of motion (ROM) using a goniometer and manual muscle testing (MMT). Some of the other commonly used assessment techniques include the Ashworth and Modified Ashworth Spasticity Scale[268]; the Barthel Index that assesses mobility, ADL, and continence[269]; the Berg Balance Scale for measuring balance and assessing the likelihood of falls[270]; the Functional Independence Measure (FIM), which assesses abilities of feeding, bathing, dressing, transfers, gait, cognitive function and social interactions; the International Classification of Functioning (ICF), which focuses on functional levels of everyday activities[271,272]; and the Tinetti Assessment Tool, which focuses on the evaluation of gait and balance.[273,274] An assessment tool specifically for people with MS is the MS Functional Composite (MSFC), which combines the results of a timed 25-feet walk test with the assessment of fine motor skills.

"It Happened in the Clinic"

*M*rs. Davis was a 65-year-old woman diagnosed with multiple sclerosis for the past 20 years. She was receiving home care physical therapy as a result of an exacerbation of her multiple sclerosis symptoms and a reduction in her mobility. She was no longer able to perform transfers from her wheelchair to the bed without assistance or to take a few steps with a walker as she had been able to do two months earlier. She had previously been able to stand at the kitchen sink for a few minutes after standing up from her wheelchair but was now unable to do so. The physical therapist was working on transfers and sit to standing with the patient. The patient's husband worked during the day, and the goal was to try and make the patient more independent. Transfers with a sliding board were progressing well for the patient. Transferring from the wheelchair to the bed was possible with minimal assistance. Because the patient was becoming very stiff in her lower extremity joints, the physical therapist was anxious to progress to standing activities as soon as possible. Passive range of motion was performed twice a day by the patient's husband for the lower extremities. The first time the physical therapist stood the patient using a gait belt, standing in front of the patient, and blocking the patient's knees with her knees. Mrs. Davis was able to stand for approximately 2 minutes with the weight supported by the physical therapist. The following day, the patient reported to the physical therapist that the standing seemed to have really been good for her. She was able to have a normal bowel movement yesterday evening, which had not been possible for the past 2 months. We often do not think about some of the effects of physical therapy intervention on other bodily functions. The normal movements and activities that people perform keep the whole body including the heart, intestinal, and respiratory systems working in a functional way. When people become immobile, their entire body systems become affected.

Near-Drowning/Drowning With Partial or Full Recovery

Drowning is the fifth leading cause of accidental death in the United States with an incidence of 2.5 to 3.5 for every 100,000 of the total population. ☻ Drowning is responsible for more than 8,000 deaths annually in the United States, 1,500 of which involve children. Up to one quarter of these deaths are in children 14 years of age or younger. For every death that occurs by drowning, another 4 people are hospitalized, and 14 are seen in the emergency department of hospitals.[275] Working in the ICU may involve working with the rehabilitation of patients who survive after a near-drowning incident. Many of those who survive near-drowning accidents are under 15 years of age and male. Drowning was redefined in 2002 at the World Congress on Drowning as primary respiratory impairment resulting from submersion in a liquid. The term "near-drowning" was recommended to be discontinued, although the term is still commonly used in U.S. hospitals. The outcomes of drowning were stated to be death, delayed death or morbidity, or life without morbidity (no ill effects).[276]

Etiology. The etiology of near-drowning usually is different for adults and children. Adults who experience near-drowning often have accidents involving water sports in rivers, lakes, and the sea. Such accidents occur in surfing, waterskiing, jet skiing, and scuba diving. ☻ The age group most affected by near-drowning is between age 15 and 24. Males are more likely to experience near-drowning than

females in both boat-related and non-boat-related incidents. Diving into shallow water associated with neck and head trauma often leads to near-drowning incidents. Alcohol consumption and the use of illicit drugs often are related to these accidents. However, other precipitating factors can include arthritis, diabetes, and neurological disorders related to weakness of muscles when swimming and seizure disorders that occur while people are in the water. Other factors that may contribute to near-drowning are depression, attempted suicide, and panic disorder.[277] Children most often experience near-drowning in family swimming pools and bathtubs. Girls are more often affected in bathtub incidents than boys. The most at risk age group for bathtub near-drowning is under 4 years.[278]

Signs and Symptoms. The characteristic long-term signs and symptoms of near-drowning range from none to severe neurological deficits and pulmonary complications. The immediate signs and symptoms include altered vital signs with hypothermia (lowered core body temperature), tachycardia (fast heart rate) or bradycardia (slow heart rate); anxiety; hypoxia (reduced levels of oxygen to tissues), dyspnea (difficulty breathing), or tachypnea (fast breathing); metabolic acidosis (altered state of the chemical balance in the body); altered levels of consciousness; and cardiopulmonary arrest. The results of near-drowning include anoxia of the brain and pulmonary damage resulting from aspiration of fluid into the lungs. Pulmonary edema and pneumonia are common results of near-drowning. Neurologically there may be seizures, coma, changes in state of awareness, and changes in mental state. Survival is often complicated by the onset of pneumonia resulting in death several days after the incident. People who survive may have extensive brain damage and pulmonary problems such as adult respiratory distress syndrome (ARDS). Infections from waterborne organisms may complicate recovery.[279]

Prognosis. Prevention of near-drowning is always the best strategy. ☻ Adults need to have other people with them when they participate in water sports, and children need to be kept under constant supervision when bathing and swimming in pools. The extent of damage to the lungs and brain depends on the length of time the individual remains in the water and the temperature of the water. In really cold water, the rate of damage to vital nerve tissues and the brain may be slowed down. Drowning accidents in children result in a 35% fatality rate, with another 33% having some neurological deficits and 11% having severe neurological impairments. The remaining percentage of children survive without any ill effects.[280]

Medical Intervention. Prevention of near-drowning is the most effective strategy. All pools and hot tubs should be fenced to prevent children from accidently falling into the water. People should avoid alcohol if they are going to swim or boat, and no one should swim alone, especially children. ⊛ Children should be closely supervised around any body of water, including the bathtub. Inside the home, toilet seats should be secured shut with a child-safety device if small children are in the house. When people are having difficulty in the water, a rescue attempt should be made without endangering the life of the rescuer. Rescue breathing may be needed during the rescue and immediately afterward. The neck or spine may be injured, so care should be taken to keep the neck in a neutral position if possible. After the person is rescued and starts breathing, he or she should be sent to the hospital or be seen by a physician.[281] If people are not revived at the scene, they will be transferred to a hospital and may require long-term rehabilitation.

Physical Therapy Intervention. PT intervention largely is focused on the neurological rehabilitation of patients who survive the first few days after the incident. The extent of the neurological damage depends on the length of time of submersion. Treatment focuses on return of functional movement and neurodevelopmental treatment techniques, which are beyond the scope of this book. Patient positioning to prevent pressure ulcers is important and also treatment of the associated impaired respiratory function. The specific precautions and considerations for PT intervention for people who have sustained a near-drowning incident involve all of those previously stated for other conditions.

Neuropathy, Peripheral Neuropathy and Polyneuropathy

Neuropathy is a term that covers disease of the peripheral nerves that affects the motor, sensory, and autonomic systems. The condition is divided into two types: mononeuropathies affecting one peripheral nerve and polyneuropathies affecting multiple peripheral nerves. The focus in this section is on polyneuropathy. More than 20 million people in the United States are affected by the condition. People of any age may experience peripheral neuropathy, but it is more common in older adults.[282]

Etiology. In approximately 30% of people with the condition, there is no known cause. In another 30%, the neuropathy is associated with diabetes mellitus (diabetic neuropathy). Guillain-Barré syndrome is a rare form of polyneuropathy that is described earlier in this chapter.

The remaining are the result of other processes, including alcoholism (alcoholic neuropathy); autoimmune disease; diseases such as cancer, kidney failure, thyroid dysfunction; environmental toxins such as heavy metals; hereditary diseases such as Charcot-Marie-Tooth; infections such as AIDS, herpes zoster (shingles), and Lyme disease; long-term use of some medications; and vitamin B deficiency or malnutrition.[283]

Signs and Symptoms. The onset of the symptoms of peripheral neuropathy may be sudden or gradual over a period of years depending on the causative factors. The symptoms are usually greater in the distal lower extremities. The symptoms of neuropathy are extensive. Many people experience pain during various phases of the disease process including regeneration of nerves. Weakness and atrophy of the muscles in the distal extremities occurs with fasciculations (involuntary muscle twitches) and muscle cramping. Altered or loss of sensation is experienced in the distal extremities often exhibited as a "stocking" or "glove" distribution of the whole of the foot or hand when multiple peripheral nerves are affected. The loss of vibratory, touch, pressure, and temperature sensation; numbness of the skin; and loss of kinesthetic awareness (position in space) lead to heat intolerance, the inability to perform fine motor tasks, and a reduction in balance, coordination, and ambulatory abilities. The loss of weight-bearing function leads to bone degeneration. General hypotension (low blood pressure) or orthostatic hypotension (lowered BP on standing) results in dizziness and further issues with poor balance. The progression of weakness to muscles of the face and torso lead to problems with swallowing and eating. Intestinal symptoms such as diarrhea or constipation and incontinence may occur if the nerves to the internal organs are involved.[284,285]

Prognosis. Neuropathy may be mild without affecting function or may be severe and debilitating. The sensory loss in the distal extremities can lead to complications such as skin breakdown and, in some severe instances, may result in the need for amputation of part of the limb. People with severe peripheral neuropathy may be unable to walk without assistive devices and may be dependent on a wheelchair for mobility.

Medical Intervention. The diagnosis of neuropathy includes ruling out other possible neurological causes, such as brain or spinal tumors, spinal stenosis, CVA with the use of CT and MRI. An MRI can detect damage to the spinal nerves caused by the neuropathy. A spinal tap and examination of the CSF can determine the presence of high levels of proteins or cortisol. When neuropathy is suspected, an electromyogram (EMG) and nerve conduction velocity tests can determine the extent of damage to the peripheral nerves.[286] The medical intervention depends on the cause of the neuropathy. A team approach to include the dietician, neurologist, nurse, occupational therapist, physical therapist, psychologist, social worker, and speech and language therapist is required for management of people with neuropathy. Whenever possible, the underlying cause is treated. People with diabetic neuropathy will be instructed how to control blood sugar levels to prevent further deterioration of the neuropathy. Good nutrition and the addition of vitamin supplements are important. People are advised to stop drinking alcohol and smoking. People with all forms of neuropathy need to be instructed how to take care of their feet to ensure the skin is in good condition and prevent skin breakdown. Orthopedic shoes with an increased depth are usually indicated for people with neuropathy to prevent rubbing of the skin. If wounds occur, they must be treated as soon as possible to prevent infection. Pharmacological intervention to reduce neuropathic pain varies but may include analgesics, antidepressants, mexiletine (a heart medication), and antiepileptic medications such as gabapentin, or carbamazepine.[287]

Physical Therapy Intervention. The physical therapy intervention depends on the manifestations of the neuropathy in people with the condition. Evaluation by the physical therapist involves extensive manual muscle testing (MMT) and skin sensation testing for vibration, touch, pressure, kinesthetic awareness, temperature, and pain. Instruction in care of the feet with the use of a long-handled mirror to observe the plantar surface of the foot is recommended. Detailed ideas regarding the management of people with diabetes and foot care are provided in Chapter 9. Orthotic devices such as ankle-foot orthoses may be required for people with weakness or paralysis of the anterior tibial muscles (foot drop). Wound treatment often is indicated if skin breakdown is evident. The prevention of joint and muscle contractures is important with instructions for the appropriate positioning of joints and the use of orthotic devices as needed. Other physical therapy interventions may include gait training including stairs and ramps; balance and coordination exercises; strengthening, stretching, and endurance exercises; a home exercise program; and general aerobic activities.

Parkinson's Disease

Parkinson's disease is a condition affecting the basal ganglia in the brain, which results in movement and behavior dysfunction. Note that some conditions affect the basal ganglia and result in similar symptoms to Parkinson's disease. This is called Parkinsonism. The basal ganglia are groups of gray matter within the cerebrum which are parts of the extrapyramidal system. The extrapyramidal system controls movement. Parkinson's disease affects approximately 1% of people over the age of 50 in the United States. At least 500,000 people are living with this disease in the United States. The condition affects men more than women and becomes more common with aging.[288]

Etiology. Considerable research is ongoing to discover the specific causes of Parkinson's disease. Primary or idiopathic disease is idiopathic (of unknown cause) and may be hereditary.[289] Genetic studies have demonstrated a link between several gene mutations and the development of the disease. Some of these gene mutations include the gene for alpha-synuclein (Lewy bodies in the substantia nigra of people with PD contain clumps of these proteins found on autopsy); parkin gene (the abnormal gene prevents the normal breakdown of proteins in nerve cells leading to a buildup of toxins that destroy the cells); DJ-1 gene; PINK1 gene (mutations may damage the nerve cell mitochondria and lower the production of energy at a cellular level); and the DRDN gene (mutations may lead to muscle tremors). Secondary Parkinson's disease can be caused by infections, drug and other toxic reactions, cerebrovascular diseases, and as a result of trauma or brain tumors affecting the basal ganglia. Primary Parkinson's disease is a progressive degenerative disease affecting the substantia nigra part of the basal ganglia. The cells of the substantia nigra are destroyed, and there is decreased production of dopamine by the caudate nucleus and putamen. As much as 80% or more of the dopamine (neurotransmitter)-producing cells in the substantia nigra of the basal ganglia in the brain are destroyed in people with Parkinson's. Lewy bodies (clumps of proteins) are present in the neurons of the substantia nigra and the brainstem of people with the disease.[290] The risk factors for PD seem to be greater in industrialized countries, especially in farmers and agricultural workers, leading to the conclusion that exposure to pesticides may be an environmental cause. Viruses may be an environmental trigger of the disease.[291]

Signs and Symptoms. The characteristic signs and symptoms of Parkinson's include a nonvoluntary resting tremor, muscle atrophy, cogwheel rigidity of muscles, bradykinesia and akinesia, difficulty initiating movements, a masklike facial expression, a shuffling gait pattern, reduced balance, retropulsion, cognitive impairments, breathing difficulties, and speech and swallowing problems. The resting tremor is exhibited as a "pill-rolling" tremor when the hands are at rest.[292] The thumbs constantly roll across the fingers, and people are unable to control the movement. When people start to use the hands functionally, the tremor either disappears or is reduced. Cogwheel rigidity of the muscles occurs. This rigidity is exhibited as a stiffness in the muscles which releases in short bursts when passive pressure is applied in much the same way as the cogs of a wheel in a machine. As a result of muscle stiffness, there is bradykinesia (slowness of movement) and akinesia (no movement), resulting in the loss of the ability to start motion. This impaired movement often results in difficulty with initiating movements such as walking. Interestingly, patients with Parkinson's do quite well climbing stairs because of the lines of the steps. The reason why ambulation is easier for these people when lines are drawn on the floor is not fully understood. In people with severe cases of Parkinson's, there is a characteristic masklike face, resulting from the muscle rigidity, which makes it difficult for patients to demonstrate facial expression. Other characteristics include a shuffling gait pattern with reduced or absent arm swing, reduced balance abilities, retropulsion (leaning backward during ambulation), cognitive impairments, breathing difficulties, and problems with speech and swallowing. The staging of Parkinson's disease using the Hoehn and Yahr staging scale is provided in Table 7-15.

Another screening tool used for people with Parkinson's disease is the Unified Parkinson's Disease Rating Scale (UPDRS), which measures all aspects of function including ADL, mobility, mental ability, and behavioral issues.

Prognosis. Although there is no cure for Parkinson's and the disease is chronic and progressive, many people with Parkinson's live a long life. Severity of the symptoms of Parkinson's disease varies greatly among people. If coping strategies and medications are provided, many patients manage to remain comparatively functional for most of the time.[293]

Medical Intervention. Medical treatment is provided through several types of medications. Levodopa is a precursor of dopamine. Unlike dopamine, Levodopa is able to pass through the blood-brain barrier into the brain. Carbidopa is often combined with the Levodopa. Carbidopa

Table 7.15 The Staging of Parkinson's Disease Using the Hoehn and Yahr Scale

STAGE	SIGNS AND SYMPTOMS ASSOCIATED WITH STAGE
Stage 1	Signs and symptoms unilateral, mild, and not disabling Tremors in one limb Slight changes in posture, mobility, and facial expression
Stage 2	Bilateral symptoms Some disability Noticeable change in posture and gait
Stage 3	Slowing of movements Balance deficits in standing and ambulation Moderately severe dysfunction
Stage 4	Severe symptoms Able to walk with difficulty Bradykinesia and rigidity present Unable to live alone
Stage 5	Muscle atrophy Feelings of generally not being well Fatigue Unable to stand or ambulate Require constant nursing care

allows the Levodopa to reach the brain before it converts into dopamine. The effects of these medications vary, and sometimes they work for a time and then stop working. Anticholinergic medications are prescribed to reduce the activity of the neurotransmitter acetylcholine and reduce tremors and muscle rigidity. Antidepressants may be required. More recent medications include COX-2 inhibitors. The COX-2 enzyme triggers inflammation in damaged cells and the COX-2 inhibitors seem to protect the nerve cells from damage.[294] Surgical intervention can involve a pallidotomy (removal of the globus pallidus part of the basal ganglia) and thalamotomy (removal of the thalamus). These surgeries are used for people with severe disease because the risk of other brain damage is fairly high. A comparatively new technique called deep brain stimulation involves the implantation of electrodes into the brain and may be helpful in reducing the tremors and movement problems. The implantation of stem cells into the substantia nigra also is being studied, with promising results. Gene therapy based on the discovery of the many genetic mutations responsible for Parkinson's disease is under research development.[295] People will benefit from physical therapy, occupational therapy, and speech and language pathology interventions. The occupational therapy focuses on ADL and coping with activities such as cooking and bathing. Speech therapy is indicated when the muscle rigidity affects the facial, speech, and swallowing muscles.

Physical Therapy Intervention. As with all physical therapy intervention, the evaluating PT must focus on the functional problems exhibited by patients. Physical therapy can be beneficial for people with Parkinson's disease. Relaxation techniques may help in the early stages of the disease, together with breathing exercises to increase the excursion of the ribs and maintain as much mobility as possible. Rehabilitation consisting of gait, balance, coordination, and strengthening exercises is extremely important. Assistive devices are used as necessary. An exercise program for increasing joint range of motion, increasing muscle strength, and improving endurance and cardiovascular function is essential. Appropriate home exercise programs should be included. Music or counting can be helpful for the patient to create a rhythm, and stepping over lines drawn on the floor can facilitate lifting up the feet. Modalities such as hot moist packs, electrical stimulation, and short-wave diathermy may be useful to reduce pain and help with relaxation. NOTE: The use of short wave diathermy is contraindicated for people who have deep brain stimulation implants.[296]

"It Happened in the Clinic"

*M*rs. Daily was 80 years old and diagnosed with Parkinson's disease. She was admitted to a rehabilitation unit after several falls for physical therapy to increase her functional abilities. She had a shuffling gait with no arm swing, severe retropulsion (leaning backward), difficulty initiating movement, cogwheel rigidity of her upper and lower extremities, a masklike facial expression as a result of rigidity of the facial muscles, and severe resting tremor of the hands. Her cognitive abilities were normal. Mrs. Daily was provided with strengthening exercises performed individually and in a group setting with other patients on the rehabilitation unit to improve her socialization skills. Ambulation with a rolling walker was proving to be difficult because of her retropulsion. The parallel bars were not helping because they provided too much support and her skills within the bars did not carry over to using the walker. She managed with standby guard on stairs with a handrail and seemed to do well when she had visual cues provided by the edge of the steps. After some trial and error and limited success with dropping bean bags in front of the patient to

encourage her to lift up her feet during ambulation, it was decided to try a new strategy. The maintenance department was asked to make some 3-foot lengths of one-inch square wood with a "T" at the end to prevent rolling of the rods. These were placed within the parallel bars at intervals of 12 inches. Mrs. Daily proceeded to walk well within the parallel bars using these visual cues, picking up her feet and leaning forward rather than backward. After a few days of practicing, her ambulation skills with the rods in the parallel bars, she was able to continue this skill with a wheeled walker without the rods

Post-Polio Syndrome

Poliomyelitis is described in Chapter 10 on infectious diseases. Post-polio syndrome is a neurological condition exhibited by some people who have had an acute episode of poliomyelitis in early life. The neurological problems associated with post-polio syndrome occur many years after the original poliomyelitis infection. Estimates are that between 28.5% and 64% of the 640,000 people who survived polio exhibit signs of postpolio syndrome approximately 35 years after the original infection.[297] The current increase in people with post-polio syndrome is attributed to the polio epidemics in the 1940s and 1950s. Post-polio syndrome is reported in all parts of the world where polio infections have occurred.

Etiology. Post-polio syndrome is exclusively exhibited in people who previously had poliomyelitis infection. Although the actual cause of the disease process is unknown, the main theory is that the motor neurons spared during the original infection become overused and stressed and stop working. This occurrence is considered an autoimmune response to the death of the neurons.[298]

Signs and Symptoms. The signs and symptoms of post-polio syndrome tend to develop slowly with muscle weakness and atrophy, general fatigue, reduced muscle endurance, loss of energy, and myalgia (pain in muscles). The fatigue may be accompanied by mental exhaustion and lack of concentration. The weakness of post-polio syndrome is called post-polio progressive muscular atrophy. The progressive weakness may occur in muscles previously affected by polio or in ones not affected. Respiratory problems may develop as a result of muscle weakness. Weakness of the muscles of the face may lead to dysphagia and dysarthria. The muscle weakness leads to joint problems and soft tissue inflammation, which can result in lack of mobility and function.[299]

Prognosis. Currently no cure exists for post-polio syndrome. However, the effects of the weakness caused by the condition can be managed.

Medical Intervention. The diagnosis of post-polio syndrome involves ruling out other possible causes of muscle weakness such as neuropathy, myopathy, or radiculopathy. No specific medical test is conclusive for post-polio syndrome. Pharmacological interventions have not proven helpful in clinical trials.[300]

Physical Therapy Intervention. The management of people with post-polio syndrome is through advice regarding changes in lifestyle to reduce excessive physical activity, the provision of assistive devices for ambulation, and lower extremity orthoses as needed. Energy conservation techniques and periods of rest are important with intermittent use of a wheelchair in some cases. If the muscle weakness is not severe, improvement of strength can be achieved through use of a low-impact aerobic and strengthening exercise program designed not to fatigue the muscles or the patient.[301]

Spinal Cord Injury

Spinal cord injury (SCI) is the term used for people who have sustained an injury to the spine that reduces or completely disrupts the spinal cord resulting in partial or complete paralysis below the level of injury. The injury may be classified as complete or incomplete spinal cord injury. A spinal cord injury is considered a medical emergency. As many as 12,000 spinal cord injuries occur in the United States annually.[302] The number of people living with a spinal cord injury in the United States is estimated to be approximately 259,000.[303] The worldwide incidence of SCI is 15 to 40 per million people. People between the ages of 15 and 25 have the greatest risk, and males with SCI outnumber females 4 to 1.[304]

Etiology. The main cause of spinal cord injury is trauma. Approximately 56% of all spinal cord injuries affect the cervical spine. Motor vehicle accidents account for 50% of injuries, falls and work-related injuries for 30%, violent crimes for 11%, and sports-related injuries for 9%.[305] The initial or primary injury affects the spinal column with possible fracture or dislocation, damages the spinal cord and blood vessels, and damages neuronal and glial (supportive matrix cells for neurons) cells. The secondary effects of the SCI include edema, ischemia, inflammation, delayed cell death, and the production of free radicals, which further damage the neurons and glial cells, and the onset of scarring.[306]

Signs and Symptoms. Injury to the cervical spine results in tetraplegia or quadriplegia, involving paralysis or weakness of all four limbs and the trunk. Injury to the thoracic or lumbar spine results in paraplegia involving the lower extremities and the trunk below the level of the lesion. The signs and symptoms of people with spinal cord injury are divided into phases. The immediate phase lasts from 0 to 2 hours after injury. During this phase, spinal shock occurs in which there is no activity below the level of the lesion. The actual mechanism involved in spinal shock is not understood fully. Edema occurs in the spinal cord, which leads to hemorrhage and death of cells in the gray and white matter leading to ischemia (loss of oxygen) of the spinal cord. The acute phase lasts from 2 to 48 hours after injury. During this phase the hemorrhage continues with an increase in inflammation and edema, the production of free radical molecules which further damage tissue, and an immune system response which results in damage to neurons and glial cells. In the subacute phase, which lasts from 2 days to 2 weeks, the phagocytes start to clean up the cell debris and destroy myelin. During this phase, the major scarring occurs, which creates a barrier for the regeneration of neuronal axons. The intermediate phase lasts from 2 weeks to 6 months, during which time the scarring matures and the neurons start to sprout axon buds. The final phase is the chronic phase, which starts at 6 months and continues for the life of the people involved. The stability of symptoms and the neurological deficits may not occur until 1 to 2 years after the accident.[307] In the long-term, people with tetraplegia are more likely to have some bone density loss related to non-weight-bearing.[308] The occurrence of pressure ulcers is more likely in individuals with tetraplegia.[309] Depression is common in people with SCI, and suicidal ideation may be noted. Some people exhibit hostility and turn to substance abuse as a result of depression and too much free time after discharge from rehabilitation.[310]

Prognosis. The prognosis for people with spinal cord injury depends on the spinal level of injury and the degree of damage to the spinal cord. Many people who sustain upper cervical-level lesions do not survive. Of those who do survive, the mortality rate tends to be higher during the first year of recovery from a spinal cord injury. The overall life expectancy for people with a spinal cord lesion is slightly lower than that of the general population with an increased likelihood of early mortality in people with more severe motor and sensory deficits.[311] A complete spinal cord lesion affects all motor, sensory, and autonomic functions below the level of the injury. If the damage is high in the cervical spine, the innervation is lost to the diaphragm (phrenic nerve), and a respirator is required. People dependent on a respirator are more likely to have respiratory infections that may lead to mortality. Bladder and bowel dysfunction is a common problem in all people with SCI, and this leads to an increased risk of urinary and bowel infections. An increased susceptibility of the respiratory and cardiac systems results in problems that also may cause death.[312]

Medical Intervention. The medical intervention for people with spinal cord injuries involves a team approach with inclusion of the neurologist, nurses, physical therapists, occupational therapists, speech and language pathologists, social workers, and psychologists/psychiatrists. The immediate care of people with a spinal cord injury is in the acute care unit (ACU) or ICU. Saving life is the initial concern, with immobilization of the spine in the presence of a fracture to reduce the risk of further damage to the spinal cord. Radiographs, CT scans, and MRI are performed to determine the extent of the injuries. The average stay in the ICU is 12 days, with an additional 37 days stay in a specialized rehabilitation unit before return to the home environment.[313] Frequent positioning changes are needed to prevent the occurrence of pressure ulcers. Wound care is important to prevent infection. If infection occurs, antimicrobial medications are prescribed specific and sufficient to destroy the infection.[314] The administration of methylprednisolone for the first 24 to 48 hours after the injury has been shown to reduce the damage from inflammation that causes the secondary effects of injury as has the use of light therapy on the spine.[315,316] Counseling for people with SCI can help to alleviate some of the stress associated with recovery. Vocational training also helps to reduce depression and restore confidence.[317]

Research is ongoing for SCI treatment. Various avenues are pursued. Neuronal stem cell research is under review.[318] Stimulating the growth of nerve axons by transplanting Schwann cells into the damaged spinal cord and giving a substance called cyclic adenosine monophosphate seems to encourage the growth factor genes in the nerve cells.[319] Inhibitory proteins including TROY and Nogo have been identified during research, which prevent the CNS neuron axons from regrowing. Blocking these myelin-inhibiting proteins may open the door to the regrowth of axons and enhance recovery from SCI, MS, CVA, and other nervous system disorders.[320] In 2009, researchers at Harvard Medical School identified the area of the neuron to which some of these growth inhibiting proteins bind. This research offers hope that a medication may be developed to block this inhibitory growth response and improve the ability of the neural axons to regrow.[321]

Physical Therapy Intervention. Physical therapy intervention for people with SCI is an essential part of the rehabilitation process. Intervention occurs during all phases of the recovery. As more research reveals the capacity of the neurological system to recover, the role of rehabilitation is likely to focus more on recovery and less on compensatory mechanisms during exercise and ambulation training.[322] Functional electrical stimulation of muscles of the lower or upper extremities may be used during the acute phase of recovery when mobility exercises are contraindicated as a result of spinal fractures.[323] The physical therapist and PTA should be vigilant in monitoring for the presence of deep venous thrombosis and heterotopic ossification when working with people who have a SCI.[324] Progressive exercises start with passive motion of joints and stretching of muscles to prevent joint and muscle contractures. However, in some instances, contractures are desired to increase function. Caution must be exercised when stretching to avoid stretching the flexors of the fingers in people with cervical lesions as this can reduce the ability for the **tenodesis grip.** Allowing the flexors to contract can enable people to use the hook grasp (tenodesis grip) to hold items and assist with propelling a wheelchair. During transfers and exercise, the hand should be held in a fist to prevent stretching of the finger flexors. As people start to recover some muscle tone, active assisted exercises are appropriate leading to active exercises. The use of PNF patterns often is helpful. Every person with a SCI has different deficits and needs to be evaluated by the physical therapist on an ongoing basis. Physical therapy will include mobility training in a wheelchair or with an ambulatory device, prescription of suitable wheelchair transportation according to the motor abilities of patients, transfer training using sliding boards and rotation transfer discs as needed, balance exercises in various body positions, and progressive exercises for bed mobility. People with cervical lesions likely will need a power wheelchair. The control mechanisms for power chairs are available as head control switches and sip and puff for people with high cervical lesions. People with some strength in their upper extremities may be able to use a joystick hand controlled wheelchair. Most people with paraplegia can manage with a standard wheelchair as long as it has removable arm rests and elevating leg rests. Light weight wheelchairs are available to reduce the difficulty of handling the chair. Strengthening of the uninvolved limbs should start as soon as possible within the restrictions of immobility of the spine during the acute phase of recovery. Resisted exercises for the upper extremities usually are appropriate for people with injury to the lumbar spine during the acute phase. The rehabilitation of people with SCI is varied, and the physical therapist should consult texts regarding specific SCI rehabilitation for further information.

Traumatic Brain Injury and Head Injury

Traumatic brain injury (TBI) or head injury (HI) is an external injury to the head that causes damage to the tissue of the brain and results in various manifestations of neurological deficits depending on the area of the brain affected. Two types of TBI exist, a closed head injury and an open head injury. National statistics are difficult to interpret because some sources cite the total number of head injuries occurring each year through the emergency rooms, and others cite only those that result in significant brain injury resulting in prolonged side effects. According to the CDC, a total of 1.4 million people are seen in emergency rooms each year with TBI. Of these, approximately 50,000 people die, 235,000 are hospitalized, and 1.1 million are treated and released. The number of people who sustain a TBI without attending the emergency room is unknown. As many as 5.3 million people in the United States have long-term effects resulting from a TBI. [325] Traumatic brain injury accounts for as many as 40% of all the deaths resulting from acute injuries in the United States. The incidence of mild TBI is calculated to be 131 per 100,000 of the population. The incidence of severe TBI is lower at 21 per 100,000 of the population. Children between the ages of 0 to 14 years experience 475,000 incidences of TBI annually. [326] 🔊

Etiology. An external injury to the head results in damage of varying degrees to the brain tissue. According to the CDC, the most common causes of a TBI are falls and road traffic accidents (RTA), also called a motor traffic accident (MTA), motor vehicle accident (MVA), or motor vehicle crash (MVC). Other causes include direct blows to the head and assaults. [327] Sports injuries account for some of these incidences of TBI, with cycling and football the most common causes. The use of head protection substantially reduces these injuries. [328] Those at highest risk for TBI are males under age 45 and specifically between ages 15 and 24 years. Other high-risk groups include children between the ages of 0 and 14, men twice as often as women, people in the military, people with low income, people from ethnic minority groups, inner-city residents, unmarried individuals, and people with a history of alcohol abuse or previous TBI. [329]

Signs and Symptoms. People recovering from a TBI fall into the categories of mild, moderate, and severe. The general characteristic signs and symptoms of people with any type of head injury may include loss of consciousness; headaches and dizziness; changes in behavior, mood swings, and sleep patterns; alterations in cognitive function, such as confusion, reduced memory, and poor concentration and attention; severe fatigue and lethargy (lack of desire to do anything); and sensory problems such as blurred vision and unusual or bad taste in the mouth. People with moderate to severe TBI may have vomiting and nausea; seizures and altered levels of consciousness, including coma; dilation of one or both pupils of the eyes; altered cognition, personality changes, and emotional disturbances; sensory deficits such as loss or reduction of skin sensation, loss of hearing, vision, taste and smell, and speech difficulties such as slurring; motor deficits with various levels of functional disability including hemiplegia, muscle weakness of the extremities, and loss of coordination of movement; and additional mental symptoms such as confusion and agitation. The long-term effects of a severe TBI may include behavior problems such as depression, personality changes, socially inappropriate behaviors, and aggression. Some people with severe TBI may remain in a persistent vegetative state (PVS) for more than a month, during which time they are minimally responsive to any stimulus. Another possibility is coma and death. [330] Another possible outcome of TBI is posttraumatic stress disorder. This condition may cause disturbances in sleep with nightmares, flashbacks to the event, outbursts of anger, and severe agitation with feelings of worry and sadness. [331]

A closed head injury may not appear to be as severe as an open head injury, but damage to the brain may be just as extensive, or may be worse, than that sustained in an open head injury. A closed head injury may cause a concussion resulting in transient symptoms of altered mental abilities including retrograde amnesia (loss of memory of incidents before the accident, which may be temporary or permanent)[332,333,334] or posttraumatic amnesia (inability to formulate new learning or ideas). The duration of posttraumatic amnesia often is used as a predictor of outcome for people with a TBI because the longer the posttraumatic amnesia lasts, the more severe tends to be the outcome. [335] Another characteristic of a closed head injury may be an external contusion demonstrated by a bruise on the head, which may be accompanied with localized edema. Other contusions may be within the brain and not manifested as an external bruise. People with an injury caused by a reverberating head injury may sustain two injuries to the brain. In a "whiplash" car accident, the head may hit the windshield or be pitched forward into extreme flexion and then be thrown backward. The brain sustains an injury where the head hits the window and also at the exact opposite aspect of the brain, from the vibration of the brain against the inside of the skull sustained in the whiplash. The damage at the initial impact site is called the coup injury, and the injury at the opposite side of the brain is called the contrecoup or countercoup injury (see Fig. 7-15). People with such injuries may have extensive problems with diffuse brain damage depending on the amount of trauma sustained. In some cases of TBI, a hematoma may form within the brain tissue. Brain hematomas can be life threatening. An epidural hematoma can form between the skull and the dura mater covering of the brain, and a subdural hematoma may form deep to the brain dura. In either case, blood within the area of the hematoma creates pressure on the tissue of the brain, resulting in ischemia of the brain tissues. In cases of hematoma, pressure must be released as soon as possible through surgical craniotomy and aspiration of the blood. Another characteristic of head injury may be edema of the actual brain tissue. This edema can cause diffuse pressure on the brain, because the skull does not allow for expansion of the brain and results in an increased intracranial pressure (ICP). Monitoring of the ICP is performed in the ICU. An ICP of greater than 40 mm Hg may result in severe brain damage with cerebral ischemia, edema, hypoxia and hydrocephalus.[336] The signs and symptoms associated with a raised ICP include severe headache, reduced heart rate and elevated blood pressure, altered levels of consciousness, nausea or vomiting, and vision disturbances such as blurred vision resulting from papilledema (pressure on the optic nerve from the brain edema). These symptoms can occur as much as several weeks after the head injury, although they are usually noted within a week of the incident.

Open head injuries cause many of the same characteristic manifestations as those of closed head injuries; however, there are usually lacerations to the head and face and considerable loss of blood. If the skull is fractured, bone fragments may directly damage brain tissue. These bone fragments need to be surgically removed before closing the wound. Facial lacerations require careful stitching to avoid undue scarring, but the immediate measures are to stop the bleeding and keep the patient alive.

People who have sustained a TBI are assessed for level of consciousness using the Glasgow Coma Scale (GCS) on admission to the emergency room (see the section earlier in this chapter on the Glasgow Coma Scale for grading criteria). The length of time a person remains in an unconscious state has been shown to indicate the long-term prognosis of the patient. The assessment scale determines the person's response to stimuli by checking general motor response, eye opening, and the ability to respond verbally to commands. Responses in the three categories can add up to a total score of 15 in the least affected to a lowest score of 3 for those severely affected. The GCS is used as an indicator of survival after TBI and to determine the level of severity. People who score

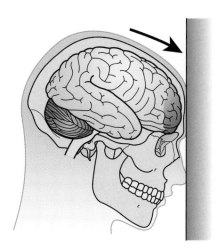

Coup

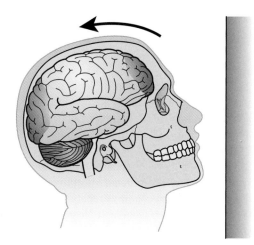

Contrecoup/countercoup

FIGURE 7.15 Coup and countercoup head injury

between 3 and 8 on the GCS and are comatose are admitted to the ICU.[337]

Prognosis. The symptoms of people with mild cases of TBI may resolve within a period of days or weeks. Mild TBI rarely results in death. Approximately 50% of people who sustain a severe TBI will require surgery to repair or remove brain hematomas.[338] People with moderate and severe TBI likely will have residual problems of varying degrees with cognitive and motor dysfunctions depending on the location of the damage to the brain.

Medical Intervention. Immediate medical intervention is required for people who have sustained a moderate or severe head injury. Many people who sustain a mild head injury do not seek medical assistance. Preservation of life is most important by maintaining oxygen levels to the brain and body. The prevention of hypoxia of the brain reduces the risk of long-term brain damage. The blood pressure is controlled and blood flow determined. The level of consciousness is determined using the GCS and the level of cognition using the Rancho Los Amigos Scale of Cognitive Functioning. Radiographs are taken of the head and neck to determine the presence of fractures. A CT scan or MRI of the head helps to determine initial damage to the brain. Surgical removal of contusions and hematomas in the brain, or removal of bone fragments and foreign objects such as bullets, may be required. During the recovery period, a team approach to rehabilitation is used consisting of physical therapy, occupational therapy, speech and language therapy, physiatry, psychiatry, pharmacy, social work, and nursing.[339] The management of certain neurological problems such as spasticity may require pharmacological management with antispasticity medications such as baclofen and botulinum toxin.[340]

Physical Therapy Intervention. Physical therapy intervention is indicated for the rehabilitation of people with moderate and severe TBI. The PT and PTA are involved in the team approach for the total rehabilitation of patients. Although the PT intervention is for the motor deficits resulting from TBI, the cognitive level of the patient must be taken into consideration. Psychological methods for behavior modification may be incorporated into physical therapy sessions to assist with the cognitive rehabilitation of patients.[341,342] People may be unable to learn new motor skills or understand simple instructions. Even people who progress well in their return to full independent ambulation may have impaired judgment. This can present problems with functional ambulation in the real world.

People may be able to walk independently but unable to determine when to safely cross the road. Other individuals may not be able to find the door to their own room despite the fact they can walk up steps independently. Many people who sustain a TBI have depression as a result of the cellular physiological response of the brain to the trauma. Behavioral problems may occur after TBI, and patients may respond inappropriately to other people. Some people become aggressive or exhibit overt sexually inappropriate actions.

In the acute care environment of the ICU, the physical therapy intervention depends on the length of time patients remain in the ICU. If patients are on a respirator as a result of brainstem involvement, the PT intervention may include bed and chair positioning for prevention of contractures and pressure ulcers, postural drainage and pulmonary hygiene procedures, active assisted exercises, bed mobility exercises, and even ambulation. The PT and PTA may be asked to instruct the nursing staff in range of motion exercises. In the longer-term rehabilitation process, a variety of physical therapy interventions are required to control spasticity and stimulate the return of muscle strength and functional movement. These interventions may include aquatic therapy; NDT, PNF, and other neurological physical therapy techniques (see Physical Therapy Interventions in this chapter); muscle strengthening, stretching, and endurance exercises; ambulation, balance and coordination exercises; and functional reeducation.[343,344] Working with the occupational therapist and speech and language pathologist during treatment sessions often is beneficial for patients. While the physical therapist works with people on gross motor activities, the occupational therapist may work on the fine motor control and the speech and language pathologist on speech volume and control. The performance of functional activities increases the breathing capacity and helps to improve voice production.

Precautions and Considerations for Physical Therapy Intervention. Precautions and considerations for PT intervention for patients with TBI on the ICU involve all those previously stated for people with a CVA plus the following:

1. Check vital signs and intracranial pressure levels prior to and throughout working with patients.
2. Speak to patients and explain what you are doing in simple, short statements, even if they appear to be in a coma. They may be able to hear you, and the stimulation may assist with return to consciousness.

3. Observe patients in a coma carefully for responses to movement such as eye flutter, pupil dilation, withdrawal responses of limbs, or any movement previously not noted.

4. Alert the nurse of any changes in patient response that seem unusual.

5. Keep treatment times fairly short, perhaps visiting patients twice a day for no more than 15 minutes at a time.

6. Involve the family in the intervention by explaining to them the reason for the intervention and the goals. However, give these explanations away from patients to avoid overstimulation. In the ICU setting, the family may not be able to be involved with the specific treatment interventions as in the subacute setting.

7. Document the PT intervention carefully and objectively in the patient's chart. Be sure to note the length of time of the intervention and any response to treatment noticed.

8. Keep in communication every day with the supervising PT because patient status is likely to change rapidly in some cases, and the plan of care may need to be updated by the PT.

CASE STUDY 7.1

This 97-year-old lady has advanced Alzheimer's disease. She fractured her right hip when she sustained a fall 3 weeks ago. She is unable to understand more than basic instructions and does not remember events that occurred even 5 minutes ago. She is not combative. Before her fall, she was independently mobile without any assistive device, able to toilet herself, but required assistance to take a bath. Owing to her other medical problems of congestive heart failure and diabetes mellitus, surgical fixation of the fracture was not an option. She spent 2 weeks in the acute care unit of a hospital and 1 week in a rehabilitation center. She has just returned to the residential home where she lives, and the physical therapist has evaluated her. The plan of care developed by the physical therapist includes strengthening exercises for the left lower extremity, bilateral upper extremity strengthening and stretching exercises, and mobility training as possible with an appropriate assistive device with nonweight-bearing on the right lower extremity. A wheelchair is provided for ease of transport. The challenge for the PTA is to help this patient to be mobile while keeping her weight off the right lower extremity.

How would you modify your intervention approach when working with this patient who has

Alzheimer's disease and has a fractured left hip with a request from the physician for non-weight-bearing activity? Consider the types of interventions that you would normally perform for people who are cognitively aware and then think about how to adjust your instructions and activities for someone who is confused when answering the following questions.

1. How would you speak to the patient so that she will understand instructions? Give examples.

2. What kind of ambulatory device might you consider using with this person? Are there any safety considerations?

3. Would you obtain a wheelchair for the patient, and if so how will you train her to use it?

4. How will you prevent the patient from ambulating and placing weight on her right lower extremity? When considering this question, bear in mind the ethical and legal issues surrounding the use of restraints.

5. What sort of strengthening exercises will you provide for this patient, and how will you ensure she performs them?

6. How will you involve the care facility staff in the rehabilitation program for this person and what kind of in-service training might you provide?

CASE STUDY 7.2

A 72-year-old man with moderate to advanced Parkinsonism is attending the outpatient physical therapy clinic to increase his mobility. The patient is oriented ×3 with normal cognitive abilities. He exhibits a shuffling gait, retropulsion (leaning backward) during ambulation, poor balance in standing and during ambulation, rigidity of upper and lower extremity muscles with no arm swing during gait, severe resting tremor in the hands, reduced strength of upper and lower extremities of 3+/5, inability to climb or descend stairs, and inability to ambulate more than 10 feet without assistance from his wife. The patient has taken L-dopa in the past but is currently not taking this medication. The physical therapist has evaluated the patient and determined the goals of independent ambulation with or without an appropriate assistive device for 100 feet to enable the patient to reach the mailbox at the end of his driveway,

(Continued)

independent ascending and descending 12 stairs using a handrail to enable safety within the home, and independent rising from a chair. The plan of care includes mobility training to achieve the goals of ambulation, stair climbing, and rising from a chair; strengthening exercises for upper and lower extremities; balance reeducation; and postural advice.

1. Detail six strengthening exercises you would recommend for the upper and lower extremities including a home exercise program. Write out the home exercise program in a format suitable for sending home with the patient including some graphics.

2. What kind of assistive ambulatory device would this patient likely need?

3. How will you ensure safety during ambulation?

4. How might you encourage better posture for this patient?

5. How would you address the problem of retropulsion?

6. What special strategies might you use for the treatment sessions for this patient in view of the diagnosis of Parkinson's disease?

7. Explain some balance reeducation exercises progressing from lying, to sitting, to standing.

8. What specific safety issues will you consider for this person?

STUDY QUESTIONS

1. Explain how a nerve impulse is transmitted along a neuron.

2. Describe the process of Wallerian degeneration.

3. Name three major types of physical therapy interventions that may be used when working with people with neurological dysfunction. (Specific techniques developed by clinicians.)

4. What kinds of neurological deficits are likely to occur if there is damage to the cerebellum?

5. Explain why people who experience a cerebrovascular accident have symptoms of weakness on the opposite side of the body to that of the damage within the brain.

6. Describe the difference between posttraumatic amnesia and retrograde amnesia.

7. Explain the use of the Glasgow Coma Scale and the Rancho Los Amigos assessment.

8. Explain what Tinel's sign and Phalen's test are used to diagnose.

9. Describe the four basic patterns of movement used in proprioceptive neuromuscular facilitation exercises.

10. Discuss the different types of spina bifida with a classmate.

11. Define amyotrophic lateral sclerosis.

12. List five characteristic signs and symptoms of Parkinson's disease.

13. Discuss strategies to help a patient with Parkinson's disease overcome the effects of difficulty initiating movement.

14. Describe three progressive neurological diseases.

15. How are you likely to be involved with the interventions for people with a traumatic brain injury during their time on the intensive care unit?

⬤ USEFUL WEB SITES

American Academy of Orthopaedic Surgeons
http://orthoinfo.aaos.org

American Chronic Pain Association
http://www.theacpa.org

American Diabetes Association
http://www.diabetes.org

American Epilepsy Society
http://www.aesnet.org

American Parkinson Disease Association
http://www.apdaparkinson.org

Amyotrophic Lateral Sclerosis (ALS) Association
http://www.alsa.org

Epilepsy Foundation of America
http://www.epilepsyfoundation.org

Guillain Barré Syndrome (GBS/CIDP) International
http://www.gbs-cidp.org

National Foundation for the Treatment of Pain
http://www.paincare.org

National Parkinson's Foundation
http://www.parkinson.org

Parkinson's Disease Foundation
http://www.pdf.org

United Cerebral Palsy
http://www.ucp.org/

Vestibular Disorders Association
http://www.vestibular.org

◉ REFERENCES

[1] Bobath, B. (1985). *Abnormal postural reflex activity caused by brain lesions*, 3rd edition. London: William Heinemann Medical Books.

[2] Nolte, J. (2002). *The human brain: an introduction to its functional anatomy*, 5th edition. St Louis, MO: Mosby, p. 3.

[3] McNeill, M. E. (1997). *Neuroanatomy primer*. Baltimore: Williams & Wilkins, p. 34.

[4] Lundy-Ekman, L. (1998). *Neuroscience: fundamentals for rehabilitation*. Philadelphia: W. B. Saunders, p. 27.

[5] Nolte, J. Ibid., p. 15.

[6] Ibid., p. 185.

[7] Ibid., p. 413.

[8] Ibid., p. 102.

[9] Ibid., p. 390.

[10] Ibid., p. 526.

[11] Ibid., p. 553.

[12] Ibid., p. 224.

[13] Lundy-Ekman, L. Ibid., p. 154.

[14] Canright, S., editor. (2009). *Human vestibular system in space*. NASA. Retrieved 4.3.10 from http://www.nasa.gov/audience/forstudents/9-12/features/F_Human_Vestibular_System_in_Space.html

[15] Sumway-Cook, A., & Woollacott, M. H. (2001). *Motor control: theory and practical application*. Philadelphia: Lippincott Williams & Wilkins, p. 76.

[16] Vestibular Disorders Association. (2009). Retrieved 4.3.10 from www.vestibular.org

[17] Hoch, D. B. (2008). Limbic system. *MedlinePlus Medical Encyclopedia*. Retrieved 4.4.10 from http://www.nlm.nih.gov/medlineplus/ency/imagepages/19244.htm

[18] Kiernan, J. A. (1998). *The human nervous system: an anatomical viewpoint*, 7th edition. Philadelphia: Lippincott-Raven.

[19] Weedman-Molavi, D. (1997). Medial temporal lobe: The limbic system. *Neuroscience tutorial*. Washington University School of Medicine. Retrieved 4.4.10 from http://thalamus.wustl.edu

[20] Zull, J. E. (2002). *The art of changing the brain: enriching the practice of teaching by exploring the biology of learning*. Stirling, VA: Stylus.

[21] Cohen, H. (1999). *Neuroscience for rehabilitation*, 2nd edition. Philadelphia: Lippincott Williams & Wilkins

[22] Quan, D., & Bird, S. J. (1999). Nerve conduction studies and electromyography in the evaluation of peripheral nerve injuries. *University Penn Orthopaed J*, 12:45–51.

[23] Beirowski, B., et al. (2005, February). The progressive nature of Wallerian degeneration in wild type and slow Wallerian degeneration (Wld) nerves. *Neuroscience*, 6:6.

[24] Hoch, D. B. (2008). Radial nerve dysfunction. *MedlinePlus Medical Encyclopedia*. Retrieved 4.4.2010 from http://www.nlm.nih.gov/medlineplus/ency/article/001434.htm

[25] Cowles, R. A. (2009). Thoracic outlet syndrome. *MedlinePlus Medical Encyclopedia*. Retrieved 4.4.2010 from http://www.nlm.nih.gov/medlineplus/ency/article/001434.htm

[26] National Institute for Neurological Disorders and Stroke, National Institutes of Health. (2008). NINDS thoracic outlet syndrome information page. Retrieved 4.3.10 from http://www.ninds.nih.gov/disorders/thoracic/thoracic.htm

[27] Petty, N. J. (2006). *Neuromusculoskeletal examination and assessment: a handbook for therapists*. Edinburgh, UK: Elsevier, Churchill Livingstone, p. 74.

[28] American Academy of Orthopaedic Surgeons. (2009). *Electrodiagnostic testing*. Retrieved 4.5.2010 from http://orthoinfo.aaos.org/topic.cfm?topic=A00270&return_link=0

[29] Teasdale, G., & Jennett, B. (1974). Assessment of coma and impaired consciousness. *Lancet*, 81–84.

[30] Ibid.

[31] Centers for Disease Control and Prevention. (2006). *Glasgow Coma Scale*. Emergency Preparedness and Response, National Center for Injury Prevention and Control (NCIPC). Retrieved 4.5.2010 from http://www.bt.cdc.gov/masscasualties/gscale.asp

[32] Agre, J. C., et al. (1987). Strength testing with a portable dynamometer: reliability for upper and lower extremities. *Arch Phys Med Rehabil* 68:454.

[33] Bohannon, R. W., & Andrews, A. W. (1987). Interrater reliability of hand-held dynamometry. *Phys Ther* 67:931.

[34] Kendall, F. P., McCreary, E. K., & Provance, P. G. (1993). *Muscles: testing and function*, 4th edition, Baltimore: Williams & Wilkins

[35] O'Sullivan, S. B., & Schmitz, T. J. (2007). *Physical rehabilitation*, 5th edition. Philadelphia: F. A. Davis, p. 181.

[36] Wadsworth, C. T. et al. (1987). Intrarater reliability of manual muscle testing and hand-held dynametric muscle testing. *Phys Ther* 67:1342.

[37] Petty, N. J. Ibid., pp. 72, 243, 332.

[38] Butler, D. S. (2000). *The sensitive nervous system*. Adelaide, Australia: Noigroup, p. 13.

[39] Petty, N. J. Ibid., p. 75.

[40] Butler, D. S. (2000). Ibid., p. 287.

[41] Ibid.

[42] Ibid., 277–285.

[43] Ibid.

[44] Ibid., pp. 313–324.

[45] Ibid., pp. 325-331.

[46] Ibid., pp. 331-336.

[47] Levin, H. S., O'Donneel, V. M., & Grossman, R. G. (1979). Galveston Orientation and Amnesia Test. *J Nerv Ment Disord* 167:675–684.

[48] Tate, R. L., et al. (2005). *Post-traumatic amnesia: an investigation into the validity of measuring instruments* [final report]. Sydney: Motor Accident Authority of New South Wales.

[49] Folstein, M., Folstein, S., & McHugh, P. (1975). "Mini-Mental State." A practical method for grading the cognitive state of patients for the clinician. *J Psychiatr Res* 12:189–198.

[50] Spreen, O., & Benton, A. L. (1977). Neurosensory center comprehensive examination for aphasia. Victoria, Canada: University of Victoria.

[51] Bushke, H., & Fuld, P. A. (1974). Evaluating storage, retention, and retrieval in disordered memory and learning. *Neurology* 24:1019–1025.

[52] Reynolds, C. R., & Bigler, E. D. (1994). *Test of memory and learning*. Texas: Pro-Ed.

[53] Rancho Los Amigos National Rehabilitation Center. (1990). Family guide to the Rancho Levels of Cognitive Functioning. Retrieved 4.6.10 from http://www.rancho.org/patient_education/bi_cognition.pdf

[54] Riddle, D. L. (1991, February 1). Reliability of measurements of cervical spine range of motion—comparison of three methods. *The*

Free Library. Retrieved 10.3.2009 from http://www.thefreelibrary.com/Reliability of measurements of cervical spine range of motion - ...-a010829235

55 Watkins, M. A., et al. (1991). Reliability of goniometric measurements and visual estimates of knee range of motion obtained in a clinical setting. *Phys Ther* 71:90–96.

56 Ellis, B., & Bruton, A. (2002). A study to compare the reliability of composite finger flexion with goniometry for measurement of range of motion in the hand. *Clin Rehabil* 16:562–570.

57 Ibid.

58 Urbano, F. L. (2000, July). Tinel's sign and Phalen's maneuver: physical signs of carpal tunnel syndrome. *Hospital Physician*. Retrieved 10.24.2010 from http://www.turner-white.com/pdf/hp_jul00_tinel.pdf

59 Ibid.

60 Cowles, R. A. (2009). Thoracic outlet syndrome. *MedlinePlus Medical Encyclopedia*. Retrieved 10.19.2010 from http://www.nlm.nih.gov/medlineplus/ency/article/001434.htm

61 Petty, N. J. Ibid., p. 222.

62 Ibid., p. 222.

63 Family Practice Notebook LLC. (2008). *Adson's test*. Retrieved 11.19.2010 from http://www.fpnotebook.com/Ortho/Exam/AdsnsTst.htm

64 Petty, N. J. Ibid., p. 222.

65 Periyasamy, R., Manivannan, M., & Narayanamurphy, V. B. R. (2008). Changes in two point discrimination and the law of mobility in diabetes mellitus patients. *J Brachial Plex Peripher Nerve Inj* 3:3.

66 Zhang, Z., et al. (2008). A quantitative method for determining spatial discriminative capacity. *Biomedical Engineering Online*, 7:12. Retrieved 11.19.2010 from http://www.pubmedcentral.nih.gov/articlerender.fcgi?artid=2292727

67 Lundborg, G., & Rosen, B. (2004). The two-point discrimination test—time for a re-appraisal? *J Hand Surg* 29:418–422.

68 Richter, R. R., & Reinking, M. F. (2005). Evidence in practice: how does evidence on the diagnostic accuracy of the vertebral artery test influence teaching of the test in a professional level physical therapist education program? *Phys Ther* 85:589–599.

69 Butler, D. S. (1991). *Mobilization of the nervous system*. Melbourne, Australia: Churchill Livingstone.

70 Ibid.

71 Ibid., pp. 3-4.

72 Ibid., p. 203.

73 Brennan, R. (n.d.). *What is the Alexander technique?* Retrieved 10.22.2010 from http://www.alexandertechnique.com/articles/brennan/

74 Brunnstrom, S. (1970). *Movement therapy in hemiplegia: a neurophysiological approach*. Hagerstown, MD: Harper & Row.

75 Taub, E., Uswatte, G., & Pidikiti, R. (1999). Constraint-induced movement therapy: a new family of techniques with broad application to physical rehabilitation—a clinical review. *J Rehabil Res Dev* 36:237–251.

76 Wolk, S. L., et al. (2006). Effect of constraint-induced movement therapy on upper extremity function 3 to 9 months after stroke. *JAMA* 296:2095–2104.

77 Gauthier, L. V. (2009). Improvement after constraint-induced movement therapy is independent of infarct location in chronic stroke patients. *Stroke* 40:2468–2472.

78 Ries, J. D., & Leonard, R. (2006). Evidence in practice. Is there evidence to support the use of constraint-induced therapy to improve the quality and quantity of upper extremity function of a 2½ year-old girl with congenital hemiparesis? *Phys Ther* 86:746–752.

79 Dahl, A. E., et al. (2008). Short and long-term outcome of constraint-induced movement therapy after stroke: a randomized controlled feasibility trial. *Clinical Rehabilitation*, 22: 436-447.

80 Taub, E., Uswatte, G., & Pidikiti, R. Ibid., p. 36.

81 Mark, V. W., et al. (2008). Constraint-induced movement therapy can improve hemiparetic progressive multiple sclerosis, preliminary findings. *Mult Scler* 14:992–994.

82 Taub, E., Uswatte, G., & Pidikiti, R. Ibid., 36.

83 Hammer, A M., & Lindmark, B. (2009). Effects of forced use on arm function in the subacute phase after stroke: a randomized, clinical pilot study. *Phys Ther* 89:526–539.

84 Bianco, T. (1999). *Craniosacral therapy: celebrate the healing power of a gentle touch*. Retrieved 11.19.2010 from http://www.spineuniverse.com/displayarticle.php/article784.html

85 Hanten, W.P., et al. (1998) Craniosacral rhythm: reliability and relationships with cardiac and respiratory rates. *J Orthop Sports Phys Ther* 27:213–218.

86 Wirth-Pattullo, V., & Hayes, K. W. (1994). Interrater reliability of craniosacral rate measurements and their relationship with subjects' and examiners' heart and respiratory rate measurements. *Phys Ther* 74:908–916; discussion 917–920.

87 International Feldenkrais Federation. (n.d.). *The Feldenkrais method*. Retrieved 11.19.2010 from http://feldenkrais-method.org/index.php?q=node/338

88 Rondoni, A., & Bertozzi, L. (2009, July). Effectiveness of the Feldenkrais method in the improvement of health status in adult patients with low back pain or at risk of developing it. *Scienza Riabilitativa* 11:5–14.

89 Vrantsidis, F., et al. (2009). Getting grounded gracefully: effectiveness and acceptability of Feldenkrais in improving balance. *J Aging Phys Activity* 17:57–76.

90 Stephens, J., et al. (2006). Lengthening the hamstring muscles without stretching using "awareness through movement." *Phys Ther* 86:1641–1650.

91 Batson, G., & Deutsch, J. E. (2005). Effects of Feldenkrais awareness through movement on balance in adults with chronic neurological deficits following stroke: a preliminary study. *Compl Health Pract Rev* 10:203–210.

92 Barnes, J. F. (2009). Myofascial release: What is myofascial release? Retrieved 11.20.2010 from http://www.myofascialrelease.com/fascia_massage/public/whatis_myofascial_release.asp

93 Barnes, J. F. (2009). Myofascial release: Treatment programs that can change your life. Retrieved 4.8.2010 from http://www.myofascialrelease.com/mfr/mfr_treatment.asp

94 Remvig, L., Ellis, R. M., & Patijn, J. (2008, March). Myofascial release: an evidence-based treatment approach? *Int Musculoskel Med* 30:29–35.

95 The Bobath Centre. (2008). *The founders and history*. Retrieved 11.20.2010 from http://www.bobath.org.uk/TheFoundersandHistory.html

96 Mayston, M. J. (2008). *The Bobath concept today*. The Bobath Centre. Retrieved 11.20.2010 from http://www.bobath.org.uk/BobathConceptToday.html

97 Adler, S. S., Beckers, D., & Buck, M. (2000). *PNF in practice: an illustrated guide*, second, revised edition. Berlin: Springer-Verlag.

98 Ibid.

99 Stallings-Sahler, S. (2007). About A. Jean Ayres. *Sensory Integration Global Network*. Retrieved 11.20.2010 from http://www.siglobalnetwork.org/index_en/index.html

100 Blanche, E. I., Botticelli, T. M., & Hallway, M. K. (1995). *Combining neuro-developmental treatment and sensory integration principles: an approach to pediatric therapy*. San Antonio, TX: Therapy Skill Builders.

101 Taylor-Piliae, R. E. (2003). Tai Chi as an adjunct to cardiac rehabilitation exercise training. *J Cardiopulm Rehabil* 23:90–96.

102 Kuramoto, A. M. (2006). Therapeutic effects of Tai Chi exercise: research review. *Wisconsin Med J* 105:42–46.

103 Ranganath, P., & Rajangam, S. (2007). Anencephaly—a review. *Perinatol J Perinatal Neonatal Care* 9:50–54.

[104] Ibid.

[105] Stemp-Morlock, G. (2007). Pesticides and anencephaly. *Environ Health Perspect* 115:78–79.

[106] Muñoz, J. B., et al. (2005). Socioeconomic factors and the risk of anencephaly in a Mexican population: a case-control study. *Public Health Rep* 120:39–45.

[107] Anencephaly. (1971). *Clin Pediatr* 10:3–4.

[108] National Institutes of Neurological Disorders and Stroke, National Institutes of Health. (2009). NINDS anencephaly information page. Retrieved 11.20.2010 from http://www.ninds.nih.gov/disorders/anencephaly/anencephaly.htm#Is_there_any_treatment

[109] Baird, P. A., & Sadonick, A. D. (1984). Survival in infants with anencephaly. *Clin Pediatr* 23:268–271.

[110] Ferdinando, C., et al. (2004). Anencephaly: MRI findings and pathogenetic theories. *Pediatr Radiol* 34, 1012–1016. Retrieved 10.24.2009 from ProQuest Health and Medical Complete. (Document ID: 1316641521).

[111] Chatzipapas, I. K., Whitlow, B. J., & Economides, D. L. (1999). The "Mickey Mouse" sign and the diagnosis of anencephaly in early pregnancy. *Ultrasound Obstet Gynecol* 13:196–199.

[112] Centers for Disease Control and Prevention. (2004). Spina bifida and anencephaly before and after folic acid mandate—United States, 1995–1996 and 1999–2000. *MMWR Morb Mortal Wkly Rep* 53:362–365.

[113] Pakzaban, P. (2010). Chiari malformation. *eMed from WebMD*. Retrieved 11.20.2010 from http://emedicine.medscape.com/article/1483583-overview

[114] Mayo Clinic. (2010). *Chiari malformation: causes*. Mayo Foundation for Medical Education and Research. Retrieved from http://www.mayoclinic.com/health/chiari-malformation/DS00839/DSECTION=causes

[115] Murray, C., et al. (2006). Arnold Chiari malformation presenting with sleep disordered breathing in well children. *Arch Dis Child* 91:342–343.

[116] Pakzaban, P. Ibid.

[117] National Institutes of Neurological Disorders and Stroke, National Institutes of Health. (2009). *NINDS Chiari malformation information page*. Retrieved 11.20.2010 from http://www.ninds.nih.gov/disorders/chiari/chiari.htm#What_is_the_prognosis

[118] Pakzaban, P. Ibid.

[119] Autism Society of America. (2008). *About autism*. Retrieved 11.20.2010 from http://www.autism-society.org/site/PageServer?pagename=about_home

[120] Ibid.

[121] National Institutes of Neurological Disorders and Stroke, National Institutes of Health. (2010). *Autism fact sheet*. Retrieved 11.20.2010 from http://www.ninds.nih.gov/disorders/autism/detail_autism.htm

[122] Autism Society of America. Ibid.

[123] Kaneshiro, N. K. (2010). Autism. *MedlinePlus Medical Encyclopedia*. Retrieved 11.20.2010 from http://www.nlm.nih.gov/medlineplus/ency/article/001526.htm

[124] National Institutes of Neurological Disorders and Stroke, National Institutes of Health. (2010). Ibid.

[125] Ibid.

[126] Ibid.

[127] Hayhurst, C. (2008). Treating kids with autism. *PT Magazine Phys Ther* 16:20–27.

[128] Nazarali, N. (2009). Movement planning and reprogramming in individuals with autism. *J Autism Dev Disord* 39:1401–1411.

[129] Petrus, C., et al. (2008). Effects of exercise interventions on stereotypic behaviours in children with autism spectrum disorder. *Physiother Can* 60:134–145.

[130] Carmichael Olson, H., et al. (2007). Responding to the challenge of early intervention for fetal alcohol spectrum disorders. *Infants Young Child* 20:172–189.

[131] American Academy of Pediatrics. (2000). Fetal alcohol syndrome and alcohol-related neurodevelopmental disorders. Committee on Substance Abuse and Committee on Children with Disabilities. *Pediatrics* 106:358–361.

[132] Carmichael Olson, H., et al. Ibid.

[133] Westcott, S. L., & Burtner, P. (2004). Postural control in children: implications for pediatric practice. *Phys Occup Ther Pediatr* 24(1/2):5-55.

[134] Osborn, J. A., Harris, S. R., & Weinberg, J. (1993). Fetal alcohol syndrome: review of the literature with implications for the physical therapist. *Phys Ther* 73:41–49.

[135] The Carter Centers for Brain Research in Holoprosencephaly and Related Malformations. (n.d.). *Information about holoprosencephaly*. Retrieved 11.20.2010 from http://www.stanford.edu/group/hpe/

[136] Solomon, B. D., Gropman, A., & Muenke, M. (2010). Holoprosencephaly overview. *GeneReviews*. Retrieved 11.20.2010 from http://www.ncbi.nlm.nih.gov/bookshelf/br.fcgi?book=gene&part=hpe-overview

[137] Ibid.

[138] The Carter Centers for Brain Research in Holoprosencephaly and Related Malformations. (n.d.). Ibid.

[139] National Institute of Neurological Disorders and Stroke, National Institutes of Health. (2007). *NINDS Holoprosencephaly information page*. Retrieved 10.15.2010 from http://www.ninds.nih.gov/disorders/holoprosencephaly/holoprosencephaly.htm

[140] The Carter Centers for Brain Research in Holoprosencephaly and Related Malformations. (n.d.). Ibid.

[141] Solomon, B. D., Gropman, A., & Muenke, M. Ibid.

[142] The Carter Centers for Brain Research in Holoprosencephaly and Related Malformations. (n.d.). Ibid.

[143] Solomon, B. D., Gropman, A., & Muenke, M. Ibid.

[144] The Mount Sinai Hospital/Mount Sinai School of Medicine. (2009, August). Mount Sinai researchers find new Alzheimer's disease treatment promising. *NewsRx Health*. ProQuest http://wf2dnvr12.webfeat.org/OKDxM1440/url=http://proquest.umi.com/pqdweb?vinst...

[145] Cassels, C. (2009, Sept). Difficulties with activities of daily living strong predictor of progression to dementia. *Arch Neurol* 66:1151–1157.

[146] National Institute of Neurological Disorders & Stroke, National Institutes of Health. (2010). *NINDS Alzheimer's disease information page*. Retrieved 11.20.2010 from http://www.ninds.nih.gov/disorders/alzheimersdisease/alzheimersdisease.htm

[147] Alzheimer's Association. (2010). *Stages of Alzheimer's*. Retrieved 11.20.2010 from http://www.alz.org/alzheimers_disease_stages_of_alzheimers.asp

[148] Kovach, C. (1996). Alzheimer's disease: long-term care issues. *Issues Law Med* 12:47–56.

[149] Alzheimer's Association. (2010). Ibid.

[150] *Cardiovascular Week* editors. (2009, July). Alzheimer's association; brain imaging and proteins in spinal fluid may improve Alzheimer's prediction and diagnosis. *Cardiovasc Week*, p. 273, NewsRx.com. Retrieved 9.9.2009 from ProQuest http://wf2dnvr12.webfeat.org/OKDcM1445/url=http://proquest.umi.com/pqdweb?vinst=PR

[151] *Medical Devices and Surgical Technology Week* editors and staff. (2009, August). Dementia: data on dementia described by researchers at University of Adelaide. *Med Devices Surg Technol Week*, ProQuest. Retrieved from http://wf2dnvr12.webfeat.org/OKDcM1436/url=http://proquest.umi.com/pqdweb?vinst=PR.

[152] Peters, R. (2009, May). The prevention of dementia. *Int J Geriatr Psychiatry* 24:452–458.

[153] University of California. (2009). Neural stem cells offer potential treatment for Alzheimer's disease. *NewsRx Health*. Retrieved 4.4.2009 from ProQuest at http://wf2dnvr12.webfeat.org

[154] The Mount Sinai Hospital/Mount Sinai School of Medicine. Ibid.

[155] Holliday-Welsh, D., Gessert, C., & Renier, C. (2009, March). Massage in the management of agitation in nursing home residents with cognitive impairment. *Geriatric Nurs* 30:108–117.

[156] Munn, Z. (2009). Physical activity programs for persons with dementia. *J Adv Nurs* 65:776–777.

[157] ALS Association. (2008). *Initial symptoms of ALS*. Retrieved 4.4.2009 from http://www.alsa.org/als/symptoms.cfm

[158] Stitham, S. O., & Hoch, D. B. (2010). *Amyotrophic lateral sclerosis*. Retrieved 11.20.2010 from http://www.nlm.nih.gov/medlineplus/ency/article/000688.htm

[159] National Institute of Neurological Disorders and Stroke, National Institutes of Health. (2010). *Amyotrophic lateral sclerosis fact sheet*. Retrieved 11.20.2010 from http://www.ninds.nih.gov/disorders/amyotrophiclateralsclerosis/detail_amyotrophiclateralsclerosis.htm#126454842

[160] Ibid.

[161] Ramirez, C., et al. (2008). Fatigue in amyotrophic lateral sclerosis: frequency and associated factors. *Amyotrophic Lateral Sclerosis* 9:75-80.

[162] ALS Association Ibid.

[163] National Institute of Neurological Disorders and Stroke, National Institutes of Health *Amyotrophic lateral sclerosis fact sheet: What are the symptoms?* Ibid.

[164] Simmons, Z. (2009). Management strategies for patients with amyotrophic lateral sclerosis from diagnosis through death. *Neurologist* 11:257–270.

[165] Corcia, P., & Meininger, V. (2008). Management of amyotrophic lateral sclerosis. *Drug* 68:1037–1048.

[166] Cleary, S., et al. (2008). Using active rehabilitation to decrease the risk of pneumonia in end-of-life amyotrophic lateral sclerosis and dementia care. *Can Nurs Home* 19:4–10.

[167] National Institute of Neurological Disorders and Stroke, National Institutes of Health. *Amyotrophic lateral sclerosis fact sheet: What are the symptoms?* Ibid.

[168] Stephenson, J. (2004). Gene therapy and ALS. *JAMA* 291:2809.

[169] ALS Association. (2008). Ibid.

[170] National Institute of Neurological Disorders and Stroke, National Institutes of Health. *Amyotrophic lateral sclerosis fact sheet: What are the symptoms?* Ibid.

[171] Ibid.

[172] Lewis, M., & Rushanan, S. (2007). The role of the physical therapist and occupational therapy in the treatment of amyotrophic lateral sclerosis. *Neurorehabilitation* 22:451–461.

[173] National Institute of Neurological Disorders and Stroke, National Institutes of Health. *Amyotrophic lateral sclerosis fact sheet: How is ALS treated?* Ibid.

[174] Surgeon General's Report. (2004). *Highlights: smoking among adults in the United States: coronary heart disease and stroke*. Centers for Disease Control and Prevention. Retrieved 4.4.2009 from http://www.cdc.gov/tobacco/data_statistics/sgr/2004/highlights/heart_disease/index.htm

[175] Turner, C. (2008). The diagnosis and initial management of stroke and transient ischaemic attack. *Primary Health Care* 18:32–36.

[176] Surgeon General's Report. Ibid.

[177] U.S. Department of Health and Human Services. *The Health Consequences of Involuntary Exposure to Tobacco Smoke: A Report of the Surgeon General—Executive Summary*. U.S. Department of Health and Human Services, Centers for Disease Control and Prevention, Coordinating Center for Health Promotion, National Center for Chronic Disease Prevention and Health Promotion, Office on Smoking and Health, 2006.

[178] Stroke guide. (2009). *WebMD*. Retrieved 4.7.2010 from http://www.webmd.com/stroke/guide/stroke-overview-facts

[179] Purroy, F., et al. (2007, Dec). Patterns and predictors of early risk of recurrence after transient ischemic attack with respect to etiological subtypes. *Stroke*, 38:3225–3229.

[180] Turner, C. Ibid.

[181] Stroke guide. Ibid.

[182] Sudlow, C. (2008). Preventing further vascular events after a stroke or transient ischaemic attack: an update on medical management. *Pract Neurol* 8:141–157.

[183] Stroke guide. Ibid.

[184] Ellis, M. D. (2009). Progressive shoulder abduction loading is a crucial element of arm rehabilitation in chronic stroke. *Neurorehabil Neural Repair* 23:862–869.

[185] Creutzfeldt-Jakob disease. (2010). *MedlinePlus Medical Encyclopedia*. Retrieved 11.20.2010 from http://www.nlm.nih.gov/medlineplus/creutzfeldtjakobdisease.html

[186] Genetics Home Reference. (2010). *Prion disease*. Retrieved 11.20.2010 from http://ghr.nlm.nih.gov/condition=priondisease

[187] National Institute of Neurological Disorders and Stroke, National Institutes of Health. (2009). Creutzfeldt-Jakob disease fact sheet. Retrieved 4.4.2010 from http://www.ninds.nih.gov/disorders/cjd/detail_cjd.htm

[188] Ibid.

[189] Genetics Home Reference. (2010). Ibid.

[190] Centers for Disease Control and Prevention. (2010). *BSE (bovine spongiform encephalopathy, or mad cow disease)*. Retrieved 11.20.2010 from http://www.cdc.gov/ncidod/dvrd/bse/

[191] National Institute of Neurological Disorders and Stroke, National Institutes of Health. Creutzfeldt-Jakob disease fact sheet. Ibid.

[192] Ibid.

[193] Meissner, B., et al. (2009). MRI lesion profiles in sporadic Creutzfeldt-Jakob disease. *Neurology* 72:1994–2001.

[194] National Institute of Neurological Disorders and Stroke, National Institutes of Health. Creutzfeldt-Jakob disease fact sheet. Ibid.

[195] Arciniegas, D. B., & Dubovsky, S. L. (2009). Dementia due to other general medical conditions and dementia due to multiple etiologies. In *Gabbard's treatments of psychiatric disorders*, 4th edition, American Psychiatric Publishing.

[196] BUPA Health Information Team. (2009). *Dementia*. Retrieved on 4.4.10 from http://hcd2.bupa.co.uk/fact_sheets/html/Dementia.html

[197] Lewy Body Dementia Association. (2009). *What is LBD?* Retrieved 4.4.2010 from http://www.lbda.org/category/3437/what-is-lbd.htm

[198] Arciniegas, D. B., & Dubovsky, S. L. Ibid.

[199] Ibid.

[200] BUPA Health Information Team. (2009). Retrieved on 11.18.10 from http://hcd2.bupa.co.uk/fact_sheets/html/Dementia.html#2 Ibid.

[201] Arciniegas, D. B., & Dubovsky, S. L. Ibid., p. 7.

[202] Edwards, K. R., et al. (2004). Efficacy and safety of galantamine in patients with dementia with Lewy bodies: a 12 week interim analysis. *Dement Geriatr Cogn Disord* 17(suppl 1):40–48.

[203] Tapus, A., Fasola, J., & Mataric, M. J. (2008). *Cognitive assistance and physical therapy for dementia patients using socially assistive robots*. University of Southern California. Retrieved 4.4.2010 from http://cres.usc.edu/pubdb_html/files_upload/578.pdf

[204] O'Hara, K. A., & Shafer, P. O. (2008). Epilepsy 101: Getting started. American Epilepsy Society archives. Retrieved on 11.18.10 from http://www.aesnet.org/go/professional-development/educational-opportunities/teleconsults/archived-programs/epilepsy-101/epilepsy-101-getting-started

[205] Mayo Clinic Staff. (2009). *Epilepsy*. Mayo Foundation for Medical Education and Research. Retrieved 4.4.2010 from http://www.mayoclinic.com/print/epilepsy/DS00342/DSECTION=all&METHOD=print

[206] Epilepsy Foundation of America. (2009). Epileptic syndromes. Retrieved on 4.4.10 from http://www.epilepsyfoundation.org/about/types/syndromes/index.cfm

[207] Mayo Clinic Staff. (2009). Epilepsy. Ibid.

[208] Ibid.

[209] National Institute of Neurological Disorders and Stroke, National Institutes of Health. (2010). *NINDS epilepsy information page*. Retrieved 11.20.2010 from http://www.ninds.nih.gov/disorders/epilepsy/epilepsy.htm

[210] Mayo Clinic Staff. (2009). Epilepsy. Ibid.

[211] Searson, B. (2008). Meeting the challenges of epilepsy. *Learn Disabil Pract* 11:29–35.

212 Epilepsy Foundation of America. (2009). Treatment options: medications. Retrieved 4.4.2010 from http://www.epilepsyfoundation.org/about/treatment/medications/

213 Karceski, S. (2009). Juvenile myoclonic epilepsy, a common epilepsy syndrome. *Neurology* 73:e64–e67.

214 Landmark, C. J., & Johanneson, S. I. (2008). Pharmacological management of epilepsy: recent advances and future prospects. *Drugs* 68:1926–1939.

215 Epilepsy Foundation of America. (2009). Treatment options: Vagus nerve stimulation. Retrieved 4.4.2010 from http://www.epilepsyfoundation.org/about/treatment/vns/

216 Boon, P., et al. (2009). Electrical stimulation for the treatment of epilepsy. *Neurotherapeutics* 6:218–227.

217 Nakase, H., et al. (2007). Long-term follow-up outcome after surgical treatment for lesional temporal lobe epilepsy. *Neurol Res* 29:588–593.

218 Chandra, P. S., et al. (2008). Hemispherectomy for intractable epilepsy. *Neurol India* 56:127–132.

219 Rogawski, M. A., & Holmes, G. L. (2009). Nontraditional epilepsy treatment approaches. *Neurotherapeutics* 6:213–217.

220 National Institute of Neurological Disorders and Stroke, National Institutes of Health. (2010). *NINDS Guillain Barré syndrome fact sheet.* Retrieved 10.29.10 from http://www.ninds.nih.gov/disorders/gbs/detail_gbs.htm

221 Haber, P., et al. (2009). Vaccines and Guillain-Barré syndrome. *Drug Safety* 32:309–423.

222 Khiani, V., et al. (2008). Acute inflammatory demyelinating polyneuropathy associated with pegylated interferon alpha 2a therapy for chronic hepatitis C virus infection. *World J Gastroenterol* 14:318–321.

223 National Institute of Neurological Disorders and Stroke, National Institutes of Health. *NINDS Guillain Barré syndrome fact sheet.* Ibid.

224 Ibid.

225 Petzold, A., et al. (2009). CSF biomarkers for proximal axonal damage improve prognostic accuracy in acute phase of Guillain-Barré syndrome. *Muscle Nerve* 40:42–49.

226 Strauss, J., et al. (2009). Plasma cortisol levels in Guillain-Barré syndrome. *Crit Care Med* 37:2436–2440.

227 Köhrmann, M., et al. (2009). Mechanical ventilation in Guillain-Barré syndrome: does age influence functional outcome? *Eur Neurol* 61:358–363.

228 Petzold, A., et al. Ibid.

229 Strauss, J. et al. Ibid.

230 National Institute of Neurological Disorders and Stroke, National Institutes of Health. *NINDS Guillain Barré syndrome fact sheet.* Ibid.

231 Walton, T., et al. (2005). Usefulness of digital gait analysis for assessing patients with Guillain-Barré syndrome. *Int J Ther Rehabil* 12:388–394.

232 Jamshidi, N., et al. (2009). Modelling of human walking to optimize the function of ankle-foot orthosis in Guillain-Barré patients with drop foot. *Singapore Med J* 50:412–417.

233 Karavatas, S. G. (2005). The role of neurodevelopmental sequencing in the physical therapy management of a geriatric patient with Guillain-Barré syndrome. *Topics Geriatr Rehabil* 21:133–135.

234 Bulley, P. (2003). The podiatron: an adjunct to physiotherapy treatment for Guillain-Barré syndrome. *Physiother Res Int* 8:210–215.

235 Bolek, J. E., & Somodi, M. (1998). Exploring opportunities for collaboration in an era of managed care: A biofeedback-assisted treatment plan. *Profess Psychol Res Pract* 29:71–73.

236 Niclis, J., et al. (2009). Human embryonic stem cell models of Huntington's disease. *Reproductive BioMed Online.* 19:106–113. Retrieved 4.4.2010 from www.rbmonline.com

237 Rego, A. C., & Periera de Almeida, L. (2005). Molecular targets and therapeutic strategies in Huntington's disease. *Curr Drug Targets CNS Neurol Disord* 4:361–381.

238 Genetics Home Reference. (2010). HTT. US National Library of Med, National Institutes of Health, Dept. of Health and Human Services. Retrieved 11.20.2010 from http://ghr.nlm.nih.gov/gene=htt

239 Mayo Clinic Staff. (2009). *Huntington's disease: symptoms.* Mayo Foundation for Medical Education and Research. Retrieved 4.4.2010 from http://www.mayoclinic.com/health/huntingtons-disease/DS00401/DSECTION=symptoms

240 Adam, O. R., & Jankovic, J. (2008). Symptomatic treatment of Huntington's disease. *Neurotherapeutics* 5:181–197.

241 Fogliani, A. M., Giogio, A., & Bonomo, V. (2003). Awareness of involuntary movements in Huntington's disease with olanzapine: a case report. *Minerva Psichiatrica* 44:189–190.

242 Mayo Clinic Staff. (2009). *Huntington's disease: symptoms.* Mayo Foundation for Medical Education and Research. Retrieved 4.4.2010 from http://www.mayoclinic.com/health/huntingtons-disease/DS00401/DSECTION=symptoms

243 Niclis, J., et al. Ibid.

244 Mayo Clinic Staff. (2010). *Huntington's disease: Tests and diagnosis.* Mayo Foundation for Medical Education and Research. Retrieved 11.20.2010 from http://www.mayoclinic.com/health/huntingtons-disease/DS00401/DSECTION=tests-and-diagnosis

245 Mayo Clinic Staff. (2009). *Huntington's disease: Treatments and drugs.* Mayo Foundation for Medical Education and Research. Retrieved 4.4.2010 from http://www.mayoclinic.com/health/huntingtons-disease/DS00401/DSECTION=treatments-and-drugs

246 De Tommaso, M., et al. (2007). Two-years' follow-up of rivastigmine treatment in Huntington's disease. *Clin Neuropharmacol* 30:43–46.

247 Mayo Clinic Staff. *Huntington's disease: Treatments and drugs.* Ibid.

248 Adam, O. R., & Jankovic, J. Ibid.

249 Niclis, J., et al. Ibid.

250 Pickett, T., Altmaier, E., & Paulsen, J. S. (2007). Caregiver burden in Huntington's disease. *Rehabil Psychol* 52:311–318.

251 Aubeeluck, A., & Buchanan, H. (2007). The Huntington's disease quality of life battery for carers: reliability and validity. *Clin Genet* 71:434–445.

252 Mayo Clinic Staff. (2009). *Huntington's disease: Coping and support.* Mayo Foundation for Medical Education and Research. Retrieved 4.6.2010 from http://www.mayoclinic.com/health/huntingtons-disease/DS00401/DSECTION=coping-and-support

253 Bosse, M. E., et al. (2008). Physical therapy intervention for people with Huntington's disease. *Phys Ther* 88:820–831.

254 Jenkins, T. M., Khaleeli, Z., & Thompson, A. J. (2008, April). Diagnosis and management of primary progressive multiple sclerosis. *Minerva Med* 99:141–155.

255 Nazario, B. (2010). What causes multiple sclerosis? *WebMD.* Retrieved 11.20.2010 from http://www.webmd.com/multiple-sclerosis/guide/multiple-sclerosis-causes

256 National Multiple Sclerosis Society. (2009). *Genetics.* Retrieved 10.11.2009 from http://www.nationalmssociety.org/about-multiple-sclerosis/who-gets-ms/genetics/index.aspx

257 Nazario, B. Ibid.

258 Nazario, B. (2009). Recognizing multiple sclerosis. WebMD. Retrieved 11.20.2010 from http://www.webmd.com/multiple-sclerosis/guide/recognizing-multiple-sclerosis

259 Miller, D. H., et al. (2008). Differential diagnosis of suspected multiple sclerosis: a consensus approach. *Mult Scler* 14:1157–1174.

260 Benedict, R., et al. (2002, Aug). Minimal neuropsychological assessment of MS patients: a consensus approach. *Clin Neuropsychol* 16:381–397.

261 Hoffman, M. (2009). Multiple sclerosis: drug therapy. *WebMD.* Retrieved 4.7.2010 from http://www.webmd.com/multiple-sclerosis/guide/ms-drug-therapy

262 Di Fabio, R. P., et al. (1997). Health-related quality of life for patients with progressive multiple sclerosis: influence of rehabilitation. *Phys Ther* 77:1704–1716.

263 Fragoso, Y. D., Santana, D. L., & Pinto, R. C. (2008). The positive effects of a physical activity program for multiple sclerosis patients with fatigue. *Neurorehabilitation* 23:153–157.

264 Dalgas, V., Stenager, E., & Ingemann-Hansen, T. (2008). Multiple sclerosis and physical exercise: recommendations for the application of resistance-, endurance- and combined training. *Mult Scler* 14:35–53.

265 Paul, L., et al. (2008, Aug). The effect of functional electrical stimulation on the physiological cost of gait in people with multiple sclerosis. *Mult Scler* 14:954–961.

266 Mark, V. W., et al. (2008). Constraint-induced movement therapy can improve hemiparetic progressive multiple sclerosis. Preliminary findings. *Mult Scler* 14:992–994.

267 Peterson, C. (2001). Exercise in 94 degrees F water for a patient with multiple sclerosis. *Phys Ther* 81:1049–1058.

268 Lee, M. C., et al. (1989). The Ashworth Scale: A reliable and reproducible method of measuring spasticity. *J Neurol Rehabil* 3:205–209.

269 Mahoney, F. I., & Barthel, D. W. (1965). Functional evaluation: the Barthel Index. *Maryland State Med J* 14:61–65.

270 Berg, K., et al. (1992). Measuring balance in the elderly: Validation of an instrument. *Can J Public Health* 2(suppl):57–11.

271 Paltamaa, J., et al. (2008). Measuring deterioration in international classification of functioning domains of people with multiple sclerosis who are ambulatory. *Phys Ther* 88:176–190.

272 Kesselring, J., et al. (2008, March). Developing the ICF score sets for multiple sclerosis to specify functioning. *Mult Scler* 14:252–254.

273 Lewis, C. (1993). Balance, gait test proves simple yet useful. *PT Bull* 2/10:9, 40.

274 Tinetti, M. E. (1986). Performance oriented assessment of mobility problems in elderly patients. *JAGS* 34:119–126.

275 Shepherd, S. M., & Shoff, W. H. (2010). Drowning: differential diagnoses and workup. *eMedicine from WebMD, Medscape*. Retrieved 11.20.2010 from http://emedicine.medscape.com/article/772753-diagnosis

276 Ibid.

277 Ibid.

278 Ibid.

279 Ibid.

280 Ibid.

281 Heller, J. L. (2009). Near-drowning. *MedlinePlus Medical Encyclopedia*. Retrieved 4.7.2010 from http://www.nlm.nih.gov/medlineplus/ency/article/000046.htm

282 The Neuropathy Association. (2009). *About peripheral neuropathy: facts*. Retrieved 4.7.2010 from http://www.neuropathy.org/site/PageServer?pagename=About_Facts

283 Understanding peripheral neuropathy. (2009). *WebMD*. Retrieved 4.8.2010 from http://www.webmd.com/brain/understanding-peripheral-neuropathy-basics

284 Ibid.

285 National Institute of Neurological Disorders and Stroke, National Institutes of Health. (2010). *Peripheral neuropathy fact sheet*. Retrieved 11.20.2010 from http://www.ninds.nih.gov/disorders/peripheralneuropathy/detail_peripheralneuropathy.htm

286 Ibid.

287 Ibid.

288 National Institute of Neurological Disorders and Stroke, National Institutes of Health. (2004, December). Parkinson's disease: challenges, progress, and promise [NIH Publication No. 05-5595].

289 Hoch, D. B. (2009). Parkinson's disease. *MedlinePlus Medical Encyclopedia*. Retrieved 10.15.2010 from http://www.nlm.nih.gov/medlineplus/ency/article/000755.htm

290 National Institute of Neurological Disorders and Stroke. Parkinson's Disease: Challenges, Progress, and Promise. NIH. NIH Publication No. 05-5595.

291 National Institute of Neurological Disorders and Stroke, National Institutes of Health. Parkinson's disease: challenges, progress, and promise. Ibid.

292 Hoch, D. B. (2009). Ibid.

293 National Institute of Neurological Disorders and Stroke, National Institutes of Health. (2009). *NINDS Parkinson's disease information page*. Retrieved 10.14.2010 from http://www.ninds.nih.gov/disorders/parkinsons_disease/parkinsons_disease.htm

294 National Institute of Neurological Disorders and Stroke, National Institutes of Health. Parkinson's disease: challenges, progress, and promise. Ibid.

295 Ibid.

296 Glass, J. (2010). Parkinson's disease: physical and occupational therapy. Cleveland Clinic. *WebMD*. Retrieved 11.20.2010 from http://www.webmd.com/parkinsons-disease/physical-occupational-therapy

297 Jubelt, B., & Agre, J. C. (2000). Characteristics and management of postpolio syndrome. *JAMA* 284:412–414.

298 Sharma, K. R., et al. (1994). Excessive muscular fatigue in the postpoliomyelitis syndrome. *Neurology* 44:642–646.

299 Jubelt, B., & Agre, J. C. Ibid.

300 Ibid.

301 Agre, J. C., Rodriquez, A. A. (1997). Muscular function in late polio and the role of exercise in post-polio patients. *Neurorehabilitation* 8:107–118.

302 Pearse, D. D., et al. (2004). cAMP and Schwann cells promote axonal growth and functional recovery after spinal cord injury. *Nat Med* 10:610–616.

303 The National SCI Statistical Center. (2009). *Facts and figures at a glance 2009*. Retrieved 4.8.2010 from https://www.nscisc.uab.edu//public_content/facts_figures_2009.aspx

304 Rowland, J. W., et al. (2008). Status of acute spinal cord injury pathophysiology and emerging therapies: epidemiology of spinal cord injury. *Neurosurg Focus* 25:E2.

305 Ibid.

306 Ibid.

307 Ibid.

308 Garland, D. E., Adkins, R. H., & Stewart, C. A. (2008). Five-year longitudinal bone evaluations in individuals with chronic complete spinal cord injury. *J Spinal Cord Med* 31:543–550.

309 Guihan, M. et al. (2008). Predictors of pressure ulcer recurrence in veterans with spinal cord injury. *J Spinal Cord Med* 31:551–559.

310 Salmons, R. (2008). A study of quality of life issues for individuals with spinal cord injury following treatment and financial settlement. *J Life Care Planning*, 7:73-83.

311 The National SCI Statistical Center. Ibid.

312 National Institute of Neurological Disorders and Stroke, National Institutes of Health. (2010). *NINDS spinal cord injury information page*. Retrieved 11.20.2010 from http://www.ninds.nih.gov/disorders/sci/sci.htm

313 The National SCI Statistical Center. Ibid.

314 Evans, C. T. (2007). *Blood stream infections in veterans with spinal cord injury*. PhD dissertation, University of Illinois at Chicago [Pub. No. AAT 3274019].

315 Bracken, M. B. et al. (1997). Administration of methylprednisolone for 24 to 48 hours or tirilazad mesylate for 48 hours in the treatment of acute spinal cord injury. *JAMA* 277:1597–1604.

316 Byrnes, K. (2003). *810 nm light treatment of spinal cord injury alters the immune response and improves axonal regeneration and functional recovery*. PhD dissertation, Uniformed Services University of the Health Sciences [Pub No. AAT 3117206].

317 Salmons, R. (2008). A study of quality of life issues for individuals with spinal cord injury following treatment and financial settlement. *J Life Care Planning* 7:73–83.

318 Cao, F. J., & Feng, S. Q. (2009). Human umbilical cord mesenchymal stem cells and the treatment of spinal cord injury. *Chinese Med J* 122:225–231.

319 Pearse, D. D., et al. (2004). Ibid.

320 Park, J. B., et al. (2005). A TNF receptor family member, TROY, is a coreceptor with Nogo receptor in mediating the inhibitory activity of myelin inhibitors. *Neuron*, 45:345–351.

321 Preidt, R. (2009). A drug to cure spinal cord injury? *MedlinePlus Medical Encyclopedia.* Retrieved 7.20.2009 from http://www.nlm.nih.gov/medlineplus/news/fullstory_90649.html

322 Behrman, A., Bowden, M. G., & Nair, P. M. (2006). Neuroplasticity after spinal cord injury and training: An emerging paradigm shift in rehabilitation and walking recovery. *Phys Ther* 86:1406–1425.

323 Wallace, L., & McQueen, J. (2008). Acute phase functional electrical stimulation for the upper limb after cervical spinal cord injury. *Int J Ther Rehabil* 15:230–234.

324 Bellby, J., & Mulligan, H. (2008). Deep vein thrombosis and heterotropic ossification following spinal cord injury—a clinical perspective for physiotherapists. *N Z J Physiother* 36:7–14.

325 National Center for Injury Prevention and Control, Centers for Disease Control and Prevention. (2009). *Injury prevention and control: traumatic brain injury?* Retrieved 11.20.2010 from http://www.cdc.gov/ncipc/tbi/TBI.htm

326 Dawodu, S. T. (2009). Traumatic brain injury (TBI)—definition, epidemiology, pathophysiology. *eMed from WebMD.* Retrieved 7.11.2009 from http://emedicine.medscape.com/article/326510-overview

327 Post-traumatic stress disorder. (2009). *MedlinePlus Medical Encyclopedia.* Retrieved 7.11.2009 from http://www.nlm.nih.gov/medlineplus/posttraumaticstressdisorder.html

328 American Association of Neurological Surgeons. (2009). *Sports-related head injury.* Retrieved 11.20.2010 from http://aans.org/Patient%20Information/Conditions%20and%20Treatments/Sports-Related%20Head%20Injury.aspx

329 Dawodu, S. T. Ibid.

330 National Institute for Neurological Disorders and Stroke, National Institutes of Health. (2010). NINDS traumatic brain injury information page. Retrieved 11.20.2010 from http://www.ninds.nih.gov/disorders/tbi/tbi.htm

331 Post-traumatic stress disorder. (2009). Ibid.

332 Reed, J. M., & Squire, L. R. (1998). Retrograde amnesia for facts and events: findings from four new cases. *J Neurosci* 18:3943–3954.

333 Gold, J. J., & Squire, L. R. (2006). The anatomy of amnesia: Neurohistological analysis of three new cases. *Learning and Memory*, 13:699-710.

334 Squire, L. R., Haist, F., & Shimamura, A. P. (1989). The neurology of memory: quantitative assessment of retrograde amnesia in two groups of amnesic patients. *J Neurosci* 9:828–839.

335 Nakase-Richardson, R., Yablon, S. A., & Sherer, M. (2007). Prospective comparison of acute confusion severity with duration of post-traumatic amnesia in predicting employment outcome after traumatic brain injury. *J Neurol Neurosurg Psychiatry* 78:872–876.

336 Dawodu, S. T. Ibid.

337 Ibid.

338 National Institute for Neurological Disorders and Stroke, National Institutes of Health. NINDS traumatic brain injury information page. Ibid.

339 Ibid.

340 Birns, J., & Fitzpatrick, M. (2008). Management of spasticity: a brief overview of educational and pharmacological therapies. *Br J Neurosci Nurs* 4:370–373.

341 Dixon, M. R., & Tibbetts, P. A. (2009). The effects of choice on self-control. *J Appl Behav Anal* 42:243–252.

342 Dixon, M. R., & Falcometa, T. S. (2004). Preference for progressive delays and concurrent physical therapy exercise in an adult with acquired brain injury. *J Appl Behav Anal* 37:101–105.

343 Katz-Leurer, M., Rotem, H., Keren, O., & Meyer, S. (2009). Balance abilities and gait characteristics in post-traumatic brain injury, cerebral palsy and typically developed children. *Dev Neurorehabil* 12:100–105.

344 Vanderploeg, P. D., et al. (2008). Rehabilitation of traumatic brain injury in active duty military personnel and veterans: Defense and Veterans Brain Injury Center randomized controlled trial of two rehabilitation approaches. *Arch Phys Med Rehabil* 89:2227–2238.

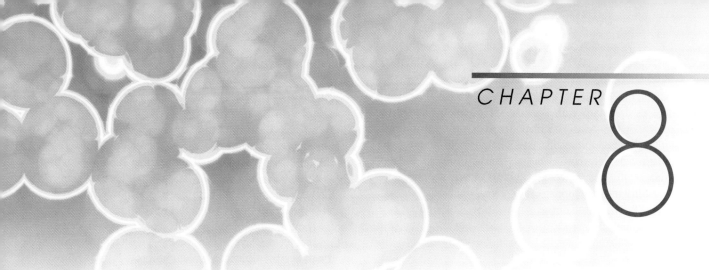

CHAPTER 8

Burns and Skin Conditions

LEARNING OBJECTIVES

After completion of this chapter, students should be able to:

- Describe the structure, anatomy, and physiology of skin
- Identify the mechanical mechanisms of burns
- Describe the pathological mechanisms of burns and other skin conditions
- Determine the classification of burns
- Analyze the relevance of the Rule of Nines in the medical management of patients with burns
- Discuss the physical therapy intervention for patients with various skin conditions
- Determine the role of the physical therapist assistant in working with patients with burns and other skin conditions
- Discuss the contraindications, precautions, and special considerations for physical therapist/physical therapist assistant intervention for patients with burns and other skin conditions

CHAPTER OUTLINE

KEY TERMS

Allograft
Arterial insufficiency/ischemic ulcer
Autograft
Cellulitis
Contact dermatitis
Débridement
Decubitus ulcer
Deep partial-thickness burns
Dermatome instrument
Eschar
Escharotomy
Full-thickness burns
Full-thickness skin graft
Keloid and hypertrophic scarring
Inosculation
Necrotizing fasciitis
Rule of Nines
Split-thickness skin graft
Subdermal burns
Superficial burns
Superficial partial-thickness burns
Venous stasis ulcer
Xenograft

Introduction

This chapter starts with a review of the anatomy and physiology of the skin. The main focus is on burn injuries. Other skin conditions discussed include cold injuries, circulatory deficit skin conditions such as arterial and venous insufficiency ulcers, decubitus ulcers, neoplasias of the skin, and infections resulting from bacteria, viruses, fungi, and vector-borne organisms. Throughout the chapter, physical therapy interventions are discussed, and the comparison is made between treatment options for venous and arterial ulcers.

Why Does the Physical Therapist Assistant Need to Know About the Anatomy and Physiology of Skin?

The physical therapist assistant (PTA) needs to have knowledge of healthy skin and its functions because skin conditions result in loss of these functions. When the epidermis, dermis, and subcutaneous layers are damaged, the whole body is at risk from several factors, such as infection, dehydration, and even death. To understand the treatment of skin conditions, particularly burns, the PTA needs to appreciate the likely ramifications when specific layers of skin are damaged. Knowledge of the site of the sensory nerve endings in the skin is also important, because damage to these nerve endings can cause impairments of sensory function, which are noted not only in skin and integumentary conditions but also in neurological diseases and orthopedic conditions.

Anatomy And Physiology of the Skin

The skin is an organ consisting of an outer epidermis and an inner layer of dermis that serves a protective function for the underlying organs and tissue (see Table 8-1 and Fig. 8-1). This fascinating body organ provides a covering for the body that prevents both the loss of body fluid and the absorption of fluids from the environment into the body; protects the blood vessels and nerves, located within the dermal layer, from damage; protects the body from damage by ultraviolet radiation; provides a defense against the invasion of bacteria and other disease-causing agents; controls the body temperature through the network of blood vessels; produces vitamin D; and provides a location for the nerve endings that protect the body against noxious external stimuli.

The skin consists of the outer epidermis and the deeper layer of dermis, each of which contain several layers. The epidermis or outermost layer of the skin is composed of five layers. The layers of epidermis are continually renewed from squamous epithelial cells formed in the stratum basale. Dead skin cells in the stratum corneum are constantly sloughed off from the surface of the skin, and cells produced in the stratum basale layer replace them. Cells produced in the stratum basale gradually migrate into the stratum corneum. This process of migration may take up to several weeks. Cells remain in the outer stratum corneum for approximately 14 days before they slough off the surface in a process called desquamation. The epidermis is being replaced constantly and any one cell lives for 45 to 75 days.[1] The epidermis does not have any blood vessels or nerves, and thus, its nutrition is provided from the dermal layer of the skin. The layers of the epidermis are detailed in Table 8-2.

Table 8.1 **Protective Functions of the Skin**

FUNCTION OF SKIN	FACTORS INFLUENCING THE FUNCTION OF THE SKIN
Prevention of loss of body fluid or absorption of fluid from the environment	Keratin, a protein, found in skin, hair, and nails. In stratum granulosum keratin prevents loss of body fluids or absorption of fluid from the external environment. Without this function, the body would swell up with water when swimming. Sebum secreted by sebaceous glands lubricates skin and hair and further reduces fluid loss. The skin is actually selectively permeable—certain medications can be absorbed by the skin.
Protection of the network of blood vessels and nerves in the dermis	Collagen fiber network in the dermis supports and protects the blood vessels and nerves.
Protection from ultraviolet radiation	Melanocytes in the epidermis produce melanin which helps to protect the skin from ultraviolet (UV) light and reduces the risk of sunburn.

Table 8.1 **Protective Functions of the Skin** (continued)

FUNCTION OF SKIN	FACTORS INFLUENCING THE FUNCTION OF THE SKIN
Defense against bacteria	Sebum secreted by sebaceous glands is acidic and thus acts as an antibacterial. Normal organisms living on the skin are antibacterial. Hair keeps infectious organisms at a distance from the skin.
Control of body temperature	Production of sweat by the sweat glands stimulates evaporation from the surface of the skin, which cools the skin. Vasodilation of cutaneous blood vessels helps to disseminate heat. Increased blood flow causes heat production in the skin and loss of warmth. Hair provides insulation by trapping air.
Production of vitamin D	Vitamin D is synthesized in the skin when exposed to sunlight (UVB radiation). Vitamin D increases the absorption of Calcium (Ca) and Potassium (P) from the intestine and promotes normal bone formation. Vitamin D deficiency leads to reduced calcium absorption and reduced bone density.
Sensation for protection from external noxious stimuli	See Figure 8-2 for the various nerve endings in the skin and Table 8-3 for the types of sensory nerve endings in the dermis and epidermis of the skin and their functions.

The deep layer of the skin is called the dermis. This dermal layer is composed of layers of collagen and elastin connective tissue, which provide the characteristics of strength, pliability, and texture to the skin. The dermis contains all the sensory nerve endings including the eccrine glands (sweat glands), free nerve endings, Krause end bulbs (cold receptors), Merkel's discs, Pacinian corpuscles, and Ruffini corpuscles (see Fig. 8-2). Also contained within the dermis are the blood vessels, hair follicles, and sebaceous glands (see Table 8-3). The dermis also contains fibroblasts, which produce collagen during the wound-healing process. Mast cells and macrophages in the dermis play a role in the inflammatory process described in Chapter 1. The dermis has two distinct layers, the more superficial papillary dermis and the deeper reticular dermis.[2] The collagen rich reticular dermal layer provides strength, elasticity, and extensibility to the skin. Deep to the dermis is a layer of subcutaneous tissue, called the subcutis, or the hypodermis, consisting of fat cells, blood vessels, lymphatic vessels, connective tissue, and sensory nerve receptors. This fatty layer provides protection for the internal organs by absorbing the impact caused by trauma and insulating the body against heat loss.[3]

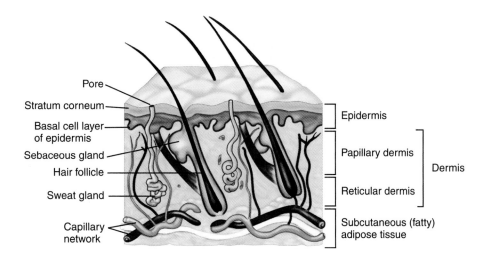

FIGURE 8.1 Cross-section of the skin.

Pore
Stratum corneum
Basal cell layer of epidermis
Sebaceous gland
Hair follicle
Sweat gland
Capillary network

Epidermis
Papillary dermis
Reticular dermis
Dermis
Subcutaneous (fatty) adipose tissue

Table 8.2 **Layers of the Epidermis of the Skin and Skin Appendages of the Epidermis With Their Characteristics**

LAYER OF SKIN	CHARACTERISTICS
Stratum basale also called the germinal layer or basement membrane	Formation of squamous epithelial cells Hair produced by this layer Contains melanocytes Contains Langerhans cells, thought to act as phagocytes and to destroy antigens Protect the deep organs from infection
Stratum spinosum	Layer of cells that lie on top of the germinal layer
Stratum granulosum	The protein keratin is deposited in this layer
Stratum lucidum	Most evident in thickened areas of skin on feet and hands
Stratum corneum	Outermost layer of dead skin cells
Hair follicles	Epithelium lining the follicle is continuous with the epidermis Plays a function in the re-epithelialization of burns unless the burn is very deep
Sebaceous glands	None on palms of hands or soles of feet Associated with the hair root Secretes sebum which lubricates skin (In burns, there may be damage to the glands and insufficient sebum produced to lubricate the skin.)
Apocrine sweat glands	Found in axilla and pubic areas Arises from the dermis
Eccrine sweat glands	Located in all body areas Concentrated in axilla, forehead, palms, and soles of feet Controlled by the hypothalamus Plays a large role in temperature regulation

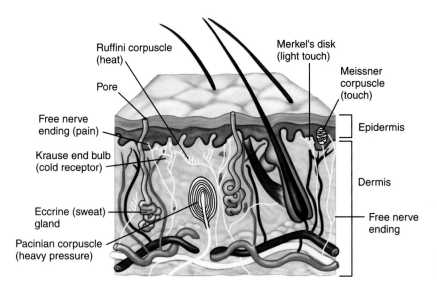

FIGURE 8.2 Various nerve endings in the skin.

Table 8.3 Types of Sensory Nerve Endings in Dermis and Epidermis of the Skin and Their Function

TYPE	FUNCTION
Free nerve endings (located in dermis and epidermis)	Pain and itching sensation; also help with discrimination in the fingers and toes
Ruffini corpuscles (found close to hair follicles in the dermis)	Pressure sensation—slow acting
Ruffini end organs	Warmth sensation
Pacinian corpuscles (deep layers of dermis)	Vibration sensation
Krause end bulb (superficial dermis)	Cold sensation
Merkel's endings	Touch sensation

Why Does the Physical Therapist Assistant Need to Know About Skin Conditions and Diseases?

The PTA needs to be familiar with some of the more common skin conditions, especially those associated with other disease processes seen in the physical therapy clinic and to be aware of some of the terms used when describing skin conditions to better understand the patient history and read the patient chart.

Physical therapy intervention for patients with severe burns is an integral part of physical therapy practice. The PTA will work with patients with burns in both inpatient and outpatient settings. Many other skin conditions are manifestations of systemic diseases, such as gout, systemic lupus erythematosus, scleroderma, Reiter's disease, rheumatoid arthritis, Kaposi's sarcoma, and syphilis. The PTA will observe many of these associated skin conditions when working with patients. Some skin conditions may be related to infectious diseases, parasitic infections, neurological diseases, carcinoma, or an allergic reaction to medications or other allergens. The skin lesions are usually characteristic of the disease process and assist the physician in diagnosis. Other skin lesions are congenital skin conditions, such as a nevus or birthmark or albinism, the latter of which is identified by a complete lack of pigmentation in the skin, eyes, and hair. A substance called melanin, produced by melanocytes in the skin, acts as a protective barrier in the skin against ultraviolet light. Melanin can be considered the body's own sunscreen. Dark skin contains more melanin that light-colored skin. People with albinism are unable to synthesize melanin and burn easily with exposure to the sun.

Skin Conditions and Diseases

HINTS ON USE OF THE GUIDE TO PHYSICAL THERAPIST PRACTICE

Burns and skin conditions fall under the *Guide to Physical Therapist Practice,* Integumentary Preferred Practice Patterns 7

- 7B "Impaired integumentary integrity associated with superficial skin involvement" (p. 601): Patients with superficial burns, cellulitis, and dermatitis are included in this pattern.
- 7C "Impaired integumentary integrity associated with partial-thickness skin involvement and scar formation" (p. 619): Patients with partial-thickness burns fit into this practice pattern.
- 7D "Impaired integumentary integrity associated with full-thickness skin involvement and scar formation" (p. 637): Patients with full-thickness burns are appropriate for this practice pattern; also included in this pattern are those with frostbite and keloid scarring formation.
- 7E "Impaired integumentary integrity associated with skin involvement extending into fascia, muscle, or bone and scar formation" (p. 655): This pattern

(Continued)

includes patients who have sustained severe electrical burns or burns that extend deeper than the skin.

PLEASE NOTE: when referencing diabetes mellitus the specific effect of the disease is what the PTA should determine before looking in the *Guide*. Where diabetes has interfered with the neuromuscular or musculoskeletal systems, those sections of the *Guide* need to be reviewed.

(From the American Physical Therapy Association, 2003. *Guide to physical therapist practice,* revised 2nd edition. Alexandria, VA: APTA. Used with permission.)

Some of the more commonly seen skin conditions in physical therapy are presented in this chapter. Skin conditions fall into several categories, including thermal injuries (heat and cold); infections; circulatory deficit skin lesions, such as arterial and venous insufficiency ulcers, and neoplasia, and congenital conditions. Healing and immune reactions are described in Chapters 1 and 2. Several of the more common types of skin lesions, which are characteristic of many skin conditions are detailed in Table 8-4. Some of these skin lesions can also be seen in Figure 8-3.

Table 8.4 **Types of Skin Lesions**

SKIN LESION	APPEARANCE
Vesicle, bulla, or blister	All names for an area of skin raised and full of fluid, including conditions such as poison ivy allergic reaction, sunburn, herpes blisters, or systemic diseases
Pustule	A localized area filled with pus such as in acne
Macule and patch	A flat area of skin of a different color, that can be of any size; can be blue, brown, purple, red, or white
Papule and nodule	Papules are areas of skin raised and up to 5 mm in diameter, and nodules are ≥5 mm diameter Warts are a kind of papule or nodule; many skin conditions fall under this classification including cysts, boils, melanoma, Kaposi's sarcoma, and the skin manifestations of systemic lupus erythematosus
Nevi/mole	Raised skin lesions that are pigmented brown, black, or red; can be classified as nodules; nevi are often large (e.g., a "birth mark")
Rash	An area of skin that erupts with any of the above lesions
Tumor	Large diameter nodule, may be benign or malignant; the skin is the major site of malignant tumors
Scales, scaly papules, and squames	Dry, scaly skin found in conditions such as dermatitis and eczema; squames are large scales.
Lichenification	Rough skin usually caused by constant rubbing
Excoriations and erosions	Damage to the skin from trauma such as a scratch; erosions are superficial areas of redness
Ulcer	A depression in the skin that penetrates to the dermis or below and results in loss of the epidermis and dermis Includes neuropathic ulcers, which are painless and found in such conditions as diabetes, polyneuropathy, syphilis, and leprosy; ischemic ulcers due to arterial disease; decubitus ulcers in immobile patients; and ulcers caused by other diseases Basal cell carcinoma may also fall under the ulcer classification
Sinus	A tunnel-like lesion that can pass from the skin into the underlying tissue or between two cavities such as between the rectum and vagina
Fissure	An opening in the skin epidermis that extends into the deep skin layers caused by fungal infections such as athlete's foot

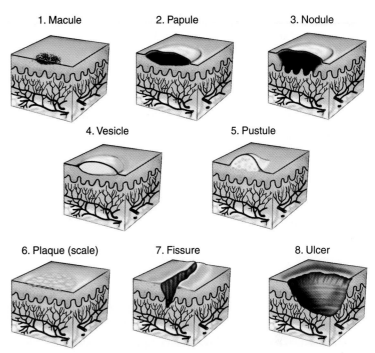

FIGURE 8.3 Appearance of various skin lesions. (1) macule: flat with a clear outline; (2) papule: small lump with a solid feel; (3) nodule: firm and elevated above the surface of the skin, extends deeply into the layers of the skin; (4) vesicle or blister: usually fluid filled with a thin covering of skin; (5) pustule: area filled with pus or exudates raised above the level of the surrounding skin; (6) plaque: scaly skin lesion; (7) fissure: a crack in tissue which may extend deeply into the dermal layer of the skin; (8). ulcer: an open cavity in tissue of varying depth.

Thermal Injuries

Thermal injuries to the skin are caused by exposure to extremes of either hot or cold temperatures. In either scenario, the damage to the body depends on the depth of injury to the skin and the underlying tissue, the length of time the skin was exposed to the damaging agent, the area covered by the damage, and the location of the problem. Burn damage to the face, genitalia, hands, and feet is considered more serious than to other areas of the body. Relatively small areas of burns in a small child or infant are potentially much more serious than in an adult as a result of the smaller surface area of the body. Burns are classified as **superficial, superficial partial-thickness, deep partial thickness, full-thickness,** and **subdermal**. Details of the various classifications of burns are included in the signs and symptoms section. The physical therapist (PT) and PTA are part of the health care team involved in the treatment of thermal injuries serious enough to require medical attention. Radiation injuries are a subset of thermal injuries. Sun exposure can produce a partial-thickness burn with blistering and scarring. Prolonged exposure to the sun causes premature aging of the skin, resulting in loss of elasticity, and a reduced ability to heal. The sun's rays are also carcinogenic and can cause tumors of the skin.

Burns

The American Burn Association estimates that more than 500,000 people each year are treated for burn injuries in the United States, and of these, approximately 4,000 die.[4] Most of the deaths are attributed to house fires, with some caused by motor vehicle or aircraft accidents, electrocution, or damage from chemicals, and hot liquids. Of the 500,000 incidents of burns, approximately 40,000 people have to be hospitalized each year.[5] The number of burns in this report does not take into consideration the many minor burns which do not require medical attention. Within the pediatric population, toddlers and infants under 4 years of age most often are at risk of burns, and this age group accounts for more than 50% of the pediatric burns seen in the United States.[6]

As already described, the skin is responsible for temperature regulation, the control of fluid loss or intake, the sensation to external stimuli, the production of vitamin D, and the secretion of lubricating oils. The skin plays a major role in the body's defense against disease. The appearance of the body must also be considered, because burns can leave scars that impact the psychological well-being of patients.

Etiology. The treatment of burn injuries has improved dramatically in since the 1990s, and special burn centers are available throughout the country. Burns can be caused by a variety of heat sources from a stove or fire, the sun, electrical shock, chemicals, or hot liquids including water and oils. Temperatures do not have to be high to cause damage to the skin. According to Sidor (2006), a water heater set at 158° Fahrenheit can produce water temperatures that can cause "full-thickness skin burns within one second."[7] The higher the temperature, the shorter the time needed to produce severe damage.

Signs and Symptoms. Burns are classified according to the depth of damage to the skin, the area of skin damaged, the length of time and type of exposure, and the area of the body affected.

An explanation of the classification of burns as superficial, superficial partial-thickness, deep partial thickness, full-thickness, and subdermal is as follows:

• **Superficial burns** (previously called first-degree burns) affect only the epidermis (see Fig. 8-4), for example, a sunburn that causes an erythema (redness) with minimal edema secondary to the inflammatory response, which resolves within a few days. This type of burn does not cause scarring of the skin.

• **Superficial partial-thickness burns** (previously called second-degree burns) destroy the epidermis and damage part of the papillary dermal layers (see Fig. 8-4).

Pressure to the affected area causes blanching (whiteness) with a fast return of pink coloration because the blood vessels remain intact. A blister forms over the burn, and pain is present due to irritation of the pain nerve endings in the dermis. The burn usually heals within 10 days by migration of epithelium from the edges of the wound and from the epithelial lining of the hair follicles. Minimal scarring occurs with the superficial partial-thickness burn, but a danger of infection is a concern.

• **Deep partial-thickness burns** (previously called third-degree burns) destroy the epidermis and damage the dermis down as far as the reticular layer (see Fig. 8-4). Because all the nerve endings except the Pacinian corpuscles are in the upper layers of dermis these as well as the blood vessels, most hair follicles and sweat glands will be damaged. Deep pressure sensation detected by the Pacinian corpuscles within the reticular layer of the dermis remains intact. These burns may be red or white looking, and when pressure is applied to the area, blanching occurs with a slow return of pink color as a result of blood vessel damage. The edema is also severe because of the leakage of blood into the tissues from the damaged blood vessels and the inability of the circulation to remove the products of inflammation as a result of the blood vessel damage. If some of the hair follicles remain intact, this

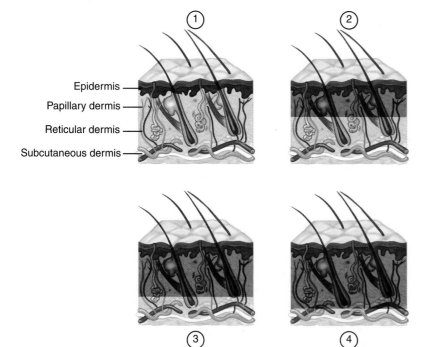

FIGURE 8.4 Depths of skin involved in various types of burn shown by shaded areas. (1) Depth of skin involved in a superficial burn. (2) Depth of skin involved in a superficial partial-thickness burn. (3) Depth of skin involved in a deep partial-thickness burn. (4) Depth of skin involved in a full-thickness burn.

Epidermis
Papillary dermis
Reticular dermis
Subcutaneous dermis

is an indication that the burn is a deep partial-thickness rather than full-thickness. These burns usually heal in 3 to 5 weeks, but the healed skin is dry and flaky as a result of the destruction of sebaceous and sweat glands.

- **Keloid** and **hypertrophic scarring** are side effects of these burns and can cause unsightly scar tissue (see Fig. 8-5). Keloid scarring is an excessive amount of healed tissue that extends beyond the parameters of the original wound. Hypertrophic scarring is a raised scar but is isolated to the area of the original wound. Both keloid and hypertrophic scarring occur as a result

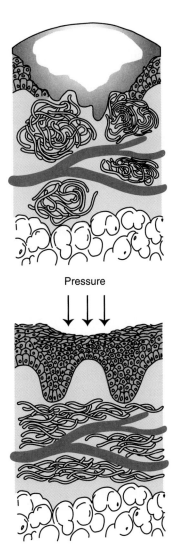

Pressure

FIGURE 8.5 Keloid or hypertrophic scarring. (Top) Collagen forms in a disorganized way in the hypertrophic or keloid scar. (Bottom) Appearance when pressure is applied to a healing wound the collagen fibers form in an organized way.

of the disorganization of collagen fibers during the healing process. The use of pressure garments during the healing process can assist in promoting reorganization of the collagen fibers to reduce the occurrence of this scarring.

- **Full-thickness burns** (previously called fourth-degree burns) destroy both epidermis and dermis and often the underlying layers of fat tissue (refer to Fig. 8-4). The main characteristic of these burns is **eschar,** which is dead tissue that looks and feels like leather with black, red, or white coloration. No sensation exists in these burns because the sensory nerves have been destroyed. Hair follicles and all the dermal glands are destroyed. Eschar must be surgically removed (**escharotomy**) otherwise the edema beneath the eschar can cause pressure damage to the deep blood vessels, restricting blood flow to the adjacent normal tissues resulting in ischemia. In addition, eschar is a breeding ground for infection and prevents the graft from adhering to the underlying tissues. Full-thickness burns do not heal without surgical graft intervention because the underlying collagen, which usually acts as the base for the development of granulation tissue, is destroyed.

- **Subdermal burns** (also previously classified as fourth-degree burns) destroy epidermis, dermis, and all underlying tissues including fat, muscle, and even bone. These burns are usually caused by a flame or electrical shock and also require surgical intervention. In many cases, an amputation of the affected limb may be required. In other instances, extensive skin grafting is needed. Such burns are often lethal, especially if the trunk is involved.

- **Electrical burns** are different from other types of burn. An electric current passes through the body following the line of least resistance, specifically the blood vessels and nerves. Damage to the body other than the place where the current entered and exited the body may not be immediately known, but the blood vessels, heart and kidneys as well as the nerves may experience extensive damage. Blood vessel damage may cause extensive ischemia to tissues resulting in gangrene. The spinal cord may also be damaged. The complete extent of damage may not be known for several days.

People with burns may have several classifications of burns simultaneously resulting from one incident. For example, small areas of full-thickness burn may be surrounded by areas of partial-thickness and superficial burns. The full-thickness burns are not painful, but the partial and superficial burns are painful. The three burn wound zones are detailed in Table 8-5.

Table 8.5   **Burn Wound Zones**

ZONE	AFFECTED TISSUE
Zone of coagulation	Cells damaged irreversibly; skin dies, eschar forms High risk of infection
Zone of stasis	Cells may die if no intervention within the first 48 hours after injury
Zone of hyperemia	Minimal cell damage and recovery in a few days

The Rule of Nines. The Rule of Nines is a further tool to classify burns according to the size and area of the body covered by the burn.[8] The Rule of Nines simply means the body is divided into nine sections of surface area that are each 9% of the total. This method of assessing burns can be useful in emergency situations to determine seriousness of the burn and the urgency of transporting the patient to hospital. An infant or small child with a head burn is much more at risk than an adult because the head is a larger proportion of the total body surface area on a child than that of the adult. In the adult, the head is 9% of the total body surface, whereas in the infant it is 17%. See Table 8-6 for Rule of Nines values in the adult, infant, and small child.

Complications. Some of the major complications of burns include the following:

• Infection: may cause death in people who otherwise seem to be recovering well
• Cardiac arrest: most often associated with electrical burns. A current of frequency between 40 and 110 Hz produces tetany (constant contraction) of skeletal muscle and falls within the range of normal household current. Such a current can cause the heart to go into asystole and may result in cardiac arrest. High-voltage injuries causing temperatures as high as 5,000° Centigrade result in severe thermal injuries and cardiac arrest. Lightning strikes may also cause asystole, central apnea (loss of blood supply to the body internal organs) and shock to the respiratory center in the brain, which can result in cardiac arrest.[9]
• Smoke inhalation: patients with burns received in building fires may also sustain smoke inhalation which causes damage to the lungs.
• Inhalation of noxious chemicals such as carbon monoxide may be toxic to the system in addition to the heat damage caused by the fire.
• Pneumonia is a common side effect of severe burns in people who require hospitalization in intensive care units. Pneumonia is particularly prevalent in people with inhalation burns and increases the risk of death. The pathogens responsible for pneumonia may be present at the time of admission or acquired in the hospital as nosocomial infections.[10]
• Hypothermia: people with burns may lose heat rapidly at temperatures normally considered comfortable. Room temperatures for patients with burns should be kept close to body temperature to prevent excessive heat loss.
• Scarring that reduces functional activity. Scar tissue can form over joint surfaces, preventing full motion of the joint as a result of the reduced extensibility of the skin. On the face, scar tissue around the mouth can prevent the mouth from fully opening and can result in difficulty with eating.

People with more serious burns require admission to a burn unit and include those patients who have inhaled fumes, or fall within any of the following categories:

• Full-thickness burns covering more than 2% to 5% of the body's total surface area

Table 8.6   **Rule of Nines Values for Adult and Infant/Small Child**

AREA OF BODY	PERCENTAGE OF BODY AREA—ADULT	PERCENTAGE OF BODY AREA—INFANT/SMALLCHILD
Head	9% (anterior 4.5%, posterior 4.5%)	17% (anterior 8.5%, posterior 8.5%)
Each upper extremity	9% (anterior 4.5%, posterior 4.5%)	9% (anterior 4.5%, posterior 4.5%)
Each lower extremity	18% (anterior 9%, posterior 9%)	13% (anterior 6.5%, posterior 6.5%)
Anterior trunk	18%	18%
Posterior trunk	18%	18%

- Burns on the face, genitalia, hands, or feet
- Partial-thickness burns covering more than 20% of the body
- Chemical or high-voltage electrical burns
- ⊛ Children, infants, and toddlers, especially those whose care providers are unable to treat the wound and those children who are suspected of being abused by intentional burning[11]
- Those at high risk of developing infections or delayed wound healing, such as people with diabetes, those who are immunocompromised, and the elderly

Wound Healing in Burns. The healing process in burns is the same as that described in Chapter 1. In partial-thickness burns, epithelium migrates across the surface of the wound and closes the area. This mechanism occurs in partial-thickness wounds as a result of the presence of epithelial tissue in the intact hair follicles. In deeper burns, the healing takes place through the process of inflammation, proliferation, and maturation, or remodeling with scar tissue formation (see Chapter 1).

Prognosis. The prognosis for people with burns depends on the amount of the body surface burned, the depth of the burn, and the physical condition of the patient. ⊛ Patients who are very young or very old are more at risk of sustaining a fatal or lethal injury. People with other disease processes such as diabetes and immunosuppressive conditions are also at greater risk of dying as a result of even a minimal injury. Since the late 1990s, the survival rate for those with extensive burns has improved. In 1996, approximately 50% of those with burns on 70% of their body surface survived.[12] In 2006, Besner and O'Connor estimated that in the under 15-year-old group, patients with 95% of their total body surface burned survived.[13] This improvement is credited to the development of more sophisticated burn management techniques, the evolution of topical antibiotics, and better immediate injury management during transit to specialized burn units.[14] Even people who survive after extensive and serious burns have scarring that affects movement and cosmetic appearance.

Medical Intervention. The treatment of the burn wound initially consists of ensuring the patient survives. Vital functions must be stabilized, fluid loss minimized, wounds cleansed and the patient transported to hospital. The main goal first is to prevent death and then to prevent infection. Wounds are **débrided** (cleaned by removing dead and nonviable tissue) and nonadherent dressings are applied to maintain the moist environment optimal for wound healing to occur. The application of antimicrobial ointments such as Silver sulfadiazine cream (Silvadene) helps to reduce the risk of infection and reduces fluid loss by the body.[15] Surgical intervention may be required to remove the thick, blackened, dead tissue called eschar. In cases in which the eschar forms all the way round the circumference of a limb, it must be removed to prevent constriction of the blood flow in the limb.[16]

Extensive and deep burns may have to be covered with a skin graft. An **autograft** uses a patient's own skin to provide wound coverage. The skin is removed from a donor site area unaffected by the burn, such as the thigh or buttocks. The donor site is often painful during healing as a result of the removal of superficial skin layers, which preserves the integrity of the pain nerve endings. A **split-thickness skin graft** involves partial-thickness removal of epidermis and some dermis using an instrument called a **dermatome**. A **full-thickness skin graft** consists of the epidermis and the dermis. Both skin graft procedures are performed under general anesthesia.[17] An **allograft** provides a graft from another human, usually a cadaver. Allografts are a good substitute for autografts but will eventually slough off when the patient's own skin has healed beneath the graft. The autograft remains in place permanently. A **xenograft** is taken from an animal. The skin of a pig is the most histologically compatible with a human. A recent development is the culture of the patient's own epithelial cells to produce a skin substitute.[18] A sheet graft is a skin graft that is processed by making meshlike cuts (fenestration) in the segment of removed skin to enable it to be stretched over a larger area. The success of a skin graft largely depends on the area grafted having sufficient blood supply and being immobilized for the first 72 hours. An adequate blood supply and sufficient immobilization does not, however, always prevent graft rejection. The process of capillaries penetrating the graft is called **inosculation.** This inosculation of the buds of the capillaries into the skin graft creating a network that attaches the graft to the area usually occurs within 48 to 72 hours after application of the graft.[19] Adequate nutrition is extremely important for individuals with burns. A high level of caloric intake is required to ensure the survival and healing for people with severe burns.

Physical Therapy Intervention. An overview of the physical therapy treatment possibilities is included here, but for further details of burn treatment, the PTA is advised to consult books specializing in burn management. PTs may perform sharp débridement with a scalpel or scissors using sterile technique to remove eschar and nonviable tissues if they have been educated in these procedures. The PTA is not encouraged to perform sharp débridement because ongoing evaluation of the wound is necessary and outside the scope of work of the PTA. Although some PTAs may be wound-care specialists the American Physical Therapy Association's (APTA) position is that PTAs should not perform selective sharp débridement. If PTAs do perform these procedures and litigation occurs, the PTA, PT, MD, and hospital could all be considered liable. The general rule is that both PTs and PTAs must practice within their scope of expertise, education, and experience, as determined by the practice act of the state in which the individual practices.

Physical therapy intervention for patients with burns is directed toward the prevention of deformity by stretching scar tissue and maintaining joint range of motion. Positioning the patient optimally to stretch the affected skin is performed by the physical and occupational therapy team.[20] The role of the PT and the PTA in wound care is also important. The PTA may provide whirlpool therapy between 98.6° and 104° Fahrenheit and pulsatile lavage during the stages of cleansing. PTAs must be aware that they cannot place the patient in a whirlpool for the first 72 hours after a graft (unless under specific instructions from the physician). Patients also must not perform excessive exercises that may produce loosening of the graft until it has had time to adhere to the graft site. Pulsatile lavage is especially useful for cleansing wounds after surgical débridement that remain heavily exudative, require more rigorous continued débridement, or for wounds that have foreign bodies implanted in them, such as battle-site wounds.[21,22] However, the importance of maintaining strict infection control procedures during the use of pulsatile lavage has been emphasized as a result of infection outbreaks in hospitals linked to the use of this equipment.[23,24,25] During the cleansing stage, the whirlpool agitation level may be quite high to promote nonspecific débridement. During the period after skin grafting, care must be taken to avoid loosening the graft. Whirlpool agitation is low and the temperature cooler to prevent damage to sensitive healing tissue. Care must be taken when changing dressings to limit the amount of bleeding. Gentle stretching of muscles, skin, and ligaments during the healing process is important. Stretching is often painful for the patient but necessary to prevent contractures. Sometimes stretching is not sufficient, and surgical release of scar tissue has to be performed. Other

factors include the prevention of muscular atrophy, cardiovascular conditioning exercises, and activities of daily living (ADL).

The creation of a sterile field and use of sterile (aseptic) technique during wound care management for people with burns is essential to reduce the risk of infection. The following is a brief overview of sterile technique:

- Set up the sterile field with all appropriate items needed for the dressing change immediately before performing the dressing change. Ensure the sterility of all equipment by checking packages are sealed and within the required shelf date. Do not turn away from the sterile field; otherwise, the field is considered contaminated. Do not leave the sterile field.
- Wash hands and don sterile gown, gloves, and mask; keep hands above the level of the sterile field in the accepted manner. Areas below the level of the waist of the person performing the aseptic technique are considered contaminated.[26]
- After completion of the dressing change remove the gown, gloves, and mask in accordance with accepted sterile procedure practice to prevent cross-contamination.

Physical therapy intervention for patients with burns is a specialized area of practice, and it is beyond the scope of this book to describe all aspects of PT intervention. If the soft tissues are splinted in an elongated position from the beginning of the intervention, the recovery for patients will be enhanced. The PT/PTA will be involved in positioning for prevention of shortening of structures in the burned area. Active exercises for stretching and strengthening are taught to patients. If patients are unconscious, passive movements must be performed to prevent contractures, and splints are provided to place the affected area on a stretch. The continual reevaluation by the PT is important, but the PTA may work with the PT to provide intervention for patients. The importance of the PT and PTA working closely together and communicating often is paramount to achieve maximal functional level. Patients with extensive burns are provided with custom-fitted pressure garments to reduce keloid or hypertrophic scarring. Patients are provided with a home exercise program, and outpatient PT may be provided for continued exercise. The PT and PTA are part of the comprehensive rehabilitation team that provides intervention for patients with burns.

PTA PRECAUTIONS FOR PATIENTS WITH BURNS

1. Use standard/universal precautions at all times when the wound is exposed to protect the patient from infection and contamination.

2. Follow the PT plan of care and physician's orders closely.

3. Check the patient's chart daily for changes in physician orders, such as alteration in topical medications used for the wound, changes in orders for PT intervention, and possible surgery performed. Notify the supervising PT of any change before commencing treatment.

4. When removing wound dressings, soak the dressing and area to make the dressing easier to remove and reduce damage to the wound to a minimum. This is not necessary if the physician's orders indicate dressing removal to assist with débridement of the wound.

5. Do not provide high agitation whirlpool to a recently grafted area; it may loosen the graft. Always check physician's orders carefully, and if a change of orders is noted, contact the supervising PT. When the physician performs any procedure on a wound, the patient must be reevaluated by the PT before the PTA can recommence treatment.

6. Be careful when changing wound dressings not to damage sensitive granulating tissue.

7. Communicate daily with the PT regarding the patient's status.

8. Provide the patient with stretching and strengthening exercises and full range of movement (ROM) of joints.

9. Ensure the patient is positioned to place the affected area on a stretch when at rest to prevent contractures. Watch for signs of vascular and neurological compromise with prolonged stretching. Report any indications of compromise to the PT and physician.

10. Provide the patient with a home exercise program and educate the family or care providers in positioning and home management techniques.

GERIATRIC CONSIDERATIONS

In an elderly patient with burns, a smaller area of burn may be more serious than in a younger adult. Elderly patients burned on comparatively small areas of the face or torso may require hospitalization to ensure sufficient hydration. Extra care has to be taken to prevent infection and other complications. If a patient lives alone, he or she may require assistance in the home for a period of time to ensure adequate nutrition and hydration for the healing process. As with any injury to an elderly person, there is the possibility of confusion particularly if dehydration and malnutrition are apparent. The burn may be related to a household accident in the kitchen or from a

fireplace, and these issues need to be addressed by a social worker before the patient returns home. A home visit may be appropriate by the PT and PTA to determine safety risks and architectural barriers and to provide solutions and recommendations to improve environmental safety.

Cold Injuries

Several conditions fall under the category of cold thermal injuries. These include immersion foot, also called "trench foot," frostbite, and hypothermia. Physical therapy intervention is not usually required in the treatment of any of these conditions, but the conditions are briefly described.

Immersion Foot or "Trench Foot"

Immersion foot received the name "trench foot" after recognition of the condition in soldiers who stood in flooded trenches during World War I. The soldiers had no means to dry their socks and boots and were at risk of severe skin compromise. The incidence of immersion foot is usually found in military personnel during war conditions and in people who participate in wilderness sports and activities.[27] Although footwear has improved significantly since World War I, soldiers in the Falklands War experienced the condition as a result of the extreme cold and damp environment.

Etiology. Immersion foot is caused by prolonged exposure of the feet to wet conditions.[28] People in the military and those who participate in outdoor extreme sports and wilderness activities are at risk for immersion foot.

Signs and Symptoms. The characteristic signs and symptoms of immersion foot include numbness, itching, pain, edema, cyanosis, and blotching of the skin. In severe cases, the condition may cause permanent dilation of the peripheral, superficial blood vessels, causing a bluish tinge to the skin resulting in necrosis of the tissues of the feet and the development of blisters and ulcers or gangrene.

Prognosis. Although some severe cases of immersion foot may result in ongoing problems with sensitivity of the feet or the need for amputation, generally the prognosis is favorable for return of full function of the feet.

Medical Intervention. The primary treatment for immersion foot is to dry the feet as soon as possible and to change socks and footwear as often as possible to avoid standing in wet shoes. In some cases, gradual warming of the feet using warm foot baths is recommended. Most intervention is focused on prevention of the condition.[29] In severe cases amputation, may be required.

Physical Therapy Intervention. None indicated unless débridement (removal of dead and necrotic tissue), wound care, or postamputation care are necessary.

Frostbite

The areas of the body most prone to frostbite are the hands, feet, and face especially the lips, nose, and ears. However, any area of the body that is exposed to subzero temperatures may be affected. A variety of people are susceptible to frostbite, including the homeless, athletes who participate in winter and high altitude sports, and people stranded in extremely cold weather without shelter.[30] Additional risk factors for developing frostbite include people with vascular compromise, such as those taking beta blocker medications; those with peripheral vascular disease, diabetes, arthritis, peripheral neuropathy, thyroid disease, infection, or Raynaud's phenomenon; and those who smoke.[31]

Etiology. Frostbite damages the skin, and sometimes underlying tissues, as a result of exposure to below freezing temperatures.

Signs and Symptoms. When exposed to cold temperatures, the superficial blood vessels dilate and are unable to adjust the blood flow to the tissues causing ischemia of the exposed areas. The tissue of the exposed area freezes and becomes pale and hard and when warmed becomes swollen, red, and painful.[32] If exposure of the skin results in necrosis of the tissues, then the tissues are black. The affected area may not recover from the insult. Sometimes gangrene occurs in the affected tissues and the person may experience spontaneous amputation of the fingers, toes, nose, or ears. Surgical amputation of necrosed tissue may be necessary. The long-term effects of frostbite may include cold sensitivity, sensory deficits, joint stiffness, and muscle atrophy.[33]

Prognosis. Frostbite is not life-threatening unless accompanied by hypothermia. Most individuals have little or no damage to the skin. In severe cases, irreversible damage may occur to the muscles, tendons, nerves, and bones requiring amputation of the limb or excision and surgical débridement of the affected area.

Medical Intervention. Slow and gradual warming of the affected area is recommended to allow the circulation to adjust to the change in temperature. Warming can be achieved by placing the body part in warm water or keeping the room temperature warm. The affected area should not be warmed if further possibility of cold exposure exists because refreezing of the tissue can increase the tissue damage.[34] Non-steroidal anti-inflammatory drugs (NSAIDs) may be recommended for reduction of the pain associated with the warming of the affected areas, and penicillin may be needed to treat infection.[35] In severe cases of frostbite, the affected part may have to be excised/débrided, or an amputation performed.

Physical Therapy Intervention. PT may be necessary depending on the extent of injury.

> NOTE: **People with Raynaud's phenomenon (refer to Chapter 3) are prone to the adverse effects of both heat and cold in the extremities. Avoid a cool therapy pool for treatment, and cold/ice packs for these individuals, because they are unable to accommodate to the cold and will have a reaction similar to that of frostbite. Any extremes of temperature will result in vascular injury in people with Raynaud's phenomenon.**

Hypothermia

Hypothermia is an emergency condition resulting from prolonged exposure to cold that causes the body to react to preserve the vital organs, shunting blood from the periphery. The body is unable to accommodate to continual exposure to cold, resulting in death. According to the Centers for Disease Control and Prevention (2006) 4,607 deaths in the United States between the years 1999 and 2002 were attributed to hypothermia.[36]

Etiology. Hypothermia is caused by exposure to the cold causing the core body temperature to drop below the level of 95° Fahrenheit. The people most at risk for hypothermia are those of advanced age or with chronic medical conditions. Others who are susceptible are individuals who abuse substances and those who are homeless.

Signs and Symptoms. The primary signs and symptoms of hypothermia include sleepiness, confusion, and numbness in the limbs. The onset of the condition is gradual and people may not realize they are becoming hypothermic.[37] Other signs may include shivering, bradypnea (very slow breathing), and slurring of the speech.[38]

Prognosis. Hypothermia is dangerous and can result in death if not treated quickly.

Medical Intervention. The medical intervention includes gradual warming of the person, placing the affected person in a warm environment when possible, avoiding massage, and removing wet or damp clothing.

Physical Therapy Intervention. PT may be necessary for any complications resulting from hypothermia.

Infectious Diseases of the Skin

Skin manifestations occur in many infectious diseases, which are beyond the scope of this book. The following section provides descriptions of some of the more common skin conditions, especially those most likely to be observed in physical therapy practice. Skin infections are caused by a variety of infectious agents including bacteria, viruses, fungi, and vector-borne pathogens, all of which are described in this section.

BACTERIAL INFECTIONS OF THE SKIN

Bacterial infections of the skin are mainly caused by *Staphylococcus* and *Streptococcus* bacteria. The bacterial skin infections described in this section include boils and carbuncles, cellulitis, and impetigo.

Boils and Carbuncles

Boils are infected individual hair follicles, and carbuncles are infected multiple hair follicles. People with chronic diseases or preexisting skin conditions, such as individuals with diabetes, a compromised immune system, acne, or dermatitis, have the greatest risk for developing boils and carbuncles.

Etiology. Boils and carbuncles both are caused by the *Staphylococcus aureus* bacteria. The bacteria, always present on the skin, enter the skin through a scratch or other break, and infect the hair follicle.

Signs and Symptoms. Boils and carbuncles start as a small lump on the skin, which becomes inflamed over a period of 1 to 2 weeks. The classic signs of inflammation such as erythema, edema, and pain are present. Both boils and carbuncles form pus and are commonly found on the neck but can be located anywhere on the body (see Fig. 8-6).

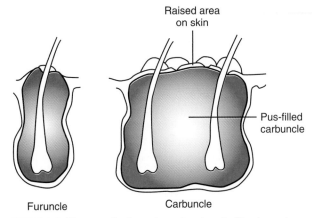

FIGURE 8.6 Diagram of a furuncle and carbuncle. The furuncle and carbuncle are caused by bacterial infection of the hair follicles. The pus-filled carbuncle is shown with several "heads."

Carbuncles also may be accompanied by systemic symptoms such as fever and fatigue. [39]

Prognosis. The prognosis is good for boils and carbuncles. Sometimes a boil, and more especially a carbuncle, may leave a scar on the skin.

Medical Intervention. Many boils and carbuncles rupture and drain after a period of about a week without any intervention. However, both boils and carbuncles may require systemic antimicrobial therapy given orally, through injection, or intravenously. Occasionally excision may be necessary.

Physical Therapy Intervention. Physical therapy intervention is not indicated for boils and carbuncles unless specific wound care is required.

Cellulitis

Cellulitis, also called erysipelas, is an infection and inflammation in the dermal and subcutaneous layers of the skin. The types of cellulitis include erysipelas, which is a superficial cellulitis, and parametritis, which affects the parametrium or tissue near the uterus. **Necrotizing fasciitis,** a severe form of infection which destroys the fascia, is also considered to be a type of cellulitis.[40] The incidence of cellulitis is higher in people with chronic diseases such as diabetes, malnutrition, ulcerated lower extremities, and individuals taking steroid medications. The incidence of cellulitis in the United States is approximately 1:1000 people per year.[41]

Etiology. Cellulitis is caused by infection with *Streptococcus pyogenes* or *Staphylococcus aureus* bacteria. Many cases of cellulitis infection are methicillin-resistant. Refer to Chapter 2 for further information regarding medication-resistant infections.

Signs and Symptoms. The characteristic signs and symptoms of the condition include a skin erythema, edema, extreme tenderness to palpation, and the presence of skin nodules. Cellulitis is seen more often in the foot and lower leg (see Fig. 8-7).

Prognosis. Cellulitis usually resolves with oral or intravenous antimicrobial medications. The more severe necrotizing fasciitis usually requires hospitalization and can be fatal if not treated.[42]

Medical Intervention. The medical intervention for cellulitis ranges between the use of antimicrobial medications for the majority of patients[43] and surgery for complicated cases.[44] Necrotizing fasciitis may require large areas of skin and underlying tissue to be excised to prevent the spread of the infection.

Physical Therapy Intervention. Cellulitis is not treated by the PT or PTA; however, it is fairly common to observe cellulitis in the physical therapy clinic. PTAs should refer the patient to the supervising PT and to the physician if they suspect the patient has developed the condition.

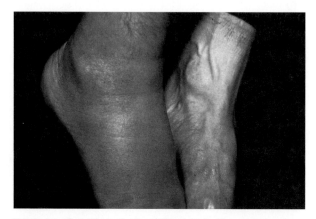

FIGURE 8.7 Cellulitis in the foot. (Reprinted with permission from Goldsmith, Lowell A., Lazarus, Gerald S., and Tharp, Michael D. *Adult and Pediatric Dermatology: A Color Guide to Diagnosis and Treatment*, 1st edition, p. 82, Philadelphia: F. A. Davis, 1997.)

Impetigo

⊛ Impetigo is a common skin infection mainly found in young children and elderly people but can occur in any person. The incidence of impetigo is prevalent in the presence of malnutrition and poor living conditions and occurs more during warmer weather.[45]

Etiology. Impetigo is an infection of the superficial layers of the skin caused by either *Staphylococcal aureus*, or *streptococcal* group A bacteria (not the same ones that cause strep throat).[46] The bacteria colonize open areas of the skin, such as cuts and insect bites. Impetigo is contagious and is spread by close contact, in schools and overcrowded housing, with either the infected pus in the sores, or through contact with the nasal secretions of the infected person.[47]

Signs and Symptoms. The signs and symptoms of impetigo are small, pus-filled pimples, surrounded by an erythema, that form on the face, arms, or legs.[48] The pustules usually cause itching. ⊛ Children spread the bacterial infection with the hands to other parts of the body, and to other people, by scratching the small pustules.

Prognosis. Impetigo is curable with antimicrobial medications.

Medical Intervention. The diagnosis of impetigo is achieved through observation of the typical skin pustules and cultures of the infected material. Antimicrobial medications are prescribed orally or in ointment form. One recently approved ointment by the Food and Drug Administration found to be effective for the treatment of impetigo is retapamulin (Altabax), which has to be used twice daily for 5 days.[49,50] A vaccine against group A *Streptococcus* is currently undergoing trials through the National Institutes of Health (NIH) and if successful will prevent impetigo, strep throat, and many other diseases caused by the streptococcal bacteria.[51]

Physical Therapy Intervention. Physical therapy intervention is not indicated for the treatment of impetigo. However, frequent hand washing and the use of protective gloves will reduce the risk of transmission of the infection if working with patients with impetigo.

FUNGAL INFECTIONS OF THE SKIN

Fungal infections of the skin are caused by infection with a variety of fungi. Two such fungal infections are described in this section, including candidiasis and tinea.

These two fungal infections are the most likely to be seen in physical therapy practice.

Candidiasis

Candida albicans is the most common of the group of fungi that cause infections known as candidiasis, candidosis, or moniliasis. ⊛ The condition affects the mucosal areas of the mouth and genital areas and areas of skin and is found mainly in children and older people. However, genital candidiasis is particularly prevalent in immune-suppressed individuals and people with diabetes.[52] *Candida albicans* affects both males and females equally.

Etiology. *Candida albicans* is a fungus normally found in the intestines. The fungus usually does not cause problems in healthy individuals. If individuals become immunologically challenged as a result of a disease process, the fungus may start colonizing areas in the mouth, genital areas, or on the skin or nails. Specific names for areas infected by *C. albicans* include oral candidiasis (oral thrush), vulvovaginal candidiasis (of the female genitalia), chronic paronychia of the nail fold, and onychomycosis of the nail plate.[53] ⊛ People at higher risk of candida infections include children and older adults; people with HIV/AIDS; people with endocrine disorders, such as diabetes mellitus; those with general debility as a result of cancer, malnutrition, or chronic disease; people taking broad-spectrum antimicrobial medications for other infectious disease processes; those with preexisting skin conditions, such as psoriasis; and people who wear nylon incontinence protection or synthetic or plastic underwear that predisposes a warm, moist environment conducive to the growth of the fungus.[54]

Signs and Symptoms. Candida infection causes lesions to break out on the mucosa of the mouth and genitalia, causing itching and discomfort, with an associated whitish discharge. When candida is produced in excess within the intestinal system the effects may include diarrhea and/or constipation, flatulence, and bloating. The infection can cause damage to the intestinal wall allowing toxins to pass into the blood and subsequently causing systemic symptoms such as muscle aches, migraine headaches, and food allergies.[55] Other signs and symptoms of systemic infection with candida include changes to the endocrine system, which may cause cystitis (inflammation of the bladder), joint pains, allergic reactions such as asthma or hayfever, and irregularities in menstruation.[56]

Prognosis. *C. albicans* infections usually resolve with the use of either topical or systemic antifungal medications. However, people with HIV/AIDS may have chronic problems with the infection because of the compromised immune system.

Medical Intervention. The diagnosis of *C. albicans* infections may be performed visually by the physician according to the signs and symptoms or may require a swab of the infected area and a culture in the laboratory for confirmation of the diagnosis.

Physical Therapy Intervention. Physical therapy intervention is not indicated for candida; however, PTAs need to be conscious of these fungal infections and use Standard Precautions if any skin lesions are present to prevent the further spread of infection.

Tinea

⊛ Tinea, also called ringworm, is a common fungal skin condition found in children and adults. The fungus thrives in damp places such as shower floors and swimming pool surrounds.

Etiology. Tinea or ringworm is caused by a fungal or dermatophyte infection. ⊛ Tinea is especially common in children over age 5 years. The infection is spread by direct contact with an infected person or through contaminated moist surfaces such as showers and swimming pools, and may also be spread by pets.[57] A study by Szepietowski et al. (2006) found that people with tinea often had a chronic toenail infection called onychomycosis.[58]

Signs and Symptoms. Tinea is a common infection that can affect the foot as tinea pedis (athlete's foot), the nails as tinea corporis, the groin as tinea cruris (jock itch), the scalp as tinea capitis, and the face as tinea faciei. Another term used for the infection is ringworm, although the condition has nothing to do with a "worm." The skin reaction caused by tinea is red, itchy, and may cause a burning sensation. In the feet, the infection tends to occur between the toes where the skin is moist and causes cracking of the skin.

Prognosis. Tinea can be cured with appropriate antifungal medications but has a tendency to recur. Some individuals seem to have a genetic tendency to be affected by the fungus.[59]

Medical Intervention. Antifungal medications in the form of sprays and ointments may be purchased with or without prescription. Some tinea infections may require the stronger topical agents (ointments and lotions) available by prescription or an oral antifungal medication.[60] Topical antifungal agents include clotrimazole, miconazole, and econazole. Oral antifungals include terbinafine, itraconazole, griseofulvin, and fluconazole.[61]

Physical Therapy Intervention. Physical therapy intervention is not indicated for the treatment of tinea. PTs and PTAs should wash the hands frequently and use protective gloves as part of the Standard Precautions when working with patients who may have tinea to prevent the spread of infection.

VIRAL INFECTIONS OF THE SKIN
Viral infections of the skin are caused by a variety of viruses. The most commonly seen viral skin infections seen in physical therapy are herpes simplex, herpes zoster, and warts or verrucae, all of which are described in this section.

Herpes simplex

Incidence of the herpes simplex virus is demonstrated by the existence of the herpes infection in 85% of the U.S. population as a result of childhood infection. Estimates of the prevalence of Type 2 herpes simplex indicate that approximately one in five people in the United States are infected with the virus.[62]

Etiology. Herpes simplex (cold sores) is caused by the herpes virus that causes type 1 (HSV-1) and type 2 (HSV-2) infections. The virus can be spread by contact with open sores. Type 2 herpes simplex is a sexually transmitted disease (STD) that can be spread via contact even when there are no apparent visible lesions.[63] Herpes simplex can be transmitted from a mother to her child during vaginal delivery. Outbreaks of herpes simplex Types 1 and 2 are prevalent in individuals who are immunosuppressed, especially those with HIV/AIDS.

Signs and Symptoms. The characteristics of Type 1 herpes simplex include a rash of small vesicles round the mouth, on the lips, or inside the mouth on the gums, which usually burns and stings. ⊛ The initial infection usually occurs in childhood and may be accompanied by fever or upper respiratory infections. Reoccurrences of the problem can arise at any age after excessive exposure to the sun, another type of viral infection, trauma to the face,

or fever. The characteristics of Type 2 herpes simplex, otherwise known as genital herpes or herpes genitalis, include crusting lesions on the genitalia of both males and females. [64] Both types of herpes manifestations resolve within a couple of weeks.

Prognosis. Type 1 herpes usually resolves on its own and is not usually treated with any specific drugs. Type 2 herpes is spread by sexual contact and may be spread to a partner even when the lesions are not present. Type 2 herpes is a chronic problem that is not curable, but it can be controlled with medications.

Medical Intervention. Pharmacological intervention for genital herpes involves systemic antiviral drugs such as acyclovir, valacyclovir, or famciclovir. In some cases, these medications may also be prescribed for severe outbreaks of oral herpes.[65]

Physical Therapy Intervention. No physical therapy intervention is indicated for herpes simplex; however, the PTA should use Standard (Universal) Precautions when working with individuals with any dermatological manifestation to prevent the potential spread of infection.

Herpes Zoster

Herpes zoster is a viral infectious disease commonly known as "shingles" from the Latin *cingulus* meaning a girdle. The virus can be spread via the rash of "shingles" and may cause an outbreak of chicken pox in people who have never been exposed to the herpes zoster virus. Incidence of the disease is usually in the population of people over 55 to 60 years of age. Herpes zoster is more common in people who are immunosuppressed, such as those with Hodgkin's disease, cancer, HIV/AIDS; those undergoing chemotherapy or radiation treatment; or those who have received an organ transplant. Between 500,000 and 1,000,000 cases of herpes zoster are recorded every year in the United States.[66,67] The disease is 3 times more prevalent in the white population than the black population.[68]

Etiology. Herpes zoster is caused by the varicella zoster virus (VZV), which also causes chicken pox. The name is derived from the skin rash of blister-like vesicles that occurs along the area of the dermatome (area of skin) supplied by the nerve root affected by the virus (refer to Chapter 7 for more information on dermatomes). The virus is stored in the posterior root ganglion of the spinal nerves after initial infection with the virus.[69] In times of emotional or physical stress such as chronic illness, the virus becomes reactivated and causes pain and a rash along the dermatome of the involved nerve root.[70]

Signs and Symptoms. The characteristic signs and symptoms of herpes zoster include intense, burning pain, hypersensitivity of the skin, and a blister-like rash (vesicles), which occur along the path of the spinal or cranial nerve involved.[71] Rashes may occur on the face, neck, thoracic spine, trunk, and occasionally in the genital area (see Fig. 8-8). Severe pain may be the first sign of a herpes zoster infection, preceding the rash by several days, and patients often seek medical advice at the onset of pain. Other signs and symptoms of herpes zoster may include headaches, malaise, lymph node swelling, joint and abdominal pain, and fever.[72] The symptoms of herpes zoster usually last approximately a month. One of the long-term side effects of herpes zoster is postherpetic neuralgia (severe nerve pain) in the area affected by the herpes zoster. Approximately 50% of people over age 60 who develop herpes zoster will also develop postherpetic neuralgia, which may continue for months or years.[73] Other complications that occasionally arise include bladder and bowel dysfunction after sacral nerve involvement. When the facial nerve is affected the condition is termed Ramsay Hunt syndrome, in which there is facial muscle paralysis, loss of hearing, and loss of taste.[74] When the herpes zoster rash becomes infected, cellulitis may occur. People do not usually have more than one episode of shingles, but sometimes an episode may occur at a different spinal nerve root level.

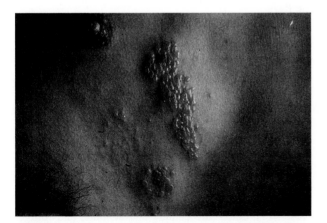

FIGURE 8.8 Herpes zoster on the anterolateral trunk showing the typical vesicles. (Reprinted with permission from Goldsmith, Lowell A., Lazarus, Gerald S., and Tharp, Michael D. *Adult and Pediatric Dermatology: A Color Guide to Diagnosis and Treatment*, 1st edition, p. 307, Philadelphia: F. A. Davis, 1997.)

Prognosis. Usually, herpes zoster is not life threatening, but the complications such as postherpetic neuralgia, Ramsay Hunt syndrome, and bladder and bowel dysfunction can be debilitating for the patient. Patients with compromised immune systems are more at risk for serious side effects of the infection.

Medical Intervention. The diagnosis of herpes zoster is through observation of the vesicle rash along a nerve root level dermatome, review of other signs and symptoms, and taking a patient history. After the skin rash appears, the diagnosis is easier to make. In some cases, confirmation of the diagnosis may be performed through a complete blood count (CBC) to reveal a raised white cell count, an immunoglobulin test to show whether there is an increased varicella antibody level, and a culture of the skin lesions for the presence of the varicella virus.[75,76] The medical treatment for herpes zoster may be to allow the virus to run its course. Antiviral medications such as acyclovir, valacyclovir, and famciclovir may be effective in reducing the incidence of postherpetic neuralgia, when started as soon as the rash appears.[77] The use of steroids and analgesic medications such as NSAIDS or narcotic analgesics help to reduce the pain and topical anti-itch lotions can alleviate the intense itching caused by the rash.[78] When postherpetic neuralgia occurs, the medications prescribed may include tricyclic antidepressants such as amitriptyline (Elavil), antiseizure medications, and lidocaine skin patches.[79] Varicella vaccinations are available for children to prevent infection with the varicella virus that causes chicken pox.[80] In 2006, a vaccine was made available for adults called Zostavax, which reduces the risk of contracting shingles by approximately 60%.[81] The vaccine does not prevent people from contracting the herpes zoster virus, but it boosts the immune system for those who already have some immunity to the disease.[82]

"It Happened in the Clinic"

A female patient in her mid-60s was referred to PT for severe pain in her thoracic spine radiating into her ribs on the right side. The physician suspected a pulled muscle. On evaluation, the PT was unable to determine the specific muscle problem and the history related by the patient was inconclusive. She had been doing some gardening during the previous 2 days, but this was not unusual for her lifestyle. PT intervention was started with hot moist packs to the affected area and gentle exercises. The report to the

(Continued)

physician related the inconclusive nature of the evaluation findings. On return to the PT department 2 days later, the patient was noted to have a red rash extending from the spine and along the space between the sixth and seventh ribs on the right side. The PT immediately called the physician, and the patient was seen again and the diagnosis made of herpes zoster (shingles). The PT was discontinued because efficacy was not determined, and the heat tended to increase rather than decrease the pain. This occurrence is not unusual because the pain of herpes zoster precedes the rash in most cases.

Physical Therapy Intervention. The pain associated with an acute episode of herpes zoster usually is not treated by physical therapy. The PT/PTA may see some of these patients for pain management prior to the skin rash appearing. After the rash or "shingles" appear, the patient must be referred back to the physician for definitive diagnosis. Physical therapy may be indicated for patients with postherpetic neuralgia. The use of chronic pain treatment methods can help to alleviate the severe pain of this side effect of herpes zoster. The PTA should use the appropriate Standard (Universal) Precautions when working with patients with herpes zoster to prevent the spread of infection.

Wart and Verruca

Warts, also called verrucae (plural of verruca), are common skin lesions. Warts are frequently found on the hands as verruca vulgaris but also may occur on the face and forehead as flat warts, on the plantar surface of the feet as verruca plantaris (plantar warts), on the nails of the hands and feet as subungual and periungual warts, and on the genital areas as condyloma acuminatum (genital or venereal warts). Condyloma acuminatum is the most common sexually transmitted disease in the United States.[83] The disease affects between 500,000 people with 1 million new cases in the United States every year. Approximately 10% to 15% of the U.S. population is infected with the human papilloma virus (HPV).[84]

Etiology. Warts/verrucae are caused by more than 120 identified human papilloma viruses (HPVs), 40 of which can cause genital warts.[85] Warts are contagious, so they can be passed from one person to another through direct contact. Condyloma acuminatum tends to be more readily contagious than other types of warts and is transmitted from person to person via sexual contact.[86] The incubation period from contact with the condyloma acuminatum to development of the wart in a person is thought to be approximately 3 months.[87]

Signs and Symptoms. Most commonly occurring warts on the hands occur either singly or in small groups. The appearance of most warts is a round, raised skin lesion that can be light colored, dark brown, or pink. Warts are usually painless, but plantar warts can become painful as a result of pressure exerted on them from walking.[88]

Prognosis. Warts are an irritation that can become painful. Genital warts are a common sexually transmitted disease. Complications from warts include scarring of the skin where a wart is removed, and occasionally keloid scarring.[89] The complications of genital warts include the development of cervical or vulvar cancer in females.

Medical Intervention. Over-the-counter medications are available to remove unsightly warts. Removal of warts by a physician may be achieved with the use of cryotherapy (freezing), electrocautery (burning off the wart), or with a laser. The newly developed Gardasil vaccine can protect young women against both cervical cancer and genital warts.[90]

Physical Therapy Intervention. The PTA should follow Standard (Universal) Precautions when working with patients exhibiting warts on areas of the body to be treated. The use of gloves helps to prevent the spread of the infection to other areas of the patient's body or to the PTA.

VECTOR-BORNE (INSECT BORNE) SKIN INFECTIONS

The two vector-borne skin infections described in this section are transmitted by insects and arachnoids and include scabies and pediculosis. These skin infections are more commonly seen in pediatric physical therapy practice settings and in group residences.

Scabies

Scabies outbreaks are fairly common in places where people are in groups such as nursing homes, hospitals, and other chronic health care settings, prisons, preschools, child-care centers and schools, and refugee camps. Poor sanitary conditions contribute to outbreaks of scabies.[91] The skin disease is also common in overcrowded conditions, especially in underdeveloped areas of the world.[92,93]

Etiology. Scabies is a highly contagious skin infection caused by the scabies mite *Sarcoptes scabiei* (a member of the spider family with eight legs), sometimes called the "itch mite." The mite is only about a third of a millimeter in size and cannot be seen without using a magnifying glass.[94] The spread of the mite that causes the skin disease can occur before the rash appears on the skin because the incubation period for the larvae to emerge from the egg is 4 to 6 weeks.[95] The parasite is transmitted through close and prolonged contact with an infected person. The sharing of clothing, bedding, and towels can increase the likelihood of infection.[96]

Signs and Symptoms. The scabies mite burrows into the epidermis of the skin and lays its eggs. After 4 to 6 weeks, the larvae hatch, rise to the surface of the skin, and then burrow into it. The larvae form tracks in the skin that may appear as dark lines. The combination of burrowing of the larvae and the deposit of feces within the skin causes inflammation, itching, and **pruritus** (a rash). The mites tend to concentrate where it is warm and moist, such as at the elbow creases, in the web spaces of the fingers, at the wrists, under the breasts, in the groin, and at the waistline. The mites are spread by contact. If the patient scratches the affected skin, the mites and their larvae can be spread to other areas of the body.

Prognosis. Scabies is not usually life threatening but in some cases can lead to glomerulonephritis (kidney disease).[97]

Medical Intervention. Treatment of scabies is through the use of a topical lotion such as 1% lindane, or a systemic medication such as ivermectin.[98,99] A topical lotion such as Elimite containing permethrin may also be used. The lotions have to be applied to the whole body and left on for several hours before washing them off. Antihistamines may also be prescribed to reduce the intensity of the itching caused by the scabies.[100]

Physical Therapy Intervention. PTs and PTAs may contract scabies if a person they are treating has an infestation. Gloves should be worn and regular hand-washing practiced to prevent the spread of the scabies.

Pediculosis (Lice)

Pediculosis is a common insect-borne infection affecting between 6 and 12 million people every year in the United States, particularly children between 5 and 11 years of age.[101] The condition occurs worldwide and is common in child-care settings and schools, where close contact between children allows the lice to travel from one child to another.

Etiology. Pediculosis is caused by contact and subsequent infestation with lice.

Signs and Symptoms. Lice infestations, otherwise called pediculosis, can occur as body lice (pediculus humanus corporis), head lice (pediculus humanus capitis), or pubic lice (pediculus pubis). Pediculus pubis is a sexually transmitted condition. The head louse (singular for lice) is the most common in the United States and may infect the eyelashes as well as the hair of the scalp. These insect parasites feed on blood and are specific to humans. The female head louse lays eggs called nits on the hair, and the lice that emerge after 6 to 10 days feed by sucking blood from the scalp (see Fig. 8-9).[102] Close contact, especially among family members or between children in a day-care or school situation, can spread the infestation. Lice particularly like clean hair because they can attach their eggs to it more easily. The body louse often clings and lays its eggs in the seams of clothing.

Prognosis. Lice can be controlled and eliminated, but there is a tendency for recurrence especially in schools and child-care centers. Lice can spread infectious diseases such as typhus, trench fever, and relapsing fever in areas of the world where these diseases are prevalent.[103]

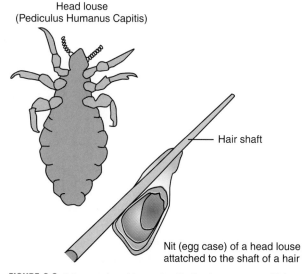

FIGURE 8.9 A human head louse (pediculus humanus capitis) and a nit (egg case) attached to a hair shaft.

Medical Intervention. Some of the medications used to treat pediculosis include lindane (Kwell) shampoos, permethrin-based solutions (Elimite, Nix), pyrethrin shampoos (RID shampoo), malathion lotions (Ovide), and oral medications such as Ivermectin.[104] Many head lice are becoming resistant to permethrin, so the lotions with malathion content such as Ovide are now more effective.[105,106] A fine-tooth comb is also used to remove any eggs from the hair. Any clothing or bed linens must be washed in very hot water and dried at high temperatures to prevent reinfestation. Combs and hairbrushes should be either thrown away or disinfected at high temperatures.

Physical Therapy Intervention. The PTA should wear rubber gloves and wash hands regularly when treating a patient with suspected or diagnosed lice. PTAs will see cases of lice infestation in the clinical setting and may need to undergo treatment, particularly if working in acute care settings or school-based practice.

OTHER SKIN CONDITIONS

This section presents other skin conditions that may be seen by the physical therapist and physical therapist assistant but do not fit within the categories previously mentioned. These skin conditions include acne vulgaris, eczema, and psoriasis.

Acne vulgaris

Acne vulgaris is a chronic condition of the skin involving the sebaceous glands. The onset of acne vulgaris is usually associated with puberty and may last into early adulthood. Between 60% and 70% of people in the United States are affected by acne at some point in their lives.[107]

Etiology. The factors that cause an individual to develop acne may include profuse sweating, heredity, poor general health, and changing hormone levels such as increased testosterone and androgen levels. Pathologically, the sebaceous glands produce excessive sebum and keratin, which block the hair follicles. The blocked hair follicles become a breeding ground for bacteria.

Signs and Symptoms. The characteristic signs and symptoms of acne include comedones consisting of either blackheads or white heads. The blocked follicles and sebaceous ducts may become infected, causing pustules. In severe cases, cysts form, resulting in scarring once these areas heal.[108] In some cases, the whole area of skin affected may be inflamed, with red or purple discoloration.

The affected areas are mainly the head, upper back, and upper chest with males affected more than females.

Prognosis. No actual cure exists for acne, but lotions, creams, laser, light therapy, and the use of antibiotic medications can reduce the severity of the condition.

Medical Intervention. People with moderate or severe acne usually need to consult a physician or dermatologist. The pharmacological intervention for acne includes the use of topical ointments to reduce infection, and solutions that prevent keratin from plugging the sebaceous ducts and hair follicles can be helpful. More recent innovations include the use of laser therapy and light therapy.[109]

Physical Therapy Intervention. When treating patients with acne, gloves should be worn to prevent the spread of infection for the patient, and hand washing should be performed diligently. If performing massage, the pustules may burst, resulting in the possibility of spreading the problem for the patient by infecting adjoining hair follicles and sebaceous ducts.

Eczema, Dermatitis, and Urticaria

The terms eczema, dermatitis, and urticaria are largely interchangeable. Eczema is a generic term applied to chronic noninfectious skin lesions of atopic dermatitis that include papules and vesicles with inflammation, pruritus, and lichenification (leathery looking areas). Scratching of the lesions causes further inflammation. One form of eczema, latex allergy, is common in health care and dental workers.[110] Atopic dermatitis occurs in as many as 10% of children worldwide.[111] The condition occurs more in children than adults and has a high association with allergic rhinitis and asthma.[112]

Etiology. Eczema can be caused by contact with allergens such as soaps, detergents, latex gloves, animal fur, clothing, cosmetics, dust, metals in jewelry, foods, and drugs, or may be of an unknown cause.[113,114] Seborrheic dermatitis on the face, scalp, ears, and chest (see Fig. 8-10) is a chronic condition of the sebaceous glands that causes scaling of the skin and the production of dandruff.[115] **Contact dermatitis** or urticaria is commonly called hives and is usually the result of irritation by an external source such as wool, poison ivy, adhesive tape, and latex or internally as a result of a drug or food allergy, causing a Type 1 hypersensitivity reaction. Contact dermatitis is a

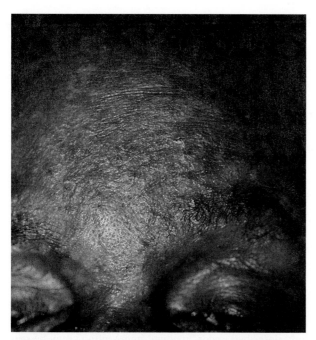

FIGURE 8.10 Seborrheic dermatitis of the forehead and eyebrows. (Reprinted with permission from Goldsmith, Lowell A., Lazarus, Gerald S., and Tharp, Michael D. *Adult and Pediatric Dermatology: A Color Guide to Diagnosis and Treatment*, 1st edition, p. 260, Philadelphia: F. A. Davis, 1997.)

common condition found on the dorsal surfaces of the hands in health care providers resulting from repeated hand washing with harsh chemicals and wearing latex gloves. Atopic dermatitis is also linked to a hereditary defect in the epidermis of the skin.[116]

Signs and Symptoms. The general signs and symptoms of eczema are erythema, edema, skin papules, and sensations of itching, stinging, and burning. If the eczema results from an allergic response, the symptoms usually start within 24 to 72 hours after contact with the offending allergen.[117] The characteristic signs and symptoms of atopic dermatitis include inflammation of the skin, which causes redness, and local irritation. In many cases, the skin can develop open areas that crack, crust, and can bleed.[118] The most common areas of skin eruptions in children are the posterior aspect of the knees, anterior aspect of the elbows, wrists, hands, ankles, and neck.[119,120] Cases of atopic dermatitis may be aggravated by the use of scented soaps or alcohol-based lotions.

Prognosis. Eczema caused by allergic reactions usually clears up with the use of topical (ointments) or systemic antihistamine medications. Atopic dermatitis may be

persistent but is often helped by keeping the skin clean and dry, and using moisturizing lotions.

Medical Intervention. The diagnosis of eczema is determined from the patient history, but in some cases, an allergic patch test may be performed to isolate the causative irritant. In cases precipitated by allergic reactions, an antihistamine is provided. In nonallergic cases, a topical (skin) ointment may be prescribed by the physician. Some topical applications may, however, actually cause the described reactions.[121] Some people with eczema are treated with a combination of oral psoralen and ultraviolet light (PUVA).[122] Advice to the patient includes the avoidance of harsh detergents on the skin and prolonged soaking in water. Mild soaps without alcohol content should be used and topical ointments and lotions to keep the skin in good condition.[123] In the case of latex allergy, avoidance of latex products is important. Occasionally ultraviolet light is used in severe cases to resolve the skin erosions.

Physical Therapy Intervention. The PTA must take care that the skin is not irritated when treating patients with lotions for ultrasound transmission, and electrode gels. Use of compression devices and splints can also cause dermatitis, and patients should be instructed to rinse off soaps from the skin carefully before applying and after removing splints. Care should also be taken to make sure the patient is not in contact with latex products to avoid latex allergy eczema. Some physical therapists perform ultraviolet light interventions for the treatment of severe and persistent atopic dermatitis.

Psoriasis

Psoriasis is a chronic, hereditary skin disease. Psoriasis is not infectious or contagious. Psoriasis affects approximately 7.5 million people in the United States and 125 million people worldwide.[124] The incidence of psoriasis in the United States is between 2% and 2.6% of the population, with 150,000 to 260,000 new cases diagnosed each year.[125] In other parts of the world, such as the United Kingdom, approximately 1% to 2% of the population are affected.[126] Females are slightly more affected, mainly between the ages of 15 and 30, and it is more prevalent in the Caucasian population.[127] As described in Chapter 6, psoriasis may be associated with psoriatic arthritis.

Etiology. Once thought to be a skin disorder, psoriasis is now considered to be autoimmune in nature.[128] Scientists have identified DNA markers that are linked to the susceptibility of developing psoriasis.[129,130] Pathologically, the skin cells in psoriatic lesions only live approximately 4 days as opposed to the normal 28 days, resulting in a rapid exfoliation of skin cells from the surface of the body. Smoking has been identified as a risk factor for the development of psoriasis.[131,132]

Signs and Symptoms. The signs and symptoms of psoriasis include patches of red scaly skin with silver areas on the elbows, knees, sacrum, and at the base of the skull in the hairline (see Fig. 8-11), although psoriasis can affect any area of the body. The nails of the feet and hands may be pitted and thickened. The symptoms of psoriasis can be exacerbated by the presence of infections or increased levels of stress.[133]

Prognosis. Psoriasis is not a life-threatening disease. However, a recent study by Gelfand et al. (2007) in the United Kingdom indicated that people with severe forms of psoriasis may have a slight reduction in life expectancy of between 3 and 4 years.[134]

Medical Intervention. Medical interventions include several over-the-counter methods, including phototherapy such as ultraviolet light, salicylic acid lotions, coal tar ointments (Doctar, Theraplex T), mild hydrocortisone

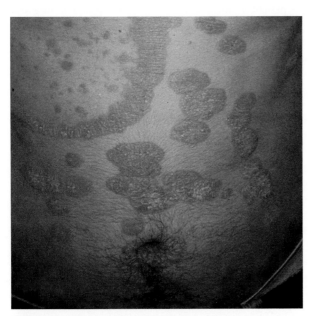

FIGURE 8.11 Typical bright red scaly plaque of psoriasis. (Reprinted with permission from Goldsmith, Lowell A., Lazarus, Gerald S., and Tharp, Michael D. *Adult and Pediatric Dermatology: A Color Guide to Diagnosis and Treatment*, 1st edition, p. 285, Philadelphia: F. A. Davis, 1997.)

creams, and NSAIDs. Some of the prescription medications for psoriasis include synthetic vitamin D creams (Dovonex), vitamin A derivatives (Tazorac), and stronger steroidal ointments (Aristocort, Kenalog, and betamethasone creams).[135] Topical retinoid medications such as Tazorac reduce the rate of skin cell production, and keratolytic agents such as anthralin smooth the skin by removing scales. Psoralen plus UV-A light (PUVA) is also used to treat psoriasis.[136]

Research opinions vary about the effectiveness of the use of orally administered PUVA in the management of psoriasis. Some studies have not demonstrated any significant benefits of the treatment,[137,138] whereas others show that ultraviolet therapy can be beneficial, and perhaps even more effective when combined with saline baths.[139-140] People with psoriasis often do not wish to expose their skin to the sun because they are embarrassed by the appearance of the skin.

Physical Therapy Intervention. The use of ultraviolet light described under "medical intervention" may be performed by the physical therapist. This modality is not available in many clinics, however. Guidelines for the recommended dosage should be followed carefully to avoid overexposure, which could lead to burns and skin cancer. Some patients may choose to use tanning beds for control of psoriasis. The use of tanning beds should be regulated by the physician or PT to prevent overexposure to the ultraviolet light.

Neoplasms of the Skin

Neoplasms of the skin are malignant tumors or cancerous areas of tissue. Numerous types of skin neoplasia exist, but the ones described in this section include basal cell carcinoma, squamous cell carcinoma, malignant melanoma, and Kaposi's sarcoma. These types of skin neoplasia are the most commonly seen in physical therapy practice.

Basal Cell Carcinoma. Basal cell carcinoma is the most common form of skin cancer in the United States. More than 900,000 people are diagnosed with basal cell carcinoma each year, with twice as many occurrences in men than women.[141] The cancer is a malignant, slow-growing skin tumor, and rarely metastasizes.[142]

Etiology. Basal cell carcinomas originate in the epidermis of the skin and outer sheath of the hair follicle.[143] The actual etiology of the tumors is not known. The most common sites are on areas of skin most exposed to sunlight or other types of ultraviolet light. The use of tanning beds has increased the incidence of this skin cancer in the younger population. These tumors are more predominant in fair-skinned, blue- or green-eyed people; those who have received overexposure to x-ray therapy; and those who are immunosuppressed.[144]

Signs and Symptoms. The areas of skin usually exposed to ultraviolet light are most at risk for basal cell carcinoma such as the face, chest, and hands (see Figure 8-12).The skin tumors are usually painless and may be almost any color. Pigmented areas of skin that have a sunken area in the middle, bleed easily, do not fully heal, or have unusual blood vessels around them may indicate a basal cell carcinoma.[145] Some basal cell carcinomas are nodular with a distinct lumpy appearance.

Prognosis. The basal cell carcinomas rarely metastasize but may grow quite large if left untreated. When the tumors are near the eyes, growth of the tumor into the surrounding tissue is more of a concern. Treated areas of basal cell carcinoma may return after removal in approximately 10% of cases. Basal cell carcinomas do not appear to affect life expectancy unless metastasis occurs.

Medical Intervention. The basal cell carcinomas are diagnosed through a skin biopsy. Surgical removal of the tumor may be performed with simple excision of the area, electrodessication with an electric current that dries out the tissue and kills the cells, cryosurgery that freezes the tissue, or Mohs micrographic surgery in which tissue is removed and observed under a microscope to ensure removal of all the cancerous tissue.[146] In some cases, an antineoplastic agent (anticancer) ointment may be used to destroy the cancerous tissue such as 5-fluorouracil (Efudex, Corac, or Fluoroplex).[147] To prevent further problems with basal cell carcinoma people should use sunscreens of SPF 15 or higher when exposed to the sun and cover exposed areas of skin with clothing such as hats, long-sleeved shirts, and long pants.

Physical Therapy Intervention. No PT intervention is indicated for basal cell carcinoma; however, wound care may be indicated after surgical removal.

Squamous Cell Carcinoma

Squamous cell carcinoma is the second most common skin cancer in the United States. More than 700,000 new cases of squamous cell carcinoma are diagnosed each year.[148] The incidence of squamous cell carcinoma is most frequent in the over-50 age group and is up to 3 times more common in men than in women.[149]

Etiology. Squamous cell carcinoma is most often caused by prolonged exposure to the sun or other sources of ultraviolet light. Other risk factors include chewing tobacco and smoking (tumors in the mouth),[150] previously burned or scarred areas of skin, contact with industrial carcinogens such as arsenic, and areas of skin with actinic keratosis, a precancerous skin condition that appears dry and scaly.[151] Other people at higher risk of developing squamous cell carcinoma include those who are fair skinned, those who are infected with the human papillomavirus, and those who are immunosuppressed, have undergone chemotherapy, have had previous episodes of skin cancer, have any of a variety of chronic inflammatory conditions, or have HIV/AIDS.[152]

Signs and Symptoms. The characteristic appearance of these tumors is similar to a nonhealing ulcer with an irregular shape. The affected area is thickened, rough, crusted, occasionally with a raised border, and may bleed.[153] Squamous cell carcinoma lesions are most often located on the face, neck, scalp, ears, lips, shoulders and arms, upper back, and trunk (see Figure 8-13). If there is any change in shape, size, color, or sudden bleeding of an existing lesion, patients should consult a physician.

Prognosis. The prognosis is good when the lesions are diagnosed early and treated. Approximately 95% of all squamous cell carcinomas are curable when removed in the early stages.[154] In some cases, the lesions will spread to the underlying bone and ligaments and may metastasize to other areas of the body. Squamous cell carcinoma

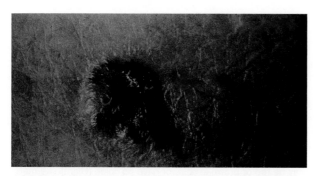

FIGURE 8.12 Basal cell carcinoma. (Reprinted with permission from Goldsmith, Lowell A., Lazarus, Gerald S., and Tharp, Michael D. *Adult and Pediatric Dermatology: A Color Guide to Diagnosis and Treatment*, 1st edition, p. 144, Philadelphia: F. A. Davis, 1997.)

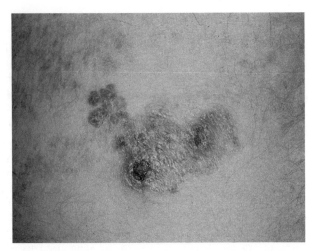

FIGURE 8.13 Squamous cell carcinoma. (Reprinted with permission from Goldsmith, Lowell A., Lazarus, Gerald S., and Tharp, Michael D. *Adult and Pediatric Dermatology: A Color Guide to Diagnosis and Treatment*, 1st edition, p. 237, Philadelphia: F. A. Davis, 1997.)

lesions located on the ears, lip, and nose are the ones most likely to metastasize.[155] People who have had one lesion of squamous cell carcinoma are more likely to recur or have another lesion. Regular skin checks are recommended to detect lesions in the early stages of development.

Medical Intervention. The medical treatments for squamous cell carcinoma lesions are similar to those for basal cell carcinoma. A tissue biopsy is taken of the lesion to confirm the diagnosis. Surgical interventions include curettage and electrodessication, cryosurgery, Mohs micrographic surgery, simple surgical excision, radiation with an electron beam, laser therapy, and systemic chemotherapy.[156] The choice of surgical intervention depends on the extent and depth of the lesion. Mohs micrographic surgery is reported to be the most effective form of surgery with the lowest recurrence rate of lesions after surgery.[157] Lesions diagnosed in the early stages of development may respond to the use of photodynamic therapy, which is a topical cream, or an injected fluid of 5-aminolevulinic acid. This treatment is also used for the treatment of actinic keratosis, a precursor to skin cancers.[158] In some cases in which extensive lesions are removed, skin grafting may be necessary.[159]

Physical Therapy Intervention. The PT and PTA may identify possible problem skin lesions when treating patients because they see areas of skin not normally exposed or those not observable by the patient. If the PTA observes a suspicious skin lesion, the supervising PT should be notified so that the patient can be advised to visit a physician and have the lesion examined.

Malignant Melanoma

Malignant melanoma is an extremely malignant, invasive form of skin cancer. Although malignant melanoma accounts for approximately only 4% of the total cases of skin cancer, it is responsible for 74% of the deaths.[160] One in 60 Americans are likely to develop malignant melanoma during their lifetime. The American Academy of Dermatology expected approximately 60,000 cases of invasive melanoma, and 50,000 cases of melanoma in situ to be reported, and 8,110 deaths to be attributed to malignant melanoma in the United States in 2007.[161]

Etiology. Overexposure to the sun, especially during childhood, is a major cause of malignant melanoma, and fair-skinned individuals are more susceptible to development of the tumor.[162] Other risk factors for the development of malignant melanoma include having a fair complexion, the presence of multiple moles, a family history of the disease, and older age. Pathologically, the source of the tumor is in the melanocytes, the cells in the skin that produce pigment. The tumor may develop from a preexisting nevus (mole) or freckle or may spontaneously appear in normal skin. See Figure 8-14 for a comparison between a mole and a malignant melanoma.

Signs and Symptoms. The types of melanoma (see Figs. 8-15 and 8-16) include lentigo melanoma and superficial spreading melanoma, which are both localized to the epidermis. These types of melanoma can turn into the

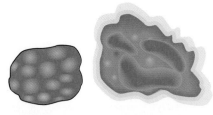

Mole (Nevus)   Malignant melanoma

FIGURE 8.14 Comparison of a mole and a malignant melanoma. (Left) The mole or nevus has smooth edges with a raised center, may be red or brown in color or have no color. (Right) The malignant melanoma is an irregular shape. Tends to be larger than a nevus and is dark red to bluish black in color. *Note:* This is not a definitive description of malignant melanoma and a variety of shapes, sizes, and colorations are possible. Carcinoma does not always follow a subscribed pattern.

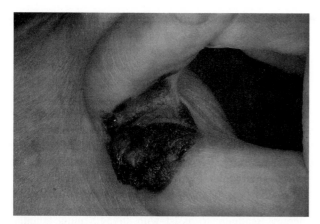

FIGURE 8.15 Malignant melanoma. (Reprinted with permission from Goldsmith, Lowell A., Lazarus, Gerald S., and Tharp, Michael D. *Adult and Pediatric Dermatology: A Color Guide to Diagnosis and Treatment*, 1st edition, p. 137, Philadelphia: F. A. Davis, 1997.)

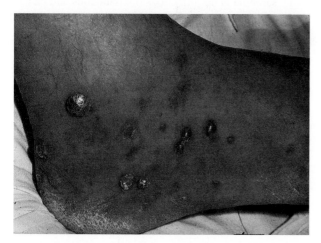

FIGURE 8.16 Kaposi's sarcoma on a foot. (Reprinted with permission from Goldsmith, Lowell A., Lazarus, Gerald S., and Tharp, Michael D. *Adult and Pediatric Dermatology: A Color Guide to Diagnosis and Treatment*, 1st edition, p. 138, Philadelphia: F. A. Davis, 1997.)

more severe type of nodular melanoma if left untreated. The nodular type of melanoma spreads rapidly into the dermis and underlying tissues. A specific type called acral lentiginous melanoma is found on the palm of the hand, the sole of the foot, and beneath the nails. Warning signs of melanoma to look for when checking the skin are skin lesions that have mixed flat and raised portions, an irregular shape, dark brown or black lesions, variations of color within the one lesion, itching, changes in any skin lesion, a mole larger than 6 mm in diameter, or bleeding of a lesion.[163,164] The sudden appearance of a mole-like lesion or a lesion with some of the previously described characteristics that is also over 6 mm in diameter are cause for concern.[165]

Prognosis. The depth of invasion of tissue by the tumor determines the classification of the stage of the tumor. A Level I tumor is a curable lesion, Level II and III tumors have spread to the upper layers of the dermis, Level IV lesions have spread to the reticular dermis, and Level V tumors have spread to the subdermal layers and metastasized.[166] Approximately 40% of patients with Level IV lesions, and 20% of those with a Level V lesion survive more than 5 years.[167,168]

Medical Intervention. Surgical excision of malignant melanoma is usually the preferred and most effective method of intervention. Excision of the lymph nodes surrounding the malignant melanoma has been effective in reducing the rate of metastasis in some people.[169] Lymph node excision may be recommended as an elective surgery. Interferon-alpha-2b, a substance that attacks tumor cells, may be prescribed after surgery. Interleukin-2 amplifies the immune response of the body to tumor cells and may also be prescribed, especially for those patients with Level V metastasizing tumors.[170]

Physical Therapy Intervention. If the PTA observes a skin lesion that is suspect, the PT should be notified and a suggestion made to patients that they see their physician. Early detection and removal of skin cancers improves the prognosis for the patient. Several videos are available that show various types of skin cancers and assist the health care provider in early detection of possible problem lesions in their patients.

Kaposi's Sarcoma

Kaposi's sarcoma is a malignant tumor originating in the blood vessels and connective tissue of the dermis of the skin, as well as the linings of the mouth, nose, throat, and other organs[171] (see Fig. 8-16). Kaposi's sarcoma is a rare cancer except in those patients with acquired immunodeficiency syndrome (AIDS). A Kaposi's sarcoma is not infectious.

Etiology. The Kaposi's sarcoma–associated herpes virus (KSHV) has been identified as a causative factor for Kaposi's sarcoma. Estimates of the number of people in the United States infected with the KSHV virus range between 3.5% and 25%, but only a few of these people actually develop Kaposi's sarcoma.[172] This virus is particularly a problem in patients with HIV.[173] In patients who are negative for HIV, the onset of Kaposi's sarcoma is occasionally connected with the use of corticosteroids[174] and is also associated with the use of immunosuppressive medications used to prevent rejection of a donor organ in patients who receive a transplant.[175] The corticosteroids tend to suppress the immune system, making the patient more susceptible to this type of cancer.

Signs and Symptoms. Kaposi's sarcoma tumors are found on the face and lower legs, although they can occur on any area of the body including the throat, nose, mouth, and other body organs. The tumors are characteristically red, purple, or brown; are of various sizes; and spread fairly rapidly in patients with AIDS. The condition may also be associated with fever, swollen lymph glands, and weight loss.[176]

Prognosis. The tumors develop slowly in patients who are not infected with HIV, and with the treatments now available for HIV/AIDS, the progression of the disease is slowed. The prognosis is not encouraging for patients with AIDS and Kaposi's sarcoma that has progressed to a later stage because the tumor can spread rapidly to underlying tissues and cause death. In a study by Spano et al, the survival time for people with progressive Kaposi's sarcoma ranged between 9 and 126 months from the date of diagnosis.[177]

Medical Intervention. The medical treatment for Kaposi's sarcoma involves radiation and chemotherapy. Patients with AIDS-related Kaposi's sarcoma are treated with a regimen of highly active antiretroviral therapy (HAART) to control the AIDS before either radiation or chemotherapy treatment.[178]

Physical Therapy Intervention. Patients with Kaposi's sarcoma and HIV/AIDS are often seen for physical therapy treatment to assist with strengthening, ambulation, endurance training, and general mobility. The PTA should follow universal precautions to reduce the risk of transmitting an infection to the already immunosuppressed patient who has AIDS and Kaposi's sarcoma. Kaposi's sarcoma is not infectious or contagious and cannot be transmitted to the PT and PTA. Wound care is not typically provided by the PT.

SKIN ULCERATIONS

Many skin ulcers are caused by arterial or venous insufficiency. Please see Table 8-7 for a comparison of the characteristics of these ulcers. Some ulcers, such as

Table 8.7   **Characteristics of Arterial and Venous Ulcers**

	ARTERIAL ULCER CHARACTERISTICS	VENOUS ULCER CHARACTERISTICS
Appearance	Rounded shape, smooth, rolled, clearly defined edges Hard black eschar covering all or part of wound Minimal granulation tissue, if any Necrotic tissue often present Deep tendons may be exposed	Irregular shape often with jagged edges Granulation tissue in base of wound
Arterial pulses	Absent or weak in dorsalis pedis and/or popliteal pulses	Intact
Causes	Diabetes Hyperlipidemia Smoking	Thrombosis of vein Venous valve insufficiency
Drainage	Minimal May be yellow and purulent	Drainage may be profuse or moderate
Edema	Dependent edema unrelieved by leg elevation; leg elevation can cause pain	Edema is reduced when legs are elevated and ankle pumps performed
Location	Inferior to ankle on lateral and dorsal aspects of foot, and ankle, heel, distal foot, and toes Anterior tibia	Mainly superior to the medial malleolus and on the medial aspect of lower leg

Table 8.7 Characteristics of Arterial and Venous Ulcers (continued)

	ARTERIAL ULCER CHARACTERISTICS	VENOUS ULCER CHARACTERISTICS
Occurrence	More common in over-50 years age group	Account for 80% of all leg ulcers
Pain	At rest When walking, intermittent claudication Increased pain when leg elevated above level of heart	Minimal or no pain Some pain on standing Pain usually relieved by elevating legs
Size	Varies; often deep	May be large; mainly superficial and shallow
Surrounding skin	Pallor of lower extremity when leg elevated; dark red or purple appearance (rubor) when leg dependent Skin cracked, dry, scaly, shiny, and cold; may be no leg hair	Darkened hyperpigmentation of skin around the ulcer ("brawny")

decubitus ulcers, are the result of pressure on the area of skin. Treatment of any skin ulceration requires that any underlying causative systemic condition of the patient be addressed by the physician. In some cases, skin ulcerations may have a mixed cause of both arterial and venous insufficiency, but usually one cause predominates.[179] Most commonly, skin ulcers are found in men over 45 and women over 55 years of age.[180]

Arterial, Ischemic, and Diabetic Ulcers

Arterial insufficiency or ischemic ulcers occur in patients with peripheral vascular disease. One form of ischemic ulcer is the diabetic ulcer, which results from the cardiovascular complications of diabetes. People with diabetes mellitus are between 15 and 46 times more likely to develop ischemic ulcers than those people without diabetes.[181] (See Chapter 9 for more information about diabetes mellitus.) Approximately 3% to 6% of Americans have diabetes. Of these people, 15% are likely to develop lower leg or foot ulcers, and 12% to 24% may have to undergo amputation.[182]

Etiology. The etiology of ischemic ulcers is complex. In each case, the actual cause of an ischemic ulcer is a reduction in oxygenation perfusion of the tissues. The resultant lack of oxygenated blood to the skin, muscles, and other tissues results in gangrene and ischemic ulcerated areas in the lower extremities. The risk factors for the development of arterial insufficiency ulcers include a hereditary tendency, smoking, high blood pressure, diabetes mellitus, hypercholesterolemia, and atherosclerosis.

Additional risk factors for the development of ischemic ulcers for patients with diabetes mellitus include peripheral neuropathy, reduced joint range of motion particularly at the ankle and knee, obesity, poor footwear, and reduced vision.[183]

Signs and Symptoms. The general signs and symptoms of ischemia in the lower extremities include the absence of arterial pulses in the lower extremity, night pain in the feet, absence of hair on the lower leg and foot, and pallor of the skin in the foot when the leg is elevated.[184] Ischemic ulcers usually form on the lower extremities of patients (see Fig. 8-17). Refer to Chapter 3 for information about peripheral vascular disease, and Chapter 9 for further information about diabetes mellitus. These

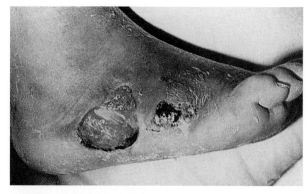

FIGURE 8.17 Ulceration secondary to arterial insufficiency. (Reprinted with permission from Goldsmith, Lowell A., Lazarus, Gerald S., and Tharp, Michael D. *Adult and Pediatric Dermatology: A Color Guide to Diagnosis and Treatment*, 1st edition, p. 223, Philadelphia: F. A. Davis, 1997.)

ischemic ulcers mainly occur distally to the ankle and on the lateral aspect of the foot or ankle, on the heel, or on the distal part of the foot under the metatarsal heads, and toes.[185] Some ischemic ulcers do, however, occur on the medial aspect of the foot and ankle. The shape of ischemic ulcers is often circular and sometimes described as having a "punched-out" appearance.[186] Ischemic ulcers rarely bleed and either are slow to heal or fail to heal. Many arterial ulcers have necrotic tissue and thick, black eschar covering the wound. Placing the leg in a dependent position (over the edge of the bed or in a sitting position) often relieves the pain associated with ischemic ulcers by allowing gravity to assist the peripheral arterial circulation. Ulcers on the lower extremities do not heal well if the circulation is insufficient to supply the needed oxygenation and nutrients to the involved area.[187]

Prognosis. The underlying cause of the poor arterial circulation needs to be addressed for patients with arterial insufficiency ulcers, particularly those that are slow to heal or are severe.[188] If the oxygenation of the tissues is restored, the arterial ulcers usually heal well, but many arterial ulcers heal either slowly, or not at all, if the oxygenation of the tissues remains poor.[189]

Medical Intervention. The diagnosis of ischemia is through observance of the skin and palpation of the lower extremity arterial pulses. Other diagnostic tools are the duplex scanner to identify blockages in the arteries, CT, and MRI.[190] Ischemic problems in the lower extremity are often treated surgically with replacement of the affected blood vessels, or the insertion of stents into the artery to maintain a patent (open) vessel. In some patients unable to undergo surgery, hyperbaric oxygen therapy (HBOT) may be used to improve the oxygenation of the tissues and increase angiogenesis (development of new blood vessels) in the hypoxic tissue (tissue with low oxygen content).[191] The HBOT is administered either through a chamber such as a room that delivers a high content of oxygen or through a machine that fits over the limb and administers a high level of oxygen to the involved area. Infection of wounds is a major problem for patients with diabetes, because they may not notice pain as a result of peripheral neuropathy. Hyperglycemia sometimes indicates infection in patients with diabetes. The débridement of necrotic tissue and eschar is performed after the arterial circulation is restored to the area of the wound.[192] Advice is provided to patients regarding the reduction of risk factors such as

smoking cessation, controlling the diabetes mellitus symptoms, reducing hypertension, and reducing hypercholesterolemia.[193] When indicated, the physician prescribes antihypertensive and cholesterol-lowering medications. In cases of nonhealing ulcers with related gangrene and ischemic tissue, an amputation of the affected part of the limb may be required.

Physical Therapy Intervention. The PTA must check the dorsalis pedis (dorsal pedal) pulse before each treatment when working with patients with arterial insufficiency or diabetes. Whirlpool treatment is not effective in stimulating circulation if the arteries are so narrowed that they cannot allow the passage of blood. Using a whirlpool that is too warm may cause burns if the circulation is insufficient to diffuse the localized heating effect on the tissues. Extreme caution must be taken when treating the arterial ulcer. See Table 8-7 for the characteristics of arterial and venous ulcers. Most patients who have an amputation of the lower extremity receive physical therapy intervention. In some cases, the intervention is for wound-care management, and in others for rehabilitation to return the patient to functional activities after amputation surgery. The PTA will be involved in preparing patients for use of a prosthesis; training patients in donning and doffing the prosthesis; gait training; teaching strengthening, mobility, and endurance exercises; teaching safe and effective use of wheelchairs; and the prevention of contractures. See the section on diabetes in Chapter 9 for advice to give to the patient with diabetes and precautions to take when treating the patient. See Chapter 14 for the implications for the elderly patient with diabetes.

Specific Physical Therapy Intervention for the Person With an Arterial (Ischemic) Ulcer. The following list does not detail a definitive treatment regimen for the person with an arterial ulcer. The PTA is directed to consult a specific wound-treatment text such as Sussman and Bates-Jenson's *Wound Care: A Collaborative Practice Manual for Health Professionals*, third edition,[194] to determine more detailed intervention techniques. The author strongly suggests that PTAs involved with extensive wound care should attend continuing education courses on the subject to increase their level of expertise.

1. The physical therapist performs a complete evaluation of the wound to include location, depth, extent, size, odor, drainage type and amount, tissue damage, infection (tissue culture taken and sent to lab), appearance, and

sensation of surrounding skin. The condition of the surrounding skin, and presence or absence of arterial pulses—dorsalis pedis, posterior tibial, and popliteal should also be noted.

2. The physical therapist develops a plan of care for the PTA to follow, and regular consultation and communication must occur between the PT and the PTA to determine progress and the need to adjust the treatment goals and interventions.

3. The PTA documents any observations of the wound before and after treatment. This includes size (be sure to use the same method as the evaluating physical therapist with either centimeters or inches), appearance, drainage type and amount noted on the removed dressing, odor (if any), patient pain level, appearance of surrounding skin, and treatment method used. Patient response to treatment should be noted.

4. The physical therapist will débride the wound if this has not been performed surgically by the physician. Effectiveness of wound-healing measures will depend on the level of circulation to the tissue. Physical therapy intervention by the following means may not be effective if the arterial blood supply is severely limited. The débridement of necrotic tissue is shown to reduce the possibility of infection in the wound because necrotic tissue contains bacteria.[195]

   A. Selective sharp débridement is performed with scalpel or scissors and is considered to be outside the scope of work for the PTA by the American Physical Therapy Association (APTA). Ongoing débridement may be necessary because the wound will not heal unless it is clear of necrotic tissue and infection.

   B. Nonselective mechanical débridement is so called because it removes necrotic tissue but also removes some sound tissue. This type of débridement can be performed using the following:
      • Wet-to-dry gauze dressings. The theory is that when the dressing is removed, the necrotic tissue adheres to the dressing and is removed with the dressing. If the dressing is not applied correctly and specifically to just the wound area, it will damage healthy/viable tissue. This method is not effective for wounds completely covered with eschar.
      • Whirlpool treatment with agitation levels as high as tolerated by the patient to loosen necrotic tissue and make it easier to remove. The agitator can be directed at the wound during treatment for maximum effect. Water temperature must not be higher than 1° Centigrade above body temperature due to the poor arterial circulation.[196] Water temperatures above body temperature can cause a burn because the circulation cannot diffuse the heating effect of the water.
      • Wound irrigation can be performed using a syringe, with a needle or catheter to insert into the wound, and filled with saline solution or a nonionic wound cleanser. This technique can be used with each dressing change. Pressure can be adjusted so that a low pressure is used on healing wounds and a high pressure on necrotic wounds. Another method is to use pulsatile lavage equipment. The pressure can be adjusted to provide different levels of debridement, and combined with suction the cleansing effect is enhanced. Pulsatile lavage has also been shown to stimulate the production of granulation tissue and promote healing.

   C. Chemical débridement with enzymes is slow acting but can be effective. The enzyme agent is applied directly to the wound. Eschar is not affected by enzyme agents unless the eschar is deeply scored with a scalpel to allow the agent to penetrate beneath the eschar.

   D. Autolytic débridement is a form of self-débridement. The wound is covered with an occlusive (sealing) or semiocclusive dressing that maintains the moisture in the wound and stimulates the white blood cells to destroy the necrotic tissue. This procedure has limited application in arterial ulcers because the wounds are generally rather dry. Also the dressings can cause maceration (softening and sloughing) of the surrounding tissue and prevent regular observation of the wound.

5. Ultrasound may be used at nonthermal doses to change the permeability of the cell membranes, and electrical stimulation may also be used to encourage healing.[197]

6. The wound dressings applied must help the dry wound to become a moist environment conducive to wound healing.[198]

7. Advise the patient to avoid elevating the leg above the level of the heart.

8. Avoid pressure dressings as the arterial circulation is unable to cope with the extra stress of pressure bandages.

9. Do _not_ use heat to the area, and advise the patient to avoid heat, because the arterial circulation is unable to cope with the extra stress of the heat, and use of heat could result in a burn. (Heat may be applied to proximal areas to improve circulation with the hope that distal circulation may be positively affected.)

10. Provide instructions on dressing changes to the patient and care provider if the patient is seen as an outpatient. Instructions must be specific giving frequency of dressing changes.

11. Provide instruction in non-weight-bearing ambulation for the affected limb (or as instructed by the physician), bed rest with the bed head raised 5°, and protection of the affected leg. Areas around the leg should be well padded to prevent further injury. A walker or other assisted device is needed for ambulation. A walker is preferable because it provides some measure of protection for the leg during non-weight-bearing status.

12. Give advice on prevention of further ulcers (see the section in Chapter 9 on Physical Therapy Advice to the Patient With Diabetes Mellitus).

Note on Physical Therapist Assistant Implications for Patients With Amputations. The PTA must be aware of correct positioning to prevent contractures in the amputated limb. When a transtibial (below knee) amputation is performed, hamstrings contractures can become a problem; therefore, positioning with the knee extended must be emphasized to prevent flexion contractures. The patient must be instructed to keep the knee straight without a pillow beneath the knee and given an explanation as to why. The explanation must include how placing a pillow under the knee causes shortening of the hip flexors and the knee flexors and how this shortening will affect the ability to use a prosthetic device. Most patients who are cognitively able to understand these issues will comply with the treatment regimen because they want to be able to walk. In the patient cognitively unable to comply with instructions, the care provider must be vigilant with the observance of positioning to reduce the likelihood of contractures. Additionally, exercises for the patient with a transtibial amputation must emphasize quadriceps activity, which are at a greater mechanical advantage because of the reduced lever arm of the lower leg, to overcome the effect of the hamstrings. In patients with a transfemoral (above-knee) amputation, the hip flexors are the strongest muscles, which tend to pull the hip into a flexed position leading to a hip flexion contracture. The patient must be positioned prone several times a day to stretch the hip flexors and perform hip extension exercises to overcome the strength of the hip flexors. Failure to follow these procedures, or noncompliance of the patient, can result in contractures, which may prevent the use of a prosthesis.

Venous Stasis Ulcers

Venous ulcers, or **venous stasis ulcers,** are most common in the over-60-year age group. The incidence of venous stasis ulcers increases with age and is slightly higher in women than men.[199] An estimated 600,000 cases of venous stasis ulcers occur per year in the United States.[200]

Etiology. Patients with venous stasis ulcers have impaired venous circulation and usually have a history of trauma to the area involved, varicose veins, or thrombosis of the deep veins. Other risk factors for development of venous stasis ulcers are heart disease, deep venous thrombosis (DVT), obesity, and genetic defects of the valves of the veins.[201]

Signs and Symptoms. Venous stasis ulcers are usually located on the medial aspect of the lower leg superior to the ankle and are irregular in shape (see Fig. 8-18). The lower extremity pulses are usually intact. Necrotic tissue in the venous stasis ulcer is frequently yellow, white, or gray and not black as it is in arterial ulcers. Most venous wounds produce significant exudate. In many cases of venous stasis, there is also lymphatic involvement causing edema. Cellulitis is a common side effect of lower extremity venous problems.

Prognosis. Although some venous stasis ulcers may remain a chronic problem, most ulcers of venous origin respond well to treatment and heal completely. According to Khachemoune and Kauffman, approximately 70% of

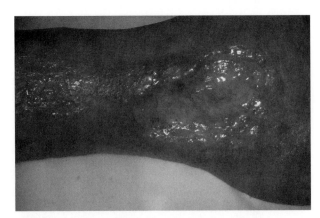

FIGURE 8.18 Venous stasis ulcer over medial malleolus. (Reprinted with permission from Goldsmith, Lowell A., Lazarus, Gerald S., and Tharp, Michael D. *Adult and Pediatric Dermatology: A Color Guide to Diagnosis and Treatment*, 1st edition, p. 454, Philadelphia: F. A. Davis, 1997.)

venous ulcers heal within 6 months.[202] However, the risk of reoccurrence of leg ulcers is high.[203]

Medical Intervention. The débridement techniques used for venous stasis ulcers are the same as those detailed for arterial wounds. The softer necrotic tissue of the venous stasis ulcer can usually be removed by using tweezers. Care must be taken to prevent pull on muscle or tendon tissue when debriding the deep venous wound. Because wounds heal more quickly when moist, not wet, dressings need to absorb some of the excessive exudate formed by the venous stasis ulcer to promote optimal healing. The ligation and stripping of both superficial and deeper veins in the lower extremities is a surgical option for people with chronic venous insufficiency ulcers that do not respond to conservative management.[204]

Physical Therapy Intervention for the Venous Stasis Ulcer. Interventions for venous stasis ulcers vary from those used for arterial ulcers. Some of the basic procedures remain the same, however. The following list is not a definitive list of physical therapy interventions.

1. The physical therapist performs a complete evaluation of the wound for location, depth, extent, size, odor, drainage type and amount, tissue damage, infection (tissue culture taken and sent to lab), appearance, and sensation of surrounding skin. The condition of the surrounding skin, and presence of arterial pulses— dorsalis pedis, posterior tibial, and popliteal should also be noted.

2. The PT develops a plan of care for the PTA to follow and regular consultation/communication must occur between the PT and the PTA to determine progress and the need to adjust the treatment goals and interventions.

3. The PTA must document any observations of the wound before and after treatment. This includes size (be sure to use the same method as the evaluating physical therapist with either centimeters or inches), appearance, drainage type and amount noted on the removed dressing, odor, patient pain level, appearance of surrounding skin, and treatment method used. Patient response to treatment should also be noted.

4. The physical therapist will débride the wound. Surgical débridement is not usually required for venous wounds, and the débridement often can be performed with tweezers rather than sharp instruments. PTAs are allowed to débride the wound if it is within their field of expertise, as long as sharp débridement is not required. Debridement procedures are the same as noted for arterial ulcers. The techniques most used for venous ulcer débridement are application of occlusive dressings such as hydrogels or hydrocolloids or the use of enzymatic preparations.

5. The use of electrical stimulation may be recommended by the physical therapist.[205,206]

6. Provide advice to the patient to elevate the leg above the level of the heart to assist venous return to the heart, especially when sleeping. Blocks of wood under the foot of the bed can be used to assist with this process.

7. The use of compression dressings such as an Unna Boot can be effective when applied over a dressing for a venous ulcer. The pressure assists venous return and promotes healing of the wound. Use of compression hose can also be effective, once the wound is healed, to reduce swelling and assist with venous return. Compression therapy continues to be one of the standards in the treatment of venous insufficiency ulcers.[207]

8. Provide instructions on wound dressing changes to the patient and care provider if the patient is seen as an outpatient. Instructions must be specific giving frequency of dressing changes.

9. Patients should be encouraged to exercise the involved leg to include ankle pump exercises, quad sets, and hamstring work to encourage the venous return. An exception to ankle pumps would be if the wound was at the level of the ankle and in performing the exercises the wound bed was disturbed enough to reduce wound healing. Moderate walking and other activity should be encouraged. Standing in one position for prolonged periods should be discouraged.

10. Provide home exercises to encourage venous return and help to prevent future problems. Although most venous stasis ulcers will heal, they heal with scarring and the resultant skin is rather fragile. Care must be taken to prevent trauma to the area, which could cause further skin breakdown. Regular elevation of the legs to reduce the effects of edema can be helpful.

Comparison of PT Treatments for Venous and Arterial Ulcers. In summary, some important differences exist between the characteristics of venous stasis ulcers and arterial insufficiency leg ulcers that have an impact on the method of treatment for the patient (see Tables 8.7 and 8.8). If the venous system is compromised, the general rules are as follows:

1. Compression of the extremity—over wound dressings if necessary.

Table 8.8   **Differences in Treatment for Arterial and Venous Ulcers**

TREATMENT CONSIDERATIONS	ARTERIAL ULCERS	VENOUS STASIS ULCERS
Tipping of bed	Bed head raised	Foot of bed raised
Clothing	**DO NOT** use support hose or TED stockings **DO NOT** use anything tight round the leg at the knee or ankle such as tight socks	Use of support hose/TED stockings Do not use anything tight round the leg at the knee or ankle, such as tight socks
Wound dressings	**DO NOT** use compression bandages	Use dressings with compression such as an Unna boot to assist healing
External compression devices	**DO NOT** use external compression devices	Use external compression devices at home and in the physical therapy clinic to reduce edema
Whirlpool	Use cool water whirlpool only	Use mild warmth whirlpool—not hot
Massage	**DO NOT** use massage	Edema massage is helpful in reducing edema

2. Elevation of the affected part above the level of the heart when resting, so that gravity assists the venous return to the heart. Patients should be encouraged to rest in this way for periods during the day.
3. Exercises to assist venous return with the effect of the muscle pump and compression of the veins as they pass over the joints. These should be performed with limb in elevation whenever possible.
4. Elevation of the foot of bed at night to assist venous return.
5. Performance of edema massage to facilitate reduction of swelling in the affected extremity.
6. Application of some mild heating to encourage venous return.

If the arterial system is compromised, the general rules are as follows:

1. DO NOT give compression of the extremity; the arteries are unable to cope, and applying more pressure would make it worse.
2. DO NOT elevate limb. Lower the limb below the level of the heart so that gravity will assist the flow of the arterial system to the extremity.
3. MONITOR level of exercises carefully for the effects of intermittent claudication—Buerger-Allen exercises may be given. Strenuous exercises should not be given.
4. ELEVATE BED HEAD at night to assist arterial circulation.
5. DO NOT do edema massage.

6. DO NOT give heat to affected limb. The arterial system is already unable to cope with the demands of the circulation and additional heat will place further stress on the arterial system.

Pressure (Decubitus) Ulcers

Pressure ulcers, **decubitus ulcers,** or bedsores are all names for the same condition. The incidence of pressure ulcers is greatest in persons who are immobile and unable to shift position in a bed or a chair (see Fig. 8-19). Therefore, the incidence of these ulcers is greater in the elderly, the immobile, the mentally impaired population who have a low nutritional status, and those with spinal cord lesions or cerebrovascular accidents. The treatment of pressure ulcers costs more than $1 billion each year in the United States.[208] (The implications for the costs and use of personnel for treatment of pressure ulcers in the elderly population are discussed further in Chapter 14.)

Etiology. Pressure ulcers are caused by prolonged pressure on tissues overlying bony prominences. Pressure is exerted between the surface of the bed or chair into the tissues against the bony prominence. The pressure compresses the blood vessels resulting in ischemia of the tissue. Lying in one position or sitting in one place too long without moving can cause pressure ulcers.[209] The compression force on the tissues, created by being sandwiched between the bone and the bed, causes occlusion of the blood vessels, and loss of nutrition to the affected tissues.

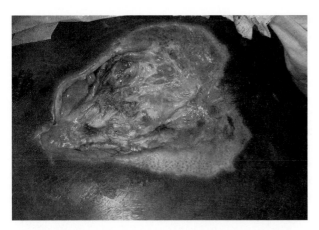

FIGURE 8.19 Decubitus (pressure) ulcer. (Reprinted with permission from Goldsmith, Lowell A., Lazarus, Gerald S., and Tharp, Michael D. *Adult and Pediatric Dermatology: A Color Guide to Diagnosis and Treatment*, 1st edition, p. 445, Philadelphia: F. A. Davis, 1997.)

If the compression lasts 2 hours or more, irreversible damage to the tissues may occur.[210] In some people with very poor nutritional status, pressure ulcers may occur in less than 2 hours. Under normal circumstances people shift their weight off the bony prominence when discomfort is felt, but when people are immobile, they are unable to move to change the pressure.

Signs and Symptoms. The areas of the body most susceptible to pressure ulcers are the sacrum, ischial tuberosities, lateral malleoli, calcaneal area of the heel, greater trochanters, scapulae, and ribs. The head and face can be at risk if the patient lies prone, and in side-lying, the ears can be affected. Some pressure areas may only look red, but the damage to the tissue beneath the skin may be extensive. These areas may open up and become seriously ulcerated over a period of a few days. Muscle tissue becomes damaged quickly by lack of blood supply. Full-thickness or Stage IV pressure ulcers tend to develop sinuses that track beneath the skin. Tunneling, lipping, and undermining of the edges of these ulcers may also occur. Undermining means that the apparent edges of the ulcer do not show the true extent of the affected area. The actual area may be considerably larger than the opening in the skin. A complication of severe, chronic pressure ulcers is the development of malignant tumors in the nonhealing skin.[211]

Classification of Pressure Ulcers. Pressure ulcers are classified into stages depending on the depth of the tissue damage:

Stage I. Area of reddened or purple colored skin. May be warm or cool to the touch and be painful or itchy.

Stage II. Partial-thickness skin loss. May be a blister or a small ulcerated area.

Stage III. Full-thickness skin loss with subcutaneous tissue necrosis.

Stage IV. Full-thickness skin loss with subcutaneous tissue necrosis and damage to muscle, tendons, ligaments, and bone.

Closed pressure ulcer. These ulcers look small on the surface, or the skin may be intact, but the underlying tissue damage is extensive and may extend to bone.

Prognosis. The prognosis for patients with early-stage pressure ulcers is good, although healing may take several weeks. Infection can become a problem in chronic pressure ulcers and the risk for further skin breakdown is always present. Preventive care is required to try to prevent additional skin damage.[212]

Medical Intervention. Treatment of the pressure ulcer follows the same principles as other wound care. However, attention needs to be given to the nutritional status of the patient. In the absence of good nutrition, healing will be delayed regardless of the type of treatment provided. A culture of the wound is taken and sent to the lab for analysis. Débridement follows the same sequence as for the other types of ulcers previously described. The concentration of treatment is to remove necrotic tissue and stimulate the production of granulation tissue as a precursor to growth of new skin, and closure of the wound. Some pressure ulcers can be large, covering the whole sacral area, and may also be full-thickness or Stage IV depth. Such wounds may not ever fully heal depending on the nutritional and health status of the patient. If these areas heal, they may be susceptible to further breakdown and should be protected from additional trauma.[213]

Prevention of decubitus ulcers is the most important method of reducing the incidence of these debilitating wounds.[214] Regular turning of patients in hospital and nursing home settings can reduce the risk of pressure ulcers but may not prevent them. The use of cushions and special padding for positioning can also reduce the risk of pressure. In people who are very sick, the skin may become fragile and more prone to breakdown. Sacral pressure ulcers are more prevalent if the patient is incontinent because the skin may remain moist and become soft and macerated. The maceration of the tissue leads to breakdown of the skin with minimal external pressure. Another factor leading to skin breakdown is shearing force. If patients are moved up the bed by sliding or slide down the bed by themselves, the skin and underlying tissues can be exposed to a shearing force that can damage the already delicate, undernourished tissue. Special beds, such as waterbeds, to reduce pressure, and intermittent pressure beds can be helpful in the prevention of pressure ulcers. Unfortunately, these beds also make performance of exercises and ambulation difficult, creating a challenge for the PT, PTA, and other health care professionals during rehabilitation.

Physical Therapy Intervention. Physical therapy treatment of the ulcer may include the following:

- Débridement
- Ice massage around the perimeter of the wound to stimulate deep circulation
- Whirlpool if the ulcer is on the lower or upper extremities or a full-body whirlpool tank for trunk areas if necessary
- Occlusive or semiocclusive dressings to maintain a moist environment optimal for healing for a dry wound
- Absorbent dressings, such as alginate dressings, for heavily draining wounds to maintain a moist, but not wet, environment conducive to healing
- Packing of areas with sinus formation, tunneling, or undermining with dressings of suitable material to encourage healing from the wound surface and not across the surface of the skin which would leave a cavity
- Wound irrigation using a syringe or pulsatile lavage unit
- Electrical stimulation to the wound bed to stimulate the healing process
- Vacuum device, with a sponge fitted into the wound cavity to remove copious exudate

Special Considerations for the Physical Therapist Assistant. As part of the health care team, the PTA must be careful to prevent adding to the problem of pressure ulcers by causing shearing forces. Care must be taken when moving patients to ensure the skin is not dragged along the bed. Encouraging patients to move themselves is preferable, providing assistance as needed. If patients are overweight and two people try to move them up in the bed, there is a strong possibility that the buttocks and sacrum will drag on the bed, causing a shearing force on the sacrum or low back. Good positioning in the bed and chair is important. If patients need to be in wheelchairs for prolonged periods of time, chairs should be fitted specifically for them. Positioning

devices should be used to prevent sliding in the chair, and if the patient is immobile, a tilt-in-space chair should be considered to provide the ability to alter the gravitational forces on the body. The management of the elderly patient to prevent pressure ulcers is discussed further in Chapter 14.

The previously discussed information is not intended to be a definitive list of possible physical therapy interventions. New innovations in wound care are discovered every year. If PTAs become involved as part of the wound-care team, they should attend regular update conferences on wound-care advancements.

CASE STUDY 8.1

A 59-year-old female is attending physical therapy for treatment of a venous stasis ulcer on her left lower leg. She has had the ulcer for more than 1 month and only recently sought medical help due to the pain caused by the ulcer. She is an administrative assistant working 8 hours a day at a desk and rarely takes a break during her working day. She normally spends a lot of time in front of the television at home in the evenings because she relates being very tired after work. She has been dressing the ulcer herself with dry gauze dressings, and it has been getting gradually larger with more copious drainage. The ulcer is located immediately superior to the medial malleolus, and measures 1 X 1.2 cm. Drainage is copious, slightly cream/yellow, but not foul smelling. The edges of the wound are irregular. No tunneling, sinus formation, or undermining is observed. The base of the wound is pink with some yellow areas, but no evidence of granulation tissue. The physical therapist has evaluated the patient and determined the plan of care to include three times weekly visits for whirlpool therapy for débridement and cleansing, appropriate wound dressings, advice to patient on wound care and lower extremity exercises, and application of compression dressings when the wound is sufficiently cleansed. Long-term goals are to reduce the wound size by 80% in 6 weeks, teach appropriate exercise regimen including a balance of ambulation and rest, return to functional activities, and provide suggestions for lifestyle changes to prevent future reoccurrence of the same problem. Short-term goals are to reduce the size of the ulcer by 30% in 2 weeks, reduce drainage of wound by 50%, teach circulatory stimulation exercises, positioning for rest, and provide advice on activities and care of the wound. The PT has asked you to treat the patient.

1. Explain what type of whirlpool treatment you will provide for this patient. Include the optimum temperature, position of agitator in relation to the wound, and length of time in the whirlpool tank.

2. Describe the possible types of dressings suitable for this copiously draining wound. How will your wound dressing of choice change as the wound drainage reduces? What kind of compression bandage system will you use? What precautions will you take?

3. Detail the exercises you will teach this patient and the positioning you will suggest during the workday, at home in the evening, and in bed at night.

4. What lifestyle changes might you suggest to this patient? Think how you will go about suggesting these changes.

5. Write a daily treatment note detailing your observations of the wound and your treatment provided.

6. What situations or changes will you communicate to your supervising PT?

CASE STUDY 8.2

A 26-year-old male sustained full-thickness burns to both arms at his place of work in a seafood restaurant when a crab boiler exploded. His wounds are healed subsequent to skin grafting. He is attending physical therapy for stretching exercises to restore his range of motion to both elbows and return to functional activities including return to work. The physical therapist has evaluated him and determined the right elbow is 15° to 100° of flexion (lacking 15° of extension), and the left elbow is 10° to 95°. Shoulders are grossly within normal limits for range of movement because he has been performing shoulder mobility exercises within pain tolerance. The manual muscle test (MMT) of right elbow flexors 3/5 and the left 4/5. Wrist flexors 4/5 bilaterally, and wrist extensors 3/5 bilaterally. Both shoulders are 4/5 in all ranges due to lack of strengthening over the past 3 months. The plan of care developed by the PT includes stretching exercises for bilateral elbows, strengthening exercises for all weak muscles, skin care, and home exercise program.

1. Develop a series of six stretching exercises for the elbows that the patient can perform in the clinic and as a home exercise program.

2. Develop six progressive strengthening exercises for each muscle group exhibiting weakness. Provide the patient with the ability to perform these at home.

3. Give the patient advice on skin care to prevent damage to the healed skin.

4. Instruct the patient in precautions to take when performing activities of daily living to prevent damage to the healed burn area.

5. Document a treatment session performed by the patient.

STUDY QUESTIONS

1. Describe a full-thickness burn.

2. What is the Rule of Nines?

3. What precautions should the PTA observe when treating a patient with herpes zoster?

4. The PTA notes that a nevus on the upper back of a patient looks unusual. What steps should the PTA employ?

5. A patient with an ischemic arterial ulcer on the lower extremity is in a lot of pain at night. What suggestions can the PTA provide to help relieve the pain?

6. Describe the differences between venous stasis ulcers and ischemic arterial ulcers.

7. Explain the differences in physical therapy management between the venous stasis ulcer and the ischemic ulcer.

8. Detail the four stages of a pressure ulcer.

9. What precautions can the PTA take to reduce the risk of causing a pressure ulcer when working with an immobile patient?

⬤ USEFUL WEB SITES

American Academy of Dermatology
http://www.aad.org

American Academy of Family Physicians
http://www.aafp.org

American Burn Association
http://www.ameriburn.org

American Osteopathic College of Dermatology
http://www.aocd.org/dermatologic

American Social Health Association
http://www.ashastd.org

Centers for Disease Control and Prevention
http://www.cdc.gov/vaccines

National Cancer Institute
http://www.cancer.gov

National Eczema Association
http://www.nationaleczema.org

National Institutes of Allergy and Infectious Diseases
http://www.niaid.nih.gov

National Institute of Arthritis and Musculoskeletal and Skin Diseases
http://www.niams.nih.gov

National Psoriasis Foundation
http://www.psoriasis.org

New Zealand Dermatological Society
http://dermnetnz.org

The Skin Cancer Foundation
http://www.skincancer.org

⬤ REFERENCES

[1] Richard, R. L., & Staley, M. J. (1994). *Burn care and rehabilitation: principles and practice*. Philadelphia: F. A. Davis.

[2] *US National Cancer Institute's Surveillance, Epidemiology and End Results (SEER) Program and Emory University*. (2005). Layers of the skin. SEERS Web-based Training Modules. Atlanta SEER Cancer Registry. Retrieved 11.20.2010 from http://training.seer.cancer.gov/melanoma/anatomy/layers.html

[3] Ibid.

[4] American Burn Association. (2007). *Burn incidence and treatment in the US: 2007 fact sheet*. Retrieved 5.6.2009 from http://www.ameriburn.org/resources_factsheet.php

[5] Ibid.

[6] Goodis, J., & Schraga, E. D. (2010). Burns, thermal. *eMedicine from WebMD*. Retrieved 11.20.2010 from http://www.emedicine.com/ped/TOPIC301.HTM

[7] Ibid.

[8] Wedro, B. C. (2008). Burn percentage in adults: Rule of Nines. *eMedicineHealth*. Retrieved 6.9.2009 from http://www.emedicine-health.com/burn_percentage_in_adults_rule_of_nines/article_em.htm

[9] Benson, B. E., et al. (2010). Electrical injuries. *eMedicine from WebMD*. Retrieved 11.20.2010 from http://www.emedicine.com/PED/topic2734.htm

[10] De la Cal, M. A. (2006). Pneumonia in patients with severe burns: a classification according to the concept of the carrier state. *Chest* 119:1160–1165. American College of Chest Physicians.

[11] Besner, G. E., & Otabor, I, A. (2009). Burns: surgical perspective. *eMedicine from WebMD*. Retrieved 5.6.2010 from http://www.emedicine.com/ped/topic2929.htm

[12] Mann, R., & Heimbach, D. (1996). Prognosis and treatment of burns. *Western J Med* 165:215–220. Retrieved 5.6.2010 from http://www.pubmedcentral.nih.gov/pagerender.fcgi?artid=1303748&pageindex=4#page

[13] Besner, G. E., & Otabor, I, A. Ibid.

[14] Mann, R., & Heimbach, D. Ibid.

[15] Besner, G. E., & Otabor, I, A. Ibid.

[16] Ibid.

[17] Weber, S. M., Ghanem, T. A., & Wax, M. K. (2010). Skin grafts, split thickness. *eMedicine from WebMD*. Retrieved 11.20.2010 from http://www.emedicine.com/Ent/topic47.htm

[18] Ibid.

[19] Magliacani, G. (1990). The surgical treatment of burns: skin substitutes. *Ann MBC* 3. Retrieved 5.7.2010 from http://www.medbc.com/annals/review/vol_3/num_3/text/vol3n3p145.htm

[20] Hawkins, E. B., & Ehrlich, S. D. (2006). *Burns*. University of Maryland Medical Center. Retrieved 5.7.2010 from http://www.umm.edu/altmed/articles/burns-000021.htm

[21] Corbett, L. Q., & Milne, C. T. (2001). Wound care in the age of PPS: tools for survival. *Home Health Care Manage Pract* 13:93–105.

[22] Keblish, D. J., & DeMaio, M. (1998). Early pulsatile lavage for the decontamination of contact wounds: historical review and point proposal. *Military Med* 163:844–846.

[23] Grassia, T. (2005). Wound care equipment linked to Acinetobacter outbreak. *Infect Dis News*. Retrieved 9.6.2009 from http://www.infectiousdiseasenews.com/200502/tools.asp

[24] Marasco, P. V., Sanga, C., Gordon, E. S., Simpson, J., Morykwas, M., & Marks, M. (2005). Prevention of aerosol contamination during pulsatile lavage. *Plastic Surgery 2005 conference*. Retrieved 9.6.2009 from http://asps.confex.com/asps/2005am/techprogram/paper_8622.htm

[25] Maragakis, L. L., et al. (2004). An outbreak of multidrug resistant *Acinetobacter baumannii* associated with pulsatile lavage wound treatment. *JAMA* 292;3006–3011.

[26] Minor, M. A. D., & Minor, S. D. (2006). *Patient care skills*, 5th edition. Upper Saddle River, NJ: Pearson, Prentice Hall, p. 58.

[27] Centers for Disease Control and Prevention. (2005). *Emergency preparedness and response. Trench foot or immersion foot*. Retrieved 11.20.2010 from http://www.bt.cdc.gov/disasters/trenchfoot.asp

[28] Centers for Disease Control and Prevention, Department of Health and Human Services. *Trench foot or immersion foot: disaster recovery fact sheet*. Ibid.

[29] Centers for Disease Control and Prevention, Department of Health and Human Services. Ibid.

[30] Mechem, C. C. (2007). Frostbite. *eMedicine from WebMD*. Retrieved 7.9.2009 from http://www.emedicine.com/emerg/topic209.htm

[31] Heller, J. L. (2010). Frostbite. *MedlinePlus Medical Encyclopedia*. Retrieved 11.20.2010 from http://www.nlm.nih.gov/medlineplus/ency/article/000057.htm

[32] Ibid.

[33] Mechem, C. C. Ibid.

[34] Ibid.

[35] Ibid.

[36] Centers for Disease Control and Prevention. (2006). Hypothermia related deaths—United Sates, 1999–2003 and 2005. *MMWR Morbid Mortal Wkly Rep* 55:282–284.

37 U.S. National Library of Medicine. (2010). Hypothermia. *Medline-Plus Medical Encyclopedia*. Retrieved 11.20.2010 from http://www.nlm.nih.gov/medlineplus/hypothermia.html

38 Mayo Clinic. (2010). *Hypothermia: first aid.* Retrieved 9.26.2010 from http://www.mayoclinic.com/print/first-aid-hypothermia/FA00017/METHOD=print

39 Mayo Clinic. (2010). *Boils and carbuncles.* Retrieved 9.26.2010 from http://www.mayoclinic.com/health/boils-and-carbuncles/DS00466/DSECTION=2

40 Gabillot-Carre, M., & Roujeau, J. C. (2007). Acute bacterial skin infections and cellulitis. *Curr Opin Infect Dis* 20:118–123.

41 Ibid.

42 Ibid.

43 Hepburn, M. J., et al. (2004). Comparison of short course (5 days) and standard (10 days) treatment for uncomplicated cellulitis. *Arch Int Med* 164:1669–1674.

44 Bellew, S. G., et al. (2003). Successful treatment of recalcitrant dissecting cellulitis of the scalp with complete scalp excision and split thickness skin graft. *Dermatol Surg* 29:1068–1070.

45 US Food and Drug Administration. (2007). *New ointment treats impetigo.* Retrieved 03.29.08 from http://www.fda.gov/consumer/updates/impetigo052107.html

46 National Institutes of Allergy and Infectious Diseases, National Institutes of Health. (2007). *Impetigo.* Retrieved 03.29.08 from http://www3.niaid.nih.gov/healthscience/healthtopics/impetigo/overview.htm

47 Ibid.

48 U.S. National Library of Medicine. (2008). Impetigo. *MedlinePlus Medical Encyclopedia.* Retrieved 03.29.08 from http://www.nlm.nih.gov/medlineplus/impetigo.html

49 U.S. Food and Drug Administration. *New ointment treats impetigo.* Ibid.

50 Oranje, A. P., et al. (2007). Topical retapamulin ointment, 1% versus sodium fusidate ointment, 2% for impetigo: a randomized, observer-blinded, noninferiority study. *Dermatology* 215:331–340.

51 National Institutes of Health. (2007). Group A streptococcal infections. Retrieved 03.29.08 from http://www3.niaid.nih.gov/healthscience/healthtopics/streptococcal/research.htm

52 New Zealand Dermatological Society. (2010). *Candida.* Retrieved 11.20.2010 from http://dermnetnz.org/fungal/candida.html

53 Ibid.

54 Ibid.

55 National Candida Society. (2010). *What is candida?* Retrieved 11.20.2010 from http://www.candida-society.org.uk

56 Ibid.

57 Tinea infections. (2008). *MedlinePlus Medical Encyclopedia.* Retrieved 03.29.08 from http://www.nlm.nih.gov/medlineplus/tineainfections.html

58 Szepietowski, J. C. (2006). Factors influencing coexistence of toenail onychomycosis with Tinea pedis and other dermatomycoses. *Arch Dermatol* 142:1279–1284.

59 American Osteopathic College of Dermatology. (n.d.). Fungus infections: preventing recurrence. *Dermatologic Database.* Retrieved 03.29.08 from http://www.aocd.org/skin/dermatologic_diseases/fungus_preventing.html

60 VisualDxHealth. (2008). *Ringworm, facial (tinea faciale): information for adults. Treatments your physician may prescribe.* Retrieved 03.29.08 from http://www.visualdxhealth.com/adult/tineaFaciale-treatments.htm

61 Ibid.

62 American Social Health Association. (2008). Herpes: signs and symptoms. Retrieved 7.25.2009 from http://www.ashastd.org/herpes/herpes_learn_symptoms.cfm

63 U.S. National Library of Medicine. (2010). Herpes simplex. *Medline-Plus Medical Encyclopedia.* Retrieved 11.18.2010 from http://www.nlm.nih.gov/medlineplus/herpessimplex.html

64 American Social Health Association. Ibid.

65 American Social Health Association. (2008). Treatment for genital herpes. Retrieved 6.9.2009 from http://www.ashastd.org/herpes/herpes_learn_treatment.cfm#1

66 Stöppler, M. C., & Shiel, W. C. (2010). Shingles (herpes zoster). *MedicineNet.com.* Retrieved 11.18.2010 from http://www.medicinenet.com/shingles/article.htm

67 Centers for Disease Control and Prevention. (2008). Vaccines and immunizations. Shingles disease—questions and answers (herpes zoster). Retrieved 6.9.2009 from http://www.cdc.gov/vaccines/vpd-vac/shingles/dis-faqs.htm

68 Krause, R. S. (2010). Herpes zoster. *eMedicine from WebMD.* Retrieved 11.19.2010 from http://www.emedicine.com/emerg/TOPIC823.HTM

69 Ibid.

70 Stöppler, M. C., & Shiel, W. C. Ibid.

71 Ibid.

72 Gandhi, M. (2006). Shingles. *MedlinePlus Medical Encyclopedia.* Retrieved 11.19.2010 from http://www.nlm.nih.gov/medlineplus/ency/article/000858.htm

73 Ibid.

74 Ibid.

75 Ibid.

76 Krause, R. S. Ibid.

77 Stöppler, M. C., & Shiel, W. C. Ibid.

78 Krause, R. S. Ibid.

79 Stöppler, M. C., & Shiel, W. C. Ibid.

80 Centers for Disease Control and Prevention. Vaccines and immunizations. Shingles disease—Questions and answers (herpes zoster). Ibid.

81 Stöppler, M. C., & Shiel, W. C. Ibid.

82 Mitka, M. (2006). FDA approves shingles vaccine: herpes zoster vaccine targets older adults. *JAMA* 296:157–158.

83 Rosen, T. (2003). Update on genital lesions. *JAMA* 290:1001–1005.

84 Higgins, R. V., Naumann, R. W., & Hall, J. (2010). Condyloma acuminatum. *eMedicine by WebMD.* Retrieved 11.18.2010 from http://www.emedicine.com/med/TOPIC3293.HTM

85 Higgins, R. V., Naumann, R. W., & Hall, J. Ibid.

86 Berman, K. (2009). Warts. *MedlinePlus Medical Encyclopedia.* Retrieved 6.5.2010 from http://www.nlm.nih.gov/medlineplus/ency/article/000885.htm

87 Higgins, R. V., Naumann, R. W., & Hall, J. Ibid.

88 Berman, K. Ibid.

89 Ibid.

90 Ibid.

91 Centers for Disease Control and Prevention. (2010). *Parasites: scabies.* Retrieved 11.18.2010 from http://www.cdc.gov/parasites/scabies/

92 Holness, D. L., DeKoven, J. G., & Nethercott, J. R. (1992). Scabies in chronic health care institutions. *Arch Dermatol* 128:1257–1260.

93 Walton, S. F., & Currie, B. J. (2007). Problems in diagnosing scabies, a global disease in human and animal populations. *Clin Microbiol Rev* 20:268–279.

94 Rockoff, A., & Stöppler, M. C. (2010). Scabies. *MedicineNet.com.* Retrieved 11.18.2010 from http://www.medicinenet.com/scabies/article.htm

95 Walton, S. F., & Currie, B. J. Ibid.

96 Centers for Disease Control and Prevention. (2010). *Parasites: scabies.* Ibid.

97 Walton, S. F., & Currie, B. J. (2007). Ibid.

98 Chouela, E. N. et al. (1999). Equivalent therapeutic efficacy and safety of ivermectin and lindane in the treatment of human scabies. *Arc Dermatol* 135:651–655.

99 Garcia, C., et al. (2007). Use of ivermectin to treat an institutional outbreak of scabies in a low-resource setting. *Infect Control Hosp Epidemiol* 28:13337–1338.

100 Rockoff, A., & Stöppler, M. C. Ibid.

101 Rubeiz, N., & Kibbi, A-G. (2009). Pediculosis. *eMedicine from WebMD*. Retrieved 6.9.2010 from http://www.emedicine.com/emerg/topic409.htm

102 Ibid.

103 Ibid.

104 Ibid.

105 Meinking, T. L. (2001). Comparative efficacy of treatments for pediculosis capitis infestations. *Arch Dermatol* 137:287–292.

106 Thomas, D. R., et al. (2006). Surveillance of insecticide resistance in head lice using biochemical and molecular methods. *Arch Dis Child* 91:777–778.

107 Fulton, J., Jr. (2010). Acne vulgaris. eMedicine from WebMD. Retrieved 11.20.2010 from http://emedicine.medscape.com/article/1069804-overview

108 Rockoff, A. (2008). Acne (pimples). *MedicineNet.com*. Retrieved 5.6.2009 from http://www.medicinenet.com/acne/article.htm

109 Fulton, J., Jr. Ibid.

110 Taylor, J. S., & Praditsuwan, P. (1996). Latex allergy. Review of 44 cases including outcome and frequent association with allergic hand eczema. *Arch Dermatol* 132:265–271.

111 Hanifin, J. M. (2008). *Research confirms genetic skin barrier linked to eczema*. American Academy of Dermatology. Retrieved 3.29.08 from http://www.aad.org/media/background/news/Releases/Research_Confirms_Genetic_Skin_Barrier_Defect_Link/

112 Becker, J. M. (2007). Allergic rhinitis. *eMedicine from WebMD*. Pediatrics, allergy and immunology. Retrieved on 03.25.07 from http://www.emedicine.com/ped/topic2560.htm

113 U.S. National Library of Medicine. (2010). Eczema. *MedlinePlus Medical Encyclopedia*. Retrieved 11.20.2010 from http://www.nlm.nih.gov/medlineplus/eczema.html

114 Atopic dermatitis. (2005). *MedicineNet.com*. Retrieved 03.25.07 from http://www.medicinenet.com/atopic_dermatitis/page6.htm

115 National Eczema Association. (2009). *All about atopic dermatitis*. Retrieved 5.6.2009 from http://www.nationaleczema.org/living/all_about_atopic_dermatits.htm

116 Hanifin, J. M. (2008). *Research confirms genetic skin barrier linked to eczema*. American Academy of Dermatology. Retrieved 4.6.2009 from http://www.aad.org/media/background/news/skinconditions_2008_02_03_research.html

117 DermNet NZ. (2010). *Allergic contact dermatitis*. Retrieved 11.20.2010 from http://www.dermnetnz.org/dermatitis/contact-allergy.html

118 Atopic dermatitis. (2005). Ibid.

119 Ibid.

120 National Institute of Arthritis and Musculoskeletal and Skin Diseases. (2003). *Atopic dermatitis*. Retrieved 07.26.07 from http://www.niams.nih.gov/hi/topics/dermatitis/#link_e

121 DermNet NZ. Ibid.

122 vanCoevorden, A. M. et al. (2004). Comparison of oral Psoralen-UV-A with a portable tanning unit at home versus hospital administered bath Psoralen-UV-A in patients with chronic hand eczema: an open-label randomized controlled trial of efficacy. *Arch Dermatol* 140:1463–1466.

123 DermNet NZ. Ibid.

124 National Psoriasis Foundation. (2010). *About psoriasis: statistics*. Retrieved 11.20.2010 from http://www.psoriasis.org/netcommunity/learn_statistics

125 Gordon, R., & Rosh, A. J. (2010). Psoriasis. *eMedicine from WebMD*. Retrieved 11.20.2010 from http://emedicine.medscape.com/article/762805-overview

126 Huerta, C., Rivero, E., & Rodriguez, L. A. G. (2007). Incidence and risk factors for psoriasis in the general population. *Arch Dermatol* 143:1559–1565.

127 Gordon, R., & Rosh, A. J. Ibid.

128 Gelfand, J. M. (2007). Long-term treatment for severe psoriasis: we're halfway there, with a long way to go. *Arch Dermatol* 143:1191–1193.

129 National Psoriasis Foundation. (2010). *About psoriasis: statistics*. Retrieved 11.20.2010 from http://www.psoriasis.org/netcommunity/learn_statistics

130 National Institute of Arthritis and Musculoskeletal and Skin Diseases. (2006). *Researchers identify gene which causes susceptibility to psoriasis*. Retrieved 3.29.08 from http://www.niams.nih.gov/News_and_Events/Spotlight_on_Research/2006/psoriasis_gene.asp

131 Huerta, C., Rivero, E., & Rodriguez, L. A. G. (2007). Incidence and risk factors for psoriasis in the general population. *Arch Dermatol* 143:1559–1565.

132 Herron, M. D., et al. (2005). Impact of obesity and smoking on psoriasis presentation and management. *Arch Dermatol* 14:1527–1534.

133 U.S. National Library of Medicine. (2010). Psoriasis. *MedlinePlus Medical Encyclopedia*. Retrieved 11.20.2010 from http://www.nlm.nih.gov/medlineplus/psoriasis.html

134 Gelfand, J. M. (2007). The risk of mortality in patients with psoriasis: results from a population-based study. *Arch Dermatol* 143:1493–1499.

135 National Psoriasis Foundation. (2008). Over-the-counter (OTC) topicals. Retrieved from http://www.psoriasis.org/netcommunity/sublearn03_mild_otc

136 Gordon, R., & Rosh, A. J. Ibid.

137 Gelfand, J. M. Long-term treatment for severe psoriasis: we're halfway there, with a long way to go. Ibid.

138 Nijsten, T., Looman, C. W. N., & Stern, R. S. (2007). Clinical severity of psoriasis in last 20 years of PUVA study. *Arch Dermatol* 143:1113–1121.

139 Borockaw, T., et al. (2007). A pragmatic randomized controlled trial on the effectiveness of highly concentrated saline spa water baths followed by UVB compared to UVB only in moderate to severe psoriasis. *J Altern Complement Med* 13:725–732.

140 Su, J., Pearce, D. J., & Feldman, S. R. (2005). The role of commercial tanning beds and ultraviolet A light in the treatment of psoriasis. *J Dermatol Treat* 16:324–326.

141 Bader, R. S. (2009). Basal cell carcinoma. *eMedicine from WebMD*. Retrieved 11.20.2010 from http://www.emedicine.com/MED/topic214.htm

142 Ibid.

143 Ibid.

144 Berman, K. (2008). Basal cell carcinoma. *MedlinePlus Medical Encyclopedia*. Retrieved from http://www.nlm.nih.gov/medlineplus/ency/article/000824.htm

145 Ibid.

146 Ibid.

147 Bader, R. S. Ibid.

148 The Skin Cancer Foundation. (2010). Squamous cell carcinoma. Retrieved 11.20.2010 from http://www.skincancer.org/squamous/index.php

149 Hess, S. D., & Schmults, C. D. (2010). Squamous cell carcinoma. *eMedicine from WebMD*. http://emedicine.medscape.com/article/1101535-overview

150 Smith, R. V. (2008). Oral squamous cell carcinoma. *Merck Manuals Online Medical Library for Healthcare Professionals*. Retrieved 4.6.2009 from http://www.merck.com/mmpe/sec08/ch093/ch093e.html

151 The Skin Cancer Foundation. Ibid.

152 Hess, S. D., & Schmults, C. D. Ibid.

153 The Skin Cancer Foundation. Ibid.

154 Kantor, J. (2009). Squamous cell skin cancer. *MedlinePlus Medical Encyclopedia*. Retrieved from http://www.nlm.nih.gov/medlineplus/ency/article/000829.htm

155 The Skin Cancer Foundation. Squamous cell carcinoma. Ibid.

156 Hess, S. D., & Schmults, C. D. Ibid.

157 National Cancer Institute. (2010). *Squamous cell carcinoma of the skin*. Retrieved 11.20.2010 from http://www.cancer.gov/cancertopics/pdq/treatment/skin/HealthProfessional/page5

158 The Skin Cancer Foundation. Ibid.

159 Kantor, J. Ibid.

160 Swetter, S. M. (2010). Malignant melanoma. *eMedicine from WebMD*. Retrieved 11.20.2010 from http://www.emedicine.com/DERM/topic257.htm

161 Ibid.

162 Ibid.

163 Ibid.

164 Melanoma. (2010). *Medline Plus*. Retrieved 11.20.2010 from http://www.nlm.nih.gov/medlineplus/melanoma.html

165 Swetter, S. M. Ibid.

166 Ibid.

167 Ibid.

168 Tan, W. W. (2010). Malignant melanoma. *eMedicine from WebMD*. Retrieved 11.20.2010 from http://emedicine.medscape.com/article/280245-overview

169 Swetter, S. M. Ibid.

170 Tan, W. W. (2010). Ibid.

171 American Cancer Society. (2006). *What is Kaposi sarcoma?* Retrieved from http://www.cancer.org/docroot/cri/content/cri_2_4_1x_what_is_kaposis_sarcoma_21.asp?sitearea=cri

172 American Cancer Society. (2006). *Do we know what causes Kaposi's sarcoma?* Retrieved from http://www.cancer.org/docroot/CRI/content/CRI_2_4_2X_Do_we_know_what_causes_Kaposis_Sarcoma_21.asp?rnav=cri

173 Abada, R., et al. (2008). SIAH-1 interacts with the Kaposi's sarcoma associated herpesvirus-encoded ORF45 protein and promotes its ubiquitination and proteasomal degradation. *J Virol* 82:3.

174 Bektas, M., et al. (2008). Colorectal involvement of Kaposi's sarcoma in a HIV negative case. *Digest Endosc* 20:96–97.

175 Serraina, D., et al. (2007). Risk of cancer following immunosuppression in organ transplant recipients and in HIV-positive individuals in southern Europe. *Eur J Cancer* 43:2117–2123.

176 American Cancer Society. What is Kaposi sarcoma? Ibid.

177 Spano, J-P., et al. (2000). Factors predictive of disease progression and death in AIDS-related Kaposi's sarcoma. *HIV Med* 1:232–237.

178 American Cancer Society. (2006). *General considerations in the treatment of Kaposi sarcoma*. Retrieved 11.22.10 from http://www.cancer.org/Cancer/KaposiSarcoma/DetailedGuide/kaposi-sarcoma-treating-general-considerations

179 Grey, J. E., & Harding, K. G. (2006). Venous and arterial leg ulcers. *BMJ* 332:347–350.

180 Ibid.

181 Armstrong, D. G., & Lavery, L. A. (1998). Diabetic ulcers: prevention, diagnosis and classification. *Am Fam Physicians*. Retrieved 05.01.08 from http://www.aafp.org/afp/980315ap/armstron.html

182 Stillman, R. M. (2010). Diabetic ulcers. *eMedicine from WebMD*. Retrieved 11.22.10 from http://emedicine.medscape.com/article/460282-overview

183 Armstrong, D. G., & Lavery, L. A. Ibid.

184 Ibid.

185 Ibid.

186 Grey, J. E., & Harding, K. G. Ibid.

187 McCulloch, S. V., et al. (2003). Healing potential of lower-extremity ulcers in patients with arterial insufficiency with and without revascularization. *Wounds* 15:390–394.

188 Ibid.

189 Hopf, H. W., et al. (2006). Guidelines for the treatment of arterial insufficiency ulcers. *Wound Repair Regen* 14:693–710, p. 702.

190 Stillman, R. M. (2010). Diabetic ulcers. *eMedicine from WebMD*. Retrieved 11.22.10 from http://emedicine.medscape.com/article/460282-overview

191 Hopf, H. W., et al. Ibid., p. 706.

192 Ibid., p. 699.

193 Ibid., p. 709.

194 Sussman, C., & Bates-Jensen, B. M. (2006). *Wound care: a collaborative practice manual for health professionals*, 3rd edition. Gaithersburg, MD: Lippincott Williams & Wilkins.

195 Hopf, H. W., et al. Ibid., p. 699.

196 Sussman, C. (1998).Whirlpool in wound care. *Wound Care Information Network*. Retrieved 11.22.10 from http://medicaledu.com/whirlpoo.htm

197 Hopf, H. W., et al. Ibid., p. 705.

198 Hopf, H. W., et al. Ibid., p. 704.

199 Venous ulcers. (2005). *The Doctor's Doctor*. Retrieved 5.01.08 from http://www.thedoctorsdoctor.com/Diseases/skin_ulcer_venous.htm

200 Khachemoune, A., & Kauffman, C. L. (2007). Management of leg ulcers. *Internet J Dermatol* 1. Retrieved 5.01.08 from http://www.ispub.com/ostia/index.php?xmlFilePath=journals/ijd/vol1n2/ulcer2.xml

201 Venous ulcers. Ibid.

202 Khachemoune, A., & Kauffman, C. L. Ibid.

203 Venous ulcers. Ibid.

204 Khachemoune, A., & Kauffman, C. L. Ibid.

205 Feedar, J. A., Kloth, L. C., & Gentzhow, G. D. (1991). Chronic dermal ulcer healing enhanced with monophasic pulsed electrical stimulation. *Phys Ther* 71:639–649.

206 Houghton, P. E., et al. (2003). Effect of electrical stimulation on chronic leg ulcer size and appearance. *Phys Ther* 83:17–28.

207 Choucair, M., & Phillips, T. J. (1998). Compression therapy. *Dermatol Surg* 24:141–148.

208 Revis, D. R. (2010). Decubitus ulcers. *eMedicine from WebMD*. Retrieved 11.22.10 from http://www.emedicine.com/med/topic2709.htm

209 Ibid.

210 Ibid.

211 Ibid.

212 Collison, D. W. (2008). Dermatologic disorders: pressure ulcers. *Merck Manuals Online Medical Library for Healthcare Professionals*. Retrieved 6.4.2009 from http://www.merck.com/mmpe/sec10/ch126/ch126a.html?qt=shear++stress&alt=sh

213 Revis, D. R. Ibid.

214 Collison, D. W. Dermatologic disorders: pressure ulcers. Ibid.

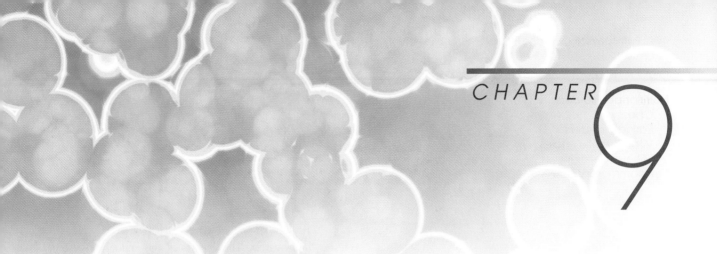

Endocrine, Metabolic, and Nutritional Disorders

LEARNING OBJECTIVES

After completion of this chapter, students should be able to:

- Review the anatomy and physiology of the endocrine system
- Describe the pathological mechanisms of endocrine diseases, metabolic diseases, and nutritional disorders
- Discuss the physical therapy interventions for patients with diabetes mellitus and other endocrine, metabolic, and nutritional disorders
- Determine the role of the physical therapist assistant working with patients with endocrine, metabolic, and nutritional disorders
- Apply contraindications, precautions, and special indications for physical therapist/physical therapist assistant intervention for patients with diabetes mellitus and other endocrine, metabolic, and nutritional disorders

KEY TERMS

Acromegaly
Addison's disease
Addisonian crisis
Autonomic neuropathy
Body mass index (BMI)
Calcimimetic medications
Cushing's disease
Dermatome
Diabetes insipidus
Diabetes mellitus
Diabetic neuropathy
Gigantism
Graves' disease
Homeostasis
Hypercalcemia
Hypercalcuria
Hyperglycemia
Myotome
Myxedema
Peripheral neuropathy
Relative weight

CHAPTER OUTLINE

CHAPTER OUTLINE (continued)

Nutritional Disorders
   Obesity
   Eating disorders
   Vitamin deficiencies
   Mineral deficiencies
   Inflammatory bowel disease

Introduction

This chapter provides a basic review of the anatomy and physiology of the endocrine and metabolic systems. Diseases and disorders of the endocrine system such as pituitary, thyroid, parathyroid, and adrenal diseases are described. Diabetes mellitus (DM) is fully discussed with the inclusion of guidelines for the physical therapist assistant (PTA) when treating people with DM. Metabolic disorders including the balance of acids and bases in the human system, phenylketonuria, and Wilson's disease are described. Some of the nutritional disorders are also included in this chapter, such as obesity, eating disorders, and vitamin and mineral deficiencies.

Why Does The Physical Therapist Assistant Need to Know About the Anatomy and Physiology of the Endocrine System?

An understanding of the anatomy and physiology of the complex endocrine system serves as a basis for the pathological disorders of this system. The normal interaction of the endocrine glands of the body maintains homeostasis (optimal functioning) within the body. Disturbances in these interactions result in the disorders of the endocrine system, which affect the levels of strength and energy available for people who participate in physical therapy interventions.

Anatomy and Physiology of the Endocrine System

The endocrine system consists of many areas of the body including the pituitary, thyroid and parathyroid glands, adrenal glands, and certain cells of the pancreas, thymus, testes, and ovaries. These parts of the endocrine system are connected through the blood circulation and act as a regulating mechanism for the functions of the body systems. Details of the endocrine glands, including their hormones and effects, are found in Table 9-1. The ductless endocrine glands produce and secrete hormones that travel through the body via the blood supply and affect other organs or body systems specific to the individual hormone. Hormones are chemicals produced by the endocrine system and may be of various types such as proteins, steroids, peptides, amino acids, or amines. All of the endocrine glands are closely related, and damage or malfunction of one affects the others. When the endocrine system works correctly, body systems work smoothly. When the endocrine system is imbalanced, with an over- or underproduction of hormones, malabsorption of the hormone by the specific organ, or a breakdown of the transport system, the body reacts adversely.

The pituitary gland, also known as the "master gland," is a small saclike organ approximately 1 cm in diameter and located at the base of the brain in the sella turcica (Turkish saddle).[1] The pituitary gland lies close to the hypothalamus. The anterior and posterior sections of the pituitary are connected to the hypothalamus by neurons, and pituitary blood vessels. The pituitary gland controls and releases trophic hormones into the blood circulation, which all have an effect on other endocrine glands, and nonendocrine structures (see Table 9-1). The posterior pituitary consists of the axons of cells located in the hypothalamus. The hypothalamus releases substances called neuroendocrine releasing factors into the pituitary, which control the functional release of the hormones produced by the pituitary. See Table 9-1 for details of the hormones released by the pituitary.

The thyroid, and four parathyroid glands, lie together in the neck. The thyroid contains follicular cells and C cells, which produce different hormones. The thyroid and parathyroids are involved with the maintenance of calcium homeostasis in the blood (see Table 9.1).

The two adrenal glands are located in the abdomen attached to the kidneys. Each of the adrenal glands has a medulla and a cortex. The cortex has three areas, which each secrete different hormones: the zona glomerulosa, zona fasciculate, and zona reticularis. The adrenocorticotropic hormone (ACTH), produced by the pituitary gland, stimulates, the adrenal cortex. See Table 9-1 for details of hormones secreted by the adrenal glands. The islets of Langerhans cells located in the pancreas produce insulin, glucagon, and somatostatin, all of which have an effect on blood glucose levels. Disorders related to these hormones are detailed later in the chapter. The testes and ovaries produce hormones, which are listed in Table 9-1, and the diseases associated with dysfunction of these hormones are described in Chapter 11. The thymus is located in the mediastinum extending toward the thyroid in the neck and is involved with the production of T-cells crucial for an intact immune system. The T-cells develop in the thymus and then migrate to the lymph glands and the spleen under the influence of the hormone thymosin produced in the thymus.

Why Does the Physical Therapist Assistant Need to Know About Diseases and Disorders of the Endocrine System?

Disorders of the endocrine system are not directly treated with physical therapy. People with endocrine disorders attend physical therapy services for treatment of many other conditions. The effects of the endocrine disorder may have an impact on the interventions provided by the PT and PTA. Knowledge of the effects of a variety of endocrine disorders assists the PT and PTA in providing optimal interventions for people with a comorbid endocrine condition.

Table 9.1 Hormones Produced by Specific Endocrine Glands and Their Effects

ENDOCRINE GLAND	HORMONE(S) PRODUCED BY THE ENDOCRINE GLAND	EFFECT OF HORMONE
Anterior pituitary or adenohypophysis	Growth hormone (GH)	Affects tissue growth
	Prolactin (PRL)	Stimulates development and growth of the female mammary glands in preparation for lactation and then promotes milk production
	Adrenocorticotropic hormone (ACTH)	Stimulates the adrenal glands to produce cortical hormones
	Gonadotropins: luteinizing hormone (LH), follicle stimulating hormone (FSH)	LH stimulates the ovaries to produce ova, estrogen, and progesterone
		FSH stimulates the testis to produce sperm and testosterone
	Thyrotropic hormone (TSH) or thyroid stimulating hormone	Stimulates the thyroid to produce thyroid hormones; regulates T3 and T4 production by the C cells of the thyroid
Posterior pituitary or neurohypophysis	Oxytocin (pitressin): produced in the hypothalamus and stored and secreted by the posterior pituitary	Stimulates contraction of the uterus for birth and stimulates lactation (milk production) by the breast after birth
	Antidiuretic hormone (ADH): produced in the hypothalamus and stored and secreted by the posterior pituitary	Stimulates reabsorption of water by the kidneys
Thyroid	Follicular cells secrete thyroxine (T4) and triiodothyronine (T3)	Metabolism
	C cells secrete calcitonin (a polypeptide)	Affects calcium homeostasis in the blood

(table continues on page 386)

Table 9.1   **Hormones Produced by Specific Endocrine Glands and Their Effects** (continued)

ENDOCRINE GLAND	HORMONE(S) PRODUCED BY THE ENDOCRINE GLAND	EFFECT OF HORMONE
Parathyroids	Polypeptide parathormone (PTH)	Regulates homeostasis of calcium and phosphate in the blood Promotes resorption of calcium from renal tubules in kidney to reduce calcium levels in urine Promotes bone resorption and release of calcium into blood Stimulates production of vitamin D in the kidney, which aids in absorption of calcium from food in intestines
Adrenal cortex	Zona glomerulosa secretes mineral corticoids such as aldosterone Zona fasciculata secretes glucocorticoids such as cortisone Zona reticularis secretes sex steroids such as estrogens and androgens	Regulate potassium and sodium levels and affect carbohydrate metabolism Regulate potassium and sodium levels and affect carbohydrate metabolism Affect sex organ function
Adrenal medulla	Epinephrine and norepinephrine (amines)	Sympathetic nervous system functions and carbohydrate metabolism Create increase in blood pressure, tachycardia, and hyperglycemia (high levels of sugar in the blood)
Islets of Langerhans (Pancreas)	Insulin, glucagon, and somatostatin (polypeptides)	Control of blood sugar levels
Gonads	Androgens produced by the Leydig cells of the testes in the male—testosterone Estrogen Progesterone produced by ovaries in female	Male sex hormone controls male sexual characteristics Secretion is controlled by the gonadotropins from the pituitary Menstrual cycle, pregnancy Affects female reproductive organs, female sexual characteristics; stimulated by pituitary gonadotropins FSH and LH Progesterone stimulates the breast tissue for lactation and prepares endometrium for implantation of the fertilized ovum
Thymus	Thymosin	Development of T-cells essential for the immune system

Endocrine System Diseases and Disorders

HINTS ON USE OF THE GUIDE TO PHYSICAL THERAPIST PRACTICE

The classification of the *Guide to Physical Therapist Practice (2001)* practice patterns is complex when dealing with diabetes due to the various manifestations of the disease process. The specific pattern that is appropriate for the patient depends on the symptoms and course the disease has taken and what the physical therapy intervention relates to at a particular time. In all cases, the appropriate pattern is based on the evaluation findings of the physical therapist. The patterns may be musculoskeletal, neurological, cardiovascular/pulmonary, or integumentary.

- 4C "Impaired muscle performance" (p. S161): If the diabetes affects the patient's ability to perform functional tasks at work or home that require muscle strength, this is the most appropriate pattern within the musculoskeletal section.

- 4J "Impaired motor function, muscle performance, range of motion, gait, locomotion, and balance associated with amputation" (p. S287): In more severe restrictions of function subsequent to amputation, this would be the appropriate pattern within the musculoskeletal practice pattern.

- 5G "Impaired motor function and sensory integrity associated with acute or chronic polyneuropathies" (p. S411): Some patients with diabetes have lower or upper extremity diabetic neuropathy and 5G is the appropriate neuromuscular practice pattern.

- 6A Primary prevention/risk reduction for cardiovascular/pulmonary disorders (p. S465): A preventive course of therapy may be based on use of the relationship of diabetes to the risk of developing heart disease and fit into the cardiovascular/pulmonary practice pattern 6A.

- 6B Impaired aerobic capacity/endurance associated with deconditioning (p. S475): If the diabetes causes multisystem problems the patient may be designated under cardiovascular/pulmonary pattern 6B.

- 7A Primary prevention/risk reduction for integumentary disorders (p. S589): In many cases, patients with diabetes are at risk for skin conditions, burns, and ulcers due to neuropathy and/or vascular insufficiency and may have preventive therapy based on integumentary pattern 7A.

- 7B Impaired integumentary integrity associated with superficial skin involvement (p. S601): If a patient with diabetes develops a diabetic ulcer that requires physical therapy intervention, the integumentary pattern involved is 7B.

(From the American Physical Therapy Association, 2003. *Guide to physical therapist practice*, revised 2nd edition. Alexandria, VA: APTA. Used with permission.)

Endocrinology is the study of the endocrine system. A physician specializing in endocrinology is called an endocrinologist. Diseases of the endocrine system are caused by imbalances of specific hormones in the body. Hormonal imbalance may be due to over- or underproduction of a hormone by a specific endocrine gland or to the lack of ability of the organ or system affected by the hormone to absorb the necessary hormone. Interruption of the transport system of the hormone from the endocrine gland to its target may also be a cause of endocrine diseases.

Pituitary Diseases

The trophic hormones of the pituitary glands influence many of the other endocrine glands. The pituitary is controlled by the hypothalamus, which produces gonadotropin releasing hormone (GnRH).

Pituitary hypofunction

Pituitary hypofunction is a comparatively rare condition that can affect any age group, and all or part of the pituitary. Complete pituitary hypofunction in the adult is called Simmonds disease. Two other types of adult pituitary hypofunction include **diabetes insipidus,** resulting from damage to the posterior pituitary, and Sheehan's syndrome, resulting from blood loss to the pituitary during pregnancy. Pituitary dwarfism is the congenital form of pituitary hypofunction.

Etiology. Pituitary hypofunction may be the result of a congenital defect or a tumor of the pituitary gland or may be caused by ischemic factors resulting from illness or surgery. Pituitary tumors can be either benign or malignant. Simmonds disease results from damage to the pituitary from tumors, trauma at the base of the skull, or infection that causes complete hypofunction of the pituitary in the adult.[2] Pituitary dwarfism, or hypogonadism, is caused by a congenital defect of the pituitary. Damage to the posterior pituitary results in diabetes insipidus and causes reduced production of the antidiuretic hormone (ADH). Damage to the pituitary gland may also occur as a result of blood loss during delivery of a baby. The blood loss restricts the blood supply to the pituitary gland and results in a type of pituitary hypofunction called Sheehan's syndrome.

Signs and Symptoms. The signs and symptoms of Simmonds disease include weakness, hypotension, weight loss, loss of energy, atrophy of the internal organs, and, in some cases, severe emaciation as a result of the depletion of fat deposits. Pituitary dwarfism is characterized by short stature, failure to grow, delayed or absent puberty, headaches, excessive thirst, and increased urine output.[3] Diabetes insipidus is characterized by production of large amounts of urine as a result of the reduced production of antidiuretic hormone.

Prognosis. The prognosis for all types of pituitary hypofunction is good with appropriate treatment to restore the normal hormonal balance.

Medical Intervention. The diagnosis of pituitary dwarfism is achieved through testing for hormone deficiencies. The pharmacological intervention for pituitary dwarfism consists of supplementary doses of a synthetic growth hormone.[4] The pharmacological treatment for Simmonds disease involves providing doses of the deficient hormones normally produced by the pituitary gland. Diabetes insipidus is effectively treated with doses of ADH.[5]

Physical Therapy Intervention. Physical therapy is not indicated for pituitary hypofunction unless the side effects of the disease process create physical deficits treatable with physical therapy.

Hyperpituitarism

⊛ Hyperpituitarism may start in childhood, although rarely before the onset of puberty.[6] The adult onset of the condition is usually between the ages of 30 and 50. The incidence of hyperpituitarism in children is rare with less than 0.1 cases per million of the pediatric population annually.[7] The incidence of acromegaly, the adult manifestation of hyperpituitarism, is 116.9 cases per million of the population per year, with a prevalence of 4,676 cases per million of the population in the United States.[8]

Etiology. Enlargement of the pituitary may be caused by adenomas and may affect any or all of the parts of the pituitary. The resulting signs and symptoms caused by the adenoma is dependent on which cells in the pituitary are affected by the tumor. Most pituitary tumors are benign, but some may cause compression of the optic chiasm and lead to blindness.

Signs and Symptoms. In both the adult and the child, the condition causes overproduction of growth hormone (GH), which upsets the normal endocrine balance for growth factors. GH stimulates the liver to produce insulin-like growth factor (IGF-1) that in turn causes body tissue growth. When high levels of IGF-1 exist the usual reaction of the pituitary is to reduce the production and release of GH, but when a tumor is present, the pituitary continues to release excessive amounts of GH. The hypothalamus produces and releases somatostatin, a hormone that also inhibits GH production and release. This system of checks and balances for the release of GH is interrupted by the pituitary tumor resulting in **acromegaly** in the adult and **gigantism** in the child.[9] ⊛ If the growth hormone cells in the anterior lobe of the pituitary are affected in the child, there is an overproduction of growth hormone, resulting in such characteristics as longitudinal growth of the bones and gigantism. In some instances, children exhibit weight gain and failure to grow as a result of adenoma growth on the pituitary.[10] Acromegaly in the adult results in large hands and feet; enlarged jaw, nose, lips, and tongue; general changes in facial appearance with thickening of the facial soft tissues; and mood swings

(see Fig. 9-1).[11] Acromegaly also causes enlargement of the internal organs including the heart, resulting in cardiomyopathy. Other problems caused by acromegaly include diabetes, hyperglycemia, hypercalcemia, hypertension, fatigue, impaired vision, headaches, and arthritis.[12,13] If pituitary tumors affect the corticotropic cells that produce ACTH, symptoms occur similar to that of **Cushing's disease.** This disease is described in the section on adrenocortical diseases.

Prognosis. Once diagnosed, the prognosis is good for both children and adults with pituitary adenomas when surgical excision of the adenoma is performed. The success of surgical excision depends on the size of the pituitary tumor and whether the whole tumor can be removed. If the tumor has grown large and encroaches on other areas of the brain, the long-term results may not be as good. Untreated acromegaly can cause death.

Medical Intervention. The diagnosis of all forms of pituitary dysfunction can be the most difficult part of the medical intervention process. Part of the diagnostic process is to check the levels of GH, IGF-1, and somatostatin in the blood. Several types of medical intervention are possible for acromegaly and gigantism. Surgical excision of the enlarged pituitary, or the tumor within the pituitary, can be performed, but changes in the bone are not reversible. Transsphenoidal surgical excision is usually performed through the nose to access the pituitary at the frontal area of the brain.[14] Radiation therapy may be performed after surgical excision if parts of the tumor remain. Pharmacological interventions include substances called somatostatin analogs (SSAs) that shrink the tumor before surgery, GH receptor agonists that interfere with the action of

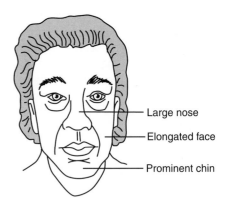

FIGURE 9.1 The face of a woman affected with acromegaly showing a thickened appearance of the tissues of the cheeks, chin, and forehead.

Large nose

Elongated face

Prominent chin

GH and normalize IGF-1 levels, and pituitary hormone replacement therapy when all of the pituitary is removed.[15]

Physical Therapy Intervention. Physical therapy is not a primary treatment for the treatment of people with hyperpituitarism. People with acromegaly may require intervention for muscle strengthening and management of the arthritic symptoms associated with the condition.

Thyroid Diseases

Thyroid diseases occur when there is an imbalance in the concentration of the thyroid producing hormones circulating in the body. The imbalance may be caused by over-or under-production of these hormones. Major causes of these disorders include autoimmune disorders, congenital absence of the thyroid, or the presence of tumors.

Hyperthyroidism

Hyperthyroidism is an autoimmune disease in which antibodies develop that mimic thyrotropic or thyroid stimulating hormone (TSH), causing the thyroid to secrete excessive amounts of thyroxine (T4) and triiodothyronine (T3) hormones.[16] **Graves' disease** is one of the more common types of hyperthyroidism and is 8 times more common in women than in men.[17] The age of onset is typically between the ages of 30 and 40.

Etiology. Several causes of hyperthyroidism exist including Graves' disease, toxic nodular goiter, hyperplasia of the thyroid, thyroiditis, and thyroid tumors. Most thyroid tumors are benign adenomas. Malignant tumors of the thyroid are extremely rare. Taking thyroid hormone supplements can also precipitate hyperthyroidism.[18] In all cases, hyperthyroidism is characterized by an overproduction of thyroid hormones, also known as thyrotoxicosis. Nodular goiter and adenomas (benign tumors) of the thyroid gland cause enlargement of part of the thyroid, whereas Graves' disease and thyroiditis cause enlargement of the whole thyroid gland.

Signs and Symptoms. The signs and symptoms of hyperthyroidism develop slowly and thus are detected only when the symptoms become more severe. Patients with Graves' disease often have a characteristic exophthalmos, a condition of bulging eyes (see Fig. 9-2). A goiter is an enlargement of the thyroid, noticeable as a horizontal swelling on the anterior of the neck. Some of the other signs and symptoms of hyperthyroidism include nervousness and tremor, depression, mood swings, fatigue, diarrhea, restlessness, tachycardia, congestive heart failure

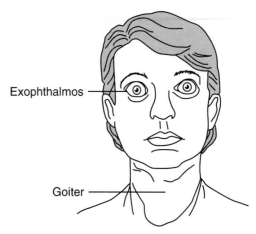

FIGURE 9.2 A patient with Grave's disease showing the typical goiter and exophthalmos, with wide open eyes, staring, or protrusion of the eyeball.

(CHF), heat intolerance, palpitations, profuse sweating, hair loss, blurred or double vision, changes in the menstrual cycle, muscle weakness, inflammation of the ligaments and tendons, and weight loss with increased appetite.[19,20,21] In severe cases, hyperthyroidism can cause blindness and osteoporosis.[22] A goiter may be present. Not all goiters have a hyper- or hypothyroid effect, and not all signs and symptoms are present in each person.

Prognosis. Most people with hyperthyroidism can be treated successfully with one of the methods detailed in the "medical intervention" section. People with severe Graves' disease may experience blindness. The condition can be fatal if left untreated.[23]

Medical Intervention. The diagnosis of hyperthyroidism may be partially achieved through blood tests. People with hyperthyroidism exhibit low levels of TSH in serum and higher than normal levels of T4 and T3.[24] Some of the laboratory medical tests performed for the diagnosis of thyroid dysfunction can be seen in Table 9-2. Several options are available for the medical treatment of the disease. Pharmacological intervention with beta blockers such as propranolol or Inderal blocks the effects of the excessive thyroid hormones produced but does not cure the actual thyroid problem. Antithyroid medications such as methimazole and propylthiouracil (PTV) reduce the production of thyroid hormones by the thyroid. The thyroid selectively absorbs iodine, and so radioactive iodine treatment can be administered to destroy the thyroid cells, thus reducing the amount of hormones produced. Surgical excision using a partial thyroidectomy or complete thyroidectomy can also

Table 9.2   **Some Thyroid Function Tests**

TEST	PURPOSE
Serum TSH	Tests for hyper and hypothyroidism
T3	Elevated levels in hyperthyroidism
Free T4	Screening for hyper or hypothyroidism
TSH receptor antibody	Positive in Graves' disease

TSH = thyroid stimulating hormone.

be performed. Surgical excision carries certain risks including damage to the recurrent laryngeal nerve that supplies the larynx in 1% of cases.[25]

Physical Therapy Intervention. The PT and PTA may treat people with hyperthyroidism if the signs and symptoms include muscle and soft tissue deficits.

Precautions for Physical Therapy Intervention. Precautions include ensuring that the patient does not become too fatigued during treatment and monitoring heart rate and blood pressure, particularly in the postsurgical patient. Patients who have received radiation treatment for thyroid cancers have contamination of their saliva. Specific precautions must be followed to prevent irradiation of the PT and PTA during physical therapy intervention, particularly during the performance of postural drainage and pulmonary hygiene techniques.

Hypothyroidism

Hypothyroidism, or underactive thyroid, is a lack of production and secretion of thyroid hormones. Several types of hypothyroidism exist including cretinism, Hashimoto's disease/Hashimoto's thyroiditis, congenital aplasia, secondary hypothyroidism, and tertiary hypothyroidism. Hypothyroidism is a common condition affecting approximately 3% to 5% of the U.S. population, and the disease is between 2 and 8 times more common in women than in men.[26,27] The incidence of the disease increases with age with between 2% and 20% of older adults experiencing symptoms of hypothyroidism.[28] Cretinism, or congenital hypothyroidism, occurs in 1 out of 4,000 newborns.[29] In congenital aplasia, the person is born without a thyroid gland.

Etiology. Hypothyroidism has several causes. Cretinism is a form of congenital hypothyroidism. People born

without a thyroid gland have congenital aplasia. Thyroiditis, inflammation of the thyroid gland, also known as Hashimoto's disease or Hashimoto's thyroiditis, causes enlargement of the thyroid. Hashimoto's is an inherited, autoimmune disease that is up to 10 times more common in women than men.[30] After the inflammation of Hashimoto's disease subsides, the thyroid may be replaced with fibrous tissue, and a shrinking of the thyroid occurs, which causes a reduction in the function of the thyroid gland. The thyroid requires iodine to synthesize thyroid hormones, thus iodine deficiency can also cause hypothyroidism by reducing the thyroid's ability to produce thyroid hormones. Secondary hypothyroidism is caused by pituitary disease, and tertiary hypothyroidism is caused by hypothalamic disease. Both the pituitary and hypothalamus secrete hormones that directly affect the thyroid. Subclinical hypothyroidism is a recognized condition that indicates the predisposition to develop hypothyroidism.

Signs and Symptoms. The characteristic signs and symptoms of hypothyroidism vary depending on the age of the patient. In children, the condition results in thyroid dwarfism associated with mental retardation. In adults, the main characteristic is **myxedema,** also known as Gull's disease, with signs and symptoms such as edema of the skin, obesity, intolerance to cold, and lack of energy. The systemic effects of hypothyroidism cause total metabolic slow down, which affects multiple body organs and systems causing reduced mental alertness, impaired memory, depression, emotional lability, weight gain, bradycardia, hypercholesterolemia, fatigue, reduced physical endurance, constipation, muscle weakness, muscle cramping, stiffness, lower extremity edema, and general body aches.[31,32] People with Hashimoto's disease tend to have other autoimmune conditions, such as diabetes or pernicious anemia. See Figure 9-3 for a comparison of hyperthyroidism and hypothyroidism. Hypothyroidism during pregnancy may increase the possibility of side effects such as preeclampsia, anemia, postpartum hemorrhage, spontaneous abortion, low birth weight, impaired cognitive function of the fetus, and fetal mortality.[33]

Prognosis. Most people with hypothyroidism can be effectively treated with medications. In some severe cases, a life-threatening myxedema coma can occur, triggered by illness, stress, trauma, or surgery. When left untreated, hypothyroidism can result in cardiomyopathy (enlarged heart), heart failure, and pleural effusion (fluid

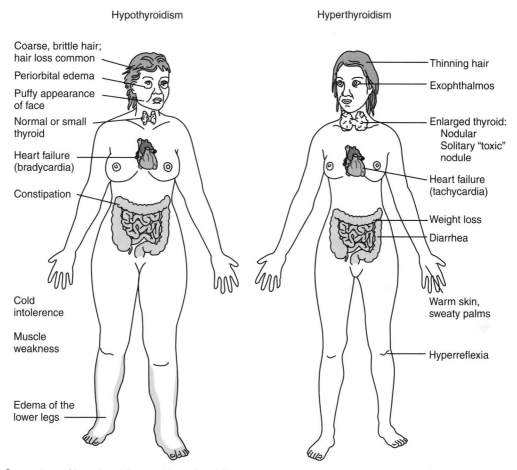

Hypothyroidism

Hyperthyroidism

- Coarse, brittle hair; hair loss common
- Periorbital edema
- Puffy appearance of face
- Normal or small thyroid
- Heart failure (bradycardia)
- Constipation
- Cold intolerance
- Muscle weakness
- Edema of the lower legs

- Thinning hair
- Exophthalmos
- Enlarged thyroid: Nodular Solitary "toxic" nodule
- Heart failure (tachycardia)
- Weight loss
- Diarrhea
- Warm skin, sweaty palms
- Hyperreflexia

FIGURE 9.3 Comparison of hypothyroidism and hyperthyroidism

filled pleura). Such adverse side effects of the disease can impact the quality of life of the individual. Hypothyroidism experienced during pregnancy can have detrimental effects on the fetus as described under Signs and Symptoms.

Medical Intervention. The diagnosis of Hashimoto's disease is achieved through detection of antibodies to the enzyme thyroid peroxidase (anti-TPO antibodies) in the blood. Hypothyroidism can also be detected through blood tests for levels of the T4 and T3 hormones. However, in the early stages of the disease, these hormone levels may be within normal limits. Detection of higher than usual TSH levels may indicate that the pituitary is providing additional TSH to stimulate the thyroid to produce hormones.[34] The pharmacological treatment is through the administration of thyroid hormone medications such as synthetic T4 in the form of Levoxyl or Synthroid,

synthetic T3 in the form of Cytomel, or both. Medications are usually required for the rest of the person's life.

Physical Therapy Intervention. Physical therapy may be indicated to help improve the patient's endurance to activity and strengthen muscles.

Parathyroid Diseases. Parathyroid diseases are the result of over- or underproduction of the parathyroid hormones and are divided into hyperparathyroid and hypoparathyroid conditions.

Hyperparathyroidism. Hyperparathyroidism is overactivity of the parathyroid glands. The three types of hyperparathyroidism are primary, secondary, and tertiary. Approximately 100,000 people in the United States develop hyperthyroidism annually, and of these women outnumber men in a 2:1 ratio. The incidence of hyperparathyroidism increases with age.[35] ⊛ Secondary hyperparathyroidism in children can result in rickets, although this is rare in the United States.[36]

Etiology. The etiology of primary hyperparathyroidism is overproduction of parathormone, also called parathyroid hormone (PTH). Primary hyperparathyroidism often results from adenoma of the parathyroid, or hyperplasia of the parathyroid, and is less commonly the result of carcinoma. In cases of primary hyperparathyroidism, too much PTH is produced by the parathyroid glands in response to the malignant growth or hypertrophy of the glands. This overproduction of PTH in primary hyperparathyroidism can also cause a reduction in phosphate levels in the body as a result of overexcretion of phosphates from the kidneys.[37] In secondary hyperparathyroidism, the overproduction of PTH is triggered in response to low levels of calcium absorption as a result of vitamin D deficiency, or poor absorption of calcium within the intestines.[38] Malnutrition can cause secondary hyperparathyroidism. In children, low levels of calcium or vitamin D (or both) cause rickets.[39] ⊛ Rickets is a condition of childhood in which low calcium levels result in malformation of the bones and bowing of the long bones. Secondary and tertiary parathyroidism are often seen in persons with chronic renal insufficiency. Chronic renal disease is one of the main causes of secondary hyperparathyroidism, although gastric bypass surgery may also cause the condition as a result of alterations in vitamin D and calcium absorption.[40] When calcium levels in the urine rise sharply, the condition is termed tertiary.

Signs and Symptoms. The signs and symptoms of parathyroid disease range from none to severe. The pathological signs of hyperparathyroidism include **hypercalcemia** (too much calcium in the blood), **hypercalciuria** (high levels of calcium in the urine), high levels of PTH in circulating blood, bone resorption by overstimulation of osteoclasts, and renal disease. If bone resorption is severe, it can result in a condition called osteitis fibrosa cystica or von Recklinghausen's disease, both of which resemble osteoporosis. This in turn causes pathological fractures, resulting in an increased thoracic kyphosis, and compression fractures of the vertebral bodies of the spine.[41] Clinically the patient with primary hyperparathyroidism shows characteristics of bowel problems, weakness, hypotonic muscles, depression, and sometimes seizures. The characteristics of secondary hyperparathyroidism include decalcification of bones resulting in fractures, renal stones due to the buildup of calcium salts, muscle weakness,

fatigue, hypertension, constipation, nausea, vomiting, and mental changes such as poor memory or confusion.[42] ⊛ Children with rickets develop bone deformities such as bowing of the tibia and femur, joint effusions, and fractures.[43]

Prognosis. The prognosis is good for primary hyperparathyroidism after surgical excision of the parathyroid glands. Only approximately 1% of people develop problems with the vocal cords as a result of damage to the accessory nerve or the recurrent laryngeal branch of the vagus nerve during surgery. Secondary hyperparathyroidism caused by malabsorption of calcium or dietary insufficiencies of calcium or vitamin D, is usually reversible with corrections of the calcium and/or vitamin D dietary intake.[44] Vitamin D is essential for the body to be able to absorb calcium (see the section on vitamin deficiencies later in this chapter). Other types of secondary hyperparathyroidism may be more difficult to treat and depend on resolution of the initiating cause of the condition. ⊛ Children with rickets may develop permanent bowing of the long bones of the lower extremity if the disease is not treated early.

Medical Intervention. The diagnosis of primary hyperparathyroidism is achieved through blood tests demonstrating increased levels of calcium in the blood and urine, high levels of phosphate in urine, and low levels of phosphate in the blood serum. High levels of parathyroid hormone may also be detected in the blood. Surgical excision of the parathyroid glands is usually necessary if the cause of the disease is either an adenoma or hyperplasia of the parathyroid glands. **Calcimimetic** medications, molecular agents that reduce the levels of parathyroid hormone release by the parathyroid glands, may also be provided to reduce the amount of calcium production in primary hyperparathyroidism.[45,46] The treatment for secondary hyperparathyroidism is correction of the lack of calcium and/or vitamin D through the use of calcium and vitamin D supplements, and dietary changes.[47]

Physical Therapy Intervention. Physical therapy for these individuals usually involves the encouragement of gentle exercise and mobility. Many people with hyperparathyroidism have joint arthritis, back pain, or loss of functional mobility. Care must be taken when working with people with hyperparathyroidism because there is an increased danger of fracture as a result of the osteoporosis or osteopenia associated with the condition. When assisting individuals with transfers and ambulation, the PTA should do so gently and carefully. Energy conservation techniques are achieved by providing adequate rest between periods of activity because people may fatigue quickly.

Hypoparathyroidism

Reduced function of the parathyroids results in hypoparathyroidism.

Etiology. This condition is rare and is usually caused by surgery for carcinoma of the neck region in which the parathyroid glands are removed. Radioactive iodine treatment for hyperthyroidism occasionally causes damage to the parathyroid glands.[48] Another cause of the condition is a congenital absence of the parathyroid glands known as DiGeorge syndrome. The condition may also be caused by an autoimmune response or malignancy or be medication induced.[49]

Signs and Symptoms. The effects of hypoparathyroidism are generally the opposite to those of hyperparathyroidism. Loss of the parathyroid hormone (PTH) causes low levels of calcium in the blood, leading to changes in nerve transmission affecting the muscles and heart. The condition is also associated with high levels of phosphate in the blood. Deposits of calcium may build up in the eyes and brain. The general signs and symptoms of the condition include muscle cramps and spasms, convulsions, pain in the abdomen, face, and lower extremities, dryness of hair and skin, brittle nails, reduced formation of tooth enamel, and cataracts.[50]

Prognosis. When diagnosed early, the prognosis for people with hypoparathyroidism is good. The changes such as brain calcifications, cataracts, and tooth enamel resulting from the condition are not reversible.[51]

Medical Intervention. The diagnosis of hypoparathyroidism is achieved through blood tests for low serum levels of calcium, high serum levels of phosphorus, and low serum levels of PTH. Computed tomography (CT) scans are used to detect brain calcifications.[52] The pharmacological treatment includes the use of PTH hormone therapy, a high-calcium diet, and calcium supplements. Restoration of the metabolic levels of calcium and phosphorus requires regular blood analysis.[53]

Physical Therapy Intervention. No physical therapy is indicated for this condition. However, physical therapists and physical therapists assistants need to be aware of the impact of this condition because they may be treating people for other conditions who have hypoparathyroidism.

Adrenal Cortex Diseases

Adrenal cortex diseases consist of those diseases that result in either hypofunction or hyperfunction of the adrenal cortex. Addison's disease is one of hypofunction of the adrenal cortex. Three main syndromes are associated with adrenocortical hyperfunction: Cushing's syndrome is caused by excessive amounts of cortisol, Conn's syndrome is the result of excessive amounts of aldosterone, and adrenogenital syndrome results from excessive amounts of androgens. Each of these conditions is described in this section.

Addison's Disease, Adrenocortical Hypofunction, Hypocortisolism, and Adrenal Insufficiency

Adrenal insufficiency conditions may be either primary, such as **Addison's disease**, or secondary, resulting from external factors. A primary disease is one resulting from a defect within the structure and not caused by an external factor. The estimates of the incidence of Addison's disease range from approximately five to six per million of the population in the United States.[54] However, secondary forms of adrenal insufficiency are more common than primary.[55,56] Addison's disease affects females more than males in a ratio of 1.5–3.5:1, and the age of onset of the condition is usually between the ages of 30 and 50, although the condition can affect all age groups.[57]

Etiology. The most prevalent cause of primary adrenocortical insufficiency is an autoimmune destruction of the adrenal glands. When the autoimmune destruction involves other glands as well as the adrenals, the condition is called polyendocrine deficiency syndrome. The polyendocrine deficiency syndrome may be Type I or Type II. ⊕ Type I occurs in children and Type II in young adults. The polyendocrine form of the disease is considered hereditary. The secondary form of adrenal insufficiency disease can result from tuberculosis, hemorrhage in the adrenal glands, infections such as cytomegalovirus, malignancy of the pituitary or hypothalamus, or be precipitated by radiation therapy administered for malignancy of the pituitary gland or the hypothalamus.[58] An Addison-like condition can be caused by trauma, surgery, infection, or postpartum. People with chronic adrenal insufficiency who do not take their steroid medication consistently may develop the condition. A temporary form of adrenal insufficiency may be caused if people suddenly stop taking a glucocorticoid hormone such as prednisone. Abrupt discontinuation of prednisone blocks the release of ACTH and corticotrophin releasing hormone (CRH) resulting in low levels of cortisol production in the body.[59]

Signs and Symptoms. The adrenal cortex produces cortisol and aldosterone, both of which control multiple organs and body systems. Cortisol in particular controls blood pressure and cardiovascular functions, inhibits the inflammatory response, and assists in the control of insulin and the regulation of protein, carbohydrate, and fat metabolism. The effects of a reduction of cortisol in the body therefore result in systemic symptoms including muscle weakness, fatigue, nausea, weight loss, diarrhea, nausea, vomiting, hypotension, and depression.[60,61] Changes in skin coloration with increased pigmentation occur as a result of the loss of inhibition of the pituitary ACTH, which increases the amount of melanocyte stimulating hormone (MSH) secreted by the anterior pituitary. Low levels of aldosterone may cause electrolyte imbalance, dehydration, hypotension, and even cardiac arrest. An acute adrenal insufficiency episode, also called an **Addisonian crisis,** results in symptoms such as acute pain in the back, abdomen, or lower extremities, severe vomiting and diarrhea, dehydration, severe hypotension, and, in some cases, loss of consciousness.[62]

Prognosis. The usual prognosis for people with Addison's disease is good when medications are taken consistently. An Addisonian crisis may result in severe metabolic failure including severe lowering of the blood pressure, reduction of blood glucose levels, and high levels of potassium and can be fatal if not treated. The mortality rate is reported to be only 1.4 deaths per million cases per year.[63]

Medical Intervention. The diagnosis of adrenal insufficiency can be difficult. Laboratory tests to determine cortisol levels can indicate low levels or lack of cortisol. Radiographs of the adrenal glands and the pituitary may be needed. An ACTH stimulation test measures the response of the body to an injection of synthetic ACTH. The normal response of the body to an injection of ACTH is a rise of cortisol in both the urine and the blood. When there is no response to an ACTH injection, the test is considered positive for adrenal insufficiency. Further testing has to be performed to determine the cause of the insufficiency. The pharmacological treatment of adrenal insufficiency is with corticosteroid medications (glucocorticoid hormones) to replace the levels of cortisol. Aldosterone replacement therapy may also be required. During an Addisonian crisis, injections and infusions are administered with fluids, salts, and glucocorticoid hormones.[64]

Physical Therapy Intervention. No physical therapy is indicated for people with the symptoms of adrenal insufficiency. People with this problem usually wear a medical alert device. They need to be monitored carefully during physical therapy interventions for other conditions to ensure the signs and symptoms of adrenal insufficiency do not occur.

Cushing's Syndrome and Cushing's Disease

Cushing's syndrome and disease are characterized by hypercortisolism (high levels of cortisol in blood, urine, and saliva). Cushing's syndrome and disease are usually diagnosed in females between the ages of 20 and 60. The prevalence of Cushing's syndrome is approximately 0.7 to 2.4/million population.[65] Approximately 85% of people with Cushing's disease have adenomas of the pituitary.[66]

Etiology. The etiology of Cushing's syndrome/disease varies. The disease may result from hyperfunction of the adrenal glands caused by hyperplasia of the adrenal glands, benign or malignant tumors of either the pituitary or adrenal cortex, or the intake of cortisol in the form of hydrocortisone medications.[67] In some cases, the increased level of cortisol arises from tumors elsewhere in the body, such as small cell lung carcinoma, that produce adrenocorticotropic hormone (ACTH) causing the adrenal glands to produce excessive amounts of cortisol.[68] When hypercortisolism occurs as a result of excessive ACTH production by the pituitary, the condition is called Cushing's disease rather than Cushing's syndrome. People with Type II diabetes, particularly those with comorbid hypertension, are also at risk for Cushing's syndrome.[69]

Signs and Symptoms. The characteristic signs and symptoms of both Cushing's syndrome and Cushing's disease include abdominal and facial obesity with the characteristic "moon face" seen in people who take steroidal medications. The "buffalo hump" appearance in the area of the upper trapezius, redness of the face, thinning of the skin which bruises easily, hypertension, hirsutism (excessive hair growth), osteoporosis, an impaired immune system, proximal myopathy (muscle weakness in the proximal extremities and shoulder and pelvic girdles), and diabetes are also present.[70] The symptoms include fatigue, muscle weakness, mental changes, and striae (discolored areas of skin resembling stretch marks). A temporary form of hypercortisolemia (hypercortisolism) is also associated with certain conditions including depression, anorexia nervosa, and alcoholism and during the late stages of pregnancy.[71]

Prognosis. Cushing's disease is fairly rare but can be life threatening if not treated. People with advanced Cushing's disease are reported to have a 5 times higher rate of mortality than the rest of the population.[72]

Medical Intervention. The diagnosis of Cushing's disease can be difficult as a result of the fluctuation of signs and symptoms.[73] The Endocrine Society released new guidelines in 2008 for testing procedures for Cushing's disease, which include testing the levels of cortisol in urine and saliva. Patients with high levels of cortisol are then referred to an endocrinologist by their physician.[74] The use of magnetic resonance imaging (MRI) and CT scans detects pituitary tumors and hyperplasia of the adrenal glands. Surgical excision of the adrenal glands, or one gland in the case of carcinoma, may be performed.

Radiotherapy for the adrenal glands or the pituitary is often performed when the Cushing's disease is the result of a malignant tumor. Medications that lower the production of cortisol, such as metyrapone and ketoconazole, may be used, but the results are inconclusive and the side effects include hirsutism.[75]

Physical Therapy Intervention. Although physical therapy is not directly prescribed for Cushing's syndrome, many patients have manifestations associated with the syndrome secondary to corticosteroid treatment for arthritic conditions. Precautions for patients with Cushing's syndrome include care of the skin, which is susceptible to tearing and bruising; care of joints; and caution with exercises and activities because the patient may be prone to fractures secondary to osteoporosis. People with Cushing's disease have a reduced ability to heal as a result of the reduced protein absorption caused by the syndrome. See Figure 9-4 for a comparison of the visual

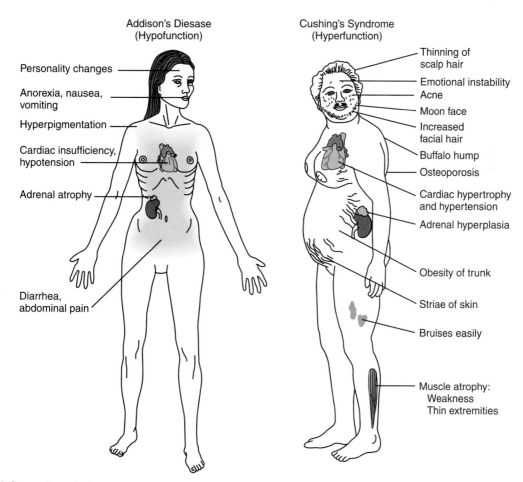

FIGURE 9.4 Comparison of adrenocortical hyperfunction (Cushing's syndrome) and hypofunction (Addison's disease).

signs of patients with adrenocortical hyperfunction and hypofunction.

Conn Syndrome

Conn syndrome, also called primary hyperaldosteronism, is the result of the hypersecretion of aldosterone by the adrenal cortex. The prevalence of the condition is approximately one case per million of the population.[76] However, the incidence of Conn's syndrome in people with hypertension is thought to be about 0.05% to 2%.[77] The condition is twice as common in women as men and usually occurs between the ages of 30 and 60.

Etiology. The etiology of Conn syndrome includes adenomas of the cortex of the adrenal glands or hyperplasia of the aldosterone-producing cells of the adrenal glands.[78]

Signs and Symptoms. The main symptom of Conn syndrome is hypertension. The condition causes changes in the mineral balance resulting in the retention of sodium and reduced levels of potassium as a result of the excess secretion from the kidneys. Other signs and symptoms may include fatigue, muscle weakness, polyuria (excessive urination), and nocturia (night-time urination).[79]

Prognosis. The side effects of Conn syndrome can be life threatening. Extreme hypokalemia (low levels of potassium) when left untreated can lead to cardiac arrhythmias that are potentially fatal. Severe and prolonged hypertension leads to heart disease, congestive heart failure, and cerebrovascular accident (stroke).[80] Such side effects make the diagnosis and treatment of Conn syndrome essential.

Medical Intervention. The medical management of Conn's syndrome resulting from adrenal adenomas is through endoscopic (via an endoscope) excision of the affected section of the adrenal gland, also called laparoscopic adrenalectomy. Adrenal hyperplasia is usually treated with medications.[81] The control of hypertension and hypokalemia is achieved with the use of antihypertensive, diuretic medications such as spironolactone (Aldacterone) or eplerenone (Inspra). Other medications may include angiotensin converting enzyme (ACE) inhibitors, calcium channel antagonists, or angiotensin II blockers.[82] People are recommended to follow a low-sodium diet even after surgical intervention.

Physical Therapy Intervention. Physical therapy intervention is not indicated for people with Conn syndrome. Some people with the side effects of the disease, such as

heart disease and stroke, will require physical therapy intervention as described in other areas of this book.

Congenital Adrenal Hyperplasia/ Adrenogenital Syndrome ⊕

Congenital adrenal hyperplasia, also called adrenogenital syndrome, and 21-hydroxylase deficiency, is a condition found in children. The condition affects both girls and boys. Prevalence of the syndrome is 1:10,000 to 18,000 births.[83,84] The condition occurs in all populations throughout the world, but the incidence is higher in certain populations such as the Yupik of Alaska (1 in 400 births) and people of Moroccan and Iranian-Jewish descent.[85]

Etiology. Congenital adrenal hyperplasia is the term used for several autosomal recessive enzymatic defects, often on gene CYP21A, that result in the lack of production of the 21-hydroxylase enzyme.[86] This lack of 21-hydroxylase results in the minimal production of cortisol and aldosterone by the adrenal glands, high levels of production of ACTH by the pituitary gland, and hyperplasia of the adrenal glands.[87] The result is an overproduction of the male sex hormones androgens.

Signs and Symptoms. The signs and symptoms associated with congenital adrenal hyperplasia are different for boys and girls. Boys tend to develop several mature male characteristics early, including a deep voice; pubic, facial, and axillary hair; a larger than usual penis; small testes; and overdeveloped muscles. Girls exhibit androgenous genitalia (a mixture of male and female external genitalia), although the internal reproductive organs are female. Girls also experience abnormal menstruation or delayed onset of menstruation, a deep voice, facial hair, and early development of pubic and axillary body hair. Both boys and girls tend to be tall for their age but are then smaller than typical adults.[88] Severe forms of the condition occur in approximately 75% of children born with congenital adrenal hyperplasia that can result in adrenal crisis. The loss of sodium and potassium salts from the body can lead to cardiac arrhythmias, severe electrolyte imbalances, dehydration, and vomiting.[89]

Prognosis. Adrenal crisis in the newborn can be fatal. Children with less serious congenital adrenal hyperplasia respond well to medications. Females may be infertile, and males have a higher risk of developing testicular cancers later in life.[90]

Medical Intervention. Genetic testing is recommended for families with a history of congenital adrenal hyperplasia.

The detection of females with the condition is easier than males because females are born with several external male genitalia characteristics. Laboratory tests for blood and urine demonstrate high levels of progesterone and dehydroepiandrosterone (DHEA) and low levels of aldosterone and cortisol. Radiographs of the bones of affected children indicate more mature bone formation than expected for the age of the child. The pharmacological management of the condition is with cortisol substitutes such as dexamethasone, fludrocortisones, or hydrocortisone. In most cases, individuals will take these medications for the rest of their lives.[91] Girls with predominantly external male genitalia may undergo surgical removal during the first few months after birth.

Physical Therapy Intervention. None indicated.

Adrenal Medulla Diseases

Two main diseases of the adrenal medulla exist, both of which are tumors.

Neuroblastomas and Pheochromocytomas

Neuroblastomas of the adrenal medulla occur mainly in young children. Approximately 500 to 600 cases of neuroblastoma occur in the United States in any given year.[92,93] These neuroblastomas account for approximately 8% to 10 % of all pediatric malignancies, with an incidence of 8.0 to 8.7 cases per million of the pediatric population.[94] Pheochromocytomas are fairly large tumors (over 3 cm in diameter) found mainly in the adult adrenal medulla. The incidence of pheochromocytomas is unknown, but they are rare. Males and females are equally affected, usually between the ages of 20 and 40.[95]

Etiology. Neuroblastomas are tumors derived from neuroblasts. Neuroblastomas tend to grow rapidly and are usually highly malignant, with rapid metastases to the bone and bone marrow. Although most neuroblastomas develop in the adrenal medulla, some develop in other areas of the body such as the abdomen, pelvis, neck, or chest. Pheochromocytomas are tumors, usually benign, in the adult adrenal medulla that cause the adrenal gland to produce excessive amounts of catecholamines (adrenaline and noradrenaline). Approximately 15% of pheochromocytoma tumors are genetic in origin, and the other 85% are of unknown origin.[96]

Signs and Symptoms. The signs and symptoms of neuroblastomas in the adrenal medulla are often rather vague with feelings of fatigue and loss of appetite.[97] ☻ Children with large neuroblastomas may experience abdominal pain. When the tumor has metastasized to the bone and bone marrow, children may limp as a result of bone pain.[98] The signs and symptoms of pheochromocytoma tumors in the adult include headaches, tachycardia or irregular heart beat, hypertension, sweating, feelings of anxiety, fear or panic, chest pain, pallor, dizziness, tremor and weight loss.[99,100]

Prognosis. Neuroblastomas are responsible for approximately 15% of the pediatric deaths from cancer each year.[101] In many cases, the diagnosis of neuroblastoma occurs after the malignancy has metastasized to the bone and bone marrow. People with pheochromocytoma who have had adrenalectomy (removal of the adrenal gland) may be susceptible to adrenal crisis at times of severe illness or stress as a result of low levels of cortisol in the body.[102] When adequately medicated, people are not at risk of death from this condition.

Medical Intervention. The diagnosis of neuroblastomas occurs anytime from in utero, with the use of sonography, to 10 years of age. The diagnosis of tumors of the adrenal medulla is made with the help of the CT or MRI. Bone marrow tests and biopsy may also be needed, especially for neuroblastomas. The medical intervention for both types of tumor is through adrenalectomy (surgical removal of the adrenal gland) or surgical excision of the medullary tumor and/or of the adrenal medulla.[103] Radiation, chemotherapy, immunotherapy, and stem-cell transplantation also are used for neuroblastomas.[104] Supplemental cortisol therapy may be necessary after removal of the adrenal gland.

Physical Therapy Intervention. None indicated. However, patients may be seen for conditions other than adrenal medulla diseases.

Why Does the Physical Therapist Assistant Need to Know About Diabetes Mellitus?

Many people with diabetes mellitus (DM) attend physical therapy clinics for multiple other reasons as well as for the treatment of diabetic ulcers. The PTA needs to be aware of the side effects of DM as they pertain to the indications, contraindications, and precautions for physical therapy interventions.

Diabetes Mellitus

Diabetes mellitus is described here separately from the other endocrine disorders because of its importance to physical therapist practice. A brief outline of the normal function of the pancreas is needed to understand the mechanism of DM. Insulin is formed by the beta cells of the islets of Langerhans in the pancreas. When high levels of glucose build up in the serum of the blood (hyperglycemia), the beta cells are stimulated to release insulin into the blood. Insulin promotes the transport of glucose to the liver, where it undergoes glycolysis and is then stored as glycogen. A reduction in insulin therefore causes hyperglycemia, and an excess of insulin causes hypoglycemia. Insulin also plays a part in the synthesis of proteins from amino acids, and fats from triglycerides. When insulin levels are reduced, fats in the body are broken down in an attempt to release more glucose, and ketone bodies form in the blood.

DM is a chronic metabolic disorder resulting from the lack of production of insulin by the pancreas, or the inability of the body to utilize insulin. Recent changes in nomenclature have been recommended. The preferred terms are now Type 1 diabetes for insulin-dependent and Type 2 for non-insulin-dependent diabetes. Type 1 diabetes was also known as juvenile-onset diabetes.

The statistics related to DM are frightening in their enormity. According to the National Diabetes Information Clearing House published by the National Institutes of Health,[105] the following 2005 statistics (the most recently published data from the 2007 fact sheet; Table 9.3) are applicable to the prevalence of DM in the United States:

Type 1 DM occurs most frequently in children. Type 2 DM is the more common form of diabetes and is particularly prevalent in African Americans, Asian Americans, Pacific Islanders, people of Latin descent, and elderly people of the total population.[106] The U.S. statistics for 2002 and 2003 (the most recent available) showed that among youth there were 15,000 diagnoses of Type 1 and 3,700 diagnoses of Type 2 DM per year. The incidence was 19 cases per 100,000 of the youth population for Type 1 and 5.3 per 100,000 for Type 2.[107] The direct costs of medical intervention for people with diabetes is estimated to be approximately $116 billion annually, and, when combined with the indirect costs of disability, loss of work hours, and premature death, the cost rises to $174 billion annually.[108]

Etiology. Type 1 diabetes mellitus is an autoimmune condition known to have a genetic component. The body destroys its own pancreatic islet of Langerhans beta cells, which produce insulin. The destruction of these cells

Table 9.3 **Prevalence of Diabetes Mellitus (DM) in the United States, 2007**

AGE GROUP	NO. OF PEOPLE WITH DM	PERCENTAGE OF POPULATION WITH DM
All ages combined	23.6 million 17.9 million diagnosed 5.7 million undiagnosed	7.8%
Under 20	186,300	0.2%
Over 20 (men and women)	23.5 million 1.6 million new cases diagnosed per year	10.7%
Over 60 (men and women)	12.2 million	23.1%
Men over 20	12 million	11.2%
Women over 20	11.5 million	10.2%
Non-Hispanic Whites over 20	14.9 million	9.8%
Non-Hispanic Blacks over 20	3.7 million	14.7%

Information from National Institute of Diabetes and Digestive and Kidney Diseases. *National Diabetes Statistics,* 2007 fact sheet. Bethesda, MD: U.S. Department of Health and Human Services, National Institutes of Health, *2008.* Retrieved from http://diabetes.niddk.nih.gov/dm/pubs/statistics/#allages.

sometimes follows an infection with a pathogen such as viral mumps or exposure to a toxic substance. The consequence of this destruction is that the pancreas produces either very little or no insulin.[109] Ten percent of people with Type 1 DM have the idiopathic form, which has no known cause. Type 2 DM is the most common form of diabetes. In Type 2 DM, the body either does not produce sufficient insulin or the body is unable to utilize what is produced.[110] The etiology of Type 2 DM is largely unknown. However, certain risk factors have been identified for the development of Type 2 diabetes, including genetic factors in certain ethnic groups such as African Americans, Asian Americans, Pacific Islanders, and people of Latin descent; age over-45; a sedentary lifestyle; hypertension; hypercholesterolemia; a history of gestational diabetes (during pregnancy); a poor diet; being overweight; and abdominal obesity. Patients with Type 2 diabetes have a resistance to insulin and an altered response to glucose, causing **hyperglycemia.**[111] See Table 9-4 for factors affecting glucose levels of the blood in patients with DM.

Signs and Symptoms. The signs and symptoms of both Type 1 and Type 2 diabetes are similar; however, the symptoms of Type 1 DM tend to occur suddenly and can be severe, whereas the symptoms of Type 2 develop more gradually over a period of months or even years. Clinically, the characteristics of DM include output of urine that contains glucose, thirst, blurred vision, weight loss, increased appetite, nausea and vomiting, abdominal pain, amenorrhea (absence of menstruation), and erectile dysfunction.[112,113]

Hypoglycemia occurs when the blood sugar levels fall below 70. The signs and symptoms of hypoglycemia may include shaking, drowsiness, sweating, headaches, dizziness, double vision, confusion, extreme hunger, general weakness, loss of coordination, and nervousness.[114] If left untreated, hypoglycemia can progress to coma and death. When ketoacidosis occurs (ketones build up in the blood as a result of the breakdown of fats in the body for energy), the signs and symptoms may include nausea, vomiting, flushing of the face, dryness of the skin and mouth, abdominal pain, tachypnea (abnormally fast breathing), and a fruity smell on the breath.[115]

The complications and long-term effects of DM include eye conditions such as glaucoma, cataracts, retinal detachment, and diabetic retinopathies[116] (see Table 9-5 for the common complications of DM). End-stage renal disease is a major complication, particularly of Type 1 DM of more than 20 years duration (see Fig. 9-5 for the long-term complications of DM). Many people with end-stage renal disease are on long-term kidney dialysis. In the United States, more than 280,000 people are on long-term kidney dialysis.[117] Kidney damage can be minimized by effective control of hyperglycemia and hypertension. **Peripheral neuropathies,** diabetic vascular disease and ischemia are severe complications that greatly increase the risk of developing gangrene of the foot. In severe cases of gangrene and ischemia with nonhealing ulceration of the affected limb, amputation may be required. Many diabetic neuropathies cause a "stocking" or "glove" paresthesia. This pattern of paresthesia is unique to a peripheral neuropathy. Usually peripheral nerve involvement causes pain and paresthesia in the area of skin or tissue supplied by the nerve root affected. These areas of nerve supply to the skin and muscles are called **dermatomes** (an area of skin supplied by a nerve

Table 9.4 **Factors Affecting Glucose Levels of the Blood in Patients With Diabetes Mellitus**

TYPE OF BLOOD GLUCOSE PROBLEM	FACTORS CAUSING GLUCOSE PROBLEMS
Hyperglycemia	Medications such as corticosteroids, diuretics, beta blockers, and calcium channel blockers Hormones such as epinephrine, glucocorticoids, and growth hormone When patient is under physical stress after extreme exercise or severe psychological stress; e.g., trauma, pregnancy, surgery, puberty, infection (and not taking sufficient insulin) Not taking insulin or missing doses of insulin Alcohol intake: insulin levels not maintained
Hypoglycemia	After exercise: insulin should not be injected close to muscles to be exercised before exercise Unexpected bouts of exercise such as running for a bus, climbing stairs because an elevator is not working, walking several blocks for therapy session Not eating before exercise Taking too much insulin

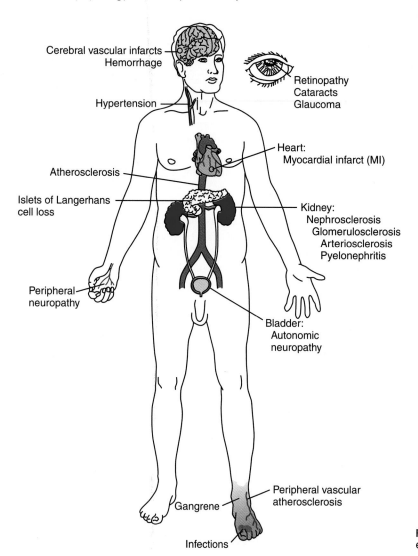

Cerebral vascular infarcts
Hemorrhage

Retinopathy
Cataracts
Glaucoma

Hypertension

Heart:
Myocardial infarct (MI)

Atherosclerosis

Islets of Langerhans
cell loss

Kidney:
Nephrosclerosis
Glomerulosclerosis
Arteriosclerosis
Pyelonephritis

Peripheral
neuropathy

Bladder:
Autonomic
neuropathy

Peripheral vascular
atherosclerosis

Gangrene

Infections

FIGURE 9.5 The long-term complications and effects of diabetes.

root) and **myotomes** (an area of muscle supplied by a nerve root). In a neuropathy, the area of involvement is the result of circulatory and sensory changes and does not follow the dermatome and myotome patterns. The sensory nerves are affected, making the foot and lower leg, or hand and forearm, insensitive to heat, cold, pain, or vibration. This makes patients susceptible to injury from tight shoes, burns, and mild trauma. People with DM must be educated to observe their feet regularly using a long-handled mirror to check the plantar surface of the foot daily. Advice on footwear with adequate toe box depth to allow for movement of the toes is essential. The feet and toes need to be dried thoroughly after bathing to prevent skin maceration. Some patients experience a very painful type of neuropathy, which can cause depression and loss of sleep. **Autonomic neuropathy** can cause general bodily problems such as constipation or diarrhea, postural hypotension, erectile dysfunction, and bladder emptying difficulties.[118] Diabetic coma may occur if people ingest too much or too little insulin, have an infection, or have a cardiovascular incident. Cardiovascular disease is a further complication of DM. Atherosclerosis may occur with associated hypertension and aneurysms of the major arteries and disease of the peripheral arteries. A major danger for those with DM remains the increased susceptibility to infection as a result of the excess glucose within the body and the delay or inability of the body to heal.

Acute Charcot's arthropathy is associated with diabetes mellitus. This unilateral arthropathy occurs in the feet of many people with peripheral neuropathy associated with DM. The symptoms include edema, erythema, and joint effusion of the foot and ankle and an increase in skin temperature over the involved area. Despite the neuropathy many people relate feeling pain in the area of the ankle and foot.[119] In the initial stages of Charcot's arthropathy, the bones undergo destruction with multiple fractures, and the joints are frequently dislocated. As the condition progresses, the joint becomes ankylosed with hypertrophy of the affected bones, resulting in loss of motion at the affected joints.[120]

Prognosis. The prognosis for patients with both Type 1 and Type 2 diabetes has improved greatly over recent years as a result of advances in the management of the disease. The education of both people with DM and their care providers improves the outcome for these patients. People with uncontrolled, long-standing diabetes mellitus are at high risk for serious complications such as peripheral neuropathy and peripheral circulatory problems, both of which can result in diabetic ulcers. Many people with diabetic ulcers experience delayed healing or nonhealing and may require amputation of the affected foot or lower extremity. In 2005, DM ranked as the seventh leading cause of death in the United States, with a total of 233,619 deaths attributed to the disease.[121] The risk for cerebrovascular accidents in people with diabetes mellitus is between 2 and 4 times higher than for the general population. DM was also ranked as the leading cause of blindness in the age group from 20 to 74 with between 12,000 and 24,000 new cases of diabetic retinopathy diagnosed each year.[122] Diabetes is also responsible for 44% of new cases of kidney failure each year, and more than 60% of nontraumatic lower extremity amputations. In 2004, approximately 71,000 lower extremity amputations were performed as a result of diabetes mellitus.[123] See Table 9-5 for common complications associated with DM.

Medical Intervention. Diabetes mellitus is diagnosed through a variety of laboratory tests. Positive tests for diabetes mellitus include the presence of glucose and ketone bodies in the urine, a fasting blood glucose test with

Table 9.5 **Common complications of diabetes mellitus**

COMPLICATION	RESULTING PROBLEMS
Diabetic neuropathy (a type of polyneuropathy)	Foot drop – weakness of tibialis anterior Susceptible to injury due to loss of sensation of skin – leads to burns, open wounds, cuts, abrasions that may be slow to heal due to reduced circulation efficiency. Increased risk of infection is present. "Stocking" or "glove" parasthesias Carpel tunnel syndrome as a result of ischemia of the median nerve which increases the sensitivity of the nerve to external stimuli Charcot's joint—a type of diabetic neuropathic arthropathy. Proprioceptive sensation in the joint is lost, the affected bone fractures, and ankylosis of the joint occurs.
Diabetic amyotrophy	A type of proximal muscle weakness found in some patients with DM
Eye problems	Glaucoma, retinopathy, cataracts
Renal disease	Reduced function of kidneys due to renal artery stenosis leading to chronic renal failure
Cardiac and vascular diseases	Cerebrovascular disease, coronary artery disease, peripheral vascular disease are common Ischemic changes in the limb. May lead to diabetic ulcerations of the leg. Healing is delayed due to impaired circulation. In severe ischemic disease amputation of the affected limb may be required Reflex sympathetic dystrophy is common Dupuyten's contracture – flexion contracture of one or more digits with associated thickening of the palmar fascia Limited joint mobility particularly of the hands and "stiff hand syndrome." Causes are a combination of vascular and neuropathic Gangrene to extremities – a mixture of vascular and neuropathic causes
Bone disease	Osteoporosis as a result of changed levels of insulin affecting bone density

more than 126 mg/dL, a nonfasting blood glucose test with over 200 mg/dL, an insulin test of the blood with very low levels of insulin, and a C-peptide test with very low levels or no C-peptide. C-peptide is a by-product of insulin production and is usually present in the blood.[124]

People with Type 1 diabetes and those with Type 2 who do not respond to other medications must take insulin. Insulin injections may have to be self-administered several times a day depending on the level of glucose in the blood.[125] Several kinds of insulin are available; some are slow acting, and others act for prolonged or intermediate lengths of time.[126] A physician must determine the correct medication for the individual patient. Insulin is introduced into the body by injection, via an insulin pump, or using an insulin jet injector. Injections are given in the abdomen, upper arms, thighs, or buttocks, and people vary the injection site to reduce the soreness. The target blood glucose levels are between 70 and 130 mg/dL before meals and less than 180 mg/dL 1 to 2 hours after a meal.[127] However, some endocrinologists are being more conservative and diagnosing people with glucose levels between 100 and 120 as prediabetic with microvascular changes already present. Pharmacological intervention other than insulin may work for some people with diabetes or be used in addition to insulin. Alpha-glucosidase inhibitors work by slowing down the digestion of carbohydrates and thus preventing blood glucose levels from rising too rapidly after eating. Some examples of alpha-glucosidase inhibitors are miglitol (Glyset) and acarbose (Precose).[128] Biguanides are prescribed for people with insulin resistance to lower the amount of glucose made by the liver. Biguanides such as metformin (Glucophage, Glucophage XR, and Riomet) also improve cholesterol levels.[129] D-phenylalanine derivatives such as nateglinide (Starlix), Dpp-4 inhibitors such as sitagliptin phosphate (Januvia), meglitinides such as repaglinide (Prandin), and sulfonylureas such as glimepiride (Amaryl), glyburide (Dia Beta), chlorpropamide (Diabinase), and glipizide (Glucotrol) all stimulate the body to produce more insulin after food intake to prevent glucose levels from elevating too high.[130]

The medical management of the patient with DM includes referral to a dietician for diet adjustment and education to reduce the intake of sugars and increase dietary fiber. Weight loss also improves the control of diabetes symptoms for people who are overweight.[131] Moderate exercise is good for people with diabetes because it helps to keep weight down and speeds up the utilization of insulin by the body. However, too much exercise can result in hypoglycemia as a result of the rapid utilization of sugars and lowering of insulin levels. The referral to a podiatrist is preferable for people with diabetes both for cutting nails and general foot care, and for advice regarding orthotics and specialized footwear to minimize the development of skin irritation and ulcerations.[132] Regular visits to the ophthalmologist are necessary to screen for visual complications.

Physical Therapy Intervention. Physical therapy intervention can play a major part in the education of both the patient and the family. Well-monitored exercise programs can effectively reduce the risk for some of the long-term side effects associated with diabetes mellitus. People with DM should receive a full physical examination by the physician before referral for physical therapy intervention. An exercise program consisting of low to moderate resistive exercises and aerobic exercise to a low or moderate intensity level, between 3 and 5 times per week, is recommended for people with DM.[133] Some physical therapists specialize in orthotics and work with the podiatrist to relieve pressure forces on the foot of the person with diabetes during ambulation.[134,135] The effects of regular exercise, particularly ambulation, are well noted to improve blood pressure, assist with weight loss, lower heart rate, lower cholesterol levels, and assist the body in utilizing insulin.[136] Most of the physical therapy intervention for patients with DM is for associated problems that develop secondary to the disease process. Many patients with DM have diabetic ulcers, which require wound care intervention. These patients often have a neuropathy with a resulting lack of sensation to hot and cold in the lower extremities, which makes them susceptible to burns and injury. Muscle weakness and various levels of functional disability are common and require strengthening exercises, functional training, and reeducation. Passive lengthening of the Achilles tendon can improve passive and active ankle dorsiflexion range and both reduce the pain of peripheral neuropathy and the ability to ambulate comfortably.[137,138] Some evidence suggests that the pain experienced with diabetic neuropathy may be improved with the use of high-frequency external muscle stimulation rather than transcutaneous neuromuscular stimulation (TENS).[139] People with end-stage renal disease (ESRD) as a result of DM require additional monitoring and adaptation of exercise programs. People with ESRD have a low tolerance to activity and reduced cardiopulmonary capacity as a result of multiple factors including decreased cardiac efficiency and output, atrophy of muscles, and anemia. Exercise programs for people with ESRD should be of low intensity, may consist of non-weight-bearing exercises, and should be closely monitored by the PT and/or PTA for signs of fatigue.[140]

Physical therapy intervention is required for people who have had amputations as a result of the long-standing complications of diabetes. Physical therapy intervention for people with amputations is beyond the scope of this book. However, the PT and PTA are involved extensively with patient care before and after surgical lower extremity amputation, including wound management, wrapping of the residual limb, teaching people self-management for wrapping of the limb, exercise programs for strengthening and stretching, prevention of contractures of the affected limb, preparing the residual limb for fitting of a prosthesis by shaping the residual limb and teaching range of motion exercises, monitoring the donning and doffing of the prosthetic limb, education for skin care of the affected and nonaffected limbs, and gait training. The PTA is encouraged to consult a text regarding specific prosthetic and orthotic management for further information.

Acute Charcot's arthropathy is managed with non-weight bearing ambulation with a variety of assistive devices to individually address patient needs.

Implications for the Physical Therapist Assistant. The PT and PTA need to be familiar with the medications taken by the patient and understand the possible changes of the patient's condition when the medication is not working correctly or has not been taken. When patients do not take their medication, delayed healing and a diabetic crisis may occur.

"It happened in the clinic"

A 50-year-old man with a diagnosis of diabetes mellitus was referred to PT for evaluation and treatment of an open wound on the plantar surface of the left foot. Evaluation by the PT revealed that the patient had diabetic neuropathy and had minimal sensation to pressure or touch in his left foot. The patient got a small stone in the left shoe, was unable to feel it, and developed a slight wound on the plantar surface of the left foot. He did not know this had occurred until 4 days later when he noticed a blood stain on his left sock and asked his wife to look at his foot. The wound was .5 inches in diameter with drainage and some bleeding. The patient went to the physician and was referred to PT. Wound care protocols were followed for the patient, but the main intervention was education of the patient and his wife to reduce the risk of a repeat of the incident. The patient was instructed in use of a long-handled mirror to inspect the plantar surface of the foot each day and given advice regarding wearing footwear with more depth and self-inspection of footwear before donning shoes.

PHYSICAL THERAPY ADVICE FOR THE PATIENT WITH DIABETES MELLITUS

1. Exercise regularly, particularly aerobic exercise, to stimulate the cardiovascular system and improve circulation. Walking is particularly good.
2. Wear shoes that provide good support but have plenty of room for the toes. A deeper toe box-depth shoe is needed to avoid rubbing of the skin. Shoes and socks should not be tight.
3. Do not wear any socks that are tight round the lower leg or knee such as knee-high socks that restrict the circulation. Cotton socks or those that wick away moisture are preferred. Generally white socks are better as dyes may irritate the skin.
4. Check feet daily, or have your care provider check them for you. A long-handled mirror is useful to see the soles of the feet. Be sure to check between the toes. Any signs of redness, rubbing, or other skin irritation should be reported to a podiatrist or physician immediately.
5. Visit a podiatrist or chiropodist regularly to have toenails cut and any foot problems resolved. If the skin is cut, there is a greater chance of infection in patients with DM and a longer healing time. Feet should not be soaked too long because this will soften the skin and make it prone to breakdown.
6. Eat a balanced diet and try to control weight.
7. Test blood sugar levels regularly and take the prescribed medicine as indicated by the physician.
8. Follow all medical advice for control of the diabetic symptoms.
9. If you experience increased occurrences of weakness, fatigue, blurred vision, or changes in bladder or bowel habits, visit your physician.
10. Dry feet well after bathing to prevent skin irritation and breakdown.
11. Use a bed cradle at night to keep the weight of the bedclothes off the feet.
12. Use light-weight bed clothes that are not tucked in. A light-weight comforter-type quilt is preferable.

13. Use an assistive device to ambulate when balance is poor. Your physical therapist will determine the appropriate device and provide instructions for proper use.
14. Exercise more in the morning than the afternoon to prevent hypoglycemic episodes during the night.
15. Do NOT exercise alone. Take a friend with you or exercise with a group of people.
16. Be aware that hypoglycemia may occur after exercise sessions and check glucose levels accordingly.
17. Do NOT sit too close to fires with your feet and do NOT place feet on a central heating radiator. Take care when using heating pads. Do NOT leave heating pads turned on when you are asleep. Do NOT sleep with a hot water bottle next to your feet.
18. When taking a bath check the water temperature with your elbow to make sure it is not too hot. You may not be able to detect the temperature with your feet and could get a burn if the water is too hot. Water for a bath should be mildly warm, not hot.
19. Do NOT walk around the house or outside without shoes. You are at risk of injuring your feet. You may not know you have stepped on something and could easily get an infection.
20. Do not exercise in very high or very low temperatures. If it is very hot outside, do not go out for a run. Try to exercise in a controlled climatic environment (e.g., taking a walk in a shopping mall rather than outside).

PRECAUTIONS FOR THE PHYSICAL THERAPIST ASSISTANT WHEN TREATING PATIENTS WITH DM

1. Do not fatigue the patient with overexertion. Too much exertion can deplete the insulin levels and lead to hyperglycemia.
2. Monitor vital signs carefully before, during, and after exercise sessions.
3. Check the dorsalis pedis pulse (pedal pulse) before each treatment session, particularly if performing treatment for lower extremity ischemic ulcers.
4. Monitor patients for signs of hypoglycemia and hyperglycemia. If a patient has an episode, administer sugar and contact the physician.
5. Beware of extreme thirst as this could be a precursor to a hyperglycemic episode.
6. When applying thermal agents, use extra insulating layers and test skin carefully for sensitivity to warmth and cold. When using hot packs, check the patient's skin every 5 minutes to ensure the skin is not too red. If arterial supply is impaired, do not use hot packs over the affected area. Consider using heat proximally

on the limb to stimulate circulation through an indirect heating effect.
7. When using aquatherapy, ensure patients have taken their required insulin and have eaten correctly. Watch the patient for signs of fatigue and hypoglycemia.
8. Keep whirlpool temperatures below body temperature to avoid stressing the impaired circulation. Generally, water temperature should be 97° Fahrenheit.
9. Warn patients that they may have hypoglycemia several hours after exercise and instruct them to monitor glucose levels carefully.
10. If you think a patient is hypoglycemic, administer some fruit juice as long as they are conscious. If the patient is actually hyperglycemic, it will not make it worse. If the patient is hypoglycemic, it could prevent a coma.
11. Do NOT provide therapy if the patient is having problems with noncontrolled glucose levels or hypertension. Refer the patient back to the physician.

Diabetic Neuropathy

Diabetic neuropathy is a fairly common side effect of long-term diabetes mellitus. The cause of the neuropathy is not fully understood. Circulation in the diabetic limb and glucose metabolism are impaired. The deposition of sorbitol, fructose, and glucose in the nerve tissues leads to electrolyte imbalances and nerve tissue dysfunction.[141] The poor circulation to the limb also results in poor circulation to the nerve tissue. In diabetes, the neuropathy is usually peripheral, affecting the peripheral (distal) lower extremities and occasionally the distal upper extremities. Many people with DM experience a burning or tingling pain, numbness, weakness, and atrophy of the lower leg muscles, leading to a foot drop, and edema of the foot, ankle, and sometimes the lower leg.[142]

GERIATRIC CONSIDERATIONS

Elderly patients with diabetes mellitus (DM) become increasingly at risk when memory loss occurs. Forgetting to take a dose of insulin or taking more than one dose because of a memory lapse are both problematic. Lack of suitable nutrition can also be a problem. Patients who live alone are especially at risk because they may not cook for themselves. Some patients may not have the ability to give themselves an insulin injection as a result of reduced range of motion or dexterity. In addition, many patients with longstanding DM have reduced vision and may be unable to care for themselves adequately. Many elderly patients require residential placement in assisted living or nursing homes sooner than would normally be necessary because of either the DM diagnosis or the lack of substantial support from family and friends.

Diabetic Coma

Coma can occur as a result of either hyperglycemic or hypoglycemic events. Coma is more commonly seen in people with hyperglycemia than hypoglycemia and in those with Type 2 diabetes.[143] Extreme thirst is one of the warning signs of hyperglycemic coma, and this condition can be brought on in people with Type 2 diabetes as a result of infections.[144] The patient with hyperglycemia will have a gradual onset of symptoms over a period of a few days (see Table 9-6). Most patients with DM are aware of the warning signs of hypoglycemia and carry something sweet with them for emergencies, thus reducing the risk of coma. Physical therapy departments often keep orange juice in the facility for emergency situations. Once a person is in a coma, you must not administer anything by mouth. Activate the emergency medical system and monitor the patient for vital signs. Administer cardiopulmonary resuscitation if necessary. Stay with the patient and continually monitor the vital signs until the emergency medical team arrives. Diabetic coma is not common in the physical therapy setting, but the PT and PTA must know the warning signs and be able to act accordingly.

Why Does the Physical Therapist Assistant Need to Know About Metabolic Diseases and Disorders?

Although the physical therapist assistant does not actually treat people for metabolic disorders some of these people attend the physical therapy clinic. An understanding of these metabolic disorders allows the PTA to better appreciate the impact of the side effects of these diseases on patients who may have reduced cognition, strength, stamina, and energy for physical therapy interventions.

Table 9.6 **Symptoms of Hyperglycemia and Hypoglycemia**

TYPE OF GLYCEMIC EVENT	SYMPTOMS
Hypoglycemia: may lead to insulin shock, which can be life threatening if untreated	Onset of symptoms is sudden Weakness, shaking Headache, blurred vision, pale skin (pallor) Confusion, nervousness Profuse perspiration Increased heart rate, palpitations Hunger Convulsions, may lead to coma Blood glucose levels below 70 mg/dl
Hyperglycemia	Gradual onset of symptoms Extreme thirst Confusion, lethargy Abdominal pain Excessive urination (*polyuria*) Dehydration Seizures leading to coma Blood glucose levels above 300 mg/dL
Diabetic ketoacidosis	Gradual onset of symptoms Fever, red face Polyuria Abdominal pain, nausea, rapid respirations, weakness Thirst, dry mouth, fruity breath odor Headache Blood glucose levels above 300 mg/dL

Metabolic Disorders

Metabolic disorders are those related to the malfunction of absorption of essential minerals and nutrients for the body or which upset the natural balance of acid and alkaline homeostasis. In some cases, the malfunction results in toxicity, and in others, it results in a reduction of essential nutrition to the cells and tissues of the body. The disorders described in this section include the balance of acids and bases, phenylketonuria, and Wilson's disease.

Balance of Acids and Bases

The balance of acids and bass (alkalines) in the body is essential for normal cell and organ function. Healthy metabolism is characterized by a pH of extracellular fluids between 7.35 and 7.45. The maintenance of this pH is called **homeostasis.** When the body is injured or diseased, the acid-base balance is disturbed, and the chemical reactions in the body cause increases (alkalosis) or decreases (acidosis) in pH. When these changes occur, all body organs are affected, including the lungs, heart, kidneys, liver, and the neuromuscular system. These metabolic effects are noted in many of the diseases described in previous chapters, such as inflammatory conditions, and systemic diseases, such as systematic lupus erythematosus (SLE). The maintenance of hydration is important for electrolyte homeostasis and normal fluid balance. People should be encouraged to drink plenty of water and eat a low-sodium diet in an attempt to preserve homeostasis and promote healing. Fluid intake should not, however, be encouraged in cases of kidney malfunction when patients are on kidney dialysis. Many patients with lower extremity edema stop drinking because of the swelling, whereas drinking more fluids will actually reduce the swelling. An adequate explanation to people regarding how good fluid intake will help to reduce swelling not increase it is important when working with people in the physical therapy clinic. Many conditions requiring physical therapy intervention such as muscular weakness and neurological symptoms can be associated with metabolic and electrolyte imbalances. If the PT or PTA suspects that the patient's symptoms do not match the expected symptoms of the physical therapy diagnosis, then the patient should be referred back to the physician. Some of the signs and symptoms associated with fluid and electrolyte imbalance include changes in skin temperature, tendon reflexes, and vital signs. Other factors regarding fluid and electrolyte imbalance are listed in Table 9-7.

Table 9.7 **Signs and Symptoms Associated With Electrolyte and Fluid Imbalance**

Vital sign changes	Changes in rate of respirations, dyspnea Tachycardia, hypertension, irregular pulse rate Postural hypotension (blood pressure drops when patient stands)
Skin changes	Altered skin temperature, may be warmer or colder than usual Edema
Muscle and nerve changes	Cramping and twitching of muscles Muscle fatigue Deep tendon reflex changes (central nervous system); may be either decreased as in acidosis or increased as in alkalosis
General changes mainly associated with central nervous system	Brain tissue changes resulting in memory loss, hallucinations, and depression

Phenylketonuria ☻

Phenylketonuria (PKU) is a comparatively rare metabolic condition.

Etiology. Phenylketonuria is an autosomal, recessive, hereditary disease characterized by a raised level of phenylalanine in the body that impairs cognitive and intellectual functions.[145] The disease affects approximately one in every 12,000 to 15,000 live births in the United States each year.[146] This hereditary disease results from a lack of the enzyme phenylalanine hydroxylase, which normally synthesizes the amino acid phenylalanine into tyrosine.[147] Tyrosine plays a role in the production of dopamine, norepinephrine and epinephrine.

Signs and Symptoms. A buildup of phenylalanine in the blood leads to the secretion of phenylpyruvic acid in the urine. High levels of phenylalanine in the system are toxic to the body. In people with undiagnosed or untreated PKU, lesions occur within the brain with atrophy of the gray matter, abnormalities of the white matter, and demyelination of the neural axons.[148] These abnormalities result in mental retardation, neuropathy, and seizures.[149] As a result of the reduced intake of protein in the diet, growth retardation is common.[150] Additional symptoms may include sweating, loss of muscular coordination, tremors (as a result of reduced amounts of dopamine normally synthesized by tyrosine), and spasticity.

Prognosis. The disease is incurable, but the effects of the disease can be controlled by a low protein, and thus low phenylalanine, diet, commencing immediately upon diagnosis. When PKU is treated consistently and a low protein diet maintained, the effects of the condition are minimized.

Medical Intervention. A screening test for PKU is mandatory in the United States within 24 hours of birth. People with phenylketonuria require medical monitoring of levels of phenylalanine in the blood plasma.[151] The low phenylalanine diet must be maintained for life.[152] People with the disease receive an amino acid dietary supplement free of phenylalanine to maintain protein intake. A medication called Kuvan (sapropterin dihydrochloride) was the first drug to be approved for the treatment of PKU by the U.S. Food and Drug Administration in December 2007.[153] Kuvan helps to further reduce levels of phenylalanine levels in blood when used with a low protein diet.[154]

Physical Therapy Intervention. The PT and PTA may become involved in the treatment of children with this condition if the disease remains undetected and the child has mental retardation. The physical therapy is directed at stimulating the developmental sequence and working with muscular coordination activities.

Wilson's Disease

Wilson's disease is a hereditary, metabolic disorder that affects the metabolism of copper by the liver resulting in toxic levels of copper building up in the liver, kidneys, brain, and eyes.[155] This rare disease has an incidence of approximately 1:30,000 of the population.[156] The disease is present from birth and may cause organ damage as early as 2 or 3 years of age.[157] ☺ Most people start to have symptoms between the ages of 5 and 35.[158,159]

Etiology. This autosomal, recessive, genetic disease is caused by mutations of the ATP7B gene that affects the ATPase 7B enzyme responsible for the transport of copper throughout the body.[160]

Signs and Symptoms. The characteristic signs and symptoms of the disease include impaired function of the liver, kidneys, circulatory system, and neurological system. Common symptoms that prompt people to seek medical

help include abdominal pain and swelling, edema of the lower extremities, vomiting blood, jaundice, fatigue, and problems with talking and swallowing such as dysarthria (speech problems due to muscle weakness), dysphasia (speech problems due to central nervous system deficits), and dysphagia (swallowing problems).[161] Women with the disease may have menstrual problems, infertility, and experience multiple miscarriages.[162] Other general signs include anemia, early-onset osteoporosis and arthritis, impaired blood clotting, and a low platelet and white blood cell count.[163] A common sign of Wilson's disease is gold or greenish-gold Kayser-Fleischer rings around the iris of the eye within the cornea caused by deposits of copper.[164] Many neurological symptoms may occur including dystonia, bradykinesia, ataxia, gait problems, hand tremors, loss of fine motor skills, and psychiatric problems such as behavioral and emotional disturbances, dementia, depression, homicidal and suicidal ideation, aggression, and psychosis.[165-166] In people with advanced stages of the disease, degeneration and atrophy are present in many areas of the brain including the basal ganglia, brainstem, midbrain, cerebellum, and cerebrum in both gray and white matter.[167] The involvement of the cerebellum results in disorders of movement.[168] In people with end-stage disease muscle atrophy, contractures, and fractures may be present.

Prognosis. When undiagnosed or untreated for a prolonged period, Wilson's disease is fatal.[169] Liver transplant is required for many people with advanced stages of the disease. With early diagnosis and treatment, the advanced effects of the disease can be prevented.

Medical Intervention. The diagnosis of Wilson's disease is difficult as a result of the wide variety of signs and symptoms exhibited by patients. MRI and single-photon emission computed tomography (SPECT) are both used for the diagnosis of Wilson's disease. Areas of focus include the brain and the liver.[170] The pharmacological management of Wilson's disease is with chelating drugs (meaning these drugs bind with metals), such as d-penicillamine (Cuprimine) and trientine hydrochloride (Syprine), which actually bind with the copper and remove it from the body. Zinc is also administered in conjunction with the chelating agents to block absorption of copper by the digestive tract.[171,172] These pharmacological treatments prevent further progression of the disease process but do not reverse the damage to organs already affected by the disease. Genetic testing for the abnormalities of the ATP7B gene are now suggested to detect the disease before the damage to vital organs has time to occur.[173] Dietary recommendations include reducing the intake of copper by avoiding ingestion of shellfish or liver.[174]

Physical Therapy Intervention. People with Wilson's disease who have neuromuscular symptoms benefit from physical therapy intervention. The literature regarding physical therapy for the treatment of people with Wilson's disease is minimal. The focus of treatment depends on the individual symptoms, but may include balance and gait reeducation, muscle strengthening exercises, functional activities, and energy conservation techniques.

Why Does the Physical Therapist Assistant Need to Know About Nutritional Disorders?

As part of the holistic (whole body) approach to physical therapy the PTA needs to be aware of some of the nutritional disorders present in people with whom they are working. Obesity is one of the disorders that leads to other major health problems including diabetes mellitus and heart conditions. As part of the Healthy People 2020 initiative,[175] obesity is one of the main foci of attention in the United States as a preventive medicine and change in lifestyle choice. The PT and PTA are in a unique position to influence the lifestyle choices of their patients through recommendations for healthy eating combined with regular exercise. People with anorexia nervosa and bulimia nervosa may have adverse side effects that impair their ability to participate in physical therapy interventions. Because the PTA works with people with all these conditions, a basic understanding of nutritional disorders is essential.

Nutritional Disorders

Nutritional disorders are discussed as they pertain to healing, wellness, and general physical condition. The PTA does not treat nutritional disorders but is often in a position of trust with the patient and can emphasize positive steps toward healthy nutrition. As part of the health care team, PTs and PTAs should emphasize healthy lifestyles including good hydration and healthy eating habits. Lack

of adequate hydration can play a major role in the disease process. During PT intervention, good hydration is essential for muscle function. Patients should be encouraged to drink plenty of water during treatment sessions unless they have a fluid intake limitation determined by the physician. If working with patients in the hospital setting, the PTA should check to see whether fluid intake is being monitored. If so, the PTA should make a note in the patient chart about the amount of fluid the patient drinks and eliminates during the PT session.

Overweight and Obesity

Obesity is a major health problem in the western world. Of particular concern is the number of overweight and obese children in the United States and throughout Europe. Every 10 years, the Department of Health and Human Services develops a new set of goals for improving the health of the American people. The Healthy People 2020 set into motion in 2010 has a major focus on nutrition and weight status. A reduction in the numbers of adults, children, and adolescents who are overweight or obese, and the promotion of healthy eating habits are goals for the next decade.[176] A rise in the childhood obesity levels demonstrated in the United Kingdom through a 2004 survey showed that more than one quarter of all children between the ages of 11 and 18 were clinically obese.[177] Estimates show that approximately 70% to 85% of children who are obese will become obese adults.[178] Diets high in protein and fats may lead to higher incidences of many diseases including myocardial infarctions, cerebrovascular accidents, and diabetes; however, genetic predisposition is also responsible for some obesity.

Complications From Obesity

The World Health Organization (WHO) estimates that the cost of obesity to the health systems in Europe is close to 1% of the gross domestic product (gross national product). This huge proportion of money needed to treat people with diseases associated with obesity has made obesity one of the top concerns for health organizations worldwide.[179] Projections for the United States are that by 2010 more than 20% of the population will be morbidly obese.[180] In 2006, the obesity levels in some states already exceeded this projection.[181]

Etiology. Obesity is caused by multiple factors, including genetics, dietary habits, sedentary lifestyles, cultural factors, and metabolic rates of individuals.[182,183] The intake of a diet high in protein and fats is a definite contributing factor to obesity. The recent finding of the link between the adenovirus-36 (Ad-36) and adenovirus-37 (Ad-37) and obesity raised the awareness of a virus associated with increased weight.[184,185] These DNA adenoviruses are part of family of viruses associated with the common cold and are prevalent in individuals who are obese.

Signs and Symptoms. No real signs and symptoms exist for obesity other than excess weight over and above the parameters determined by the WHO and the Centers for Disease Control and Prevention (CDC). The signs and symptoms of concern are those of the comorbid conditions associated with obesity. These signs and symptoms can be found in the sections of this book concerning the individual diseases mentioned in the introduction to obesity.

Prognosis. According to the CDC, the combination of a high waist measurement and a greater **body mass index (BMI)** increases the risk of people having obesity-related diseases.[186] These include hypertension, cholesterolemia (high low-density lipoprotein, low high-density lipoprotein, high triglycerides), Type 2 diabetes, coronary heart disease, cerebrovascular accident, gallbladder disease, osteoarthritis, sleep apnea, respiratory insufficiency, and certain cancers such as breast, colon, and endometrial.[187] Recent research has shown that obesity may be related to delayed diagnosis of breast cancer rather than to an increased risk for breast cancer.[188] A 1995 study, published by the *New England Journal of Medicine,* of 115,195 U.S. women between the ages of 30 and 35 in 1976 and followed for the next 16 years, showed a correlation between increased weight and a higher risk of death from obesity-associated diseases in middle age.[189] In 2004, a report in Doctors Lounge cited CDC information that indicated that obesity was becoming second only to smoking as the leading preventable cause of death in the United States.[190]

Medical Intervention. Several scales are used to determine body fat ratios. No scale is completely accurate, and they can only be used as a guide. **Relative weight** (RW) is the weight of the individual divided by the optimal weight for the height in inches of the person (as determined by a scale produced by the U.S. government), multiplied by 100. The body mass index (BMI) is more complex to calculate. To find the BMI, the body weight, measured in kilograms, is divided by the height in meters squared.[191] This value is considered to be more accurate in determining body fat levels because the relative weight does not distinguish between fat and muscle weight

values. According to the CDC, the normal values for BMI are between 18.5 and 24.9 kg/m^2, an overweight BMI is between 25 and 29.9 kg/m^2, Class I obesity is between 30 and 34.9 kg/m^2, Class II obesity between 35 and 39.9 kg/m^2, and Class III obesity over 40 kg/m^2.[192] An additional factor to take into consideration is the waist measurement when calculating the BMI. The measurement of skinfold thickness with special calipers is sometimes used to assess the levels of body fat but is less accurate than using the BMI. Other methods of determining the level of fat in the body are by measuring and weighing the body under water and computerized tomography. These methods are less readily available and more expensive than the more usual method of calculating the BMI and are rarely used.[193] ⊛ When calculating the BMI for children and adolescents, the same calculations are used as the adult, but the values are adjusted according to gender and age.

The pharmacological approach to control of obesity includes the use of lipase inhibitors such as Orlistat that inhibit the absorption of fats within the intestine. The main side effects of lipase inhibitors are changes in bowel habits, including gas, diarrhea, and intestinal cramps.[194] Behavior modification can be provided to help individuals identify faulty eating habits, develop more healthy eating habits, and provide support groups.[195] In extreme circumstances, surgery is performed to bypass the intestine or reduce the size of the stomach. These surgeries are usually performed only if people have a life-threatening medical problem associated with obesity.

Physical Therapy Intervention. Physical therapy intervention can play a major role in behavior modification to increase daily exercise and activity, but people who are overweight require ongoing encouragement to maintain weight loss and may benefit from participating in weight loss groups and other social support mechanisms. Exercise alone will not always produce the necessary amount of weight loss, but when combined with a low-fat, low-caloric intake diet, exercise can help people lose weight.[196] The PT and PTA can be influential in the reduction of obesity in the young. Exercise instruction sessions provided to children in school systems can explain exercise, posture, and eating habits. Physical education within the school curriculum is becoming less important in schools across the country in favor of more academics. This deemphasis of physical education may result in a population that does not understand the value of exercise. Coupled with the amount of time children spend in front of the TV, computer, and playing sedentary games, this devaluing of exercise does not auger well for the future health of these children as they grow to adulthood. Recess in schools does not encourage outside play, and many children cannot play outside at home because of unsafe environments. Physical therapy professionals need to become involved more in the prevention of obesity, and education about the awareness of the need for physical activity.

Prevention of obesity is the best way of reducing the risks of comorbid, life-threatening diseases in adulthood. The prevalence of both overweight and obesity is increasing among children and young adults. Hlaing, Nath, and Huffman reported that "weight gain during college years is considerably greater than that observed in the general population over the same time frame" (p. 83).[197] This weight gain places college students at increased risk of cardiovascular diseases. Hlaing et al. suggested that the college years set the stage for patterns of behavior in adulthood, making this an ideal venue for the involvement of the physical therapy profession.[198] In addition, physical therapy interventions for increased pulmonary function can help people with a reduction in lung volumes as a result of obesity.[199] Fitness programs for people who are obese may need to take into consideration the extra amount of energy expenditure required by those who are overweight. When assessing the cardiovascular fitness of people who are obese the 12-minute walk/run test seems to offer the most accurate data.[200] According to Ohtake (2008), 20 minutes of moderate exercise, such as brisk walking, on most days may not be suitable for people who are obese because it may raise the heart rate too much. Ohtake's recommendation for people who are overweight, particularly when starting an exercise program, is to walk at a slower pace for a little longer. Ohtake suggested that a slower speed of ambulation encourages compliance to the routine of exercise and reduces the stress on weight-bearing joints, already overburdened by the increased weight.[201] These ideas are actually in line with the CDC recommendations for people who are obese to start to walk for approximately 10 minutes per day 3 days a week and build up to 20 to 30 minutes 5 days a week. The total time of walking or other similar activity may be split up into several 10-minute sessions rather than one long session.[202]

Eating Disorders

The two eating disorders described in this section include anorexia nervosa and bulimia nervosa. Both these conditions result in lack of nutrition of the body that can lead to severe impairment in the musculoskeletal system as well as cognitive dysfunctions and organ disease.

Anorexia Nervosa

Anorexia nervosa is both a psychiatric and a nutritional disease. This serious eating disorder predominantly affects young females during and immediately after the onset of adolescence. However, 5% of those affected by the disorder are male.[203] The prevalence of anorexia nervosa is approximately 3 to 5 in 1,000 of the general population.[204] Some estimates are that 1 in every 100 adolescent girls has the disorder, and that between 0.5% and 3.7% of all women will have anorexia at some time during their lives.[205] Girls who are Caucasian and come from middle and upper socioeconomic groups seem to be more at risk for the disorder.[206]

Etiology. The etiology of anorexia nervosa is unknown. A variety of factors play a role in the development of the condition including social, psychological, and endocrinal. The hormones that are involved with appetite are thought to play a significant role in the onset of the disorder.[207] Appetite control hormones include serotonin (monoamines released by the hypothalamus), neuropeptides such as cholecystokinin, and leptin leading to the theory that dysfunction of the hypothalamus may cause the disorder.[208] Recent findings also suggest that areas of the brain, mainly in the cerebrum, may atrophy and precipitate the onset of the condition.[209]

Signs and Symptoms. The main characteristic signs and symptoms of the condition are that people believe they are overweight and have a fear of remaining overweight. In many instances, the body weight is below 85% of the expected body weight, and so the person is not overweight at all.[210] The sense of body image is affected in an obsessive way. The condition causes cessation of menstruation in the female and a lower than expected body weight, resulting in malnutrition. The signs, symptoms, and complications of anorexia nervosa include constipation, depression, osteoporosis, intolerance to cold, hypoglycemic coma, renal failure as a result of dehydration and rhabdomyolysis (breakdown of muscle fibers), cardiac arrhythmia, and temporary cognitive deficits including reduced levels of concentration.[211-212] A correlation has been determined between migraine headaches and anorexia nervosa with 75% of people with anorexia experiencing migraine headaches as opposed to approximately 12% of the general population. Migraine headaches in adolescent females may be one of the precursors of anorexia nervosa.[213]

Prognosis. The early diagnosis and treatment of people with anorexia nervosa greatly improves the prognosis. Approximately 50% of people with anorexia nervosa recover completely, and 20% remain chronically ill for the rest of their lives.[214] In people with prolonged anorexia nervosa, cardiac arrhythmia and renal failure may occur. Osteoporosis and osteopenia are complications of the disorder that may continue into adulthood even if the disorder is resolved.[215] The mortality rate for people with the disorder is much higher than for the rest of the population. Between 6% and 10% of people with anorexia nervosa will die as a result of the condition.[216] Deaths result mainly from kidney failure, cardiac complications, electrolyte imbalances, and suicide.[217]

Medical Intervention. Medical intervention for people with anorexia nervosa involves the whole family and a variety of health care providers. ☻ The parents and siblings of the affected adolescent are required to be part of the counseling process to understand how they can help to support the person through recovery, both emotionally and physically. Typically those involved with treatment include a physician, a psychologist, psychiatrist, and a licensed counselor, a nurse, and a dietician.[218] People with anorexia nervosa may need to be hospitalized if they are extremely dehydrated, or have become emaciated as a result of malnutrition. Group therapy and the use of support groups with other people with the condition are helpful as part of the counseling program. The psychological intervention for people with anorexia nervosa is a prolonged program in which patients have to build a level of trust with the health care provider.[219] Antidepressant medications are used in conjunction with counseling.

Physical Therapy Intervention. Although physical therapy intervention is not specifically indicated for people with anorexia nervosa, the condition is so prevalent that people with the disorder will be seen in the physical therapy clinic while treated for other conditions. The PTA should be aware of the implications of anorexia nervosa when providing interventions for physical therapy diagnoses. People with anorexia nervosa may fatigue rapidly or tend to over-exercise in an attempt to lose weight. Close monitoring of the exercise programs of people with the disorder is required to ensure compliance with the home exercise program especially after surgery or injury. Because many people with anorexia nervosa are in denial that they have an eating disorder, the recovery process may be complicated.

Bulimia Nervosa

Bulimia nervosa is a chronic eating disorder more common in females than males. The age of onset of bulimia nervosa is slightly higher than for anorexia, between the ages of 16 and 35.[220]

Etiology. The etiology of bulimia nervosa is unknown, but like anorexia nervosa, a strong psychological component and possible multiple contributing factors exist. The theories regarding the etiology of bulimia nervosa include a hereditary tendency and a behavioral component of impulsivity. People with bulimia nervosa demonstrate feelings of low self-worth and often are overinfluenced by peer and societal pressures to be thin.[221] Approximately 50% of people with anorexia nervosa develop bulimia nervosa.[222]

Signs and Symptoms. Patients with bulimia nervosa binge-eat vast quantities of food followed by purging of the food by self-induced vomiting or through the use of laxatives or diuretics (increase urine output), in an attempt to prevent any weight gain. People with bulimia have a compulsive concern about body weight and shape, even when their body weight is within the expected normal for their height and age, but may not be emaciated like those people with anorexia nervosa.[223] Bulimia causes a reduced nutritional status, which can affect the pancreas, intestine (constipation, hemorrhoids), teeth (cavities, gum infections, enamel erosion), and esophagus, and create electrolyte imbalances and dehydration.[224] The constant regurgitation of food, with the accompanying stomach acid, can permanently damage the esophagus.[225] Depression and anemia are both common in people with this condition. Migraine headaches are associated with bulimia, as they are with anorexia, and may be one of the precursors of the condition.[226] Approximately 84% of people with both anorexia and bulimia nervosa have migraine headaches that start before or at the same time as the eating disorder, compared to 12.5% of the general population who have migraine headaches.[227]

Prognosis. Many people with bulimia nervosa have reoccurrences of binging and vomiting episodes throughout their lives even when they are initially able to control their symptoms.[228] Unlike anorexia nervosa, bulimia nervosa is not usually life threatening.

Medical Intervention. The diagnosis of bulimia nervosa may be difficult. People with bulimia keep the episodes of binge eating and vomiting a secret, and even close family members may be unaware of the problem. People affected with the disorder may appear to be eating normally and then self-induce vomiting. The medical intervention for people with bulimia nervosa includes cognitive behavior therapy and the use of antidepressant medications.[229] The antidepressant prescribed for bulimia is fluoxetine (Prozac), a selective serotonin reuptake inhibitor (SSRI), which treats the symptoms of depression and may lower the frequency of binging and vomiting episodes.[230]

Physical Therapy Intervention. Physical therapy intervention is not indicated for bulimia nervosa, but the PT and PTA may treat people for other problems and recognize the warning signs of this eating disorder. In many cases, the PT and/or PTA develop a good rapport with individuals and may be taken into the confidence of the person with bulimia nervosa. Talking to the individual may allow the PT or PTA to suggest that the patient seek medical help. If the patient is a minor, the therapist should speak to the parent or guardian. The PT may also include the subjective findings regarding bulimia in the correspondence sent to the physician.

Vitamin Deficiencies. Vitamin deficiencies occur as a result of poor diet, reduced absorption of vitamins by the body, alcoholism, or metabolic disorders. Excessive amounts of a particular vitamin absorbed by the body can also lead to medical problems. The Food and Drug Administration (FDA) has established optimum levels of individual vitamin intake per day. See Table 9-8 for recommended daily intake of various vitamins and minerals. Some vitamins require the presence of other substances to be effective; for example, vitamin D is essential for the absorption of calcium. A balanced diet supplies all the vitamins necessary for a healthy body; however, many people in the Western world do not eat sufficient fresh fruits and vegetables, meat, and cereals to provide the necessary nutrients. A balance of proteins, carbohydrates, and fats is necessary for a balanced diet. Table 9-9 shows the functions of the main vitamins and the medical problems resulting from deficiency of the vitamin. Vitamin deficiencies are also thought to reduce the ability of the body to fight off infection. Vitamin supplements are popular, but naturally occurring vitamins found in foods may be more readily absorbed and utilized by the body. Toxicity due to high intake of vitamins is mainly found in the fat-soluble vitamins (see Table 9-9). The water-soluble vitamins are excreted by the kidneys and thus do not build up in the body.

(text continues on page 414)

Table 9.8　Dietary Daily Intake Recommendations of Vitamins and Minerals

VITAMIN OR MINERAL	RECOMMENDED DAILY ALLOWANCE—MALES	RECOMMENDED DAILY ALLOWANCE—FEMALES	RECOMMENDED DAILY ALLOWANCE DURING PREGNANCY
Vitamin A	900 µg	700 µg	750–770 µg
Vitamin B$_1$ (thiamin)	0.9–1.2 mg	0.9–1.1 mg	1.4 mg
Vitamin B$_2$ (riboflavin)	1.1 mg	0.9 mg	1.2 mg
Vitamin B$_6$	1.1–1.4 mg	1.0–1.3 mg	1.6 mg
Vitamin B$_{12}$ (cobalamin)	1.8–2.4 µg	1.8–2.4 µg	2.6 µg
Niacin	12 mg	11 mg	14 mg
Folate (folic acid)	400 µg	400 µg	400 µg
Vitamin C (ascorbic acid)	45–90 mg	45–75 mg	80–85 mg
Vitamin D (calciferol)	5–15 µg	5–15 µg	5 µg
Vitamin E (a-tocopherol)	12 mg	12 mg	12 mg
Vitamin K	60–120 mg	60–90 mg	75–90 mg
Calcium	1,000–1,200 mg	1,000–1,200 mg	1,000–1,300 mg
Chromium	25–35 µg	20–25 µg	29–30 µg

Table 9.8 Dietary Daily Intake Recommendations of Vitamins and Minerals (continued)

VITAMIN OR MINERAL	RECOMMENDED DAILY ALLOWANCE—MALES	RECOMMENDED DAILY ALLOWANCE—FEMALES	RECOMMENDED DAILY ALLOWANCE DURING PREGNANCY
Copper	700–900 µg	700–900 µg	1,000 µg
Fluoride	2–4 mg	2 -3 mg	3 mg
Iodine	120–150 µg	120–150 µg	220 µg
Iron	8–11 mg	8–18 mg	27 mg
Magnesium	240–420 mg	240–320 mg	350–400 mg
Manganese	1.9–2.3 mg	1.6–1.8 mg	2.0 mg
Phosphorus	700–1,250 mg	700–1,250 mg	700–1,250 mg
Selenium	40–55 µg	40–55 µg	60 µg
Zinc	8–11 mg	8 mg	11–12 mg

(Information compiled from data published by National Academy of Sciences (2005), Institute of Medicine, Food and Nutrition Board. *Dietary reference intake: Vitamins; Dietary reference intakes: elements; Dietary reference intakes: and Estimated average requirements for groups.* Retrieved from http://www.iom.edu. Also from Centers for Disease Control and Prevention at www.cdc.gov.

Table 9.9 Vitamin Functions and Deficiencies

VITAMIN	FUNCTION	SOURCE OF VITAMIN	RESULTS OF DEFICIENCY
Vitamin A–retinol (fat soluble)	Regulation of cell growth and differentiation in mucous membranes, synthesis of visual protein, immunity to infection May help to prevent cancer Embryonic development	Fish, eggs, dairy products, liver Carotenoids such as beta-carotene (precursors of Vit A) found in spinach, carrots and other green leafy vegetables Stored in the liver	Night-vision deficits, reduced immunity to infection in children Vitamin A toxicity may occur and produce headaches, vomiting, dry skin, hair loss
Vit B_1—thiamine (water soluble)	Nervous system health and nerve conduction, synthesis of adenosine triphosphate (ATP), metabolism of carbohydrates	Naturally occurring foods (not found in white flour or white sugar) Whole grains and enriched breads	Wet (cardiac disease) and dry Beriberi (peripheral neuropathy) Wernicke-Korsakoff syndrome (ataxic gait, confusion, nystagmus, reduced energy) Often a result of alcoholism
Vit B_2—riboflavin (water soluble)	Antioxidant, blood health, metabolism of nucleic acid	Meat, organ meats, vegetables, dairy products, breads	Eye problems (Mainly found in alcoholics, cancer or other chronic diseases)
Vit B_6—Pyridoxine (water soluble)	Formation of pyridoxal-5-phosphate Metabolism of amino acids	Cereals, organ meats, soy products	Dermatitis, keratitis, peripheral neuropathy Sometimes seen during pregnancy; supplements needed for the mother May be caused by medications including oral contraceptives and alcoholism

(table continues on page 414)

Table 9.9   **Vitamin Functions and Deficiencies** (continued)

VITAMIN	FUNCTION	SOURCE OF VITAMIN	RESULTS OF DEFICIENCY
Vit B$_{12}$—Cyanocobalamin/cobalamin (water soluble)	Nucleic acid synthesis, nervous system health, blood health	Meat and dairy products, fish, poultry	Pernicious anemia, mental confusion
Niacin (water soluble)	Lowers plasma low-density lipoprotein, cell metabolism	Peas and beans, grains, seed oils, meat Also synthesized from the amino acid tryptophan	Pellagra (dermatitis, diarrhea and dementia)
Folate—folic acid (water soluble)	Nucleic acid and amino acid synthesis	Fresh fruits and vegetables	Megaloblastic anemia
Vit C–ascorbic acid (Water soluble)	Antioxidant, collagen synthesis, wound healing, drug metabolism	Citrus fruits, tomatoes, potatoes, green vegetables, strawberries	Scurvy (delayed wound healing, bleeding into joints, gum disease, loss of teeth)
Vit D—calciferol (fat soluble)	Facilitates calcium and phosphorus absorption by the intestines Works with parathyroid hormone to take calcium from bone when the vitamin is in short supply	Produced in the skin in response to ultraviolet rays Fish, grains and plants, fortified milk, eggs, fish liver oils	Osteomalacia, rickets
Vit E–a-tocopherol (fat soluble)	Antioxidant, needed for nervous system health, reproductive health	Nuts, whole grains, nut and vegetable seed oils, green vegetables, fruit, dairy products, fish and meat	Neural syndromes affecting spine and cerebellum (may be a side effect of cystic fibrosis) Vitamin E toxicity is rare, but can cause nausea and diarrhea
Vit K (Fat soluble)	Affects prothrombin production and development of other clotting factors of VII, IX and X, protein synthesis, bone metabolism, protein synthesis	Bile from the gallbladder and common bile duct required for Vit K absorption by the intestine Green vegetables and plant oils	Deficits in blood clotting mechanism including hemorrhagic disease of the newborn

Mineral Deficiencies

The most important minerals required by the body are calcium, iron, potassium, sodium, zinc, magnesium, chloride, and iodine. As described in Chapter 6, calcium is crucial to bone formation and general bone health. A lack of calcium in the body leads to the conditions of osteomalacia in the adult, and rickets in the child. Iron is essential for hemoglobin synthesis. Iron is stored mainly in the erythrocytes, liver, and spleen. A lack of iron in the body results in anemia. Iron is needed in the daily diet because it is excreted from the body in the urine, in the blood during menstruation, and in sweat and feces. During exercise, iron is lost through excessive sweating. Iodine is necessary for thyroid health. Potassium, sodium, chloride, zinc, and magnesium are all needed for nerve transmission, muscle function, cardiac function, healing, and protein synthesis.

Inflammatory Bowel Disease

The inflammatory bowel diseases are described in Chapter 14. This group of diseases is mentioned here due to the malabsorption of nutrients from foods caused by these diseases as a result of diarrhea. People with inflammatory bowel disease may need to take vitamin and mineral supplements to prevent the onset of the symptoms caused by reduced intake, or absorption, of these essential dietary elements.

CASE STUDY 9.1

A 60-year-old female patient attends the physical therapy clinic. She has a diagnosis of diabetes mellitus (DM) and has a peripheral neuropathy of the right lower extremity. The PT has evaluated the patient and determined the plan of care. The patient has difficulty ambulating as the result of a foot drop caused by the peripheral neuropathy. You are designated by the PT to treat the patient. Treatment is to include lower extremity strengthening exercises, gait training with an appropriate assistive device, a home exercise program, advice on suitable footwear, and precautions to take at home to prevent complications from the diabetes.

1. Develop a strengthening exercise program for the right lower extremity taking into consideration the peripheral neuropathy and associated lack of skin sensation.

2. Develop a home exercise program the patient can perform independently.

3. Choose an appropriate assistive device for ambulation.

4. Detail the precautions the patient needs to take at home to prevent foot problems secondary to the peripheral neuropathy and DM. Develop a list suitable for giving to the patient to take home regarding these precautions.

STUDY QUESTIONS

1. List three hormones produced by the anterior pituitary gland.

2. Name a disease process caused by pituitary hypofunction.

3. Name a disease caused by pituitary hyperfunction.

4. What are some of the characteristics of hyperthyroidism?

5. What precautions should the PTA be aware of when treating the patient with hyperthyroidism?

6. What is Addison's disease?

7. What is Cushing's syndrome and what is its relevance to the PTA?

8. Describe the pancreatic dysfunction mechanism in diabetes mellitus (DM).

9. Complications of DM are many. Name three of the most common complications the PTA may see in the clinic and explain the significance of a knowledge regarding DM for the PTA.

10. Detail advice the PT/PTA should provide to the patient with DM.

11. Describe precautions the PTA should take when treating the patient with DM.

12. Obesity is a common problem in the United States and the Western world. Why should PTs and PTAs be concerned about this problem, and what can they do to help reduce the incidence of obesity?

⊙ USEFUL WEB SITES

American Diabetes Association
http://www.diabetes.org

Centers for Disease Control and Prevention
http://www.cdc.gov

eMedicine from WebMD
http://www.emedicine.com (Requires registration to obtain log in information. No cost)

Mayo Clinic
http://www.mayoclinic.com

MedlinePlus, U.S. National Library of Medicine, National Institutes of Health
http://www.nlm.nih.gov/medlineplus

Memorial Sloan-Kettering Cancer Center
http://www.mskcc.org

National Endocrine and Metabolic Diseases Information Service

National Institutes of Diabetes and Digestive and Kidney Diseases, National Institutes of Health

http://www.endocrine.niddk.nih.gov

U.S. Food and Drug Administration

U.S. Department of Health and Human Services

http://www.fda.gov

WebMD

http://www.webmd.com

● REFERENCES

[1] Pituitary disorders. (2010). *MedlinePlus Medical Encyclopedia.* Retrieved 11.23.10 from http://www.nlm.nih.gov/medlineplus/pituitarydisorders.html

[2] Kattah, J. (2009). Pituitary tumors. *eMedicine from WebMD.* Retrieved 11.23.10 from http://www.emedicine.com/NEURO/topic312.htm

[3] Kaneshior, N. K. (2010). Growth hormone deficiency. *MedlinePlus Medical Encyclopedia.* Retrieved 11.23.10 from http://www.nlm.nih.gov/MEDLINEPLUS/ency/article/001176.htm

[4] Kattah, J (2009). Pituitary tumors. *eMedicine from WebMD.* Retrieved 11.23.10 from http://www.emedicine.com/NEURO/topic312.htm

[5] Zieve, D. (20010). Diabetes insipidus. *MedlinePlus Medical Encyclopedia.* Retrieved 11.23.10 from http://www.nlm.nih.gov/medlineplus/ency/article/000377.htm

[6] Ferry, R. F. Jr., & Shim, M. (2006). Hyperpituitarism. *eMedicine from WebMD.* Retrieved 6.3.2008 from http://cancerweb.ncl.ac.uk/cgi-bin/omd?hyperpituitarism

[7] Ibid.

[8] Acromegaly.org. (2010). *Acromegaly.* Retrieved 11.23.10 from http://www.acromegaly.org/

[9] National Endocrine and Metabolic Diseases Information Service. (2008). *Acromegaly.* Retrieved 9.6.2009 from http://www.endocrine.niddk.nih.gov/pubs/acro/acro.htm#treat

[10] Ferry, R. F. Jr., & Shim, M. Hyperpituitarism. *eMedicine from WebMD.* Ibid.

[11] Center for Cancer Education. (2007). *Hyperpituitarism.* University of Newcastle upon Tyne. Retrieved 6.3.2008 from http://cancerweb.ncl.ac.uk/cgi-bin/omd?hyperpituitarism

[12] Acromegaly.org. Ibid.

[13] National Endocrine and Metabolic Diseases Information Service. *Acromegaly.* Ibid.

[14] Ibid.

[15] Ibid.

[16] Hyperthyroidism. (2010). *MedlinePlus Medical Encyclopedia.* Retrieved 11.23.10 from http://www.nlm.nih.gov/MEDLINEPLUS/ency/article/000356.htm

[17] Norman, J. (2010). *Hyperthyroidism.* EndocrineWeb.com. Retrieved 11.23.10 from http://www.endocrineweb.com/hyper4.html

[18] Ibid.

[19] Ibid.

[20] *Mayo Clinic Staff.* (2010). Hyperthyroidism (overactive thyroid gland). Retrieved 11.23.10 from http://www.mayoclinic.com/health/hyperthyroidism/DS00344

[21] Hyperthyroidism. (2010). Ibid.

[22] Mayo Clinic. *Hyperthyroidism (overactive thyroid gland).* Ibid.

[23] Mayo Clinic. Ibid.

[24] Hyperthyroidism. Ibid.

[25] Norman, J. Ibid.

[26] Mathur, R., et al. (2010). Hypothyroidism. *MedicineNet.com.* Retrieved 11.23.10 from http://www.medicinenet.com/hypothyroidism/page5.htm

[27] Bharaktiya, S., et al. (2010). Hypothyroidism. *eMedicine from WebMD.* Retrieved 11.23.10 from http://www.emedicine.com/med/TOPIC1145.HTM

[28] Ibid.

[29] Ibid.

[30] Mathur, R. Ibid.

[31] Ibid.

[32] Bharaktiya, S., et al. Ibid.

[33] Ibid.

[34] Mathur, R. Ibid.

[35] National Endocrine and Metabolic Diseases Information Service. (2006). *Hyperparathyroidism.* Retrieved 9.6.2008 from http://www.endocrine.niddk.nih.gov/pubs/hyper/hyper.htm

[36] Kaneshiro, N. K. (2010). Rickets. *MedlinePlus, MedlinePlus Medical Encyclopedia.* Retrieved 11.23.10 from http://www.nlm.nih.gov/medlineplus/ency/article/000344.htm

[37] National Endocrine and Metabolic Diseases Information Service. *Hyperparathyroidism.* Ibid.

[38] Eckman, A. S. (2010). Hyperparathyroidism. *MedlinePlus, MedlinePlus Medical Encyclopedia.* Retrieved 11.23.10 from http://www.nlm.nih.gov/medlineplus/ency/article/001215.htm

[39] Eckman, A. S. (2010). Secondary hyperparathyroidism. *MedlinePlus Medical Encyclopedia.* Retrieved 11.23.10 from http://www.nlm.nih.gov/medlineplus/ency/article/000318.htm

[40] Clements, R. H., et al. (2008). Hyperparathyroidism and vitamin D deficiency after laparascopic gastric bypass. *Am Surg* 74:469–475.

[41] Mayo Foundation for Medical Education and Research (2010). *Hyperthyroidism.* Retrieved 11.22.10 from http://www.mayoclinic.com/health/hyperparathyroidism/DS00396/DSECTION=symptoms

[42] Ibid.

[43] Eckman, A. S. Secondary hyperparathyroidism. Ibid.

[44] Eckman, A. S. Hyperparathyroidism. Ibid.

[45] National Endocrine and Metabolic Diseases Information Service. *Hyperparathyroidism.* Ibid.

[46] Goodman, W. G. (2002). Calcimimitic agents and secondary hyperparathyroidism: treatment and prevention. *Nephrology, Dialysis, and Transplant* 17:204–207. Retrieved 9.6.2008 from http://ndt.oxfordjournals.org/cgi/content/full/17/2/204

[47] Eckman, A. S. Hyperparathyroidism. Ibid.

[48] Ibid.

[49] Wallace, D. J., & Gliwa, A. (2009). Hypoparathyroidism. *eMedicine from WebMD.* Retrieved 4.12.2010 from http://www.emedicine.com/emerg/TOPIC276.HTM

[50] Eckman, A. S. Hypoparathyroidism. Ibid.

[51] Eckman, A. S. Hypoparathyroidism. Ibid.

[52] Wallace, D. J., & Gliwa, A. Ibid.

[53] Eckman, A. S. Hypoparathyroidism. Ibid.

[54] Liotta, E. A., & Elston, D. M. (2010). Addison disease. *eMedicine from WebMD.* Retrieved 11.22.10 from http://www.emedicine.com/derm/topic761.htm

[55] National Institute of Diabetes and Digestive and Kidney Diseases. (2009). *Adrenal insufficiency and Addison's disease.* Retrieved 4.6.2010 from http://endocrine.niddk.nih.gov/pubs/addison/addison.htm

[56] Seibel, J. A. (2009). Understanding Addison's disease. *WebMD.* Retrieved 6.4.2010 from http://www.webmd.com/a-to-z-guides/understanding-addisons-disease-basics

[57] Liotta, E. A., & Elston, D. M. Addison disease. *eMedicine from WebMD.* Ibid.

[58] National Institute of Diabetes and Digestive and Kidney Diseases. (2009). *Adrenal insufficiency and Addison's disease.* Ibid.

[59] Ibid.

[60] Ibid.

61 Addison's disease. (2010). *MedlinePlus Medical Encyclopedia.* Retrieved 11.23.10 from http://www.nlm.nih.gov/medlineplus/addisonsdisease.html

62 National Institute of Diabetes and Digestive and Kidney Diseases. (2009). *Adrenal insufficiency and Addison's disease.* Ibid.

63 Liotta, E. A., & Elston, D. M. (2010). Addison disease. *eMedicine from WebMD.* Retrieved 11.22.10 from http://www.emedicine.com/derm/topic761.htm

64 National Institute of Diabetes and Digestive and Kidney Diseases. (2009). *Adrenal insufficiency and Addison's disease.* Ibid.

65 Newell-Price, J. (2008). Cushing's syndrome. *Clin Med* 8:204–208, p. 204. Retrieved 8.20.2008 from ProQuest Health and Medical Complete database (Document ID: 1455084331).

66 Ibid., p. 207.

67 Usdan, L., & Lee, S. L. (2008, July). Cushing syndrome and bilateral adrenal enlargement. *Endocr Today* 6:14. Retrieved 8.20.2008 from ProQuest Health and Medical Complete database (Document ID: 1521905311).

68 Kola, B., & Grossman, A. B. (2008). Dynamic testing in Cushing's syndrome. *Pituitary* 11:155–162, p. 155. Retrieved 8.20.2008 from ProQuest Health and Medical Complete database (Document ID: 1473306071).

69 Newell-Price, J. Ibid., p. 204.

70 Ibid., p. 204.

71 Ibid., p. 204.

72 Ibid., p. 204.

73 Kola, B., & Grossman, A. B. Ibid., p. 155.

74 Haigh, C., & Bell, D. S. H. (2008, August). Guidelines released for Cushing's syndrome. *Endocr Today* 6L11. Retrieved 8.20.2008 from ProQuest Health & Medical Complete database (Document ID: 1534872741).

75 Newell-Price, J. Ibid., p. 207.

76 Chew, S. (2008). Conn's syndrome. *Cushing's Help and Support.* Retrieved 8.20.2008 from http://www.cushings-help.com/conns_syndrome.htm

77 Jabbour, S. A. (2009). Conn syndrome. *eMedicine from WebMD.* Retrieved 4.6.2010 from http://www.emedicine.com/med/topic432.htm

78 Walz, M. K., et al. (2008). Retroperitoneoscopic adrenalectomy in Conn's syndrome caused by adrenal adenomas or nodular hyperplasia. *World J Surg* 32:847–853. Retrieved 8.20.2008 from ProQuest Health and Medical Complete database (Document ID: 1470821451). p. 847.

79 Chew, S. Ibid.

80 Jabbour, S. A. Ibid.

81 Walz, M. K., et al. Ibid.

82 Jabbour, S. A. Ibid.

83 Haldeman-Englert, C. (2010). Congenital adrenal hyperplasia. *MedlinePlus Medical Encyclopedia.* Retrieved 11.23.10 from http://www.nlm.nih.gov/medlineplus/ency/article/000411.htm

84 Genetics Home Reference. (2010). *21-hydroxylase deficiency.* Retrieved 11.22.2010 from http://ghr.nlm.nih.gov/condition=21hydroxylasedeficiency

85 Wilson, T. A. (2010). Congenital adrenal hyperplasia. *eMedicine from WebMD.* Retrieved 11.22.2010 from http://www.emedicine.com/ped/topic48.htm

86 Ibid.

87 Hernanz-Schulman, M., Brock, J. W., & Russell, W. (2002). Sonographic findings in infants with congenital adrenal hyperplasia. *Pediatr Radiol* 32:130–137. Retrieved 8.20.2008 from ProQuest Health and Medical Complete database (Document ID: 1316644811), p. 130.

88 Haldeman-Englert, C. Ibid.

89 Ibid.

90 Ibid.

91 Ibid.

92 Memorial Sloan-Kettering Cancer Center. (2005). *Neuroblastoma.* Retrieved 8.22.2008 from http://www.mskcc.org/mskcc/html/2868.cfm?utm_source=AdWords

93 West, S. F., et al. (2008). Neuroblastoma. *eMedicine from WebMD.* Retrieved 8.8.2008 from http://www.emedicine.com/radio/topic472.htm

94 Ibid.

95 Krishan, A., & Shirkhoda, A. (2007). Pheochromocytoma. *eMedicine from WebMD.* Retrieved 6.5.2008 from http://www.emedicine.com/RADIO/topic552.htm

96 University of Texas, MD Anderson Cancer Center. (2010). *Pheochromocytoma.* Retrieved 11.22.2010 from http://www.mdanderson.org/patient-and-cancer-information/cancer-information/cancer-types/adrenal-disease/pheochromocytoma.html

97 Memorial Sloan-Kettering Cancer Center. Ibid.

98 West, S. F., & Correa, J. D. Ibid.

99 Pheochromocytoma. (2010). *MedlinePlus Medical Encyclopedia.* Retrieved 11.23.2010 from http://www.nlm.nih.gov/medlineplus/pheochromocytoma.html

100 University of Texas, MD Anderson Cancer Center. Ibid.

101 West, S. F., & Correa, J. D. Ibid.

102 University of Texas, MD Anderson Cancer Center. (2010). Ibid.

103 Ibid.

104 Memorial Sloan-Kettering Cancer Center. (2005). *Neuroblastoma.* Retrieved 8.22.2008 from http://www.mskcc.org/mskcc/html/2868.cfm?utm_source=AdWords

105 National Institute of Diabetes and Digestive and Kidney Diseases. (2008). *National Diabetes Statistics, 2007 fact sheet.* Bethesda, MD: U.S. Department of Health and Human Services, National Institutes of Health. Retrieved 4.8.2009 from http://diabetes.niddk.nih.gov/dm/pubs/statistics/#allages

106 American Diabetes Association. (n.d.). *Type 2 diabetes.* Retrieved 8.22.2008 from http://www.diabetes.org/type–2-diabetes.jsp

107 National Institute of Diabetes and Digestive and Kidney Diseases. Ibid.

108 Ibid.

109 Eckman, A. S. (2010). Type 1 diabetes. *MedlinePlus Medical Encyclopedia.* Retrieved 11.23.10 from http://www.nlm.nih.gov/medlineplus/ency/article/000305.htm

110 American Diabetes Association. (n.d.). *Type 2 diabetes.* Retrieved 8.22.2008 from http://www.diabetes.org/type–2-diabetes.jsp

111 Juhn, G., Eltz, D. R., & Stacy, K. A. (2007). Type 2 diabetes. *MedlinePlus Medical Encyclopedia.* Retrieved 8.22.2008 from http://www.nlm.nih.gov/MEDLINEPLUS/ency/article/000313.htm

112 Eckman, A. S. Ibid.

113 Juhn, G., Eltz, D. R., & Stacy, K. A. Ibid.

114 Eckman, A. S. Ibid.

115 Ibid.

116 Ibid.

117 Silberberg, C. (2010). End stage renal disease. *MedlinePlus Medical Encyclopedia.* Retrieved 11.23.10 from http://www.nlm.nih.gov/medlineplus/ency/article/000500.htm

118 National Diabetes Information Clearinghouse. (2009). *Diabetic neuropathies: The nerve damage of diabetes.* Retrieved 6.4.2010 from http://diabetes.niddk.nih.gov/dm/pubs/neuropathies/

119 Armstrong, D. G., & Lavery, L. A. (1998). Acute Charcot's arthropathy of the foot and ankle. *Phys Ther* 78:74–80. Retrieved 8.20.2008, from Research Library Database (Document ID: 25457769).

120 Ibid.

121 National Institute of Diabetes and Digestive and Kidney Diseases. *National Diabetes Statistics, 2007 fact sheet.* Ibid.

122 Ibid.

123 Ibid.

124 Eckman, A. S. (2010). Ibid.

[125] National Diabetes Information Clearinghouse. (2010). *What I need to know about diabetes medications.* Retrieved 11.23.10 from http://diabetes.niddk.nih.gov/dm/pubs/medicines_ez/

[126] Ibid.

[127] National Diabetes Information Clearinghouse. (NDIC) (2008). *What targets are recommended for blood glucose levels?* Retrieved from http://diabetes.niddk.nih.gov/dm/pubs/medicines_ez/#targets

[128] National Diabetes Information Clearinghouse. (NDIC) (2008). *Alpha-glucosidase inhibitor.* Retrieved 4.6.2009 from http://diabetes.niddk.nih.gov/dm/pubs/medicines_ez/insert_D.htm

[129] National Diabetes Information Clearinghouse. (NDIC) (2008). *Biguanide.* Retrieved from 4.6.2009 http://diabetes.niddk.nih.gov/dm/pubs/medicines_ez/insert_E.htm

[130] National Diabetes Information Clearinghouse. (NDIC) (2008). *D-phenylalanine derivatives.* Retrieved 4.6.2009 from http://diabetes .niddk.nih.gov/dm/pubs/medicines_ez/insert_F.htm

[131] Redmon, J. B., et al. (2005). Two-year outcome of a combination of weight loss therapies for Type 2 diabetes. *Diabetes Care* 28:1311–1115. Retrieved 8.20.2008 from Research Library Database (Document ID: 879526371).

[132] Mueller, M. J., et al. (2006). Efficacy and mechanism of orthotic devices to unload metatarsal heads in people with diabetes and a history of plantar ulcers. *Phys Ther* 86:833–842. Retrieved 08.20.08 from Research Library Database (Document ID: 1049783691).

[133] Evans, N., & Forsyth, E. (2004). End-stage renal disease in people with Type 2 diabetes: systemic manifestations and exercise implications. *Phys Ther* 84:454–463. Retrieved 8.20.08, from Research Library Database (Document ID: 637163041).

[134] Mueller, M. J., et al. Ibid.

[135] Mueller, M. J., et al. (1999). Use of computed tomography and plantar pressure measurement for management of neuropathic ulcers in patients with diabetes. *Phys Ther* 79:296–307. Retrieved 8.20.08 from Research Library Database (Document ID: 39904265).

[136] Di Loreto, C., et al. (2005). Make your diabetic patients walk: long-term impact of different amounts of physical activity on Type 2 diabetes. *Diabetes Care* 28:1295–1302. Retrieved 8.20.08 from Research Library Database (Document ID: 879526431).

[137] Salsich, G. B., et al. (2005). Effect of Achilles tendon lengthening on ankle muscle performance in people with diabetes mellitus and a neuropathic plantar ulcer. *Phys Ther* 85:34–43. Retrieved 8.20.08 from Research Library Database (Document ID: 776363931).

[138] Salsich, G. B., Mueller, M. J., & Sahrmann, S. A. (2000). Passive ankle stiffness in subjects with diabetes and peripheral neuropathy versus an age-matched comparison group. *Phys Ther* 80:352–362. Retrieved 8.20.08 from Research Library Database (Document ID: 52943170).

[139] L. Reichstein, et al. (2005). Effective treatment of symptomatic diabetic polyneuropathy by high-frequency external muscle stimulation. *Diabetologia* 48:824–828. Retrieved 8.20.08 from ProQuest Health and Medical Complete Database (Document ID: 841206241).

[140] Evans, N., Forsyth, E. Ibid.

[141] Quan, D., & Soliman, E. (2006). Diabetic neuropathy. *eMedicine from WebMD.* Retrieved from http://www.emedicine.com/neuro/topic88.htm

[142] National Diabetes Information Clearinghouse. (2009). *Diabetic neuropathies: the nerve damage of diabetes.* Retrieved 4.6.2010 from http://diabetes.niddk.nih.gov/dm/pubs/neuropathies/#cause

[143] Hurd, R. (2006). Diabetic hyperglycemic hyperosmolar coma. *MedlinePlus Medical Encyclopedia.* Retrieved 7.18.2008 from http://www.nlm.nih.gov/medlineplus/ency/article/000304.htm

[144] Hurd, R. (2006). Diabetic hyperglycemic hyperosmolar coma. Ibid.

[145] Longo, N., et al. (2007). Noninvasive measurement of phenylalanine by iontophoretic extraction in patients with phenylketonuria. *J Inherited Metabol Dis* 30:910–915. Retrieved 8.20.08 from ProQuest Health and Medical Complete Database (Document ID: 1397839691).

[146] US Food and Drug Administration. (2007). *FDA approves Kuvan for treatment of phenylketonuria (PKU).* Retrieved 8.16.2008 from http://www.fda.gov/bbs/topics/NEWS/2007/NEW01761.html

[147] Longo, N., et. al. Ibid., p. 911.

[148] *Pathophysiology in PKU.* (n.d.). Retrieved 8.16.2008 from http://www.pku.com/HCP/PKUBiochemistry/Pathophysiology.aspx

[149] Yu, Y. G., et al. (2007). Effects of phenylalanine and its metabolites on cytoplasmic free calcium in cortical neurons. *Neurochem Res* 32:1292–1301. Retrieved 8.20.08 from ProQuest Health and Medical Complete Database (Document ID: 1294986381).

[150] Huemer, M., et al. (2007). Growth and body composition in children with classical phenylketonuria: results in 34 patients and review of the literature. *J Inherited Metab Dis* 30:694–699. Retrieved 8.20.08 from ProQuest Health and Medical Complete Database (Document ID: 1367597761).

[151] Longo, N., et al. Ibid.

[152] Ibid., p. 911.

[153] US Food and Drug Administration. Ibid.

[154] *Pathophysiology in PKU.* (n.d.). Retrieved 8.16.2008 from http://www.pku.com/HCP/PKUBiochemistry/Pathophysiology.aspx

[155] Lopez Morra, H. A., Debes, J. D., & Dickstein, G. (2007). Wilson's disease: what lies beneath. *Digest Dis Sci* 52:941–942. Retrieved 8.20.08 from ProQuest Health and Medical Complete Database (Document ID: 1244569101).

[156] Schmidt, H. H.-J. (2007). Introducing single-nucleotide polymorphism markers in the diagnosis of wilson disease. *Clin Chem* 53:1568–1569. Retrieved 8.20.08 from ProQuest Health and Medical Complete Database (Document ID: 1337241531).

[157] Ibid.

[158] Wilson's Disease Association International. (2009). *About Wilson's disease.* Retrieved 11.23.10 from http://www.wilsonsdisease.org/about-wilsondisease.php

[159] National Digestive Diseases Information Clearinghouse. (2009). *Wilson disease.* Retrieved 11.23.10 from http://digestive.niddk.nih.gov/ddiseases/pubs/wilson/

[160] Schmidt, H. H.-J. Ibid.

[161] National Digestive Diseases Information Clearinghouse. Ibid.

[162] Wilson's Disease Association International. (2009). Ibid.

[163] National Digestive Diseases Information Clearinghouse. Ibid.

[164] Ibid.

[165] Lopez Morra, H. A., Debes, J. D., & Dickstein, G. Ibid.

[166] National Institutes of Neurological Disorders and Stroke. (2007). *NINDS Wilson's disease information page.* Retrieved 8.16.2008 from http://www.ninds.nih.gov/disorders/wilsons/wilsons.htm

[167] Sinha, S., et al. (2006). Wilson's disease: cranial MRI observations and clinical correlation. *Neuroradiology* 48:613–621. Retrieved 8.20.08 from Research Library Database (Document ID: 1131634181).

[168] Piga, M., et al. (2008). Brain MRI and SPECT in the diagnosis of early neurological involvement in Wilson's disease. *Eur J Nucl Med Molec Imaging* 35:716–724. Retrieved 8.20.08 from ProQuest Health and Medical Complete Database (Document ID: 1451763451).

[169] National Digestive Diseases Information Clearinghouse. Ibid.

[170] Piga, M., et al. Ibid.

[171] Schmidt, H. H.-J. Ibid.

[172] National Digestive Diseases Information Clearinghouse. Ibid.

[173] Schmidt, H. H.-J. Ibid.

[174] National Digestive Diseases Information Clearinghouse. Ibid.

[175] U.S. Department of Health and Human Services. (2009). *Healthy People 2020.* Retrieved 11.23.10 from http://www.healthypeople.gov/HP2020/

[176] Ibid.

[177] Rising levels of childhood obesity a "public health time bomb"? (2007). *Health Hygiene* 28:8. Retrieved 8.20.08 from Research Library Database (Document ID: 1289071661).

[178] Ibid.

[179] Europe weighs the cost of obesity. (2007). *J Royal Soc Promotion Health* 127:3. Retrieved 8.20.08 from Research Library Database (Document ID: 1215151481).

[180] Jones, R. L., & Nzekwu, M-M. U. (2006). The effects of body mass index on lung volumes. *Chest* 130:827–833. Retrieved 8.20.08 from ProQuest Health and Medical Complete Database (Document ID: 1146094411).

[181] Ohtake, P. J. (2008). The impact of obesity on walking: implications for fitness assessment and exercise prescription. *Cardiopulm Phys Ther J* 19:52–53. Retrieved 8.20.08 from ProQuest Nursing & Allied Health Source Database (Document ID: 1502909031).

[182] Afridi, A. K., & Khan, A. (2004). Prevalence and etiology of obesity—an overview. *Pakistan J Nutr* 3:14–25.

[183] Racette, S. B., Deusinger, S. S., & Deusinger, R. H. (2003). Obesity: overview of prevalence, etiology, and treatment. *Phys Ther* 83:276–288. Retrieved 8.20.08 from Research Library Database (Document ID: 323784881).

[184] DeNoon, D. J. (2007). Obesity virus: more, bigger fat cells. Common virus boosts fat-cell production—and makes fat cells fatter. *WebMD.* Retrieved 4.8.2008 from http://www.webmd.com/diet/news/20070820/obesity-virus-more-bigger-fat-cells

[185] Afridi, A. K., & Khan, A. Ibid.

[186] Centers for Disease Control and Prevention. (2008). About BMI for adults. Department of Health and Human Services. Retrieved 5.7.2009 from http://www.cdc.gov/nccdphp/dnpa/healthyweight/assessing/bmi/adult_BMI/about_adult_BMI.htm

[187] Ibid.

[188] Majed, B., et al. (2008). Is obesity an independent prognosis factor in woman breast cancer? *Breast Cancer Res Treat* 111:329–342. Retrieved 8.20.08 from Research Library Database (Document ID: 1518968131).

[189] Manson, J. E., et al. (1995, September). Body weight and mortality among women. *New Engl J Med* 333:677–685.

[190] Fouad, T. (2004). CDC: Obesity approaching tobacco as top preventable cause of death. *Doctor's Lounge.* Retrieved 8.16.2008 from http://www.doctorslounge.com/primary/articles/obesity_death/

[191] Partnership for healthy weight management. (n.d.). Body mass index (BMI). Retrieved 6.4.2008 from http://www.consumer.gov/weightloss/bmi.htm

[192] Centers for Disease Control and Prevention (2008). Ibid.

[193] Ibid.

[194] Orlistat. (2010). *MedlinePlus Medical Encyclopedia.* Retrieved 11.22.10 from http://www.nlm.nih.gov/medlineplus/druginfo/medmaster/a601244.html

[195] Racette, S. B., Deusinger, S. S., & Deusinger, R. H. Ibid.

[196] Ibid.

[197] Hlaing, W. W., Nath, S. D., & Huffman, F. G. (2007). Assessing overweight and cardiovascular risks among college students. *Am J Health Educ* 38:83–90. Retrieved 8.20.08 from ProQuest Nursing & Allied Health Source Database (Document ID: 1264042291).

[198] Ibid.

[199] Jones, R. L., & Nzekwu, M-M. U. Ibid.

[200] Drinkard, B., et al. (2001). Relationships between walk/run performance and cardiorespiratory fitness in adolescents who are overweight. *Phys Ther* 81:1889–1896. Retrieved 8.20.08 from Research Library Database (Document ID: 94621716).

[201] Ohtake, P. J. Ibid.

[202] Office of the Surgeon General, Centers for Disease Control and Prevention, US Department of Health and Human Services. (2007). Overweight and obesity: what you can do. Retrieved 8.20.2008 from http://www.surgeongeneral.gov/topics/obesity/calltoaction/fact_whatcanyoudo.htm

[203] Dryden-Edwards, R. (2010). Anorexia nervosa. *MedicineNet.com.* Retrieved 11.22.2010 from http://www.medicinenet.com/anorexia_nervosa/article.htm

[204] Ostuzzi, R., et al. (2008). Eating disorders and headache: coincidence or consequence? *Neurol Sci Suppl* 29:S83–87. Retrieved 8.20.08 from ProQuest Health and Medical Complete Database (Document ID: 1497356841).

[205] Dryden-Edwards, R. Anorexia nervosa. Ibid.

[206] Dryden-Edwards, R. Ibid.

[207] Ostuzzi, R., et al. bid.

[208] Ibid.

[209] Mühlau, M., et al. (2007). Gray matter decrease of the anterior cingulate cortex in anorexia nervosa. *Am J Psychiatry* 164:1850–1857. Retrieved 8.20.08 from Research Library Database (Document ID: 1393735941)

[210] Ostuzzi, R., et al. Ibid.

[211] Russell, J., et al. (2007). Anorexia nervosa and the brain. *J Psychosom Obstetr Gynecol* 28:17 [Abstracts from the XV International Congress of ISPOG]. Retrieved 8.20.08 from ProQuest Health and Medical Complete Database (Document ID: 1426331391).

[212] Legroux-Gérot, I., et al. (2007). Evaluation of bone loss and its mechanisms in anorexia nervosa. *Calcif Tissue Tiss Int* 81:174–182. Retrieved 8.20.08 from ProQuest Health and Medical Complete Database (Document ID: 1332000911).

[213] Ostuzzi, R., et al. Ibid.

[214] Dryden-Edwards, R. Ibid.

[215] Mika, C., et al. (2007). A 2-year prospective study of bone metabolism and bone mineral density in adolescents with anorexia nervosa. *J Neural Transm* 114:1611–1618. Retrieved 8.20.08 from ProQuest Health and Medical Complete Database (Document ID: 1394687861).

[216] Merrill, D. B. (2010). Anorexia nervosa. *MedlinePlus Medical Encyclopedia.* Retrieved 11.23.10 from http://www.nlm.nih.gov/medlineplus/ency/article/000362.htm

[217] Signorini, A., et al. (2007). Long-term mortality in anorexia nervosa: a report after an 8-year follow-up and a review of the most recent literature. *Eur J Clin Nutr* 61:119–122. Retrieved 8.20.08 from Research Library Database (Document ID: 1178316861).

[218] Anorexia nervosa—treatment overview. (2009). *WebMD.* Retrieved 11.22.10 from http://www.webmd.com/mental-health/anorexia-nervosa/anorexia-nervosa-treatment-overview

[219] Grohol, J. M. (2010) Anorexia nervosa treatment. *PsychCentral.* Retrieved 11.22.10 from http://psychcentral.com/disorders/ sx2t.htm

[220] Ostuzzi, R., et al. Ibid.

[221] Mayo Clinic. (2010). *Bulimia nervosa.* Mayo Foundation for Medical Education and Research. Retrieved 11.22.10 from http://www.mayoclinic.com/health/bulimia/DS00607/DSECTION= treatments-and-drugs

[222] Ostuzzi, R., et al. Ibid.

[223] Ibid.

[224] Ballas, P. (2010). Bulimia. *MedlinePlus Medical Encyclopedia.* Retrieved 11.22.10 from http://www.nlm.nih.gov/medlineplus/ency/article/000341.htm

[225] Ibid.

[226] Ostuzzi, R., et al. Ibid.

[227] Ibid.

[228] Ballas, P. Ibid.

[229] Hall, M. N., Friedman, R. J., II, & Leach, L. (2008). Treatment of bulimia nervosa. *Am Fam Physician* 77:1588, 1592. Retrieved 8.20.08 from Research Library Database (Document ID: 1486040891).

[230] Mayo Clinic. *Bulimia nervosa.* Ibid.

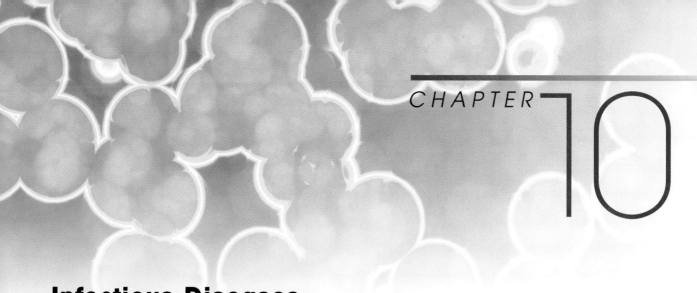

CHAPTER 10

Infectious Diseases

LEARNING OBJECTIVES

After completion of this chapter, students should be able to:

- Delineate the pathology and transmission of various types of hepatitis
- Describe the pathological mechanisms of various sexually transmitted diseases (STDs) including AIDS/HIV
- Discuss physical therapy interventions for people with AIDS/HIV
- Analyze the significance of the pathology and transmission of hepatitis to the physical therapist assistant
- Describe the pathology of various vector-borne infectious diseases in the United States
- Describe the pathology of other infectious diseases and their relationship to health care employees
- Determine the role of physical therapy intervention in the management of people with infectious diseases
- Apply protective measures to prevent contraction and spread when managing individuals with infectious diseases

CHAPTER OUTLINE

Introduction
Hepatitis
    Hepatitis A
    Hepatitis B (HBV)
    Hepatitis C (HCV)
    Hepatitis D, E and G
    Alcoholic Hepatitis
Human Immunodeficiency Virus and Acquired Immune Deficiency
    Syndrome
Sexually Transmitted Diseases
    Chancroid
    Chlamydia

KEY TERMS

AIDS dementia complex
Candidiasis (thrush)
Chlamydia
Cytomegalovirus (CMV)
Epstein-Barr virus (EBV)
Hantaviruses
Hepatitis B
Highly active antiretroviral therapy
    (HAART)
HIV/AIDS
Necrotizing fasciitis
Nosocomial infections
Opportunistic infections
Pertussis
Pneumocystis carinii
Pneumocystic jiroeci pneumonia
Poliomyelitis
Portal hypertension
Post-poliomyelitis syndrome
Reverse transcriptase
Reye's syndrome
Tabes dorsalis
Varicella (chickenpox)
West Nile virus

C H A P T E R O U T L I N E (continued)

Introduction

With the increasing incidence of infectious diseases in the United States, physical therapist assistants (PTAs) will most likely treat people who have these conditions. In some cases, the infection will have been identified, whereas other infections may remain undiagnosed at the time of treatment. People with some infectious diseases may exhibit characteristic signs and symptoms that may require physical therapy intervention. Physical therapy interventions for people with infectious diseases require the use of Standard (Universal) Precautions to protect both the patient and the provider of care. All health care workers are required to be immunized or demonstrate

immunity to certain infectious diseases, according to the Centers for Disease Control and Prevention (CDC) guidelines for control of infectious diseases.

The general basis of infective agents is described in Chapter 2. Many infectious diseases are described throughout the text in relation to specific body systems. The infectious diseases in this chapter are limited to those not related to a specific organ system described elsewhere in this book. Others may be of note to increase awareness of the potential of the spread of infection and the likelihood of the PTA coming into contact with persons with the infection. Sexually transmitted diseases are also detailed in this chapter. Diseases with specific bone, joint, cardiac, or respiratory symptoms may have been mentioned in previous chapters. Several of the diseases described in this chapter fall under the classification of blood-borne pathogens, including HIV/AIDS and hepatitis. This chapter is in no way a definitive description of all infectious diseases. The PTA should refer to an infectious disease text for details of diseases not discussed and for further details of the described diseases.

Why Does the Physical Therapist Assistant Need to Know About Hepatitis?

Knowledge regarding hepatitis is vital for the physical therapist assistant (PTA) for several reasons. Hepatitis B is one of the blood-borne pathogens that is more likely to be contracted by health care workers. The virus responsible for hepatitis B (HBV) is transmitted via blood and body fluids of an infected individual. The virus remains viable in these fluids even when outside the body. Spills of blood can remain contaminated for many hours, increasing the risk of heath care workers coming into contact with the virus. Health care workers can be protected from contracting this virus by a series of hepatitis B vaccinations. Knowledge of the pathology of hepatitis B can help the PTA to make informed decisions regarding vaccination options and ensure the use of Standard (Universal) Precautions and spill cleanup protocols when working with all patients to prevent the spread of the infection.

Hepatitis

Hepatitis is a group of liver infections and diseases caused by a variety of viruses. Several types of **hepatitis** exist, including **hepatitis A** (HAV), **hepatitis B (HBV)**, **hepatitis C** (HCV), **hepatitis D** (HDV), **hepatitis E** (HEV), **hepatitis G** (HGV), and **alcoholic hepatitis**. Health care providers have the greatest risk of being exposed to hepatitis B as a result of its prevalence and presence in the clinical setting.[1] The hepatitis B virus can live outside the body for extended periods of time, and thus the risk of contracting HBV is much greater for the health care provider. All health care workers are encouraged to have the hepatitis B vaccinations series unless they are allergic to any of the substances contained in the vaccine, such as yeast, or are advised not to do so by their physician. The hepatitis B vaccine does not contain the live virus; therefore, the risk

of contracting the disease from the vaccine is eliminated. In the United States, the blood supply for transfusion is checked for the presence of all types of hepatitis. The risk of contracting hepatitis from a blood transfusion has therefore been reduced to a minimum in recent years.[2]

All blood spills should be cleaned up using the recommendations from the CDC and the Occupational Safety and Health Administration (OSHA) regulations (Standards 29CFR), blood-borne pathogens section 1910.1030.[3] This regulation states that all spills must be "immediately contained and cleaned up by [people] . . . properly trained and equipped to work with potentially concentrated infectious materials" (Section 1910.1030 (e)(2)(ii)(K)). PTAs should be adequately trained in cleaning up spills of body fluids. Such training is particularly important for those PTAs working in wound care. In the clinical setting, the PTA should follow the guidelines developed by the institution for clean-up of body fluids. Guidelines include the use of Universal Precautions with gloves, masks, and gowns when necessary and the use of a solution of one part sodium hypochlorite (bleach) diluted in 10 parts water. The bleach should be sprayed and left on the contaminated area for 20 minutes to ensure the elimination of infective substances. All materials used to clean up spills of blood and body fluids should be disposed of in a bag (usually red) designated for contaminated substances.

Hepatitis A

Hepatitis A (HAV) is an acute liver disease also known as the traveler's virus because it is prevalent in underdeveloped countries where sewage treatment facilities are either nonexistent or poor or where human excrement is used for fertilizing vegetables. ⊛ Children particularly are at risk for contracting the disease. In 2006, the CDC stated that 3,579 new cases of acute hepatitis A were reported. When the numbers were adjusted to account for underreporting of the infection, the CDC estimated the number of new infections in the United States in 2006 to be 32,000. The incidence of the disease in 2006 was approximately 1.2 per 100,000 of the population, the lowest it had been for some years.[4]

Etiology. Hepatitis A (HAV) is an RNA virus transmitted through contact with body fluids, feces, and ingestion of contaminated food and drinking water.[5] The virus can remain viable (able to transmit infection) outside the body for several months. Once inside the body, the disease incubates within an average of 28 days within the liver and large quantities of the HAV virus are excreted in the feces.[6]

Signs and Symptoms. The characteristic signs and symptoms of hepatitis A include vomiting, loss of appetite, fatigue, abdominal pain, diarrhea, fever, joint pains, dark-colored urine, clay-colored feces, and jaundice.[7] Usually the symptoms of the disease resolve within 2 months without liver damage. However, the severity of the symptoms tends to increase with the age of the person.[8] ⊛ Medical recommendations from the CDC suggest that children over 1 year of age, those traveling to high-risk areas of the world, individuals working in health care, and people working with children should have the HAV vaccine.[9]

Prognosis. The prognosis for people with Hepatitis A is good. The condition does not lead to liver damage or chronic forms of hepatitis. People at greater risk for contracting the disease include those with clotting factor disorders, men who have sex with men, people with chronic liver disease, those who use illicit drugs, and people who work with primates such as chimpanzees and gorillas.[10]

Medical Intervention. The diagnosis of HAV is made through a blood test for the HAV virus. The best intervention for HAV is prevention. A vaccination is available provided in a two-dose series and can be administered to anyone over 1 year of age. Chlorination of water as practiced in the United States is effective in killing the virus. Hand washing before and after food preparation and after toileting and changing babies' diapers are some of the most effective methods of prevention of transmission of the disease. No medication is provided for the condition once contracted but immunoglobulin (Ig) can help to strengthen the immune system and reduce the effects of the infection.[11]

Physical Therapy Intervention. No direct physical therapy intervention is provided for people with hepatitis A. The PTA should practice regular hand washing to reduce the risk of either contracting the disease or transmitting it to others. If working with children, particular care should be taken to wash hands after changing diapers. All blood and body fluid spills should be cleaned up using the recommendations from OSHA and the CDC detailed in the general section regarding hepatitis.

Hepatitis B (HBV)

The reported incidence of hepatitis B in the United States is 1.6 in 100,000 of the population, but the CDC estimates that the actual incidence is up to 10 times higher.[12] In 2006, a reported 46,000 people in the United States were newly infected with HBV with rates of infection the highest in males between the ages of 25 and 44. The CDC estimates that between 800,000 and 1.4 million people in the United States live with chronic hepatitis as a result of HBV infection. Worldwide, chronic hepatitis affects 350 million people with 620,000 deaths attributed to HBV related liver disease each year.[13] The risk of contracting hepatitis B is extremely high for those individuals with HIV or other immunosuppressive disorders. Health care workers also are at risk of contracting the disease. ⊛ Since 1991, the CDC has recommended that all children and health care workers have the three series of vaccinations to protect them from this extremely virulent form of hepatitis. The number of people affected each year has reduced significantly since then. The HBV virus can remain viable (able to infect a person) outside the body for prolonged periods of time, thus increasing the risk of contact. HBV in contaminated blood on the surface of a table or equipment can remain viable for as long as 7 days.[14] All blood and body fluid spills should be cleaned up using the recommendations from OSHA and the CDC detailed in the general section regarding hepatitis.

Etiology. Hepatitis B (HBV) is a DNA virus and more serious than hepatitis A. HBV is a blood-borne pathogen transmitted through contact with contaminated blood, blood products, or through sexual contact. Specific methods of transmission may include blood transfusions; direct contact with the blood from an infected person into the eyes or a skin cut; contaminated instruments from such things as acupuncture, tattoos, and piercings; needle sharing when taking illicit drugs; unsafe sex; and from an infected mother to her child during the birthing process.[15] The incubation period between transmission of the virus and the appearance of symptoms can be anywhere from 6 weeks to 6 months.[16]

Signs and Symptoms. The characteristic signs and symptoms of HBV include loss of appetite, nausea and vomiting, weakness, fatigue, a low-grade fever, joint and muscle pains and aching, and a possible skin rash. Damage to the liver resulting from the infection may cause jaundice to develop with additional signs and symptoms of yellowing of the skin and dark-colored urine.[17]

Prognosis. In the majority of people infected with the virus, the acute symptoms subside a few weeks after they appear, and the liver returns to normal function within a period of a few months. Chronic hepatitis with liver failure may develop in approximately 5% of adults, and develops in approximately 95% of infants, and 50% of children aged 1 to 5 years with the infection.[18] Liver cirrhosis[19] and higher rates of liver cancers are reported long-term complications of hepatitis B. Approximately 1% of those infected with hepatitis B die.[20]

Medical Intervention. Prevention of hepatitis B is the most effective medical intervention. A series of vaccinations is available to prevent hepatitis B. This vaccination with a recombinant hepatitis B vaccine (derived from yeast cells and not from the actual disease) is also effective in preventing newborns from infection with the virus from an infected mother.[21] The classic method of vaccination is with a series of three injections at Days 0, 30, and 60. Some research has shown that accelerating the time with doses at 0, 10, and 30 days is just as effective for protecting health care workers against the HBV virus.[22] The CDC now recommends vaccination of all children in the United States and for all health care workers who do not demonstrate immunity to the condition.[23] Immunity to HBV can be determined through a blood titer to detect antibodies to HBV. The latest CDC recommendations (2008) are that booster shots for HBV are only needed for people with compromised immune systems or who are on kidney dialysis. Booster shots prolong the length of time of immunity to HBV.[24] Some pharmacological agents used to treat people with chronic HBV include HBV inhibitors such as adefovir dipivoxil (Hypsera) and entecavir (Baraclude) and antiviral medications such as interferon and lamivudine. The use of interferons or nucleoside/nucleotide analogues is successful in reducing virus reproduction in as many as 90% of people with chronic HBV infection.[25]

Physical Therapy Intervention. Physical therapy intervention is not indicated directly for HBV. However, many people treated by the PTA will have either been in contact with HBV or have the condition. The importance of following Standard Precautions when working with all people cannot be over emphasized. Because the HBV virus remains viable for so long outside the body, all blood or body fluids should be treated as if they are contaminated. Receiving immunization for HBV is not mandatory but should be carefully considered for self-protection against this virulent and serious disease.

Hepatitis C (HCV)

Hepatitis C is a viral infection affecting the liver prevalent among people who use intravenous drugs. More than 85% of people who contract HCV develop the chronic form of the disease. Over 4 million people in the United States and approximately 180 million worldwide have chronic hepatitis C.[26] This chronic form of HCV is considered to be underreported and on the increase both in the United States and worldwide.

Etiology. Hepatitis C (HCV) is an RNA virus transmitted via infected blood that is most common in persons who use intravenous illicit drugs or have multiple sexual partners.[27] Currently, six genotypes of the virus have been identified, with a total of 50 subtypes.[28] Hepatitis C has been reported after blood transfusion, but since 1992, the blood supply in the United States has been tested for the virus, and the chances of infection from this source are minimal. In more rare instances, hepatitis C may develop as a nosocomial infection in people who are catheterized or may also be passed from mother to child during delivery.[29]

Signs and Symptoms. The incubation period for HCV is approximately 6 or 7 weeks; however, in some people the disease exists for years without any outward signs or symptoms. Once the signs and symptoms appear, they are usually mild; however, many people with HCV develop a chronic form of the condition, which may last their whole life. The signs and symptoms of acute HCV include a reduction in appetite, fatigue, abdominal pain and tenderness on palpation over the region of the liver in the right upper quadrant of the abdomen, and muscle and joint pains.[30] Chronic HCV may cause liver cirrhosis in those who are immunosuppressed as a result of HIV or alcoholism or may lead to an increased risk of liver cancer.[31] The signs and symptoms of cirrhosis of the liver include an enlarged liver and spleen, jaundice, atrophy of muscles, skin abrasions or a rash, ascites (abdominal edema), ankle edema, and occasionally neuropathy in the distal lower extremities. Other complications associated with HCV include glomerulonephritis, a seronegative form of arthritis, Sjögren's syndrome, non-Hodgkin's lymphomas, and fibromyalgia.[32]

Prognosis. The prognosis for people with HCV depends on the severity of the infection. People with chronic HCV are at risk for liver failure, which can be life threatening.

Medical Intervention. Prevention is the best course of action for HCV by avoiding the risk behaviors for the condition described in the etiology section. No vaccine exists for the prevention of HCV. Most people with HCV do not get better without treatment; however, many people have a mild form of the disease that may not affect their health. The diagnostic testing for HCV includes checking hepatic function with a liver function test (LFT). The LFT is a group of several blood tests to detect abnormalities in the liver chemistry.[33] The specific diagnosis of HCV is achieved through other blood tests such as the anti-HCV test and the HCV-RIBA test, which detect the presence of antibodies to HCV. A viral load test determines the concentration of the virus in the blood, and the viral genotyping indicates which of the six types of HCV is causing the infection. The treatment options are governed by the type of HCV virus, because some of the viruses are more difficult to treat.[34] A liver biopsy may be performed to determine the level of damage of the liver, including necrosis, fibrosis, and inflammation, but is not considered part of the diagnosis. The pharmacological intervention is limited to those with progressive forms of HCV and consists of antiviral medications such as alpha interferon or ribavirin.[35] In people with severe liver disease, a liver transplant may be indicated.

Physical Therapy Intervention. Physical therapy intervention is often indicated for people with HCV-associated arthritis or fibromyalgia. Both of these conditions are chronic and result in functional deficits. The type of intervention is individually based on the results of the evaluation by the PT but is focused on improving functional ambulation and activities of daily living (ADL), increasing joint mobility, muscle strength, and endurance, as well as teaching energy conservation techniques.

Hepatitis D, E and G

Some less common forms of hepatitis include hepatitis D (HDV), hepatitis E (HEV), and hepatitis G (HGV). Approximately 15 million people worldwide are infected with HDV, with the prevalence greater in adults than children.[36] Approximately 2% to 5% of the population are carriers for hepatitis G.[37]

Etiology. Hepatitis D (HDV or delta agent) is a fairly rare RNA virus found in relation to HBV. The HDV virus relies on the HBV virus to replicate.[38] The virus is a bloodborne pathogen, usually transmitted through sexual activity, blood transfusion, or intravenous drug use. People infected with HBV or HDV are thought to be at increased risk of hepatic carcinoma. Hepatitis E (HEV) is another RNA virus spread in contaminated food and drinking water in parts of Asia, Africa, and South America. People who travel in parts of the world where HEV is common are at risk for this disease.[39] Pregnant women in particular are at risk because 20% develop a severe form of hepatitis E, which causes hepatic necrosis. Hepatitis G (HGV) virus also called GB virus-C, is transmitted through skin

wounds and is most prevalent in people who use intravenous drugs and people undergoing hemodialysis. HGV is often found in people who have HCV. This form of hepatitis is less serious than other forms of hepatitis.

Signs and Symptoms. The general signs and symptoms of HDV and HEV include jaundice, fatigue, abdominal pain, diarrhea, nausea, vomiting, loss of appetite, headache, dark-colored urine, and fever. Occasionally, an encephalopathy develops in HDV, causing confusion.[40] Absence of any signs and symptoms are characteristic of HGV.

Prognosis. In rare cases, HDV can be life threatening as a result of end-stage liver disease. HEV usually resolves over the course of weeks or months with no lasting effects. HGV occurs in the presence of other forms of hepatitis and does not seem to be a dangerous form of the disease.

Medical Intervention. The detection of any of the types of hepatitis follows the same diagnostic pattern as for HAV, HBV, and HCV. The HBV vaccination protects against HDV because the viruses occur together. No Food and Drug Administration–approved vaccination currently exists to prevent HGV or HEV. Pharmacological treatment for HDV is with antiviral medications such as interferon alpha (Roferon). When HDV remains untreated and liver failure occurs, a liver transplant may be indicated.[41] People with HEV infection do not usually require any pharmacological intervention. The prevention of HEV is achieved through avoidance of drinking tap water or eating contaminated food such as uncooked foods that have been washed in tap water. No treatment is indicated for people with HGV.

Physical Therapy Intervention. Physical therapy intervention is not indicated for people with hepatitis D, G, or E. Regular hand washing and avoidance of at-risk behaviors are the best prevention against transmission of the diseases.

Alcoholic Hepatitis

Alcoholic hepatitis is a chronic and serious condition of the liver precipitated by extreme alcohol intake. Alcoholic hepatitis usually develops in people who either drink heavily or binge drink, but in some cases people who drink moderately develop the disease. Not all people who drink heavily develop the disease. Women are more susceptible than men to alcoholic hepatitis. Alcoholic liver disease affects more than 2 million people in the United States.[42] The disease can affect any age group, but the peak incidence is between the ages of 20 and 60. The most recent statistics available from the CDC are for 2007 data published in 2009. The preliminary report for 2007 data showed that cirrhosis of the liver remained one of the top 15 causes of death in the United States in 2005, with 28,504 deaths attributable to the disease.[43]

Etiology. Heavy intake of alcohol is associated with alcoholic hepatitis, but genetic markers are thought to increase the risk for the disease because not all people who drink heavily actually acquire the disease. Malnutrition, immunological factors, and the presence of other forms of hepatitis are also considered to be involved with the onset of the disease.[44] The damage to the liver is caused by acetaldehyde, one of the toxic by-products of the breakdown of ethanol (alcohol) by the liver.[45]

Signs and Symptoms. The signs and symptoms of alcoholic hepatitis include pain and tenderness in the abdomen, ascites (abdominal edema), nausea, fever, loss of appetite, fatigue, excessive thirst, dry mouth, pallor, rapid and unexplained weight gain, tachycardia, anemia (alcohol suppresses the formation of red blood cells by the bone marrow), thrombocytopenia (reduced number of platelets in blood), and mental confusion resulting from encephalopathy.[46] The complications of alcoholic hepatitis include **portal hypertension** (increased blood pressure in the portal vein), varices (enlarged and distended veins), ascites (edema in the abdomen), an increased tendency to bruise and bleed with bleeding in the gastrointestinal tract, cirrhosis of the liver, and hepatic encephalopathy as a result of the buildup of ammonia in the brain.[47]

Prognosis. The main predictor of severity of alcoholic hepatitis is the presence of hepatic encephalopathy. In people with hepatic encephalopathy, the mortality rate is much higher. Alcoholic hepatitis may lead to liver necrosis and cirrhosis (see Chapter 14). People with less severe disease may recover over several months if they stop consuming alcohol. The predicted mortality rate for people hospitalized for alcoholic hepatitis is 40% in the first year after admission. This statistic assumes the severity of those requiring hospitalization.[48] In some cases, death occurs after a period of heavy drinking.

Medical Intervention. The diagnosis of alcoholic hepatitis is determined through blood tests for the presence of elevated levels of liver enzymes such as gamma-glutamyltransferase (GGT), aspartate aminotransferase (AST), and alanine aminotransferase (ALAT). Other diagnostic techniques include liver function tests for levels of albumin and bilirubin, ultrasound scans of the liver and liver biopsy. People with hepatic hepatitis have an enlarged liver apparent on ultrasound scan. The medical interventions include advice on refraining from the use of alcohol, nutritional consultations, weight loss programs if needed, and, in severe cases, a liver transplant. Some medications such as corticosteroids and antioxidants may be prescribed on a temporary basis to reduce the inflammation in the liver.[49]

Physical Therapy Intervention. Physical therapy intervention is not indicated for the treatment of alcoholic hepatitis. Some of the signs and symptoms associated with the disease may affect physical therapy interventions for patients attending physical therapy for other conditions.

Why Does the Physical Therapist Assistant Need to Know About HIV/AIDS?

Many people with advanced stages of AIDS infection require physical therapy interventions for improving mobility and strength. The PTA will work with people with HIV/AIDS in most clinical settings. Additionally, a clear knowledge regarding the disease helps to dispel some of the common myths about it. Health care workers are at a low risk for infection with HIV through needle sticks and blood-borne pathways. The risk of contracting HIV from a needle stick contaminated with HIV positive blood is approximately 0.3%.[50] Infection is not transmitted through casual contact, and the PT and PTA are at minimal risk for contracting AIDS in the workplace when treating a patient with HIV or AIDS even when they are exposed to blood products or have a sharps contact. The risk of contracting HIV from contact with mucous membranes is estimated at 0.09%.[51] Prevention of a blood-borne pathogen exposure is of primary importance. Standard (Universal) Precautions should always be utilized when treating any patient with open wounds or when the risk of contact with blood or body fluids is present. Because the PT and PTA do not always know when a patient has HIV or any other infectious disease, Standard (Universal) Precautions should be used with all patients when appropriate. If a needle stick occurs, the PT/PTA should follow the protocol of the site in

(Continued)

which they are working. PTA students should also follow the protocols set by their educational program. The most recent guidelines published by the CDC in 2005 detail the recommendations for medical management of postexposure prophylaxis for health care workers. The general guidelines indicate use of one or two of the reverse transcriptase inhibitor pharmacologic agents approved by the CDC for a period up to 4 weeks. The prescription of appropriate medications is provided by the medical personnel in the health care facility. Each health care facility is required to have a plan in place for the management of workers exposed to blood-borne pathogens defined by OSHA.[52]

Human Immunodeficiency Virus and Acquired Immune Deficiency Syndrome

HINTS ON USE OF THE GUIDE TO PHYSICAL THERAPIST PRACTICE

Patients with acquired immune deficiency syndrome (AIDS) receive physical therapy intervention for various manifestations of the disease.

- 4C "Impaired muscle performance" (p. 161): If the patient has reduction in muscle strength and is having difficulty performing work- or home-related tasks, he or she could be placed under the Musculoskeletal Preferred Practice Pattern 4C.
- 5E "Impaired motor function and sensory integrity associated with progressive disorders of the central nervous system (p. 375): Advanced cases of AIDS can result in central nervous system involvement affecting coordination, balance, and sensation; under such circumstances the Preferred Practice Pattern used would likely be the Neuromuscular pattern 5E.
- 6B "Impaired aerobic capacity/endurance associated with deconditioning" (p. 475): If the level of endurance and cardiovascular function is reduced the Cardiovascular/Pulmonary pattern 6B could be used.
- 6H "Impaired circulation and anthropometric dimensions associated with lymphatic system disorders" (p. 569): In cases in which there is loss of skin sensation and edema in the limbs, perhaps associated with pain, the appropriate pattern could be the Cardiovascular/Pulmonary pattern 6H.

- 7C "Impaired integumentary integrity associated with partial thickness skin involvement and scar formation" (p. 619): If the patient has Kaposi's sarcoma, the indicated pattern could be Integumentary Preferred Practice Pattern" 7C.
- 7E "Impaired integumentary integrity associated with skin involvement extending into fascia, muscle, or bone and scar formation" (p. 655): This is an alternative integumentary practice pattern for patients with Kaposi's sarcoma.

(From the American Physical Therapy Association, 2003. *Guide to physical therapist practice,* revised 2nd edition. Alexandria, VA: APTA. Used with permission.)

Human Immunodeficiency virus (HIV)/**Autoimmune deficiency syndrome** (AIDS) is a sexually transmitted viral disease. The worldwide prevalence of HIV/AIDS is a major health concern. The cumulative number of deaths attributed to AIDS worldwide is approximately 25 million people, and in 2008 the number of people throughout the world living with HIV/AIDS was thought to be approximately 33.4 million.[53] Approximately 95% of the total numbers of people with AIDS in the world live in developing countries. The areas of major concern for the World Health Organization (WHO) are Africa and Asia. AIDS is a leading cause of death in Africa, and almost two thirds of all people with HIV/AIDS live in sub-Saharan Africa, totaling 28 million people.[54]

Data for the incidence of HIV infection released by the CDC indicated 56,300 new infections of HIV in the United States in 2006. Of these new infections, 53% were homosexual and bisexual men, and 43% were African American men and women.[55] A total of 31% of new infections were heterosexual people and 12% were people who abused drugs. The total estimated number of people living with HIV/AIDS in the United States and its dependent countries and territories in 2003 was between 1,039,000 and 1,185,000. Of these, approximately 24% to 27% of people were not aware they had the infection. In 2006, the number of people living with AIDS in the United States and its dependent countries and territories was approximately 448,871. According to the CDC, the total number of people living within the United States with full-blown AIDS in 2006 was 37,852, and of these 26,989 were men and 9,801 women.[56] The cumulative estimate of the number of deaths resulting from AIDS through 2006 in the United States is 565,927.

NOTE: *AIDS and HIV are not notifiable diseases in the United States as a result of the possible discrimination that could occur if the privacy of people with the condition was breached. This means that physicians are not required to notify the CDC of the names of people affected by the virus. The numbers of cases diagnosed by physicians are reported for statistical purposes and used in efforts to prevent the spread of the disease. The 1996 Health Insurance Portability and Accountability Act (HIPAA) increased the regulations regarding privacy of medical information especially for electronically transmitted information. These laws affect the delivery of physical therapy and all health care providers. When discussing patients for case study purposes no identifiable factors, such as age or ethnicity, may be used. In addition, the only people allowed access to medical records are those directly involved with the care of the patient. Each state in the United States has laws pertaining to privacy of medical records and many of these state laws are even more strict than the HIPAA laws. As with all patient information, the PTA must ensure the privacy of the information and not discuss the patient's medical condition with anyone not directly involved in the treatment of the patient. In some cases, the condition is not noted in the medical chart at all to preserve privacy. If the PTA is informed by patients that they have AIDS, this information must be kept confidential.*

Etiology. AIDS is a blood-borne pathogen caused by the human immunodeficiency virus (HIV). Initial infection with HIV may remain undetectable in the bloodstream for several weeks. Even though detectable in the blood, the HIV virus may not produce any symptoms for prolonged periods of time. Acquired immune deficiency syndrome is different from the autoimmune diseases described in Chapter 8. In AIDS, the body fails to develop antibodies to infecting organisms, rather than attacking its own cells. This lack of defense leaves the body susceptible to **opportunistic infections** that take advantage of the body's lowered immunity. The body fails to recognize or defend itself against these foreign invaders, and therefore infections that a healthy individual fights off easily become life threatening to people with AIDS.

Pathologically, HIV is an RNA retrovirus, which attaches to the CD4 receptor on the T-lymphocytes. The retrovirus requires the presence of **reverse transcriptase** to be able to multiply within the invaded cells.[57] Several

HIV viruses exist, including HIV 1 and 2. HIV 2 is found mostly in Africa, and the onset of AIDS is not as rapid in this form of the viral infection. Recent reports indicate that more virulent and drug-resistant strains of the AIDS virus are developing, partly as a result of the mixture of pharmaceutical therapy required and the inconsistency of following the physician-specified instructions for taking these medications.[58] The virus gradually attacks more and more of the T-lymphocytes over time. The T-lymphocytes are the white blood cells of the immune system that destroy cells infected with viruses and other cells recognized as foreign to the body such as cancer cells. The rate of progression of the disease depends on the rate of attack and destruction of these T-lymphocytes. A mean latency period of between 10 and 15 years occurs between initial infection with HIV and the development of the symptoms of full-blown AIDS. The virus is a blood-borne pathogen transmitted through intimate contact with blood products or infected semen. Sexual transmission can occur with unprotected sex in heterosexual and homosexual relationships when micro-tears occur in the walls of the vagina or rectum, allowing the virus to gain entry to the cells and blood. Reduction of the spread of the virus can be effected by the use of condoms, which can prevent blood contact when used correctly. Other means of transmission include shared hypodermic needles in people using illegal drugs and transmission of the virus from mother to child during pregnancy, during the birthing process, and through breast milk. During the initial stages of HIV detection in the early 1980s, some people were infected through the blood supply after receiving blood transfusions or through transplantation with an infected donor organ. This risk has now been largely eradicated in the United States as a result of screening the blood of donors.[59]

Signs and Symptoms. The characteristic signs and symptoms of HIV infection may include initial symptoms of a flulike nature, which may remain undetected. These include fever, sweating, diarrhea, headaches, joint or muscle pain, fatigue, blurred vision, swollen lymph glands, shortness of breath, cough, and a rash; however, some patients never experience any of these initial symptoms.[60,61] The reason patients seem to have a latency period of months or years before onset of the symptoms of AIDS is not known. Other longer-term signs and symptoms of AIDS include weight loss, chronic diarrhea, chronic fatigue, generalized and progressive weakness, and joint arthritis. Many neurological problems are associated with AIDS. **AIDS dementia complex** is a recognized group of signs and symptoms associated with advanced AIDS and may include encephalitis, behavioral changes, meningitis, a reduction in cognitive function, psychological and neuropsychiatric disorders, central nervous system lymphomas, and brain tumors. Other neurological symptoms can include pain, peripheral neuropathy, stroke, seizures, herpes zoster, spinal cord problems, cerebellar atrophy resulting in loss of coordination of movement and gait disorders, depression, loss of vision, brain damage, and coma.[62]

Secondary infections that may become life threatening in people with AIDS do not normally cause such virulent infections in a healthy person because the body is able to fight off the infection. These secondary, or opportunistic, infections include pneumonia caused by *Pneumocystis carinii,* now also called **pneumocystic jiroeci pneumonia;** tuberculosis or *Mycobacterium avium,* a bacterium related to tuberculosis; salmonellosis; herpes simplex (cold sores) and herpes zoster (shingles); non-Hodgkin's lymphoma; and **cytomegalovirus** (CMV). Seemingly inconsequential fungal infections such as **candidiasis** (thrush) can become a severe problem for the patient with AIDS (see Fig. 10.1). The fungus can attack the mucous membranes of the mouth, throat, trachea, lungs, and genital areas and may be resistant to treatment.[63] Herpes simplex, described in Chapter 8, can also be a chronic problem resistant to pharmaceutical intervention. Kaposi's sarcoma (see Chapter 8) is a malignant blood-vessel and skin condition present in many people with AIDS but rare in the general population. Women infected with HIV have a high incidence of vaginal candidiasis, malignancies of the cervix, and pelvic inflammatory disease.

Prognosis. No cure currently exists for HIV/AIDS. The prognosis for patients with AIDS has improved somewhat

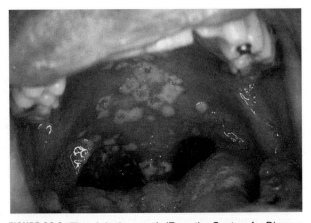

FIGURE 10.1 Thrush in the mouth (From the Centers for Disease Control and Prevention/Sol Silverman, Jr., DDS).

It Happened in the Clinic

A young man in his 20s was receiving inpatient treatment and was referred to the PT department in the acute care hospital for mobility rehabilitation and strengthening. His diagnosis was advanced AIDS/HIV with dementia. Evaluation by the PT determined that the patient was unable to follow multiple-level commands. Balance was poor, he exhibited ataxia during ambulation, and overall muscle strength was diminished with upper and lower extremity strength 3+/5. The patient was instructed in the use of a walker and given a home exercise program, which was written on an instruction sheet for the patient to take home. Stair climbing was unsafe, and the care provider was instructed not to allow the patient to use the stairs without assistance and to use a gait belt for all ambulatory activities. The patient was returning home and was provided with hospice care organized by the social worker.

in recent years as a result of improvements in pharmaceutical therapy. The disease was the fifth leading cause of death in the United States in 2006 as opposed to the number one cause of death in 1995. The most recent statistics available from the CDC are that in 2006, 14,627 people died as a result of AIDS in the United States.[64] The cumulative estimate for deaths related to AIDS through 2006 is 565,927 in the United States and its dependent countries and territories. As medications are developed for the treatment of AIDS the possibilities of increased life expectancy after onset of HIV infection are increased. Research is ongoing to find an immunization for HIV, as well as a cure. At the moment, the best defense against the disease is prevention through safe sex, not sharing needles, taking adequate precautions when handling used needles (i.e., not recapping needles), and the use of Standard Precautions when there is potential for contact with blood or body fluids. The virus does not live for more than a few seconds when outside the body, so the potential risk of transmission is far less than for hepatitis B, which was discussed earlier in this chapter.

Medical Intervention. The diagnosis of HIV is performed through the detection of the HIV virus in the blood. The diagnosis of AIDS is performed through laboratory blood tests for the presence of the HIV virus plus a CD4 T-lymphocyte count below 200/mm³ (normal level 600–1,200/mm³), and/or a percentage of CD4 lymphocytes to the total number of lymphocytes of approximately 25% (normal value 40%), and the length of time since detection of the HIV virus in the blood.[65,66] Additionally, the presence of one of the common opportunistic infections detailed under "signs and symptoms" usually indicates that people with HIV have progressed to a phase of lowered immune system defense and full-blown AIDS.[67] The pharmacology for HIV and AIDS consists of a drug "soup." A commonly used combination of medications called **highly active antiretroviral therapy** (HAART) improves the T-cell count, suppresses the replication of the HIV virus, and reduces the incidence of onset of secondary opportunistic infections.[68] When the HIV virus remains suppressed and the CD4 lymphocyte count is maintained over 200, patients have a longer life expectancy and a better quality of life. However, people must take the medications every day to prevent becoming resistant to the combination of drugs. Some of the side effects of this potent mixture of medications include headaches, weakness, malaise, and fat accumulation around the upper back and abdomen.[69] The regimen of medications used for the treatment of people with AIDS is constantly changing. Other medications are prescribed as necessary to treat the symptoms of opportunistic infections as they arise. The *Guidelines for Prevention and Treatment of Opportunistic Infections in HIV-Infected Adults and Adolescents* was published in 2009 by the CDC, the National Institutes of Health, and the HIV Medicine Association of the Infectious Diseases Society of America and is available from http://www.aidsinfo.nih.gov. A category of drugs used in the treatment of HIV/AIDS is called reverse transcriptase inhibitors and includes zidovudine (Hivid), stavudine (Zerit), didanosine (Videx), and lamivudine (Epivir). Some of these medications are used for prophylaxis after a needle stick and for pregnant women with AIDS to reduce the risk of spread of the virus to the fetus.[70] Many trials for newly developed medications are underway, and the research into both a vaccination against HIV and a cure are ongoing worldwide.

Physical Therapy Intervention. PT intervention is frequently required for people with AIDS. In the later stages of the disease, as previously described, manifestations of muscle weakness and atrophy, fatigue, peripheral neuropathy, coordination problems, and AIDS dementia complex are present. All or any of these symptoms can be indications for physical therapy intervention. Evaluation by the PT, and subsequent treatment by the PTA, may include exercise programs for strengthening, balance, coordination, and endurance, general aerobic conditioning within patient tolerance, gait training and functional mobility training with the use of specific assistive devices, bed mobility exercises, breathing exercises, and energy-conservation techniques. The education of the care providers is essential for transfers and ambulation assistance and exercise supervision. Instruction in the use of a mechanical lift may also be necessary for in-home use. When providing physical therapy intervention for people with AIDS, it is important to remember that AIDS/HIV cannot be transmitted through touch. Many people with AIDS feel isolated by their condition, and the value of touch in the therapeutic setting cannot be overestimated.

Why Does the Physical Therapist Assistant Need to Know About Sexually Transmitted Diseases?

Although health care workers are not usually at risk for most sexually transmitted diseases in the workplace, these diseases are increasingly present in the general community. Some of the sexually transmitted diseases may also be transmitted through blood and body fluids and precautions against these diseases include the use of Standard (Universal) Precautions when working with people especially if there is a risk of exposure to blood or body fluids. Some of the signs and symptoms in people with sexually transmitted diseases that are not treated may include joint, muscle, and mobility problems, which may be an indication for physical therapy interventions. Knowledge of these sexually transmitted diseases assists the PT and PTA in developing and administering appropriate exercise programs and other physical therapy interventions for people with these symptoms and in reducing the possibility of infection or cross-infection.

Sexually Transmitted Diseases

The sexually transmitted diseases described in this section include chancroid, chlamydia, cytomegalovirus, gonorrhea, human papillomavirus, and syphilis. This is not a complete list of sexually transmitted diseases but encompasses the ones most commonly seen in the United States.

Chancroid

Chancroid is a sexually transmitted bacterial disease and should not be confused with the chancre ulceration of syphilis. Chancroid is fairly rare in the United States, with most people infected when traveling overseas in developing countries. An estimated 6 million people are diagnosed with chancroid worldwide, with most cases occurring in Africa, Asia, and the Caribbean. Chancroid ulcerations are more prevalent in men than women in a 3.25:1 ratio and are more common in men who have not been circumcised.[71] The mean age of onset for chancroid is 30.[72]

Etiology. The etiology of chancroid is the sexually transmitted *Haemophilus ducreyi* bacillus. The incubation period between infection and onset of symptoms is between 1 and 14 days.[73] Chancroid is often found in association with other sexually transmitted diseases, such as chlamydia and gonorrhea.

Signs and Symptoms. The characteristic signs and symptoms of chancroid start with a small papule that turns into a pustule and then opens up into a painful skin ulceration on the genitalia with peripheral inflammation and a necrotic wound base. The ulceration varies in size from about an eighth of an inch to 2 inches or more in diameter. Men usually have one or two ulcerations, whereas women may have as many as four. Fever and general feelings of malaise may develop, as well as inflammation of the inguinal lymph nodes. The lymph nodes and ulcerations often become abscesses, which either rupture or require surgical drainage.[74]

Prognosis. Chancroid is curable with treatment and also recovers without treatment, although the recovery may be prolonged and cause considerable pain. People with chancroid are at greater risk of infection with HIV.[75] Complications from chancroid include scarring and the formation of fistulas.[76]

Medical Intervention. The diagnosis of chancroid is achieved through a culture of the tissue within the chancroid ulcers. Infected lymph nodes are drained with a needle or excised under local anesthesia.[77] The pharmacological intervention is with antimicrobial medications such as azithromycin, ceftriaxone, ciprofloxacin, or erythromycin. Cleansing of the ulcerations and soaking of the affected areas are required for wound care.[78]

Physical Therapy Intervention. Physical therapy intervention usually is not indicated for people with chancroid. Occasionally, people with open, slow-healing ulcerations may require wound care intervention. Physical therapy clinicians should follow Standard Universal Precautions procedures when treating chancroid wounds.

Chlamydia

Chlamydia is one of the most common sexually transmitted diseases in the United States In 2006, the CDC reported 1,030,911 infections with chlamydia from all 50 states and the District of Columbia. An estimated 2,291,000 people in the United States are infected with chlamydia between the ages of 14 and 29.[79]

Etiology. Chlamydia is caused by the parasitic organism *Chlamydia trachomatis*. The disease is transmitted through vaginal, oral, and anal sexual intercourse.[80]

Signs and Symptoms. Approximately 75% of infected women and 50% of infected men do not have any signs or symptoms associated with chlamydia infection. In women, the infection attacks the cervix and urethra and can spread to the rectum and the throat. Any signs and symptoms associated with chlamydia appear between 1 and 3 weeks after infection. The symptoms in women can include vaginal discharge and burning sensations during urination. If the infection remains undetected and untreated, the symptoms become more severe with abdominal pain, low back pain, fever, vaginal bleeding, and dyspareunia (pain during sexual intercourse). Long-term infection with chlamydia can cause pelvic inflammatory disease (PID), resulting in chronic pelvic pain, infertility and possible ectopic pregnancy (development of the fetus outside the uterus). Approximately 40% of women who are not treated for chlamydia develop PID. Delivery of a premature infant is more likely in women with chlamydia, and women with the infection are 5 times more likely to contract HIV. [81] The signs and symptoms in men infected with chlamydia include burning sensations during urination, discharge from the penis, and burning and itching of the skin of the penis. Both men and women can have rectal pain and discharge and bleeding from the rectum, as well as infection in the throat. A rare side effect of chlamydia infection is Reiter's syndrome, a disease consisting of a triad of symptoms, including skins lesions, and inflammation of the eye and urethra. Newborn infants with chlamydia are prone to pneumonia and conjunctivitis.[82]

Prognosis. Chlamydia is curable with antimicrobial medications. Women with chlamydia infection who are untreated may develop pelvic inflammatory disease and become infertile or develop ectopic pregnancy, which is life threatening.[83]

Medical Intervention. Testing for chlamydia is performed through a laboratory culture of swab from the cervix or from a urine sample. The pharmacology for chlamydia is with antimicrobials such as doxycycline or azithromycin. Unlike other STDs, chlamydia does not seem to have developed resistance to current antimicrobial medications. Reinfection with chlamydia is common. Newborns are treated with antimicrobial eyedrops to protect against chlamydia.[84] Medical advice includes counseling regarding the practice of safe sex and reduction of at-risk sexual behaviors, such as multiple partners.[85] Annual screening for all sexually active women, especially those aged 25 and younger, is recommended. Women who are pregnant should also be tested.

Physical Therapy Intervention. No physical therapy intervention is indicated for people with chlamydia infection.

Cytomegalovirus ⊜

Cytomegalovirus (CMV) is a common sexually transmitted viral infection in adults, with between 50% and 80% of adults infected by age 40. The virus is the most common congenital virus infection in the United States and is a worldwide phenomenon. Each year approximately 40,000 infants in the United States are born with the disease. Overall, 1 in 150 infants are born with CMV, and 1 in 5 of these infants and 1 in 750 of all children born will develop permanent disability as a result. In the United States, 5,000 children each year have permanent disability resulting from CMV.[86]

Etiology. The cytomegalovirus (CMV) is related to the herpes viruses. The virus is present in all body fluids of an infected person including the saliva, blood, tears, semen, vaginal fluids, breast milk, and urine. Transmission of the virus occurs through close personal contact with infected body fluids such as sexual contact, direct contact with blood products, or close personal contact in day-care centers. The disease may be passed onto the fetus during pregnancy or through breast milk from an infected mother.[87]

Signs and Symptoms. Often adults with CMV infection do not exhibit signs and symptoms. If signs and symptoms are present, they may mimic mild influenza and include fever, fatigue, and general feelings of malaise, joint and muscle pains, sore throat, lymph node inflammation, thrombocytopenia, and splenomegaly (an enlarged spleen). The characteristic signs and symptoms of the newborn with the neonatal syndrome of CMV include a low birth weight and size, microcephaly (small brain), respiratory problems, mental retardation, motor delay and movement coordination deficits, seizures, hearing and vision loss, jaundice,

splenomegaly, hepatomegaly (an enlarged liver), and central nervous system problems.[88] Some of these symptoms may not be apparent at birth but may take several months to develop or may not occur at all.[89] CMV may cause many problems in people who are immunocompromised, including gastrointestinal problems, such as colitis; pulmonary infections, including pneumonia; encephalitis; neuropathy; and retinitis. People undergoing organ transplantation surgery are at a particularly high risk of infection from cytomegalovirus. The symptoms of the disease in these people can be mistaken for organ rejection.[90]

Prognosis. The general prognosis for people with cytomegalovirus is good. Adults with CMV are generally not at risk of permanent health issues unless they are immunocompromised. The main concern is for children born with the disease. Women who have recently become infected with CMV immediately before pregnancy or who become infected during pregnancy are most at risk for passing the virus to the unborn child.[91] However, the risk of passing the virus to a child during pregnancy is generally low. In children, the permanent motor and cognitive deficits and hearing and vision loss cause lifelong disability. Children severely affected can die as a result of the infection, although this is rare.

Medical Intervention. The presence of the disease in women can be detected by a screening blood test for CMV IgG antibodies. The recommendations from the CDC do not include testing of CMV for all pregnant women.[92] No vaccine is currently available for CMV, although research is ongoing to create one.[93,94,95] The treatment of infants with ganciclovir (antiviral medication) has shown some promising results for the prevention of progression of hearing loss caused by central nervous system disease.[96] Antiviral medications are also used in the treatment of people undergoing transplant surgery who have complications resulting from cytomegalovirus.[97]

Physical Therapy Intervention. When providing physical therapy interventions for people with comorbid CMV or working with children, the use of Standard Precautions should be followed carefully. Hand washing is particularly important, as is the use of gloves when necessary to prevent exposure to body fluids.

Gonorrhea

Gonorrhea is a common bacterial sexually transmitted disease caused by *Neisseria gonorrhoeae*. The incidence of gonorrhea in the United States is estimated to be

700,000 new cases per year consisting of both males and females. The prevalence is 120.9 cases per 100,000 of the population. ⚕Gonorrhea infections are common among teenagers but can occur in any age group.[98] The incubation period for the bacteria ranges from a few days to 30 days before signs and symptoms become apparent.

Etiology. Gonorrhea is a curable STD caused by the gram-negative bacteria *N. gonorrhoeae*.[99] The transmission of the bacteria can occur through sexual intercourse and from a mother to a baby during delivery. Infection with the bacteria can occur more than once even after successful treatment for the condition. As in all STDs, the use of a condom can significantly reduce the risk of spread of the infection. If the disease remains undetected and untreated, the infected person can continue to transmit the infection.

Signs and Symptoms. The characteristic signs and symptoms of the disease include urethritis in men, and cervicitis in women. The urethritis starts with a burning sensation and whitish discharge on urination and progresses to painful inflammation associated with a yellow or green discharge. The infection may include the rectum and prostate, and occasionally the eye. The testes may also become swollen and painful. Epididymitis (inflammation of the epididymus in the testicular sac) is a complication of untreated gonorrhea in the male and can lead to infertility. Women may experience a purulent urethral discharge associated with urinary urgency, frequency, or dysuria (inability to urinate). Vaginal discharge and inflammation of the cervix leads to involvement of the uterus and ovaries. Women may not exhibit outward symptoms and the disease may go unnoticed. Serious complications include pelvic inflammatory disease in females, which leads to the development of internal organ abscesses, chronic pelvic pain, and infertility or the likelihood of an ectopic pregnancy (development of the fetus outside the uterus), which also may be life threatening.[100] Both males and females may have rectal discharge and bleeding, anal itching and soreness, and painful bowel movements.

Prognosis. Antimicrobial resistant *N. gonorrhoeae* is an evolving problem throughout the world.[101] [102] According to statistics from the CDC, 16.4% of gonorrheal infections in the United States in 2003 were resistant to penicillin, tetracycline, or both.[103] Some bacteria are also developing resistance to spectinomycin and fluoroquinolones. The long-term complications of untreated disease can be life threatening, affecting the blood and joints of those infected. People with gonorrhea are more susceptible to contracting infection with HIV.[104]

Medical Intervention. Antimicrobial medications are used to treat gonorrhea. Testing the bacteria for resistance to specific antimicrobial medications is necessary as a result of the rise of resistant forms of the bacteria. A simple gram staining of a culture, also called a gram culture test (GC test) taken from people suspected of having gonorrhea can enable viewing of the bacteria under a microscope.[105] A more sensitive test for gonorrhea is the nucleic acid amplification test (NAAT) that amplifies the DNA present in *N. gonorrhoeae*.[106] Many people with gonorrhea also have chlamydia infection (see section on chlamydia), and both infections are usually treated at the same time.[107]

Physical Therapy Intervention. No physical therapy intervention is indicated for gonorrhea infection. Standard precautions should be followed when providing interventions for female or male pelvic disorders.

Human Papillomavirus

Human papillomavirus (HPV) is the most common sexually transmitted infection in the United States. More than 20 million people in the United States are infected with human papillomavirus (HPV), and each year an additional 6.2 million become infected.[108,109]

Etiology. HPVs cause condylomata acuminata (warts) by stimulating skin cells to undergo metaplasia (change to another type of cell). Genital warts caused by these viruses are highly contagious. More than 100 types of HPV exist, some of which are classified as "low-risk" because they only cause warts, and others are "high-risk" because they cause cancer. High-risk HPV viruses are also called oncogenic or carcinogenic. The types of HPV that cause most genital warts are HPV-6 and HPV-11. The two HPV viruses that cause most cervical cancers are HPV-16 and HPV-18.[110] These viruses are associated with an increased risk of carcinomas of the rectum, cervix, vulva, and other genital areas infected. These viruses are also included in the list of opportunistic infections associated with HIV and AIDS.[111]

Signs and Symptoms. Many people infected with HPV do not know they have the disease because they do not have any signs or symptoms. In some people, warts are visible on the external genitalia; in other cases, internal warts are discovered during medical examinations. Warts may occur on any area of the female or male genitalia.[112]

Prognosis. Approximately 90% of people with HPV are able to eradicate the infection within 2 years with no long-term effects. However, people with compromised immune systems, including those with HIV/AIDS, can be severely affected by the disease. In cases in which the HPV leads to cancer, the disease can be life threatening.[113] The National Cancer Institute estimated that in 2007, approximately 11,000 women in the United States would be diagnosed with cervical cancer, and 4,000 of those diagnosed would die. Worldwide, cervical cancer affects half a million women with over a quarter of a million deaths annually.[114]

Medical Intervention. The diagnosis of HPV warts is mainly achieved through visual examination. A Pap smear (scraping of the cervical tissue) is diagnostic for early signs of cervical cancer. In most cases, early detection of cervical cancer reduces the mortality rate. Condylomata may be surgically excised with cryotherapy (freezing), loop electrosurgical excision procedure (LEEP; also called electrocautery), laser, or with conventional surgery.[115] The condylomata also may be treated with a medication in cream or solution form or left for resolution with the body's own immune system. Treatment options for cervical cancer include surgery, radiation therapy, and chemotherapy depending on the staging of the cancer. Routine Pap smears are recommended for women for early detection of cervical cancer. ⊛ The HPV/cervical cancer vaccination Gardasil is recommended for all girls 11 to 12 years of age and for women aged 13 to 26 who have not received the vaccination previously.[116,117] Gardasil protects against HPV-6 and HPV-11, which cause condylomata, and HPV-16 and HPV-18, which cause 70% of all cervical cancers.[118]

Physical Therapy Intervention. Physical therapy is not indicated for people with HPV. Standard precautions should be used when providing female or male pelvic therapy.

Syphilis

Syphilis is a sexually transmitted bacterial disease. The most recent data revealed that 36,000 people were diagnosed with syphilis in the United States in 2006. ⊛ Congenital syphilis (infants born with syphilis) accounted for 349 cases, and the incidence was highest in women aged between 20 and 24 years, and men aged between 35 and 39.[119] The risk for contracting syphilis is underestimated. Syphilis is also described in Chapter 6 in relation to a form of arthritis associated with later stages of the disease called tertiary, or late-stage, syphilis. A national plan to eliminate syphilis in the United States was started in 1999, led by the CDC in liaison with federal, state, and local health departments. Although awareness of the disease has been raised, the incidence of syphilis continues to be a national issue.[120]

Etiology. Syphilis is caused by the spirochete bacteria *Treponema pallidum*. The transmission of the infection is through sexual intercourse contact with the chancre (open sores) on the genitalia, vagina, anus, rectum, lips, and inside the mouth. Other modes of transmission are more mundane and include contact with contaminated surfaces and environments such as toilet seats, doorknobs, swimming pools, hot tubs, bath tubs, eating utensils, and clothing.

Pathologically, the disease can be transmitted to others after the first 3 weeks of incubation and during the first year and then becomes latent in the body. ⊛ Transmission to a fetus is possible after the 10th week of pregnancy and causes congenital syphilis in the child.[121]

Signs and Symptoms. The characteristic signs and symptoms of syphilis vary with the stage of the disease. In some instances, no signs or symptoms manifest for many years after infection. Many of the chancres are small, or are internally located, so that they are not noticed. Congenital syphilis is infectious via the skin rash, nasal discharge, or oral lesions. The main signs and symptoms of primary syphilis are painless and infectious chancres on the skin of the genitalia, anus, lips, or mouth which appear between 10 and 90 days after infection (see Fig. 10.2). The chancre is usually small, round, and painless and is similar to the skin ulceration of herpes simplex (see Chapter 8 for details of herpes simplex II, also called genital herpes). This chancre heals without any treatment, making diagnosis of the disease difficult once healed. If undetected and untreated, the disease goes into the secondary stage of syphilis approximately 1 year after initial infection. During the secondary stage, a rough, reddish brown rash develops on the soles of the feet and palms of the hands, as well as other parts of the body.

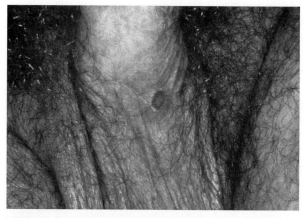

FIGURE 10.2 Syphilis infection showing a chancre on the proximal penile shaft (From the Centers for Disease Control and Prevention/Dr. N. J. Fiumara and Dr. Gavin Hart).

The rash is also infectious.[122] Additional signs and symptoms of secondary syphilis include fever, sore throat, headaches, weight loss, hair loss, swollen lymph glands, fatigue, and muscle aches. All the symptoms of secondary stage syphilis resolve regardless whether treatment is provided. Many people with undetected syphilis may go into a latent stage in which the infection lies dormant within the body for many years. Tertiary syphilis, also called late-stage syphilis, occurs when the disease goes undetected and untreated and affects internal organs, such as the brain and nervous system, heart, circulatory system, liver, eyes, bones, and joints. Syphilitic infection of the spinal cord takes the form of **tabes dorsalis,** also called progressive locomotor ataxia or syphilitic spinal sclerosis, which destroys sensory nerve axons and causes personality changes and dementia. The resulting signs and symptoms of tabes dorsalis include incoordination movement disorders, such as an ataxic gait, paralysis, weakness, numbness, blindness, deafness, severe pain, and even death.[123] Joint problems can be manifested as a severe form of syphilitic arthritis of the spine and hips, which causes erosion of bones and joints. These tertiary symptoms may occur as much as 25 years after infection with the bacteria and are not curable.

Prognosis. Syphilis is life threatening without diagnosis and treatment. The prognosis for people diagnosed and treated during the primary and secondary stages of syphilitic infection is good. Those who remain undiagnosed and untreated and enter the tertiary/late stage can still be treated, but damage to internal organs, bones, and joints cannot be reversed. ⊛ The transmission of syphilis from an infected mother to the fetus can result in a still birth or an infected child. If children born with syphilis are not diagnosed and treated immediately after birth the disease can result in developmental delay, seizures, or death.[124] People with syphilis are at greater risk of contracting or transmitting HIV. As a result of the HIV/AIDS epidemic late-stage syphilis in the form of tabes dorsalis is becoming more common.[125]

Medical Intervention. The diagnosis of syphilis is achieved through cultures taken from the chancre or rash. A dark-field microscope detects the *T. pallidum* bacteria. Blood tests for detection of antibodies to the bacteria are also performed, although these antibodies may not become apparent until up to 3 months after initial infection.[126] The medical management of syphilis is straightforward during the primary stage. Penicillin or other antimicrobial medications are administered by intramuscular injection. The disease is transmissible to other people as long as the chancre, or rash, are present. People are cautioned that it is possible to become infected with syphilis multiple times and to avoid at risk behaviors and to practice safe sex with the use of condoms. Regular screening for the presence of syphilis is recommended for people who are at highest risk of contracting the disease.[127]

Physical Therapy Intervention. During the primary and secondary stages of syphilis, no physical therapy is indicated. People who develop late stage/tertiary syphilis may require intervention for the musculoskeletal disorders associated with the condition.

GERIATRIC CONSIDERATIONS

AIDS/HIV and sexually transmitted diseases (STDs) affect all age groups. Sexually transmitted diseases are often considered to be diseases of the young, but elderly people can also be affected. Some older patients who have joint problems may have contracted syphilis in early life that either remained undetected or was not treatable before the development of antibiotics. Syphilis that is untreated can result in severe arthritic changes in the spine and hips. Although rarely seen today, these conditions can be very painful. PTs and PTAs working in less well-developed countries may see more arthritis type problems caused by STDs because of the lack of availability of antibiotics and medical treatment.

Why Does the Physical Therapist Assistant Need to Know About Nosocomial Infections?

The transmission of nosocomial infections acquired in the health care setting creates a risk for both patients and care providers. Physical therapist assistants work in many practice settings, such as nursing homes and hospitals, where these infections are commonly found. The reduction of spread of these infections is extremely important for the welfare of patients. Simple precautions such as regular hand washing between interventions with different patients can effectively prevent the spread of nosocomial infections. As part of the health care team, the responsibility for reducing the spread of these infections lies with the physical therapist assistant.

Nosocomial Infections

Nosocomial infections, also called hospital-acquired or health care–associated infections, are those that are acquired while the patient is in the hospital or other health care, setting such as a nursing home. The topic of nosocomial infections is also briefly described in Chapter 2. The CDC had a National Nosocomial Infections Surveillance System (NNIS) that was developed in the 1970s to help track the number of nosocomial infections and to help in the development of ways to combat the problem. The NNIS was replaced by the National Healthcare Safety Network (NHSN) in 2006, which now completes the reporting for nosocomial infections throughout the country.[128]

Complications of Nosocomial Infections

The percentage of patients acquiring these infections in the United States is 5% of those people admitted for acute-care hospitalization. The incidence is 5 infections for every 1,000 patient days in the hospital. More than 2 million people each year are affected by nosocomial infections in the United States, with a similar pattern throughout other Western countries. The infections result in an additional 26,250 deaths per year at a cost of $4.5 billion annually.[129] The statistics concerning these infections are one of the reasons to decrease the length of hospitalization to a minimum whenever possible.

Etiology. The causes of nosocomial infections are viruses, bacteria, and fungi. Historically, the most common causative agents of most nosocomial infections are *Streptococci*, *Staphylococcus aureus*, *Enterococci*, *Pseudomonads*, *Escherichia coli*, *Enterobacter* species, and pseudomonas types of bacteria. The intensive care units in hospitals are associated with the most cases of illness and death from nosocomial infections and seem to be the central place in hospitals for emerging antimicrobial resistance.[130] The risk factors for health care–associated infections are divided into three groups. Patient-related risk factors include the seriousness of the illness, whether the immune system is compromised, and the length of stay necessary. The longer the hospital stay, the more likely people are to acquire a nosocomial infection. Some of the organizational risk factors include contamination of air-conditioning or water systems, how close together the patient beds are located, and the nurse-to-patient ratio. The greater the patient to nurse ratio, the higher the likelihood of transmission of infection from nurse to patient and from patient to patient.

So-called iatrogenic risk factors are associated with the pathogens present on the hands of medical personnel. These factors are increased when invasive procedures are performed, such as indwelling catheters, intravenous lines, intubation, and mechanical ventilation.[131]

Signs and Symptoms. The general signs and symptoms for nosocomial infections are the same as for other infections and include fever, skin rash, fatigue and general malaise, and tachycardia. People who did not have a fever before they entered the hospital but develop one are suspected of having a nosocomial infection. The site of the infection is often related to the type of invasive procedure. Infections in the bloodstream may result from an intravenous line; urinary tract infections may be the result of bacteria entering through an indwelling catheter; pneumonia may be related to the use of a ventilator; and a surgical incision with a drain may result in incision infection.

Prognosis. People who develop nosocomial infections have approximately double the mortality and morbidity risk of other patients in the hospital. Neonates, especially those with a low birth weight, are particularly vulnerable to the infections.[132]

MEDICAL INTERVENTION

A sample of the infection must be sent to the laboratory to test for sensitivity to specific drugs so that the correct drug can be administered to fight the infection. Identification of the infective organism is determined by laboratory studies with blood cultures and fungal cultures. A broad-spectrum antimicrobial medication may be started before the identification of the pathogenic organism.[133] When the organism is antimicrobial resistant, it does not necessarily mean that the infection is worse than the nonresistant type, but it is more difficult to treat, and people with compromised immune systems are more at risk. When specific sites are infected, the diagnostic tests may include radiographs, oximetry, sputum sample analysis for chest infections, throat cultures, and stool testing for gastrointestinal infections. The treatment for nosocomial infections includes the removal of indwelling catheters or intravenous lines whenever possible, if these are considered to be the source of the infection. Antimicrobial medications, antivirals such as ganciclovir and voriconazole, and antifungals such as fluconazole, and voriconazole are prescribed.

Prevention of nosocomial infections is the most important intervention. Standard (Universal) Precautions are the most effective way of reducing the risk of nosocomial infections. As explained in Chapter 2, hand washing plays a huge part in the reduction of the spread of these infections. Other ways to reduce the risk of infection are for medical staff to only use indwelling catheters, intravenous lines, and other invasive procedures when absolutely necessary, and to remove them from the patient as quickly as medically possible. Everyone in the intensive care unit (ICU) is responsible for meticulous hand washing and ensuring that the rooms are clean and clear of infection.

Physical Therapy Intervention. As part of the health care team, the physical therapist and PTA are responsible for using standard precautions and practicing regular hand washing to prevent the spread of infections. Hand washing should occur between each patient intervention and whenever handling catheter tubes or intravenous lines.

> ### Why Does the Physical Therapist Assistant Need to Know About Vector- and Animal-Borne Infectious Diseases?
>
> Vector (insect)-borne and animal-borne infections are common throughout the world. Several of these infectious diseases are found in the United States Some of these diseases, such as Lyme disease, cause signs and symptoms that may require physical therapy intervention. Physical therapists and assistants travel worldwide both for pleasure and to provide medical interventions in other countries. A knowledge of these diseases is advisable to take preventive measures to prevent contraction of these infections.

Insect (Vector)- and Animal-Borne Infectious Diseases

Vector-borne infectious diseases are those diseases transmitted to humans through the bite of insects. Many insect- or vector-borne, diseases exist throughout the world. Some of these viruses and bacteria originated in other countries and are now found in the United States. Other vector-borne diseases have existed in the United States for a long time. Some of the more common ones in the news in the United States are Lyme Disease (described in Chapter 5), Rocky Mountain spotted fever, and **West Nile virus.** Dengue fever (also called Dengue hemorrhagic fever), malaria, plague, typhus, and yellow fever are found in other parts of the world, with some instances occurring within the United States. Because many people now travel to distant places, the incidence of these diseases in other

countries is cause for concern. The PTA is quite likely to see patients with these diseases particularly if the symptoms include joint and muscular pains. These diseases are not directly infectious to others unless a transmitting insect is in the area. Various blood-sucking insects are associated with the spread of these diseases.

Animal-borne diseases transmitted to humans within the United States include the two most commonly known: hantaviruses, transmitted through rodents, and rabies, transmitted through the bite of an infected animal. Both diseases are relatively rare in the United States, but prompt medical intervention can prevent the severe outcomes including death from these infections.

Dengue Fever and Dengue Hemorrhagic Fever

Dengue fever is a potentially dangerous viral infectious disease transmitted to humans by the *Aedes aegypti* mosquito. Dengue fever is common in tropical and subtropical areas of the world where the climate is hot and humid. The disease is common in Southeast Asia, China, Thailand, Vietnam, Singapore, Malaysia, and East Africa. Other areas prone to outbreaks of the disease include the Caribbean, Puerto Rico, Cuba, Central America, Australia, Tahiti, and other South and Central Pacific islands.[134,135] Each year, between 100 and 200 cases of Dengue fever are introduced into the United States by travelers.[136] Worldwide an estimated 50 million people are infected each year, and 500,000 people have the more severe form of Dengue hemorrhagic fever.[137]

Etiology. Dengue fever is a virus transmitted by the *Aedes aegypti* mosquito. The mosquito lays its eggs in standing water, and the adult mosquitoes emerge within 8 days. The virus is transmitted through the bite of an infected mosquito. Four types of the virus have been identified. One person possibly could contract Dengue fever up to four times, with each of the strains of the virus.

Signs and Symptoms. The incubation period of the disease is from 3 to 15 days after the mosquito bite. The acute phase of Dengue fever last from a few days to 2 weeks, but some symptoms last for several weeks. The symptoms include fever up to 104°F, bradycardia, hypotension, fatigue, headaches, myalgia (muscle pains) and arthralgia (joint pains), nausea and/or vomiting, edema of hands and feet with erythema, profuse sweating, and skin rash.[138] ☻ Occasionally the more severe form of the disease, called Dengue hemorrhagic fever, occurs, particularly in people with compromised immune systems and children aged under 10 years. Symptoms of the hemorrhagic form of the disease include chills, high temperature, severe headache, severe abdominal pain, backache, depression, sore throat, and signs of hemorrhage such as nose and gum bleeding, petechiae (red or purple blisters beneath the skin), blood in the stools, and unusual bruising.[139] People with Dengue hemorrhagic fever can go into shock with circulatory system collapse.[140]

Prognosis. The prognosis for Dengue fever is usually good. Dengue hemorrhagic fever can be life threatening or fatal, and most people with the condition require hospitalization.[141] The mortality rate from dengue hemorrhagic fever averages 5%.[142]

Medical Intervention. Prevention of mosquito bites is the best way to deter Dengue fever. In areas where Dengue fever is prevalent, people should use mosquito nets over their beds, spray insecticides around and in the house, remove standing water containers that are breeding grounds for the mosquitoes, use mesh screens in windows and doors, and generally avoid mosquito bites. In most cases, the treatment for the infection involves plenty of rest, high fluid intake, and the use of over the counter analgesics/antiinflammatories such as paracetamol or acetaminophen. The use of aspirin and ibuprofen should be avoided because these medications can cause ulcerations and bleeding within the digestive tract.[143] No vaccination is currently available for Dengue fever.

Physical Therapy Intervention. None indicated.

Hantaviruses

Hantaviruses are a group of related viruses that cause disease worldwide especially in poor housing conditions with infestations of mice and rats. Several types of hantavirus have been identified in the United States, South America, and parts of Asia. In the United States, the disease is called hantavirus pulmonary syndrome (HPS). Hantavirus infection is rare in the United States, with approximately 100 cases reported in total.[144]

Etiology. Hantaviruses are RNA viruses transmitted by contact with infected rodents or with rodent urine or feces. Estimates are that most people contract the virus by inhaling dust when sweeping infrequently visited sheds, cabins, and houses. HPS is a rare but deadly form of the disease found across the United States.[145]

Signs and Symptoms. This group of viruses causes hemorrhagic fever (bleeding in internal organs), which can result in kidney damage, pulmonary symptoms, and death. The incubation period is from 1 to 5 weeks. The initial symptoms of hantavirus pulmonary syndrome are fatigue, fever, headache, dizziness, nausea and vomiting, diarrhea, abdominal pain, and muscle aches in the lower extremities and low back. In the later stage, the symptoms worsen with hypoxia, hypotension, severe shortness of breath and cough, and acute respiratory distress syndrome (ARDS).[146,147]

Prognosis. More than 50% of people infected with hantavirus die of respiratory failure.[148]

Medical Intervention. The medical intervention is focused on prevention of the disease through extermination of rodents in and around housing.[149] Diagnostic testing for hantavirus includes a complete blood count (CBC), which detects an increase in white blood cell count. The platelet count decreases to below 150,000 and continues to fall. Chest x-rays show lung congestion and fluid content, the liver enzymes are elevated, serum albumin is decreased, red blood cell numbers are increased, and antibody tests detect the hantavirus. Most people with hantavirus require hospitalization for respiratory support.[150] No current pharmacological treatment is available to treat persons with hantaviruses.

Physical Therapy Intervention. None indicated.

Malaria

Malaria is a serious infectious disease transmitted to humans by the plasmodium parasite via the female *Anopheles* mosquito. Malaria infects an estimated 190 million to 311 million people worldwide each year. Approximately 1 million people die as a result of malaria annually, mainly in Africa. Malaria is still endemic in parts of the world with tropical and subtropical climates including Mexico, South America, Africa, and India. The higher temperatures in these countries increase the rate of the parasitic growth. According to the CDC in 2008 between 708,000 and 1,003,000 people died from malaria mainly in sub-Saharan Africa.[151]

Etiology. The etiological agent of malaria is the plasmodium parasite transmitted by the female Anopheles mosquito. Although more than 350 species of *Anopheles* mosquito exist, only 30 to 50 of the species actually transmit the disease. The parasite is transmitted via the mosquito from one person to another as the mosquito feeds. The mosquito serves as a vector but is not affected by the parasite. The parasites grow in the liver of the human host and then spread to the red blood cells where they multiply and destroy the red cells. The blood cell stage of the parasite is the gametocyte. This stage of the parasite is the one transmitted to the female mosquito when it feeds. The gametocyte form of the parasite is the one that causes the signs and symptoms of malaria.[152] The continuation of the life cycle of the plasmodium takes place in the salivary glands of the mosquito. After 10 to 18 days, the parasites develop into sporozoites and are injected into another human host when the mosquito feeds.

Signs and Symptoms. The plasmodium parasite attacks the liver, causing the characteristic signs and symptoms of malaria which occur approximately 6 to 9 days after a bite from an infected mosquito. The symptoms may mimic influenza and include bouts of chills and fever, profuse sweating, gastrointestinal disturbances, dizziness, backache, muscle and joint pains, and cough. Intermittent acute episodes of the disease may occur years after initial infection. Severe complications of the disease include anemia, kidney failure, and cerebral malarial infection.[153]

Prognosis. Although four types of *Plasmodium* exist, the *Plasmodium falciparum* is responsible for most of the deaths throughout the world. This form of *Plasmodium* is estimated to kill between 700,000 and 2.7 million people each year. ☻ Young children in Africa are most susceptible. Other *Plasmodium* species cause disease that can lie dormant in the liver for many years and cause repeated exacerbations of signs and symptoms for the rest of a person's life.[154]

Medical Intervention. Prevention of the spread of infection is the main way to control outbreaks of malaria. Preventive measures involve prevention of mosquito bites and include the use of over-the-bed nets, window and door screens, insect repellents containing Deet, and the use of clothing to cover the skin.[155] Pharmacological prevention includes taking antimalarial medications such as chloroquine, mefloquine (Lariam), doxycycline, or atovaquone/proquanil (Malerone) before visiting infested areas, as well as during and after return. The CDC maintains recommendations for travelers to areas of the world endemic for malaria, including the effective preventive and suppressive medications.[156] Malaria is diagnosed through laboratory tests with blood smears placed under a microscope stained with Giemsa to highlight the parasite,

immunochromatography rapid diagnostic tests (RDTs) to detect antibodies, and the detection of plasmodium nucleic acids using polymerase chain reactions (PCR). In countries that are endemic for malaria, the resources for costly diagnostic tests are frequently not available.[157] In the United States, the disease is no longer endemic, so the diagnosis of infection is often delayed because physicians are not expecting a diagnosis of malaria.

Physical Therapy Intervention. Although malaria usually is not found in the United States, the PTA may see cases of the disease in people from other countries or those who have traveled to endemic regions of the world. Any case of flulike symptoms should be cause for concern if there is a possibility the person was exposed to malarial infection.

Plague

Plague is an infectious bacterial disease affecting animals and humans. In the United States, isolated cases of plague tend to appear. The last epidemic of plague in the United States was in Los Angeles in 1924–1925. Each year approximately 10 to 15 cases of plague are reported in the United States. Most occurrences are in New Mexico, northern Arizona, southern Colorado, California, far west Nevada, and southern Oregon. Worldwide the World Health Organization reports that between 1,000 and 3,000 people are infected annually by the disease.[158] The pneumonia caused by plague causes death if not treated. The "black death" described in Europe in the 14th century was so-called because of the black spots that developed on the skin in severe cases. This skin manifestation often preceded death. Recent increased interest in the plague has resulted from the possibility of use of the infection by terrorists.[159]

Etiology. Three different forms of plague are recognized: bubonic plague, pneumonic plague, and septicemic plague. The etiological agent of plague in humans is the plague bacillus *Yersinia pestis* found in rodents, domestic cats and dogs, sheep, and camels. The bacillus can be transmitted to humans by direct contact with the infected animal, a bite from an infected rodent flea, or from person to person through airborne droplets coughed by the person infected with pneumonic plague.[160] Most cases of plague are found in areas with poor sanitary conditions and overcrowding, or where there is likely to be direct contact with wild animals.[161]

Signs and Symptoms. Specific signs and symptoms are associated with each type of plague. Bubonic plague is characterized by lymphadenopathy (swollen lymph glands), called "bubo," mainly of the groin and axilla. The bubo become inflamed, necrotic, and hemorrhagic. The bacillus then infects most organs of the body if untreated. Pneumonic plague results in multilobe pneumonia, with rapid onset of bacteremia and septicemia. Septicemic plague results from bacteria directly introduced into the vascular system and causes rapid onset of septicemia (general body infection). Other general signs and symptoms of plague include fever, severe headaches, delirium, tachycardia, and meningitis. People infected with plague who have pneumonia are isolated because of the risk of spreading the disease to others. All people with plague usually are hospitalized.[162]

Prognosis. In the United States, 14% (one in seven) of people infected with *Y. pestis* die. Once in the body, the bacteria multiply and spread rapidly, causing extensive disease, which if treated quickly is curable.[163] The mortality rate for bubonic plague is 1% to 15% if treated, and 40% to 60% if untreated. Septicemic plague is fatal in 40% of cases when treated, and 100% of cases when untreated. The worst prognosis is for pneumonic plague, with 100% fatality if not treated within the first 24 hours of infection.[164]

Medical Intervention. Diagnosis of the disease is important for survival of the infected person. Laboratory testing of the infected tissue from the bubo is the most reliable method of diagnosis.[165] Prevention of infection can be provided by taking prophylactic antimicrobials medications such as tetracyclines or sulfonamides for people likely to be in contact with the infection for a short period of time.[166] People who are diagnosed with plague are treated with antimicrobial medications such as streptomycin, gentomycin, tetracyclines, or chloramphenicol.[167]

Physical Therapy Intervention. None indicated.

Rabies

Rabies is the most well-known animal transmitted viral disease in humans but is fairly rare in the United States. Worldwide, approximately 55,000 people die each year from rabies infection. Most of these deaths occur in Asia and Africa.[168] The animals most associated with the spread of rabies in the United States are raccoons, skunks, bats, and foxes. Domestic animals rarely transmit the disease because all pet dogs and cats must be vaccinated against rabies in the United States. In 2006 (the most recent data available), the 49 continental U.S. states, Washington DC, and Puerto Rico had a total number of 6,940

reported cases of animals with rabies. Hawaii remains free of rabies. Only three cases of human infections were reported in the same year. The average number of deaths from rabies each year in the United States is two or three.[169] According to the CDC, the costs of treatment for exposure to rabies is roughly $1,000, but the costs for follow-up and prevention range between $10,000 and $100 million depending on the level of control of animals and the area affected by the disease.[170]

Etiology. Rabies is a type of encephalitis virus transmitted through contact with the saliva of an infected animal. Animals associated with the infection in the United States include bats, raccoons, skunks, and foxes. Domestic animals can be infected and therefore immunization is required for pets in the United States. The virus travels to the brain via the nerves and is then transmitted to other areas of the body including the salivary glands. Once the salivary glands are infected, a bite from an infected animal can transmit rabies to a human or another animal. The average incubation period between infection and the appearance of symptoms of the disease is 3 to 7 weeks, although it can be much longer.[171]

Signs and Symptoms. Once the incubation period ends and symptoms appear, the earliest symptoms include pain and paresthesia at the site of the bite, fever, headache, and general malaise similar to the symptoms of influenza. The later characteristic signs and symptoms are associated with encephalitis and myelitis. The neurological signs include mental confusion, paralysis, and hallucinations, as well as difficulty swallowing, hypersalivation, and hydrophobia (fear of water). Pathologically, Negri bodies (inclusion bodies) are found in the cytoplasm of neuronal cells in the hippocampus and cerebellum.

Prognosis. Once rabies affects the brain, the disease is fatal.[172] People infected with the rabies virus who are not treated usually die a few days after the onset of the later symptoms, perhaps many weeks after the initial animal bite.[173] In the United States, people who are treated after exposure do not develop rabies symptoms.[174]

Medical Intervention. People bitten by a wild animal may require postexposure prophylaxis, which includes administration of the rabies immune globulin around the area of the bite and several doses of the rabies vaccine.[175] An immunization also exists for people at high risk of being bitten during their work or leisure activities. Prevention measures against rabies include having domestic pets immunized against rabies infection and avoiding touching wild or stray animals.

Physical Therapy Intervention. None indicated.

Rocky Mountain Spotted Fever

Rocky Mountain spotted fever is one of the most severe and frequently reported rickettsia-related illnesses in the United States.[176] Between 250 and 1,200 cases of the disease are reported annually in the United States ⊛ The prevalence of the disease is 3.1 per million people with the highest rate of infection in older adults between the ages of 60 and 69 and children between the ages of 5 and 9.[177] The main areas of distribution are in the South Atlantic States of Delaware, Maryland, Virginia, West Virginia, North Carolina, and Washington D.C. Other states where the prevalence is highest are Arkansas, Louisiana, Oklahoma, and Texas. Over two thirds of the cases of the disease are reported in children aged under 15 years. Other countries reporting cases of rickettsia include Argentina, Brazil, Colombia, Costa Rica, Mexico, and Panama.[178]

Etiology. Rocky Mountain spotted fever is caused by the *Rickettsia ricketsii* bacteria transmitted to humans through tick bites. The ticks involved with transmission of the disease are usually the American dog tick, *Dermacentor variabilis*, the Rocky Mountain wood tick, and the *Dermacentor andersoni*.[179] Most infections occur during the months between April and September when the ticks are most prevalent. People who live or work close to woods seem to be at a higher risk of contracting the disease. The bacteria causes necrosis of cells with hemorrhage resulting in the profuse skin rash associated with the disease, and damage to internal organs and tissues.[180]

Signs and Symptoms. The early characteristic signs and symptoms of the disease are similar to those of influenza with the sudden onset of headaches, muscle pain, fever and chills, cough and respiratory symptoms, and occasionally coma. A skin rash may appear on the wrists and ankles spreading to the whole body a few days after infection.[181] Later signs and symptoms include a diffuse rash especially located on the soles of the feet and palms of the hands in 80% of the people with the disease, although approximately 15% never have a rash. Abdominal pain, joint pain, and diarrhea are also common. Long-term complications of the disease can include gangrene, loss of bowel and bladder control, movement disorders, hearing loss, and even partial paralysis of the lower extremities.[182] Neurological complications can include encephalitis, seizures, cranial nerve damage, blindness, and deafness. Lung involvement can cause pulmonary edema, interstitial pneumonia, and adult respiratory distress syndrome (ARDS). Other problems can include myocarditis, renal disease, and severe intestinal bleeding that can be life threatening.[183]

Prognosis. The disease is occasionally fatal, especially in the elderly, with a current mortality rate of 1.4%.[184] Severe complications can include debilitating disease with neurological, intestinal, or respiratory system problems. Many people with the disease have to be hospitalized for treatment.[185]

Medical Intervention. Prevention of Rocky Mountain spotted fever is through the use of tick repellents containing DEET and protective clothing. People in tick-infested areas should wear long-legged pants, with pants tucked into socks to prevent ticks from crawling onto the skin. Wearing light-colored clothing allows the ticks to be seen more easily. After return home, people should check their body for ticks and remove them with tweezers. The diagnosis of Rocky Mountain spotted fever is made by laboratory tests of blood. Laboratory tests may include antibody titers, kidney function tests, platelet count, prothrombin time (PT), red blood cell count, urinalysis to check for the presence of blood and protein in the urine, and skin biopsy taken from an area with the rash.[186] Positive laboratory findings may include an abnormal white cell count, thrombocytopenia (low platelet count), hyponatremia (low sodium levels in blood), and elevated liver enzymes. An immunofluorescence assay (IFA) test can also detect antibodies to the bacteria in blood.[187] Treatment includes the administration of antimicrobial medications such as tetracycline, doxycycline, and chloramphenicol.[188] People with severe cases of the disease may require hospitalization and emergency room procedures such as intubation, intravenous hookups, blood transfusions for severe gastrointestinal bleeding, or platelet transfusions if thrombocytopenia is severe.[189]

Physical Therapy Intervention. None indicated.

Typhus

Typhus is an acute infectious disease transmitted to humans by fleas and lice. Typhus is mainly found in areas of overcrowding. Areas at high risk for infection include refugee camps and wartime locations. Many people imprisoned in concentration camps during World War II contracted the disease and experienced a relapse of symptoms years later.[190] Endemic typhus is rare in the United States with only approximately 15 cases reported in total. Murine typhus is occasionally diagnosed in the southern and southeastern states during the summer and fall. Worldwide, typhus is reported in Central and South America, Africa, northern China, and parts of the Himalayas.[191]

Etiology. Typhus is a group of acute infectious diseases caused by a variety of *Rickettsia* organisms transmitted to humans by fleas and lice. Epidemic typhus, the more serious, is caused by *Rickettsia prowazekii* found in *Pediculus corporis* (the human body louse) and is also linked with fleas and lice from the flying squirrel. *R. prowazekii* also causes Bill-Zinsser disease, which is a form of typhus that reactivates months, or even years, after the initial infection. Endemic and murine typhus are both caused by *Rickettsia typhi* transmitted by animal fleas.[192]

Signs and Symptoms. The characteristic signs and symptoms of all forms of typhus include fever up to 105°F, headache, arthralgia (joint pains), abdominal pain, cough, "flulike" symptoms such as nausea and vomiting, pneumonia, cardiac, and circulatory problems. People with endemic typhus may experience delirium, hypotension, myalgia, and acute light sensitivity.[193] The symptoms last for approximately 2 to 3 weeks. The most serious symptoms are found in people with epidemic typhus and can include gangrene, central nervous system dysfunction, involvement of multiple organs, and even death. However, most of these symptoms are prevented by treatment.

Prognosis. Because typhus is rare in the United States, the mortality rate is not an issue of great concern. The mortality rate for people with untreated epidemic typhus worldwide ranges from 20% to 60%, but when treated, that rate drops to 3% to 4%. The mortality rate for treated murine typhus is between 1% and 4%. The overall prognosis for people with typhus is excellent when treatment is provided.[194]

Medical Intervention. Prevention is the best defense against typhus. Preventive measures include avoidance of endemic areas whenever possible; avoidance of overcrowded, unsanitary conditions; the use of insect repellents; wearing protective clothing; controlling body lice; and regular bathing. A vaccine for typhus is no longer available or considered necessary in the United States[195] Typhus is diagnosed through blood tests such as a complete blood count (CBC). Positive signs for typhus may include anemia, thrombocytopenia, hyponatremia (low levels of sodium), raised liver enzymes, mild kidney failure,

and the presence of typhus antibodies. The pharmacological intervention for typhus is with antimicrobial medications, such as tetracycline, doxycycline, and chloramphenicol. Intravenous fluids also may be needed.[196]

Physical Therapy Intervention. None indicated.

West Nile Virus or West Nile Encephalitis

The West Nile virus (WNV) is a potentially serious viral infection that affects humans, mammals, and birds. WNV was first discovered in Uganda in 1937 with outbreaks in several parts of the world since that time. Since detection of the virus in the United States in 1999, cases have been documented in all of the 48 continental states. The virus is also prevalent in seven of the Canadian provinces, Mexico, Puerto Rico, and some of the Caribbean islands.[197] In an attempt to track the numbers of cases, several states have Web sites that publish data about WNV within their state and also from around the country. California updates its Web site every week, and Pennsylvania places information every day.[198,199] In 2007, 3,630 cases of WNV were diagnosed, and 124 of those were fatal.[200] In the United States, 833 human cases of WNV were reported by September 23, 2008, with 18 fatalities.[201]

Etiology. WNV is an RNA virus and one of a group of *Flavivirus* associated with the Japanese encephalitis virus. The virus infects birds and mammals as well as humans. This group of viruses was identified in the United States in 1999 as a newly occurring arboviral (virus borne by arthropods) encephalitis. WNV is transmitted from birds by mosquitoes (see Fig. 10.3). The birds carry reservoirs of the live virus for several days before either dying or becoming immune. The birds carry the live virus the mosquitoes can pick up the virus during a bite and transmit the virus to humans and other animals. Humans and animals do not hold reservoirs of live virus. A small number of cases of WNV have been associated with organ transplantation, blood transfusion, and mother-to-infant transmission through breast milk. Such cases are extremely rare.[202]

Signs and Symptoms. The incubation period from infection to development of signs and symptoms for WNV is between 2 and 14 days. Only 20% of people who are infected with WNV actually develop any symptoms. Most of the 20% who develop symptoms have a comparatively mild form of West Nile fever. The signs and symptoms of West Nile fever include fever, headache, and occasionally

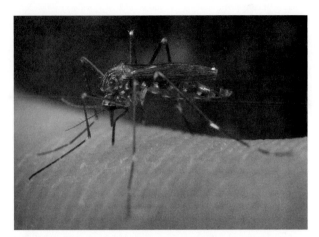

FIGURE 10.3 The *Aedes japonicas* mosquito, one of the mosquitoes responsible for the transmission of the West Nile virus (From the Centers for Disease Control and Prevention/Frank Collins, PhD).

lymphadenopathy (swollen lymph nodes), skin rash, and eye pain. A minority of people with West Nile fever actually have neurological involvement. The symptoms of this neuroinvasive WNV can range from severe headaches and fever to meningitis and encephalitis. Approximately 60% to 75% of people with neuroinvasive WNV develop encephalitis or meningitis with wide-ranging symptoms of altered mental state, headaches, stiffness of the neck (typical of meningitis), confusion, lethargy, coma, cranial nerve palsies, paralysis of the limbs, tremors, movement disorders such as ataxia, weakness, and gastrointestinal symptoms. A rare form of WNV is WNV poliomyelitis. Symptoms of this form include fever, headaches, limb weakness or paralysis, and respiratory muscle paralysis resulting in respiratory failure.[203]

Prognosis. More than 80% of the people who are infected with WNV have a mild form with no symptoms. The disease can be especially dangerous for the elderly and those who are immunosuppressed. Older age seems to be related to a higher incidence of death as a result of encephalitis and meningitis.[204]

Medical Intervention. People can protect themselves from WNV by using insect repellent sprays and wearing long sleeves and long-leg trousers when visiting insect infested areas. All doors and windows should have screens to prevent mosquitoes entering the home or workplace, and any standing water should be removed to prevent mosquitoes from laying eggs.[205] Gloves should be worn when handling dead wild animals and birds.[206] No vaccination is available for the WNV, but travelers to Asia can be vaccinated against the Japanese B encephalitis.

Physical Therapy Intervention. Physical therapy intervention may become necessary in advanced stages of the disease when physical and mental abilities are impaired and physical function is adversely affected. Although the WNV is not usually transmitted from one person to another, Standard (Universal) Precautions should be practiced when working with people with the virus.

Yellow Fever

Yellow fever is a viral infectious disease affecting humans and monkeys. The yellow fever virus causes epidemics in South and Central America and Africa, especially in areas of tropical climate close to the equator. According to WHO, yellow fever is once again becoming a "serious public health issue" in Africa and South America. Some of the programs that control mosquito populations have become underfunded, and mosquitoes are thriving increasing the number of outbreaks of yellow fever. An estimated 200,000 people each year are infected with the yellow fever virus, and of these 30,000 die.[207]

Etiology. The yellow fever virus is one of the flavivirus group, transmitted to humans and monkeys by several types of the *Aedes* and *Haemagogus* mosquitoes. The mosquitoes act as the reservoir of infection and pass the virus on to the next generation of mosquitoes in their eggs. These insects are found around houses and in jungles. Three types of yellow fever have been identified. Sylvatic (jungle) yellow fever is found in tropical rain forests affecting monkeys. Humans are infected when mosquitoes bite an infected monkey and then bite a human, passing on the virus. Intermediate yellow fever is common in Africa and may affect several villages. This type of yellow fever does not cause many deaths. The urban form of yellow fever causes large epidemics. Most commonly, this occurs when migrating infected people move into a densely populated area, and the *Aedes* mosquito transmits the infection.[208]

Signs and Symptoms. The incubation period from infection with the yellow fever virus to development of signs and symptoms is from 3 to 6 days. A large percentage of people who are infected do not develop any symptoms. In the initial acute phase symptoms include fever, headache and backache, muscle pains, loss of appetite, nausea and vomiting, and a slow pulse. In the 15% of people who develop a toxic phase of the disease, the signs and symptoms may include fever, jaundice, abdominal pain, vomiting, kidney problems ranging from reduced function to kidney failure, severe hepatitis, and hemorrhagic fever with bleeding from the mouth, nose, eyes, and stomach.[209]

Prognosis. Most people infected with yellow fever either have no symptoms or have an illness for a few days and recover quickly. Approximately 15% develop a toxic phase of the disease. In this group, 50% die within 10 to 15 days, and the other 50% fully recover.[210] Complete recovery from the toxic phase of yellow fever can require a year or more.[211]

Medical Intervention. The best approach for prevention of yellow fever is through vaccination. One dose of vaccination provides immunity for more than 10 years. If 80% of the population in an at-risk area were vaccinated yellow fever, outbreaks could be prevented. Vaccination is also recommended for those traveling to areas known to have infected mosquitoes. The usual precautions are taken to prevent insect bites including the use of insect repellants, covering body parts with clothing, using nets over beds, and installing screens on windows and doors. Mosquito control programs are also important to prevent yellow fever. The diagnosis of yellow fever is complicated because the symptoms resemble those of many other diseases. Laboratory blood and serum immunoassay tests for IgG yellow fever antibodies are used to confirm the diagnosis. A complete blood count (CBC) may identify leukopenia and thrombocytopenia.[212] No specific treatment is available for people infected with yellow fever. Prevention of dehydration is important. Constant care is necessary during the acute stages of the illness. In developing countries, the resources often are not available for either vaccination programs or adequate care of people infected.[213]

Physical Therapy Intervention. None indicated.

Why Does the Physical Therapist Assistant Need to Know About Infectious Disease Immunity?

Physical therapist assistants and other health care workers are exposed to many infectious diseases during clinical practice. Many of these infections can be prevented by vaccination. In most health care settings, the proof of immunity to the more common infectious diseases is a mandatory requirement for employment. Prevention of infection with these diseases protects both the health care provider and the people with whom they work.

Preventable Infectious Diseases for Which Health Care Workers Are Required to Have Immunity

This section provides information regarding the infectious diseases that health care workers in the United States are required to demonstrate immunity against as a condition of employment. Many of these recognized infectious diseases are preventable through vaccination. People who work in the health care setting are expected to demonstrate immunity to several of these diseases. Blood titers are taken to determine the presence or absence of antibodies in the blood. If a titer reveals that a person does not have immunity to a disease, the person must be vaccinated. This level of prevention with health care workers helps to reduce the risk and spread of infectious diseases. OSHA (www.osha.gov) and the CDC (www.cdc.gov) have guidelines for the demonstration of immunity to the following diseases by health care personnel. Some of these infectious diseases are caused by gram-negative or gram-positive bacteria, which are listed in Table 10-1. The following are described diseases preventable with vaccination: diphtheria, mumps, pertussis, poliomyelitis, rubella, rubeola, tetanus, and varicella.

Diphtheria

Diphtheria is an acute infectious disease that now is rare in most of the Western world. Fewer than five people per year are reported to have diphtheria in the United States. The risks of contracting diphtheria are increased in crowded living conditions, poor public health hygiene and sanitation, and lack of immunization. The disease remains endemic in many developing countries throughout the world where vaccination programs are not consistent. The disease is reportable to the CDC, which means that when someone is diagnosed, the physician must file a report with the CDC.

Etiology. Diphtheria is an acute infectious disease caused by the *Corynebacterium diphtheriae* bacteria. This unusual bacterium becomes infected with a virus that causes production of toxins. The toxins create a reaction with the lining of the tonsils, pharynx, or nasal cavity that causes a characteristic pseudomembrane to form across the pharynx that can prevent breathing.[214] The bacterium is spread from person to person through respiratory droplets from an infected individual coughing and sneezing or through contaminated food or drinks.[215]

Table 10.1 **Diseases Caused by Gram-Negative and Gram-Positive Bacteria**

GRAM-NEGATIVE BACTERIA	GRAM-POSITIVE BACTERIA
Whooping cough: *Bordetella pertussis*	Anthrax: *Bacillus anthracis*
Meningitis: *Neisseria meningitidis*	"Strep" throat: Streptococcal infections
Legionnaire's disease: *Legionella pneumophila*	Wound infections and urinary tract infections: Enterococcal infections
Salmonella: *Salmonellosis enterica*	Pneumonia, meningitis: Pneumococcal infections
Typhoid fever: *Salmonellosis*	Skin infections such as boils, osteomyelitis, toxic shock syndrome: *Staphylococcus aureus* infections
Gastroenteritis: *Escherichia coli* or *Entameba coli*	Botulism: *Clostridium botulinum*
Cholera: *Vibrio cholerae*	Diphtheria: *Corynebacterium diphtheriae*
Brucellosis: *Brucella*	
Pneumonia: *Haemophilus influenza*	
Chancroid: *Haemophilus ducreyi*	
Plague: *Yersinia pestis*	

Signs and Symptoms. The incubation period from infection to the onset of symptoms is between 2 and 5 days. Tests performed for the diagnosis of diphtheria include throat cultures and gram staining of tissue to identify the diphtheria bacterium. The characteristic signs and symptoms of the disease include the pseudomembrane already described, which blocks the airways and can cause breathing difficulties or cessation of breathing. Other symptoms include cough, low-grade fever and chills, sore throat, edema of the neck, painful swallowing, drooling, hoarseness, and changes in the color of the skin as a result of hypoxia. Complications from the disease can involve systemic symptoms such as myocarditis (inflammation of the heart), temporary paralysis, and damage to the kidneys from the toxins.[216] One form of diphtheria can infect the skin and causes fewer complications than the respiratory infection.

Prognosis. Untreated diphtheria is potentially life threatening as a result of the pseudomembrane that forms across the trachea and prevents breathing. The death rate among people who develop diphtheria is 5% to 10%.[217] Diphtheria has largely been eradicated as a health hazard in most of the Western world through immunization with DTaP (Diphtheria, tetanus toxoids, and acellular pertussis vaccine) against the disease in childhood. As a result, the disease is rare.[218]

Medical Intervention. The vaccine is administered to children in four doses before age 6 years. The immunity from the vaccination is thought to last approximately 10 years, thus requiring that adults receive boosters.[219] When a person is diagnosed with diphtheria, the diphtheria antitoxin is injected directly into a muscle or delivered through an intravenous line. Antimicrobial medications such as penicillin or erythromycin are prescribed. When the illness is severe, hospitalization may be necessary for intravenous fluids, supplemental oxygen therapy, bed rest, cardiac monitoring, intubation, and removal of the airway blockage. All people in contact with the infected person should receive booster diphtheria vaccinations.[220]

Physical Therapy Intervention. None indicated.

Mumps

Mumps is an acute, viral infection, usually affecting children. As a result of vaccination programs, the disease is rare in the United States, with fewer than 1,000 people affected each year.[221] The disease is reportable to the CDC.

Etiology. The cause of mumps is the paramyxovirus, which is transmitted through respiratory droplets from an infected person who coughs or sneezes or through contact with urine. Transmission also can occur from touching contaminated toys or table surfaces.[222]

Signs and Symptoms. The incubation period between infection and the onset of the symptoms ranges from 12 to 25 days, with the disease usually lasting from a few days to 2 weeks. The most infectious stage is 3 days before and the first 5 days after the onset of parotitis (inflammation and tenderness of the parotid salivary glands).[223] The characteristic signs and symptoms of mumps include parotitis, fever, fatigue, muscle aching, and loss of appetite. Serious complications are rare but may include pancreatitis, meningitis, orchitis (inflammation of the testes), mastitis (inflammation of the breasts), oophoritis (inflammation of the ovaries), and spontaneous abortion of the fetus if a mother is infected during early pregnancy.[224,225] The parotitis causes swelling of the face, which often occurs on one side and then develops on the other after the first side has resolved.

Prognosis. The outcome for people with mumps is usually good. Serious complications from the disease are rare in the United States.

Medical Intervention. The attenuated (weak, live vaccine) MMR vaccination (measles, mumps, and rubella vaccine) reduces the risk of contracting mumps. Regular hand washing can also minimize the risk of transmission.[226] Laboratory testing for mumps includes tissue swabs of nasopharyngeal secretions, urine, or blood to identify the mumps virus. A blood test for mumps-specific IgG antibodies may also be performed.[227] No specific treatment exists for someone with mumps other than ensuring hydration and keeping the person comfortable. If serious illness occurs, the person may have to be hospitalized.

Physical Therapy Intervention. None indicated.

Pertussis (Whooping Cough)

Pertussis, also known as whooping cough, is a highly infectious bacterial upper respiratory tract infection. The disease mainly affected children under age 2 before a vaccine was available. Most cases of pertussis are seen in adults or adolescents.[228] In 2004 (the most recent data available at the time of this writing), approximately 25,827 cases of pertussis in the United States were reported to the CDC.[229]

Etiology. Pertussis is caused by the gram-negative bacteria *Bordetella pertussis* or *Bordetella parapertussis*.[230]

Transmission of the disease from person to person is through respiratory droplets from coughing or sneezing. The bacteria attach to the cilia of the respiratory tract epithelial cells causing inflammation and paralysis of the cilia, which prevents effective expelling of the mucus.[231]

Signs and Symptoms. The incubation period between the infection and the onset of symptoms is usually 7 to 10 days but can range anywhere from 4 to 21 days. The characteristic signs and symptoms of pertussis are divided into three stages, with the first stage, often called the catarrhal stage, including coldlike symptoms such as sneezing, a low-grade fever, and a mild cough. This stage lasts approximately 1 to 2 weeks. After 2 weeks, the cough becomes more severe with a hacking quality and consists of episodes or paroxysms of coughing with production of thick mucus. Cyanosis (blue coloration of the skin) may occur during coughing paroxysms as a result of an oxygen deficit to the tissues and may be followed by vomiting, diarrhea, and exhaustion. This paroxysmal stage lasts between 1 and 6 weeks.[232] The cough tends to be worse at night. The inspiratory phase of the cough has a whooping noise, which gives the disease its name. Choking can occur in infants with the disease.[233] The third stage, the recovery stage of the disease, can last for several weeks or months with respiratory tract infections common during this phase. Complications from the disease include bacterial pneumonia, which occurs in only approximately 5.2% of people with pertussis infection, and, more rarely, neurological deficits such as seizures and encephalopathy resulting from hypoxia during coughing episodes. Dehydration may also be a concern particularly in infants with the disease.[234] Adults may experience sleeping disorders, urinary incontinence, pneumonia, and rib fractures as a result of the disease.

Prognosis. Areas of the world where the vaccine is not readily available have the highest death rates from pertussis. WHO reported a total of 294,000 deaths from pertussis in 2002 in developing countries.[235] In the United States, a total of 66 deaths were reported to the CDC between 2004 and 2005, and of those, 85% were infants under age 3 months.[236] Young infants are more susceptible because they have not received all of the doses of the vaccinations. The DTaP (infant form) and TDaP (adolescent and adult from) vaccines provide protection against the disease and reduce the risk of spreading the infection. In some cases, the vaccine does not prevent the disease but reduces the severity of the symptoms and prevents serious illness. Receiving the vaccination or contracting pertussis do not provide lifelong immunity to the disease, and booster vaccinations are necessary if outbreaks of pertussis are reported.[237]

Medical Intervention. The diagnosis of pertussis is achieved through cultures of infected mucus, and complete blood count (CBC) laboratory tests to detect an increased lymphocyte count. Antimicrobial therapy with erythromycin or amoxicillin is effective for people with the disease and reduces the likelihood of spreading the infection. Other medical intervention may include intravenous fluids and sedatives. Infants with the disease may need to be hospitalized because they may stop breathing during coughing episodes or become dehydrated. Prevention of the disease is preferable. Immunization against pertussis is provided by the DTP, or more recent DTaP vaccine given to infants in four doses, which provides immunity against a combination of diseases including diptheria, tetanus, and pertussis. Booster vaccinations are given at age 11 or 12 years in the form of Tdap and also may be administered to adults in contact with infected people.[238]

Physical Therapy Intervention. Chest physical therapy may be indicated during hospitalization, especially when a mucus sample is required for testing in the laboratory.

Poliomyelitis and Post-Polio Syndrome

Poliomyelitis (polio) is an acute viral infectious disease affecting humans. Physical therapy originated as a result of the polio outbreaks in the late 1800s and early 1900s in the United States. The treatment of people with polio led to the formation of reconstruction aides, with the subsequent development of physical therapy as a profession. The effects of polio have been largely eradicated in the developed world since the development of the polio vaccination in the 1950s. However, poliomyelitis remains endemic in India, Pakistan, Africa, Southeast Asia, and parts of the Middle East. In 2007, 1,315 people were reported to have poliomyelitis worldwide, with up to 98% of all cases occurring in India, Pakistan, and Nigeria. In 2008 a polio outbreak occurred in Nigeria causing an increase of cases worldwide to 1,652.[239] Currently, the disease is rare in the United States, with no reported cases since 1999.[240] Most people who become infected with polio have not been immunized and have traveled to parts of the world where polio outbreaks are common.[241] A more recently detected condition is **post-poliomyelitis syndrome (post-polio syndrome).** This condition occurs in individuals who had paralytic poliomyelitis many years previously

and later experience worsening of their symptoms. The impact of post-polio syndrome may be a far-reaching health care concern because approximately 12 to 20 million people in the world have survived polio infection.[242]

Etiology. Poliomyelitis is caused by the poliomyelitis virus. The virus is transmitted through direct person-to-person contact with nasal or oral secretions, infected mucus, or infected feces. The virus enters the body through the mouth or nose and multiplies within the throat and intestines. The infection is absorbed into the circulatory and lymphatic systems and transmitted throughout the body.[243] ⊛ The people most at risk of contracting the virus include children, the elderly, and pregnant women.

Post-polio syndrome occurs in people who previously had paralytic poliomyelitis. Although the actual etiology of post-polio syndrome is unknown, theories exist. One is that during the original polio infection when the virus causes irreversible damage to the neurons of the anterior horn cells in the spinal cord, the neurons develop new sprouts. The increased muscle weakness manifested in post-polio syndrome is thought to be the result of degeneration of the sprouts of these enlarged motor units.[244]

Signs and Symptoms. The incubation period between infection and the onset of symptoms is usually 7 to 14 days but can range from 5 to 35 days. The signs and symptoms of poliomyelitis vary from minor to severe. Three types of poliomyelitis are recognized: subclinical, nonparalytic, and paralytic. The nonparalytic and paralytic forms affect the nervous system and the brain. The symptoms of subclinical poliomyelitis include mild fever, general malaise, headache, sore and inflamed throat, and vomiting. Some people with subclinical polio do not have any symptoms. The symptoms usually last approximately 72 hours. Nonparalytic poliomyelitis causes symptoms of pain, stiffness, muscle tenderness, and spasm in the lumbar and cervical spines, lower and upper extremities, and abdomen. Other symptoms include fever, headaches, diarrhea, fatigue, skin rash, and vomiting. The symptoms of nonparalytic polio last between 1 and 2 weeks. The paralytic form of the disease causes more severe neurological symptoms. A particularly severe form of paralytic polio is called bulbar polio because it destroys the motor neurons of the brainstem, causing swallowing, breathing, and speech difficulties.[245] Symptoms of paralytic polio include altered skin sensation; respiratory distress as a result of paralysis of the respiratory muscles, including the diaphragm; urinary hesitancy (difficulty starting the flow of urine); drooling as a result of facial nerve involvement; mood swings and loss of control of temper; rapid-onset, asymmetrical (one-sided) muscle weakness; hypersensitivity to touch; muscle pain; stiffness and spasms in the lumbar and cervical spines and lower extremities; and swallowing difficulties. Other symptoms include headache, abdominal bloating, and constipation. The symptoms of paralytic polio may be temporary or permanent.[246]

Post-polio syndrome develops in people who previously had paralytic poliomyelitis with associated muscle atrophy and weakness and gained either partial or complete functional recovery. The symptoms of the syndrome develop many years after the original disease. The syndrome is characterized by the development of either gradual or sudden onset of a progressive new muscle weakness and muscle fatigue in the muscles originally affected by the disease. People complain of reduced endurance to activity and muscle and joint pains. To be significant for diagnosis, the symptoms have to be present for at least a year.[247] Other signs and symptoms may include intolerance to extremes of heat and cold, sleeping problems, reduced ability to perform activities of daily living (ADLs), and, more rarely, breathing and swallowing problems.[248]

Prognosis. People with subclinical poliomyelitis usually have a full recovery. When the brain and spinal cord are involved, paralysis and death can occur. Paralytic polio is considered a medical emergency. Only 1 out of every 200 people infected with poliomyelitis develops paralysis, and of those approximately 5% to 10% die from respiratory muscle paralysis.[249] Most people with paralytic polio have long-term disabilities associated with the effects of the disease.[250] Some of the long-term complications of poliomyelitis may include aspiration pneumonia and other respiratory problems such as pulmonary edema, cor pulmonale, hypertension, paralytic ileus (paralysis of the intestinal muscles of peristalsis), permanent paralysis, and frequent urinary tract infections, which may result in the development of kidney stones.[251] Little is known about the long-term effects of postpoliomyelitis syndrome, although research studies are ongoing.[252]

Medical Intervention. The best prevention of poliomyelitis in the United States is the inactivated polio vaccine (IPV). The oral polio vaccine (OPV) is still used in parts of the world where polio is common because it is more effective at reducing the transmission of the disease from one person to another which is not a problem in the United States.[253] ☺ Children are given a course of four injections at 2 months, 4 months, 6 to 18 months, and 4 to 6 years of age.[254,255] Poliomyelitis is diagnosed through viral cultures of the feces, cerebrospinal fluid, and throat swabs. Blood tests to detect the presence of polio antibodies also are helpful. The medical management of people with poliomyelitis depends on the form of the disease. People with subclinical polio may not have any symptoms or may think they have a case of the flu and not go to the physician. People with nonparalytic and paralytic forms of the disease may require a variety of interventions. Symptoms of urinary retention may require medications such as bethanechol. Headaches, muscle pains, and muscle spasms may be treated with moist heat and analgesics. Urinary tract infections are treated with antimicrobial medications. People with paralytic poliomyelitis require long-term rehabilitation, including extensive physical therapy, corrective shoes, orthotics, and bracing, and may require orthopedic surgery.[256] Those with bulbar polio require respiratory support from positive pressure ventilators, either temporarily or permanently.[257]

Physical Therapy Intervention. PT intervention for people with poliomyelitis includes the reeducation of patients in ADLs, ambulation, and strengthening exercises. Many people with post-poliomyelitis syndrome are seen in the physical therapy clinic. Specific interventions are currently being formulated to help reduce the effects of the condition. People with this condition should not overfatigue the involved muscles. Excessive fatigue of the muscles can result in the reduced functional abilities of patients for the next few days, and recovery of the involved muscles may be slow. Physical therapy intervention should therefore include advice on lifestyle changes and adaptations to optimize function, create energy conservation, and reduce fatigue. According to Post Polio Health International research studies have shown that an exercise program specifically developed for the individual with post-polio syndrome by a health care professional can be effective.[258] Programs should consist of low- to moderate-intensity exercise, a slowly progressing exercise routine, and a combination of stretching, aerobic, strengthening, and endurance exercises.[259-260]

Rubella (German Measles) ☺

Rubella is a viral, infectious disease once fairly common in children but now more prevalent in young adults who have not been immunized. Rubella is particularly dangerous when contracted by a pregnant woman during the first 20 weeks of pregnancy because it can cause fetal defects.

Etiology. Rubella, also called German measles, is an infectious virus transmitted in air droplets from an infected person. The rubella virus is a rubivirus of the togaviridae family.[261] The incubation period from infection with rubella to the onset of symptoms is between 14 and 23 days.[262] People with rubella are infectious 1 week before and 1 week after development of the rash. In some cases, infants with rubella continue to have infected urine and nasal secretions for many months.[263]

Signs and Symptoms. The characteristic signs and symptoms of rubella, a systemic disease, are similar to those of influenza and usually are rather mild. Some people with rubella have no symptoms. Adults with rubella tend to have more severe symptoms than children. The symptoms include a low-grade fever, headaches, lymphadenopathy in the cervical region (swollen lymph glands), rhinitis with coryza (runny nose), conjunctivitis, and a skin rash with pink or red spots on the face spreading to the trunk and limbs (see Fig. 10-4).[264] Adults with the disease sometimes have arthralgia (joint pains) and joint edema. The main symptoms of rubella last for approximately 3 days, but lymphadenopathy may last for over a week, and arthralgia may persist for more than a few weeks.[265] Adults with rubella tend to take much longer to recover from the disease than children. Congenital rubella can cause congenital rubella syndrome consisting of any or all symptoms including congenital heart defects, microcephaly, mental retardation, motoric and growth retardation, hearing problems, cataracts, glaucoma, and liver,

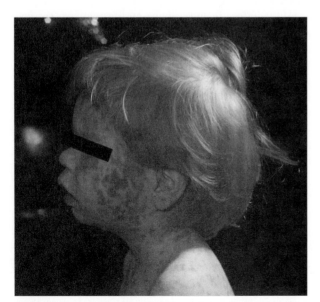

FIGURE 10.4 A young boy with the maculopapular rash characteristic of rubella (German measles) (From the Centers for Disease Control and Prevention).

spleen, and bone marrow abnormalities.[266] Such defects in the child are permanent.

Prognosis. Rubella is usually a mild infectious disease with no long-standing effects. However, rubella can cause congenital defects in a fetus if the mother is infected during the first 20 weeks of pregnancy.[267] Estimates are that 25% of infants born to mothers who were infected with rubella during the first trimester of pregnancy develop congenital rubella syndrome.[268]

Medical Intervention. No specific pharmacological treatment exists for rubella. Prevention of the disease through immunization with the MMR (measles, mumps, and rubella) vaccine is provided to all children in the United States in two doses. The first dose is at between 12 and 15 months and the second dose at 4 to 6 years.[269] Young women of childbearing age should receive an antibody titer for rubella to ensure immunity against the infection before considering pregnancy.[270] Pregnant women should avoid close contact with people infected with rubella and should not receive the vaccine.

Physical Therapy Intervention. Physical therapy intervention may be required for the child with motor delay or mental retardation caused by congenital rubella. Health care workers, including PTAs, are required to demonstrate immunity to rubella before working in a health care setting.

Rubeola (Measles)

Rubeola is a highly infectious viral disease. This disease is now rare in the United States because of the development of a vaccine in 1963. Before the development of the vaccine for rubeola, 3 to 4 million people, mainly children, were affected by the disease every year in the United States, with 500 deaths per year.[271] In 2005, there were 66 reported cases of rubeola, which occurred in people who were not vaccinated or had become infected through travel to other countries. Worldwide, the disease affects approximately 50 million people and causes up to 1 million deaths each year.[272] In 2008 between January 1 and July 31, an increase was noted in the number of children in the United States reported to have rubeola; most had not received vaccinations because of parent objections.[273]

Etiology. Rubeola is caused by a single-strand RNA *Morbillivirus* known as paramyxoviridae transmitted from nose, throat, and oral secretions spread through droplets in the air, by coughing and sneezing. The virus replicates in the lymph nodes and then spreads to the rest of the body.[274] The incubation period is between 7 and 21 days, with a general average of 10 to 14 days.[275] The infectious period of the disease is 4 days before the rash appears until 4 days after it appears. The virus can remain in the air for up to 2 hours and continues to be infectious. ⊛ The people most at risk for infection with the rubeola virus are infants under 12 months of age because they cannot be vaccinated until that age, as well as people who have never been vaccinated or were vaccinated with a previous form of vaccine between 1963 and 1967.[276] Of the people who are not immunized against rubeola, 90% become infected if they are in contact with someone with rubeola.

Signs and Symptoms. The characteristic signs and symptoms of rubeola last for about 10 days and include a bright red skin rash, which starts on the face and progresses to the rest of the body lasting more than 3 days, a fever, photophobia (sensitivity to light), cough, coryza (runny nose), and conjunctivitis. The main signs and symptoms are often called the 3 Cs of rubeola: cough, coryza, and conjunctivitis.[277] Koplik's spots (crystal-like deposits surrounded by a red ring) may occur on mucous membranes of the mouth and genitalia, and a yellow exudate may exist on the tonsils. Approximately 30% of the people infected with rubeola develop some complication. Complications can vary in severity from diarrhea and ear infections, to immunosuppression, pneumonia, encephalitis, and vitamin A deficiency, which leads to blindness.[278,279] The signs and symptoms of encephalitis include a severe headache, fever, vomiting, seizures, stiffness of the neck, drowsiness, and sometimes coma. Women who are pregnant and become infected with rubeola have a higher risk of death and an increased risk of delivering the infant prematurely, having a stillborn infant, or having a miscarriage. Unlike rubella, no known birth defects associated with rubeola exist.[280] ⊛ A modified form of rubeola occurs in infants who have some immunity from the disease from their mother. The incubation period for modified rubeola is longer, and the symptoms are milder and last a shorter amount of time. Atypical rubeola is severe and develops in people who received vaccination between 1963 and 1967. This older version of the vaccination did not provide immunity to the disease. The symptoms of atypical rubeola include pneumonia, pleural effusions, edema of the extremities, and a rash that starts on the ankles and wrists rather than the head.[281]

Prognosis. Although pneumonia and encephalitis are rare, they are life-threatening. Of the people with rubeola who develop encephalitis, the death rate is 15%.[282] The MMR vaccination provided in the United States prevents many of these serious complications. ⊛ Blindness resulting from rubeola infection affects 60,000 children a year in developing countries. In developing countries without vaccination, death rates from measles can be as high as 10%.[283]

Medical Intervention. The prevention of severe cases of rubeola through immunization is extremely important. ⊛ In the United States children are vaccinated with MMR (measles, mumps and rubella) at 12 months and again at 4 years of age.[284] The vaccine provides individuals with approximately 98% immunity from contracting rubeola. People who have actually had the rubeola infection develop immunity for life.[285] The rubeola part of the vaccine is a live attenuated (weakened) virus. All health care workers have to demonstrate immunity to rubeola through a titer or receive the vaccination against the disease. The diagnosis of rubeola mainly involves taking a clinical history. The presence of Koplik's spots in the mouth may help with the diagnosis and blood tests for the presence of IgM antibodies to rubeola may confirm the diagnosis.[286] The medical intervention for people with rubeola consists of bed rest, plenty of fluids to prevent dehydration, and isolation from other people to avoid spreading the disease.[287]

Physical Therapy Intervention. None indicated. Isolation precautions must be followed when contact with a person infected with rubeola is unavoidable.

Tetanus

Tetanus is an acute bacterial disease. The disease is rare in the United States with fewer than 50 cases per year reported. In other parts of the world where the immunization is either limited or absent, the disease is more common and results in fatalities. The worldwide annual incidence of the disease is 0.5%, which equates to approximately 1 million cases per year. In 2002, 213,000 people died throughout the world as a result of tetanus infection.[288] Most people who contract the infection have not been adequately vaccinated.

Etiology. The cause of tetanus, also known as lockjaw, is via spores of the *Clostridium tetani* bacteria found in soil, house dust, and in the intestines of both animals and humans. The spores of *C. tetani* can remain viable (alive) in the soil for more than 40 years and are resistant to heat, desiccation, and most disinfectants.[289,290] When the spores enter the body through an open wound, they reproduce and excrete an extremely toxic neurotoxin called tetanospasmin that attacks the central nervous system by interfering with neurotransmission across the synapses.[291,292] The types of wounds most likely to be susceptible to the tetanus bacteria include deep puncture wounds, insect bites, burns, self-performed tattooing or body piercing, and intravenous illicit drug sites.[293] 🖐 Infants who contract the disease soon after birth are usually infected through the residual of the umbilical cord when hygiene is not adequate. The incubation period between infection and the onset of symptoms is between 2 days and 2 months, with an average of 14 days.

Signs and Symptoms. The characteristic signs and symptoms of tetanus include tetany (involuntary tonic/tetanic muscle spasms) that starts near the site of the wound and progresses to the whole body. Spasms of the jaw muscles are particularly common causing the trismus (tightness of the mouth and jaw muscles) that gives the disease the name "lockjaw." The tonic spasms include the muscles of respiration, making swallowing and breathing difficult. The muscle spasms can be severe enough to cause spinal fractures and muscle tears. A total arching of the spine into extension as a result of the muscle tetany is called opisthotonos, caused by contraction of both agonist and antagonist muscles.[294,295] Other signs and symptoms may include fever, excessive sweating, neck stiffness, headaches, irritability, incontinence of bowel and bladder, and severe body extensor muscle spasms, causing rigidity and convulsions.[296,297] The recovery period from tetanus occurs slowly over several months.

Prognosis. People who are infected with the *C. tetani* bacteria usually do not have any long-standing neurological effects from the disease once recovered. However, some people may continue to have hypertonia after recovery from the infection.[298] As a result of the tetanic contractions of the respiratory muscles, the disease is often fatal if untreated. The mortality rate worldwide for people infected with tetanus is 45%. In the United States, the mortality rate is 6% for those who received some level of immunization and 15% for those with no immunizations. When people require mechanical ventilation, the mortality rate is increased to 30%.[299] With adequate intervention, the death rate is reduced to less than 10%.[300] Respiratory infections resulting from the reduced respiratory function also pose a danger of death.[301] Muscle spasms of the throat can result in hypoxia and permanent brain damage in rare instances.[302]

Medical Intervention. Detection and diagnosis of the disease may be symptomatic. No laboratory tests are available for diagnosis of tetanus. A spatula test can indicate infection. A spatula is touched to the oropharynx and a bite down on the spatula is considered positive. The usual response to this test is the gag reflex; however, the gag reflex is paralyzed by the tetanus toxin.[303] 🖐 The disease can be prevented by immunization with the DTaP vaccine in the infant. Four doses of the DTaP are given before age 2 and a booster shot at age 4 to 6 years. After that, booster shots are given every 10 years, or within 5 years when an injury occurs that is likely to transmit the disease.[304] Most people and infants with tetanus infection are hospitalized in the intensive care unit on bed rest to monitor respiratory functions. The wound that provided the portal of infection may be surgically débrided.[305] Antimicrobial medications such as penicillin G, metronidazole, or doxycycline and antitoxins to neutralize the effect of the toxins produced by the bacteria are given to people with tetanus infection. Muscle tetanic contractions are controlled with sedatives such as diazepam, phenobarbitol, baclofen, or dantrolene or by neuromuscular blocking agents such as vecuronium.[306] These sedatives effectively paralyze the muscles requiring a mechanical ventilator.[307] Passive immunization with tetanus immunoglobulin (TIG) is sometimes administered as part of the postexposure tetanus prophylaxis.[308] People who are infected with tetanus need an immunization upon recovery because having the active disease does not provide immunity. The immunization is given into the muscle near the wound and also the buttocks when the early symptoms of tetanus are recognized.[309]

Physical Therapy Intervention. PT intervention may be necessary during the ventilator stages of treatment to provide instruction to hospital personnel regarding passive range of motion and position changes to prevent pressure ulcers. Intervention may be necessary during the recovery phase to instruct the individual in breathing exercises and to provide mobility and strengthening rehabilitation exercises to return the person to full function.

Varicella (Chickenpox)

Varicella is a common, highly infectious viral disease. Outbreaks of varicella are comparatively rare in the United States. Before vaccination programs, varicella caused between 50 and 100 deaths per year in the United States. Currently, an average of 10 people die per year as a result of varicella infection, and most of these deaths occur in people who have not been vaccinated.[310]

Etiology. The etiology of varicella, more commonly known as chickenpox, is infection with the herpes zoster virus.[311] 🖐 The same virus causes both chickenpox in children and shingles in the adult. (See Chapter 8 for details regarding shingles.) The incubation period of the virus is 10 to 21 days, and it is highly contagious during a period from 2 days before the rash appears until 5 days after the rash appears. The infection is transmitted through infected respiratory droplets or by contact with the open rash.[312] The varicella virus infects the respiratory tract and multiplies within the lymph nodes. A small proportion (2%) of children born to women who contracted varicella during the first two trimesters of pregnancy have congenital varicella syndrome as a result of the virus passing from the mother to the fetus via the placenta.[313]

Signs and Symptoms. The characteristic signs and symptoms of varicella include mild fever, headache, anorexia, cough, coryza (runny nose), sore throat, general malaise, and a rash. The rash causes small but intensely irritating, blisterlike ulcerations, especially on the face, scalp, mouth, chest, and trunk. The number of ulcerations can vary from hundreds to several thousand. The lower and upper extremities also may be affected with the rash. The rash lasts approximately 2 weeks, and children with the disease are isolated from other children.[314] Adults and adolescents are more likely to have severe illness associated with varicella. People who have been vaccinated may get mild forms of the infection. Secondary infections that can occur with varicella include bacterial infections of the skin, encephalitis, and pneumonia.[315] The signs and symptoms of congenital varicella syndrome include microcephaly, cataracts, and growth retardation.[316]

Prognosis. ⊛ Most children with varicella recover fully with no complications unless they have some other comorbid condition causing a compromised immune system. Approximately 1 in every 50 people who contract varicella develop some sort of complication. The mortality rate in the United States is low with 2 deaths per 100,000 people with varicella between the ages of 1 and 14.[317]

Medical Intervention. ⊛ Vaccination is provided in two doses to children over age 1 year in the United States, if children have not had the disease and developed immunity. All health care workers are tested for the presence of the varicella antibody and are provided with immunization if the tests are negative.[318] The pharmacological intervention for people with varicella may consist of antiviral medications such as acyclovir if the infection is severe. Antipyretic medications, such as acetaminophen and ibuprofen, are prescribed to reduce fever, and antihistamines such as diphenhydramine (Benadryl) help to reduce itching and to help children sleep. Chest radiographs may be necessary if the person is having respiratory symptoms.[319] Children with varicella may wear mittens to prevent scratching the blisters and causing skin infections.

Physical Therapy Intervention. None indicated. All health care personnel are required to provide proof of immunity to varicella. The recommendations from the CDC vary from year to year, so PTAs working in the health care setting need to keep up to date with the current requirements.[320]

Why Does the Physical Therapist Assistant Need to Know About Other Infectious Diseases?

The knowledge of some other infectious diseases not covered in previous sections is important for the PTA. Some of these diseases, such as anthrax and variola (smallpox), are of importance in the preparedness of all health care workers for the possibility of use in a terrorist attack. Other infections are commonly observed in health care, and even though the associated signs and symptoms may not be an indication for physical therapy interventions, the PTA may need to take precautions against transmission of these diseases.

Other Infectious Diseases

The following section discusses some of the infectious diseases not previously described. These diseases include anthrax, botulism, infectious mononucleosis, influenza, Legionnaire's disease, meningitis, toxic shock syndrome, and variola (smallpox). All these diseases have the potential for serious illness and mortality.

Anthrax

Interest in the anthrax bacteria has been heightened in recent years as a result of the possibility of use during a terrorist attack. The CDC keeps up-to-date information on this and all other infectious diseases on its Web site at www.cdc.org. The anthrax bacterium is commonly found in herbivorous (plant-eating) domestic animals, such as cattle, sheep, goats, camels, and deer. The most common areas of the world for anthrax are those with agricultural economies such as South and Central America, Southern and Eastern Europe, Asia, Africa, the Caribbean, and the Middle East. Although anthrax infections occur in the United States every year in livestock and deer, human infection is rare.[321]

Etiology. Anthrax is a highly infectious disease caused by a spore-producing bacteria called *Bacillus anthracis.* Three distinct forms of the disease occur: cutaneous, inhalation, and intestinal. Most human infections result from handling the meat or products of infected animals such as wool, leather, or meat, eating the undercooked meat of infected animals, or inhaling anthrax spores. Approximately 95% of all people infected with anthrax develop it through cutaneous transmission.[322]

Signs and Symptoms. The characteristic signs and symptoms of the disease vary with the mode of transmission. When the bacteria is transmitted through a skin lesion, the initial lesion looks like an insect bite and then develops into an ulceration with a necrotic center. The area surrounding the site becomes edematous and the lymph nodes become inflamed. In rare instances, the symptoms may progress to general sepsis and meningitis. The initial signs and symptoms of inhaled anthrax are similar to the common cold but develop into severe pulmonary problems and systemic shock. If the anthrax bacteria is ingested, it causes intestinal symptoms, including anorexia, fever, vomiting, severe diarrhea, and abdominal pain with vomiting of blood. Other symptoms may include a sore throat, dysphagia (inability to swallow), edema of the neck, and lymphadenopathy.[323]

Prognosis. The intestinal form of anthrax is fatal in approximately 25% to 60% of the cases (CDC).[324] Inhaled anthrax is usually fatal if not treated. When antimicrobial medications are provided, people with intestinal anthrax still have a 45% mortality rate. The cutaneous form of anthrax is usually well controlled with antimicrobial medications, but if people remain untreated, approximately 20% will die.[325]

Medical Intervention. Prevention of anthrax is preferable by avoiding contact with animal products and meat in countries with a high incidence of infected animals. The use of respirators is recommended for people who regularly handle animal products in parts of the world where anthrax is common. A vaccine is available for people at risk of exposure to the disease including laboratory workers, military personnel, and people handling animals in

areas of high incidence or who work with animal products such as leather or fur imported from countries where anthrax is common. The vaccine is 93% effective in preventing anthrax infection upon exposure.[326,327] The diagnosis of anthrax infection is achieved through blood tests for antibodies to *B. anthracis,* and cultures of blood, skin lesion secretions, respiratory secretions, and spinal fluid for the presence of the bacteria. People diagnosed with anthrax are placed on antimicrobial medications such as penicillin G, doxycycline, amoxicillin, ampicillin, ciprofloxacin (Cipro), or levofloxacin.[328] Chest radiographs may be necessary for people with suspected inhaled anthrax. Early treatment with antimicrobials improves the outcome, but unfortunately, most people do not know they have anthrax, which delays the treatment.[329,330]

Physical Therapy Intervention. No physical therapy is indicated for people with anthrax. The infection is not spread from person to person, so the risks of contracting the disease from an infected person are minimal. In the event of a terrorist attack with anthrax, the PTA may be involved in the general emergency response as part of the Emergency Action Plan (EAP) within the hospital. All hospital personnel should be familiar with the EAP for their facility.[331]

Botulism

Botulism is a potentially dangerous bacterial infection, also known as food poisoning. The bacterium is found all over the world in soil and untreated water systems.[332] Approximately 145 people a year are diagnosed with botulism in the United States, mainly infants. The diagnosis of botulism is considered a medical emergency.[333]

Etiology. Botulism is caused by the *Clostridium botulinum* bacteria. The bacteria may be found in improperly bottled, canned, and pre-prepared foods but is usually found in home-canned foods. The extremely potent toxins produced by the spores of the bacteria prevent the release of acetylcholine at the neural synapse, causing paralysis of the muscles.[334]

Signs and Symptoms. The incubation period for botulism ranges from 6 hours to as much as 10 days. Most people infected with the bacteria have symptoms within 36 hours of eating contaminated food.[335] The characteristic signs and symptoms include abdominal cramping, double vision, dry mouth, nausea, respiratory problems that can lead to respiratory failure, vomiting, visual disturbances, dysphagia (inability to swallow), dysphasia (speech impairment), and weakness and paralysis. Weakness and other neurological symptoms may last for up to a year after the recovery from botulism.[336]

Prognosis. People with severe untreated cases of the disease can have paralysis of the respiratory system, resulting in death. Early medical treatment improves the outcome for people with botulism. The mortality rate for people with botulism in the United States is 3% to 5%. The weakness and paralysis and respiratory problems caused by the disease can last a few years and result in disability.[337]

Medical Intervention. The likelihood of contracting botulism can be reduced by throwing away any canned foods that have bulging lids and any foods that do not smell right. The diagnosis of botulism is achieved through a stool culture for evidence of the bacteria. Pharmacological intervention is with the botulinus antitoxin. The use of antimicrobial medications seems to have little effect on the bacteria. Patients with respiratory problems have to be hospitalized and may need to be placed on mechanical ventilators during the respiratory failure stage of the disease. If dysphagia is present, intravenous fluids and feeding through a gastric tube may be necessary.[338]

Physical Therapy Intervention. Physical therapy is indicated for people with botulism during the acute phase if respiratory therapy is needed. During the recovery from severe cases of botulism people may require neurological rehabilitation for the weakness and paralysis associated with the condition. [339]

Infectious Mononucleosis

Infectious mononucleosis is an infectious disease most commonly found in teenagers and young adults. In other parts of the world, including Europe and the United Kingdom, the disease is called glandular fever.

Etiology. Infectious mononucleosis, also known as the "kissing disease," is an acute disease caused by the **Epstein-Barr virus (EBV)** or the cytomegalovirus (CMV), both of which are types of herpes virus.[340,341] The disease is spread via saliva. The incubation period for the virus is between 4 and 6 weeks. EBV is one of the most common human viruses, and 95% of adults have acquired the infection by age 40. When the EBV virus infects adolescents and young adults, 35% to 50% have a chance of contracting mononucleosis.[342] After people contract HBV, the virus remains in the body for the rest of their life, and they can pass on the infection even though they are not

symptomatic. This dormant infection is also thought to play a part in the development of Burkitt's lymphoma and nasopharyngeal carcinoma.[343]

Signs and Symptoms. Some people who contract EPV do not have any symptoms. The characteristic signs and symptoms of mononucleosis include fever, sore throat, loss of appetite, headache, general feelings of fatigue, muscle aching and stiffness, and lympadenopathy especially in the neck. Some people develop a measles-like skin rash.[344] Complications associated with the disease include hepatitis and inflammation of the spleen. Although the symptoms of mononucleosis usually only last between 1 and 2 months, on occasion, they can last several months.[345]

Prognosis. The prognosis for mononucleosis is usually good. The disease resolves itself within a few months. Complications from the disease are rare.[346] After people have completely recovered from mononucleosis, a repeat infection is not possible. However, if people return to normal activities before the infection is completely resolved, a recurrence of the symptoms may occur.

Medical Intervention. The diagnosis of mononucleosis is achieved through the clinical symptoms and laboratory tests to identify the virus. Specific tests include the mononucleosis monospot test for antibodies present as a result of the infection and an EBV antibody titer.[347] The white blood cell count is usually raised, and liver function tests may show some abnormalities.[348] No specific treatment is available for the condition, although the use of steroid medications may help to reduce the inflammation of the throat and tonsils.[349] General nonsteroidal anti-inflammatory medications may be recommended to reduce the pain and fever. Gargling with warm saline solution, plenty of rest, and sufficient fluids all help to ease the discomfort of the disease.[350] People who develop inflammation of the spleen are advised to avoid participation in contact sports because rupture of the spleen could occur.[351]

Physical Therapy Intervention. No physical therapy intervention is indicated for mononucleosis.

Influenza (Flu)

In the United States, between 5% and 20% of the population each year contract influenza. More than 200,000 people are hospitalized each year, and approximately 36,000 people die from the disease. ☻ The most susceptible people are older adults, young children, and people with other chronic diseases.[352]

Etiology. Influenza (flu) is an acute viral disease affecting the upper respiratory tract caused by influenza viruses A and B.[353] The virus is spread from person to person through air droplets from coughing or sneezing or by direct contact with the virus and mucous membranes of the eyes and mouth. The virus is infectious from 1 day before and 5 days after the start of symptoms.[354] Transmission of influenza directly from animals to humans is rare. Wild birds act as a reservoir of infection for influenza A virus. Other animals such as horses and pigs can also get influenza. Occasionally an animal will be infected with both a human and an avian influenza virus and develop a combined form of the disease, which can then be transmitted to humans and be very infectious.[355] The types of influenza virus are constantly changing, which means that antibodies to one strain of influenza do not protect against a different strain.[356] The viral pneumonia caused by the virus may be made worse by a secondary bacterial infection.

Signs and Symptoms. The characteristic signs and symptoms of influenza range from mild to severe and include cough, high fever, sore throat, dyspnea, muscle aching, headache, diarrhea and vomiting, and general debility. People with chronic diseases such as asthma, heart disease, or diabetes can have exacerbation of the symptoms of these other diseases when they have influenza.[357] Complications arising from influenza infection include pneumonia, bronchitis, sinus infections, and ear infections.

> 🕮 NOTE: In children, a rare condition called **Reye's syndrome** can result from several types of viral infections. This condition causes encephalopathy and hepatic (liver) failure and can be fatal. The risk of contracting Reye's syndrome is increased with using aspirin during a viral disease in children.[358]

Prognosis. Many types of flu are mild, but severe forms of the virus exist that cause pneumonia and even death. The elderly, the very young, and people with comorbidities are most susceptible to the more serious forms of the disease.[359]

Medical Intervention. Prevention of influenza is improved through vaccination with the influenza vaccine. This vaccine is different each year, and an annual vaccination is now recommended by the CDC for all people above the age of 6 months between October and December.[360,361] The symptoms of flu last up to a week. Because it is a virus, little can be given to relieve the symptoms. The main recommendations are plenty of rest, fluids, and the avoidance of alcohol and smoking.[362] People who develop pneumonia may require sputum cultures, blood cultures, and a complete blood count (CBC) to verify the diagnosis. If bacterial infection occurs in addition to the viral infection, the use of antimicrobials can resolve the resulting symptoms.[363]

Physical Therapy Intervention. No physical therapy is generally indicated for influenza unless pneumonia develops and chest physical therapy is needed. All health care workers are recommended to have the vaccination unless a medical condition contraindicates the use of vaccine. Health care workers who are not immunized pose a risk of infection for susceptible populations, such as the elderly and the very young in neonatal units.[364]

Legionellosis/Legionnaire's Disease

Legionellosis, also called Legionnaire's disease and Pontiac fever, is also mentioned in Chapter 4 with the different types of pneumonia. Between 8,000 and 18,000 people are hospitalized each year as a result of legionellosis. The disease is named after an outbreak in a group of people from the American Legion in Philadelphia in 1976.[365]

Etiology. Legionnaire's disease is a respiratory disease and a type of pneumonia caused by the *Legionella* bacteria. The incubation period from becoming infected with the bacteria and starting with symptoms is between 2 and 14 days. *Legionella* bacteria occur naturally in warm water supplies. Transmission of the bacteria is via water droplets inhaled into the lungs. The most common method of transmission of the bacteria to humans is through contaminated water supplies in shower heads, hot tubs, and air-conditioning and heating systems in large buildings. The bacteria cannot be transmitted from one person to another.[366] The people most at risk of infection are those with compromised immune systems, chronic lung disease, smokers, and those over age 65 years.

Signs and Symptoms. The bacterium causes a type of pneumonia with high fever, a productive cough, chills, headache, and muscle aches. A milder form of the disease caused by the same bacteria is called Pontiac fever.[367]

Prognosis. Legionellosis is a serious disease that results in the death of between 5% and 30% of people who are infected. Antimicrobial medications are effective in treating the condition, but people who are immunocompromised are at greater risk of mortality.[368]

Medical Intervention. The diagnosis of legionellosis is through the cultures of sputum, blood, and urine for evidence of the *Legionella* bacteria. Antibody levels in blood are also diagnostic tools. Chest radiographs are used to determine signs of pneumonia. Pharmacological intervention is with antimicrobial drugs.[369]

Physical Therapy Intervention. Physical therapy may be indicated for chest percussion, postural drainage, and other pulmonary hygiene interventions in severe cases of pneumonia related to legionellosis.

Meningitis ☻

Meningitis most commonly occurs in children and young adults under age 30, although people over 60 years are also at risk for the disease. The incidence of the disease is between 2 and 3 per 100,000 people in the United States. Meningitis is endemic in several parts of Africa and India and in other developing countries.[370]

Etiology. The causes of meningitis are varied and include viruses, bacteria, fungi, brain tumors, and drug allergies. The most common causative agents are viruses. The enteroviruses that also cause a lot of intestinal illnesses are often responsible for the infection. Other viruses that cause meningitis include the herpes simplex virus and West Nile virus. The many types of bacterial meningitis include cryptococcal, *Escherichia coli*, meningococcal, pneumococcal, staphylococcal, streptococcal, syphilitic, and tuberculous.[371]

Signs and Symptoms. Meningitis causes inflammation of the meninges of the brain and spinal cord. Viral meningitis tends to be a milder form of the disease that lasts up to 2 weeks. Bacterial meningitis can develop suddenly over a period of less than 24 hours and can be serious, resulting in increased intracranial pressure that can cause pressure on the brain and neural tissues. The general signs and symptoms of meningitis include fever, nausea, vomiting, photophobia (sensitivity to light), severe headaches, meningismus (stiffness of the neck), altered levels of consciousness, seizures, tachypnea, agitation, opisthotonus (severe extensor muscle spasms), and reduced appetite.[372]

Prognosis. Viral meningitis usually is not a serious illness and resolves within 2 weeks. Bacterial meningitis can be serious and sometimes fatal. A diagnosis of bacterial meningitis is considered a medical emergency. An early diagnosis and treatment intervention improves the outcome for people with bacterial meningitis. Those with bacterial meningitis are more likely to have long-term brain or other neurological damage and may have hearing or vision loss, and hydrocephalus.[373]

Medical Intervention. Prevention of some types of meningitis is possible through vaccination with the pneumococcal conjugate vaccine and the meningococcal vaccine.[374] These vaccines are recommended for children about to enter high school and for college students who are going to be residing in a residence hall. People who travel to countries where meningitis is prevalent may also receive the vaccines.[375] The diagnosis of meningitis involves a complete blood count (CBC), chest radiographs, computed tomography scans or magnetic resonance imaging of the head, and lumbar puncture to obtain samples of cerebrospinal fluid (CSF) for measurement of glucose levels, cell count, and culture to detect the causative bacteria. The bacterial type of the disease is treated with antimicrobials depending on the causative bacteria. Viral meningitis is not treatable with medications but usually resolves within 2 weeks without treatment. In people with severe meningitis, usually bacterial, hospitalization may be needed with intravenous fluids and antiseizure medications.[376]

Physical Therapy Intervention. Physical therapy intervention may be indicated for people recovering from bacterial meningitis who have neurological deficits. The physical therapy focuses on functional rehabilitation, prevention of contractures and deformities, and ADL.

Toxic Shock Syndrome

Toxic shock syndrome is a form of sepsis, a bacterial infection that affects the whole body. The incidence of toxic shock syndrome in the United States is between 2.4 and 16 people per 100,000 of the population. Strains of methicillin resistant *Staphylococcus aureus* (MRSA) are increasing the incidence of the syndrome.

Etiology. The etiology of toxic shock syndrome is an infection with either staphylococcal or streptococcal bacteria. The shock to the body is caused by the response of the immune system to the exotoxins, collectively called pyrogenic toxin superantigens (SAgs), produced by the bacteria. Toxic shock syndrome has been linked with many kinds of bacterial infection with the staphylococcal and streptococcal bacteria including pneumonia, osteomyelitis, and skin and gynecological infections, as well as infections from the use of tampons in women.[377]

Signs and Symptoms. The characteristic signs and symptoms of the disease include high fever, hypotension, tachycardia, cardiac arrhythmias, diarrhea with abdominal pain, vomiting, sore throat, altered mental status including confusion, headaches, arthralgia and myalgia, and a body rash.

Prognosis. Toxic shock syndrome caused by streptococcal bacteria tends to be more serious than staphylococcal and results in approximately a 70% mortality rate. Fortunately, the streptococcal form of the syndrome is not as common. In most cases of toxic shock syndrome, prompt treatment with antimicrobial medications can resolve the infection.[378]

Medical Intervention. The diagnosis of toxic shock syndrome involves many tests and requires that the signs and symptoms involve at least three body systems, such as the gastrointestinal tract, respiratory system, and muscular system. A complete blood count reveals an increased white blood cell count, mild anemia, and thrombocytopenia. Electrolyte tests usually show hypocalcemia, hypokalemia, and hyponatremia. Renal and liver function tests are abnormal, urine analysis reveals protein, glucose, and red cells in the urine, and arterial blood gases are positive for acidosis and hypoxia. The pharmacological intervention is with antimicrobial medications, and steroids to reduce the inflammation.[379]

Physical Therapy Intervention. Physical therapy is not indicated for people with toxic shock syndrome.

NOTE: *Streptococcal Infections*

Streptococcus bacteria are responsible for several skin conditions including cellulitis or erysipelas and impetigo, all of which are described in Chapter 8. Streptococcal infections can also cause many other conditions including "strep throat," pneumonia, streptococcal toxic shock syndrome, meningitis, and a type of infection that destroys the deep muscle fascia called **necrotizing fasciitis.** The pneumonia associated with streptococcal infections is particularly serious and may cause endocarditis.

Variola (Smallpox)

Smallpox was eradicated from the world in its natural form in 1977 (CDC) as the result of a massive worldwide vaccination campaign by the WHO. However, because some specimens of the virus were preserved in laboratories around the world, the risk of the use of the virus in acts of terrorism has resulted in a renewed interest in the disease.

Etiology. Smallpox is caused by the variola virus. The disease is extremely infectious and spread by saliva droplets and by secretions from the skin rash on bedding and clothing.

Signs and Symptoms. The signs and symptoms of variola include a high fever, severe headaches and backaches, and a rash that starts off pink or red and turns into pus filled spots which then crust over. Vomiting, severe diarrhea, hemorrhage, and extreme fatigue are also present. The virus resulted in pneumonia and encephalitis in many people, and in some necrosis of internal organs such as the lungs and intestine. Survivors of the virus were often deeply scarred with pox marks on the skin from the rash.[380]

Prognosis. Infection with the variola major virus resulted in a 30% mortality rate before the eradication of the disease. The less severe variola minor virus resulted in a 1% mortality rate.

Medical Intervention. Diagnostic tests for variola include blood analysis to reveal an initial low white blood cell count and later high count and a low platelet count. Antibody tests for variola are performed. Up to 1977, the smallpox vaccination was administered to prevent the spread of the disease. Since 1977, the smallpox vaccination has not been used. However, some laboratories are involved with developing smallpox vaccination in case of a terrorist attack using the virus. Treatment of people infected with variola involves administration of the vaccine within the first 4 days after exposure to the virus and isolation of the infected person and close contacts to prevent the spread of the disease.[381]

Physical Therapy Intervention. No physical therapy intervention is indicated for people infected with variola. In the event of an outbreak of variola as the result of a terrorist attack, the hospital emergency plan may be initiated, and the PTA could be involved to the extent determined by the specific site.

CASE STUDY 10.1

A 45-year-old man attends physical therapy with the diagnosis of early-stage AIDS dementia complex with associated functional limitations and reduced ambulatory abilities. The patient is able to follow simple commands but becomes somewhat confused with complicated instructions. Evaluation findings by the physical therapist include generalized weakness in upper and lower extremities of between 3+/5 and 4/5 strength. His range of motion in all joints is within functional limits. Balance in sitting is normal, but in standing and ambulation, it is fair. He has difficulty rising from a chair and requires moderate assistance of one person to ambulate without an assistive device. Transfers onto his bed are difficult. He is unable to bathe independently because he cannot get in and out of the bathtub. He has a home health aide who is only available 2 hours each day, but in the evenings, he has a family member who is available and lives in the same house. The PT designates to the PTA to provide PT intervention for the patient. The plan of care includes progressive strengthening exercises for upper and lower extremities with a home exercise program; balance reeducation; ambulation training, with appropriate assistive device to include stairs; and transfer training, including chair to bed, into the car, and in and out of the bathtub. Frequency of intervention is to be twice a week for 4 weeks to optimize function and return to as much independence and safety as possible.

1. Develop a progressive strengthening exercise program within the plan of care developed by the PT for the patient for the upper and lower extremities for the next four weeks. Keep in mind the patient's

level of cognition and ability to follow commands. Keep instructions to as few words as possible.

2. Develop a series of progressive balance exercises to increase the balance in standing and ambulation of the patient.

3. What ambulatory device would you choose for the patient, and what precautions would you need to be aware of for this patient?

4. Decide what kinds of transfers you will perform with the patient. What level of assistance will be needed, and what training will you need to give to the care providers?

5. What level of independence might you expect with this patient?

6. What specific safety issues will you concentrate on during your physical therapy intervention sessions?

7. Write a treatment note for the patient in either a subjective, objective, assessment, plan (SOAP) format or narrative form consistent with the SOAP categories.

8. Develop a home exercise program in writing to give to the patient. Consider the level of cognition of the patient.

STUDY QUESTIONS

1. What are the symptoms of hepatitis B, and why is this disease of importance in the health care field?

2. Name the causative virus of AIDS and describe any particular characteristics of the virus.

3. Describe three symptoms of AIDS.

4. Discuss with other members of your class or other PTs or PTAs the appropriate strategy for treating patients with AIDS who have requested that no one except the treating therapist know about their diagnosis because their partner does not know. Consider all legal and ethical issues involved in this situation

including patient privacy. Keep in mind that AIDS is not a notifiable disease.

5. Name three sexually transmitted diseases other than AIDS.

6. Name five infectious diseases that health care workers are required to demonstrate immunity to by OSHA.

7. Discuss post-poliomyelitis syndrome and the implication of this condition for physical therapy intervention.

8. Describe three insect-borne infectious diseases found in the United States.

⬤ USEFUL WEB SITES

AIDS information, National Institutes of Health
http://aidsinfo.nih.gov

American Association for Clinical Chemistry
Lab Tests Online
http://labtestsonline.org

American College of Rheumatology
http://www.rheumatology.org

Arthritis Foundation
http://www.arthritis.org

Centers for Disease Control and Prevention
http://www.cdc.gov

MedicineNet.com
http://www.medicinenet.com

MedlinePlus
http://www.nlm.nih.gov

National Digestive Diseases Information Clearing House
http://digestive.niddk.nih.gov

National Institute of Allergy and Infectious Diseases
http://www3.niaid.nih.gov/

National Institute of Neurological Disorders and Stroke
http://www.ninds.nih.gov

World Health Organization (WHO)
http://www.who.int

⬤ REFERENCES

[1] Centers for Disease Control and Prevention. (2009). *Hepatitis B: FAQs for health professionals.* Retrieved 11.23.10 from http://www.cdc.gov/hepatitis/HBV/HBVfaq.htm#treatment

[2] Longstreth, G. F. (2009). Hepatitis B. *MedlinePlus Medical Encyclopedia.* Retrieved 11.24.10 from http://www.nlm.nih.gov/medlineplus/ency/article/000279.htm

[3] Occupational Safety and Health Administration. (1992, updated 2006 & 2008). Regulations (Standards – 29 CFR). Bloodborne pathogens section 1910.1030. Retrieved 11.24.10 from http://www.osha.gov/pls/oshaweb/owadisp.show_document?p_table=STANDARDS&p_id=10051

[4] Centers for Disease Control and Prevention. (2008). *Hepatitis A.* Retrieved 5.7.2009 from http://www.cdc.gov/hepatitis/HAV/HAVfaq.htm#general

[5] Hepatitis A. (2008). *MedlinePlus Medical Encyclopedia.* Retrieved 5.7.2009 from http://www.nlm.nih.gov/medlineplus/hepatitisa.html

[6] Centers for Disease Control and Prevention. *Hepatitis A.* Ibid.

[7] National Institutes of Allergy and Infectious Diseases. (2007). *Hepatitis A.* Retrieved 5.7.2009 from http://www3.niaid.nih.gov/topics/hepatitis/hepatitisA/treatment.htm

[8] Ibid.

[9] Centers for Disease Control and Prevention. *Hepatitis A.* Ibid.

[10] Ibid.

[11] National Institutes of Allergy and Infectious Diseases. *Hepatitis A.* Ibid.

[12] Centers for Disease Control and Prevention. *Hepatitis B: FAQs for health professionals.* Ibid.

[13] Ibid.

[14] Ibid.

[15] Longstreth, G. F. (2009). Hepatitis B. *MedlinePlus Medical Encyclopedia.* Retrieved 11.24.10 from http://www.nlm.nih.gov/medlineplus/ency/article/000279.htm

[16] Centers for Disease Control and Prevention. (2008). *Hepatitis B.* Retrieved 5.7.2009 from http://www.cdc.gov/hepatitis/HBV.htm

[17] Longstreth, G. F. Ibid.

[18] Centers for Disease Control and Prevention. *Hepatitis B: FAQs for health professionals.* Ibid.

[19] Longstreth, G. F. (2009). Cirrhosis. Retrieved 11.24.10 from http://www.nlm.nih.gov/medlineplus/ency/article/000255.htm

[20] Longstreth, G. F. Hepatitis B. Ibid.

[21] Lee, C., et al (2006). Effect of hepatitis B immunization in newborn infants of mothers positive for hepatitis B surface antigen: systematic review and meta-analysis. *BMJ* 332:328–336.

[22] Tarhan, M. O., et al (2006). Accelerated versus classical hepatitis B virus vaccination programs in healthcare workers: accelerated vs classical HBV vaccination. *Med Sci Monitor Int Med J Exp Clin Res* 12:CR467–470.

[23] Longstreth, G. F. Hepatitis B. Ibid.

[24] Centers for Disease Control and Prevention. *Hepatitis B: FAQs.* Ibid.

[25] MedicineNet.com. (2009). *Hepatitis B: What is new in the treatment of hepatitis virus?* Retrieved 11.24.10 from http://www.medicinenet.com/hepatitis_b/page10.htm

[26] National Institutes of Allergy and Infectious Diseases. (2008). *Hepatitis C: Overview.* Retrieved 5.7.2009 from http://www3.niaid.nih.gov/healthscience/healthtopics/HepatitisC/overview.htm

[27] National Institutes of Allergy and Infectious Diseases. (2008). *Hepatitis C: transmission.* Retrieved 5.7.2009 from http://www3.niaid.nih.gov/topics/hepatitis/hepatitisC/transmission.htm

[28] National Digestive Diseases Information Clearing House. (2010). *Chronic hepatitis C: current disease management.* Retrieved 11.24.10 from http://digestive.niddk.nih.gov/ddiseases/pubs/chronichepc/#a

[29] National Institutes of Allergy and Infectious Diseases. *Hepatitis C: transmission.* Ibid.

[30] National Digestive Diseases Information Clearing House. *Chronic hepatitis C: current disease management.* Ibid.

[31] Hepatitis C. (2008). *MedlinePlus Medical Encyclopedia.* Retrieved 5.7.2009 from http://www.nlm.nih.gov/medlineplus/hepatitisc.html#cat5

[32] National Digestive Diseases Information Clearing House. *Chronic hepatitis C: current disease management.* Ibid.

[33] American Association for Clinical Chemistry. (2010). Liver panel. *Lab Tests Online.* Retrieved 11.24.10 from http://www.labtestsonline.org/understanding/analytes/liver_panel/glance.html

[34] American Association for Clinical Chemistry. (2010). Hepatitis C. *Lab Tests Online.* Retrieved 11.24.10 from http://www.labtestsonline.org/understanding/analytes/hepatitis_c/test.html

[35] National Digestive Diseases Information Clearing House. *Chronic hepatitis C: current disease management.* Ibid.

[36] Lacey, S. R. (2010). Hepatitis D. *eMedicine from WebMD.* Retrieved 11.24.10 from http://www.emedicine.com/med/topic994.htm

[37] Public Health Agency of Canada. (2004). *Hepatitis G fact sheet.* Retrieved 5.7.2009 from http://www.phac-aspc.gc.ca/hcai-iamss/bbp-pts/hepatitis/hep_g-eng.php

[38] Centers for Disease Control and Prevention. (2010). *Viral hepatitis.* Retrieved 11.24.10 from http://www.cdc.gov/hepatitis/index.htm

[39] National Digestive Diseases Information Clearinghouse. (2008). *Viral hepatitis: A through E and beyond.* National Institute of Diabetes and Digestive and Kidney Diseases, National Institutes of

Health. Retrieved 5.7.2009 from http://digestive.niddk.nih.gov/ddiseases/pubs/viralhepatitis/index.htm

[40] National Digestive Diseases Information Clearinghouse. *Viral hepatitis: A through E and beyond.* Ibid.

[41] Lacey, S. R. Ibid.

[41] Centers for Disease Control and Prevention. *Viral hepatitis.* Ibid.

[42] Mihas, A. A., Hung, P. D., & Heuman, P. D. (2009). Alcoholic hepatitis. *eMedicine from WebMD.* Retrieved 11.24.10 from http://www.emedicine.com/MED/topic101.htm

[43] Xu, J., Kochanek, K. D., & Tejada-Vera, B. (2009). Deaths: preliminary data for 2007. *National Vital Statistics Report,* 58. Centers for Disease Control and Prevention. Retrieved 4.6.2010 from http://www.cdc.gov/nchs/data/nvsr/nvsr58/nvsr58_01.pdf

[44] Longstreth, G. F. (2009). Alcoholic liver disease. *MedlinePlus Medical Encyclopedia.* Retrieved 11.24.10 from http://www.nlm.nih.gov/MEDLINEPLUS/ency/article/000281.htm

[45] Mayo Clinic. (2008). *Alcoholic hepatitis.* Retrieved 5.7.2009 from http://www.mayoclinic.com/health/alcoholic-hepatitis/DS00785/DSECTION

[46] Ibid.

[47] Ibid.

[48] Mihas, A. A., Hung, P. D., & Heuman, D. M. Alcoholic hepatitis. Ibid.

[49] Mayo Clinic. *Alcoholic hepatitis.* Ibid.

[50] Cichocki, M. (2006). Are health care workers at risk of getting HIV on the job? *About.com: AIDS/HIV.* Retrieved 5.10.2009 from http://aids.about.com/od/technicalquestions/f/healthrisk.htm

[51] Panlilio, A. L., et al. (2005). Updated United States Public Health Service guidelines for the management of occupational exposures to HIV and recommendations for postexposure prophylaxis. Centers for Disease Control and Prevention. *MMWR Mortal Morbid Wkly Rev* 54(RR09):1–17.

[52] Panlilio, A. L., et al. Ibid.

[53] Dugdale, D. C., III, & Vyas, J. M. (2010). AIDS. *MedlinePlus Medical Encyclopedia.* Retrieved 11.24.2010 from http://www.nlm.nih.gov/medlineplus/ency/article/000594.htm

[54] World Health Organization. (2008). *HIV/AIDS.* Retrieved 5.11.2009 from http://www.who.int/immunization/topics/hiv/en/index.html

[55] Centers for Disease Control and Prevention. (2008). *HIV incidence.* Retrieved 5.11.2009 from http://www.cdc.gov/hiv/topics/surveillance/incidence.htm

[56] Centers for Disease Control and Prevention. (2008). *HIV/AIDS statistics and surveillance: basic statistics.* Retrieved 5.11.2009 from http://www.cdc.gov/hiv/topics/surveillance/basic.htm#hivest

[57] AIDS Info. (2005). *The HIV life cycle.* Retrieved 5.11.2009 from http://aidsinfo.nih.gov/contentfiles/HIVLifeCycle_FS_en.pdf

[58] Centers for Disease Control and Prevention. (2007). *Human immunodeficiency virus type 2.* Retrieved 5.11.2009 from http://www.cdc.gov/hiv/resources/factsheets/hiv2.htm

[59] Dugdale, D. C., III, & Vyas, J. M. Ibid.

[60] World Health Organization. HIV/AIDS. Ibid.

[61] Dugdale, D. C., III, & Vyas, J. M. Ibid.

[62] National Institute of Neurological Disorders and Stroke. (2008). *Neurological complications of AIDS information page.* Retrieved from http://www.ninds.nih.gov/disorders/aids/aids.htm

[63] Dugdale, D. C., III, & Vyas, J. M. Ibid.

[64] Centers for Disease Control and Prevention. *HIV/AIDS statistics and surveillance: basic statistics.* Ibid.

[65] Cichocki. M. (2008). Understanding absolute CD4 count and CD4 percentage. *About.com: AIDS/HIV* Retrieved 11.24.10 from http://webcache.googleusercontent.com/search?q=cache:http://aids.about.com/od/aidsfactsheets/a/cd4percent.htm

[66] Begtrup, K., et al. (1997). Progression to acquired immunodeficiency syndrome is influenced by CD4 T-lymphocyte count and time since seroconversion. *Am J Epidemiol* 145:629–635.

[67] Dugdale, D. C., III, & Vyas, J. M. Ibid.

[68] Franceschi, S., et al. (2008). Kaposi sarcoma incidence in the Swiss HIV Cohort Study before and after highly active antiretroviral therapy. *Br J Cancer* 99:800–804. Retrieved 9.2.2008 from ProQuest Health and Medical Complete Database (Document ID: 1541578591).

[69] Dugdale, D. C., III, & Vyas, J. M. Ibid.

[70] Zidovudine, (azt) – oral, Retrovir. (2010). *MedicineNet.com from WebMD.* Retrieved 11.24.2010 from http://www.medicinenet.com/zidovudine_azt-oral/article.htm

[71] Hall, M. A. (2010). Chancroid. *eMedicine from WebMD.* Retrieved 11.24.10 from http://www.emedicine.com/derm/topic71.htm

[72] Mehta, N., & Silverberg, M. A. (2009). Chancroid. *eMedicine from WebMD.* Retrieved 4.4.2010 from http://www.emedicine.com/emerg/TOPIC95.HTM

[73] Vorvick, L. J. (2009). Chancroid. *MedlinePlus Medical Encyclopedia.* Retrieved 4.4.2010 from http://www.nlm.nih.gov/medlineplus/ency/article/000635.htm

[74] Ibid.

[75] Hall, M. A. Ibid.

[76] Mehta, N., & Silverberg, M. A. Ibid.

[77] Vorvick, L. J. Ibid.

[78] Hall, M. A. Ibid.

[79] Centers for Disease Control and Prevention. (2010). *Chlamydia—CDC fact sheet.* Retrieved 11.24.2010 from http://www.cdc.gov/std/Chlamydia/STDFact-Chlamydia.htm

[80] Ibid.

[81] Ibid.

[82] Ibid.

[83] Vorvick, L. J. (2010). Chlamydia. *MedlinePlus Medical Encyclopedia.* Retrieved 11.24.2010 from http://www.nlm.nih.gov/medlineplus/ency/article/001345.htm

[84] Stöppler, M. C. (2008). Chlamydia in women. *MedicineNet.com.* Retrieved 5.11.2009 from http://www.medicinenet.com/chlamydia_in_women/page3.htm

[85] Centers for Disease Control and Prevention. *Chlamydia—CDC fact sheet.* Ibid.

[86] Centers for Disease Control and Prevention. (2010). *Cytomegalovirus (CMV) and Congenital CMV infection.* Retrieved 11.24.2010 from http://www.cdc.gov/cmv/trends-stats.html

[87] Centers for Disease Control and Prevention. (2006). *Cytomegalovirus: about CMV, general information.* Retrieved 11.24.2010 from http://www.cdc.gov/cmv/overview.html

[88] Akhter, K., & Wills, T. S.(2010). Cytomegalovirus. *eMedicine from WebMD.* Retrieved 11.24.2010 from http://www.emedicine.com/MED/topic504.htm

[89] Centers for Disease Control and Prevention (2006). *Cytomegalovirus: signs and symptoms of CMV.* Retrieved 11.24.2010 from http://www.cdc.gov/cmv/signs.htm

[90] Akhter, K., & Wills, T. S. Ibid.

[91] Centers for Disease Control and Prevention. (2010). *Cytomegalovirus (CMV) and congenital CMV infection: pregnant women.* Retrieved 11.24.2010 from http://www.cdc.gov/cmv/risk/preg-women.html

[92] Ibid.

[93] Griffiths, P. D., McLean, A., & Emery, V. C. (2001). Encouraging prospects for immunization against primary cytomegalovirus infection. *Vaccine* 19:1356–1362.

[94] Arvin, A. M., Fast, P., Myers, M., Plotkin, S., Rabinovich, R., & National Vaccine Advisory Committee. (2004, July). Vaccine development to prevent cytomegalovirus disease: report from the National Vaccine Advisory Committee. *Clinical Infectious Diseases,* 39: 233-239.

[95] Zhong, J., & Khanna, R. (2007). Vaccine strategies against human cytomegalovirus infection. *Expert Rev Antiinfect Ther* 5:449–459.

[96] Kimberlin, D. W., et al. (2003). Effect of ganciclovir therapy on hearing in symptomatic congenital cytomegalovirus disease

involving the central nervous system: a randomized controlled trial. *J Pediatr* 143:16–25.

[97] Akhter, K., & Wills, T. S. Ibid.

[98] Centers for Disease Control and Prevention. (2010). *Gonorrhea—CDC fact sheet.* Retrieved 11.24.2010 from http://www.cdc.gov/std/gonorrhea/stdfact-gonorrhea.htm

[99] Gonorrhea. (2008). *MedlinePlus Medical Encyclopedia.* Retrieved 5.11.2009 from http://www.nlm.nih.gov/medlineplus/gonorrhea.html

[100] Centers for Disease Control and Prevention. *Gonorrhea—CDC fact sheet.* Ibid.

[101] WHO Western Pacific gonococcal antimicrobial surveillance programme (2008, March). Surveillance of antibiotic resistance in *Neisseria gonorrhoeae* in the WHO Western Pacific Region, 2006. *Commun Dis Intelligence* 32:48–51. Retrieved from http://www.ncbi.nlm.nih.gov/sites/entrez?Db=pubmed&Cmd=Search&Term=%22WHO%20Western%20Pacific%20Gonococccal%20Antimicrobial%20Surveillance%20Programme%22%5BCorporate%20Author%5D&itool=EntrezSystem2.PEntrez.Pubmed.Pubmed_ResultsPanel.Pubmed_DiscoveryPanel.Pubmed_RVAbstractPlus

[102] National Institute of Allergy and Infectious Diseases. (2010). Antimicrobial (Drug) resistance: *Neisseria gonorrhoeae.* Department of Health and Human Services, NIH. Retrieved 11.25.2010 from http://www.niaid.nih.gov/topics/antimicrobialResistance/Examples/neisseria/Pages/default.aspx

[103] Centers for Disease Control and Prevention. (2008). *Antimicrobial resistance and Neisseria gonorrhoeae—CDC fact sheet.* Retrieved 5.11.2009 from http://www.cdc.gov/std/gonorrhea/arg/stdfact-resistant-gonorrhea.htm

[104] Centers for Disease Control and Prevention. *Gonorrhea—CDC fact sheet.* Ibid.

[105] American Association for Clinical Chemistry. (2010). Gonorrhea. *Lab Tests Online.* Retrieved 11.24.2010 from http://www.labtestsonline.org/understanding/analytes/gonorrhea/test.html

[106] Hitt, E. (2010). Nucleic acid amplification testing detects extragenital STIs missed by cultures in young HIV-infected patients. *Medscape Today from WebMD.* 2010 National STD Prevention Conference. Retrieved 11.25.2010 from http://www.medscape.com/viewarticle/718391

[107] Centers for Disease Control and Prevention. (2010). *Gonorrhea—CDC fact sheet.* Ibid.

[108] Centers for Disease Control and Prevention. (2009). *Genital HPV infection—CDC fact sheet.* Retrieved 5.16.2010 from http://www.cdc.gov/STD/HPV/STDFact-HPV.htm

[109] National Institute of Allergy and Infectious Diseases. (2010). *Human papillomavirus and genital warts.* Retrieved 11.24.2010 from http://www3.niaid.nih.gov/topics/genitalWarts/

[110] National Cancer Institute. (2008). *Human papillomaviruses and cancer: questions and answers.* Retrieved 5.11.2009 from http://www.cancer.gov/cancertopics/factsheet/risk/HPV

[111] Centers for Disease Control and Prevention. *Genital HPV infection—CDC fact sheet.* Ibid.

[112] Ibid.

[113] Ibid.

[114] National Cancer Institute. *Human papillomaviruses and cancer: questions and answers.* Ibid.

[115] National Institute of Allergy and Infectious Diseases. *Human papillomavirus and genital warts.* Ibid.

[116] Centers for Disease Control and Prevention. (2009). *Genital HPV infection—CDC fact sheet.* Ibid.

[117] U.S. Food and Drug Administration. (2006). *Product approval information—licensing action. Gardasil® questions and answers.* Retrieved 11.24.2010 from http://www.fda.gov/BiologicsBloodVaccines/Vaccines/ApprovedProducts/ucm111283.htm

[118] National Cancer Institute. *Human papillomaviruses and cancer: questions and answers.* Ibid.

[119] Centers for Disease Control and Prevention. (2010). *Syphilis—CDC fact sheet.* Retrieved 11.24.2010 from http://www.cdc.gov/std/syphilis/STDFact-Syphilis.htm

[120] Centers for Disease Control and Prevention. (2007). *Syphilis elimination effort (SEE), The National plan to eliminate syphilis from the United States—Executive summary.* Retrieved 5.11.2009 from http://www.cdc.gov/stopsyphilis/SEEexec2006.htm

[121] Centers for Disease Control and Prevention. *Syphilis—CDC fact sheet.* Ibid.

[122] Ibid.

[123] National Institute of Neurological Disorders and Stroke. (2007). *NINDS tabes dorsalis information page.* Retrieved 5.11.2009 from http://www.ninds.nih.gov/disorders/tabes_dorsalis/tabes_dorsalis.htm

[124] Centers for Disease Control and Prevention. Syphilis—CDC fact sheet. Ibid.

[125] National Institute of Neurological Disorders and Stroke. *NINDS Tabes dorsalis information page.* Ibid.

[126] American Association for Clinical Chemistry. (2010). Syphilis. *Lab Tests Online.* Retrieved 11.24.2010 from http://www.labtestsonline.org/understanding/analytes/syphilis/test.html

[127] Centers for Disease Control and Prevention. *Syphilis—CDC fact sheet.* Ibid.

[128] Edwards, J. R., et al. (2007). National Healthcare Safety Network (NHSN). Report, data summary for 2006. *Am J Infect Contr* 35:290–301.

[129] Mirza, A., & Custodio, H. T. (2010). Hospital-acquired infections. *eMedicine from WebMD.* Retrieved 11.24.2010 from http://emedicine.medscape.com/article/967022-overview

[130] Weinstein, R. A (1998). Nosocomial infections update. *Emerging Infectious Diseases,* 4. National Center for Infectious Diseases, Centers for Disease Control and Prevention. Retrieved 11.23.10 from http://www.cdc.gov/ncidod/eid/vol4no3/weinstein.htm

[131] Mirza, A., & Custodio, H. T. Ibid.

[132] Ibid.

[133] Ibid.

[134] Cunha, J. P. (2010). Dengue fever. *MedicineNet.com.* Retrieved 11.24.2010 from http://www.medicinenet.com/dengue_fever/article.htm

[135] National Institute of Allergy and Infectious Diseases. (2010). *Dengue fever.* Retrieved 11.24.2010 from http://www.niaid.nih.gov/topics/denguefever/understanding/pages/overview.aspx

[136] Centers for Disease Control and Prevention. (2009). *Dengue: frequently asked questions.* Retrieved 11.24.2010 from http://www.cdc.gov/dengue/fAQFacts/index.html

[137] Cunha, J. P. Ibid.

[138] Centers for Disease Control and Prevention. *Dengue: frequently asked questions.* Ibid.

[139] Cunha, J. P. Ibid.

[140] Centers for Disease Control and Prevention. (2007). *Dengue and Dengue hemorrhagic fever: information for health care practitioners.* Retrieved 5.12.2009 from http://www.cdc.gov/ncidod/dvbid/dengue/dengue-hcp.htm

[141] Cunha, J. P. Ibid.

[142] Centers for Disease Control and Prevention. *Dengue:frequently asked questions* Ibid.

[143] Centers for Disease Control and Prevention. (2009). *Dengue: Prevention: How to reduce your risk of dengue infection.* Retrieved 11.24.2010 from http://www.cdc.gov/dengue/prevention/index.html

[144] Dugdale III, D. C. (2009). Hantavirus. *MedlinePlus Medical Encyclopedia.* Retrieved from http://www.nlm.nih.gov/medlineplus/ency/article/001382.htm

[145] Centers for Disease Control and Prevention. (2006). *Hantavirus pulmonary syndrome (HPS).* Retrieved 4.8.2008 from http://www.cdc.gov/ncidod/diseases/hanta/hps/

146 Centers for Disease Control and Prevention. (2004). *All about han-taviruses. What are the symptoms of HPS?* Retrieved 4.8.2008 from http://www.cdc.gov/ncidod/diseases/hanta/hps/noframes/symptoms.htm

147 Dugdale III, D. C. Hantavirus. Ibid.

148 Ibid.

149 Centers for Disease Control and Prevention. *Hantavirus pulmonary syndrome (HPS).* Ibid.

150 Smith, D. S. (2007). Ibid.

151 Centers for Disease Control and Prevention. (2010). *Malaria* Retrieved 11.24.2010 from http://www.cdc.gov/Malaria/

152 Centers for Disease Control and Prevention. (2010). Malaria: *Biology.* Retrieved 11.24.2010 from http://www.cdc.gov/malaria/about/biology/index.html

153 Ibid.

154 Ibid.

155 Ibid.

156 Centers for Disease Control and Prevention. (2010). *Malaria and travelers: choosing a drug to prevent malaria.* Retrieved 11.24.2010 from http://www.cdc.gov/malaria/travelers/drugs.html

157 Centers for Disease Control and Prevention. (2010). *Malaria: diagnosis and treatment in the United States.* Retrieved 11.24.2010 from http://www.cdc.gov/malaria/diagnosis_treatment/index.html

158 Centers for Disease Control and Prevention. (2009). *CDC Plague home page.* Retrieved 5.11.2010 from http://www.cdc.gov/ncidod/dvbid/plague/

159 Dufel, S. E., & Cronin, D. (2009). CBRNE—Plague. *eMedicine from WebMD.* Retrieved 11.24.2010 from http://www.emedicine.com/emerg/topic428.htm

160 Centers for Disease Control and Prevention. *CDC Plague home page.* Ibid.

161 Dufel, S. E., & Cronin, D. Ibid.

162 Ibid.

163 Centers for Disease Control and Prevention. (2005). *Plague: epidemiology.* Retrieved 4.8.2008 from http://www.cdc.gov/ncidod/dvbid/plague/epi.htm

164 Dufel, S. E., & Cronin, D. Ibid.

165 Centers for Disease Control and Prevention. (2005). *Plague: diagnosis.* Retrieved 4.8.2008 from http://www.cdc.gov/ncidod/dvbid/plague/diagnosis.htm

166 Centers for Disease Control and Prevention. (2005). *Plague: prevention and control.* Retrieved 4.8.2008 from http://www.cdc.gov/ncidod/dvbid/plague/prevent.htm

167 Centers for Disease Control and Prevention. (2009). *Questions and answers about plague.* Retrieved 11.24.2010 from http://www.cdc.gov/ncidod/dvbid/plague/qa.htm

168 World Health Organization. (2008). *Rabies: key facts.* Retrieved 5.11.2009 from http://www.who.int/mediacentre/factsheets/fs099/en/

169 Centers for Disease Control and Prevention. (2007). *Rabies: epidemiology.* Retrieved 4.8.2008 from http://www.cdc.gov/rabies/epidemiology.html

170 Centers for Disease Control and Prevention. (2010). *Rabies: cost of rabies prevention.* Retrieved 11.24.2010 from http://www.cdc.gov/rabies/location/usa/cost.html

171 Ibid.

172 Centers for Disease Control and Prevention. (2010). *Rabies: the path of the virus.* Retrieved 11.24.2010 from http://www.cdc.gov/rabies/transmission/body.html

173 Centers for Disease Control and Prevention. (2010). *Rabies: what are the signs and symptoms of rabies?* Retrieved 11.24.2010 from http://www.cdc.gov/rabies/symptoms/index.html.

174 Rabies: outlook. (2005). *eMedicineHealth from WebMD.* Retrieved 4.11.2008 from http://www.emedicinehealth.com/rabies/page11_em.htm

175 Centers for Disease Control and Prevention. *Rabies: what are the signs and symptoms of rabies?* Ibid.

176 Centers for Disease Control and Prevention. (2010). *Rocky mountain spotted fever: home.* Retrieved 11.24.2010 from http://www.cdc.gov/ncidod/dvrd/rmsf/index.htm

177 Amitai, A., & Sinert, R. (2009). Tick-borne diseases, Rocky Mountain spotted fever. *eMedicine from WebMD.* Retrieved 11.24.2010 from http://www.emedicine.com/EMERG/topic510.htm

178 Centers for Disease Control and Prevention. (2010). *Rocky mountain spotted fever: statistics.* Retrieved 11.24.2010 from http://www.cdc.gov/ticks/diseases/rocky_mountain_spotted_fever/statistics.html

179 Amitai, A., & Sinert, R. Tick-borne diseases, Rocky Mountain spotted fever. *eMedicine from WebMD.* Ibid

180 Centers for Disease Control and Prevention. (2010). *Rocky mountain spotted fever: the organism.* Retrieved 11.26.2010 from http://www.cdc.gov/ncidod/dvrd/rmsf/Organism.htm

181 Centers for Disease Control and Prevention. *Rocky mountain spotted fever: home.* Ibid.

182 Centers for Disease Control and Prevention. (2010). *Rocky mountain spotted fever: questions and answers.* Retrieved 11.25.2010 from http://www.cdc.gov/ticks/diseases/rocky_mountain_spotted_fever/faq.html

183 Amitai, A., & Sinert, R. Ibid.

184 Ibid.

185 Centers for Disease Control and Prevention. Rocky mountain spotted fever: questions and answers. Ibid.

186 Dugdale, D. C. (2009). Rocky Mountain spotted fever. *MedlinePlus Medical Encyclopedia.* Retrieved 11.25.2010 from http://www.nlm.nih.gov/medlineplus/ency/article/000654.htm

187 Centers for Disease Control and Prevention. (2005). *Rocky mountain spotted fever: laboratory detection.* Retrieved 4.9.2008 from http://www.cdc.gov/ncidod/dvrd/rmsf/Laboratory.htm

188 Centers for Disease Control and Prevention. *Rocky mountain spotted fever: questions and answers.* Ibid.

189 Amitai, A., & Sinert, R. Ibid.

190 Vyas, J. M. (2010). Typhus. *MedlinePlus Medical Encyclopedia.* Retrieved 11.25.2010 from http://www.nlm.nih.gov/medlineplus/ency/article/001363.htm

191 Okulicz, J. F., et al. (2008). Typhus. *eMedicine from WebMD.* Retrieved 5.11.2009 from http://www.emedicine.com/MED/topic2332.htm

192 Vyas, J. M. Ibid.

193 Ibid.

194 Okulicz, J. F., et al. Ibid.

195 Ibid.

196 Vyas, J. M. Ibid.

197 US Geological Survey's National Wildlife Health Center. (2008). *Wildlife disease information node: West Nile virus.* Retrieved 5.12.2009 from http://westnilevirus.nbii.gov/

198 Pennsylvania's West Nile Virus Surveillance Program. (2010). *Surveillance maps.* Retrieved 11.25.2010 from http://www.westnile.state.pa.us/surv.htm

199 California West Nile Virus Website. (2010). *Latest West Nile virus activity in California.* Retrieved 11.25.2010 from http://www.westnile.ca.gov/

200 Centers for Disease Control and Prevention. (2008). *West Nile virus: statistics, surveillance, and Control. 2007 West Nile virus activity in the United States.* Retrieved 5.13.2009 from http://www.cdc.gov/ncidod/dvbid/westnile/surv&controlCaseCount07_detailed.htm

201 Ibid.

202 Centers for Disease Control and Prevention. (2004).*West Nile virus: epidemiological information for clinicians.* Retrieved 4.21.2008 from http://www.cdc.gov/ncidod/dvbid/westnile/clinicians/epi.htm#agent

203 Ibid.

204 Ibid.

205 Centers for Disease Control and Prevention. (2010). *West Nile virus: fight the bite!* Retrieved 11.26.2010 from http://www.cdc.gov/ncidod/dvbid/westnile/index.htm

206 Centers for Disease Control and Prevention. *West Nile Virus: epidemiological information for clinicians.* Ibid.

207 World Health Organization. (2009). *Yellow fever.* Retrieved 11.26.2010 from http://www.who.int/mediacentre/factsheets/fs100/en/

208 Ibid.

209 Centers for Disease Control and Prevention. (2007). *Yellow fever.* Retrieved 5.14.2008 from http://www.cdc.gov/ncidod/dvbid/yellowfever/index.html

210 World Health Organization. (2009). *Yellow fever.* Ibid.

211 Loeb, M., et al. (2008). Prognosis after West Nile virus infection. *Ann Int Med* 149:134.

212 Nichols, E. M., & Gleyzer, A. (2010). Yellow fever. *eMedicine from WebMD.* Retrieved 11.26.2010 from http://www.emedicine.com/emerg/topic645.htm

213 World Health Organization. *Yellow fever.* Ibid.

214 Centers for Disease Control and Prevention. (2005). *Diphtheria.* Retrieved 5.14.2008 from http://www.cdc.gov/ncidod/dbmd/diseaseinfo/diptheria_t.htm

215 Dugdale, D. C. (2009). Diphtheria. *MedlinePlus Medical Encyclopedia.* Retrieved 11.26.2010 from http://www.nlm.nih.gov/medlineplus/ency/article/001608.htm

216 Ibid.

217 Centers for Disease Control and Prevention. *Diphtheria.* Ibid.

218 Centers for Disease Control and Prevention. (2008). Recommended immunization schedules for persons aged 0–18 years—United States, 2008. *MMWR* 57:Q1–Q4.

219 Ibid.

220 Dugdale, D. C. Diphtheria. Ibid.

221 Mumps. (2010). *MedicineNet.com.* Retrieved 11.26.2010 from http://www.medicinenet.com/mumps/article.htm

222 Ibid.

223 Ibid.

224 Mumps. (2010). *MedlinePlus Medical Encyclopedia.* Retrieved 11.26.2010 from http://www.nlm.nih.gov/medlineplus/mumps.html#cat59

225 Mumps. *MedicineNet.com.* Ibid.

226 Ibid.

227 Carmody, K. A., & Sinert, R. (2009). Mumps. *eMedicine from WebMD.* Retrieved 11.26.2010 from http://www.emedicine.com/emerg/topic324.htm

228 Kaneshiro, N. K. (2009). Pertussis. *MedlinePlus Medical Encyclopedia.* Retrieved 11.26.2010 from http://www.nlm.nih.gov/medlineplus/ency/article/001561.htm

229 Centers for Disease Control and Prevention. (2006). *Pertussis Pinkbook.* Retrieved 5.14.2008 from http://www.cdc.gov/vaccines/pubs/pinkbook/downloads/pert.pdf

230 Kaneshiro, N. K. Ibid.

231 Centers for Disease Control and Prevention. *Pertussis Pinkbook.* Ibid.

232 Ibid.

233 Kaneshiro, N. K. Ibid.

234 Centers for Disease Control and Prevention. *Pertussis Pinkbook.* Ibid.

235 Ibid.

236 Ibid.

237 Guinto-Ocampo, H., McNeil, B. K., & Aronoff, S. C (2010). Pertussis. *eMedicine from WebMD.* Retrieved 11.26.2010 from http://www.emedicine.com/ped/TOPIC1778.HTM

238 Kaneshiro, N. K. Ibid.

239 Global Polio Eradication Initiative, World Health Organization. (2010). The disease and the virus. Retrieved 11.26.2010 from http://www.polioeradication.org/disease.asp

240 *Morbidity and Mortality Weekly Report* (MMWR) (2005, April 22). *CDC's summary of notifiable diseases—United States, 2003, 52. Summary* Retrieved from Post Polio Health International. Retrieved 5.14.2008 from http://www.post-polio.org/ir-usa.html

241 Vorvick, L. (2010). Poliomyelitis. *MedlinePlus Medical Encyclopedia.* Retrieved 11.26.2010 from http://www.nlm.nih.gov/medlineplus/ency/article/001402.htm

242 Post Polio Health International. (n.d.). *Information about the late effects of polio for the health professional.* Retrieved 5.14.2008 from http://www.post-polio.org/edu/pabout3.html#hea

243 Vorvick, L. Ibid.

244 A statement about exercise for survivors of polio. (2003, Spring). *Post Polio Health,* 19. Retrieved 5.14.2008 from http://www.post-polio.org/edu/pphnews/pph19-2a.html

245 Global Polio Eradication Initiative, World Health Organization. (n.d.). *The disease and the virus.* Retrieved 5.14.2008 from http://www.polioeradication.org/disease.asp

246 Vorvick, L. Ibid.

247 A statement about exercise for survivors of polio. Ibid.

248 Post Polio Health International. (n.d.). *Information about the late effects of polio for the health professional.* Ibid.

249 Global Polio Eradication Initiative, World Health Organization. *The disease and the virus.* Ibid.

250 Vorvick, L. Ibid.

251 Ibid.

252 Post Polio Health International. Ibid.

253 Centers for Disease Control and Prevention. (2000). *Polio vaccine: what you need to know.* Retrieved 5.14.2008 from http://www.cdc.gov/vaccines/pubs/vis/downloads/vis-ipv.pdf

254 American Academy of Family Physicians. (2006). *Polio vaccine.* Retrieved 5.14.2008 from http://familydoctor.org/online/famdocen/home/healthy/vaccines/333.printerview.html

255 Centers for Disease Control and Prevention. *Polio vaccine: what you need to know.* Ibid.

256 Vorvick, L. Ibid.

257 Global Polio Readication Initiative, World Health Organization. *The disease and the virus.* Ibid.

258 Post Polio Health International. Ibid.

259 Ibid.

260 Jones, D. R., et al. (1989). Cardiorespiratory responses to aerobic training by patients with post-poliomyelitis sequelae. *JAMA* 261:3255–3258.

261 Ezike, E., & Ang, J. Y. (2009). Rubella. *eMedicine from WebMD.* Retrieved 11.25.2010 from http://www.emedicine.com/ped/TOPIC2025.HTM

262 Nemours Foundation. (2009). Infections: rubella (German measles). *KidsHealth.* Retrieved 11.26.2010 from http://kidshealth.org/parent/infections/bacterial_viral/german_measles.html#

263 Ibid.

264 Rubella. (2010). *MedlinePlus Medical Encyclopedia.* Retrieved 11.25.2010 from http://www.nlm.nih.gov/medlineplus/rubella.html

265 Nemours Foundation. Ibid.

266 Rubella. *MedlinePlus Medical Encyclopedia.* Ibid.

267 Ibid.

268 Kaneshiro, N. K. (2009). Rubella. *MedlinePlus Medical Encyclopedia.* Retrieved 4.5.2010 from http://www.nlm.nih.gov/MEDLINEPLUS/ency/article/001574.htm

269 Centers for Disease Control and Prevention. (2008). Measles, mumps, and rubella (MMR) vaccines: what you need to know. Retrieved 3.14.2009 from http://www.cdc.gov/vaccines/pubs/vis/downloads/vis-mmr.pdf

270 Nemours Foundation. Ibid.

271 Hooker, E. (2008). Measles (rubeola). *MedicineNet.com*. Retrieved 3.14.2009 from http://www.medicinenet.com/measles_rubeola/page1.htm

272 Taylor, G. A. (2010). Measles, rubeola. *eMedicine from WebMD*. Retrieved 11.25.2010 from http://www.emedicine.com/derm/topic259.htm

273 MedlinePlus. (2008). Measles cases highest since 1996. *HealthDay*. Retrieved 5.14.2009 from http://www.nlm.nih.gov/medlineplus/news/fullstory_68419.html

274 Taylor, G. A. Ibid.

275 Hooker, E. Ibid.

276 Ibid.

277 Taylor, G. A. Ibid.

278 Hooker, E. Ibid.

279 Taylor, G. A. Ibid.

280 Ibid.

281 Hooker, E. Ibid.

282 Ibid.

283 Taylor, G. A. Ibid.

284 Centers for Disease Control and Prevention. Measles, mumps, and rubella (MMR) vaccines: what you need to know. Ibid.

285 Hooker, E. Ibid.

286 Ibid.

287 Ibid.

288 Dire, D. J. (2010). Tetanus. *eMedicine from WebMD*. Retrieved 11.26.2010 from http://www.emedicine.com/emerg/topic574.htm

289 Dugdale, D. C., III, & Zieve, D. (2008). Tetanus. *MedlinePlus, Medical Encyclopedia*, Retrieved 3.14.2009 from http://www.nlm.nih.gov/medlineplus/ency/article/000615.htm

290 Dire, D. J. Ibid.

291 Nemours Foundation. (2007). Tetanus. *KidsHealth*. Retrieved 3.14.2008 from http://kidshealth.org/parent/infections/bacterial_viral/tetanus.html

292 Dire, D. J. Ibid.

293 Perlstein, D. (2007). Tetanus (lockjaw and tetanus vaccination). *MedicineNet.com*. Retrieved 3.14.2008 from http://www.medicinenet.com/tetanus/article.htm

294 Dugdale, D. C., III, & Zieve, D. Ibid.

295 Dire, D. J. Ibid.

296 Perlstein, D. Ibid.

297 Dugdale, D. C., III, & Zieve, D. Ibid.

298 Dire, D. J. Ibid.

299 Ibid.

300 Dugdale, D. C., III, & Zieve, D. Ibid.

301 Perlstein, D. Ibid.

302 Dugdale, D. C., III, & Zieve, D. Ibid.

303 Dire, D. J. Ibid.

304 Nemours Foundation. Tetanus. Ibid.

305 Dugdale, D. C., III, & Zieve, D. Ibid.

306 Dire, D. J. Ibid.

307 Perlstein, D. Ibid.

308 Nemours Foundation. Tetanus. Ibid.

309 Perlstein, D. Ibid.

310 Mehta, P. N., & Chatterjee, A. (2010). Varicella. *eMedicine from WebMD*. Retrieved 11.25.2010 from http://www.emedicine.com/ped/topic2385.htm

311 Centers for Disease Control and Prevention. (2008). *Vaccines and preventable diseases: varicella (chickenpox)*. Retrieved 3.14.2009 from http://www.cdc.gov/vaccines/vpd-vac/varicella/in-short-adult.htm

312 Mehta, P. N., & Chatterjee, A. Ibid.

313 Ibid.

314 Ibid.

315 Centers for Disease Control and Prevention. *Vaccines and preventable diseases: varicella (chickenpox)*. Ibid.

316 Mehta, P. N., & Chatterjee, A. Ibid.

317 Ibid.

318 Immunization Action Coalition. (2008). *Healthcare personnel vaccination recommendations*. Retrieved 3.14.2009 from http://www.immunize.org/catg.d/p2017.pdf

319 Mehta, P. N., & Chatterjee, A. Ibid.

320 Immunization Action Coalition. Ibid.

321 Centers for Disease Control and Prevention. (2008). *Anthrax*. Retrieved 3.15.2009 from http://www.cdc.gov/nczved/dfbmd/disease_listing/anthrax_gi.html

322 Ibid.

323 Ibid.

324 Ibid.

325 Ibid.

326 Ibid.

327 Anthrax. (2008). *MedlinePlus Medical Encyclopedia*. Retrieved 3.15.2009 from http://www.nlm.nih.gov/medlineplus/anthrax.html

328 Cunha, B. A. (2008). Anthrax. *eMedicine from WebMD*. Retrieved 3.15.2009 from http://www.emedicine.com/MED/topic148.htm

329 Centers for Disease Control and Prevention. Anthrax. Ibid.

330 Anthrax. Medline Plus Medical Encyclopedia. Ibid.

331 Occupational Safety and Health Administration. (n.d.). *Anthrax: protecting the worksite against terrorism*. Retrieved 3.15.2009 from http://www.osha.gov/SLTC/etools/anthrax/credible_risk.html#Action

332 Vorvick, L. J. (2010). Botulism. *MedlinePlus Medical Encyclopedia*. Retrieved 11.26.2010 from http://www.nlm.nih.gov/medlineplus/ency/article/003029.htm

333 Centers for Disease Control and Prevention. (2008). *Botulism*. Retrieved 3.15.2009 from http://www.cdc.gov/nczved/dfbmd/disease_listing/botulism_gi.html

334 Vorvick, L. J. Botulism. *MedlinePlus Medical Encyclopedia*. Ibid.

335 Centers for Disease Control and Prevention. *Botulism*. Ibid.

336 Vorvick, L. J. Ibid.

337 Centers for Disease Control and Prevention. *Botulism*. Ibid.

338 Vorvick, L. J. Ibid.

339 Centers for Disease Control and Prevention. *Botulism*. Ibid.

340 Vorvick, L. J. (2010). Mononucleosis. *MedlinePlus Medical Encyclopedia*. Retrieved 11.25.2010 from http://www.nlm.nih.gov/MEDLINEPLUS/ency/article/000591.htm

341 Omori, M. S. (2007). Mononucleosis. *eMedicine from WebMD*. Retrieved 3.16.2009 from http://www.emedicine.com/EMERG/topic319.htm

342 Centers for Disease Control and Prevention. (2008). *Epstein-Barr virus and infectious mononucleosis*. Retrieved 3.16.2009 from http://www.cdc.gov/ncidod/diseases/ebv.htm

343 Ibid.

344 Vorvick, L. J. Mononucleosis. Ibid.

345 Centers for Disease Control and Prevention. *Epstein-Barr virus and infectious mononucleosis*. Ibid.

346 Ibid.

347 Alexander, D. R. (2007). Mononucleosis spot test. *MedlinePlus Medical Encyclopedia*. Retrieved 3.16.2009 from http://www.nlm.nih.gov/MEDLINEPLUS/ency/article/003454.htm

348 Omori, M. S. Ibid.

349 Centers for Disease Control and Prevention. *Epstein-Barr virus and infectious mononucleosis*. Ibid.

350 Vorvick, L. J. Mononucleosis. Ibid.

351 Omori, M. S. Ibid.

352 Centers for Disease Control and Prevention. (2008). *Influenza: the disease*. Retrieved 5.12.2009 from http://www.cdc.gov/flu/

353 Centers for Disease Control and Prevention. (2008). *The influenza (flu) viruses*. Retrieved 5.12.2009 from http://www.cdc.gov/flu/about/viruses/index.htm

354 Centers for Disease Control and Prevention. (2008). *Influenza symptoms*. Retrieved 5.12.2009 from http://www.cdc.gov/flu/symptoms.htm

355 Centers for Disease Control and Prevention. (2009). *Transmission of influenza from animals to people.* Retrieved 6.4.2010 from http://www.cdc.gov/flu/about/viruses/transmission.htm

356 Centers for Disease Control and Prevention. (2008). *How the flu virus can change: "drift" and "shift."* Retrieved 5.12.2009 from http://www.cdc.gov/flu/about/viruses/change.htm

357 Centers for Disease Control and Prevention. *Influenza symptoms.* Ibid.

358 National Institute of Neurological Disorders and Stroke. (2009). *NINDS Reye's syndrome information page.* Retrieved 6.4.2010 from http://www.ninds.nih.gov/disorders/reyes_syndrome/reyes_syndrome.htm

359 Centers for Disease Control and Prevention. Influenza: the disease. Ibid.

360 Centers for Disease Control and Prevention. (2010). 2010–2011 influenza prevention and control recommendations. Retrieved 11.26.2010 from http://www.cdc.gov/flu/professionals/acip/primarychanges.htm

361 National Foundation for Infectious Diseases. (2007). *Influenza.* Retrieved from http://www.nfid.org/influenza/

362 Lentnek, A. L. (2007). The flu. *MedlinePlus Medical Encyclopedia.* Retrieved 5.12.2009 from http://www.nlm.nih.gov/medlineplus/ency/article/000080.htm

363 Ibid.

364 National Foundation for Infectious Diseases. (2007). *Influenza: unimmunized health care workers put patients at risk.* Retrieved 5.12.2009 from http://www.nfid.org/influenza/professionals_workersflu.html

365 Centers for Disease Control and Prevention. (2008). *Patient facts: learn more about Legionairres' disease.* Retrieved 5.12.2009 from http://www.cdc.gov/legionella/patient_facts.htm

366 Ibid.

367 Ibid.

368 Ibid.

369 Ibid.

370 Lazoff, M. (2010). Meningitis. *eMedicine from WebMD.* Retrieved 11.25.2010 from http://www.emedicine.com/EMERG/topic309.htm

371 Dugdale, D. C. III. (2010). Meningitis. *MedlinePlus, Medical Encyclopedia.* Retrieved 11.26.2010 from http://www.nlm.nih.gov/medlineplus/ency/article/000680.htm

372 Ibid.

373 Ibid.

374 Centers for Disease Control and Prevention. (2010). *Pneumococcal conjugate vaccine.* Retrieved 11.26.2010 from http://www.cdc.gov/vaccines/pubs/vis/downloads/vis-pcv.pdf

375 Centers for Disease Control and Prevention. (2008). *Meningococcal vaccination.* Retrieved 5.12.2009 from http://www.cdc.gov/vaccines/vpd-vac/mening/

376 Lentnek, A. L. Meningitis. Ibid.

377 Totten, V. Y., & Brenner, B. E. (2010). Toxic shock syndrome. *eMedicine from WebMD.* Retrieved 11.26.2010 from http://www.emedicine.com/emerg/TOPIC600.HTM

378 Ibid.

379 Ibid.

380 Levy, D. (2009). Variola/smallpox. *MedlinePlus Medical Encyclopedia,* Retrieved 11.10.2010 from http://www.nlm.nih.gov/medlineplus/ency/article/001356.htm

381 Ibid.

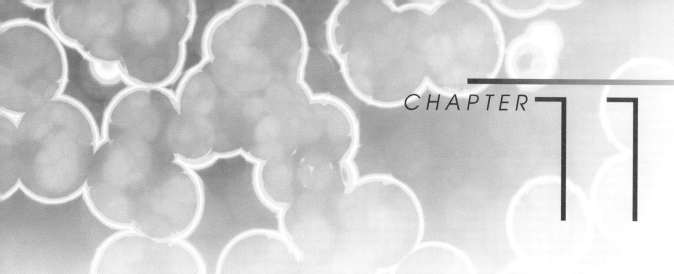

CHAPTER 11

Female and Male Reproductive System Conditions

LEARNING OBJECTIVES

After completion of this chapter, students should be able to:

- Review the anatomy and physiology of the female and male reproductive systems
- Discuss the physiological changes of the female during pregnancy
- Describe the stages of labor and the common complications of labor and pregnancy
- Discuss the pathological mechanisms of common pregnancy related conditions, menopause, and female reproductive diseases
- Discuss the pathological mechanisms of male reproductive diseases
- Determine the role of physical therapy interventions for females and males with reproductive-related conditions and diseases
- Analyze the contraindications and precautions relevant to physical therapist/physical therapist assistant intervention for patients with female and male reproductive diseases
- Determine the contraindications and precautions for physical therapy interventions for women during pregnancy

KEY TERMS

Braxton-Hicks uterine contractions
Cerclage
Caesarean section
Ectopic pregnancy
Endometriosis
Fibrocystic disease of the breast
Gestational diabetes
Leiomyomas (fibroids)
Multipara
Multigravida
Nulliparous
Pelvic floor incompetence/ weakness
Preeclampsia
Primigravida
Rectus abdominis diastasis
Respiratory distress syndrome of the newborn

CHAPTER OUTLINE

Introduction

This chapter is divided into sections regarding conditions and disease processes of both the female and male reproductive systems. The anatomy and physiology of the female and male reproductive systems is included. Other main chapter topics include pregnancy and menopause. Both the female and male reproductive diseases and conditions described in this section are intended to provide an overview of those most commonly observed in physical therapy practice.

Female reproductive system diseases and conditions include dyspareunia, endometriosis, infertility, menstrual cycle problems, carcinomas, pelvic floor incompetence and pelvic inflammatory disease, conditions of the uterus, and diseases of the breast. The section on pregnancy includes an overview of the anatomy and physiology of the female body during pregnancy, the appropriate physical therapy intervention precautions associated with women who are pregnant, pregnancy-related conditions, the stages of labor, the delivery process, some of the complications of labor and postpartum issues and problems. The physiological process of menopause is also described. The diseases of the male reproductive system include congenital abnormalities, erectile dysfunction, infertility, prostate diseases, and testicular diseases.

Why Does the Physical Therapist Assistant Need to Know About the Anatomy and Physiology of the Female Reproductive System?

Women's health has become a large part of the practice of physical therapy. The physiology of the female, including past pregnancy, has an impact on health issues experienced by women. To understand the implications of pathological conditions of the female reproductive system and the changes that occur with pregnancy, the PTA must have knowledge of the nonpathological state.

Anatomy and Physiology of the Female Reproductive System

The study of the female reproductive system and its associated diseases is called gynecology, whereas obstetrics is the study of the pregnant female, the fetus, and all aspects of the delivery and postpartum process. Physicians working with this patient population are called gynecologists or obstetricians or may specialize in both areas.

When considering diseases of the female reproductive system, the student needs to understand the normal bony and soft tissue anatomy of the female pelvis, abdomen, and breasts. (The physiology of pregnancy is considered separately later in this chapter). The pelvis is the bony support for the muscles of the pelvic floor. In the female, the bones of the pelvis provide a wide base, and potential opening, for delivery of a fetus. The bones of the pubis, ischium, ilium, and sacrum form the rim of the pelvis. The joints of the pelvis are the sacroiliac joints and the symphysis pubis (see Fig. 11-1). All of these joints are usually stable to provide the support needed for protection of the pelvic contents.

The contents of the female pelvis include the reproductive organs, the bladder, rectum, and sections of the

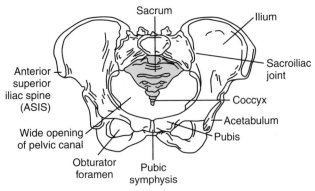

FIGURE 11.1 The bony pelvis.

small and large intestines (see Chapter 12 for the anatomy of the digestive system). Students are reminded that many muscles, nerves, and blood vessels pass through the pelvis and are therefore contents of the pelvis. The structures specific to the reproductive system contained within the female pelvis include the uterus, cervix, vagina, ovaries, and fallopian tubes. The close proximity of the bladder to the uterus should be noted (see Fig. 11-2). The uterus is hollow with muscular walls; is approximately 7.5 cm long, 5 cm wide, and 2.5 cm thick; and weighs between 30 and 40 grams. The structure lies almost horizontally above the bladder. The area of the uterus closest to the vagina is called the cervix. The uterus is a mobile structure able to adjust to changes in shape of the bladder and other internal organs. The uterus is supported in place by the surrounding abdominal viscera and, before pregnancy or abdominal surgery, by the broad and round ligaments. The blood vessels that supply the uterus are the uterine and ovarian arteries and veins. The nerve supply is derived from the hypogastric and ovarian plexuses and sacral nerve roots 3 and 4.[1]

The vagina is the passage from the exterior to the uterus situated between the bladder and the rectum within the pelvis. The vagina is directed superiorly and posteriorly and forms an angle of more than 90°, where it joins with the uterus. The walls of the vagina consist of an inner mucous membrane lining, an outer tunica muscularis (muscular layer), and a layer in between them of erectile tissue rich in blood vessels.[2]

The ovaries are oval structures approximately 4 cm long, 2 cm wide, and 8 mm thick, weighing 2 to 3.5 grams located on either side of the uterus. They are supported by the ovarian ligament, which stretches from the ovary to the uterus, and the broad ligament which is a sheet of ligament that stretches across the inside of the pelvic cavity suspending the ovaries and also assists with support of the uterus. The surface layer of the ovaries is composed of columnar cells and the internal section of connective tissue cells that resemble smooth muscle. Within the ovaries the Graafian follicles (ovisacs) contain the ova. During the childbearing years, these follicles migrate to the surface of the ovary and release their ova during the monthly menstrual cycle.[3] The two fallopian tubes extend from the uterus to each ovary acting as passageways through which the ova developed in the ovaries pass to the uterus. Fertilization of the ova by sperm occurs within the ideal environment created by the fallopian tubes.[4] Each fallopian tube terminates near the ovary in the fimbriae. These are fingerlike projections that play a part in attracting the ova into the fallopian tube for transport to the uterus for implantation. The external female genitalia include the clitoris and the labia minora and majora (see Fig. 11-3). The area of the external pelvic floor consisting of the labia, clitoris, and the openings of the urethra and vagina is sometimes called the vulva or pudendum. The clitoris is composed of erectile tissue, which responds to sexual stimulation, and the labia maintain the moisture of the mucous membranes of the vagina and urethra.

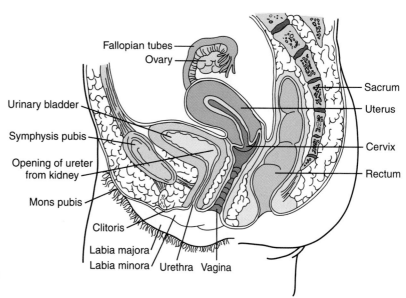

FIGURE 11.2 Contents of the female pelvis.

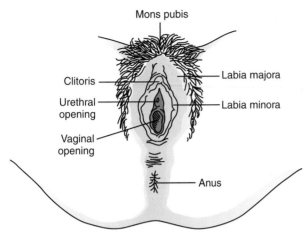

FIGURE 11.3 Female external genitalia shown in anterior view of the perineum.

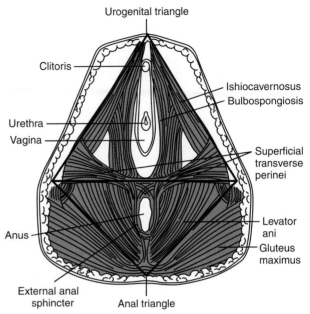

FIGURE 11.4 The urogenital and anal triangles of the pelvic floor musculature.

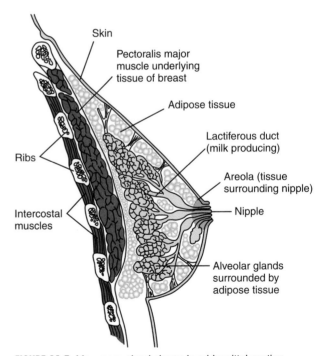

FIGURE 11.5 Mammary gland shown in midsagittal section.

The integrity of the pelvic contents is provided by the support from muscles of the perineum. The muscles of the pelvic floor are complex. The following description provides an overview only of the main muscles of the floor of the perineum. The description provides some basic muscular anatomy for the understanding of pregnancy and pathological problems of the female reproductive system. Two main layers of muscle compose the floor of the pelvis. The inner layer, or diaphragm, consists of the coccygeus and levator ani muscles. These muscles attach to the inner aspect of the ischial spines, the pubic rami, part of the obturator fascia, the raphe or perineal body between the openings of the vagina and rectum, and another raphe posterior to the rectal opening. The levator ani muscle is composed of three sections named for their attachments. These are the pubococcygeus, iliococcygeus, and puborectalis. This diaphragm forms the sphincters of the rectum and provides support for the openings of both the vagina and rectum.[5] A second layer of more superficial muscles exists called the urogenital diaphragm. This area is sometimes explained as two triangles, the urogenital triangle and the anal triangle. The anal triangle is the most posterior and surrounds the anus. The urogenital triangle consists of several layers of fascia and muscle and surrounds the openings of the urethra and vagina (see Fig. 11-4).[6]

The breasts, or mammary glands, are an integral part of the female reproductive system (see Fig. 11-5). The breasts function to provide lactation (milk) for the infant. Structurally the mammary glands lie superficial to the pectoralis major muscle and are composed of a mixture of adipose, glandular, and fibrous tissue and an intricate network of blood and lymph vessels and nerves. The lactiferous ducts within the breast transmit milk to the nipple.[7] The mammary glands are influenced by the hormones estrogen and progesterone during pregnancy causing growth of the lactiferous ducts and the glandular cells that secrete milk. After delivery, the mammary glands are influenced by prolactin and oxytocin, which prompt the production and release of milk.[8]

The physiology of the female reproductive system is an essential part of gaining an understanding of the related pathology. Hormones secreted by the ovaries and uterus, the hypothalamus and the pituitary regulate all reproductive functions (see Table 11-1).

The menstrual cycle is a normal part of the physiology of the human reproductive system. This, too, is under the influence of hormones. The uterus develops a menstrual cycle of approximately 28 days, during which time the walls of the uterus thicken in preparation for the implantation of a fertilized ovum. If implantation of an ovum does not occur, the endometrium (wall of the uterus) starts to reduce in thickness and menses (also called menorrhea or menstruation) occurs. The bleeding of menses is the sloughing off of unwanted cells from the endometrium.

The first time this menses occurs in a female is called menarche.[9] The menstrual cycle is divided into three phases: the follicular phase, the ovulatory phase, and the luteal phase. The beginning phase or follicular phase involves the stimulation of the ovum in the ovary to develop and mature. At the same time, the uterus is stimulated to produce extra blood vessels and starts to thicken in preparation for implantation of the ovum. Follicle stimulating hormone (FSH) produced by the pituitary and estrogen are the primary hormones involved in this phase. The ovulatory phase is when the ovum is released from the ovary and lasts between 16 and 32 hours approximately in the middle of the menstrual cycle. In the last or luteal phase, luteinizing hormone (LH), produced by the pituitary, stimulates the ovum, now the corpus luteum, to secrete progesterone, which further increases the development of blood vessels in the wall of the uterus. If the ovum is not fertilized, the progesterone levels fall, and menstruation or menses occurs.[10]

Table 11.1 Hormones Affecting the Reproductive System

HORMONE	ORGAN THAT PRODUCES HORMONE	EFFECTS
Estrogen	Ovary, uterus, placenta	Stimulates the development of female secondary sexual characteristics Maintains healthy reproductive organs Stimulates growth of an ovum Proliferation of blood vessels in the endometrium in preparation for implantation of the ovum Keeps the placenta healthy
Progesterone	Ovary, uterus, placenta	Proliferation of the endometrium in preparation for pregnancy Preparation of mammary glands for lactation Causes ligamentous laxity required to enable birth
Gonadotropin releasing hormone (GnRH)	Hypothalamus	Stimulates pituitary to produce gonadotropins of FSH and LH
Follicle stimulating hormone (FSH)	Anterior pituitary	Stimulate ovary to produce estrogen or progesterone
Luteinizing hormone (LH)	Anterior pituitary	Stimulate ovary to produce estrogen or progesterone In men, stimulates the production of testosterone from the testes
Prolactin	Anterior pituitary	Production of milk after birth in the alveolar glands
Oxytocin	Posterior pituitary	Causes release of milk from lactiferous ducts Stimulates uterus to contract in preparation for delivery of the fetus
Human chorionic gonadotropin (hCG)	Placenta after fertilization of the ovum	Prevents menstruation Helps to keep endometrium thickened

Why Does the Physical Therapist Assistant Need to Know About Diseases and Conditions of the Female Reproductive System?

Several of the signs and symptoms of female reproductive system diseases provide indications for physical therapy interventions. Probably the most commonly recognized female diseases requiring the use of physical therapy interventions are breast cancer and pelvic floor incompetence. Other female reproductive diseases cause signs and symptoms that may create precautions or contraindications for certain physical therapy interventions.

Diseases and Conditions of the Female Reproductive System

The diseases described in this section include those of both the internal and external reproductive structures and of the breast. Sexually transmitted diseases (STDs) are described in Chapter 10.

HINTS ON USE OF THE GUIDE TO PHYSICAL THERAPIST PRACTICE

Patients with various female and male reproductive diseases can be designated within the following *Guide to Physical Therapist Practice, Second revised edition, APTA,* Musculoskeletal Preferred Practice Patterns:

- 4A "Primary prevention/risk reduction for skeletal demineralization" (p. 133): Women going through menopause or hormonal changes such as those after a hysterectomy may fit most appropriately under preferred practice pattern 4A due to the increased risk of osteoporosis.
- 4B "Impaired posture" (p. 145): During pregnancy, a woman may have a physical therapy consultation under preferred practice pattern 4B.
- 4C "Impaired muscle performance" (p. 161): Pelvic floor dysfunction in both males and females is classified under preferred practice pattern 4C.
- 4D "Impaired joint mobility, motor function, muscle performance, and range of motion associated with connective tissue dysfunction" (p. 179): During

pregnancy, a woman may have a physical therapy consultation under preferred practice pattern 4D.

- 4E "Impaired joint mobility, motor function, muscle performance, and range of motion associated with localized inflammation" (p. 197): Prenatal or postnatal inflammation may be designated under preferred practice pattern 4E.
- 4G "Impaired joint mobility, muscle performance, and range of motion associated with fracture" (p. 233): This practice pattern may be used if there is fracture due to postradiation therapy for carcinoma of the female or male reproductive systems.
- 6H "Impaired circulation and anthropometric dimensions associated with lymphatic system disorders" (p. 569): The patient with lymphedema postmastectomy or postradiation therapy could be associated with "Cardiovascular/Pulmonary" preferred practice pattern 6H.

(From the American Physical Therapy Association, 2003. *Guide to physical therapist practice,* revised 2nd edition. Alexandria, VA: APTA. Used with permission.)

Dyspareunia

Dyspareunia is pain in the female related to intercourse. The causes of dyspareunia may be physical or psychological, or both. Dyspareunia may be caused by adhesions secondary to endometriosis (see endometriosis). Frequently dyspareunia is complicated by vaginismus, which is tightness of the vagina resulting from spasm of the pubococcygeus muscles. Other causes are pelvic inflammatory disease, postpartum trauma, physical and psychological trauma resulting from sexual assault, tumors within the vagina or cervix, vaginal inflammation or infection, urinary tract infection (UTI), and vaginal atrophy or dryness. Extreme cases of dyspareunia result from female genital mutilation practiced in various parts of the world as an initiation rite, in which the external female genitalia are removed and scar tissue forms, making sexual intercourse either painful or extremely difficult.[11] Women with dyspareunia should be referred to a physician.

Physical Therapy Intervention. Physical therapists and assistants working in women's health clinics and specialty practices often treat women with dyspareunia. These physical therapists usually work closely with psychologists and psychiatrists to treat the associated psychological causes of dyspareunia.

Endometriosis

The endometrium is tissue that lines the inside of the uterus. **Endometriosis** is a condition in which endometrial tissue starts to grow in other areas of the internal organs, such as around the ovaries, in the peritoneal cavity, and on the pelvic ligaments. Approximately 5% to 10% of women in the United States have endometriosis, with 5.5 million women affected.[12] Endometrial tissue may also grow around the heart and lungs. The ectopic (out of the usual location) endometrial tissue follows the same cycle as that within the uterus. When the ectopic endometrial tissue sloughs, the waste products are deposited in the area of the ectopic tissue and cause irritation to the surrounding structures, which may lead to inflammation and pain.

Etiology. The cause of endometriosis is unknown, but the condition sometimes occurs after a caesarean section, and it is thought that opening of the uterus may cause cells to migrate into the abdominal cavity. Another theory is that during menstruation blood flows back up into the fallopian tubes and enters the abdominal cavity.

Signs and Symptoms. Endometriosis may cause severe pain and excessive bleeding, as well as painful bowel movements and urination during menstruation; it is also responsible for many cases of infertility.[13] The pelvic pain of endometriosis may become chronic and referred into the sacral and coccygeal areas.[14] Scar tissue often occurs in areas where endometrial tissue grows within the abdominal cavity. The adhesions formed in the pelvic area as a result of endometriosis may also cause dyspareunia, which is pain related to intercourse. The pelvic adhesions may pull the vagina and its supporting ligaments into an abnormal position or cause the uterus to be retroverted.

Prognosis. No cure exists for endometriosis. Approximately 30% to 40% of women with the condition become infertile.[15]

Medical Intervention. Although endometriosis may be suspected as the cause for chronic pelvic pain in women, the definitive diagnosis is achieved by performing an exploratory laparoscopy. Women who have severe, prolonged pelvic pain caused by endometriosis have the option of oophorectomy (surgical excision of the ovaries) and hysterectomy surgeries.[16] Excision of endometrial tissue without hysterectomy is sometimes performed, but the need for further surgery is common.[17] Some women have relief of pain with the use of oral contraceptive medications.

Physical Therapy Intervention. Physical therapy intervention may be sought for pain in the pelvic, sacral, and coccygeal areas caused by endometriosis. In cases of severe menstrual pain, the PT and PTA may use transcutaneous electrical nerve stimulation (TENS) or other electrical stimulation modalities and heat to relieve symptoms.

Infertility

Infertility is described as the lack of pregnancy when a couple has attempted sexual intercourse without the use of contraception for a year. Women who have multiple, continued miscarriages may also be classified as infertile.[18] The possibility of infertility in women increases with age, particularly beyond age 30. A low sperm count (reduced numbers of sperm under 20 million per milliliter) or reduced sperm mobility in the male accounts for approximately one-third of the cases of infertility. Causes of infertility in the female include sickle cell anemia, infection with chlamydia or syphilis, scarring of the fallopian tubes from endometriosis, pelvic inflammatory disease, and polycystic ovary syndrome (PCOS).[19] In some cases, no known cause of infertility exists. A woman is most fertile within 24 hours of ovulation, and the average female age of highest rate of fertility is 24 years. The average age for highest male fertility is 25 years. The treatment for infertility varies with the cause and can be a highly complex set of procedures beyond the scope of this book to describe. Couples will select an assistive reproductive technology (ART) program.[20] Surgery may be required to remove scar tissue within the abdomen if endometriosis is determined to be the cause of the infertility. Women who are not ovulating may be placed on ovulation stimulating medications such as clomiphene citrate, on follicle stimulating hormone (FSH), or on human chorionic gonadotrophin (hCG).[21] In vitro fertilization (IVF) may be performed by removing ova from the female and sperm from the male, fertilizing within the laboratory, and then implanting the fertilized embryo in the uterus of the woman.[22] In many cases, a combination of these treatments is needed. Success rates depend on many factors including the age of the woman at the time of IVF, but in some cases, multiple pregnancies result from IVF due to the implantation of several fertilized ova at a time.

Physical Therapy Intervention. No physical therapy intervention is currently indicated for infertility.

Menstrual Cycle Problems

Disturbances in the normal menstrual cycle are comparatively common. They are frequently caused by hormonal imbalances of estrogen and progesterone. Dysmenorrhea is pain in the abdomen, low back, and medial thighs, related to menstruation and usually occurs immediately before the onset of menstruation. The prevalence has been estimated to be between 45% and 95% of all women of reproductive age. The pain varies in length of duration from a few hours to a few days and may be accompanied by other symptoms such as nausea, dizziness, fainting, and headache. Dysmenorrhea may be primary, meaning it is part of the normal process of menstruation, or it may be as a result of other conditions such as endometriosis, fibroid tumors of the ovaries or uterus, or pelvic inflammatory disease (PID).[23] Amenorrhea is the absence of menstruation. Primary amenorrhea occurs when a woman does not start to menstruate by age 16. Primary amenorrhea is rare in the United States with an incidence of less than 1%. The etiology of primary amenorrhea is complex and can include dysfunction of the hypothalamus resulting in low levels of gonadotropin releasing hormone (GnRH) and thus lack of release of FSH from the pituitary; tumors of the pituitary; genetic disorders, such as fragile X syndrome and Turner's syndrome; excessive weight loss and malnutrition; the presence of chronic medical conditions; excessive amounts of exercise; and psychiatric disorders, including depression.[24] Amenorrhea is a normal state in menopause, but when it occurs after the onset of menses, it is considered to be secondary amenorrhea resulting from diseases of the uterus or ovaries or dysfunction of either the hypothalamus or pituitary gland. Other causes include the abuse of drugs and psychiatric disorders such as depression. In some females, excessive exercise or dieting may induce secondary amenorrhea.[25] Oligomenorrhea is the term used either for very light menstruation or menstruation that occurs less than every 35 days which is less frequently than usual. Cryptomenorrhea is when the menstrual blood flow remains in the uterus due to a defect in the cervix that does not allow the blood to exit via the vagina. The buildup of the waste products can be transmitted through the wall of the uterus and may cause peritonitis.[26] **Menorrhagia** or **hypermenorrhea** are terms used for either very heavy blood flow or an excessive length of menses during menstruation. If symptoms continue for a prolonged period, there is a high risk of anemia. Secondary causes of menorrhagia may include benign or malignant tumors of the uterus.

Premenstrual Syndrome

Premenstrual syndrome (PMS), sometimes called premenstrual stress syndrome or premenstrual tension, occurs in females after the age of onset of menses. The incidence of PMS shows that it affects approximately 80% of all menstruating women to some extent, but in about 10% of women of reproductive age, the symptoms are severe enough for them to seek medical intervention.[27]

Etiology. The onset of PMS coincides with ovulation. The actual cause of PMS is still under debate. The condition is related to the menstrual cycle and ovulation, but it is not known why some women experience PMS and others do not. Hormonal activity is thought to be the culprit, but which hormone has not been fully determined. One theory is that reductions in estrogen levels immediately before menstruation result in the inhibition of dopamine and serotonin receptors resulting in increased painful stimuli.[28]

Signs and Symptoms. The characteristic symptoms of PMS usually occur at the same time each month during the menstrual cycle for an individual woman. Symptoms of the condition occur approximately midway through the menstrual cycle and may become worse up to and beyond the start of menstruation. The onset of PMS is associated with the period of ovulation. Several definitions of PMS exist, but the general idea is that the symptoms interfere in some way with the normal lifestyle of the individual each month. Many symptoms are associated with PMS. These include headaches, low back ache, depression, low levels of concentration, mood swings, skin irritations such as acne, disturbed sleep, tender breasts, joint and muscle pains, fatigue, ankle edema resulting from fluid retention, and constipation or diarrhea. A severe form of PMS known as premenstrual dysphoric disorder (PMDD) is diagnosed when the symptoms include severe depression, anger, anxiety, and lack of concentration.[29]

Prognosis. Many women who have PMS can control symptoms using medications. Prescription medications may be needed for severe symptoms such as depression.

Medical Intervention. Most of the symptoms of PMS can be relieved to some extent with the use of nonsteroidal anti-inflammatory (NSAIDs) pain medications. Although changes in diet to include reduction of caffeine intake, reduction of the amount of alcohol, and reduction of foods high in sugar or salt are often recommended, research is limited to support these measures. The relief of symptoms varies for each person. Medical intervention may include prescription of antidepressants, diuretics (reduce fluid retention), or oral contraceptives.[30,31]

Physical Therapy Intervention. Physical therapy intervention may be sought for pain relief. The effects of regular exercise have been proved to have an effect on reducing the pain of PMS.[32] Other pain-relieving modalities such as electrical stimulation, heat, or ice may be of use. Exercise programs can be developed by the physical therapist to meet the needs of the individual. Aerobic exercise has been shown to be of particular help, so walking, swimming, and biking programs are recommended. Jogging is often recommended by the medical texts but can cause problems due to vibration affecting the internal organs and irritating the already tender breasts.

Carcinomas of the Female Reproductive System

Carcinomas of the breast are detailed in a later section in this chapter under the heading of diseases of the breast.

Carcinoma of the Cervix

One of the highest incidences of cancer of the female reproductive system is carcinoma of the cervix. Cervical cancer is most prevalent in women aged between 35 and 55 years. Approximately 11,000 women are diagnosed with cervical cancer each year, and of those 4,000 die as a result of the condition.[33]

Etiology. The etiology of carcinoma of the cervix is not known. Risk factors that have been identified with the development of cervical cancer include women who participate in sexual intercourse at an early age, those who have multiple sex partners, those who smoke, and those who have acquired STDs such as chlamydia, gonorrhea, herpes simplex virus 2 (HSV-2), human papillomavirus (HPV), HIV/AIDS, or syphilis.[34] Sexually transmitted diseases are discussed in Chapter 10. Most cervical carcinomas are squamous cell carcinoma. Early detection of a lack of maturity of the squamous epithelial cells within the cervix is called dysplasia. The dysplasia may progress into invasive carcinoma of the underlying layers of the cervix. Classification of the depth of effect of the cancer is called staging and helps to determine the treatment required and the likely prognosis of the patient by the physician. Table 11-2 shows cervical cancer staging. Tumors are either exophytic (grow into the vagina) or endophytic (grow into the cervix itself). These tumors generally grow slowly over a number of years, which makes early diagnosis and treatment of the carcinoma more successful.

Signs and Symptoms. In the early stages of the cervical cancer, there may be no symptoms. Any pain, vaginal

Table 11.2 **Staging of Carcinoma of the Cervix**

STAGE OF CERVICAL CARCINOMA	CHARACTERISTICS OF THE CARCINOMA STAGE
Dysplasia and carcinoma in situ (CIS) or cervical intraepithelial neoplasia Grades I and II (CIN I and II)	Early detection of precancerous/cancerous cells
Stage 0	Carcinoma limited to the squamous cell mucosa of the lining of the cervix called CIS or CIN III Otherwise known as preinvasive carcinoma
Stage I	Invasive carcinoma located only in the tissue of the cervix
Stage II	Invasive carcinoma that has started to go beyond the cervical tissue and has infiltrated the upper end of the vagina
Stage III	Invasive carcinoma that extends to the wall of the pelvis and has infiltrated into the lower end of the vagina
Stage IV	Carcinoma has metastasized and extends into the whole of the pelvis and into the abdominal organs which may include the rectum and bladder

discharge, or vaginal bleeding may not occur until the tumor is in an advanced stage and unable to be treated. Regular Pap smears detect precancer dysplasia of the cells of the walls of the cervix.[35]

Prognosis. Prognosis for cervical carcinoma varies with the staging. Persons with Stage I have an 85% chance of survival for more than 5 years, whereas those with Stage IV have a 10% survival rate of more than 5 years.[36] The death rate from cancer of the cervix has reduced because of early detection and treatment of the condition.

Medical Intervention. A recent advance in the prevention of cervical cancer has been the development of Gardasil, a vaccination against HPV types 6, 11, 16, and 18, shown to be the main causes of cervical cancer. The vaccination is indicated for girls and women between the ages of 9 and 26 and is given in three injections over the course of a year.[37] The vaccine was approved for use by the Food and Drug Administration (FDA) in 2006.[38] Some of the diagnostic tests for detection of cervical cancer are shown in Table 11-3. Recent findings suggest that the detection of the presence of human papillomavirus (HPV; refer to Chapter 10) by DNA tests is an excellent way to detect women at risk of developing cervical cancer. The Pap smear is the most commonly used screening tool for this disease. Medical intervention may involve surgical resection of localized carcinomas with a surgical sharp instrument, freezing (cryotherapy), laser, or electrical

cauterization. A total hysterectomy may be performed for removal of the uterus, cervix, and surrounding fascia to ensure the invaded tissue is excised. In the more advanced stages, treatment consists of radiation therapy and chemotherapy and possible extensive surgery. Early detection of cervical cancer enables the prevention of progression of the disease.[39]

Physical Therapy Intervention. PTAs may be asking why they need to know about carcinoma of the cervix. The author's belief is that knowledge of the more common diseases and their prevention and detection is an important aspect for all health care personnel. By being well informed, the health care provider can extend that knowledge to the patient and assist with the encouragement of the patient to seek screening tests. Many physical therapists and physical therapist assistants are working in women's health settings and will be asked questions about standard medical procedures. Knowledge of these procedures may help to save a life.

Carcinoma and Nonmalignant Tumors of the Ovaries

A variety of types of ovarian cysts and tumors exist, many of which are benign. Ovarian cysts usually are small sacs filled with fluid within the ovaries; however, some cysts can become as large as 12 inches in diameter. Many benign cysts develop from the ovarian follicles, which protect the developing ovum (egg), and from the corpus luteum, which is the remains of the follicle after release of the ovum from the ovary. Ovarian cysts are common and occur at any age after puberty.[40] See Table 11-4 for some of the types of benign ovarian cysts. Ovarian carcinoma is diagnosed in approximately 22,000 women each year in the United States. The incidence of ovarian carcinoma is 15 in 100,000 women annually.[41] Women of northern European descent are affected more than other populations.

Etiology. The etiology of ovarian cysts is unknown. Occasionally benign cysts such as dermoid cysts may become cancerous. The risk factors associated with ovarian carcinoma include a family history of the disease, older age, white race, and having a history of infertility, breast cancer, or nulliparity (no children). Ovarian carcinoma may be precipitated by excessive amounts of gonadotropin hormones, which sometimes occurs during treatment for infertility, or as a result of medications such as tamoxifen, which are taken by women at high risk for breast cancer, or who have been diagnosed with breast cancer.[42,43]

Table 11.3 **Some Diagnostic Tests Used for Detection of Cervical Carcinoma**

DIAGNOSTIC TEST FOR CARCINOMA OF THE CERVIX	EXPLANATION OF TEST
Pap smear (Papanicolaou test)	Cells of the wall of the cervix are removed via the vagina with a cotton tip and sent for laboratory analysis for detection of dysplasia of the squamous cells
Colposcopy	A type of microscope, the colposcope is inserted into the vagina and takes an image of the outer surface of the cervix. The normal cervix looks smooth; when abnormal; there is roughness
Biopsy Punch biopsy	A small tissue sample of the cervix is removed with a sharp instrument to send for laboratory analysis
Cone biopsy	A wedge of cervical and adjoining tissue is removed surgically for laboratory analysis (rarely used)
Computed tomography, magnetic resonance imaging, positron emission tomography	Scans of the pelvic region can determine early changes in cells of the cervix
HPV DNA test	A blood test that detects the presence of the HPV virus that is responsible for an increased risk of development of cervical cancer

Table 11.4   **Types of Benign Ovarian Cysts**

NAME OF CYST	DESCRIPTION	SIGNS AND SYMPTOMS	TREATMENT
Corpus luteum cyst	Benign cyst forming from corpus luteum when ovulation fails to occur	Usually none	Often resolves without treatment
Cystadenoma	Large, benign Grows up to 12 inches in diameter Develops directly from the ovarian tissue	Abdominal pain or no symptoms Frequency of micturition as a result of pressure on the bladder Abdominal bloating, indigestion as a result of pressure on abdominal structures Cyst palpable in the abdomen	Surgical excision
Dermoid cyst	Large, benign Consist of a variety of types of tissue, including fat, bone, cartilage, or hair Grows up to 6 inches in diameter Affects mainly younger women May develop into carcinoma	Severe abdominal pain or no symptoms Dyspareunia (painful intercourse) Frequency of micturition as a result of pressure on the bladder Cyst palpable in the abdomen	Surgical excision
Endometrioma/ endometrioid cyst	Benign Forms from endometrial issue as a result of endometriosis	Chronic pelvic or abdominal pain Menstruation-associated symptoms such as dyspareunia, dysmenorrheal (painful menses), and menorrhagia (heavy bleeding)	Surgical excision may be needed
Follicular cyst	Benign Forms from follicle when ovulation fails to occur	Abdominal pain or no symptoms	Often resolves without treatment
Polycystic appearing ovary/polycystic ovary syndrome	Enlarged ovary with multiple cysts	Abdominal pain during menstruation or no symptoms If associated with polycystic ovary syndrome, symptoms may include infertility and oligomenorrhea	May resolve without treatment Excision may be necessary

Signs and Symptoms. The characteristic signs and symptoms of ovarian cysts can include abdominal pain, dyspareunia, urinary retention, frequency of micturition, or stress incontinence, and low back pain. In a majority of cases, there are no symptoms.[44] The signs and symptoms of ovarian carcinoma depend on the stage of the tumor. Women in advanced stages of ovarian cancer have weight loss, lymphadenopathy (enlarged lymph nodes), cachexia (atrophy of muscles combined with weight loss), anorexia, possible abdominal pain and dyspnea as a result of pressure of the tumor on internal organs. The mass may be palpable by the physician.

Prognosis. The prognosis for women with ovarian cysts is excellent, because these benign structures either resolve without treatment or respond well to surgical removal. Ovarian cancer is one of the most common gynecological carcinomas and is responsible for the majority of deaths from female reproductive system cancers, partly as a result of diagnosis of most ovarian cancers in the later stages. Approximately 16,000 women a year in the United States die from ovarian cancer. The overall 5-year survival rate for women after surgery for ovarian cancer is 41.6%. However, if the carcinoma is detected in the early stages, this survival rate increases to 82%.[45]

Medical Intervention. Prevention measures against ovarian carcinoma involve annual gynecological examinations by the physician. The use of contraceptive medications has been demonstrated to reduce the risk of development of ovarian carcinoma. Women at a high risk for ovarian cancer may have an oophorectomy (removal of the ovaries) performed as a prophylactic (preventive) measure.[46] No definitive diagnostic procedures are used for ovarian cysts unless the cysts are very large. An endovaginal ultrasonography scan (a thin ultrasound probe placed within the vagina) may reveal the size of the cyst. Diagnostic tests for ovarian carcinoma include ultrasonography and magnetic resonance imaging (MRI) scans with gadolinium to provide contrast on the images. Conclusive diagnosis can only be performed by histological analysis of the surgically excised ovary or tumor. Surgical procedures are performed using a laparoscopy (small incisions for microscopic surgery) or a laparotomy (full surgical incision to remove a larger tumor).[47]

Physical Therapy Intervention. Postsurgical physical therapy may be indicated for a strengthening exercise program for the abdominal muscles.

Carcinoma of the Uterus (Endometrial Carcinoma)

The usual occurrence of uterine carcinoma is in women over 45 and most often between the ages of 55 and 74, after menopause. The American Cancer Society predicted that in 2010, there would be 43,470 women diagnosed with endometrial cancer, and 7,950 would die as a result.[48] Since the mid-1970s, the rate of endometrial cancer has declined by 25%.[49]

Etiology. The etiology of endometrial carcinoma is largely unknown. Several known risk factors exist, but not all women with even several of these factors actually develop the disease. Women on hormone replacement therapy (HRT) and those who have taken oral contraceptives with high doses of estrogen and without progestin have been shown to be at higher risk of developing this cancer. However, the low-estrogen-dose contraceptives are known to reduce the risk of endometrial cancer. Other risk factors include women who started menstruating before age 12; obesity, because fat tissue actually produces estrogens; taking tamoxifen for breast cancer increases the growth of the uterus;[50] polycystic ovarian syndrome (PCOS); eating a high animal-fat diet; preexisting diabetes; breast or ovarian cancers; and previous pelvic radiation therapy.[51]

Signs and Symptoms. The characteristic symptoms of endometrial carcinoma include vaginal bleeding or vaginal discharge not associated with pain, pelvic pain, dyspareunia (pain during intercourse), and problems with urination.[52] In later stages, the tumor may be palpated externally through the abdomen. The carcinoma usually begins as a hyperplasia of the tissue of the uterus, which gradually develops into a slow-growing carcinoma. Some of the carcinomas remain localized within the uterus, whereas others extend into the adjacent cavity. Table 11-5 shows the grading and staging of endometrial carcinoma.

Prognosis. The prognosis is good when the diagnosis is made early and the carcinoma has remained comparatively localized. Prognosis is related to the stage of the carcinoma. Statistics concerning survival rates from endometrial cancer vary, but the 5-year survival rate ranges from 99% for Stage 1A through 5% for Stage IV cancers.[53,54]

Medical Intervention. Detection of endometrial carcinoma can be determined using endometrial biopsy, hysteroscopy, or dilatation and curetage (D & C) testing. In a biopsy, a catheter is inserted into the uterus through the cervix; a hysteroscopy involves a scope inserted into the uterus; and for a D & C, the physician takes a scraping of the endometrium and sends it for laboratory diagnosis.[55] Other tests include a computed tomography (CT) scan, MRI, and ultrasound imaging. Medical intervention for this carcinoma usually involves hysterectomy (removal of the uterus) and radiation therapy and/or chemotherapy.

Table 11.5 **Staging of Endometrial Carcinoma**

STAGE OF ENDOMETRIAL CARCINOMA	CHARACTERISTICS OF THE CARCINOMA STAGE
Stage I	Tumor cells are localized to the uterus
Stage II	Tumor cells are located in the uterus and the cervix
Stage III	Tumor cells are found in the uterus and the pelvis, in the fallopian tubes, ovaries, or vagina
Stage IV	Tumor has metastasized to lymph nodes and other organs such as the bladder, rectum, bone, and lung tissue

Physical Therapy Intervention. PT intervention may be requested for patients who have had abdominal surgery to encourage ambulation and early mobility. Teaching lateral costal and diaphragmatic breathing exercises to patients postoperatively is beneficial in the prevention of emboli and return to early activity because it encourages circulatory improvement in the major vessels and increase of the venous return from the extremities. If the PT and PTA are involved in chest physical therapy, the patient should be encouraged to support the surgical incision when coughing.

Carcinoma of the Vagina

Carcinoma of the vagina is much rarer than the other types of cancer described in this chapter. Several types of vaginal cancer exist. Women diagnosed with vaginal cancer account for roughly 2% or 3% of all cancers of the female reproductive system. Approximately 2,000 women are diagnosed annually with vaginal cancer in the United States.[56] The most common form of vaginal carcinoma develops in the squamous cells of the epithelial lining of the vagina and generally occurs in women over age 60 years.[57] This squamous cell type accounts for between 85% and 90% of all vaginal carcinomas. Other forms of vaginal cancer include adenocarcinoma usually diagnosed in younger women, malignant melanoma, sarcomas, and a rare rhabdomyosarcoma typically found in girls under age 3 years.[58]

Etiology. The etiology of the majority of primary vaginal cancer (cancer originating in the vagina) is not known. In many women with vaginal cancer, the origination of the cancer is in the cervix or the uterus, with spread to the vagina. Women with adenocarcinoma of the vagina were often born to mothers who received diethylbestrol (DES) during pregnancy in the 1950s to prevent miscarriage.[59]

Signs and Symptoms. Usually, no symptoms are present in the early stages of precancerous lesions of the vagina. Most precancerous lesions are found when a routine Pap smear is performed. In the later stages of vaginal cancer symptoms may include an abnormal vaginal bleeding or discharge, dyspareunia (pain during sexual intercourse), a detectable mass within the vagina, or pain on urination. Other later symptoms may include constipation and pelvic pain.[60]

Prognosis. This rare form of female cancer accounts for approximately 700 to 800 deaths per year in the United States. Advanced cancers of the vagina usually result in metastases to the lungs and liver. Diagnosis of women in the early stages of the disease improves the life expectancy.[61] When diagnosed in the precancerous stage, women can be effectively treated and not progress to cancerous lesions.

Medical Intervention. In 2008, the FDA approved the use of Gardasil immunizations for the prevention of vaginal and vulvar cancers, as well as cervical cancer.[62] Screening for precancerous, atypical squamous cells, also called precancerous areas of vaginal intraepithelial neoplasia (VAIN), in the lining of the cervix and vagina with a Pap smear test can lead to an early diagnosis and treatment of the condition. VAIN is divided into three diagnostic stages, 1, 2, and 3, with 3 the deepest. Women positive for VAIN may undergo further testing, including biopsy, colposcopy (observation of the epithelium of the vagina and cervix under magnification), and CT, MRI, or PET scans. If the cancer is in an advanced stage, a sigmoidoscopy to examine the rectum and sigmoid colon and a cystoscopy to examine the bladder may be performed to determine how far the cancer has spread.[63] Treatment options for precancerous or cancerous lesions of the vagina vary depending on the level of the diagnosis. Loop electrosurgical excision procedure (LEEP) removes the affected tissue with an electrical current; topical chemotherapy medications such as Efudex can be applied to the vagina internally over a period of several weeks, and laser therapy can be aimed at the specific affected cells.[64] In women with more advanced cancer, a partial vaginectomy (removal of part of the vagina) or a radical vaginectomy (removal of the vagina and surrounding tissue) may be performed. Women who have a radical vaginectomy can have a reconstruction of the vagina performed. Radiation therapy and laser surgery are other options, either instead of other treatment or after completion of another type of treatment.[65] [66]

Physical Therapy Intervention. No physical therapy intervention is indicated for vaginal cancer. Urinary incontinence problems resulting from surgery may be treated with electrical stimulation and biofeedback modalities.

Carcinoma of the Vulva

Carcinoma of the vulva includes any area of the external female genitalia but predominantly affects the labia and the clitoris. This rare condition mainly affects women over age 50 years, but up to 15% of affected women are under the age of 40 years. Most primary vulvar cancers (originate in the vulva) start in the squamous epithelial cells, but other types include adenocarcinomas, basal cell carcinomas, melanomas, and sarcomas.

Etiology. The actual etiology of vulva cancer is unknown. However, the predisposing risk factors for the development of carcinoma of the vulva include a history of infection with the human papillomavirus (HPV; genital warts) or syphilis, a history of cervical or vaginal cancer, diabetes, hypertension, or obesity.[67]

Signs and Symptoms. Characteristics of vulva carcinoma may include itching, but this is not always apparent, and itching may be caused by other conditions. Many women with vulva cancer lesions do not have any symptoms. Other signs and symptoms may include skin ulcerations on the external genitalia, bleeding of the area, pain with urination, and an unusual odor.[68]

Prognosis. Most of these carcinomas are localized, rarely metastasize, and can be excised effectively. In women who have vulva cancer as a secondary site of cancer as metastases from the cervix, uterus, or vagina, the prognosis may not be as good. A recurrence of the cancer may appear near the original excised tumor so regular follow-up with a physician is recommended.

Medical Intervention. Because the risk factors for vulvar cancer include sexually transmitted infections a preventative measure is through the practice of safe sexual contact. Regular pelvic examinations by a physician are effective in the early detection of vulvar cancer. Self-examinations of the pelvic area are also helpful. Diagnosis is confirmed through a biopsy of the suspicious tissue. The medical management depends on the staging of the cancer and may entail a simple excision of localized tissue, or a more extensive surgical excision with removal of local lymph nodes.[69]

Physical Therapy Intervention. No physical therapy intervention is indicated for carcinoma of the vulva.

Leiomyoma of the Uterus (Fibroids)

Leiomyomas, or fibroids are common, usually slow-growing, benign tumors that develop in the uterus. The tumors may be very small or become very large, and they usually exist in multiple numbers. Women over 30, but before menopause, are at the greatest risk for developing fibroids. The prevalence of fibroids is greater in African American than Caucasian women. Fibroids are estimated to exist in between 20% and 50% of all women aged over 30 years.[70]

Etiology. The exact etiology of fibroids is unknown, but the growth is related to estrogen hormone levels. They often develop during pregnancy and then diminish in size after delivery. Most fibroids shrink after menopause without intervention as a result of the reduction in estrogen levels. [71]

Signs and Symptoms. Fibroids may cause no symptoms. If the fibroids become large they may develop a cyst-like necrotic center, which can burst causing acute abdominal pain. General signs and symptoms of fibroids include menorrhagia (heavy bleeding) with blood clots, irregular bleeding, bleeding between menstrual periods, and pelvic and low abdominal pain. If the fibroids are large enough to press on the bladder or intestine, frequency of micturition, constipation, and rectal pain can develop.[72,73]

Prognosis. Uterine fibroids are not life threatening. However, one of the side effects includes infertility if the fallopian tubes are blocked or the uterus contains so many fibroids that implantation of the ovum is impossible. Women with extensive fibroids that develop during pregnancy may have a premature delivery or require a caesarean section.[74] In very rare instances, a fibroid may develop into a malignant sarcoma.[75]

Medical Intervention. The diagnosis of uterine fibroids may be made during a pelvic examination. A transvaginal (via the vagina and cervix) or a pelvic ultrasound may confirm the diagnosis. Other diagnostic procedures include an MRI or a CAT scan.[76] In some cases, a pelvic laparoscopic surgery, or an endometrial biopsy (biopsy of the tissue of the lining of the uterus), may be performed to rule out the possibility of cancer. Most women with fibroids will be merely monitored to ensure the fibroids do not become too large. Pharmacological intervention may include oral contraceptives to reduce menorrhagia, and nonsteroidal anti-inflammatory medications for pain. Iron supplements may be required if the blood loss is great enough to produce anemia. Surgical options include resection of the fibroids by a laparoscope via the cervix, surgical removal of the fibroids with a myomectomy, or a hysterectomy.[77] Gonadotropin-releasing hormone analogs or agonists (GnRHa) may be prescribed to reduce the size of the uterus and the fibroids before a vaginal approach hysterectomy.[78]

Physical Therapy Intervention. No physical therapy is indicated for uterine fibroids.

Pelvic Floor Incompetence and Weakness

The anatomy of the pelvic floor is described earlier in this chapter. Because the muscles of the pelvic floor provide support for the sphincters that control the anus and the urethra, it makes sense that when these muscles become weak through stretching, weakness or lack of use a lack of control of the bladder and bowel results. Most major symptoms caused by weakness of the pelvic floor musculature occur in older people, particularly women. Urinary continence is a common condition in women of all ages. Between 17% and 55% of older women have symptoms of incontinence, and between 12% and 42% of younger to middle-aged women.[79] Estimates are that approximately 13 million Americans are affected by stress urinary incontinence (SUI), with 85% of them women.[80] Worldwide, more than 200 million people have urinary incontinence.[81]

Etiology. A variety of causes exist for female pelvic floor incompetence or weakness. Some women have genetically weak pelvic floor muscles. Pregnancy places pressure and stress on the pelvic floor musculature, which is increased during vaginal delivery. Women who have multiple deliveries are more at risk of weakness of the pelvic floor as a result of stretching during the delivery process. Other factors leading to the onset of weakness may include obesity, chronic coughing as a result of smoking or respiratory diseases, constant heavy lifting, and straining during bowel motions. Surgery to the pelvic floor or abdomen such as a hysterectomy, tumors of the pelvis, and direct injuries to the pelvis may also cause weakness of the muscles.[82] In some instances weakness is the result of injury to nerves and this cannot be corrected. A study of 519 women by Sartore et al. in 2004 also demonstrated that an episiotomy during delivery was associated with a reduction in pelvic floor muscle strength.[83]

Signs and Symptoms. The stretching of the pelvic floor muscles from pregnancy and delivery may cause a temporary problem with urinary incontinence. If the ligaments supporting the uterus and pelvic floor musculature are severely damaged, more permanent incontinence problems may result. In a few cases, the damage to the pelvic floor musculature including the anal sphincter may cause fecal incontinence. Many women develop stress incontinence, which is brought on by exertion and effort such as coughing, sneezing, laughing, exercising, or lifting heavy weights, all of which cause increased intraabdominal pressure reflected down onto the weakened pelvic floor. Urge incontinence, sometimes called overactive bladder, is characterized by the sudden urge to void resulting in leakage of urine.[84] The weakened sphincters of the pelvic floor are unable to withstand the increased intraabdominal pressure. Other conditions caused by weak pelvic floor muscles include rectal prolapse and uterine prolapse.[85] Uterine prolapse is discussed later in this chapter.

Prognosis. Women with severe pelvic floor weakness as a result of nerve damage may have permanent problems with bladder or bowel incontinence, or both. However, most women can improve pelvic floor function through medical and physical therapy interventions.

Medical Intervention. The diagnosis of pelvic floor weakness and the associated problems of urinary and fecal incontinence, frequency of micturition, rectal prolapse, and uterine prolapsed, is largely through examination of the pelvis by the physician. Some symptomatic relief of urge incontinence may be obtained with the use of anticholinergic medications, which block the nerves that control the bladder muscles, allowing them to relax, such as oxybutynin and tolterodine.[86,87] Radiographic studies of the pelvis using MRI have set standards for the normal pelvic musculature for comparison to the weakened pelvis.[88] Thus, in women with severe instances of prolapse that require surgical intervention, an MRI can help to confirm the diagnosis and provide helpful images of any abnormalities before surgery.[89] A variety of surgeries are performed for stress incontinence, but most fall into two main categories called bladder neck suspension and sling procedures. In a bladder neck suspension, the neck of the bladder is stitched to part of the ligaments of the pelvis to keep the bladder in position. Sling procedures use a variety of materials to provide sling support to the bladder to maintain an optimum functional position. Injections of "bulking" materials may also be used in the area around the urethra to assist with tightening of the sphincter to prevent urine leakage.[90]

Physical Therapy Intervention. Physical therapy intervention with the use of electrical stimulation and biofeedback to the pelvic floor area can assist with reeducation of the muscles to reduce incontinence.[91,92]A vaginal or rectal electrode can be used, or pad electrodes can be situated on the inner thigh in a crossfire pattern to effect the necessary contraction. Muscle reeducation for the pelvic floor has proved successful in reducing the effects of both stress and urge incontinence.[93] The use of resistance for muscles is an important part of a strengthening exercise program. Special vaginal weighted inserts have been developed to assist in pelvic floor exercises. The PT and PTA can instruct women in the use of these inserts for home use on a regular exercise schedule. An explanation to patients that the incontinence is largely due to muscle weakness and that the muscles of the pelvic floor can be reeducated just like any other muscle is helpful. Kegel exercises or similar regimes of pelvic floor exercises are also useful in reeducation of the pelvic floor area.[94] Advice to patients should include avoid drinking coffee, which acts as an irritant to the bladder and causes more frequent urination. Educating patients includes not always emptying the bladder at the first sensation of wanting to urinate so that the bladder is retrained not to send messages to the brain quite as frequently. Placing women on a prescribed timetable for passing urine, with gradual increase of the time between bathroom visits, also helps to retrain the bladder.[95]

Pelvic Inflammatory Disease

Pelvic inflammatory disease (PID) is the name used for infections of the female reproductive system, particularly the uterus and fallopian tubes. Inflammation of the cervix (cervicitis), uterus (endometritis), fallopian tubes (salpingitis), and ovaries (oophoritis) may be involved. This condition is common in women under 25 years of age. More than 1 million women per year have symptoms of PID in the United States.[96]

Etiology. The etiology of PID includes diseases such as gonorrhea, chlamydia, and streptococcal infections. The use of intrauterine contraceptive devices (IUD) that are contaminated with bacteria may also cause the problem. Occasionally the condition will result from childbirth. Regular use of condoms or oral contraception seems to reduce the risk of contracting the disease. PID is more common in young **nulliparous** women (not had a child) and those who have had multiple sexual partners. Further risk factors include smoking and regular douching. The disease is common in women infected with HIV.[97]

Signs and Symptoms. The characteristic signs and symptoms of the disease may include lower abdominal pain, low back pain, fever, fatigue, anorexia, nausea, cervical tenderness, abdominal tenderness, frequency of urination,

and a purulent vaginal discharge. However, some women do not have any symptoms. The condition increases the risk of chronic abdominal pain, pelvic abscess, peritonitis, ectopic pregnancy, infertility, abdominal cavity scar tissue, and dyspareunia (painful sexual intercourse).[98]

Prognosis. Women who are treated quickly for the infection can avoid the serious complications of the disease. More than 100,000 women become infertile as a result of the disease each year in the United States. PID is also the most common cause of ectopic pregnancy.[99]

Medical Intervention. The diagnosis of PID is often difficult. The procedures for diagnosis may include a pelvic examination, pelvic ultrasound, a CT scan, and a history of any symptoms. In women with severe symptoms, a laparoscopy may be performed. Blood tests including a white blood cell count (WBC) to detect infection, an erythrocyte sedimentation rate (ESR), and an endocervical culture to detect the causative organism can determine which pharmacological intervention to prescribe.[100] Treatment of PID includes oral or intravenous antimicrobial medications. Sexual partners should also be treated with antimicrobial medications to prevent reinfection. The prevention of serious complications from PID can be achieved through the use of condoms, early treatment if symptoms occur, and an annual test for chlamydia infection for women under 25 years of age.

Physical Therapy Intervention. No physical therapy intervention is indicated for PID.

Uterine prolapse

A uterine prolapse is defined as a herniation or descent of the uterus into or beyond the vagina. The condition is comparatively common in women who have had several vaginal deliveries (multiparous) and those after the onset of menopause. Some women may have the condition during pregnancy, particularly with a multiple fetus pregnancy.[101] Uterine prolapse may also occur in older women as a result of lax support of the uterine structures within the pelvis. Uterine prolapse is categorized into several degrees.

- A first-degree uterine prolapse is one in which the uterus descends partly into the vagina.
- A second-degree uterine prolapse is one in which the uterus descends all the way into the vagina.
- A third-degree uterine prolapse is one in which the uterus and cervix protrude outside the external vaginal opening.

Etiology. Uterine prolapse is the result of weakness of the pelvic floor support structures including the muscles, ligaments, and fascia. Some women have a congenital weakness in the pelvic floor. The stretching of the pelvic floor structures during vaginal delivery and the reduction of estrogen levels after menopause are major risk factors for the development of uterine prolapse. The condition may also occur during pregnancy, especially in a multiple fetus pregnancy. Other risk factors include those that increase the intraabdominal pressure placing a strain on the pelvic floor such as obesity or coughing caused by chronic respiratory conditions, such as asthma and chronic obstructive airways disease (COPD).[102]

Signs and Symptoms. The signs and symptoms of uterine prolapse include low back pain exacerbated by prolonged standing and walking. Most women will feel pain at the end of the day, especially if they are on their feet for extended periods of time. Pelvic pain and dyspareunia are also common. Other symptoms may include constipation, nausea, and urinary symptoms of urgency, frequency, or incontinence.[103]

Prognosis. The danger of premature delivery exists when a woman has a prolapsed uterus. Most pregnant women with a prolapsed uterus are placed on bed rest in a Trendelenburg position (foot end of the bed raised).[104,105] A caesarean section may be required in women with severe uterine prolapse. After delivery the uterus occasionally inverts. In this condition, the uterus turns inside out and extends beyond the vaginal opening. A risk of complications exists after surgery for uterine prolapse including hemorrhage and damage to the pudendal nerve resulting in incontinence. Such complications are rare.[106] The risk of urinary incontinence is high as a result of weak pelvic floor musculature for any woman with uterine prolapse.[107]

Medical Intervention. The conservative management of uterine prolapse consists of topical estrogen to the exposed part of the vagina or uterus, vaginal pessaries to retain or correct the position of the uterus, and pelvic floor exercises. The pessaries may be ring-shaped or donut-shaped. Some of the types of pessaries used include Gehring, Gellhorn, Smith-Hodge, and Risser.[108] Surgical intervention for a prolapsed uterus often involves a hysterectomy. A hysterectomy may be a partial hysterectomy in which the uterus is excised, or the removal of the uterus and the ovaries in a total hysterectomy. Alternative surgeries include a sacral colpopexy or sacral uteropexy. These surgeries, commonly referred to as "suspensions," reposition the upper vagina and the uterus into their normal position by attaching them to the sacrum and the presacral fascia, or the sacrospinous ligament, at the level of the third sacral vertebra. The surgeries can be performed through the vagina or the abdomen. Difficulty with sexual intercourse may be a side effect of the surgery. After surgery, women have to be careful not to increase the intra-abdominal pressure. Medical advice includes no lifting of weights, no smoking, continuation of estrogen replacement therapy (ERT), and reducing the risk of constipation.[109]

Physical Therapy Intervention. With either conservative or surgical management of a prolapsed uterus, physical therapy may be indicated for strengthening of the pelvic floor musculature. However, exercises will not reverse the effects of uterine prolapse.[110] The causative factors leading to a prolapsed uterus include weakness of the pelvic floor, thus the likelihood of urinary incontinence, frequency, or stress incontinence is high. Strengthening of the pelvic floor musculature includes the use of electrical stimulation using a vaginal or rectal electrode, biofeedback, strengthening exercises, and progressive resistive exercises using vaginal weights.

Intrauterine Devices and Their Significance in Physical Therapy Intervention

The PT and PTA need to determine whether the patient has an intrauterine device in place before performing several procedures and modalities. If the PT is conducting an evaluation for low back pain and there is evidence of low abdominal pain, or the evaluation findings are inconsistent with the usual musculoskeletal pattern of signs and symptoms, the possibility of contraceptive device malfunction should be ruled out. Occasionally an intrauterine device can pierce the uterus and cause pain and inflammation. When performing short wave diathermy in the region of the pelvis or low back, it is essential to check for the presence of any metal, including intrauterine devices.

Diseases of the Breast

Regular self-examination of the breasts is recommended for all women to help in early detection of lumps or palpable changes in the breast tissue. If women perform regular examinations, they become familiar with the normal feel of the tissue and are more easily able to detect changes. Some lumps are benign, but others are malignant and require immediate medical attention. Additionally, mammography is used for early detection screening of breast tissue abnormalities. The American Cancer Society updated their guidelines for the early detection of cancer in 2010. The recommendations included an annual mammogram for all women starting at the age of 40 years, a clinical medical breast examination every 3 years for those women between the ages of 20 and 30 years and an annual examination for women over 40 years of age; breast self-examinations starting at 20 years, and an annual MRI for women at high risk (greater than 20% lifetime risk) of developing breast cancer as a result of family history or genetic tendency.[111]

Benign fibroadenoma

Benign fibroadenoma is a common, benign tumor of breast tissue that mainly occurs in women younger than 40 years, although women older than 40 may be affected. In approximately 10% to 15% of women with the condition multiple tumors exist.[112] The tumor most often affects the distal end of the lactation ducts of the breast. Approximately 50% of all biopsies of breast tissue reveal a diagnosis of benign fibroadenoma.[113]

Etiology. The cause of benign fibroadenoma is unknown. Approximately 10% of fibroadenomas resolve on their own without treatment or excision. Others stop growing when they reach the size of 2 to 3 cm. These benign tumors often grow rapidly during pregnancy but resolve after the delivery. Growth of fibroadenomas may also increase during the use of hormone replacement therapy (HRT) and when women are immunosuppressed.[114]

Signs and Symptoms. Unlike fibrocystic disease nodules, these tumors usually are not tender or painful. They are usually round, or oval, rubbery in texture, easily moveable, and encapsulated. The size varies between 1 and 15 cm in diameter, and the tumors may or may not be palpable.[115]

Prognosis. The prognosis for women with benign fibroadenoma is good. The risk of a fibroadenoma becoming malignant is low at 3%. Some sources indicate the risk of malignancy rises to between 8% and 10% for women over age 40 years.[116]

Medical Intervention. The diagnosis of benign fibroadenoma involves a variety of tests to ensure the tumor is not cancerous. For women of childbearing age, the preferred method of diagnosis is ultrasonography to avoid exposure to radiation. Other diagnostic procedures include

mammography, MRI, needle aspiration of the tumor, and image-guided biopsy.[117,118] Although some women choose to have benign fibroadenomas surgically removed, most will resolve after the onset of menopause.

Physical Therapy Intervention. No physical therapy intervention is indicated.

Breast carcinoma

Breast carcinoma is the second-most common cancer in women in the United States, and creates the second highest risk of death for women from cancer. The highest risk is from lung cancer. The incidence of breast cancer is 1 in 8 (12%) for women to develop cancer during their lifetime. As much as 80% of breast cancers occur in women over age 50 years.[119] The death rate from breast cancer in the United States is approximately 40,000 per year. In 2010, the American Cancer Society estimated that there would be approximately 207,090 new cases of invasive breast cancer in the United States, and an additional 54,010 new cases of cancer in situ, the less invasive kind of cancer.[120]

Etiology. A higher risk of breast cancer exists for those women who have a close relative, such as a sister or mother, who has had the disease. However, in 75% of women with breast cancer, there is no family history of the problem. In 5% to 10% of women who develop breast cancer, there is an inherited factor. These women have breast cancer gene 1 (BRCA1) or breast cancer gene 2 (BRCA2). The presence of these genes increases the risk for developing both breast and ovarian cancer.[121] The risk of breast cancer is higher for Caucasian women than Asian or black women. The risks are also greater for women who

- are in higher socioeconomic groups
- live in urban rather than rural areas
- are overweight, postmenopausal, and have a high density of breast tissue
- had early menarche (onset of menstruation) and late onset of menopause
- are nulliparous (do not have children)
- were older when they became pregnant
- were exposed to large amounts of radiation during childhood and adolescence
- smoke
- consume large amounts of alcohol, are using hormone replacement therapy, or oral contraceptives[122,123]

Research performed by Trichopoulos et al. demonstrated that the risk for developing breast cancer is also linked with hormone levels and the numbers of mammary tissue–specific stem cells present in the breast, factors that are present at birth.[124] Many breast lumps are detected by women when they perform a self-examination.

Signs and Symptoms. The characteristic signs and symptoms of breast cancer tumors include a palpable lump, discharge from the nipple (which may be clear or bloody), retraction or inversion of a normally prominent nipple, itching, a rash, or enlargement of the nipple. Other symptoms include enlargement or reduction in size of the breast; a change of shape of the breast, such as flattening or indentation; redness of the skin of the breast, or pitting of the skin of the breast.[125] Most carcinomas of the breast are unilateral rather than bilateral and nontender to palpation. In some women, tumors are not detected until there are gross changes of the breast tissue or palpable lymph nodes in the axilla. In such instances, the tumor usually is quite far advanced.

Prognosis. The prognosis for women with breast carcinoma depends on the stage, type, and growth rate of the cancer, and on the age and general health of the woman. The prognosis is not as good if the incident is a recurrence of a previous tumor.[126] If there are no metastases, the survival rate after 5 years is 97% according to the American Cancer Society. If the cancer is more widespread, the survival rate after 5 years is reduced to 75%. In cases in which metastases are widespread, the survival rate after 5 years is reduced to 10%. The chances of a woman's death resulting from breast cancer is 1 in 35. More than 2.5 million women are survivors of breast cancer, including those undergoing treatment and those who have completed treatment. The early diagnosis and treatment of breast cancer through annual screenings has greatly improved the survival rate for women.[127]

GERIATRIC CONSIDERATIONS

Elderly women are not exempt from the problems of breast cancer. The rehabilitation for women after radical mastectomy is important for all age groups. Maintaining upper extremity range of motion and assisting the patient to return to full upper extremity function is of paramount importance. Note that males also can have breast cancer.

Medical Intervention. Mammography screening can provide early detection of breast cancer. Controversy exists regarding what age women should start having mammography screening. The general rule is to have a screening performed for a baseline at age 40 years and then every year particularly after age 50.[128] The choices of diagnostic tests performed to determine the nature of a tumor include different types of biopsy. An excisional biopsy involves excision of the tumor; in an incisional biopsy, a section of the tumor is removed; and in a core biopsy, a large-bore needle is used to remove a core of tissue. A fine-needle aspiration may also be performed to remove tissue from the center of a tumor. A recent addition is biopsy of the sentinel lymph node. The sentinel lymph node is the first node of drainage from a tumor and indicates the degree of metastasis of the tumor.[129] An MRI is used for diagnosis and blood tests to determine estrogen and testosterone receptors may indicate whether the use of hormone therapy would be useful to stop the growth of the tumor. The medical intervention for breast cancer tumors involves a wide variety of surgeries that include breast-conserving surgeries and total mastectomies (removal of the breast). See Table 11-6 for details of possible surgeries for breast cancer. Radiation therapy, chemotherapy, and hormone therapy are all possible adjuvant treatments used after surgery. New experimental adjuvant treatments used after surgery include the administration of high doses of chemotherapy combined with stem-cell transplantation; tyrosine kinase inhibitors, which block signals to the tumor slowing or stop the growth; and the use of monoclonal antibodies, which attack the cancer cells.[130]

Physical Therapy Intervention. PT intervention may be required for women who have a total radical mastectomy when the lymph nodes are removed. In such cases, exercises for the upper extremity are needed to ensure range of motion is not lost, as are instruction in elevating the upper extremity to reduce the risk of edema. Strengthening exercises are also essential for the return of full upper extremity function. PT intervention may be needed in long-term cases of lymphedema resulting from mastectomy, in which the arm swells, and hand and shoulder function are reduced. The management of lymphedema is a specialized intervention that involves a total program known as "complex physical therapy" (CPT) or "complete decongestive therapy."[131] This includes special types of massage, compression techniques of bandaging or the use of compression garments, the use of compression pumps, specific exercises, and hydrotherapy, combined with the use of medical interventions such as medications,

Table 11.6   **Types of Surgery for Breast Carcinoma**

TYPE OF SURGERY	DESCRIPTION OF SURGERY
Lumpectomy	Breast-conserving surgery: excision of the lump or tumor without removal of any other tissue
Partial mastectomy	Breast conserving surgery: excision of the tumor and possible affected surrounding tissue from part of the breast
Lymph node dissection	Breast conserving surgery: excision of the lymph nodes affected by the carcinoma; often involves excision of the tumor and the associated lymph nodes
Total or simple mastectomy	Excision of the breast and lymph nodes involved with the carcinoma
Modified radical mastectomy	Excision of the whole breast, the axillary lymph nodes, and part of the muscles of the chest wall
Radical mastectomy (Halstead radical mastectomy)	Excision of the whole breast, chest wall muscles, and all axillary lymph nodes
Breast reconstruction	The reconstruction of a breast after mastectomy; may be performed at the same time as the mastectomy or later The reconstruction uses the woman's own tissue, a silicone gel implant, or a saline-filled implant to form a new breast

nutritional advice, and surgery. The specific physical therapy is extensive and beyond the scope of this book.[132,133]

Fibrocystic Disease

Physical therapists and physical therapist assistants do not treat **fibrocystic disease** of the breast, but because they play a role in patient education, knowledge of this condition is important. Fibrocystic disease is a benign condition of the breast, common in women 30 to 50 years of age, affecting as many as 60% of all women.[134]

Etiology. The etiology of these cysts is thought to be hormonal, and largely due to estrogen and progesterone, because the lumps tend to increase in size immediately before menstruation and decline after the onset of menopause.[135] The tendency to develop fibrocystic disease is increased with a family history of the condition. Other risk factors include a high fat diet and a high caffeine intake.

Signs and Symptoms. The characteristic signs and symptoms of the disease include painful and possibly tender lumps, usually in both breasts; fullness of the breasts that fluctuates throughout the menstrual cycle; general breast discomfort; and occasionally discharge from the nipple.[136] These benign cysts may alter in size regularly, and in some instances, the cysts become fibrosed (see Fig. 11-6).

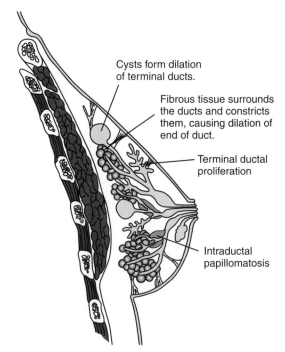

Cysts form dilation of terminal ducts.

Fibrous tissue surrounds the ducts and constricts them, causing dilation of end of duct.

Terminal ductal proliferation

Intraductal papillomatosis

FIGURE 11.6 Fibrocystic changes in the breast. Nodules may be palpated and calcifications may occur that show up on mammography.

Prognosis. Fibrocystic disease is benign and generally creates no increased risk of developing breast cancer. However, the increased density of the breast tissue caused by fibrocystic disease may impede identification of early forms of breast carcinoma on mammography or MRI.[137]

Medical Intervention. Diagnostic medical tests include a mammogram (x-ray of the breast tissue) and needle aspiration to make sure the lesion is not malignant (see Breast Carcinoma earlier in the chapter). Women with this condition should be closely monitored by their physician and be encouraged to perform regular monthly self-examinations of the breasts. No medical treatment is given to women with this condition. In some cases, patients are encouraged to reduce the amount of caffeine intake may help to reduce symptoms, but no definitive medical study demonstrates that this is effective. The effects of alternative herbal medications, such as evening primrose oil or vitamin E, is controversial and unproved. However, some women find these herbal medications effective in reducing the signs and symptoms of the condition.[138]

Physical Therapy Intervention. No physical therapy intervention is indicated.

> ### Why Does the Physical Therapist Assistant Need to Know About Pregnancy?
>
> Understanding the anatomical and physiological status of the pregnant female enables the PTA to determine the precautions and contraindications required when working with women who are pregnant. Many women who are pregnant require physical therapy intervention, and the physiological changes within the body affect the types and choice of appropriate interventions.

Pregnancy

Conception occurs when a sperm fertilizes an ovum within the fallopian tube. The implantation of this fertilized ovum (zygote) in the endometrium of the uterus starts the period of pregnancy, causing many physiological changes within the female. During the first 8 weeks, the embryo rapidly develops organs through a process called organogenesis. This period of development is crucial to the health of the developing child and the fetus is most susceptible to damage. Spontaneous abortions occur during this period as a result of injury to the embryo. After 8 weeks, the embryo is classified as a fetus.[139] The 9-month period of human pregnancy is divided into 3 trimesters, each consisting of 3 months. Pregnancy testing is achieved through a urine or blood sample, which tests for the presence of human chorionic gonadotropin hormone (hCG) produced by the developing placenta when the ovum implants in the endometrium of the uterus.[140] The normal period of gestation for the human baby is 40 weeks from the time of the last menstrual period (LMP). However, the actual age of the fetus at delivery is usually 38 weeks. The following information is used to determine the estimated date of delivery (EDD) by using Nägele's Rule:

EDD = First day of last menstrual cycle − 3 months + 7 days.

A woman pregnant for the first time is said to be **primigravida,** and a woman who has had several pregnancies is referred to as **multigravida**. **Multipara** means that the woman has delivered more than one viable child. Multiple pregnancies are when more than one fetus develop at the same time within the uterus. The usual incidence of a multiple pregnancy is approximately 1 in 80 births. Twins are more common than triplets or quadruplets. Twins may be either monozygotic (identical) in which one fertilized ovum divides into two, or dizygotic (nonidentical) in which two separate ova are fertilized and implanted. The risk of premature labor with a multiple birth is higher than for a singleton (single birth). The use of fertility technology increases the numbers of multiple pregnancies to as much as 25% to 30% for twins and 5% for triplets.[141]

Many physiological changes occur in the female body during pregnancy. The cervix becomes softened soon after conception, and the glands surrounding the cervix excrete mucous, which plugs the cervix opening to protect the developing fetus. The vagina becomes more elastic in nature with less connective tissue, in preparation for passage of the fetal head during delivery. **Braxton-Hicks uterine contractions**, or so-called false labor pains, are common throughout the second and third trimester of pregnancy. Unlike true labor contractions, the Braxton-Hicks contractions do not become stronger or more frequent.[142] Frequency of micturition (frequent urination) is often a symptom during pregnancy. This frequency of micturition is the result of an increased renal blood flow of up to 80% and also may be due to direct pressure on the bladder from the fetus. To relieve this symptom, the pregnant woman may lie on her left side. The basal metabolic rate (BMR) is altered during pregnancy as a result of the demands of the fetal circulation and nutritional needs. An increase in blood volume of up to 50% above the normal level occurs in the female during pregnancy. Cardiac output may increase up to 50% by Week 32 of the pregnancy. In the early stages of pregnancy, the stroke volume increases, but this stroke volume later levels out and the higher cardiac output is sustained by tachycardia. The heart rate in pregnancy can be as much as 15 beats per minute higher than the usual for the individual woman. The needs of the fetus require an increased oxygen uptake of 14% and progesterone causes hyperventilation to meet this need.[143] The well-known symptoms of pregnancy, such as nausea and vomiting in the early morning (morning sickness) and constipation, are usually present during the first trimester. Some women experience morning sickness, whereas others have symptoms throughout the day. Maternal weight gain is the result of the added weight of the placenta, amniotic fluid, hypertrophied uterus, the increased volume of blood and fluids, increased fat stores in breast tissue, and the fetus itself. The average weight gain during pregnancy is recommended to be approximately 25 to 35 pounds and up to 45 pounds with twins. Losing weight during pregnancy is considered to be detrimental to the fetus.[144] During the latter stages of pregnancy, fluid retention is common. Some women experience calcium and iron deficiencies, and iron supplements are prescribed to prevent the anemia caused by pregnancy.

Lactation

Lactation is milk production in the mammary glands after delivery of the infant. Several factors influence the production of milk. Before milk production, the breast produces a clear fluid called colostrum. The colostrum contains high levels of antibodies, minerals, and vitamins to protect the infant. The breast produces transitional milk for the first 2 weeks after delivery and then milk with a high fat content to satisfy the nutritional needs of the rapidly growing infant. Estrogen and progesterone influence secretion of milk and darken the areolar tissue surrounding the nipple. When the infant suckles on the nipple and the surrounding areolar tissue, it stimulates the pituitary gland to produce prolactin and oxytocin, which in turn stimulates the production of milk by allowing the "letdown" reflex to occur, starting the flow of milk. In most cases, lactation lasts approximately 6 months to 1 year, but if the infant continues to nurse (feed), it may last longer.[145]

Monitoring of the Fetus During Pregnancy

Various ways of monitoring the health of the fetus exist. One of the most commonly used methods is a diagnostic ultrasound scan of the pregnant woman's abdomen. Ultrasound is performed to check fetal growth, detect abnormalities, determine the size and number of babies, and identify the gender of the fetus. A relatively new technique called 3D and 4D scanning shows actual three-dimensional pictures of the fetus, and, in the 4D mode, movement of the fetus in real time. The scans are detailed enough to show facial expressions, such as blinking and winking and thumb sucking.[146] A simple check of the fetal heart rate is performed with a stethoscope over the woman's abdomen. An external fetal heart monitoring device may be used when the mother visits the physician's office during pregnancy. The machine is either a handheld Doppler device that is passed over the woman's abdomen and records the fetal heart rate or electrodes are attached to the woman's abdomen, with the results visible on a computer screen. The typical fetal heart rate (FHR) is between 120 and 160 beats per minute. When closer monitoring of the fetal heart rate is required during delivery contractions, an internal fetal heart monitoring device may be used. An electrode is attached to the head of the fetus through the maternal dilated cervix, and the results show both the FHR and the strength of maternal contractions.[147] CT scans, MRI, and radiographic imaging are avoided whenever possible during pregnancy, but in some cases when severe complications are suspected, a CT scan may be used.

Blood tests are taken regularly during pregnancy to monitor the health of both the mother and the fetus. During the first trimester, blood samples are taken to test for the levels of glucose, iron, and hemoglobin of the mother. Fetal health is monitored during the first trimester with maternal blood tested for pregnancy-associated plasma protein (PAPP-A) and human chorionic gonadotropin (hCG). High levels of both these factors may indicate an increased risk of fetal chromosome abnormalities and usually are followed up with further testing. During the second trimester, maternal blood is checked for levels of alpha-fetoprotein (AFP). Abnormally high levels of AFP may indicate neural tube defects, such as spina bifida, or other chromosome abnormalities, such as Down syndrome. However, the AFP is also high in the presence of a multiple pregnancy.[148] If first trimester or second trimester blood tests provide higher that expected levels of any hormone, the next step is usually an amniocentesis or a chorionic villus sampling. In addition, amniocentesis may be recommended for women over 35 and for those who have a family history of genetic defects. An amniocentesis is an invasive procedure in which a sample of amniotic fluid is taken by inserting a needle into the amniotic sac via the woman's abdomen. The position of the fetus is determined by an ultrasound scan prior to inserting the needle to ensure the fetus is not touched by the needle. A chorionic villus sample is taken from the placenta of the fetus by either passing a catheter through the abdominal wall of the woman or up through the vagina and cervix. Ultrasound visualization is used to guide the catheter. Both the amniotic fluid sample and the chorionic villus samples can be tested for genetic abnormalities and provide more specific and accurate information than a maternal blood test.[149]

"It Happened in the Clinic"

Working on the postnatal wards of an obstetric hospital in the late 1970s, the author experienced some incidents that will not be forgotten. In the mid-1950s, some pregnant women used the drug thalidomide for the control of pregnancy-related nausea, and the results were catastrophic. The babies of these women were born with deformities of the limbs. Some had a hand attached at the shoulder, and others did not have an upper extremity at all. Some were born without legs. During the late 1970s, several mothers who had been affected by this problem gave birth to their own babies. These women were amazing in their ability to care for their infants. One mother cradled the baby within her legs and was able to feed the baby independently. Another used her toes to dress and undress the child. These women were a tribute to coping with the altered abilities of people affected by physical disabilities. They turned a problem into a challenge and a triumph.

Precautions and Contraindications for PT Intervention During Pregnancy

The PTA must understand the contraindications for physical therapy intervention when a woman is pregnant. Part of the general questions asked before any physical therapy intervention should include whether a female patient is pregnant or suspects she may be pregnant. The PT will have asked the patient about the status of pregnancy during the initial evaluation, but a change in status may occur during the course of treatment, so it is always safer to inquire before each treatment session. The PTA should notify the supervising PT immediately with any change in status of the patient. In some cases, this may mean not treating the patient that day. Precautions or contraindications exist for most modalities during pregnancy. The literature is lacking regarding the use of modalities during pregnancy, probably because it is neither ethical nor sound professional practice to perform research that might in any way affect the fetus. As a result of this, therapeutic ultrasound is generally considered contraindicated around the spine and abdomen during pregnancy, and many clinicians prefer not to provide any ultrasound during pregnancy to be absolutely safe. Care should be taken not to overheat the area of the lower abdomen and lumbar spine; therefore the use of any form of heat should be avoided in these areas. Most clinicians do not use electrical stimulation during pregnancy, although the use of TENS during the delivery process is sometimes used for pain management. Mobilizations of joints are not recommended as a result of the ligamentous laxity changes caused by hormones. Craniosacral techniques may be contraindicated because of their effect on the autonomic nervous system and the possible effects of relaxation on ligaments and muscles. Shortwave diathermy should not be used anywhere in the region of the abdomen, and again many clinicians choose not to use it at all. The use of gentle massage is one of the few modalities that can be safely used for pain relief during pregnancy. Even this should be carefully monitored for any unexpected side effects and discontinued where indicated. Ice packs may be used as a modality for pain control during pregnancy for minor sprains and muscle aches.

The degree of safe exercise during pregnancy is a highly controversial issue. Recent studies such as Barakat et al.[150] and Juhl et al.[151] have shown that moderate, supervised exercise does not adversely affect women with a singleton pregnancy, and indeed may improve heart function for both mother and child. Safe levels of metabolic, cardiac and respiratory rates should not be exceeded. In the later stages of pregnancy, the mother requires a greater recovery period after exercise. The position of the fetus prevents the mother from using the diaphragm to increase the depth of breathing, and much of the increased depth is achieved by costal expansion of the chest. In general, advice given to the mother should be to exercise to moderate levels and not push to maximal levels. Women who exercised before pregnancy can safely exercise during pregnancy unless advised not to do so by the physician. Women who did not exercise regularly can be encouraged to walk and swim starting with a few minutes per day and increasing to approximately 30 minutes per day. Avoidance of overstretching or sudden twisting movements should be emphasized to prevent damage to joints and muscles with lax ligaments. As the pregnancy progresses, the level of exercise should be monitored to ensure safe levels of heart, respiratory, and metabolic function. In addition, the mother should be instructed not to lie supine for more than a few minutes in the later stages of pregnancy, including when performing exercises, because this may create pressure on the vena cava from the fetus.[152,153] When pressure is placed on the vena cava, a reduction in venous return to the heart occurs that can reduce the cardiac output causing low blood pressure. In some women, pressure is exerted on the lower aorta when in supine, and this can result in reduced blood flow to the kidneys and lower extremities, and lack of sufficient gaseous exchange to the fetus.[154]

Pregnancy-Related Conditions

The pregnancy related conditions described in this section include those that may affect the woman during pregnancy, such as low back pain and gestational diabetes, and those that may affect both the woman and the developing fetus.

Ectopic Pregnancy

An **ectopic pregnancy** occurs when fertilization of the ovum takes place but the ovum does not pass into the uterus. The ovum may become implanted in the fallopian tube, the abdominal cavity, or within the ovary itself. The frequency of ectopic pregnancy is between 1 in 40 and 1 in 100 pregnancies.[155]

Etiology. Several factors increase the risk of ectopic pregnancy, including a past ectopic pregnancy, a past infection of the fallopian tubes or salpingitis (inflammation of the fallopian tubes), and pelvic inflammatory disease (PID). Other predisposing factors may include endometriosis, previous pelvic surgery, having in vitro fertilization, and using birth control hormone pills. Any of these conditions may cause scarring of the fallopian tube, which prevents the ovum passing down the tube to the uterus.[156]

Signs and Symptoms. Many of the symptoms associated with ectopic pregnancy can mimic normal pregnancy, such as amenorrhea (cessation of menses), breast tenderness, low back pain, and nausea. Other symptoms may include pain in the abdomen or pelvis or abnormal vaginal bleeding. When the area involved in the ectopic pregnancy ruptures, severe pain may be experienced, and shock can occur. These symptoms are considered a medical emergency.[157]

Prognosis. As a result of the timely medical intervention for most women with ectopic pregnancy, the mortality rate is less than 0.1% in the United States. Infertility may occur in between 10% and 15% of women who have an ectopic pregnancy.[158] The chances of a woman having another ectopic pregnancy are 15%.[159]

Medical Intervention. Testing for an ectopic pregnancy can include a pregnancy test for human chorionic gonadotropin hormone (hCG), transvaginal or abdominal ultrasound, and blood tests. Surgical procedures may include a laparoscopy, laparotomy, or a D & C. After the diagnosis is confirmed, the ectopic zygote must be removed to preserve the life of the mother, and in some cases, the blocked fallopian tube must also be removed. If shock occurs, intravenous fluids, a blood transfusion, and supplemental oxygen may be needed. Ectopic pregnancy is not a preventable condition. However, avoiding STDs and seeking medical attention for pelvic and abdominal infections can reduce the risk of abdominal scar formation.[160]

Physical Therapy Intervention. No physical therapy intervention is indicated for ectopic pregnancy.

Gestational diabetes

In the United States, between 3% and 8% of all pregnant women have **gestational diabetes,** which is classified as diabetes that occurs during pregnancy that was not present before the pregnancy. Women who have diabetes before pregnancy must monitor blood glucose levels carefully.[161]

Etiology. The inability of the maternal system to process glucose from carbohydrates during the stress of pregnancy is not fully understood. However, during pregnancy hormones prevent the usual action of insulin in processing glucose to ensure that the fetus receives sufficient glucose for growth. In response, the mother's body needs to produce more insulin and may be unable to do so. When insufficient insulin is produced, glucose builds up in the blood, causing gestational diabetes.[162]

Signs and Symptoms. No external signs or symptoms may be evident. Often high levels of blood glucose are the only indication of gestational diabetes.

Prognosis. Most women return to pre-pregnancy status after delivery and do not have diabetes. However, gestational diabetes is a risk factor for the development of diabetes later in life. Maternal gestational diabetes that is uncontrolled can result in fetal problems, such as macrosomia (large size), hypoglycemia (low levels of blood glucose), jaundice, and respiratory distress syndrome.[163] Fortunately close medical monitoring of women with gestational diabetes prevents these complications in most instances. Usually, the mother and infant do not have any side effects as a result of gestational diabetes.

Medical Intervention. Gestational diabetes is usually detected during routine prenatal physician visits through a simple glucose test. If gestational diabetes is suspected, an oral glucose tolerance test may be performed. This test entails fasting for 4 to 8 hours and then having a blood test for glucose levels. A sugary drink is then taken, and another glucose test is administered 2 hours later. If the glucose levels in the blood are still high after the 2 hours, this is considered a positive test for gestational diabetes.[164] In some women, insulin may have to be administered to maintain glucose at acceptable levels, but usually a combination of exercise, a healthy diet, weight control, and regular testing of blood glucose levels is sufficient. Blood glucose levels usually return to normal levels within a few weeks after delivery.

Physical Therapy Intervention. Physical therapy intervention may be indicated to provide advice and instruction regarding an appropriate exercise program for women during pregnancy in order to control gestational diabetes.

Low Back Pain in Pregnancy

Low back pain (LBP) during pregnancy is fairly common. An average of 50% of pregnant women experience back pain at some time during pregnancy with an incidence of between 24 and 90% depending on the source of the information. Approximately 67% of pregnant women experience some discomfort in the lumbar spine during the night. Perhaps of economic significance is that approximately 30% of pregnant women take sick leave as a result of low back pain during pregnancy.[165] Sacroiliac pain and dysfunction are common during pregnancy as a result of the ligamentous laxity.

Etiology. In some cases, the etiology may be the result of ligamentous laxity produced by hormonal changes, such as the production of relaxin, which cause sacroiliac or symphysis pubis pain. Occasionally the coccyx becomes dislocated. Muscular pain in the lumbar region can be caused by the altered center of gravity due to the weight of the fetus anteriorly. This causes an increased lordosis of the lumbar spine and results in muscular imbalances that can cause pain. The stretching of the abdominal muscles and weakness in the abdominal muscles before pregnancy contributes to the lack of support of the lumbar spine. The actual additional weight during pregnancy may overstress the muscles, especially when the abdominal muscles are weak. Additional theories point to pressure on the aorta and vena cava from the uterus causing ischemia of the muscles which leads to pain.[166] Other known causes of low back pain include pain referred to this area from compression on the inferior vena cava and the lumbosacral plexus, kidney infection, and sacroiliac joint dysfunction.[167]

Signs and Symptoms. A variety of low back pain symptoms are described by women who are pregnant. The pain may be in the lumbar spine, in the pelvic floor area, or radiate into the buttocks and legs. A thorough evaluation of women during pregnancy may be limited because of precautions regarding overstretching of joints and muscles. Low back pain occurs in some women after delivery, not only in those women who had pain during pregnancy.[168] Women who had sacroiliac pain during pregnancy often continue to have the pain and dysfunction after delivery.

Prognosis. The low back pain associated with pregnancy usually disappears after delivery. However, in some women, the back pain continues to cause problems and physical therapy intervention is required post partum. In a few cases, the back pain may result from a radiculopathy (spinal nerve entrapment) and may require medical diagnostic testing after delivery.

Medical Intervention. The medical testing for women during pregnancy is limited by the potential damage to the fetus from imaging studies, CT scans, and MRI. Some physicians prescribe acetaminophen, whereas others prefer that women avoid all medications during pregnancy. Moderate exercise and resting in a left-side-lying position may be the only avenues available to reduce the pain.

Physical Therapy Intervention. The lack of sufficient research studies regarding exercise and pregnancy means that best practices are not yet defined. Further research studies are sorely needed by physical therapists. PT intervention may focus on use of pregnancy back supports such as sacroiliac belts or abdominal binders made specifically for women during pregnancy, postural reeducation, and postural exercises. Muscle testing of the abdominals must be performed with caution due to the possibility of a **rectus abdominis diastasis.** This is a separation of the rectus abdominis muscle at the linea alba and is a contraindication to strenuous abdominal exercises. Other contraindications to exercise routines may include chronic diseases such as diabetes, although exercise can assist with controlling diabetes. Women who are pregnant should be under medical observation during pregnancy. Physical therapy intervention postpartum (after delivery) is often beneficial in reducing low back pain. Abdominal and pelvic-floor strengthening exercises, aerobic programs, posture reeducation, aquatherapy, and resting in prone lying may all be part of the rehabilitation sequence.[169]

Placenta Accreta

Placenta accreta is the embedding of the placenta more deeply than usual in the wall of the uterus, making the separation of the placenta after delivery impossible without additional assistance. Under normal circumstances, a membrane forms in the wall of the uterus dividing the placenta from the deep wall of the uterus. In placenta accreta, the membrane does not form, and the placenta embeds deeply in the myometrium (the deep muscular layer) of the uterus, causing it to remain fixed to the uterus after delivery. This condition occurs in approximately 1 in every 2,500 deliveries.[170]

Etiology. The etiology of placenta accreta is unknown. However, an increased incidence of the condition is noted when there is a preexisting placenta previa and in women with a history of previous caesarean sections or uterine surgery.[171] The incidence of placenta accreta can be as high as 25% for women who have placenta previa and have had two or more caesarean sections.[172]

Signs and Symptoms. Women with placenta accreta may have hemorrhaging during the third trimester of pregnancy or may have no symptoms.

Prognosis. Placenta accreta may lead to premature delivery of the infant. In some women, severe hemorrhage occurs during delivery, which can be life threatening. Women who hemorrhage may require a blood transfusion.

Medical Intervention. Placenta accreta may be diagnosed through transvaginal ultrasound in cases in which the mother has hemorrhaging during pregnancy. In some instances, placenta accreta may not be suspected until delay of more than 45 minutes of the delivery of the placenta occurs. In other cases, placenta accreta may be suspected because of the presence of risk factors previously described. Surgical removal of the placenta after delivery

is often necessary and is usually associated with a hysterectomy to prevent medical complications for the mother.

Physical Therapy Intervention. As part of the prenatal health team, the physical therapist may be involved with providing advice for adequate rest and positioning for helping to delay the onset of delivery. After hysterectomy, rehabilitation may include an exercise program and posture reeducation.

Placenta Previa

Placenta previa is development of the placenta either partially or totally over the internal opening of the cervix. This positioning creates complications when contractions start because the contractions of the uterus tend to loosen the placenta from the wall of the uterus. Placenta previa occurs in between 0.03 and 0.05 pregnancies in the United States and is one of the leading causes of hemorrhage during the third trimester of pregnancy.[173]

Etiology. The actual etiology of placenta previa is unknown. The risk factors for placenta previa include multiple gestations (multiple fetuses), multiparity (a women with the second or later pregnancy), a maternal age over 35 years, infertility treatments, previous surgery of the uterus, smoking, a history of recurrent abortions, and use of illicit drugs, particularly cocaine.[174,175]

Signs and Symptoms. Some loss of blood may occur in some women, especially during the third trimester when contractions of the uterus occur. Some women do not have any symptoms.

Prognosis. Women with placenta previa are at a higher risk of needing a caesarean delivery or blood transfusion and requiring a hysterectomy at the time of caesarean delivery. The risk of septicemia and thrombophlebitis is also increased. The mortality rate for the fetus in women with placenta previa is between 2% and 3%. Maternal mortality rate for women with the condition is approximately 0.03% in the United States.[176] Pre-term delivery occurs in 50% of women with placenta previa. The risk of fetal congenital abnormalities is also increased.

Medical Intervention. Diagnosis of placenta previa is achieved most frequently through transvaginal ultrasound, although ultrasound scanning over the abdomen or an MRI may be used.[177] An early diagnosis allows for the planning for possible complications during delivery and the delay of delivery until as close to the due date as possible. In some cases women who have hemorrhaging as a result of placenta previa may be hospitalized until delivery or admitted for an immediate caesarean section if the pregnancy is beyond 34 weeks.[178] Tocolytic medications that prevent contractions, and preterm labor may be prescribed. Women with placenta previa must undergo regular medical checks. A caesarean section delivery may be required, as well as a blood transfusion, if a severe hemorrhage occurs. Some women will also require a hysterectomy at the time of delivery.

Physical Therapy Intervention. No specific physical therapy intervention is indicated for placenta previa. Physical therapy may be provided to the mother in the postpartum phase for recovery from hysterectomy.

Postdate Pregnancy

A postdate pregnancy, also called postterm pregnancy or postmaturity syndrome, is one that extends up to 42 weeks or beyond. Approximately 3% to 12% of all pregnancies fall under this category. However, many instances of postterm pregnancy are the result of inaccuracy of due dates of delivery in women who have irregular menstrual cycles or who have some hemorrhaging during pregnancy.[179]

Etiology. Most postdate deliveries are the result of the cervix not being dilated to enable labor and delivery. The identified risk factors for a postterm delivery include women who have had a previous postterm delivery, a woman in primiparity (first baby), and a male fetus.

Signs and Symptoms. The woman extends beyond the usual 40 weeks of pregnancy and on ultrasound scan the fetus appears to be mature. The maturity of the fetus is the real factor in whether labor will be induced.

Prognosis. If pregnancy advances beyond 42 weeks, the risk of danger increases for the fetus. The placenta tends to lose its viability after 40 weeks and does not supply enough oxygen and nutrients to the fetus. A fetus who is postterm delivery may have macrosomia (be larger than usual), making the delivery process more difficult for both the fetus and the mother. Some of the complications resulting from a fetus with macrosomia include shoulder dystocia, meconium aspiration (inhalation of fecal matter into the lungs), and an increased risk of death during delivery. The mother is at risk for injury to the perineum, and is more likely to require caesarean section delivery.[180]

Medical Intervention. Determining the level of maturity of the fetus affects the decision whether to induce labor in women who are postterm. Ultrasound scans of the fetus are performed to determine the size of the fetus. Monitoring of the fetal heart rate is important to ensure that the fetus is not in circulatory distress. Labor may be induced in the mother if the fetus is considered mature and truly beyond 41 weeks gestation. The decision to induce labor is controversial with some studies showing that it may increase the risks to the fetus, whereas others saying induced labor has no significant effect on the fetal outcomes.[181,182] Medications containing prostaglandin may be administered vaginally in gel form or orally by tablet to stimulate the cervix to dilate. Mechanical dilation may be used.

Physical Therapy Intervention. Physical therapy intervention for the mother postpartum follows the same sequence as other deliveries. The risk for episiotomy and caesarean delivery is higher for a larger baby and may be an indication that the mother needs assistance with the healing process and pelvic floor muscle reeducation postpartum.

Preeclampsia

Preeclampsia, sometimes called toxemia of pregnancy, is a potentially dangerous disorder in the mother during pregnancy, or immediately postpartum (after delivery). This condition is characterized by hypertension and proteinuria (protein in the urine) and affects multiple body systems. The condition occurs in approximately 5% to 8% of all pregnancies.[183]

Etiology. The etiology of preeclampsia is unknown. Theories regarding the etiology include circulatory problems to the uterus, or in general in the maternal system, a poor diet, or an immune system dysfunction. The risk factors for preeclampsia are primigravida (first pregnancy), women having multiple fetuses, a woman with a prior history of preeclampsia or a history within the family, a maternal age over 35 years, obesity of the mother, gestational diabetes, and preexisting maternal conditions, such as hypertension, diabetes, systemic lupus erythematosus, or kidney disease.[184]

Signs and Symptoms. Preeclampsia usually occurs at about 20 weeks of gestation. Some women do not have any symptoms associated with the condition, whereas others have a variety of problems, including hypertension; proteinuria (protein in the urine); nausea and vomiting;

edema of face, hands, and feet; severe headaches; vision problems; dizziness; unusual weight gain; and reduced urine output.[185] The complications of preeclampsia can include placenta abruption (premature separation of the placenta from the inner wall of the uterus); reduced circulatory flow to the placenta, which may result in a reduced birth weight of the fetus, a premature birth, or a stillbirth; HELLP syndrome, which is an acronym for the first letters of a life-threatening condition causing hemolysis (destruction of the red blood cells), elevated levels of liver enzymes, and a low platelet count; and, in severe cases, eclampsia, which is characterized by all the symptoms of preeclampsia plus seizures and can result in coma, brain damage, and death of the mother and fetus if not treated.[186]

Prognosis. The presence of preeclampsia has implications for delivery and may be one reason for a caesarean delivery. Preeclampsia is a leading cause of mortality in both women and infants with 76,000 maternal deaths and 500,000 infant/fetal deaths attributed to the condition each year in the United States alone.[187]

Medical Intervention. Preeclampsia is diagnosed during routine prenatal physician visits. When the maternal blood pressure readings are consistently higher than 140/90 mm Hg and proteinuria is detected, preeclampsia is suspected. When diagnosed, the mother and fetus have to be monitored closely. The growth of the fetus is monitored with regular ultrasound scans and the detection of fetal movement.[188] If the condition becomes severe, the baby may have to be delivered prematurely to preserve the life of both the mother and baby. The delivery may be through caesarean section.

Physical Therapy Intervention. If the physical therapist is part of the prenatal team, monitoring of the maternal blood pressure is a regular procedure. Consistently high blood pressure over 140/90 is reason for the mother to seek the physician's advice. In cases of premature delivery of an infant, the physical therapist and PTA may be involved with intervention for the premature infant and ongoing intervention for developmental delay problems of the child.

Premature Birth ☹

Premature birth occurs when an infant is delivered less than 37 weeks into the pregnancy. Babies born prematurely are often called "preemies" and have a low birth weight. Approximately 8% to 10% of babies are born prematurely.[189]

Etiology. In many cases, the cause of premature delivery is unknown. An **incompetent cervix** is weak and dilated and can cause premature effacement and labor, leading to a premature delivery of the fetus. Premature rupture of the amniotic sac can also cause premature delivery. Placenta previa, placenta accreta, and abruptio placenta can all cause premature delivery. Abruptio placenta is a condition in which the placenta loosens from the wall of the uterus before the fetus is delivered and precipitates early delivery. Abruptio placenta usually occurs at about Week 20 of pregnancy and is more common in multigravidae. The presence of multiple fetuses carries a high likelihood of a premature delivery. Other causes may be trauma to the mother or illness. Risk factors when predicting the possibility of a premature birth include maternal smoking, drinking alcohol, or using illicit drugs; maternal conditions such as diabetes or hypertension: under- or overweight women; urinary or genital tract infections; previous multiple miscarriages or abortions or previous preterm labor; and severe stress during pregnancy.[190,191]

Signs and Symptoms. A variety of symptoms can indicate the possibility of premature delivery. Daily multiple uterine contractions, lumbar pain, pelvic pain or feelings of increased pressure in the pelvis, vaginal bleeding or discharge, and diarrhea may all herald the early onset of labor.[192]

Prognosis. The earlier in the gestation an infant is born, the greater the risk for complications. In the very immature fetus, the organs may not be completely developed, and there may be esophageal atresia in which the esophagus is not connected to the stomach. **Respiratory distress syndrome of the newborn,** a lung immaturity resulting from lack of lung surfactant in infants below 34 weeks of gestation, results in the need for a respirator. The production of lung surfactant occurs between weeks 34 and 37 in the fetus. The lungs are unable to remain inflated without the presence of surfactant. The risk for respiratory distress syndrome is most prevalent when infants are born under 28 weeks of gestation. In 2005 (the most recent available data), 16,268 babies were affected by respiratory distress syndrome in the United States.[193] Other complications for the infant can include apnea (cessation of breathing), cerebral palsy, intracranial hemorrhage or hydrocephalus, developmental delay and learning disabilities, and intestinal and vision problems. A condition called retinopathy of prematurity (ROP) often affects very low birth weight babies of 2.75 pounds and under 31 weeks gestation. This bilateral eye condition affects between 14,000 and 16,000 infants per year and causes legal blindness in approximately 400 to 600 annually.[194] Initially the infant may have jaundice, anemia, and hypotension.

Medical Intervention. Regular medical checks during pregnancy are essential to monitor the progress of the mother and fetus. Advice on the prevention of premature delivery may include cessation of the use of smoking, alcohol, and illicit drugs during pregnancy; maintaining a healthy diet; and keeping chronic medical conditions, such as diabetes and hypertension, under control.[195] When women have any of the signs and symptoms previously described, the physician will check for dilation of the cervix and an intact amniotic sac. An ultrasound of the cervix can indicate the status of the cervix, and a swab of the cervix can be tested for presence of fetal fibronectin, which is present during labor.[196] In the case of an incompetent cervix, the mother may be placed on bed rest, or a suture may be used in the cervix known as **cerclage** to prevent delivery of the fetus. When placenta previa, placenta accreta, or abruptio placentae are present, a caesarean section may be required to save the life of the premature infant. Premature infants are placed in the pediatric intensive care unit (PICU) on life-sustaining measures for feeding and breathing until the body organs mature sufficiently to function independently.

Physical Therapy Intervention. Intervention for the infant may be necessary in the neonatal intensive care unit (NICU) for assistance with pulmonary hygiene techniques and postural drainage. Physical therapy intervention is commonly provided for premature infants both in early childhood intervention programs and during the school years if necessary. The developmental delays associated with prematurity can be addressed by a team of rehabilitation professionals, including the physical therapist and assistant, occupational therapist, and speech and language pathologist. When working with children born prematurely, the use of a "corrected age" may be used for the first year or two after birth. This correction makes allowances for the developmental age of the child by subtracting the number of weeks prematurity from the actual birth age.[197]

Rh Incompatability

Rh incompatibility, or hemolytic disease of the newborn (HDN), is described in Chapter 2. This occurs when the mother is rhesus negative and the baby rhesus positive. During the first pregnancy, there is usually no problem, but at delivery of the placenta or the fetus, the blood of the baby may mingle with that of the mother causing antibodies to form to the rhesus-positive blood. In a subsequent pregnancy, these antibodies cause a reaction in the fetus that can result in destruction of fetal red blood cells. This reaction causes anemia, jaundice, and possibly death of the fetus. When incompatibility of blood types between the mother and the fetus is known, the mother can be given Rh immunoglobulin (RhoGAM) immediately after birth to prevent the formation of antibodies in her blood.

Spontaneous Abortion and Miscarriage

Spontaneous abortion, or termination of a pregnancy before the 20th week, often called miscarriage, occurs in up to 20% of known pregnancies in the United States.[198] The incidence tends to be higher during a first pregnancy.

Etiology. The etiology of miscarriage is largely unknown and unpredictable, but some cases are caused by fetal or placental abnormalities. Others may be the result of incomplete implantation of the ovum in the uterus or a maternal infection or illness. Low levels of folate (folic acid) in the mother are attributed to a higher risk of miscarriage.[199] Other risk factors for miscarriage include an incompetent (lax) cervix, smoking during pregnancy, the use of illegal drugs or high alcohol intake, chronic disease of the mother, maternal infections, and an older maternal age.[200]

Signs and Symptoms. The characteristics of miscarriage include vaginal discharge or bleeding and abdominal pain or cramps. In some cases, the woman may not even realize she has been pregnant.[201]

Prognosis. Many women who have a miscarriage can have a later successful pregnancy. Reducing the risk factors involved by smoking cessation, not drinking alcohol or using illicit drugs, having treatment for chronic diseases, exercising regularly, and eating a healthy diet can reduce the risk of further miscarriage. Many physicians recommend women to start taking between 400 and 600 micrograms of folic acid per day up to 2 months before conception if possible and to continue taking the supplement during the pregnancy.[202] Folic acid is a B vitamin essential for cell growth. When taken by women who are pregnant, folic acid can reduce the risk of some of the major spine and brain birth defects such as spina bifida.[203] A daily multivitamin may also be recommended during pregnancy.

Medical Intervention. The presence of thyroid autoantibodies in the blood has been associated with an increased risk of miscarriage during the first trimester of pregnancy.[204] A 2004 study is also promising for predicting when a miscarriage may occur. This study demonstrated low levels of an immune system protein called macrophage inhibitory cytokine 1 (MIC-1) in women who miscarried, compared with women who delivered at full term. Low levels of MIC-1 may be a predictor of potential miscarriage.[205] In 2007, a study reported by Stephenson in the *Journal of the American Medical Association* showed that a newly discovered substance called D6, normally produced by the placenta, reduced inflammation and helped to protect the fetus from miscarriage in mice. The study is showing promise for the treatment of women at risk for miscarriage (p. 686).[206] In women who have an incompetent cervix a surgical procedure called cerclage, or stitching the mouth of the cervix closed, may be performed.

Physical Therapy Intervention. Physical therapy intervention usually is not indicated after miscarriage. However, in some cases, abdominal strengthening exercises, pelvic floor exercises, and an aerobic exercise program may be indicated.

Labor

The process of labor includes the complete delivery of the fetus and placenta and the period after delivery. Physical therapy interventions are commonly used during pregnancy, labor, and after delivery. A discussion of labor is included here to facilitate the PTA's understanding of the usual and unusual effects of the labor process on the body of the woman as well as on the fetus.

STAGES OF LABOR

Labor is separated into four stages: first, second, third, and postpartum. (Some sources do not include the fourth phase, which is the postpartum). Labor is classified as the series of events leading up to, and including, birth of the fetus, expulsion of the placenta, and the postpartum phase (see Fig. 11-7).

• During the first stage of labor, the cervix dilates to allow for the passage of the fetal head and the uterus starts to contract to push the head into the cervix. The mucus plug that formed during the pregnancy to keep the cervix sealed is expelled, sometimes with evidence of a little blood, but often eliminated without notice when using the toilet. The contractions become stronger, longer, and more frequent as the baby gets closer to delivery. The amniotic sac ruptures (the "water" breaks), and the cervix becomes prepared to act as the birth canal. This stage lasts approximately 8 to12 hours. If this stage lasts longer than 24 hours, the physician usually intervenes to speed up delivery.[207]

• The second stage of labor is the actual delivery of the infant. The uterus contracts strongly under the influence of the hormone oxytocin released by the pituitary gland. During this stage of delivery a determination must be made whether the mother can deliver vaginally or requires a **caesarean section.** Consideration is given to the size of the pelvic opening and the condition of the baby. If the heartbeat of the fetus is monitored and appears to be in distress, the decision may be made to perform a caesarean section. The caesarean section involves abdominal surgery performed to remove the fetus. In some cases, the baby may be delivered with the help of forceps. For a vaginal delivery, the cervix must dilate 10 cm before actual delivery of the head of the baby. The thinning of the cervix that takes place is called effacement, and when the cervix is dilated 10 cm, it is said to be complete effacement or 100% effacement.[208] The fetus usually descends through the birth canal head first, and the neck rotates to cause the normal presentation with the face pointing toward the spine of the mother. The appearance of the head of the fetus at the opening of the vagina is called crowning. In some cases the contractions do not lead to cervical dilation, and this is called dystocia, or delay in labor. The term dystocia is also applied to any complication in the delivery process that might require surgical intervention with a caesarean section.[209,210] The second stage of labor takes approximately 50 minutes for primigravidas and 20 minutes for multiparas. During this delivery stage, the mother's perineum becomes stretched, which produces a natural anesthetic effect that dulls the sensation of pain. The pressure of the head of the fetus stimulates nerve receptors in the pelvic floor of the mother, causing the Ferguson's reflex, which makes the mother want to push down and facilitate delivery of the fetus. [211]

• The third stage of labor is the delivery of the placenta. This occurs almost immediately after the birth of the baby as a result of continued uterine contractions and lasts approximately 15 to 30 minutes. In some cases, assistance is necessary for expulsion of the placenta. The placenta must be examined to make sure it is complete to ensure none of the material remains within the uterus of the mother to cause infection.[212]

• The fourth and final stage of labor is postpartum literally meaning "after delivery."

First stage of labor

Second stage of labor begins

Second stage of labor continues

Second stage of labor ends

Birth

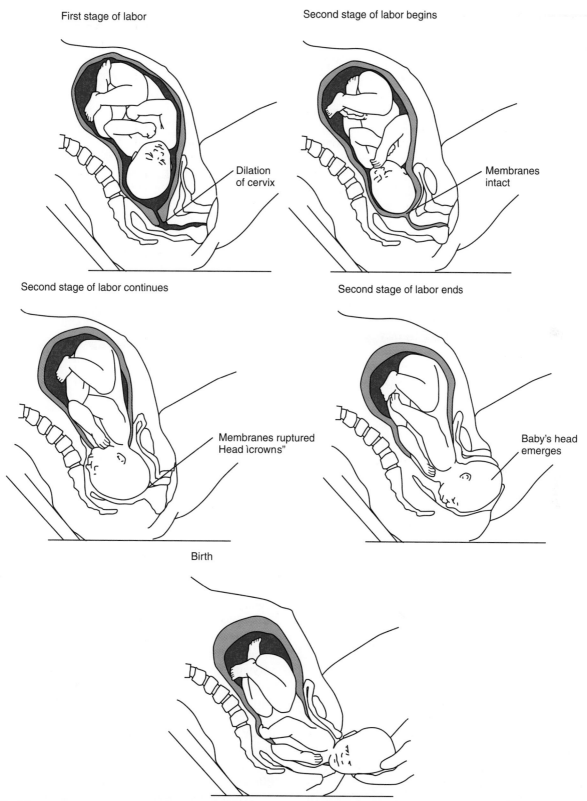

FIGURE 11.7 The stages of labor: (A) During the first stage of labor, the fetal head is in the effacement position and the cervix starts to dilate. (B) As the second stage of labor begins, the baby's head turns and progresses down the birth canal. (C) During the later part of the second stage of labor, the membranes rupture and the baby's head "crowns." (D) As the second stage of labor ends, the baby's head emerges. (E) During birth, the baby's head turns sideways and the shoulders rotate to enable the baby to exit the birth canal.

PHYSICAL THERAPY INTERVENTION FOR THE NEW MOTHER

PT intervention can be helpful after delivery to assist with the prevention of thromboembolisms by encouraging early mobilization and activity and providing pelvic floor and gentle progressive abdominal exercises to reeducate these muscles. During the first stage of labor, the PT and PTA can assist the mother with breathing correctly and relaxing in order to avoid pushing too soon, before the cervix is fully dilated. Physical therapy intervention during pregnancy may include prenatal exercise regimes, pelvic floor exercises, breathing exercises, and coaching for delivery breathing strategies. Advice for the postpartum phase to help the mother return to normal full function after delivery of the baby may also be included.

Complications of Labor

A brief description of some of the complications of labor is provided. The physical therapy interventions associated with the complication are included, where appropriate, as an overview of how the PT and PTA may be involved in the obstetrics setting.

Breech Delivery

A breech presentation is when any other part of the fetus besides the fetal head presents in the cervix during the first stage of labor. Breech births occur in 4% of all pregnancies.[213,214] Several types of breech presentation may occur and are described by the way in which the lower extremities appear in the birth canal (see Table 11-7 and Fig. 11-8). The risk factors for having a breech delivery include a fetus that is delivered before full-term, multiple fetuses, placenta previa, hydrocephalus of the fetus, women who have had breech deliveries before, and women with abnormalities of the uterus. Because the mortality

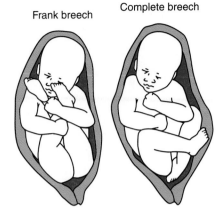

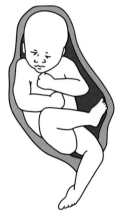

FIGURE 11.8 Types of breech presentations. (A) Frank breech in which the buttocks are presented to the cervix and the legs are extended. (B) Complete or full breech in which the buttocks are presented to the cervix and the legs are crossed. (C) Single footling breech in which one leg exits the birth canal first and the other leg is flexed within the uterus.

rate for breech delivered babies is approximately 3 times that of normal deliveries, and the risk of injury to the fetus and the mother are both greater than for a cephalic delivery (head first), the physician has to evaluate whether to perform a caesarean section.[215] Most of the damage to the fetus results from the head being delivered through a cervix that is not fully dilated. If the fetus is very small, it may be possible to deliver the baby safely vaginally. In some cases, the fetus can be turned within the uterus before delivery and a normal presentation of the head can be effected. In other cases, the fetus may be turned but turns back again to a breech presentation immediately before delivery.

Physical Therapy Intervention. No physical therapy intervention is indicated during a breech delivery. However,

Table 11.7 **Types of Breech Presentation**

TYPE OF BREECH PRESENTATION	DESCRIPTION
Frank breech	Legs extended, hips flexed, feet round chin; buttocks delivered first
Complete breech	Legs crossed in tailor sitting position
Single footling breech	One foot in birth canal
Double footling breech	Both feet in birth canal

if an episiotomy was performed to allow vaginal delivery of a breech presentation fetus, physical therapy intervention may be indicated for the mother postpartum. (See section on episiotomy for details.)

Caesarean Section Delivery

Caesarean section is the surgical removal of the fetus through the abdomen of the mother. In the United States in 2006 (the most recent data available at this writing), there were 1,367,340 caesarean section deliveries, accounting for 32% of all babies delivered.[216] The incision is either transverse across the lower abdomen (bikini,-type scar) or vertical. Many reasons exist for performing a caesarean section delivery. The chances of requiring a C-section are higher if the mother has previously had a C-section. Other reasons for caesarean delivery include the mother's pelvis being too small for the vaginal delivery of the fetus; multiple babies are present; the baby is in a breech position; the presence of a condition such as placenta previa, abruptio placentae, or preeclampsia; if the umbilical cord is wrapped round the neck of the fetus; the fetus is in respiratory distress; or the mother has undergone trauma or illness that endangers the fetus.[217] Other reasons for caesarean section include mothers who have diabetes mellitus, genital herpes, HIV, or rhesus incompatibility or if the fetus has a congenital condition such as spina bifida or hydrocephalus.[218] The caesarean section may be performed under a general anesthesia or an epidural anesthesia through the spine. An epidural anesthesia numbs the nerves below the waist so that the mother cannot feel pain. The mortality rate for infants is lower with this intervention, but the morbidity and mortality rates for the mother are higher. Complications for the mother may include a risk of uterine and surgical site infection, increased possibility of bleeding, blood clots, and urinary tract infections.[219]

Physical Therapy Intervention. PT interventions for the mother after caesarean delivery may include a progressive abdominal exercise program, pelvic floor exercises, ambulation training, and the use of TENS or other electrical modalities to reduce the effects of pain.

Episiotomy

An **episiotomy** is a commonly used incision of the maternal perineum to enlarge the opening of the vagina to assist the delivery of the fetus and reduce uncontrolled tears of the maternal perineum (see Fig. 11-9). The incision is made in the midline between the opening of the vagina and the rectum or mediolaterally into the muscle mass. The theory that if a tear occurs naturally during delivery, it may cause damage to more structures than an episiotomy is slowly changing. Many U.S. health institutions and the World Health Organization now recommend an episiotomy only be used in cases in which the fetus is in danger, the mother has extensive scarring from a previous surgery of birth, or birth complications such as a breech delivery or the need for forceps assisted delivery occur.[220,221] Natural tears of the perineum during the birthing process are categorized in four levels: a first degree, in which the tear is superficial; a second degree, which includes damage to the layers of muscle of the perineum; a third degree, which includes damage to sphincters; and a fourth degree, which may include extensive damage to the vagina, perineum, external genitalia, and the wall of the rectum. Tears have to be stitched after delivery. An episiotomy is nevertheless becoming an increasingly controversial procedure because the size of the episiotomy is usually greater than that of a tear produced

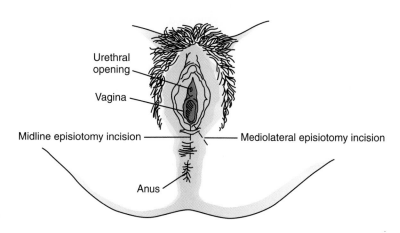

Urethral opening
Vagina
Midline episiotomy incision
Mediolateral episiotomy incision
Anus

FIGURE 11.9 Commonly used episiotomy incisions.

by the birthing process. A study by Bodner-Adler et al. in 2001 determined that midline incision episiotomy was associated with an increased risk of Grade 3, severe anal and sphincter tears.[222] Obviously, an episiotomy is preferable to a third- or fourth-degree tear because it may avoid excessive damage to pelvic floor structures. An episiotomy potentially controls the direction of the damage and prevents damage to structures that may otherwise take a long time to heal. Most episiotomies heal without problem after stitching.

Physical Therapy Intervention. The research results regarding massage of the perineal floor during both pregnancy and delivery have been mixed. Although some studies have shown massage to be effective in stretching the muscles and reducing the necessity for an episiotomy and the incidence of perineal floor damage, other studies have found no difference between the outcomes for those women who practiced massage compared to those who did not.[223,224] Self-massage of the perineal floor can be taught to pregnant women in preparation for the delivery process. PT intervention may be required to assist in the healing process of the episiotomy. Such intervention may also be applied to tears. The use of heat and electrical stimulation may relieve pain and stimulate the healing process. Pelvic floor exercises and electrical stimulation may also be indicated to reeducate the muscles and prevent complications such as urinary frequency or incontinence and fecal incontinence. Use of these modalities in cases of existing pelvic floor musculature weakness can also assist with return of function and relief of incontinence.

Forceps-Assisted Delivery

The use of forceps to assist delivery is not used as often today as a result of the increased use of the caesarean section since the mid-1960s. However, during the second stage of labor, when the fetus is delivered, the use of forceps to assist the delivery may be used when the progress of the delivery is very slow. The forceps are placed around the head or pelvis of the infant and gentle traction is applied. Other indications for the use of forceps include distress of the fetus; maternal distress with exhaustion; or preexisting maternal complications, such as hypertension, cardiac disease, or severe preeclampsia in which the effort of delivery would endanger the mother. Forceps may also be used during a breech vaginal delivery to protect the head of the fetus.[225] An episiotomy is often performed to facilitate the use of forceps in such cases. (See section on episiotomy for details.)

Physical Therapy Intervention. No physical therapy intervention is indicated during a forceps delivery. However, in cases of episiotomy, electrical stimulation, heat modalities, and progressive pelvic floor exercises may be used for rehabilitation of the pelvic floor musculature.

Multiple Births

According to the National Center for Health Statistics (2009) the incidence of twins in 2007 (most recent available data at this writing) was 32.2 per 1,000 births with a total number of twin births of 138,961 in the United States. The incidence of triplets or a higher numbers of infants was 148.9 per 100,000 live births.[226] When more than one fetus is present, the delivery is often premature. Labor often occurs between Weeks 37 and 38 for twins and even sooner when there are more than two fetuses. Twins may present in different ways. One fetus may present normally and the other breech. The multiple fetuses may become entwined or try to descend into the neck of the cervix at the same time. Caesarean section delivery may be necessary to reduce the risk of injury to the infants.[227]

Physical Therapy Intervention. Physical therapy intervention may be indicated for women with episiotomy or after a caesarean delivery as a result of the birth of multiple infants.

Postpartum Issues and Problems

Some of the following postpartum conditions often require the use of physical therapy interventions for resolution. These conditions include those affecting the muscles, ligaments, and joints of the pelvis.

Muscle Tone, Ligamentous Laxity, and Injuries

Postpartum (after delivery), the abdominal muscles are stretched, and the pelvic ligaments are lax as a result of the hormonal changes present from the childbirth. Laxity of the rectus abdominis muscle in addition to the stretch placed on the muscle by the weight of the fetus may cause a rectus diastasis in which the muscle separates from the linea alba fascial band that runs down the center of the muscle. Rectus diastasis may also occur during labor when the mother is pushing. A rectus diastasis is classified as a gap of more than two fingertips, width between adjacent sides of the rectus abdominis muscle at the level of the umbilicus when the muscle is contracted. The presence of a rectus abdominis diastasis contraindicates excessive abdominal exercises.

The internal ligaments that support the uterus and ovaries can also become damaged and stretched during delivery. This can cause uterine or cervical prolapse (projection of the structure beyond its normal boundaries), resulting in the tissue of these structures projecting through the external vaginal opening. This process may begin after delivery but may not become a real problem until menopause, when surgery is required. Sometimes the bladder projects into the vagina through a cystocele (bulge into the vagina), and coughing or lifting heavy objects will make it worse. Such conditions require surgery because they may cause difficulty with urination. After delivery, some women experience stress incontinence, which may or may not resolve.

An additional complication for women after childbirth is stretching of the pelvic floor musculature. The constant stress of supporting the weight of the fetus, placenta, and amniotic fluid stretches the muscles of the pelvic floor, causing weakness after delivery. In addition, an episiotomy or pelvic floor tear may increase the weakness of the muscles. This weakness can result in different levels of urinary incontinence. Frequency of micturition (the need to pass urine frequently) and stress incontinence (incontinence when the intra-abdominal pressure increases during coughing, sneezing, or laughing) are the most common problems.[228]

Physical Therapy Intervention. Postpartum PT intervention for the patient with rectus diastasis can include simple isometric abdominal exercises with the patient in a well-supported position such as supine, but no curls, rotations, or lower abdominal exercises involving lowering of the legs should be performed until the diastasis is healed. Women are at risk for low back injury until the abdominal muscles have returned to their pre-pregnancy state because the muscles are unable to create the positive intra-abdominal pressure necessary for good lumbar spine support. Women should also be instructed in how to sit up from supine by rolling onto their side first and using their arms to push into sitting. They should be cautioned about not sitting straight up from a supine position, which could cause further injury to the back and an increase in the rectus diastasis. If there is no rectus diastasis, women can start progressive strengthening of the abdominal muscles within a day of delivery with the permission of the physician. The PTA should be aware of rectus diastasis when providing postpartum exercises. The PT performing the evaluation should note the presence of the diastasis, and the PTA must be fully aware of the contraindications for exercise and adapt the exercise program appropriately within the plan of care.

Physical therapy intervention for pelvic floor weakness and associated urinary incontinence, either frequency of micturition or stress incontinence, may include pelvic floor muscle exercises, the use of vaginal weights to strengthen the muscles of the pelvic floor, and biofeedback therapy using a vaginal electrode to reeducate the muscles.

Pelvic Joint Injuries

The main joints injured as a result of delivery are the symphysis pubis, sacroiliac joints, and the coccyx. A small amount of symphysis pubis separation is normal during delivery, but if the baby is large, ligamentous damage can occur, causing joint subluxations and dislocations. Damage to the symphysis pubis and sacroiliac joints causes extreme pain in the areas of these joints, which is made worse by walking. Damage to the bladder may also occur during delivery, resulting in blood in the urine. Fracture or dislocation of the maternal coccyx can occur during delivery, leading to severe pain when sitting.

Physical Therapy Intervention. PT intervention for symphysis pubis and sacroiliac joint problems may include heat to reduce pain, postural advice, and instruction to reduce the risk for further injury until the joints heal. A sacroiliac binder is usually used to immobilize and stabilize the sacroiliac and symphysis pubis joints. In the case of a fracture or dislocation of the coccyx, the physical therapist may be able to perform manual therapy to correct the problem. The PTA may be involved with using modalities to reduce the pain and give advice on positioning for comfort.

Postpartum Depression and Psychosis

Some level of postpartum depression occurs to various degrees in approximately 20% of women.[229] A study by Benoit et al. (2007) found a relationship between levels of depression in women postpartum and both low income and the poor level of medical support services during pregnancy (p. 719).[230] Another study by White et al. (2006) found that a different dimension of postpartum depression included a posttraumatic stress disorder linked to particularly difficult birthing experiences.[231] Feelings of emotional upset are common due to the normal stresses of having a child. Physiologically, changes in body chemistry transpire as the woman returns to her pre-pregnant state. Hormonal changes and fluid balance changes occur. Psychologically the mother also has to adapt to the presence of a dependent infant and a change in the family dynamics. The depression can take the form of a "postpartum blues," which usually lasts only a few days. However, the depression may last several weeks and require constant care of both the mother and child. When the depression turns into a bipolar disorder, the condition is called postpartum psychosis. Women who develop postpartum psychosis are more likely to have had episodes of depression or bipolar disorder prenatally and require a full psychiatric examination and treatment.[232,233] The awareness of severe postpartum psychoses has been raised as a result of publicity in the news media of women who have murdered their children during periods of postpartum psychosis. The onset of feelings of suicide or urges to kill children, or others, requires immediate referral to a psychiatrist. The actual cause of postpartum psychosis is not yet known.

Why Does the Physical Therapist Assistant Need to Know About Menopause?

The recognition of the common effects of menopause has an impact on the understanding of these effects on the choice of physical therapy intervention and the suitability of the person for treatment. The PTA needs to be able to make appropriate clinical decisions to refer the patient back to the physical therapist or the physician.

Menopause

Menopause is the normal process of reduction and eventual cessation of menses in a woman. Menopause is not a disease but is discussed in this chapter as a result of the various medical ramifications for women. The average age of onset of menopause is between 45 and 51 years. True menopause is verified after 1 year without menstruation, although at the start of menopause the menstrual cycle may become less frequent (oligomenorrhea). The period of 1 year after the final menstruation is called menopausal transition or perimenopause.[234] In some women, the cycle stops and never starts again (amenorrhea). The onset of menopause is directly related to the end of ovulation by the ovaries. In some cases, early menopause is precipitated by an oophorectomy (surgery for removal of the ovaries) or a hysterectomy. Smoking has

also been shown to cause early menopause in some women.[235] Menopause is characterized by a lack of production of estrogen and progesterone. Some women may be advised, and choose, to take hormone replacement therapy (HRT), sometimes called estrogen replacement therapy (ERT), to reduce the symptoms of menopause. A variety of studies have demonstrated conflicting results about whether HRT reduces the risk of heart disease in some women.[236,237] A definitive answer has not been found. The same controversy exists regarding whether HRT reduces the risk of developing Alzheimer's disease.[238]

The characteristic signs and symptoms of menopause include changes in the lining of the vagina and cervix, resulting in reduced lubrication, reduced elasticity, and dryness. Difficulties with sexual intercourse may result from these changes. The wall of the uterus starts to thin, and the supporting ligaments and muscles of the uterus become reduced in tone. This may result in uterine prolapse and stress incontinence described earlier in this chapter. Flushing, commonly called hot flashes, may occur during the day or night, causing profuse sweating. Prescription antidepressants may effectively control hot flashes if they interfere with everyday life.[239] Other symptoms include headaches and insomnia (trouble sleeping). These symptoms vary in intensity and duration. Some women only experience symptoms for a short time, whereas others may have them for several years. Other effects of menopause include mood swings, lack of concentration, and thinning of the hair.[240] In some women, the physiological changes associated with menopause include reduced thyroid function and reduction in insulin production. Severe effects may include neurological changes, which may cause confusion, and memory loss. Balance may be affected resulting in a high incidence of falls. Probably the most drastic effect of the reduction of estrogen is the bone loss associated with osteoporosis (see Chapter 5). The incidence of hip, spine, and forearm fractures in older women is largely the result of osteoporosis. This bone loss is related to the reduction of estrogen production. Additional protection against osteoporosis recommended by the International Osteoporosis Foundation is a calcium supplement intake of 1,000 mg per day for women between age 19 years and menopause. Postmenopausal women are recommended to take 1,300 mg per day.[241] The National Osteoporosis Foundation in the United States recommends women over age 50 years take 1,200 mg of calcium per day, and 800 to 1,000 IU of vitamin D per day. Vitamin D enhances the absorption of calcium by the body.[242] Elemental calcium is the most readily absorbed by the body. Taking vitamin D assists with the absorption of calcium. A healthy diet rich in calcium is extremely crucial to bone health in children and adolescents. Many children do not have a high enough intake of calcium, and this puts them at risk of developing osteoporosis later in life. The greater the bone density in early life, the less will be the effect of losing half the bone density with age. Regular weight-bearing exercise, particularly walking, is also beneficial in maintaining healthy, strong bones.[243]

Why Does the Physical Therapist Assistant Need to Know About the Anatomy and Physiology of the Male Reproductive System?

An understanding of the male reproductive anatomy, which is closely linked with the urinary system, is important when discussing the diseases of the reproductive system. Physical therapist assistants are expected to recognize the medical terminology used regarding the male reproductive system to converse with other medical personnel.

Male Reproductive Anatomy

The reproductive and urinary systems of the male are closely linked to each other, thus the disease symptoms of these systems are often associated. The male reproductive system consists of the external structures of the penis, scrotum, and testes and the internal system, which includes the prostate gland, seminal vesicle, and ejaculatory duct (see Fig. 11-10).

The testes are located external to the body within the scrotal sac. This position maintains the temperature of the testes slightly below body temperature at about 96° Fahrenheit to keep the sperm healthy and motile (actively moving). The testes develop inside the body and descend to the outside of the body immediately prior to birth. Each testis is approximately 1.5 × 1 inches and consists of lobes containing seminiferous tubules in which the sperm develop. The seminiferous tubules are each approximately 250 meters long.[244] Testosterone is produced within the testes. Each sperm consists of a head with an acrosome and a nucleus containing the 23 chromosomes, a central portion containing mitochondria, and a tail or flagellum for propulsion (see Fig. 11-11). A sperm takes approximately 74 days to mature. Attached to each testis is a muscular tube approximately 6 meters in length called the

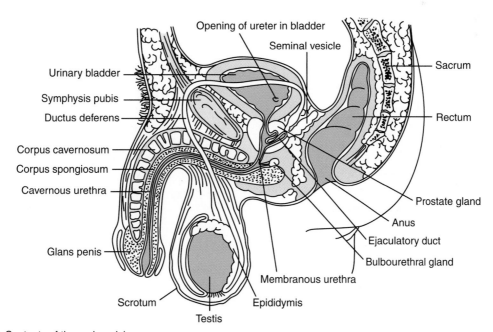

FIGURE 11.10 Contents of the male pelvis.

Mature sperm cell

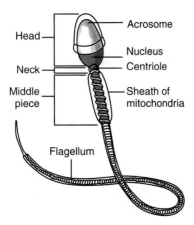

FIGURE 11.11 The structure of a mature sperm cell.

epididymis, which is looped against the posterior aspect of the testis (see Fig. 11-12). The sperm mature in the epididymis and are then propelled into the 35-cm-long ductus deferens, or vas deferens, and through the urethra by ejaculation, to fertilize the egg within the female during sexual intercourse. The ductus deferens enters the pelvis through the inguinal canal adjacent to the inguinal nerves and blood vessels, where it loops around the bladder and into the seminal vesicle and becomes the ejaculatory duct. The ejaculatory ducts enter the urethra. The prostate gland is situated just distal to the bladder and encloses the urethra. Both the seminal vesicles and the prostate gland secrete fluids that assist sperm motility. Another gland called the bulbourethral gland is located near the prostate and also produces lubricating fluid. The ductus deferens, ejaculatory ducts, prostate glands, penis, and pelvic floor muscles all play a part in ejaculation of the sperm. The ejaculation fluid consists of alkaline secretions, which neutralize the acid content of the female uterus to enable implantation of the sperm in the uterine wall. The penis contains the urethra, which acts as the opening duct for both urine, and semen. The tip of the penis is called the glans penis and is covered by the foreskin when the male is not circumcised. The walls of the penis consist of erectile tissue consisting of connective tissue and smooth muscle, with a rich blood supply. Sexual arousal causes these blood vessels to dilate under the control of the parasympathetic nervous system, causing erection of the penis. The ejaculate fluid is called semen, and contains between 20 million and 150 million sperm per milliliter.[245] Ejaculate fluid consists of fluid formed by the seminal vesicles, bulbourethral glands, and the prostate. Several hormones are responsible for sexual function in the male. Follicle-stimulating hormone (FSH) is produced by the anterior pituitary gland in response to the release of gonadotropin-releasing hormone (GnRH) from the hypothalamus. FSH stimulates the testes to produce sperm. Luteinizing hormone (LH), also produced in the anterior pituitary, stimulates the testes to produce testosterone, which in turn stimulates sex drive, secondary sexual male characteristics such as body hair growth, and muscular development and assists with the maturity of the sperm.[246] Both FSH and LH are necessary for the maturation of sperm.[247]

Why Does the Physical Therapist Assistant Need to Know About Diseases of the Male Reproductive System?

Some knowledge of male reproductive diseases is advisable for the PTA because inevitably patients with difficulties may talk to their PT or PTA. Sexually transmitted diseases are described in Chapter 10. PTAs need to know when to suggest the patient consult with the physician.

Diseases of the Male Reproductive System

Diseases of the male reproductive system are usually treated by a physician specializing in urology because of the close relationship of the male genital and urinary

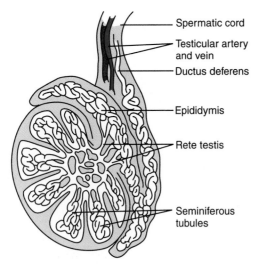

FIGURE 11.12 Midsagittal section of a testis.

systems. However, specialized physicians exist who work with both male and female infertility. Men should perform self-examinations of the scrotum regularly and understand the risks of carcinoma of the testes. Regular annual medical screening for prostate conditions is recommended for males over age 50 years.[248]

Congenital Abnormalities 🐾

Congenital abnormalities of the male reproductive system include those affecting the testes. An absence of any testes is called anorchia, and multiple testes is polyorchidism. Both these conditions are comparatively rare. A more common abnormality, occurring in approximately 3% of male newborns, is cryptorchidism, in which the testes either do not descend, or only partially descend, into the scrotal sac. In such cases, the testes remain in the abdominal cavity within the inguinal canal. The risk factors are mainly a family history of the condition or low birth weight.[249] Often the testes descend during the first year after birth, but sometimes surgery has to be performed to assist the testes to descend and to close the inguinal canal to prevent herniation of the abdominal contents through the gap.

Erectile Dysfunction

Erectile dysfunction (ED), sometimes called impotence, is defined as the inability to achieve and/or maintain an erection for sufficient time to partake in sexual intercourse, in 25% to 50% of attempts. The condition can occur at any age. Statistically, 5% of men by age 40, and 15% to 25% of men aged over 65 years experience ED.[250] However, many men who have the problem are over age 75 years. The incidence in the older age group is largely as a result of chronic medical conditions and prescription or over the counter medications that affect sexual function.

Etiology. The etiology of ED may be complex. Many men with the condition have a combination of factors, and the problem may indicate an undiagnosed medical condition. Any disruption to part of the sexual arousal system consisting of the brain, nerves, muscles, circulatory system, hormones, or emotional system can cause the problem. Men with chronic health conditions such as heart disease, atherosclerosis, hypertension, diabetes, hypercholesteremia (high cholesterol levels), and neurological conditions such as Parkinson's, cerebrovascular accident, spinal cord injury, and multiple sclerosis may be prone to the problem.[251] Erectile dysfunction may also be a side effect of prostatectomy (removal of the prostate in the presence of

prostate cancer), bladder, or rectal surgery, resulting in damage to the nerve supply to the penis or the result of a rare condition called Peyronie's disease that causes scar tissue formation within the penis.[252] Other causes and risk factors include heavy alcohol use, smoking tobacco or marijuana, use of illicit drugs, and use of certain medications, including antidepressants, antihistamines, antihypertensives, diuretics, NSAIDs, and tranquilizers.[253] Psychological problems that lead to ED can include depression and anxiety disorders.[254] [255]

Signs and Symptoms. Erectile dysfunction is a symptom in itself. The symptom may start suddenly or develop over a period of time.

Prognosis. The prognosis depends on the etiology of the condition. If the cause is an underlying medical problem, this needs to be treated in order to cure the erectile dysfunction. So many causes are possible that identification of the cause can result in an appropriate medical intervention to treat the condition. Unfortunately, many insurance companies do not provide coverage for the treatment of ED even after radical prostatectomy surgery. Efforts are now under way to rectify this issue.[256]

Medical Intervention. The diagnostic tests used to determine the cause of erectile dysfunction include blood tests for hormone levels, and to rule out other medical problems. Such tests involve a complete blood count (CBC), lipid profiles to check cholesterol and triglyceride levels, thyroid function tests, liver and kidney function tests, and urinalysis.[257] A review of the prescription medications by the physician may identify a specific medication that could be causing the problem. After initial screening, specific tests may be performed, including a complete neurological evaluation, a diagnostic ultrasound of the blood vessels of the penis, a procedure called dynamic infusion cavernosometry and cavernosography (DICC) in which a dye is injected into the blood vessels of the penis to enable radiographic viewing, and a nocturnal tumescence test in which a special tape that breaks when stretched is wrapped around the penis before sleep to see if an erection occurs during sleep. These tests can help to determine the possible physical or psychological cause of the ED.[258]

The medical treatments for erectile dysfunction vary according to the cause. Pharmacological intervention may be through the use phosphodiesterase inhibitors, which effectively increase the blood flow the muscles of the penis. Examples of these medications include sildenafil

(Viagra), tadalafil (Cialis), and vardenafil (Levitra). However, men with several other chronic conditions including heart disease, cerebrovascular event, hypotension, and uncontrolled hypertension or diabetes cannot take these phosphodiesterase inhibitors. Some men may require hormone replacement treatment (HRT). Testosterone may be taken orally, or a synthetic version of prostaglandins (Alpostadil) may be administered directly into the penis by injection or by a very small suppository into the urethra. Other types of medical intervention may include surgically inserted inflatable penile prosthetics (implants) for men with neurological damage; vascular surgery to unblock blood vessels; the use of vacuum constriction devices, also called penile pumps, for men with circulatory problems causing ED;[259] and possible counseling and sex therapy.[260,261]

Physical Therapy Intervention. None is indicated.

Infertility in the Male

The definition of infertility is the inability for a woman to become pregnant after 12 months of trying to conceive. Infertility is estimated to affect up to 15% of couples. Male infertility is responsible for approximately one-third of all infertility problems with couples, with approximately 1 in 25 men affected.[262] However, for the majority of couples, a combination of factors from both the male and the female result in infertility problems.[263] Of the men who have infertility problems, 90% are the result of either oligospermia (low sperm count) or poor quality of the semen.[264] The control of sexual functions in the male, including ejaculation and sperm production, is mediated by a closed-loop reflex system between the hypothalamus and the pituitary gland in the brain and the testes. The release of multiple hormones from this system is responsible for the normal regulation of factors affecting fertility.

Etiology. Male infertility may be the result of a variety of factors. Oligospermia (a reduced number of sperm, low sperm count), reduced motility (mobility) of the sperm, or abnormalities of the sperm themselves may reduce the effectiveness of the sperm to penetrate the female egg. Cryptorchidism (undescended testes) may cause an increase in the temperature of the scrotum and the testes, resulting in reduced sperm production by the testes. Another relatively common cause of infertility is varicocele, in which dilation of the veins in the scrotum causes heating of the testes resulting in reduced spermatogenesis (production of the number of sperm by the testes).[265] A blockage of the epididymis may reduce the quantity of

semen and affect fertility. Many hormones are involved with fertility in men. The hypothalamus produces thyrotropin-releasing hormone (TRH) and vasoactive intestinal peptide (VIP), both of which stimulate the release of prolactin from the pituitary, and dopamine, which inhibits the release of prolactin. Follicle stimulating hormone (FSH), and luteinizing hormone (LH) are both produced by the pituitary. All of these hormones affect the fertility of the male, and any identified changes in the concentrations may be the cause of the infertility problem.[266] Chronic medical problems such as diabetes, undiagnosed STD, pulmonary infections, stress, and neurological diseases may also reduce male fertility. Other risk factors for male infertility include a previous infection with mumps that may have caused atrophy of the testes; previous trauma to the testes including testicular torsion (twisting of the testes); exposure to radiation; previous bladder surgery; a history of urinary tract infections (UTIs); and developmental delay or delayed onset of puberty that may result in deficiency of the hypothalamus, pituitary, or testes. The use of certain medications or drugs such as opiates, antimicrobials, calcium channel blockers, and other anti-inflammatories including steroids may also affect the development of sperm.[267] In addition, the acid-to-alkali level of the semen can affect fertility rates. The normal pH of semen (ejaculate) is alkaline between 7.05 and 7.8. In some men infertility may be the sign of a serious disease such as cancer of the testes, pituitary, or hypothalamus, tumors that produce hormones, or liver or kidney failure.

Signs and Symptoms. The only usual sign of infertility is the lack of ability for the woman to become pregnant after a 12-month period.

Prognosis. With advances in medical interventions for couples who have fertility problems, the prognosis for improving fertility is promising. The results of the intervention depend greatly on the cause of the infertility. In some men, infertility is the sign of a serious problem, such as cancer. Seeking medical help for the problem of infertility may lead to the early diagnosis of cancers of the hypothalamus, testes, or pituitary gland, or of liver or kidney disease.[268]

Medical Intervention. The diagnosis of infertility can be complex. The following is only an overview of some of the options available for intervention for male infertility. The first approach to diagnosis lies in a complete medical history for signs of risk factors, a physical examination by the physician, blood tests to identify hormone levels, and analysis of the semen to identify the motility and numbers of sperm and the pH levels. The infertility problems in men are often identified during this initial screening. The possible treatment options fall into several categories depending on the cause of the problem. If the causative factors are hormonal, the administration of medications may correct the defect. Such medications include androgens, such as testosterone; estrogen receptor blockers to increase the secretion of the hypothalamic hormones; dopamine antagonists to inhibit the release of prolactin from the pituitary, because prolactin can cause erectile dysfunction; and gonadotropins that stimulate the production of gonadal hormones.[269] When the quality of the semen is affected, semen processing may be used to cleanse the semen before insemination into the female. Any identified infections must be treated with antimicrobials medications. A variety of surgical procedures may be performed, including a varicocelectomy for ligation of the dilated veins present in a varicocele in the scrotum; a vasovasostomy microsurgery to correct blockages of the epididymis; a transurethral resection of the ejaculatory ducts if blockage is apparent; or sperm retrieval through a biopsy of the testes or a microsurgical removal of sperm from the epididymis. After sperm are retrieved, artificial insemination of the female occurs through an intracervical insemination (ICI), in which the sperm are directly placed into the cervix, or an intrauterine insemination (IUI), directly into the uterus.[270]

Physical Therapy Intervention. None is indicated.

Prostate Diseases

The prostate diseases described in this section include the common condition of benign prostatic hyperplasia, as well as prostate cancer and prostatitis.

Benign Prostatic Hyperplasia

Benign prostatic hyperplasia (BPH) is a noncancerous, nonmalignant, hyperplasia (enlargement) of the prostate tissue, usually in the interior of the structure close to the urethra (see Fig. 11-13). Because the prostate surrounds the urethra, distal but close to the bladder, any enlargement of the gland as a result of hyperplasia can compress the urethra causing constriction and prevent emptying of the urine from the bladder. The prostate starts to enlarge as early as age 30 years, but symptoms of BPH are most prevalent in men over age 50. Approximately 50% of all men over 50 having some symptoms of BPH.[271]

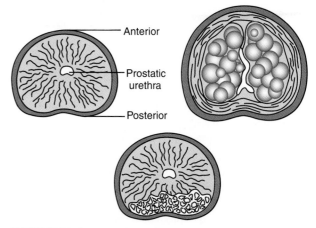

FIGURE 11.13 Cross sections of the prostate showing (A) normal prostate, (B) benign prostatic hyperplasia, and (C) carcinoma of prostate.

Etiology. The etiology of BPH is unknown, although theories suggest it is the result of altered levels of testosterone and estrogen hormones in the aging male, which stimulate prostate growth. Aging may also reduce the ability of the prostate to produce dihydrotestosterone (DHT) from testosterone. This substance is thought to have an inhibitory effect on the growth of prostate tissue, although some research indicates that the lack of DHT may be a beneficial factor for the size of the prostate.[272] A genetic predisposition to develop the condition exists in some men.

Signs and Symptoms. The characteristic signs and symptoms of prostatic hyperplasia are usually related to the inability or difficulty with urination. The prostate surrounds the urethra, thus when hypertrophy occurs, it constricts the urethra, resulting in bladder retention, slow urine flow, urge incontinence, nocturia, urinary tract infections, or blocks the urethra and prevents urination. Constriction of the urethra for a prolonged period of time can lead to chronic infections of the bladder and kidney, causing damage to these structures.[273]

Prognosis. BPH does not predispose men to prostate cancer. The condition usually responds well to medical treatment and frequently does not require any treatment.

Medical Intervention. BPH is diagnosed initially by rectal examination. Other testing includes the use of a cystoscope up into the urethra via the penis to observe the urethra and the bladder, urine flow rate, urinalysis, urine culture to rule out infection, a postvoid residual urine test to determine whether urine remains in the bladder after urination, and a possible prostate-specific antigen test to determine the likelihood of prostate cancer.[274] Many men with BPH are merely monitored by the physician for growth of the prostate and symptomatic problems. Some pharmacology interventions include the use of medications such as alpha blockers that relax the muscles of the prostate to reduce the urethral obstruction. Examples of alpha blockers include tamsulosin (Flomax), alfuzosin (Uroxatral), and terazosin (Hytrin). Another type of medication used to reduce the size of the prostate is 5-alpha reductase inhibitors such as finasteride (Proscar) and dutasteride (Avodert).[275] To provide temporary relief for urethral obstruction, a dilation of the urethra can be produced by passing a catheter through the area of the enlarged prostate pressing on the urethra. A variety of surgical interventions are possible:[276,277]

- transurethral prostate resection (TURP)—removal of part of the prostate via the urethra
- transurethral incision of the prostate (TUIP)—an incision made in the prostate via a urethral scope to enlarge the opening available for the urethra
- transurethral microwave therapy (TUMT)—microwave heat delivered to areas of the prostate via a catheter to destroy prostate cells
- transurethral needle-ablation therapy—low-level radio frequency energy delivered through needles to burn away parts of the prostate
- laser
  - photoselective vaporization of the prostate (PVP)—delivered via the urethra
  - interstitial laser coagulation—a probe placed directly into the prostate tissue to destroy cells
  - high intensity focused ultrasound—ultrasound delivered through a probe into the urethra (This procedure is in the developmental stages.)

Physical Therapy Intervention. None indicated.

Prostate Cancer

The prostate gland encloses the urethra distal to the bladder. The external surface of the prostate is palpable through the rectum. Most men diagnosed with prostate cancer are over age 65 years.[278] Carcinoma of the prostate is fairly common in older males with a lifetime 1 in 6, or 16% chance, of men having prostate cancer (see Fig. 11-13).[279] The most recent 2010 statistics from the American Cancer Society predicted approximately 32,050 men were expected to die of prostate cancer in 2010 in the United States, and 217,730 would be newly diagnosed with the condition. More than 2 million men are living with the diagnosis of prostate cancer.[280]

Etiology. The etiology of prostatic cancer is unknown. Because prostatic cancer tends to be a disease of older men, it becomes more prevalent as the average male life expectancy rises. Further risk factors associated with prostate cancer include a family history of the problem, heavy alcohol consumption, obesity, a high fat diet, and race.[281] Statistically, African Americans have a higher risk of developing prostate cancer than whites; Asian, Hispanic, and Native American men have the lowest risk.[282]

Signs and Symptoms. Unfortunately, there are few signs and symptoms associated with the early stages of most of these cancers because they tend to develop in the outer areas of the prostate, which does not cause compression of the urethra. Many older men already have some symptoms as a result of benign prostatic hyperplasia and do not notice any difference in their symptoms if cancer develops. Some specific symptoms may include hematuria (blood in the urine); frequency of urination and nocturia (the need for night-time urination); change in urine flow, such as a weak or interrupted flow; painful urination; the loss of ability to urinate; and pain in the low back, pelvis, or upper thighs. However, many men with prostate cancer do not have these symptoms.[283]

Prognosis. Prostate cancer is the second leading cause of death from cancer in men. The leading cause of cancer death is lung cancer. The risk of death from prostate cancer is 1 in 35 of those men with the disease.[284] When diagnosed early, the chances for survival are very good, and many men with the disease die from other causes. The 5-year survival rate for men diagnosed with prostate cancer is 100%, the 10-year survival rate is 91%, and the 15-year survival rate is 76%.[285]

Medical Intervention. The diagnosis of prostate cancer is improved with regular screening of the prostate. However, the decision to undergo regular screening is not an absolute because no screening test is perfect at the moment, and false-positive results may occur.[286] The recommendations for screening vary but usually involve annual screening of all men over age 50 years and screening for younger men who are at a higher risk. Screening tools include a blood test for detection of high levels of prostate-specific antigen (PSA), which may indicate a prostate condition, although not necessarily cancer, and a digital rectal examination (DRE). The normal level of PSA in the blood is usually 4 ng/mL or below, although in some men the normal level is higher.[287] A baseline measurement of the normal PSA at age 50 enables a comparison to be made with later testing. If the PSA value is raised significantly, it may indicate cancer, prostatitis, or prostate hyperplasia. However, in some cases of prostate cancer, the PSA level is not raised.[288] Another regular method of screening is a DRE by the physician. The DRE is performed via the rectum. Palpable changes in size, shape, and feel of the prostate can be effective in the initial diagnosis of prostate cancer because there are frequently no detectable signs and symptoms noted by the patient.[289] If prostate cancer is suspected, further testing is performed using transrectal ultrasound, with an ultrasound probe inserted into the rectum to visualize the prostate, and a needle biopsy of the prostate for laboratory analysis. When detected in the early stages, men with prostate cancer may not have any treatment other than regular checking to ensure the size of the tumor does not increase. A variety of other treatment options are available, including surgery with a radical prostatectomy (total excision of the prostate), radiation therapy either external or brachytherapy (internal radiation therapy) with the implantation of small radioactive pellets close to the prostate, hormone therapy to slow down the rate of growth of the prostatic tumor, or cryotherapy to freeze the cancer cells. When prostate cancer is in the advanced stages, no treatment may be possible. Advanced stages of the carcinoma cause metastases into the surrounding tissues of the bladder, rectum, and pelvis, which may extend as far as the lungs and heart. The most frequent side effects of medical treatment, particularly surgery, are pain, impotence, and incontinence.[290]

Physical Therapy Intervention. No physical therapy intervention is indicated. If male patients mention difficulty in voiding the bladder to the PTA during a therapy session, they should be directed to consult their physician.

Prostatitis

Several types of prostatitis exist. Acute prostatitis is associated with infection, and chronic prostatitis may be associated with infection. Men with chronic prostatitis tend to have recurring inflammation of the prostate.[291] The condition may occur in men of any age.

Etiology. The etiology of acute prostatitis results from a bacterial infection of the prostate often caused by a urinary tract infection (UTI) or an STD. The cause of chronic

prostatitis is often unknown but occasionally may be associated with benign prostatic hyperplasia.[292]

Signs and Symptoms. The characteristic signs and symptoms of acute prostatitis may include frequency or urgency of urination, dysuria (difficulty or pain during urination), low back pain, groin pain, low abdominal pain, and fever. The symptoms of chronic prostatitis are similar to those of acute prostatitis, occasionally with the addition of pelvic, testicular, or rectal pain.[293,294]

Prognosis. Prostatitis usually resolves with appropriate pharmacological intervention. Chronic prostatitis tends to recur.

Medical Intervention. The diagnosis of prostatitis entails a physical examination for detection of inflammation of the testes or epididymis, urinalysis and urine culture to determine infection or increased white cell count, and possibly an ultrasound scan, x-rays, or a CT scan. The pharmacological intervention for acute and chronic bacterial prostatitis is with antimicrobials for both the patient and sexual partners. Chronic noninfective prostatitis is usually treated with anti-inflammatory medications such as ibuprofen. Antidepressants are frequently prescribed to men with chronic prostatitis. Men with prostatitis should also drink plenty of liquids to maintain hydration levels.[295,296]

Physical Therapy Intervention. Physical therapy may be indicated for the control of the pain associated with chronic noninfective prostatitis. The interventions used are based on the relief of pain and teaching relaxation techniques.[297]

Testicular Diseases

The diseases discussed in this section include some of the more commonly diagnosed conditions related to the external male genitalia such as epididymitis, orchitis, testicular cancer, and cancer of the penis.

Epididymitis

Each epididymis is an approximately 6-meter-long muscular tube coiled around each testicle, which passes from the testes to the vas deferens. Sperm, formed in the testes, mature within the epididymis and are then passed along the epididymis to the vas deferens for ejaculation.[298] Epididymitis may be either acute or chronic and is inflammation of the epididymis. The condition affects up to

600,000 men in the United States each year.[299] Men between ages 18 and 50 years are most likely to have the condition, and 1 in every 1,000 men between these ages is affected annually.[300]

Etiology. The etiology of acute epididymitis is usually related to infection from the urethra or bladder. Common causes are sexually acquired diseases such as gonorrhea, or chlamydia, or systemic infections such as *Staphylococcus*, *Streptococcus*, *Escherichia coli*, or *Mycobacterium tuberculosis* (TB). Other causes include the use of an antiarrhythmia heart medication called amiodarone and a chemical epididymitis resulting from backflow of urine into the epididymis brought on by heavy lifting or benign prostatic hyperplasia with blockage of the urethra.[301] Some men may experience epididymitis after trauma to the area.[302] The risk factors associated with the incidence of epididymitis include the use of indwelling catheters for prolonged periods of time, men with structural malformations of the genitourinary system or those who are not circumcised, recent surgery in the pelvic area, benign prostatic hyperplasia, and men who are in nonmonogamous relationships and practice unprotected sex.[303,304] Chronic epididymitis may be a continuation beyond 6 weeks of the symptoms of acute epididymitis or of unknown cause. Men with chronic epididymitis tend to be over 50 years of age.[305]

Signs and Symptoms. The characteristic signs and symptoms of the condition are usually unilateral and may include dysuria, frequency, or urgency of micturition (urination); palpable "lumps" on the testicle, particularly where the epididymis attaches to the testicle; severe pain in the testis with radiating pain into the groin, more severe with bowel movements and possibly aggravated by walking; tenderness, erythema, and swelling of the scrotum, testicle, and groin; a urethral discharge and blood in the semen; enlarged inguinal lymph nodes; and fever.[306,307] Men with chronic epididymitis usually do not continue to have inflammation, but the pain may continue.

Prognosis. Acute epididymitis usually resolves with appropriate antimicrobial medications but may recur. Chronic forms of the condition may be more difficult to treat.

Medical Intervention. A physical examination by the physician may reveal palpable swelling, tenderness, and erythema of one scrotal sac. Medical tests performed to confirm the diagnosis include urinalysis and urine culture to determine the infective organism; tests for sexually transmitted infections, such as chlamydia or gonorrhea; a complete blood count (CBC); and a Doppler ultrasound to ensure the problem is not caused by a testicular torsion, which is a medical emergency requiring immediate surgery. Pharmacological intervention with antimicrobial medications usually is required, and sexual partners should also be treated. Analgesics and anti-inflammatory medications may be prescribed for pain and inflammation reduction. Bed rest, with elevation of the scrotal area and ice packs, may be needed until the symptoms subside.[308]

Physical Therapy Intervention. None is indicated.

Orchitis

Orchitis is inflammation of one or both of the testes. Orchitis occurs at any age but is common in boys who have mumps and in men over the age of 45 years with a history of epididymitis or benign prostatic hyperplasia.

Etiology. Orchitis may occur at the same time as epididymitis or as a result of a viral infection such as mumps. Bacterial infections are a less likely cause of the condition. Approximately 20% to 30% of boys develop orchitis between 4 and 6 days after the onset of mumps.[309] Other infections that can lead to orchitis include brucellosis, infectious mononucleosis, varicella, and STDs such as chlamydia and gonorrhea.[310,311] Some of the risk factors for developing orchitis include lack of immunization for mumps; a history of STDs; long-term use of an indwelling catheter; recent genitourinary surgery; a history of recurrent urinary tract infections; age over 45 years, especially if they have epididymitis or benign prostatic hyperplasia; and men who have unprotected sex with multiple partners.[312] Men with compromised immune systems as a result of HIV/AIDS are also at risk for orchitis caused by opportunistic infections.

Signs and Symptoms. The characteristic signs and symptoms of orchitis include pain, tenderness, and edema of the testicle and groin area on the same side; dysuria; penile discharge; painful ejaculation and blood in the semen; enlarged inguinal lymph nodes; and fever, fatigue, headache, malaise, and nausea.[313,314]

Prognosis. Approximately 33% of boys who develop orchitis as a result of mumps have atrophy of the testes. This atrophy may result in reduced levels of fertility or, in rare cases, sterility. Men who have had orchitis may also develop chronic epididymitis (see section on epididymitis). In rare instances, orchitis may cause infarction (death) of the testis requiring surgical excision. Other rare side effects include abscesses in the scrotum or the development of fistulas within the scrotum.[315]

Medical Intervention. The diagnosis of orchitis is achieved through the use of urinalysis, urine cultures, smear tests of the urethra for STDs, a complete blood count (CBC), Doppler ultrasound, and nuclear medicine scans of the testicle. If the orchitis is due to the mumps virus, no effective medical treatment exists other than anti-inflammatory medications, but if the cause is bacterial, antimicrobials are prescribed. Bed rest with elevation and icing of the scrotal area is recommended for the relief of pain. Prevention measures for orchitis include adequate immunization against mumps and protected sexual behaviors.[316]

Physical Therapy Intervention. Physical therapy intervention usually is not indicated for men with orchitis. However, if an abscess develops in the scrotum as a side effect of the condition, physical therapy wound care may be indicated.

Testicular Carcinoma

The incidence of testicular carcinoma in the United States is low with only 2 per 100,000 males affected each year. The condition occurs mainly in young and middle-aged men. Two main types of testicular cancer are recognized: seminomas, which grow slowly, and nonseminomas, which grow more quickly. Testicular cancer is comparatively rare and constitutes only 1% of all cancers in American men. However, the incidence of this cancer has increased by about 3% to 6% over the past 50 years, especially in men between the ages of 15 and 34 years.[317] The estimated number of men diagnosed with testicular cancer in the United States for 2010 was 8,480.[318] White males are at a higher risk of developing testicular cancer than either African American or Asian males.

Etiology. The etiology of testicular cancer is largely unknown. Statistical studies suggest a higher risk for those who had congenital cryptorchidism, have experienced previous trauma to the testes, have had testicular cancer in one testicle, or have a family history of testicular cancer. Men with HIV infection are at a higher risk of developing testicular cancer. Most testicular cancers develop from germ cells (sperm) within the testes.[319] More recently, the use of marijuana has been linked with as much as a 70% increased risk of developing testicular cancer.[320]

Signs and Symptoms. The characteristic signs and symptoms of testicular carcinoma may include edema or palpable "lumps" in the testis with or without pain, enlargement of the testicle, low back pain or lower abdominal pain, or no symptoms at all. Some men may be diagnosed with testicular cancer after seeking help with infertility problems.[321]

Prognosis. The recovery rate from testicular cancer depends on the staging of the tumor on diagnosis. In 2008, the National Cancer Institute (www.cancer.gov) attributed 380 deaths to the disease.[322] However, most testicular cancers, especially seminomas, are treatable with between a 90% and 100% cure rate. Between 2% and 5% of men will develop cancer in the other testicle within 25 years of the first diagnosis.[323] Some men may develop side effects from the treatment provided, including temporary or permanent infertility, erectile dysfunction resulting from damage to the nerves, or secondary cancers as the result of radiation therapy.[324]

Medical Intervention. A physical examination by the physician may not reveal any palpable tumor of the testicle. CT scans are usually used in the diagnosis of testicular carcinomas to observe inguinal lymph nodes and any tumor within the testicle. Blood tests for the serum markers for alpha fetoprotein (AFP), human chorionic gonadotrophin (beta hCG), and lactic dehydrogenase (LDH) can detect small tumors not visible by any other method. A chest radiograph may be used to check for metastases to the lungs, and an ultrasound of the scrotum may be able to detect tumors. The staging of testicular cancer follows similar guidelines to those of other types of carcinoma. A Stage I tumor is localized within the testicle, a Stage II tumor has spread to abdominal lymph nodes, and a Stage III tumor has metastasized beyond the abdominal lymph nodes to areas such as the lungs and the liver.[325] No screening tests exist for testicular cancer, but regular self-examinations can alert men to changes in the feel of the testes and prompt them to seek medical help to ensure early detection of any problems. Seminomas of the testicle are usually treated with radiation therapy. Surgical intervention of nonseminoma type carcinomas may be through orchiectomy (removal of the testes) and chemotherapy.[326] Ongoing medical follow-up is needed for men who have been treated for testicular cancer.

Physical Therapy Intervention. None is indicated.

Carcinoma of the Penis

Carcinoma of the penis is rare in the United States and Europe, accounting for only 0.4% to 0.6% of all cancers in men in the United States.[327] This cancer is more common in Asia, Africa, and South America. A higher incidence of the cancer is found in areas where sanitary conditions are poor.

Etiology. Squamous cell carcinoma is the most common type of penile cancer. Most penile carcinomas occur in men who are not circumcised. The human papillomavirus (HPV), responsible for many cervical cancers in women may also be a causative factor in penile carcinoma. Older men, especially those aged over 60 years, are at a higher risk of developing penile cancer. The lack of personal hygiene is a known factor in the development of this cancer.[328] Other risk factors exist for the development of penile carcinoma, including smoking, having multiple sex partners, and having a condition called phimosis in which the prepuce (foreskin) cannot be pulled back from the glans penis.[329]

Signs and Symptoms. Most carcinomas of the penis are located on the glans penis or the prepuce (foreskin). The characteristic signs and symptoms of penile carcinoma may be nonhealing lesions, reddened areas, or small papules. Men who have not been circumcised may not notice these lesions. Often no pain is experienced with cancerous lesions of the penis.[330] Occasionally, itching and burning sensations may be noticed.[331]

Prognosis. If penile cancer remains untreated, it is almost always life threatening. Many men delay seeking medical help. The earlier the cancer is diagnosed, the better the prognosis. The 5-year survival rate for men treated for penile carcinoma is 93% for Stage I, 55% for Stage II, and 30% for Stage III.[332] After the cancer has metastasized, the invasion of the inguinal, pubic, and lower abdominal lymph nodes leads to skin necrosis, general sepsis, and chronic infections, which usually result in death within 2 years.[333]

Medical Intervention. The most effective prevention of penile cancer is the circumcision of neonate boys. Circumcision performed in puberty or adulthood does not have any preventive effect. Options for the treatment of penile carcinoma vary with the staging. Radiation therapy, chemotherapy, surgical excision of a localized area of carcinoma, or partial or total penectomy (removal of the penis) are all options. Some small, superficial tumors can be removed with laser therapy, and tumors localized to the prepuce can be treated with circumcision. A Mohs micrographic surgery may be used for excision of small, superficial tumors.[334] In many instances, lymphadenectomy (removal of lymph nodes) of the inguinal nodes is also necessary.[335]

Physical Therapy Intervention. No physical therapy is indicated.

CASE STUDY 11.1

A 23-year-old female is attending your clinic with complaints of low back pain (LBP). The examination and evaluation by the PT reveals that the patient is 3 months pregnant, and the LBP is a reoccurrence of an old problem. In the past, the patient has received ultrasound, traction, electrical stimulation, and therapeutic exercises, which have relieved the pain within a few weeks. The patient is otherwise healthy with normal range of motion and strength in all extremities. She is unable to forward bend the spine more than 50% and is limited by 50% in left and right rotation and left and right side bending. She has great difficulty sitting in a chair. She is able to walk up to 3 miles at a time without too much difficulty. Her work entails prolonged sitting at a computer table, and it is difficult for her to complete her workload as a result of the LBP. The evaluating PT has determined that the plan of care will include gentle heat to the lumbar spine area, massage of the lumbar paraspinal musculature, posture education, back exercises, and advice on work and home adaptations to improve function.

1. What precautions will you need to take when applying heat to the low back in this patient?

2. Detail a suitable exercise regimen of five exercises for this patient to perform at home (include diagrams for a handout).

3. Detail the postural advice you will provide for this patient.

4. What advice will you give the patient for adaptations of her environment at work and at home to help improve her function?

5. Are there any particular things you need to bear in mind when performing the massage on this patient?

STUDY QUESTIONS

1. What is Nagele's Rule, and what is the calculation associated with it?

2. Describe the meaning of the term "multigravida."

3. What are Braxton-Hicks uterine contractions?

4. How does the maternal heart rate change during pregnancy?

5. What impact does the change in heart beat have on the physical therapy intervention and advice to the mother during pregnancy?

6. Describe an ectopic pregnancy.

7. What types of physical therapy treatment can be safely provided to reduce low back pain in a pregnant woman?

8. List the stages of labor with a short description of each stage.

9. How can performance of an episiotomy be justified?

10. List three maternal/fetal complications that can occur during pregnancy with a short description of each (do not list congenital abnormalities).

11. Describe one carcinoma of the female reproductive system.

12. Imagine you have an 82-year-old female patient with a prolapsed uterus. How would you describe this condition to the patient in terms she can understand, assuming she has no medical background?

13. How would you discuss the importance of regular breast self-examinations and mammography to a patient under your care?

14. Describe four effects of menopause.

15. Describe the various types of cancer experienced by men and the possible medical interventions.

16. Explain to another student the effects of benign prostatic hyperplasia in men, including the etiology, signs and symptoms, and medical treatment.

USEFUL WEB SITES

American Cancer Society
http://www.cancer.org

American Pregnancy Association
http://www.americanpregnancy.org

American Society for Reproductive Medicine
http://www.asrm.org

American Urological Association
http://www.auanet.org

March of Dimes
http://www.marchofdimes.org

National Cancer Institute
http://www.cancer.gov

National Center for Health Statistics
http://www.cdc.gov/fastats

National Institute of Child Health and Human Development
http://www.nichd.nih.gov

World Health Organization
http://www.who.int

REFERENCES

[1] The uterus. *Gray's Anatomy*. (Online version, 2000). Bartleby.com. Retrieved 5.16.09 from http://education.yahoo.com/reference/gray/subjects/subject/268

[2] The vagina. *Gray's Anatomy*. (Online version, 2000). Bartleby.com. Retrieved 5.16.09 from http://education.yahoo.com/reference/gray/subjects/subject/269

[3] XI Splanchnology. *Gray's Anatomy*. (Online version, 2000). The ovaries (ovaria). Bartleby.com Retrieved 5.16.09 from http://education.yahoo.com/reference/gray/subjects/subject/266

[4] Boyle, K. I., & Colon, J. M. (2008). Fallopian tube reconstruction. *eMedicine from WebMD*. Retrieved 5.16.09 from http://www.emedicine.com/med/topic3317.htm

[5] Herschorn, S. (2004). Female pelvic floor anatomy: the pelvic floor, supporting structures, and pelvic organs. *Rev Urol* 6(suppl 5): S2–S10.

[6] Mercer, S., & Hay-Smith, E. J. (2005). Anatomy in practice: the ischiorectal fossa. *N Z J Physiother* 33:61–64.

[7] Stephenson, R. G., & O'Connor, L. J. (2000). *Obstetric and gynecologic care in physical therapy*, 2nd edition. Thorofare, NJ: Slack Incorporated, p. 15.

[8] O'Reilly, D. (2007). Breast milk. *MedlinePlus Medical Encyclopedia*. Retrieved 5.16.09 from http://www.nlm.nih.gov/medlineplus/ency/article/002451.htm

[9] Stöppler, M. C. (2008). Vaginal bleeding. *MedicineNet.com*. Retrieved 5.16.09 from http://www.medicinenet.com/vaginal_bleeding/article.htm

[10] Rosenblatt, P. L. (2007). Menstrual cycle. *Merck Manuals Online Medical Library*. Retrieved 5.16.09 from http://www.merck.com/mmhe/sec22/ch241/ch241e.html

[11] Dyspareunia: painful sex for women. (2008). *Familydoctor.org*. American Academy of Family Physicians. Retrieved 5.16.2009 from http://familydoctor.org/online/famdocen/home/women/reproductive/sex-dys/669.html

[12] Wellbery, C. (1999). Diagnosis and treatment of endometriosis. *Am Fam Physician* 60, 1753–62, 1767–8. Retrieved 11.9.08 from Pro-Quest Nursing & Allied Health Source Database (Document ID: 45885241).

[13] National Institute of Child Health and Human Development. (2010). *Endometriosis*. Retrieved 11.26.2010 from http://www.nichd.nih.gov/health/topics/endometriosis.cfm

[14] Ortiz, D.D. (2008). Chronic pelvic pain in women. *Am Fam Physician* 77:1535–1542. Retrieved 11.8.08 from ProQuest Nursing & Allied Health Source Database (Document ID: 1486041031).

[15] National Institute of Child Health and Human Development. *Endometriosis*. Ibid.

[16] Wellbery, C. Ibid.

[17] Endometriosis; women hospitalized for endometriosis surgery have increased risk for future surgeries. (2006, February). *Med Devices Surg Technol Week* 197. Retrieved 11.9.08 from ProQuest Nursing & Allied Health Source Database (Document ID: 984116421).

[18] Infertility. (2008). *MedlinePlus*. Retrieved 11.9.2008 from http://www.nlm.nih.gov/medlineplus/infertility.html

[19] Brassard, M., AinMelk, Y., & Baillargeon, J. P. (2008). Polycystic ovary syndrome (PCOS). *Med Clin North Am* 92:1163–1192.

[20] Centers for Disease Control and Prevention. (2010). *Assisted reproductive technology (ART)*. Retrieved 11.26.2010 from http://www.cdc.gov/ART/

[21] American Society for Reproductive Medicine. (2006). *Medications for inducing ovulation*. Retrieved 11.26.10 from http://www.asrm.org/uploadedFiles/ASRM_Content/Resources/Patient_Resources/Fact_Sheets_and_Info_Booklets/ovulation_drugs.pdf

[22] American Pregnancy Association (2007). *In vitro fertilization*. Retrieved 5.16.09 from http://www.americanpregnancy.org/infertility/ivf.html

[23] Holder, A., Edmundson, L. D., & Erogul, M. (2009). Dysmenorrhea. *eMedicine from WebMD*. Retrieved 11.26.10 from http://www.emedicine.com/emerg/topic156.htm

[24] Popat, V., et al. (2009). Amenorrhea, primary. *eMedicine from WebMD*. Retrieved 11.26.10 from http://www.emedicine.com/med/TOPIC117.HTM

[25] Ibid.

[26] Chandran, L., & Puccio, J. A. (2008). Outflow obstructions. *eMedicine from WebMD*. Retrieved 5.16.09 from http://www.emedicine.com/ped/TOPIC514.HTM

[27] Tiemstra, J. D., & Patel, K. (1998). Hormonal therapy in the management of premenstrual syndrome. *J Am Board Fam Practice* 11:378–381.

[28] Ibid.

[29] Mayo Clinic Staff. (2007). *Premenstrual syndrome (PMS)*. Retrieved from http://www.mayoclinic.com/health/premenstrual-syndrome/DS00134/DSECTION=symptoms

[30] Premenstrual syndrome. (2008). *MedlinePlus Medical Encyclopedia*. Retrieved 11.9.08 from http://www.nlm.nih.gov/medlineplus/ency/article/001505.htm

[31] Kubba, A. A. (1985). The benefits of oral contraceptives. *J Royal Soc Promotion Health* 105:73.

[32] Premenstrual syndrome. (2008) Ibid.

[33] Zeller, J. L., & Lynm, C. (2007). Carcinoma of the cervix. *JAMA* 298:2336.

[34] Ibid.

[35] Saksouk, F. A. (2008). Cervix, cancer. *eMedicine from WebMD*. Retrieved 11.9.08 from http://www.emedicine.com/radio/topic140.htm

[36] Ibid.

[37] Merck Vaccinations. (2010). Gardasil: indications. Retrieved 11.26.10 from http://www.merckvaccines.com/Products/Gardasil/Pages/home.aspx?WT_mc.id=GL0AR

[38] U.S. Food and Drug Administration. (2006). *FDA licenses new vaccine for prevention of cervical cancer and other diseases caused by human papillomavirus*. Retrieved 11.9.08 from http://www.fda.gov/bbs/topics/NEWS/2006/NEW01385.html

[39] Saksouk, F. A. Ibid.

[40] Stoppler, M. C. (2008). Ovarian cysts. *eMedicine Health*. Retrieved 11.9.08 from http://www.emedicinehealth.com/ovarian_cysts/article_em.htm

[41] Helm, C. W. (2008). Ovarian cysts. *eMedicine from WebMD*. Retrieved 11.9.08 from http://www.emedicine.com/med/TOPIC1699.HTM

[42] Ibid.

[43] American Cancer Society. (2010). *Medicines to reduce breast cancer risk*. Retrieved 11.26.10 from http://www.cancer.org/docroot/CRI/content/CRI_2_6X_Tamoxifen_and_Raloxifene_Questions_and_Answers_5.asp

[44] Helm, C. W Ibid.

[45] Ibid.

[46] Ibid.

[47] Ibid.

[48] American Cancer Society. (2010). *What are the key statistics about endometrial cancer?* Retrieved 11.26.10 from http://www.cancer.org/docroot/cri/content/cri_2_4_1x_what_are_the_key_statistics_for_endometrial_cancer.asp

[49] National Cancer Institute. (2010). *Endometrial cancer prevention: incidence and mortality*. Retrieved 11.26.10 from http://www.cancer.gov/cancertopics/pdq/prevention/endometrial/HealthProfessional/27.cdr#Section_27

[50] Ibid.

[51] American Cancer Society. (2010). *What are the risk factors for endometrial cancer?* Retrieved from http://www.cancer.org/Cancer/EndometrialCancer/DetailedGuide/endometrial-uterine-cancer-risk-factors

[52] Uterine cancer. (2010). *MedlinePlus Medical Encyclopedia*. Retrieved 11.26.10 from http://www.nlm.nih.gov/medlineplus/uterinecancer.html

[53] American Cancer Society. *What are the key statistics about endometrial cancer?* Ibid.

[54] American Cancer Society. (2010). *How is endometrial cancer staged?* Retrieved 11.26.10 from http://www.cancer.org/Cancer/EndometrialCancer/DetailedGuide/endometrial-uterine-cancer-staging

[55] American Cancer Society. (2010). *How is endometrial cancer diagnosed?* Retrieved 11.26.10 from http://www.cancer.org/docroot/cri/content/cri_2_4_3x_how_is_endometrial_cancer_diagnosed.asp

[56] American Cancer Society. (2010). *What are the key statistics about vaginal cancer?* Retrieved 11.26.10 from http://www.cancer.org/Cancer/VaginalCancer/DetailedGuide/vaginal-cancer-key-statistics

[57] Vaginal cancer. (2010). *MedlinePlus Medical Encyclopedia*. Retrieved 11.26.10 from http://www.nlm.nih.gov/medlineplus/vaginalcancer.html

[58] American Cancer Society. (2010). *What is vaginal cancer: detailed guide?* Retrieved 11.26.10 from http://www.cancer.org/Cancer/VaginalCancer/DetailedGuide/vaginal-cancer-what-is-vaginal-cancer

[59] Nanda, R. (2006). Vaginal tumors. *National Cancer Institute* Retrieved 11.26.10 from http://www.medhelp.org/medical-information/show/425/Vaginal-tumors

[60] American Cancer Society. (2010). *How is vaginal cancer diagnosed?* Retrieved 11.26.10 from http://www.cancer.org/Cancer/VaginalCancer/DetailedGuide/vaginal-cancer-diagnosis

[61] American Cancer Society. *What are the key statistics about vaginal cancer?* Ibid.

[62] U.S. Food and Drug Administration. (2008, Sept). FDA approves expanded use of Gardasil to include preventing certain vulvar and vaginal cancers. *FDA News*. Retrieved 11.10.08 from http://www.fda.gov/bbs/topics/NEWS/2008/NEW01885.html

[63] American Cancer Society. *How is vaginal cancer diagnosed?* Ibid.

[64] Women's Cancer Network. (2008). Treatment options for precancerous lesions in the vagina. *Gynecologic Cancer Foundation.* Retrieved 5.17.09 from http://www.wcn.org/articles/types_of_cancer/vaginal/precancerous_lesions/index.html

[65] American Cancer Society. (2010). *Treating vaginal cancer topics: laser surgery.* Retrieved 11.26.10 from http://www.cancer.org/Cancer/VaginalCancer/DetailedGuide/vaginal-cancer-treating-laser-surgery

[66] American Cancer Society. (2010). *Treating vaginal cancer topics: radiation therapy.* Retrieved 11.26.10 from http://www.cancer.org/Cancer/VaginalCancer/DetailedGuide/vaginal-cancer-treating-radiation-therapy

[67] Dugdale, D. C. (2008). Cancer—vulva. *Medline Plus, MedlinePlus Medical Encyclopedia.* Retrieved 5.17.09 from http://www.nlm.nih.gov/medlineplus/ency/article/000902.htm

[68] Ibid.

[69] Ibid.

[70] Storck, S. (2009). Uterine fibroids. *MedlinePlus Medical Encyclopedia.* Retrieved 11.26.10 from http://www.nlm.nih.gov/medlineplus/ency/article/000914.htm

[71] Ibid.

[72] Storck, S. Ibid.

[73] Thomason, P. (2008). Ibid.

[74] Storck, S. Ibid.

[75] Robboy, S. J., et al. (2000). Pathology and pathophysiology of uterine smooth-muscle tumors. *Environ Health Perspect Suppl* 108(S5). National Institute of Environmental Health Sciences. Retrieved 5.16.09 from http://www.ehponline.org/members/2000/suppl-5/779–784robboy/robboy-full.html

[76] Thomason, P. (2008). Uterine leiomyoma (fibroid) imaging. *eMedicine from WebMD.* Retrieved from http://emedicine.medscape.com/article/405676–overview

[77] Storck, S. Ibid.

[78] Robboy, S. J., et al. Ibid.

[79] Wellbery, C. (2008). Distinguishing types of urinary incontinence in women. *Am Fam Physician* 78:3–4.

[80] Medical devices; uroplasty receives US FDA approvable letter for implant for female stress incontinence. (2006). Medical letter on the CDC and FDA. *NewsRx.com,* p. 69.

[81] Norton, P., & Brubaker, L. (2006). Urinary incontinence in women. *The Lancet,* 367:57–67.

[82] McNeeley, S. G. (2008). Pelvic floor disorders. *Merck Manuals Online Medical Library for Healthcare Professionals.* Retrieved 11.26.10 from http://www.merck.com/mmhe/sec22/ch249/ch249a.html

[83] Sartore, A., et al. (2004). The effects of mediolateral episiotomy on pelvic floor function after vaginal delivery. *Obstetr Gynecol* 103:669–673.

[84] Wellbery, C. Ibid.

[85] Flowers, L. K. (2009). Rectal prolapse. *eMedicine from WebMD.* Retrieved 11.26.10 from http://emedicine.medscape.com/article/776236–overview

[86] Tonks, A. (2008, March). Pelvic floor and bladder training reduces urinary incontinence in women. *BMJ* 336:473.

[87] Choo, M-S., Doo, C. K., & Lee, K.-S. (2008). Satisfaction with tolterodine: assessing symptom-specific patient-reported goal achievement in the treatment of overactive bladder in female patients (STARGATE study). *Int J Clin Practice* 62:191.

[88] Fielding, J. R., et al. (2000). MR based three-dimensional modeling of the normal pelvic floor in women: quantification of muscle mass. *Am J Roentgenol* 174:657–660.

[89] Fielding, J. R. (2002). Practical MR imaging of female pelvic floor weakness. *Radiographics* 22:295–304.

[90] Mayo Clinic. (2009). Urinary incontinence surgery: when other treatments aren't enough. *Women's Health.* Retrieved 11.26.2010 from http://www.mayoclinic.com/health/urinary-incontinence-surgery/WO00126

[91] Borello-France, et al. (2007). Pelvic floor muscle function in women with pelvic organ prolapse. *Phys Ther* 87:399–407.

[92] Rett, M. T., et al. (2007, Feb). Management of stress incontinence with surface electromyography-assisted biofeedback in women of reproductive age. *Phys Ther* 87:136–142.

[93] Borello-France, D. F., et al. (2006) Effect of pelvic-floor muscle exercise position on continence and quality of life outcomes in women with stress urinary incontinence. *Phys Ther* 86:974–986.

[94] Kegel exercises: benefits. (2008). *WebMD.* Retrieved 5.19.09 from http://women.webmd.com/tc/kegel-exercises-topic-overview

[95] Aslan, E., et al. (2008). Bladder training and Kegel exercises for women with urinary complaints living in a rest home. *Gerontology* 54:224–231.

[96] Centers for Disease Control and Prevention. (2008). *Pelvic inflammatory disease—CDC fact sheet.* Retrieved 5.19.09 from http://www.cdc.gov/std/PID/STDFact-PID.htm

[97] Ibid.

[98] Storck, S. (2009). Pelvic inflammatory disease. *MedlinePlus Medical Encyclopedia.* Retrieved from http://www.nlm.nih.gov/medlineplus/ency/article/000888.htm

[99] Centers for Disease Control and Prevention. (2008). *Pelvic inflammatory disease—CDC fact sheet.* Ibid.

[100] Storck, S. Pelvic inflammatory disease. Ibid.

[101] Barsoon, R. S., & Sinert, R. H. (2009). Uterine prolapse. *eMedicine from WebMD.* Retrieved from http://emedicine.medscape.com/article/797295–overview

[102] Ibid.

[103] Ibid.

[104] Guariglia, L., et al. (2005). Uterine prolapse in pregnancy. *Gynecol Obstetr Invest* 60:192–194.

[105] Daskalakis, G., et al. (2007). Uterine prolapse complicating pregnancy. *Arch Gynecol Obstetr* 276:391–2.

[106] Lazarou, G., Grigorescu, B. A., & Scotti, R. J. (2010). Uterine prolapse: treatment. *eMedicine from WebMD.* Retrieved 11.26.10 from http://emedicine.medscape.com/article/264231–treatment

[107] Ibid.

[108] Ibid.

[109] Ibid.

[110] Ibid.

[111] American Cancer Society. (2010). *American Cancer Society guidelines for the early detection of cancer.* Retrieved 11.26.10 from http://www.cancer.org/docroot/PED/content/PED_2_3X_ACS_Cancer_Detection_Guidelines_36.asp?sitearea=PED

[112] Roubidoux, M. A. (2009). Breast, fibroadenoma. *eMedicine from WebMD.* Retrieved 11.26.10 from http://emedicine.medscape.com/article/345779–overview

[113] Greenberg, R., Skornick, Y., & Kaplan, O. (1998). Management of breast fibroadenomas. *J Gen Int Med* 13:640–645. Retrieved 5.20.09 from http://www.pubmedcentral.nih.gov/articlerender.fcgi?artid=1497021

[114] Roubidoux, M. A. Ibid.

[115] Ibid.

[116] Ibid.

[117] Ibid.

[118] Greenberg, R., Skornick, Y., & Kaplan, O. Ibid.

[119] Mayo Clinic Staff. (2009). *Breast cancer: risk factors.* Retrieved 3.14.10 from http://www.mayoclinic.com/health/breast-cancer/DS00328/DSECTION=risk-factors

[120] American Cancer Society. (2010). *What are the key statistics for breast cancer?* Retrieved 11.26.10 from http://www.cancer.org/docroot/CRI/content/CRI_2_4_1X_What_are_the_key_statistics_for_breast_cancer_5.asp?sitearea=

[121] Mayo Clinic Staff. (2009). *Breast cancer: causes.* Retrieved 11.26.10 from www.mayoclinic.com/health/breast-cancer/DS00328/DSECTION=causes

122 Trichopoulos,D., Lagiou, P., & Adami, H.-O. (2005). Towards an integrated model for breast cancer etiology: the crucial role of the number of mammary tissue-specific stem cells. *Breast Cancer Res* 7:13–17.

123 Mayo Clinic Staff. *Breast cancer: risk factors.* Ibid.

124 Trichopoulos, D., Lagiou, P., & Adami, H.-O. Ibid.

125 Mayo Clinic Staff. (2009). *Breast cancer: symptoms.* Retrieved 11.26.10 from www.mayoclinic.com/health/breast-cancer/DS00328/DSECTION=symptoms

126 National Cancer Institute. (2010). *Breast cancer homepage.* Retrieved 11.26.10 from www.cancer.gov/cancertopics/pdg/treatment/breast/patient

127 American Cancer Society. *What are the key statistics for breast cancer?* Ibid.

128 American Cancer Society. (2010). *American Cancer Society guidelines for the early detection of cancer.* Retrieved 11.26.10 from http://www.cancer.org/docroot/PED/content/PED_2_3X_ACS_Cancer_Detection_Guidelines_36.asp?sitearea=PED

129 National Cancer Institute. *Breast cancer homepage.* Ibid.

130 Ibid.

131 Kelly, D. G. (2002). *A primer on lymphedema.* Upper Saddle River, NJ: Pearson Education (Prentice Hall).

132 Casley-Smith, J. R., & Casley-Smith, J. R. (1997). *Modern treatment for lymphoedema,* 5th revised edition. Malvern, Australia: The Lymphedema Association of Australia.

133 Casley-Smith, J. R. (1999). *Exercises for patients with lymphoedema of the arm, a guide to self-massage and hydrotherapy exercises,* 6th revised edition. Malvern, Australia: The Lymphedema Association of Australia.

134 Wechter, D. G. (2009). *Fibrocystic breast disease. MedlinePlus Medical Encyclopedia.* Retrieved from http://www.nlm.nih.gov/medlineplus/ency/article/000912.htm

135 Ibid.

136 Ibid.

137 Ibid.

138 Ibid.

139 *Taber's cyclopedic medical dictionary*, 20th edition. (2005). Philadelphia: F. A. Davis. Company, p. 790.

140 Human chorionic gonadotropin. (2008). *WebMD.* Retrieved 5.20.09 from http://www.webmd.com/baby/human-chorionic-gonadotropin-hcg

141 Bennington, L. K. (2006). Multiple pregnancy. *Healthline.* Retrieved 11.26.10 from http://www.healthline.com/galecontent/multiple-pregnancy?utm_term=multiple%20pregnancy&utm_medium=mw&utm_campaign=article

142 Nihira, M. A. (2009). Labor contractions: Braxton-Hicks or true labor? *WebMD.* Retrieved 11.26.10 from http://www.webmd.com/baby/guide/true-false-labor

143 Lof, M., et al. (March, 2005). Changes in basal metabolic rate during pregnancy in relation to changes in body weight and composition, cardiac output, insulin-like growth factor I and thyroid hormone and in relation to fetal growth. *Am J Clin Nutr* 81:678–685.

144 Nihira, M. A. (2010). Pregnancy and weight gain. *WebMD.* Retrieved 11.26.10 from http://www.webmd.com/baby/guide/healthy-weight-gain

145 Stephenson, R. G., & O'Connor, L. J. (2000). *Obstetric and gynecologic care in physical therapy,* 2nd edition. Thorofare, NJ: Slack, p. 268.

146 Baby Scanning Ltd. (n.d.) *Baby and pregnancy ultrasound scanning 3D and 4D.* Retrieved 11.25.10 from http://www.babyscanning.co.uk/

147 Vorvivk, L. J. (2010). Fetal heart monitoring. *MedlinePlus, US national Library of Medicine, National Institutes of Health.* Retrieved 11.26.10 from http://www.nlm.nih.gov/MEDLINEPLUS/ency/article/003405.htm

148 Lancaster General Hospital, Pennsylvania. (2010). *Common tests during pregnancy.* Retrieved 11.26.10 from http://www.lancastergeneralhealth.org/LGH/HWI/Health-Information-Library/Documents.aspx?OperationMode=DocumentDisplay&contentId=P01241&ContentTypeId=85

149 Ibid.

150 Barakat, R., Stirling, J. R., & Lucia, A. (2008). Does exercise training during pregnancy affect gestational age? A randomized controlled trial. *Br J Sports Med* 42:674–678.

151 Juhl, M., et al. (2008). Physical exercise during pregnancy and the risk of preterm birth: a study within the Danish national birth cohort. *Am J Epidemiol* 167:859–867.

152 Exercise during pregnancy: myth vs. fact. *WebMD.* (2009). Retrieved 11.26.10 from http://www.webmd.com/baby/features/exercise-during-pregnancy-myth-vs-fact

153 Stephenson, R. G., & O'Connor, L. J. Ibid, p. 129

154 Ciliberto, C. F., & Marx, G. F. (2008). Physiological changes associated with pregnancy. *Update Anaesthes* (online journal) Issue 9. Retrieved 5.21.09 from http://www.nda.ox.ac.uk/wfsa/html/u09/u09_003.htm

155 Vorvick, L. J. (2010). Ectopic pregnancy. *MedlinePlus Medical Encyclopedia.* Retrieved 11.26.10 from http://www.nlm.nih.gov/medlineplus/ency/article/000895.htm

156 Stöppler, M. C. (2010). Ectopic pregnancy. *MedicineNet.com.* Retrieved 11.26.10 from http://www.medicinenet.com/ectopic_pregnancy/page3.htm

157 Vorvick, L. J. Ibid.

158 Ibid.

159 Stöppler, M. C. Ibid.

160 Vorvick, L. J. Ibid.

161 Diabetes and pregnancy. (2010). MedlinePlus Medical Encyclopedia. Retrieved 11.26.10 from http://www.nlm.nih.gov/medlineplus/diabetesandpregnancy.html

162 Bupa Health Information Team. (2010). *Diabetes in pregnancy.* Retrieved 11.26.10 from http://hcd2.bupa.co.uk/fact_sheets/html/diabetes_in_pregnancy.html

163 Shriver, E. K. (2008). *Gestational diabetes.* Retrieved 5.21.09 from http://www.nichd.nih.gov/health/topics/Gestational_Diabetes.cfm

164 Ibid.

165 Sneag, D. B., & Bendo, J. A. (2007). Pregnancy-related low back pain. *Orthopedics* 30:839–845.

166 Ibid.

167 Fitzgerald, C.M., & Le, J. (2007). Back pain in pregnancy requires practitioner creativity—although this common condition isn't always treated, nonsurgical approaches can provide relief. *Biomechanics* 14:39. Retrieved 11.9.08, from ProQuest Nursing & Allied Health Source Database (Document ID: 1391914391).

168 Mantle, J., Haslam, J., & Barton, s. (2004). *Physiotherapy in obstetrics and gynaecology,* 2nd edition. Edinburgh, UK: Butterworth Heinemann.

169 Fitzgerald, C.M., & Le, J. Ibid.

170 March of Dimes. (2010). *Pregnancy complications: placental conditions.* Retrieved 11.26.10 from http://www.marchofdimes.com/professionals/14332_1154.asp

171 Ibid.

172 Dulay, A. T. (2010) Gynecology and obstetrics: placenta accreta. *Merck Manuals Online Medical Library for Healthcare Professionals.* Retrieved 11.26.10 from http://www.merck.com/mmpe/sec18/ch264/ch264l.html

173 Joy, S., & Lyon, D. (2008). Placenta previa. *eMedicine from WebMD.* Retrieved 5.21.09 from http://www.emedicine.com/med/topic3271.htm

174 Ibid.

175 March of Dimes. Ibid.

176 Joy, S., & Lyon, D. Ibid.

177 Oyelese, Y., & Smulian, J. C. (2006). Placenta previa, placenta accrete, and vasa previa. *Obstetr Gynecol* 107:927–941.

178 March of Dimes. Ibid.

179 Caughey, A. B., & Butler, J. R. (2010). Postterm pregnancy. *eMedicine from WebMD*. Retrieved 11.26.10 from http://www.emedicine.com/med/topic3248.htm

180 Ibid.

181 Alexander, J. M., McIntire, D. D., & Leveno, K. J. (2000). Forty weeks and beyond: pregnancy outcomes by week of gestation. *Obstetr Gynecol* 96:291–294.

182 Crowley, P. (2000). Interventions for preventing or improving the outcome of delivery at or beyond term. *Cochrane Database System Rev* CD000170. Retrieved 5.21.09 from http://www.medscape.com/medline/abstract/10796167

183 Preeclampsia Foundation. (2010). *About preeclampsia*. Retrieved 11.26.10 from http://www.preeclampsia.org/about.asp

184 Mayo Clinic Staff. (2009). *Preeclampsia: risk factors*. Retrieved 4.12.10 from http://www.mayoclinic.com/health/preeclampsia/DS00583/DSECTION=risk-factors

185 Mayo Clinic Staff. (2009). *Preeclampsia: symptoms*. Retrieved 4.12.09 from http://www.mayoclinic.com/health/preeclampsia/DS00583/DSECTION=symptoms

186 Mayo Clinic Staff. (2009). *Preeclampsia: complications*. Retrieved 4.12.09 from http://www.mayoclinic.com/health/preeclampsia/DS00583/DSECTION=complications

187 Preeclampsia Foundation. Ibid.

188 Mayo Clinic Staff. (2009). *Preeclampsia: tests and diagnosis*. Retrieved 4.12.09 from http://www.mayoclinic.com/health/preeclampsia/DS00583/DSECTION=tests-and-diagnosis

189 Premature babies. (2010). *MedlinePlus Medical Encyclopedia*. Retrieved 11.26.10 from http://www.nlm.nih.gov/medlineplus/prematurebabies.html

190 Mayo Clinic Staff. (2009). *Pregnancy: premature birth*. Retrieved 3.14.10 from http://www.mayoclinic.com/health/premature-birth/DS00137

191 American Pregnancy Association. (2007). *Premature labor*. Retrieved 4.12.09 from http://www.americanpregnancy.org/labornbirth/prematurelabor.html

192 Mayo Clinic Staff. Pregnancy: Premature birth. Ibid.

193 American Lung Association. (2008). *Premature babies. Respiratory distress syndrome of the newborn fact sheet*. Retrieved 4.12.09 from http://www.lungusa.org/site/apps/nlnet/content3.aspx?c=dvLUK9O0E&b=2060721&content_id={552A7003–4621–43E5–82B4–1678D9A6D963}&notoc=1

194 National Eye Institute. (2008). *Retinopathy of prematurity*. Retrieved 4.12.09 from http://www.nei.nih.gov/health/rop/

195 American Pregnancy Association. *Premature labor*. Ibid.

196 Mayo Clinic Staff. Pregnancy: premature birth. Ibid.

197 Tecklin, J. S. (1999). *Pediatric physical therapy*, 3rd edition. Philadelphia: Lippincott Williams and Wilkins, p. 85.

198 Torpy, J. M. (2002). Miscarriage. *JAMA* 288:1936.

199 Ibid.

200 Ibid.

201 Ibid.

202 Nihira, M. A. (2009). Understanding miscarriage—prevention. *WebMD*. Retrieved 3.16.10 from http://www.webmd.com/baby/understanding-miscarriage-prevention

203 Centers for Disease Control and Prevention. (2010). *Women need 400 micrograms of folic acid every day*. Retrieved 11.26.10 from http://www.cdc.gov/Features/FolicAcid/

204 Stagnaro-Green, A., et al. (1990). Detection of at-risk pregnancy by means of highly sensitive assays for thyroid autoantibodies. *JAMA* 264:1422–1425.

205 Stephenson, J. (2004). Miscarriage. Clue? *JAMA* 291:813.

206 Stephenson, J. (2007). Miscarriage and inflammation. *JAMA* 297:686.

207 Stephenson, R. G., & O'Connor, L. J. Ibid., p. 225

208 American Pregnancy Association. (2007). *Effacement*. Retrieved 4.13.09 from http://www.americanpregnancy.org/labornbirth/effacement.html

209 Joy, S., Scott, P. L., & Lyon, D. (2009). Abnormal labor. *eMedicine from WebMD*. Retrieved 11.26.10 from http://emedicine.medscape.com/article/273053-overview

210 Forouzan, I., & Bonilla, M. M. (2004). Dystocia. *eMedicine from WebMD*. Retrieved 6.22.08 from http://www.emedicine.com/med/topic3280.htm

211 Mantle, J., Haslam, J., & Barton, S. Ibid., p. 71.

212 Ibid., p. 73.

213 Stephenson, R. G., & O'Connor, L. J. Ibid., p. 248.

214 Jenis, A. (2009). Pregnancy: Breech delivery. *eMedicine from WebMD*. Retrieved 11.26.10 from http://www.emedicine.com/emerg/TOPIC868.HTM

215 Ibid.

216 National Center for Health Statistics. (2009). Births: final data for 2007, table 8. Retrieved 11.26.10 from http://www.cdc.gov/nchs/fastats/delivery.htm

217 Cesarean section. (2010). *MedlinePlus Medical Encyclopedia*. Retrieved 11.26.10 from http://www.nlm.nih.gov/medlineplus/cesareansection.html

218 March of Dimes, Pregnancy and Newborn Health Education Center. (2008). *C-section: medical reasons*. Retrieved 4.15.09 from http://www.marchofdimes.com/pnhec/240_1031.asp

219 Mayo Clinic Staff. (2010). C-section. Retrieved 11.26.10 from http://www.mayoclinic.com/print/c-section/PR00078/METHOD=print

220 World Health Organization. (2003). *Managing complications in pregnancy and childbirth. A guide for midwives and doctors. Procedures: episiotomy*. Retrieved 6.24.08 from http://www.who.int/reproductive-health/impac/Procedures/Episiotomy_P71_P75.html

221 Mayo Clinic Staff. (2010). Episiotomy: When it's needed, when it's not. Retrieved 11.26.10 from http://www.mayoclinic.com/health/episiotomy/HO00064

222 Bodner-Adler, B., et al. (2001). Risk factors for third-degree perineal tears in vaginal delivery, with an analysis of episiotomy types. *J Reprod Med* 46:752–756.

223 Shipman, M. K., et al. (1997). Antenatal perineal massage and subsequent perineal outcomes: a randomized controlled trial. *Br J Obstetr Gynaecol* 104:787–791.

224 Mei-dan, E., et al. (2008). Perineal massage during pregnancy: a prospective controlled trial. *Isr Med Assoc J* 10:499–502.

225 Mantle, J., Haslam, J., & Barton, S. Ibid., p. 80.

226 National Center for Health Statistics. (2009). Births: final data for 2007, table H, 39. *Faststats*. Centers for Disease Control and Prevention, Department of Health and Human Services. Retrieved 11.26.10 from http://www.cdc.gov/nchs/fastats/multiple.htm

227 Twins, triplets, multiple births. (2010). *MedlinePlus Medical Encyclopedia*. Retrieved 11.26.10 from http://www.nlm.nih.gov/medlineplus/twinstripletsmultiplebirths.html

228 Mantle, J., Haslam, J., & Barton, S. Ibid., p. 207.

229 Leeds, L., & Hargreaves, I. (2008). The psychological consequences of childbirth. *J Reprod Infant Psychol* 26:108. Retrieved 11.9.08 from ProQuest Nursing & Allied Health Source Database (Document ID: 1467253101).

230 Benoit, C., et al. (2007). Social factors linked to postpartum depression: A mixed-methods longitudinal study. *J Ment Health* 16:719. Retrieved 11.9.08 from ProQuest Nursing & Allied Health Source Database (Document ID: 1426371941).

231 White, T., et al. (2006). Postnatal depression and post-traumatic stress after childbirth: Prevalence, course and co-occurrence. *J Reproductive and Infant Psychology*, 24, 107–120. Retrieved 11.9.08 from ProQuest Nursing & Allied Health Source Database (Document ID: 1041316271).

232 Postpartum Psychiatric Disorders. (2007, July). *Nutrition Health Review*, 13. Retrieved 11.9.08 from ProQuest Nursing & Allied Health Source Database (Document ID: 1416435691).

233 Leeds, L., & Hargreaves, I. Ibid.

234 National Institute on Aging. (2008). Menopause. *National Institutes of Health*. Retrieved from http://www.nia.nih.gov/HealthInformation/Publications/menopause.htm

235 Ibid.

236 Fogoros, R. N. (2010). Hormone replacement therapy and heart disease. About.com. Retrieved 11.25.10 from http://heartdisease.about.com/library/weekly/aa072300a.htm

237 Bouchez, C., & Chang, L. (2007). HRT: revisiting the hormone decision. *WebMD*. Retrieved 11.26.10 from http://www.webmd.com/menopause/features/hrt-revisiting-the-hormone-decision

238 Chang, L. (2009). Alzheimer's disease therapy options. *WebMD*. Retrieved 11.26.10 from http://www.webmd.com/alzheimers/guide/alzheimers-disease-therapy-options?page=2

239 Mayo Clinic Staff. (2009). *Hot flashes*. Retrieved 4.16.10 from http://www.mayoclinic.com/print/hot-flashes/HQ01409/METHOD=print

240 Menopause. (2009). *MedlinePlus Medical Encyclopedia*. Retrieved 4.5.10 from http://www.nlm.nih.gov/medlineplus/menopause.html

241 International Osteoporosis Foundation. (2010). *Calcium*. Retrieved 11.26.10 from http://www.iofbonehealth.org/patients-public/about-osteoporosis/prevention/nutrition/calcium.html

242 National Osteoporosis Foundation. (2010). *About osteoporosis: build strong bones now*. Retrieved 11.26.10 from http://www.nof.org/aboutosteoporosis/whatwomencando/teen-women

243 American Osteopathic Association. (2009). *Exercise in postmenopausal women*. Retrieved 4.20.09 from http://www.osteopathic.org/index.cfm?PageID=you_exerfs

244 Rubenstein, J., & Brannigan, R. E. (2010). Infertility, male. *eMedicine from WebMD*. Retrieved 11.26.10 from http://emedicine.medscape.com/article/436829–overview

245 Puscheck, E. E. (2009). Obstetrics and gynecology: reproductive endocrinology and infertility: infertility. *eMedicine from WebMD*. Retrieved 11.26.10 from http://emedicine.medscape.com/article/274143-overview

246 Holt, E. H. (2010). Testosterone. *MedlinePlus Medical Encyclopedia*. Retrieved 11.26.10 from http://www.nlm.nih.gov/medlineplus/ency/article/003707.htm

247 Jabbour, S. A. (2007). Follicle-stimulating hormone abnormalities. *eMedicine from WebMD*. Retrieved 6.23.09 from http://emedicine.medscape.com/article/118810-overview

248 Centers for Disease Control and Prevention. (2010). *Prostate cancer: informed decision making: how to make a personal health care choice*. Retrieved 11.25.10 from http://www.cdc.gov/cancer/Prostate/publications/decisionguide/

249 Sumfest, J. M., Kolon, T. F., & Rukstalis, D. B. (2009). Cryptorchidism. *eMedicine from WebMD*. Retrieved 3.5.10 from http://emedicine.medscape.com/article/438378–overview

250 Baird, J. M., editor. (2007). Erectile dysfunction guide: overview and facts. *WebMD*. Retrieved 6.25.08 from http://www.webmd.com/erectile-dysfunction/guide/erectile-dysfunction-basics

251 Mayo Clinic Staff. (2010). *Erectile dysfunction: causes*. Retrieved 11.24.10 from http://www.mayoclinic.com/health/erectile-dysfunction/DS00162/DSECTION=causes

252 Baird, J. M., editor. Erectile dysfunction guide: overview and facts. Ibid.

253 Baird, J. M. (2007). Drugs linked to erectile dysfunction. *WebMD*. Retrieved 11.26.10 from http://www.webmd.com/erectile-dysfunction/guide/drugs-linked-erectile-dysfunction

254 Mayo Clinic Staff. *Erectile dysfunction: causes*. Ibid.

255 Mayo Clinic Staff. (2010). *Erectile dysfunction: symptoms*. Retrieved 11.24.10 from http://www.mayoclinic.com/health/erectile-dysfunction/DS00162/DSECTION=symptoms

256 American Urological Association (2008, May). *AUA 2008: legislation needed to provide coverage for ED treatment after prostatectomy*. Retrieved 4.30.09 from http://www.auanet.org/content/press/press_releases/article.cfm?articleNo=39

257 Baird, J. M., editor. (2007). Erectile dysfunction guide: diagnosing erectile dysfunction. *WebMD*. Retrieved 6.25.08 from http://www.webmd.com/erectile-dysfunction/guide/diagnosing-erectile-dysfunction

258 Mayo Clinic Staff. (2010). *Erectile dysfunction: tests and diagnosis*. Retrieved 11.26.10 from http://www.mayoclinic.com/health/erectile-dysfunction/DS00162/DSECTION=tests-and-diagnosis

259 Baird, J. M., editor. (2007). Erectile dysfunction guide: vacuum constriction devices. *WebMD*. http://www.webmd.com/erectile-dysfunction/guide/vacuum-constriction-devices

260 Mayo Clinic Staff. (2010). *Erectile dysfunction: treatments and drugs*. Retrieved 11.26.10 from http://www.mayoclinic.com/health/erectile-dysfunction/DS00162/DSECTION=treatments-and-drugs

261 Baird, J. M., editor. (2007). Erectile dysfunction guide: penile prosthesis. *WebMD*. Retrieved 6.25.08 from http://www.webmd.com/erectile-dysfunction/penile-prosthesis

262 Rubenstein, J., & Brannigan, R. E. (2010). Infertility, male. *eMedicine from WebMD*. Retrieved 11.26.10 from http://emedicine.medscape.com/article/436829–overview

263 American Academy of Family Physicians. (2010). *Male infertility*. Retrieved 11.23.10 from http://familydoctor.org/online/famdocen/home/men/reproductive/766.html

264 Rubenstein, J., & Brannigan, R. E. (2010). Ibid.

265 American Academy of Family Physicians. *Male infertility*. Ibid.

266 Rubenstein, J., & Brannigan, R. E. Ibid.

267 Ibid.

268 Ibid.

269 Rubenstein, J., & Brannigan, R. E. (2010). Infertility, male: treatment and medications. *eMedicine from WebMD*. Retrieved 11.23.10 from http://emedicine.medscape.com/article/436829–treatment

270 Ibid.

271 Gerber, G. (2008). Benign prostatic hyperplasia (BPH, enlarge prostate). *WebMD*. Retrieved 8.24.09 from http://www.medicinenet.com/benign_prostatic_hyperplasia/article.htm

272 National Kidney and Urologic Diseases Information Clearinghouse. (2006). *Prostate enlargement: benign prostatic hyperplasia*. Retrieved 6.26.08 from http://kidney.niddk.nih.gov/kudiseases/pubs/prostateenlargement/

273 Ibid.

274 Enlarged prostate. (2007). *MedlinePlus Medical Encyclopedia*. Retrieved 6.26.08 from http://www.nlm.nih.gov/medlineplus/ency/article/000381.htm

275 Gerber, G. Ibid.

276 National Kidney and Urologic Diseases Information Clearinghouse. (2006). Ibid.

277 Enlarged prostate. (2007). Ibid.

278 Mayo Clinic Staff. (2010). *Prostate cancer screening: should you get a PSA test?* Retrieved 11.26.10 from http://www.mayoclinic.com/health/prostate-cancer/HQ01273

279 Centers for Disease Control and Prevention. (2010). *Prostate cancer: informed decision making: how to make a personal health care choice*. Retrieved 11.25.10 from http://www.cdc.gov/cancer/Prostate/publications/decisionguide/

280 American Cancer Society. (2010). *Detailed guide: prostate cancer. What are the key statistics about prostate cancer?* Retrieved 11.26.10 from http://www.cancer.org/Cancer/ProstateCancer/DetailedGuide/prostate-cancer-key-statistics

281 National Cancer Institute. (2010). *Prostate cancer screening: summary of evidence*. Retrieved 11.26.10 from http://www.cancer.gov/cancertopics/pdq/screening/prostate/HealthProfessional

282 Centers for Disease Control and Prevention. Prostate cancer: informed decision making: how to make a personal health care choice. Ibid.

283 Ibid.

284 American Cancer Society. *Detailed guide: prostate cancer. What are the key statistics about prostate cancer?* Ibid.

285 Ibid.
286 National Cancer Institute. (2010). *Prostate cancer screening: summary of evidence*. Retrieved 11.26.10 from http://www.cancer.gov/cancertopics/pdq/screening/prostate/HealthProfessional
287 Ferrini, R., & Woolf, S. H. (1997). *Screening for prostate cancer in American men: American College of Preventive Medicine Practice Policy Statement*. Retrieved 6.27.08 from http://www.acpm.org/prostate.htm
288 Centers for Disease Control and Prevention. *Prostate cancer: informed decision making: how to make a personal health care choice*. Ibid.
289 Ibid.
290 Ibid.
291 Wedro, B. C. (2008). Prostatitis. *MedicineNet.com.* Retrieved 4.24.09 from http://www.medicinenet.com/prostatitis/article.htm
292 Gerber, G. Ibid.
293 Ibid.
294 Wedro, B. C. Ibid.
295 Gerber, G. Ibid.
296 Wedro, B. C. Ibid.
297 Ibid.
298 Dugdale, D. C. III. (2010). Pathway of sperm. *MedlinePlus Medical Encyclopedia.* Retrieved 11.24.10 from http://www.nlm.nih.gov/medlineplus/ency/imagepages/19073.htm
299 Dugdale, D. C. III. (2010). Epididymitis. *Medline Plus, MedlinePlus Medical Encyclopedia.* Retrieved 11.26.10 from http://www.nlm.nih.gov/medlineplus/ency/article/001279.htm
300 Sabanegh, E. S., Konety, B. R., & Ching, C. B. (2010). Epididymitis. *eMedicine from WebMD.* Retrieved 11.26.10 from http://emedicine.medscape.com/article/436154–overview
301 Mayo Clinic Staff. (2009). Epididymitis: causes. Retrieved 5.6.10 from http://www.mayoclinic.com/health/epididymitis/DS00603/DSECTION=causes
302 Sabanegh, E. S., Konety, B. R., & Ching, C. B. (2008). Epididymitis. *eMedicine from WebMD.* Retrieved from http://emedicine.medscape.com/article/436154–overview
303 Dugdale, D. C. III. Epididymitis. Ibid.
304 Mayo Clinic Staff. (2009). *Epididymitis: symptoms.* Retrieved 3.12.10 from http://www.mayoclinic.com/health/epididymitis/DS00603/DSECTION=symptoms
305 Sabanegh, E. S., Konety, B. R., & Ching, C. B. Ibid.
306 Dugdale, D. C. III. Epididymitis. Ibid.
307 Mayo Clinic Staff. Epididymitis: symptoms. Ibid.
308 Dugdale, D. C. III. Epididymitis. Ibid.
309 Mycyk, M. B. (2010). Orchitis. *eMedicine from WebMD.* Retrieved 11.26.10 from http://emedicine.medscape.com/article/777456–overview
310 Vorvick, L. J. (2010). Orchitis. *Medline Plus, MedlinePlus Medical Encyclopedia.* Retrieved 11.27.10 from http://www.nlm.nih.gov/medlineplus/ency/article/001280.htm
311 Mycyk, M. B. (2010). Orchitis. *eMedicine from WebMD.* Retrieved 11.26.10 from http://emedicine.medscape.com/article/777456–overview
312 Vorvick, L. J. Orchitis. Ibid.
313 Ibid.
314 Mycyk, M. B. Ibid.
315 Vorvick, L. J. Orchitis. Ibid.
316 Ibid.
317 Marijuana linked to aggressive testicular cancer. (2009). *MedlinePlus Medical Encyclopedia.* Retrieved 10.12.09 from http://www.nlm.nih.gov/medlineplus/news/fullstory_75550.html
318 National Cancer Institute. (2010). *Testicular cancer.* Retrieved 11.27.10 from http://www.cancer.gov/cancertopics/types/testicular/
319 Dugdale, D. C. III. Testicular cancer. *MedlinePlus Medical Encyclopedia.* Retrieved 11.27.10 from http://www.nlm.nih.gov/medlineplus/ency/article/001288.htm
320 Marijuana linked to aggressive testicular cancer. (2009). *MedlinePlus Medical Encyclopedia.*
321 Dugdale, D. C. III. Testicular cancer. Ibid.
322 National Cancer Institute. *Testicular cancer.* Ibid.
323 National Cancer Institute. (2010). *Testicular cancer treatment: general information about testicular cancer.* Retrieved 11.27.10 from http://www.cancer.gov/cancertopics/pdq/treatment/testicular/HealthProfessional/page1
324 Dugdale, D. C. III. Testicular cancer. Ibid.
325 Ibid.
326 National Cancer Institute. (2010). *Testicular cancer treatment: general information about testicular cancer.* Retrieved 11.27.10 from http://www.cancer.gov/cancertopics/pdq/treatment/testicular/HealthProfessional/page2
327 Eastham, J. A. et al. (2002). Squamous cell carcinoma of the penis: a retrospective review of forty-five patients in Northwest Louisiana. Southern Medical Association. *South Med J* 95:822–825.
328 Brosman, S. A. (2010). Penile cancer: treatment. *eMedicine from WebMD.* Retrieved 11.27.10 from http://emedicine.medscape.com/article/446554–treatment
329 Medical Staff of the National Cancer Institute. (2010). Penis cancer. *MedicineNet.* Retrieved 11.27.10 from http://www.medicinenet.com/penis_cancer/article.htm
330 Brosman, S. A. Ibid.
331 Draper, R. (2010). Penile carcinoma. *Patient UK.* Retrieved 11.27.10 from http://www.patient.co.uk/showdoc/40024645/
332 Ibid.
333 Brosman, S. A. Ibid.
334 Draper, R. Ibid.
335 Brosman, S. A. Ibid.

CHAPTER 12

Diseases of the Digestive and Urinary Systems

LEARNING OBJECTIVES

After completion of this chapter, students should be able to:

- Review the anatomy and physiology of the digestive and urinary systems
- Discuss the pathological mechanisms of common diseases of the digestive and urinary systems
- Describe diagnostic tests for diseases of the digestive and urinary systems
- Determine physical therapy intervention for patients with digestive and urinary system diseases
- Delineate the role of physical therapy intervention in the management of people with digestive and urinary system diseases
- Analyze the contraindications, precautions, and special considerations for physical therapist/physical therapist assistant intervention for patients with urinary and digestive system diseases

CHAPTER OUTLINE

KEY TERMS

Barium enema

Barium swallow

Chronic inflammatory bowel disease (Crohn's disease and ulcerative colitis)

Colonoscopy

Detrusor muscle

Diverticulosis/diverticulitis

Endoscopic ultrasound

Glomerular filtration rate (GFR)

Hemodialysis

Icterus

Indwelling catheter/Foley catheter

Inguinal hernia

Intravenous pyelogram (IVP)

Irritable bowel syndrome

Jaundice

Micturition

Neurogenic bladder

Peritoneal dialysis

Texas catheter

Transurethral resection

Upper gastrointestinal series (UGI)

Introduction

This chapter is divided into two main sections. In the first section the digestive system is described and in the second the urinary system. An overview of the anatomy and physiology of the digestive and urinary systems is provided. The relevance of the knowledge of the various aspects of the digestive and urinary systems to the physical therapist assistant is delineated. Some of the most commonly performed diagnostic tests and procedures for diseases of the digestive and urinary systems are outlined. The diseases of the digestive system are divided into sections for diseases of the esophagus, mouth and pharynx, stomach, small intestine, large bowel, liver and gallbladder and the pancreas. The urinary system diseases are similarly divided into those affecting the urinary bladder and those associated with the kidneys.

Why Does the Physical Therapist Assistant Need to Know About the Anatomy and Physiology of the Digestive System?

Physical therapy assistants (PTAs) need to have knowledge of the basic anatomical structure and physiology of the digestive system to understand and recognize the pathological state. Many patients have comorbid diagnoses in addition to the musculoskeletal and neurological problems treated with physical therapy interventions. Without knowledge of the normal physiology of these systems, the PTA may not realize when it is appropriate to refer the patient back to the physical therapist (PT) or the physician, or when to discontinue or defer treatment. Recognition of the medical terminology detailed in the patient chart is crucial to the provision of physical therapy intervention. Some medical diagnoses will affect the ability of patients to participate in physical therapy intervention.

Anatomy and Physiology of the Digestive System

The digestive system consists of the mouth, tongue, pharynx, esophagus, stomach, small intestine, large intestine (colon), appendix, rectum, and anus. The purpose of the digestive system is to process food taken in at the mouth into usable chemicals and nutrients that can be absorbed by the alimentary tract. Other structures included in this system are the liver, pancreas, gallbladder, and spleen.

The taking in of food via the mouth is called ingestion. The mouth is the entry point for food to the digestive system, alternatively called the digestive tract or alimentary canal. Mastication (chewing) of food into smaller particles by the teeth is assisted by the tongue moving food into the chewing area between the teeth. The salivary amylase enzyme, also called ptyalin, produced by the salivary glands in the mouth starts the process of digestion by breaking down the starches and glycogen in food into maltose and glucose sugars. The saliva assists with lubrication of the food particles to facilitate swallowing. The tongue is attached to the floor of the mouth by the frenulum and also to the hyoid bone in the neck. The tongue is a muscle covered with papillae (small projections) that has a root (most posterior in the mouth), a body, and a tip, which can be extended beyond the mouth cavity. The normal adult mouth consists of 32 teeth, including 4 incisors, 2 canines, 4 premolars, and 6 molars on both the upper and lower jaw. An intact dentition (full set of teeth) is needed for efficient mastication (chewing action). If a tooth is missing, there is no opposing tooth to chew against. In some cases, when teeth on the upper and lower jaw do not match well, problems with the temporomandibular joint occur, as discussed later in this chapter. The infant develops 20 deciduous teeth by age 2 years, and these fall out and are replaced with an adult set of teeth at about 6 years. Each tooth has a crown, a neck, and a root. The root is normally enclosed in the bone of the jaw, and the neck is covered by the gingiva (the gum tissue). The crown is the exposed part of the tooth seen in the mouth that does all the grinding of food. An extremely hard material called enamel covers the crown of the tooth. The neck of the tooth is composed of dentin, with a coating of cementum. Where the tooth fits into the socket within the jaw, there is a covering of periodontal membrane. The center of each tooth consists of a cavity containing blood vessels and nerves.

The mouth contains three pairs of salivary glands. The largest are the parotid glands, which have their openings close to the temporomandibular joints. The submandibular and sublingual glands open into the floor of the mouth beneath the tongue. Saliva consists of mucous, which acts as a lubricant for food to be formed into a bolus for ease of swallowing and also contains the enzyme salivary amylase, which starts the process of digestion.

The pharynx is actually the posterior aspect of the mouth leading into the esophagus and the trachea. The esophagus is a tube approximately 10 inches long connecting the pharynx to the stomach. Squamous epithelium cells and a mucous membrane line the walls of the esophagus. The wall of the esophagus also contains smooth muscles controlled by the autonomic nervous system. The smooth muscle is responsible for peristalsis (waves of contraction), which assist in propelling the food into the stomach. The peristalsis continues throughout the intestines. The stomach (see Fig. 12-1) empties its contents via the pyloric sphincter into the duodenal section of the small intestine. Digestion, and most of the absorption of nutrients, takes place within the small intestine. The small intestine measures approximately 1 inch in diameter and 20 feet in length. The internal surface area of the small intestine available for absorption of nutrients is greatly increased by the presence of villi (fingerlike projections) and even further increased by microvilli of the villi. (See Fig. 12-2.) The small intestine is divided into three sections: the duodenum attached to the stomach, a central jejunum, and a distal ileum, which attaches to the colon (large intestine). The exact mechanism of absorption of chemicals by the intestine is beyond the scope of this book. The reader is directed to consult a physiology text for further information.

The appendix is a small pouchlike structure, approximately 5 to 10 cm long and 0.5 to 1 cm wide, located at the junction of the small and large intestines as an extension of the cecum. Once thought to be merely a vestigial organ (no longer of any functional use), the appendix is now considered to be part of the immune system. The

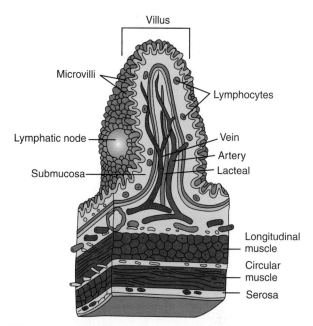

FIGURE 12.2 Internal lining of the small intestine showing villi.

appendix is largely composed of lymphatic tissue and acts as a storage container for the good bacteria needed for digestion within the intestine. When infection occurs in the intestine, the good bacteria can be destroyed. When this occurs, the appendix is able to release new colonies of bacteria into the intestines to restore the balance.[1] The colon, larger in diameter than the small intestine, approximately 2.5 inches in diameter and 5 feet in length. The cecum turns into the ascending colon (see Fig. 12-3) on the right side of the abdomen; the transverse colon, which travels horizontally across the superior aspect of the abdomen; and then the descending colon on the left side of the abdomen. The distal end of the descending colon is termed the sigmoid colon, which includes the rectum, and finally the anal canal, or anus, where the waste products of digestion exit the body. The colon does not play a part in digestion. By the time the waste materials of digestion reach the colon, there are only a few vitamins and minerals that can be reabsorbed in the colon. Water is removed from the feces (waste products of digestion) within the colon, and the colon produces mucus to facilitate the passage of feces to the anus. The colon also contains flora, which produce vitamins that are absorbed by the colon, particularly vitamin K. The mechanism that causes expulsion of feces from the anus is a defecation reflex.[2] This reflex consists of a loop reflex system from the spinal cord, which can be overridden by voluntary control. The internal anal sphincter is composed of smooth muscle,

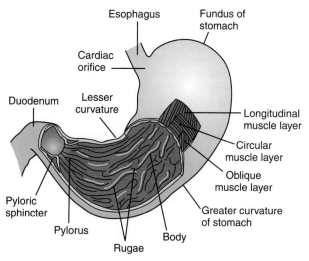

FIGURE 12.1 Anterior view of the stomach sectioned to show layers of muscle.

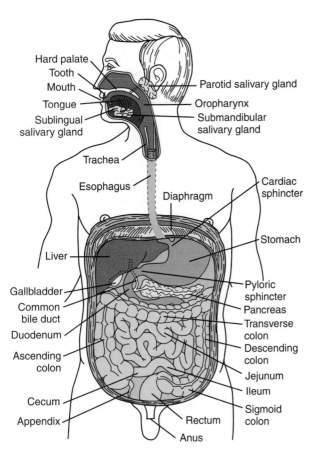

Hard palate
Tooth
Mouth
Tongue
Sublingual salivary gland
Parotid salivary gland
Oropharynx
Submandibular salivary gland
Trachea
Esophagus
Diaphragm
Cardiac sphincter
Liver
Stomach
Gallbladder
Common bile duct
Duodenum
Ascending colon
Pyloric sphincter
Pancreas
Transverse colon
Descending colon
Jejunum
Ileum
Cecum
Appendix
Sigmoid colon
Rectum
Anus

FIGURE 12.3 The digestive organs in anterior view.

which relaxes when the defecation reflex is stimulated by the peristalsis action of the intestines and allows the feces to be eliminated. The external anal sphincter provides the voluntary control mechanism. This sphincter is composed of skeletal muscle (under voluntary control), which can be tightened to prevent defecation when necessary. Muscles of the external anal sphincter can be strengthened because they are skeletal muscles. Strengthening of these muscles can, and should be, included in pelvic floor muscle reeducation programs. The inability of people to relax the pelvic floor muscles and/or the external anal sphincter can lead to difficulty with defecation.

Digestion of food is progressive throughout the digestive system. (See Table 12-1 for the enzymes and secretions that aid in digestion.) Digestive chemicals include bile secreted by the liver, via the gallbladder, into the small intestine. The pancreas secretes bicarbonates. Gastrin is secreted by the mucosa of the stomach, and in turn stimulates the release of hydrochloric acid by the stomach to start to break down the food contents of the

stomach. Both of the hormones secretin and cholecystokinin are produced by the duodenum in response to the presence of chyme, the semiliquid breakdown products of digestion. These hormones stimulate contraction of the gallbladder to release bile into the intestine.

Several factors are necessary for the digestive system to function fully. The system must be open all the way from the mouth to the anus. Any blockage prevents the digestive system working fully. Absorption through the walls of the system must be functional, and the nerve and blood supplies, and endocrine system must be intact. The blood supply to the gastrointestinal tract is from the upper and lower mesenteric arteries. The lymphatic and venous system for the intestines combines into the venous portal system, which consists of a complicated system of venous and lymphatic vessels that drain into the thoracic duct.

The liver is a large, two-lobed (right and left) structure weighing approximately 3 pounds and is located in the right side of the abdomen deep to the lower ribs, and immediately inferior to the diaphragm.[3] The liver produces bile, which is transmitted to the small intestine via the common bile duct. The duct is called "common" because it also derives from the gallbladder. The bile carries excess cholesterol and bilirubin to the intestines to be eliminated in the feces. Bile also emulsifies fats within the small intestine, aiding in fat digestion. The liver serves many other functions in the body. The liver is a major waste disposal and storage system, breaking down unwanted substances so that they can be eliminated, or detoxified, to prevent damage to other body tissues and organs. This includes the breakdown of alcohol and certain drugs and medications to prevent toxic levels forming within the body and the metabolism of hormones. The liver also regulates blood glucose levels, produces amino acids, synthesizes plasma proteins such as albumin, and the clotting factors of Factor 8, prothrombin, and fibrinogen. The phagocytes in the liver destroy bacteria from the colon venous portal system before they can be transmitted to other areas of the body. The liver is also a storage area for several vitamins, such as A, B12, D, E and K, and minerals, such as copper and iron. In addition, the liver converts ammonia, a waste product of metabolism that is toxic to the body, into urea, and diverts it to the kidneys for excretion.[4]

The gallbladder is located on the inferior surface of the right lobe of the liver. This organ acts as a storage sac for bile produced by the liver. The gallbladder consists of smooth muscle and is approximately 3 inches in diameter. The release of bile from the gallbladder is stimulated by the production of the hormone cholecystokinin by the

Table 12.1 **Enzymes and Secretions That Aid in Digestion**

ENZYME/SECRETION	WHERE PRODUCED	FUNCTION	WHERE THE ENZYME ACTS ON FOOD
Amylase	Salivary amylase present in saliva Pancreatic amylase produced by pancreas	Conversion of starches to maltose	Mouth
Bile salts	Liver (released through the gallbladder)	Fat emulsification	Small intestine
Hydrochloric acid (HCL)	Stomach	Maintains acid pH balance in the stomach to kill pathogens	Stomach
Lactase	Small intestine	Turns lactose to glucose and galactose	Small intestine
Lipase	Pancreas	Turns fats into fatty acids and glycerol	Small intestine
Maltase	Small intestine	Turns maltose to glucose	Small intestine
Pepsin	Stomach	Proteins broken down into polypeptides	Stomach
Peptidases	Small intestine	Turns peptides into amino acids	Small intestine
Sucrase	Small intestine	Turns sucrose into glucose and fructose	Small intestine
Trypsin	Pancreas	Breaks down polypeptides to peptides	Small intestine
Trypsinogen	Pancreas	Is converted to trypsin in the intestine	Small intestine

duodenum (small intestine) when food is taken into the mouth.[5]

The pancreas is a diffuse organ of approximately 6 inches in length situated within the abdomen, close to the spleen and duodenum, and posterior to the stomach. The islets of Langerhans cells are the functional units of the pancreas. The beta cells of the islets of Langerhans secrete insulin, which controls carbohydrate metabolism and the level of sugars within the blood. The alpha cells of the islets of Langerhans secrete glucagon, which counters the action of insulin and helps to preserve a balance. The pancreas also produces bicarbonates and the enzymes amylase, lipase, and trypsinogen. These substances are transmitted to the small intestine via the pancreatic duct, which joins with the common bile duct from the gallbladder and liver. (See Table 12.1 for functions of enzymes.) As with the release of bile from the common bile duct, the release of the enzymes is stimulated by other hormones—in this case, secretin and cholecystokinin.[6]

Diagnostic Medical Tests for Digestive System Diseases

Several medical tests are used to diagnose diseases of the digestive system. Although PTs and PTAs do not perform these tests, patients often ask questions about the tests they are scheduled to have performed. Having knowledge of some of the basic tests and procedures performed to diagnose digestive system diseases can be helpful in allaying the fears of patients. The diagnostic tests and procedures described in this section include radiographic studies, including barium enemas and swallows and other radiographic tests; blood, fluid, and tissue tests and esophageal pH tests; colonoscopy, sigmoidoscopy, and endoscopy; digital rectal examinations; and laparoscopic exploratory surgery.

Barium Tests

A **barium enema** is used to detect lesions in the colon, such as polyps, colon cancer, inflammatory bowel disease, or diverticula (pockets within the wall of the intestine). The preparation of patients is similar to that for the colonoscopy with a liquid diet and intestinal cleansing for 48 hours before the test. A barium enema preparation is then used, which coats the lining of the colon with an opaque medium that allows the internal outline of the colon to be visualized with a radiograph (x-ray). In a single contrast study, the colon is filled with a barium solution and then radiographed. With a double-contrast procedure, the colon is filled with a barium solution, emptied of the solution, and then filled with air. In the double-contrast study, the lining of the colon is highlighted, and the detail is better than in the single contrast. The physician performing the radiographic test can determine differences in the contours of the colon. Contraindications for this test include any medical indication that there may be a perforation of the wall of the colon because the barium solution might be absorbed into the colon or sensitivity to barium.[7,8]

A **barium swallow** for upper digestive system disorders, often called an **upper gastrointestinal series (UGI)**, may be performed. In this test, patients swallow a barium mixture solution, and radiographs are taken as the liquid enters the esophagus, stomach, and the small intestine. The procedure is painless. A physician can detect irregularities in the contours of the areas outlined by the barium liquid. Photographs of the radiographs are captured on a machine and can be printed out.[9]

Blood, Fluid, and Tissue Tests

A variety of blood, fluid, and tissue tests are performed for digestive system disorders. The most commonly requested blood test is a complete blood count (CBC). The CBC consists of testing for the red blood cell count (RBC or RCC), white blood cell count (WBC or WCC), the hematocrit levels of the blood (the fraction of the blood that is made up of red blood cells), the hemoglobin content of the blood and of each red blood cell, the mean corpuscular volume (size of the red blood cells), and the platelet count.[10] A bilirubin blood test may be performed if liver or gallbladder dysfunction is suspected. A bilirubin test measures the amount of bilirubin present in the blood serum (liquid part of the blood) and amounts are high in liver and gallbladder diseases.[11] The rate at which blood coagulates is measured using the prothrombin time (PT) and the partial thromboplastin time (PPT). Increases in these values may indicate liver or gallbladder disease, although these tests are performed for many other conditions.[12] Blood tests used in the diagnosis of specific intestinal diseases are noted within the medical intervention section for that disease.

Blood and fluid culture tests are performed to detect bacteria, parasites, or other pathogens. Cultures require several days to see whether samples produce bacterial growth when placed in a nutrient medium. People with ascites may have fluid extracted from the abdomen with a needle and sent for culture to make sure no bacteria are present. Tissue samples from biopsy are sent for histological examination. Tissue samples may be taken during any endoscopic procedure or may be obtained with a needle biopsy through the skin into the organ. A liver biopsy is usually taken with a needle.

The fecal occult blood test is a hematology test performed on feces. The presence of blood in the feces may indicate the presence of a lesion in the intestines, such as cancer, polyps, or hemorrhoids, because these may result in blood loss from the rectum. The test may be performed every year, or every 2 years, to screen those people who have a family history of colon, or intestinal cancer. People to be tested are advised to stop eating meat, fish, and root vegetables such as turnips and not to use nonsteroidal anti-inflammatory drugs (NSAIDs) or aspirin for 72 hours before the test to prevent a false-positive result. If blood is detected in the feces, more extensive testing may be performed to determine the nature of the problem.[13] When people have gastroenteritis a stool culture test may be required to examine the feces (stool) for bacteria or parasites.

Colonoscopy and Sigmoidoscopy

In 2008, updated guidelines for the screening of colon cancer were published by the American Cancer Society in conjunction with the U.S. Multi-Society Task Force on Colorectal Cancer and the American College of Radiology. These recommendations for the prevention of colon cancer screening stated that people over 50 should be routinely screened for colon cancer. If there is a history of colon cancer in the immediate family, usually parents, siblings, or children, these tests should be started at an earlier age.[14] People experiencing abdominal symptoms may also be tested to rule out certain pathological conditions such as carcinomas. People at average risk for colon cancer are screened every 5 to 10 years, whereas those at high risk may be screened annually or every other year. The new guidelines suggested several methods of screening including colonoscopy, sigmoidoscopy, barium enema, and virtual colonoscopy provided by computed tomography (CT) colonography.

A **colonoscopy** is performed as a screening and investigative procedure for people at risk of colon cancer.

Colonoscopy involves passing a flexible fiberoptic tube with a camera through the rectum into the colon looking at the descending, transverse, and ascending colons. If polyps are found they are usually removed during the procedure, and biopsies of the wall of the colon can be taken and sent for histological testing.[15] Preparation for the test includes a cleansing of the intestinal system starting approximately 48 hours before the test with an intestinal cleansing solution, a liquid diet, and oral laxatives. Some physicians place the patient under general anesthesia, and others provide mild sedation during the procedure. The early detection and removal of suspicious lesions in the colon reduces the mortality rate from colon cancer. Many insurance companies, as well as Medicare, do not pay for a screening colonoscopy unless there are abdominal symptoms, such as bleeding from the rectum. It is hoped that the reduction in mortality and overall costs from treating colon cancer will encourage these companies to start paying for this preventive care.

The flexible sigmoidoscopy is a test similar to the colonoscopy but only checks the rectum and sigmoid colon, which is the last one-third of the colon. The sigmoidoscopy is used less frequently because many cancers are located beyond the sigmoid colon and are therefore not detected by this procedure.[16]

The virtual colonoscopy is performed using a CT scanner. Preparation for the scan involves the use of laxatives. A small tube is inserted into the anus to inject air into the colon for better viewing during the CT scan. This screening test is not as accurate as traditional colonoscopy, because cancerous lesions that are flattened areas in the wall of the colon may be overlooked. In addition, polyps cannot be removed during this procedure.[17]

DIGITAL RECTAL EXAM

A digital rectal examination (DRE) is a screening test performed by a physician to determine abnormalities of the lower rectum and anus. A gloved, lubricated finger is inserted into the rectum to palpate the walls of the rectum. The detection of an abnormally large prostate in the male is also possible using this test.[18]

ENDOSCOPY

Endoscopy involves the insertion of a flexible tube containing a camera into the body. Small surgical instruments can be inserted through the endoscope to enable removal of tissue when needed. Endoscopic procedures for the upper part of the digestive system usually involve inserting the endoscope through the mouth and esophagus, with the person sedated. However, occasionally the endoscope is inserted into the body through a small incision, in which

case the person is placed under general anesthetic. The procedure performed with an endoscope is named after the structures to be examined.[19] Some of the more commonly performed endoscopic procedures for the digestive system, in addition to the colonoscopy and sigmoidoscopy previously described, include an anoscopy inserted through the anus to view the rectum and anal areas; an esophagoscopy to view the esophagus; an esophagogastroduodenoscopy (EGD) to view the esophagus, stomach, and duodenum (first part of the small intestine); a laryngoscopy to view the larynx; and a proctoscopy to view the anal, rectum, and part of the descending colon. An additional procedure called an endoscopic retrograde cholangiopancreatography involves passing the endoscope through the mouth and esophagus into the duodenum and then passing a small catheter through the endoscope and into the common bile duct. Contrast medium (dye) is then inserted into the common bile duct and radiographic images are taken. During this procedure, a small stent may be placed in the common bile duct to keep it patent (open).

ESOPHAGEAL pH MONITORING AND ESOPHAGEAL ACIDITY TESTING

A test used for people with esophageal acid reflux to determine the amount of acid entering the esophagus during a 24-hour period. A catheter with an acid sensor on the end is inserted into the esophagus via the mouth and left in place for 24 hours. The catheter and sensor is then removed and analyzed to see how often acid has refluxed into the esophagus from the stomach.[20]

LAPAROSCOPIC EXPLORATORY SURGERY

Laparoscopic exploratory surgery is mainly used for conditions of the abdomen and pelvis. The laparoscope is a flexible tube containing a camera that allows the surgeon to see inside the abdomen. This type of procedure may be used for exploratory internal examinations and also for laparoscopy-assisted surgery. The advantages of laparoscopy are that only several small incisions are needed, rather than the larger incisions of traditional surgical methods, resulting in reduced healing time. People are sedated with general anesthesia for this procedure.[21]

RADIOGRAPHIC AND IMAGING TESTS

Angiography, or arteriography, is an invasive (something inserted into the body) radiographic test performed to see whether the arteries are blocked. In this procedure, a contrast medium is injected into the arteries of the area to be examined, and a radiographic image is taken of the blood vessels. When angiography is performed for the pancreas, a catheter is passed through the femoral artery in the area of the groin to the pancreatic ducts. In some cases, instruments can be inserted through the catheter to remove tissue or insert a stent into the artery.[22]

A computerized axial tomography (CAT) scan, more often called CT scan, is a type of radiographic imaging machine with a circular hole through which the patient lies on a table. The machine rotates round the body and takes cross-sectional images of the body. People have to remain still during the scan. The benefits of the CT scan are that the images produced include the internal organs, bones, blood vessels, and other soft tissues not visible on a conventional radiographic image. The CT scan may be performed with, or without, the injection of contrast medium to highlight specific areas of interest.[23]

A liver scan, also known as a liver-spleen radionuclide scan, nuclear scan, or technetium scan, is another imaging technique used to diagnose diseases and conditions of the liver and spleen. Radioactive isotopes are injected into the veins, which are then absorbed by the liver and spleen. Images are taken of the liver and spleen, which show any abnormalities in these structures. This test is usually used in conjunction with an abdominal ultrasound, and a CT scan, to determine the diagnosis.[24]

A nuclear medicine bone scan is sometimes used for people with digestive system carcinomas to detect bone metastases. A radioactive substance called a tracer, often consisting of glucose, is injected into the circulatory system. This tracer is absorbed into the bone. A nuclear scan is then taken of the bones, which provides an image of the skeleton.[25]

Positron emission tomography (PET), sometimes called a nuclear medicine scan, is an imaging technique provided via a machine somewhat like a CT scanner. The patient has to lie within the machine on a platform and remain still during the procedure. The images from the PET scan are not as detailed as those of a CT scan or an MRI. The radioactive tracer is absorbed more in areas of increased blood supply such as cancerous tumors and areas of metastases throughout the body. These areas of increased vascularity are visible on the images. Sometimes a PET scan and a CT scan are combined in a PET/CT scan.[26]

Magnetic resonance imaging (MRI) uses magnets and radiowaves to take images called "slices" of the body, either cross-sectional or longitudinally. This machine does not use radioactivity. A contrast medium dye may or may not be used during the procedure. The strong magnets cause an alignment of hydrogen atoms in the body that creates an image of the tissues, with each type of tissue identifiably different. The images may be printed on radiographic film or stored as computer images. The MRI machine looks like a tunnel, and the person lies on a platform within the machine for the test, which can last about an hour. The magnets make a loud noise as they rotate around the machine and the body. Some people may feel claustrophobic during an MRI. A more open MRI machine is available in some medical centers to accommodate people who are either too large to use the smaller machines or who are too claustrophobic. People with certain types of metal implants such as cardiac pacemakers and some artificial heart valves are unable to have an MRI. No metals objects are allowed in the area of the machines because of the strong magnetic field created by the machine.[27]

Percutaneous transhepatic cholangiography is a procedure in which dye is injected directly into the liver and the bile ducts with a long needle inserted through the abdominal wall. A radiographic image is then taken of the liver and bile ducts.

Ultrasonography uses sound waves from a transducer head to produce images of internal abdominal organs. An abdominal ultrasound is a noninvasive technique performed with the ultrasound head passed over the external surface of the abdomen. This test is used in the detection of a variety of diseases of the abdominal organs including the liver, pancreas, and rectum. **Endoscopic ultrasound** is a special technique performed using a small ultrasound probe on the end of an endoscope. The patient is sedated, and the ultrasound probe is introduced into the area to be examined via the endoscope through the mouth and the esophagus and can take close-up images of the involved organ. This technique is mainly used for the detection of diseases in the upper part of the digestive system accessible through the esophagus.

Why Does the Physical Therapist Assistant Need to Know About Diseases of the Digestive System?

The PTA comes into contact with people with many types of digestive system diseases when providing physical therapy interventions. Some of these diseases are of minimal significance to the PTA, but others may create contraindications for certain treatment modalities or prevent the patient from participating fully in rehabilitation. For many patients with carcinoma, there may be severe debilitation and inability to tolerate more than short periods of physical therapy intervention. Some PTAs may be involved with treatment of people in hospice care, and knowledge of the following pathological conditions may be important. The main aim of intervention for patients in a hospice setting is quality of life and achieving of as much independence as possible. This may involve ambulation with appropriate assistive devices, positioning for comfort and prevention of pressure areas, teaching of family and caregivers for transfers, movement and exercise protocols to improve strength, and endurance and balance training. Not all of the following pathologies are cancerous in nature. Some involve conditions that cause general debility over a prolonged period. Such patients may seek the advice of a PT to help them achieve a level of independence in their daily life. In all cases, the PTA must practice rigorous hand washing techniques to minimize the spread of infection. Patients who are debilitated with chronic disease are much more susceptible to the transmission of infection. Care should be taken to practice Standard (Universal) Precautions with all patients. Attention to the level of fatigue with treatment is essential so as not to overtax patients and reduce the effectiveness of the physical therapy interventions.

Diseases of the Digestive System

Hints on use of the Guide to Physical Therapist Practice

Patients with internal organ disease may require physical therapy intervention as a result of general deconditioning, reduced muscle strength, or balance problems. Many practice patterns may be used for patients with deconditioning.

- 4A "Primary prevention/risk reduction for skeletal demineralization (p. 133): Patients who have become inactive and prone to reduced bone density may fall within the "Musculoskeletal" Preferred Practice Pattern 4A.
- 4C "Impaired muscle performance" (p. 161): Patients who have become inactive may fall within this "Musculoskeletal" Preferred Practice Pattern 4C.

- 4G "Impaired joint mobility, muscle performance, and range of motion associated with fracture" (p. 233): Patients with general debility could also be categorized under "Musculoskeletal" Preferred Practice Pattern 4G; patients with fractures may also be included in this pattern.
- 5A "Primary prevention/risk reduction for loss of balance and falling" (p. 307): In cases in which patients have a history of falls, dizziness, poor balance, or prolonged inactivity, the most appropriate pattern could be the "Neuromuscular" Preferred Practice Pattern 5A.
- 5G "Impaired motor function and sensory integrity associated with acute or chronic polyneuropathies" (p. 411): Patients with renal disease who have neuropathy would come under the "Neuromuscular" Preferred Practice Pattern 5G.
- 6B "Impaired aerobic capacity/endurance associated with deconditioning" (p. 483): If a patient was undergoing chronic total body system failure they may well be assigned the "Cardiovascular/Pulmonary" Preferred Practice Pattern 6B.
- 7A "Primary prevention/risk reduction for integumentary disorders" (p. 589): If patients are malnourished due to advanced disease they may have skin breakdown which would then classify them under the "Integumentary" Preferred Practice Pattern 7A.
- 7B "Impaired integumentary integrity associated with superficial skin involvement" (p. 601): The appropriate classification of a patient with debilitation and superficial skin involvement would be the "Integumentary" Preferred Practice Pattern 7B.
- 7C "Impaired integumentary integrity associated with partial-thickness skin involvement and scar formation" (p. 619): The appropriate classification of a patient with debilitation secondary to an internal organ failure and associated partial-thickness skin involvement and scar formation would be "Integumentary" Preferred Practice Pattern 7C.
- 7D "Impaired integumentary integrity with full-thickness skin involvement and scar formation" (p. 637): The appropriate classification of a patient with debilitation secondary to an internal organ failure and associated with full-thickness skin involvement and scar formation would be "Integumentary" Preferred Practice Pattern 7D.

(From the American Physical Therapy Association, 2003. *Guide to physical therapist practice*, revised 2nd edition. Alexandria, VA.)

In general, the signs and symptoms of many of the diseases of the digestive system include abdominal pain, excessive flatulence, nausea, vomiting, diarrhea, and constipation. Nausea is a feeling of impending vomiting, which may or may not result in actual vomiting. Vomiting is controlled by a center in the medulla of the brain in response to the body's need to eliminate toxic substances, and should not necessarily be prevented by using antivomiting medications. Vomiting is an involuntary reflex, which results in the elimination of the contents of the stomach, and sometimes the intestine, through involuntary contraction of the abdominal muscles and relaxation of the gastroesophageal sphincter. If vomiting continues for a prolonged period, it can cause dehydration. When vomiting occurs over a prolonged period, it is usually a sign of a serious condition and medical advice must be sought. Vomiting may also occur as a result of severe stress or pain, bad smells, or after experiencing a traumatic event. A neurological cause of vomiting may occur as a result of an increase of intracranial pressure in the brain. Usually these neurological cases cause projectile vomiting not associated with eating and are cause to seek immediate medical attention. Diarrhea may be defined as either a frequent need to eliminate stools or having excessive amounts of fluid stools. Diarrhea is sometimes associated with abdominal pain. The term *constipation* refers to stools that are hard and difficult to eliminate from the body. Each person has a different pattern of normal bowel habits. Some people may have problems with chronic patterns of either diarrhea or constipation, and others may alternate between the two. Others may not have either of these problems. In most cases, signs of disease or problems with the intestinal system are indicated when there is a change in the usual pattern of bowel movements for that individual. Chronic diarrhea can lead to malnutrition and fluid and electrolyte imbalances as a result of the lack of absorption time for the food in the intestines and is cause to seek medical attention.

Diseases of the Esophagus

Some inflammatory diseases of the esophagus such as esophagitis may be caused by infections, but most are caused by irritations from allergic substances, or from esophageal reflux of ingested material in the stomach regurgitating into the esophagus. Esophageal cancer is one of the more common carcinomas.

Esophageal Cancer

Two types of cancer are most common in the esophagus. Squamous cell carcinoma develops from the squamous epithelial cells lining the esophagus, and adenocarcinoma derives from the mucus-producing cells. The condition occurs mainly in people in the 50 to 70 age range. The incidence of the disease is from 2 to 7 times higher in people who consume large amounts of alcohol and those who smoke and is lower when the diet includes plenty of fresh vegetables especially broccoli, cauliflower, cabbage, and other green or yellow vegetables or fruit.[28] The cancer is more common in males than females, and African Americans are affected more often than Caucasians. However, the incidence and death rates have been declining since the 1990s.[29] Estimates from the National Cancer Institute included 16,640 new diagnoses and 14,500 deaths from this disease in 2010.[30]

Etiology. The etiology of esophageal cancer is largely unknown, but chronic use of alcohol and tobacco products, infection with the human papillomavirus (HPV), and malnutrition all seem to increase the risk for cancer, with alcohol and tobacco most associated with squamous cell carcinoma.[31] Another predisposing factor for adenocarcinoma of the esophagus is long-standing gastroesophageal reflux disease (GERD), in which stomach contents regurgitate into the esophagus causing irritation of the lining of the esophagus. Barrett esophagus is a condition of the esophagus that predisposes toward adenocarcinoma. In Barrett esophagus, the columnar epithelial cells of the lining of the esophagus undergo metaplasia into abnormal cells.

Signs and Symptoms. Most adenocarcinoma tumors occur in the lower third of the esophagus. Squamous cell carcinomas may occur in any part of the esophagus. The early stages of the carcinoma are often not associated with any symptoms. Dysphagia (difficulty swallowing) and weight loss are usually only apparent when the cancer is quite advanced.[32] Other signs and symptoms associated with more advanced stages of the disease may include chronic hiccups, hoarseness of the voice, and pain on swallowing food or fluids.[33]

Prognosis. Prognosis in these patients is poor because many carcinomas are not detected early enough to be treated effectively. The staging of the carcinoma follows similar guidelines to other types of malignancy. A combination of tumor type, lymph node metastasis, and the level of metastasis to other structures determines the stage of the carcinoma. This staging ranges from a Stage 0 to a Stage IVB, with IV the most invasive and extensive.[34] The overall 5-year survival rate for people with esophageal carcinoma is between 5% and 30%. However, people who are diagnosed early have a much better survival rate.[35]

Medical Intervention. The diagnosis of esophageal cancer is often difficult because many people are asymptomatic until the cancer has become well advanced. People with long-standing GERD may be screened for changes in the lining of the esophagus and Barrett esophagus using an upper gastrointestinal test, such as a barium swallow or an esophagoscopy (endoscopy of the esophagus). Other tests may include an MRI or a CT scan to determine the level of invasiveness of the tumor and an ultrasound device attached to the end of the endoscope.[36] The appropriate medical treatment may include surgical resection of the affected area of the esophagus and/or radiation and chemotherapy.[37] Surgery may be preventive in people who have Barrett esophagus to prevent cancer. Surgical procedures may be performed with traditional open surgery, minimally invasive procedures, a laparoscopic device, or laser techniques.[38,39]

Physical Therapy Intervention. PT intervention is rarely sought. A speech and language pathologist and occupational therapist specializing in swallowing and esophageal motility may be helpful in assisting with dysphagia (swallowing difficulties).

GASTROESOPHAGEAL REFLUX DISEASE
Gastroesophageal reflux disease (GERD, also known as acid reflux or heartburn, is a common condition in which the acidic contents of the stomach and the intestine regurgitate up into the lower esophagus.

Etiology. The cause of GERD may be a defect in the lower esophageal sphincter where the esophagus joins the stomach. The muscles of the sphincter may be weak or may relax at the wrong times. Another cause may be a slow emptying of the stomach contents into the intestines. Some people with GERD also have a hiatal hernia, in which part of the stomach herniates through the diaphragm.[40] Other factors that increase the risk of GERD include pregnancy; obesity, and scleroderma.

Signs and Symptoms. The usual signs and symptoms of GERD are of a burning sensation or pain in the central part of the anterior chest deep to the sternum. This sensation may occur after meals and is often worse when in a supine position at night.[41] Other symptoms may include belching, nausea, vomiting, sore throat, and difficulty swallowing.[42]

Prognosis. Chronic, severe GERD can lead to carcinoma of the esophagus if it continues over a prolonged period of time. Barrett esophagus can be a precancerous condition of the esophagus (see section on esophageal cancer).

Medical Intervention. The diagnosis of GERD is often achieved through a history of the symptoms. An upper gastrointestinal endoscopy may be performed to confirm the diagnosis. This test will reveal any esophagitis (inflammation), ulcerations, or erosions on the lining of the esophagus.[43] Esophageal acid testing performed over a 24-hour period, with a catheter inserted into the esophagus with an acid sensor on the tip, can detect the number of times acid content occurs in the esophagus. Another test is a gastric-emptying study that can detect how quickly the contents of the stomach empty into the intestines. In this test, a meal is eaten with radioactive isotope content, which can be monitored by an external Geiger counter to determine the rate of stomach emptying. The medications prescribed for GERD are usually proton pump inhibitors such as Prilosec, Prevacid, Protonix, or Nexium. These medications reduce the acidic content of the stomach and prevent the irritation of the esophagus and may even prevent the reflux.[44] Lifestyle changes that help to reduce the effects of GERD include raising the head end of the bed or sleeping on a wedge; avoiding intake of alcohol, chocolate, caffeine, and mint; and smoking cessation.[45]

Physical Therapy Intervention. Many people undergoing physical therapy intervention may indicate problems with esophageal reflux. The PT and PTA should encourage people with the condition to seek medical advice.

Diseases of the Mouth and Pharynx
The two diseases discussed in this section are carcinoma of the mouth and temporomandibular joint (TMJ) dysfunction. People with both these conditions frequently require physical therapy interventions in the recovery phase.

Carcinoma of the Mouth and Oral Carcinoma

Carcinomas of the mouth are fairly common. Estimates by the American Cancer Society were that in 2010 25,800 people would be diagnosed with oral carcinomas and 5,830 people would die. The rate of both new cases of oral cancer and the death rate has been declining since the 1970s.[46] Men are affected twice as often as women, and most cancers of the throat and mouth are diagnosed in people over age 40.[47,48] The areas of the mouth affected mainly include the lips and tongue, but any part of the oral cavity may be involved. The salivary glands can also be affected by tumors, although most of these tumors are benign. Inflammation of the salivary glands is called sialadenitis and is usually caused by viruses, such as mumps, or bacterial as a result of infection with *Staphylococcus aureus* or *Streptococcus viridans*.[49]

Etiology. The exact etiology of mouth cancers is unknown, although many start with precancerous lesions. Two common types of precancerous lesions occur in the mouth. Leukoplakia is a white area of tissue, and erythroplakia is a red area of tissue. Both types of tissue can become malignant over time, but the erythroplakia tends to be more likely to change and become cancerous. Squamous cell carcinomas are the most common, occurring in 90% of all oral carcinomas. Other types of carcinoma include salivary gland tumors and lymphomas.[50] People who smoke and drink heavily are at as much as 100 times greater risk for oral carcinomas than those who do not.[51] Pipe smoking increases the risk of cancer of the lips, and smokeless tobacco (chewing tobacco and snuff) causes cancer of the gums, the inside of the cheeks, and inner surface of the lips. Other risk factors for the development of oral cancers include a combination of smoking and alcohol use; exposure to ultraviolet light on the lips, such as those people who work outside; human papillomavirus (HPV); and chewing Betel nuts popular in several Asian countries. People whose diet is low in fruits and vegetables may also be at risk. [52,53]

Signs and Symptoms. The signs and symptoms of mouth cancers are not specific to cancer but may be caused by other problems. Some of these symptoms may include lumps in the mouth; sores that do not heal on the cheeks, roof of the mouth, on the gums, or on the tongue; white or red patches of tissue anywhere in the mouth; bleeding or pain in the mouth for no known reason; problems with the voice; or difficulty with chewing, and possibly ear pain.[54]

Prognosis. As with any carcinoma the prognosis depends on the stage of the cancer when diagnosed. The earlier the diagnosis, the better is the outcome from treatment for oral cancer. People who receive treatment for mouth cancers have an overall 5-year survival rate of 56%, and a 10-year survival rate of 41%.[55]

Medical Intervention. The initial diagnosis of oral cancers is often made by the dentist during a regular checkup appointment. Further testing for diagnosis may involve a biopsy of the suspected lesions, a laryngoscopy (a flexible tube with a fiberoptic tip linked to a camera), CT scan, MRI, and nuclear medicine bone scans. Treatment for mouth carcinomas is usually with radiation or surgical excision. Chemotherapy may be required in certain instances.[56]

Physical Therapy Intervention. Patient rehabilitation after surgical removal of tumors in the mouth may require reeducation of the muscles of the mouth. A familiarity with the muscles of the face is essential for any PT or PTA involved in this type of intervention. Treatment intervention from a speech and language pathologist and/or occupational therapist specializing in swallowing and eating disorders may also be indicated after extensive surgery as a result of the associated speech, eating, and swallowing problems.[57]

Temporomandibular Joint Dysfunction as a Result of Periodontal Disease

Physical therapist and PTAs are rarely involved with direct intervention for periodontal disease. However, disorders of the temporomandibular joint (TMJ) can be caused by periodontal disease, and physical therapy is indicated for these disorders.

Etiology. If teeth have been removed because of periodontal disease such as gingivitis (acute inflammation of the gums) or periodontitis, (inflammation of the periodontal membrane causing loosening of teeth and the destruction of bone in severe cases), this can precipitate TMJ problems. Dental caries (cavities) can also mean tooth extraction, which can lead to imbalances in the bite between the upper and lower jaw teeth, and this in turn, can cause TMJ problems. Other causes of TMJ dysfunction are arthritis, muscle spasms, and teeth clenching during sleep.

Signs and Symptoms. The characteristic signs and symptoms of TMJ dysfunction include facial, neck, and jaw pain, stiffness of the muscles of the neck and jaw, limited ability to open the mouth, and painful motion of the TMJ including clicking and grinding sensations.[58]

Prognosis. TMJ dysfunction often resolves without any intervention. Some people may have chronic pain associated with the TMJ problem that requires intervention from a pain specialist, such as a physical therapist who specializes in the TMJ.

Medical Intervention. Surgery for TMJ problems is rarely performed. Sometimes the bite will be adjusted by a dentist to align the teeth in the hope that the TMJ problem will be reduced. Home remedies such as heat, anti-inflammatory medications, and eating soft foods are often recommended. Mouth inserts to prevent tooth grinding during sleep are sometimes provided by a dentist or periodontist.

Physical Therapy Intervention. Noninvasive intervention for TMJ dysfunction, including physical therapy, is the preferred initial treatment for people with TMJ dysfunction.[59] Many physical therapists work in association with dentists and periodontists to provide intervention for patients with TMJ problems. Chronic headaches are often associated with TMJ dysfunction and respond to physical therapy intervention.[60] A review of studies performed on people with TMJ dysfunction indicated that an approach including several components works best for resolution of the problem. The most effective treatment strategies included a combination of exercise, manual therapy, relaxation, and postural advice, and correction.[61] Physical therapy intervention may include mobilizations to the TMJ and anti-inflammatory procedures such as electrical stimulation, iontophoresis, phonophoresis, and ultrasound on the area of skin overlying the TMJ.[62] Other PT interventions include exercise protocols for the mouth and neck muscles, relaxation training, advice on avoidance of the types of eating and chewing that aggravate the condition, and use of prostheses such as bite guards for use during the night to reduce tooth grinding.

Diseases of the Stomach

The diseases described in this section include only those most commonly encountered during physical therapy practice such as cancer of the stomach, gastritis, and gastroenteritis.

Carcinoma of the Stomach

The worldwide incidence of stomach cancer is 1 million people per year. The highest incidence of stomach cancer is reported to be in Japan, South America, the Middle Eastern Countries, and parts of Eastern Europe. Worldwide, stomach cancer is the second leading cause of death resulting from cancer.[63] Carcinoma of the stomach continues to affect approximately 21,000 people in the United States each year. Estimates from the National Cancer Institute for 2010 were for 21,000 people to be newly diagnosed with stomach cancer, and 10,570 deaths attributable to the disease. Men are more than twice as likely to be affected than women.[64] The incidence is greater in people of Asian, Pacific Islander, Hispanic, and African American descent than in white Americans. The incidence of gastric carcinoma has reduced during the last 75 years in the United States. The condition is rarely seen in people under age 40, and more usually in people over age 65 years.[65]

Etiology. The cause of cancer of the stomach is largely unknown. Some factors that may increase the possibility of developing stomach carcinoma include being age greater than 72 years; eating a diet high in smoked, pickled, and salty foods; smoking; a history of gastritis or previous stomach surgery; pernicious anemia; and infection with *Helicobacter pylori*.[66]

Signs and Symptoms. Unfortunately most carcinomas of the stomach remain undetected until they are in an advanced stage. Symptoms may not occur until the later stages of the disease, and may include weight loss, dyspepsia, nausea, vomiting, and minimal abdominal pain.[67]

Prognosis. The prognosis for people with cancer of the stomach is generally poor unless it is diagnosed and treated in the early stages. If people are diagnosed with localized stomach tumors, the likelihood of a cure is 50%. However, if the cancer has metastasized, the outlook is poor. The 5-year survival rate for people with cancer of the proximal part of the stomach is only between 10% and 15%.[68]

Medical Intervention. The tests performed to detect carcinoma of the stomach involve an upper gastrointestinal series such as endoscopy or barium swallows. Further studies such as a biopsy through the endoscope, complete blood count, radiographs of the chest, CT scan, and laparoscopic exploratory surgery may also be performed if stomach cancer is suspected. Staging of the carcinoma is similar to those previously described for other carcinomas from Stage I through Stage IV. If a lesion is found, it may be possible to surgically excise the area if the tumor is in Stage I or II.[69] The usual course of treatment for people with stomach cancer is surgical excision of the affected part of the stomach, and the associated lymph nodes, combined with radiation therapy and chemotherapy.[70]

Physical Therapy Intervention. Physical therapy intervention may be required for mobility training as a result of reduced ambulatory and functional status before or after surgical intervention. Teaching of the use of mechanical transfer lifts for families and caregivers is also provided for people in the terminal stages of the disease.

Gastritis and Peptic Ulcer Disease

Gastritis is an inflammation of the lining of the stomach. The main types of gastritis are erosive and nonerosive. In erosive gastritis, hemorrhage may occur. Nonerosive gastritis is also called chronic gastritis. The incidence of gastritis increases with age and affects males and females equally.[71] A more commonly used term for erosive gastritis is an ulcer or peptic ulcer disease (PUD). Peptic or gastric ulcers are smooth, craterlike lesions in the lining mucosa of the stomach, duodenum, or even the lower part of the esophagus (see Fig. 12-4 for common locations of these ulcers). After lesions occur, the digestive acids are able to further break down the area and cause even more irritation. In some cases, the ulceration actually perforates the stomach, duodenum, or esophagus. The incidence of gastric ulcers is highest in men beyond middle age but can occur in either sex at any age.

Etiology. Several causes exist for the erosive type of gastritis. The use of NSAIDs or other medications that irritate the lining of the stomach such as aspirin, heavy alcohol consumption, gastroesophageal reflux disease, smoking, viruses, ingested poisons, or the stress caused by illness, surgery, or portal hypertension may all cause the condition.[72] Most people with cases of nonerosive gastritis have no known cause. However, some are caused by an infection with the *H. pylori* bacteria, and others may be a result of pernicious anemia.[73] Estimates are that approximately between 50% and 60% of people over age 60 are infected with the *H. pylori* bacteria.[74,75]

Signs and Symptoms. The characteristic signs and symptoms of erosive gastritis include abdominal pain, particularly after eating spicy foods, and general dyspepsia (indigestion), anorexia (lack of appetite), nausea, vomiting, and signs of bleeding resulting in dark-colored stools.[76] After a peptic ulcer develops, substances such as caffeine and spicy foods may cause further irritation. In some cases, there is hemorrhage with large amounts of blood lost from the upper digestive system through vomiting. Iron-deficient anemia may also indicate the presence of an ulcer.

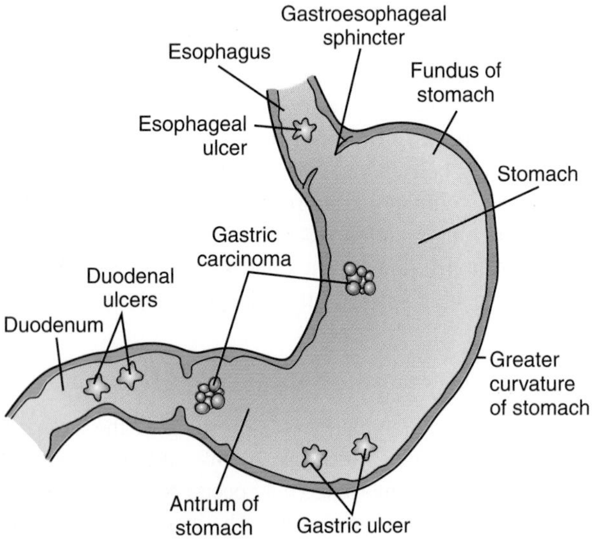

Prognosis. The prognosis for most people with gastritis is good. Most people's symptoms resolve with the use of appropriate medications and lifestyle changes.

Medical Intervention. The diagnosis of gastritis may be achieved with an upper gastrointestinal test such as a barium swallow or an endoscopy. After diagnosis, people with gastritis are treated for the cause of the condition, if one is identified. If *H. pylori* bacteria is a causative factor, the treatment involves a combination of antimicrobial medications and proton pump inhibitors such as Prevacid or Prilosec. *H. pylori* can be difficult to eliminate and frequently requires a prolonged regimen of antimicrobial therapy. Medications that coat the inside of the digestive system such as Tagamet or Zantac may also relieve the symptoms of peptic ulcers. Changes in eating habits may be recommended to try and reduce the risk of further ulcers. This advice usually includes reduction of caffeine intake, which acts as an irritant to the mucosal lining of the digestive system.[77]

Physical Therapy Intervention. Physical therapy intervention is not generally part of the treatment for gastritis. Relaxation exercises may help to reduce overall feelings of stress.

Gastroenteritis

Gastroenteritis is a generalized inflammation of the stomach and intestine caused by a variety of agents including bacteria, viruses, and parasites. The condition is extremely common because it spreads easily from person to person, especially if regular hand washing is not practiced.[78]

Etiology. The etiology of gastroenteritis may be from bacterial, viral, or parasitic infections. Symptoms may also be the result of an allergic reaction to foods or medications. Gastroenteritis symptoms are common among travelers, in association with gastric influenza, and food poisoning. The viral form of the disease is common and is usually caused by one of two viruses known as the rotavirus, or norovirus (formerly called the Norwalk virus). Water contamination is a problem in certain countries, and travelers need to be careful not to drink water or uncooked foods in areas of the world that do not have a clean water supply,

FIGURE 12.4 Diagram of some common locations of esophageal, gastric, and duodenal ulcers.

or where vegetables are fertilized with human feces.[79] Bacterial causes of gastroenteritis include *Staphylococcus aureus, Escherichia coli, Salmonella, Campylobacter, Shigella,* and *Clostridium difficile.* Parasites that cause the condition are usually Giardia and cryptosporidium.[80]

Signs and Symptoms. The characteristic signs and symptoms of gastroenteritis may include diarrhea, abdominal pain, fever, sweating, nausea, vomiting, abdominal bloating, flatulence, fatigue, headache, and dehydration.[81]

Prognosis. Many people with gastroenteritis recover without treatment. Some people infected with bacteria or parasites require medications but usually fully recover with treatment.

Medical Intervention. The incidence of the disease can be greatly reduced if precautions are taken when preparing food such as regular washing of hands and cooking meats well. Medical treatment requires identification of the causative organism through blood or stool cultures so that an appropriate medication may be prescribed. Stool culture tests include those for bacteria and an ova and parasite (O & P) exam to detect parasites.[82] During symptoms of vomiting and diarrhea, an adequate fluid intake is important to prevent dehydration. Antimotility or antidiarrheal medications may also be prescribed. Young children have to be closely monitored for fluid intake because a comparatively small amount of fluid loss can constitute a high percentage of their total body fluid, resulting in severe dehydration. Elderly people are also at risk for fluid imbalance, particularly if they are not very mobile, because it may be difficult for them to reach a supply of fluids to restore or maintain adequate hydration.

Physical Therapy Intervention. No physical therapy is indicated for the treatment of gastroenteritis. However, physical therapists and PTAs can help to reduce the spread of the infection through regular hand washing to prevent cross-infection.

Diseases of the Small Intestine

Several types of disease of the small intestines exist. Most of these diseases will not be described in great detail because physical therapy intervention is not usually required. A basic understanding of disease process and the names of the diseases is, however, advisable for the PTA. Bowel syndromes such as diarrhea and constipation are common conditions and may not always be abnormal. Many people have regular patterns of bowel motion that

include loose stools or constipation, and this pattern is normal for them. Changes in normal bowel patterns are more important to note when determining diseases of the alimentary tract. Problems with bowel incontinence may become of major importance to the PTA during physical therapy intervention for other conditions. Some of these issues are discussed further in Chapter 14.

Appendicitis

Appendicitis is an inflammation of the vermiform ("wormlike") appendix. The condition is usually of an acute nature, with a sudden onset. The appendix is attached to the cecum at the distal end of the small intestine and connects with the colon. Appendicitis can occur at any age but is more common in people between ages 10 and 30 years.[83] Appendectomy (excision of the appendix) is performed on 1 in every 2,000 people in the United States.[84] Acute appendicitis occurs in approximately 25 out of 10,000 people each year in the United States for a total of 680,000 people.[85]

Etiology. The initial cause of the problem may be due to a blockage of the appendix with a fecalith (fecal material that hardens into a rocklike consistency), a tumor, or, in some cases, parasites such as intestinal worms. Another cause is inflammation of the lymphatic tissue of the appendix, which blocks the appendix. After the appendix is blocked, bacteria can invade the internal wall of the appendix and cause further inflammation, and even perforation.[86] If the appendix is perforated or ruptures, an abscess may form. This pus-filled abscess can be an ongoing site of infection.

Signs and Symptoms. The characteristic signs and symptoms of acute appendicitis are at first generalized pain in the abdomen, leading to intense right, lower abdominal pain in an area known as McBurney's point (see Fig. 12-5). If the appendix ruptures, the pain may once again become more generalized to the whole abdomen. Other symptoms include diarrhea or constipation, nausea, vomiting, and anorexia (loss of appetite).[87,88]

Prognosis. Most people with appendicitis fully recover with no side effects. Occasionally, the blockage and infection of the appendix may cause necrosis of the appendix, and if the appendix is perforated, the infection can enter the abdomen and pelvis causing peritonitis. In severe, but rare, instances, sepsis may occur in which the infection invades the whole body. Both peritonitis and sepsis are serious conditions that can result in death if not treated.[89]

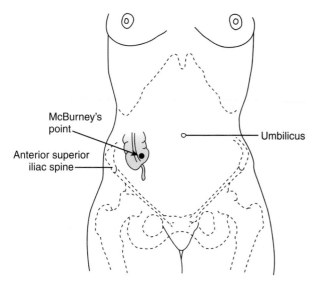

FIGURE 12.5 Position of McBurney's point in appendicitis.

Medical Intervention. The diagnosis of appendicitis may involve a variety of tests. The right lower abdomen may be tender to palpation, and the temperature is usually elevated because of infection. The white blood cell count is usually elevated as a result of infection, but this is not specific for appendicitis. Radiographic studies may include an abdominal radiograph to highlight a fecalith, an ultrasound scan to identify an enlarged appendix or an appendiceal abscess, a barium enema, a CT scan, an MRI for people who are allergic to the contrast medium administered for a CT scan, and an exploratory surgery using laparoscopy.[90,91] The use of a laparoscope is helpful because if the appendix is found to be inflamed, it can be removed during the procedure.[92]

People with appendicitis are prescribed antimicrobial medications. Some people with milder forms of appendicitis may respond to this medication and not require surgery. In most cases of acute appendicitis, an appendectomy (surgical excision of the appendix) is required. The appendectomy is usually performed using the laparoscope (a flexible tube with a light and camera through which surgical instruments can be used to remove the appendix). If an appendiceal abscess has formed as a result of a ruptured appendix, the drainage of the abscess may be performed by inserting a drainage tube into the abscess. The tube will allow drainage of the pus through the opening made in the skin of the abdomen. After the abscess has cleared and the infection has resolved, an appendectomy is then performed.[93]

Physical Therapy Intervention. Physical therapy intervention is not indicated for people with appendicitis.

Celiac Sprue (small intestine malabsorption)

Celiac sprue, otherwise called adult celiac disease or gluten enteropathy, is a malabsorption disease specific to the small intestine resulting from intolerance to a protein called gluten in the diet. Many malabsorption conditions, including those caused by gastric, liver, pancreatic, cardiovascular, and endocrine diseases, are described elsewhere in this text. Any malabsorption disease results in nutrient deficiencies of vitamins and minerals to the body and can cause major organ and body system problems. The protein gluten is found in wheat, rye, oats, and barley products. Intolerance to gluten causes damage to the lining of the small intestine in susceptible individuals, which interferes with the absorption of nutrients from food. Those people with this disorder can usually eat corn and rice products, which do not contain gluten. Some people with celiac sprue may also be allergic to lactose products such as milk and dairy products. The incidence of celiac sprue tends to run in families. Women are affected by the condition slightly more than men. Many people with the condition are diagnosed in childhood, but symptoms may not develop until adulthood. The prevalence of celiac sprue in North America is approximately 1 in every 3,000 people. However, this prevalence is thought to be underestimated.[94,95] In certain European countries such as Austria, Finland, Ireland, Italy, and Sweden the prevalence is as high as 1 in 300 people.[96]

Etiology. Celiac sprue is a chronic, immunological disease. People with the condition are allergic to a protein in gluten called gliadin, which sets up a toxic reaction in the small intestine that damages the mucosal lining, destroying the intestinal villi.[97] This damage reduces the ability of the small intestine to absorb nutrients from ingested food. The destruction of the villi results in malabsorption of fats and carbohydrates. Lactase, the enzyme that breaks down lactose (complex sugars) into glucose and galactose, is situated on the surface of the villi of the small intestine. Thus, when the villi are destroyed, lactase is not produced.[98] The disease also has a genetic component, with close family members having a 10% likelihood of developing the condition.[99] Recent research published by Symith et al. at the University of Cambridge (2008) identified that there may be a common genetic allele (location of a gene on the chromosome) for the tendency to develop both type 1 diabetes and celiac sprue.[100] Some evidence is also now coming to light that indicates chronic celiac sprue may be associated with the development of intestinal cancers.[101]

Signs and Symptoms. Early in the disease process, there may be no symptoms of celiac sprue. The characteristic later signs and symptoms of the condition may include diarrhea, odoriferous (foul-smelling) feces, flatulence, abdominal bloating, weight loss, anorexia, and steatorrhea (fat in the stools) causing feces to be light colored and float. When the disease causes malnutrition the symptoms become more severe. The advanced malnutrition caused by long-standing and severe celiac sprue can result in anemia due to low intestinal absorption of vitamin B12 and iron; edema of the distal lower extremities resulting from low levels of protein in the blood, which leads to passage of fluid into the tissues by osmosis; infertility and amenorrhea (cessation of menses) in women; muscle weakness and peripheral neuropathy due to low levels of potassium and magnesium; and osteoporosis resulting from low calcium absorption.[102] Some people with celiac sprue also have a dermatitis skin condition.[103]

Prognosis. Although there is no cure for celiac sprue, the symptoms may resolve after a few weeks on a gluten-free diet. The damage to the villi of the small intestine may not be reversible.

Medical Intervention. The diagnosis of celiac sprue is achieved through a biopsy of the small intestine using an esophagogastroduodenoscopy (EGD) via the mouth into the duodenum. Blood tests are also used to detect the antibodies produced in celiac sprue. Endomysial antibodies and antitissue transglutaminase antibodies destroy the person's own tissues, and antigliadin antibodies develop as a response to allergy to the protein gliadin in gluten.[104] Medical treatment of the condition depends on the ability to diagnose effectively. A gluten-free diet is recommended but may not always reverse existing damage. Some people have relief of the symptoms associated with celiac sprue within a few weeks of following a gluten-free diet, whereas others need several years of a gluten-free diet to quell the symptoms of the disease. A gluten-free diet is much more complicated than it may seem. Gluten is not only found in wheat, rye, oats, and barley but is used in canned foods, preserves such as tomato ketchup and mustard, processed meats such as luncheon meat and sausage, in medications as a filling agent, and in cosmetics including lipstick. Vitamin and mineral supplements are necessary for most people with celiac sprue to counteract the effects of the malabsorption.[105]

Physical Therapy Intervention. No physical therapy intervention is indicated for people with celiac sprue.

Ileus and Small Intestinal Obstruction

Obstruction of the small intestine is called ileus. The main types of ileus are obstructive ileus, and paralytic ileus. Some of the causes of ileus are related to other diseases or conditions seen in people treated by the PTA.

Etiology. Paralytic ileus may be caused by paralysis such as that caused by spinal cord injury or other trauma. In people who have a traumatic injury the nerves of the intestines are damaged or made ineffective, and the lack of peristalsis action in the intestines causes the contents to back up and create an obstruction. Other causes of paralytic ileus may include medications such as narcotics, ischemia of the intestines or the abdominal viscera, inflammation of the abdominal viscera or peritonitis, myocardial infarction, and pneumonia.[106] In obstructive ileus, there is an obstruction in the small intestine resulting from adhesions or material actually blocking the lumen of the intestine. In as many as 60% of people with obstructive ileus the cause is postoperative adhesions.[107] The blockage may be caused by ingested foreign objects, tumors, impacted feces, or volvulus (twisting of the intestines), hernias, or Crohn's disease. When a herniation of the intestine through the abdominal wall causes an obstruction it is usually the result of the small intestine protruding through the inguinal canal in the presence of an **inguinal hernia,** through the femoral canal in a femoral hernia, through the area around the umbilicus in a periumbilical hernia, or through the diaphragm into the thoracic cavity in a hiatal hernia.[108] However, in most cases of obstructive ileus the individual previously had abdominal surgery, which caused adhesions to develop in a circular manner around a section of the intestine. In people with obstructive ileus, the lumen of the intestine is smaller, and if food is not chewed fully or is present in large amounts, it may become blocked at the narrowed area of intestine. The adhesions prevent the intestine from expanding with the presence of large amounts of this ingested material.[109]

Signs and Symptoms. In people with acute cases of ileus the characteristic signs and symptoms include fever, tachycardia, severe abdominal cramping, with abdominal pain and distention, anorexia (loss of appetite), vomiting, diarrhea or constipation, and bad breath odor.[110,111]

Prognosis. In any type of ileus, the intestine can become constricted, and if the blood supply is compromised, gangrene may occur. Infection is a possible complication of ileus and the intestine may become perforated if the pressure builds up for a prolonged period of time.[112] In so-called strangulated obstructions in which the bowel is twisted and ischemia occurs, death occurs if surgical treatment is not performed.[113]

Medical Intervention. In people with severe cases of ileus, surgical resection of the intestine is required, usually performed as an emergency procedure. The surgical repair of hernias may be necessary to prevent the so-called incarceration or strangulation of the intestine. Occasionally the pressure within the intestines can be relieved using a nasogastric tube and suction. This relief of gas may reduce the need for abdominal surgery in a few people, but usually is performed before surgery.[114] Patients are usually prescribed antimicrobial, analgesic, and antiemetic (stop vomiting) medications at the same time as relief of pressure with a nasogastric tube. Fluid replacement is required with intravenous therapy, and the heart and blood pressure are monitored closely.[115]

Physical Therapy Intervention. None indicated.

Whipple's Disease

Whipple's disease is a rare bacterial, infectious disease most commonly diagnosed in men between ages 40 and 60. The main reason to include the disease here is that it causes malabsorption and can result in an arthritis-type condition.[116] People with the associated arthritis may be seen in the physical therapy department.

Etiology. Whipple's disease is caused by *Tropheryma whippelii* bacteria. These bacteria usually settle in the small intestine, but they can affect other areas of the body, including the brain, joints, heart, and lungs.[117] The bacteria damage the villi of the internal surface of the small intestine resulting in a reduced ability to absorb nutrients from food.

Signs and Symptoms. The characteristic signs and symptoms of the disease include fever without known cause, arthritis, intestinal malabsorption, diarrhea, abdominal pain, anorexia, weight loss, weakness, fatigue, and neurological and cardiac symptoms.[118]

Prognosis. The condition can be fatal if undiagnosed or untreated. People treated for the condition may take up to 2 years to recover, and the changes to the small intestine villi may not be reversible.

Medical Intervention. The medical diagnosis is determined through biopsy of the duodenum and microscopic examination to detect the causative bacteria. Patients are given antibacterial therapy medications for a prolonged period of time. Nutritional supplements are also needed to prevent malnutrition as a result of the malabsorption.[119]

Physical Therapy Intervention. Physical therapy for people with the arthritic symptoms associated with Whipple's disease follows the same path as other arthritic conditions. The concentration of rehabilitation is on improving independence through mobility reeducation, endurance activities, activities of daily living (ADL), reduction of pain and inflammation, and improvement of joint mobility.

Diseases of the Large Bowel and Large Intestine

The diseases described in this section include those most commonly seen in physical therapy practice associated with other comorbid conditions treated by physical therapy interventions. In some cases, people with diseases of the large bowel and intestines will have signs and symptoms that require physical therapy interventions. The diseases described include colorectal cancer; diverticula disease of the colon; the inflammatory bowel diseases, including Crohn's disease and ulcerative colitis; irritable bowel syndrome, ischemic bowel disease, and intestinal polyps; hemorrhoids; peritonitis; and rectal prolapse.

Colorectal Carcinoma

Most colorectal carcinomas are of the adenocarcinoma type, and the majority are situated in the sigmoid colon or rectum. Colorectal cancer of the large intestine is the most common malignant tumor of the intestinal tract and the fourth most common cancer in the United States.[120] Adenocarcinoma of the colon is more common in the Western world than in Asia or Africa, suggesting that there may be a relationship to diet. Most adenocarcinomas of the large intestine occur in people over age 50, with the risk increasing with age.[121] According to the National Cancer Institute (2010), estimates for 2010 were that 102,900 new cases of colon cancer and 39,670 new cases of rectal cancer would be diagnosed and 51,370 people would die of the disease in the United States.[122]

Etiology. The cause of colorectal cancer may be related to diet and heredity. New studies are revealing genetic markers for a predisposition to developing colon cancer, and even the likelihood of the type of colon cancer that might occur. However, it is important to note that just because someone has the genetic marker for a disease does not mean that they will develop the disease. The combination of genetic and controllable factors may help to reduce the incidence of colon cancer in the future.[123] Other risk factors for the development of colon cancer include the presence of polyps (fingerlike growths) in the wall of the colon, consumption of a high fat diet, a family or personal history of colon cancer, and a personal history of Crohn's disease or ulcerative colitis.[124]

Signs and Symptoms. The characteristic signs and symptoms of intestinal cancer are variable. No symptoms may be apparent in the early stages of the disease. In some people, there may be constipation or narrow feces as a result of obstruction of the intestine. Blood in the feces, stomach pain, unusual and unexplained weight loss, fatigue, changes in appetite, and, most important, a change in bowel habits are often indicative of a colon problem, and should be checked to rule out colon cancer.[125,126]

Prognosis. Colorectal cancer is the second most common cause of cancer-related death in the United States.[127] The survival rate for people with colorectal cancer depends on the stage of the tumor. The early detection of intestinal tumors through regular screening tests such as colonoscopy, is the key to prevention and survival. The staging of colorectal cancer follows the same guidelines as other cancers with Stages 0 through 4, with 4 the most invasive. The American Joint Committee on Cancer (TNM) staging system is used to describe the cancer. The "T" indicates the state and extent of the actual tumor, the "N" notes the extent of the spread of the cancer to the regional lymph nodes, and the "M" is the extent of metastases.[128]

Medical Intervention. Regular colonoscopy is recommended for people after age 50 to enable early detection of possible tumors (see the section on colonoscopy and sigmoidoscopy). Occult blood tests on feces detect blood in the stool, which may also provide early indications of intestinal disease. Other tests used to detect intestinal tumors include a barium enema, or swallow, and computerized axial tomography (CT scan). Polyps detected on colonoscopy are removed using the laparoscope, as a preventive measure. The medical treatment for detected carcinomas of the intestines is surgical removal of the section of intestine depending on the stage of the tumor and a combination of chemotherapy and radiation therapy.[129] Specific surgeries performed for colorectal cancer are found in Table 12-2.

Physical Therapy Intervention. None indicated.

Diverticula Disease of the Colon

A diverticulum (plural: diverticula) is a pouchlike process within the wall of the intestine, usually in the colon. These diverticula form where the bands of circular and longitudinal muscle of the wall of the colon meet to provide passage for blood vessels. The number of diverticula may vary between a few and many. People who have diverticula in their colon are said to have **diverticulosis**, whereas people who have diverticula that have become inflamed have **diverticulitis**. Diverticula disease is fairly common in the Western world. In the United States, 10% of Americans over age 40 have diverticula and 50% of people over age 60. Of those people who have diverticulosis, up to 25% will develop diverticulitis.[130]

Etiology. The actual cause of diverticula in the colon is not known. Possible risk factors for the development of the condition include a diet low in fiber and lack of exercise. Because the condition is common in developed countries and rare in Asia and Africa, the consumption of processed foods is thought to be a risk factor. Diverticula may be present as diverticulosis or become filled with feces (stool) or bacteria, which can cause diverticulitis (inflammation).[131]

Signs and Symptoms. Diverticulosis may not cause any symptoms, but may be a precursor to the development of diverticulitis. Acute attacks of diverticulitis can cause severe abdominal pain, anorexia (loss of appetite), constipation, diarrhea, fever, flatulence, nausea, vomiting, and changes in bowel habits. Diverticulitis can lead to infection, bleeding, and partial or complete blockages of the colon. The complications of diverticulitis can include perforations of the colon resulting from infection, which can develop into an abdominal abscess and peritonitis. When infections resolve, the healing process may cause adhesions that connect the colon to other abdominal structures such as the bladder, small intestine, or the skin. In such instances, a fistula (a tube) may form between the structures causing further infection. Adhesions may also form around the colon or the small intestine constricting the intestines and causing a blockage.[132]

Prognosis. The symptoms of diverticulosis usually resolve with the use of a high-fiber diet.[133] People who have severe episodes of diverticulitis that do not respond to treatment may require surgery for colon resection (removal of a

Table 12.2 **Types of Surgical Procedures Used for the Treatment of Colorectal Cancer**

SURGERY	DESCRIPTION
Colon	
Colectomy/hemicolectomy	Removal of part of the colon and associated lymph nodes when indicated May or may not require a temporary colostomy
Colostomy	The attachment of part of the colon to the abdominal wall with a stoma (opening) to the external surface of the abdomen A removable collecting bag is attached over the stoma for elimination of waste In rare instances in which a large portion of colon is removed, the colostomy may be permanent
Colostomy reversal	Reattachment of the ends of the surgically resected colon
Polypectomy and local excision	Removal of polyps in the colon and the superficial underlying cancerous tissue. Usually performed during a colonoscopy
Rectum	
Abdominoperineal (AP) resection	Surgical excision of the rectum, anus, and external anal sphincter muscles for later stages of rectal cancer A permanent colostomy is needed after this surgery
Local transanal resection	Excision of early stage rectal cancers by instrumentation introduced through the anus—no abdominal excision
Low anterior resection	Excision of affected areas of the rectum
Rectal excision with a colorectal anastomosis	Excision of the whole of the rectum in more advanced stages of rectal cancer The colon is attached to the anus in a procedure called coloanal anastomosis A colostomy is not required after this procedure
Pelvic exenteration	Extensive surgery for excision of the pelvic organs in very advanced stages of rectal cancer with involvement of pelvic organs including the uterus, bladder, and prostate A colostomy is required after this surgery and often a urostomy
Urostomy	The diversion of urine to a stoma in the abdominal wall after removal of the bladder A removable collecting bag for urine is attached to the abdominal wall

section of the colon), fistula excision or removal of an intestinal blockage.[134] A complete intestinal blockage is considered a medical emergency.

Medical Intervention. The diagnosis of diverticulosis usually occurs when people have a colonoscopy screening. If diverticulitis is suspected, other tests may include a digital rectal exam, a CT scan, abdominal ultrasound scan, and occult blood tests. The medical treatment for diverticulosis usually requires a change in diet. People with the condition may be referred to a dietician and are advised to eat fresh fruit, vegetables, cereals, and whole grains rich in dietary fiber. A fiber drink such as methylcellulose (Citrucel) or psyllium (Metamucil) may also be prescribed.[135] The use of probiotics is now becoming common in the treatment of the condition.[136] These probiotics contain cultures of bacteria that help to restore or enhance the normal bacterial flora of the intestine. Probiotics are found in certain foods such as yogurt and soy drinks.[137] If an acute or prolonged episode of diverticulitis occurs, bed rest, antimicrobial medications, and a liquid diet are usually prescribed. Some people may require colon resection surgery, with or without the use of a colostomy.[138]

Physical Therapy Intervention. Although physical therapy intervention is not usually indicated for people with diverticulitis, advice on an exercise program can help to improve the condition.

Hemorrhoids

Hemorrhoids are actually normally occurring nodules of veins located inside the distal end of the rectum or the anus. They are thought to aid in the normal function of elimination of waste from the rectum. However, the term "hemorrhoid" is used to refer to the inflammation and enlargement of these veins when they become a problem. Hemorrhoids may either be internal in the rectum or anus or become protruding hemorrhoids that extend beyond the anal opening. Hemorrhoids are common, with 50% of people developing them by age 50. Approximately 75% of people will have hemorrhoids at some time during their lives.[139] However, only approximately 4% of the population have problematic hemorrhoids that require treatment. The prevalence of hemorrhoids is greatest for people between the ages of 45 and 65 and for women during pregnancy.[140]

Etiology. Hemorrhoids become enlarged as a result of several factors such as chronic diarrhea or constipation, pregnancy, childbirth, obesity, muscle weakness, anal intercourse, and straining to eliminate stools. All of these factors increase the venous pressure around the rectum and anus causing break down of the hemorrhoids.[141]

Signs and Symptoms. The characteristic signs and symptoms of inflamed hemorrhoids include bleeding from the rectum and itching. Because the blood is fresh, it is bright red and noticeable when the individual passes stools. Protruding hemorrhoids may become painful and sore when more severe.[142]

Prognosis. The prognosis is good. Most hemorrhoids resolve with treatment. Surgical intervention is reserved for chronic, painful hemorrhoids.

Medical Intervention. The diagnosis of hemorrhoids may be coincidental when a colonoscopy is performed. If a person has problems with bleeding from the rectum, the physician may perform a digital examination or use a proctoscope or anoscope to observe the inside of the rectum.[143] Medical treatment depends on the severity of the hemorrhoids. In mild cases, alteration of the diet to include more fluids and fiber or the use of stool softeners or laxatives may resolve the problem by preventing constipation. The use of special suppositories, lotions, creams, and ointments, such as Anusol, may also be effective. These preparations may contain a local anesthetic, a vasoconstrictor

such as epinephrine, an antiseptic, and a moisturizing agent such as cocoa butter or lanolin.[144] After the hemorrhoids become chronically inflamed, a hemorrhoidectomy (surgical removal of hemorrhoids) may be performed. Other minor surgical procedures performed in a physician's office include sclerotherapy (injections directly into the hemorrhoid with a sclerosing agent) to harden and necrose the tissue; rubber band ligation in which a rubber band is placed round the base of the hemorrhoid to cut off the circulation, causing the hemorrhoid to wither; and infrared coagulation, which burns off the tissue.[145]

Physical Therapy Intervention. Specific physical therapy research is lacking for people with hemorrhoids. However, because regular exercise seems to help reduce the incidence of hemorrhoids, physical therapy intervention may be indicated. Strengthening of the pelvic floor muscles can also help to reduce the problems associated with hemorrhoids after childbirth or those exacerbated by weak pelvic floor musculature.

Inflammatory Bowel Disease (Crohn's Disease and Ulcerative Colitis)

The term **chronic inflammatory bowel disease (IBD)** covers a range of diseases, but mainly refers to Crohn's disease and ulcerative colitis. These diseases are chronic autoimmune intestinal conditions. Crohn's disease mainly affects the small intestine but can affect any part of the digestive system, whereas ulcerative colitis affects only the rectum, and colon. Both Crohn's disease and ulcerative colitis are found equally in males and females. However, Crohn's disease is usually identified in teenagers and ulcerative colitis in early adulthood. Ulcerative colitis is more common than Crohn's disease. According to the Centers for Disease Control and Prevention approximately 1.4 million people have IBD in the United States.[146] Between 1 and 10 people per 100,000 of the population each year are newly diagnosed with IBD.[147]

Etiology. A combination of risk factors are thought to contribute to the development of inflammatory bowel diseases. A mutation of the CARD15/NOD2 gene is known to increase the risk of developing Crohn's disease by 10 to 40 times that of the rest of the population. This genetic mutation is more common in the white population, particularly those of Jewish ethnicity.[148,149] These chronic diseases may also be triggered by a strain of *Escherichia coli* bacteria, causing the immune system, specifically the

Type 1 and 2 T helper cells, to destroy its own intestinal flora and damage the internal surface of the intestines.[150,151] These diseases are also more common in whites than African Americans, or Asians. Another contributing factor in the development of IBD is heavy smoking. IBD may also be associated with some autoimmune diseases such as ankylosing spondylitis and arthritis and is thought to be affected by emotional stress.[152]

Signs and Symptoms. The severity of the characteristic signs and symptoms of both ulcerative colitis and Crohn's disease varies greatly. Both diseases cause diarrhea with blood and possibly mucus, urgency of bowel movements, anemia, anorexia, malnutrition, and weight loss and are associated with exacerbations and remissions. Crohn's disease may also cause right lower abdominal pain. Additional symptoms of ulcerative colitis include fever and severe pain with cramping during the passage of feces. The malabsorption of nutrients in the intestines resulting from the disease process and the effects of diarrhea is typical of IBD and leads to anorexia and malnutrition with reduced levels of protein, minerals, and vitamins. This in turn may lead to osteoporosis.[153] In Crohn's disease, inflammation of the small intestine wall causes ulcers to form, which over time become thickened and fibrosed and make the walls of the intestine rigid, creating a narrowed lumen. This narrowing of the lumen can lead to ileus (obstruction of the small intestine). The chronic inflammatory response may also cause adhesions to form between loops of intestine or fistulas (connecting holes or tubes between two structures) to develop between loops of the intestine or between the intestine and the bladder. Some people with Crohn's disease develop fistulas between the intestine and the perianal (adjacent to the anus) skin area.[154] Ulcerative colitis affects the rectum and colon rather than the small intestine. Ulcerations form in the wall of the rectum and colon, which are in a constant state of healing. The resulting tissue is delicate and tends to bleed easily. The condition impedes the normal absorption of fluids in the colon.[155] Other less common complications of IBD may include a toxic megacolon (dilation of the colon), which is considered a medical emergency and requires a surgical colectomy; skin conditions; inflammation of the eye; and kidney disease.[156]

Prognosis. Some indications derived from research studies associate an increased risk of developing colorectal neoplasia (cancer) with severe and long-standing inflammatory bowel disease.[157] These chronic IBD conditions can lead to other more serious problems such as osteoporosis resulting from the malabsorption of nutrients.

Medical Intervention. The diagnosis of IBD involves any or all of the following: blood tests for anemia, barium swallows for upper a gastrointestinal series, a barium enema, sigmoidoscopy or colonoscopy, and CT scans.[158] The medical treatment of IBD consists of a multiple approach to control the inflammation with anti-inflammatory medications, reduce diarrhea with antimotility medications, and identify stressful situations that may precipitate an acute exacerbation of the condition. Nutritional advice plays a large role in the control of the conditions as a result of the malnutrition. In people with severe cases, surgical intervention may be needed. A colostomy or ileostomy may be performed in which an opening from the colon or ileum is made to the skin of the abdomen. This may serve as a temporary measure to give the area of the involved intestine a rest from the irritation of food. A reversal of the procedure is performed after the intestine has been given time to heal. People with ulcerative colitis may require a colectomy (excision of the colon).[159]

Physical Therapy Intervention. Physical therapy may be indicated for people who have arthritis as a result of IBD. The treatment of the arthritic condition follows the same pattern as other kinds of arthritis with improving function and mobility, reducing inflammation and pain, strengthening muscles, and increasing endurance to activity and cardiovascular fitness.

Intestinal Polyps

Intestinal polyps are small, fingerlike projections in the wall of the intestines. Intestinal polyps can be either benign or malignant. The incidence of polyps increases with age, particularly in people over age 50. Many polyps are located in the sigmoid colon and are more common in males than females.[160]

Etiology. Benign polyps are usually associated with IBD. Most of these polyps do not cause any problems, although certain types may have a tendency to turn into neoplastic tumors. Neoplastic polyps are composed of abnormal epithelial tissue and may develop into malignant tumors.[161] Risk factors for colorectal polyps include a close family member who has been diagnosed with them or who has had colon cancer.[162]

Signs and Symptoms. Most people who have intestinal polyps have no symptoms. Occasionally, rectal bleeding and blood on the feces may be present, and if the bleeding is excessive, it may result in anemia and associated symptoms of fatigue. Abdominal pain resulting from polyps is rare.[163]

Prognosis. The prognosis is good if polyps are removed. Polyps discovered during a colonoscopy are removed to prevent them turning into malignant tumors. Most polyps are slow growing, but they are sometimes precursors to cancerous tumors.

Medical Intervention. The detection of benign polyps usually occurs during a sigmoidoscopy or colonoscopy. Any polyps detected during these procedures are removed as a precautionary measure and sent for laboratory analysis. Polyps may also be identified during a barium enema or a CT scan. If polyps are found to be malignant a colectomy (removal of part of the colon) may be performed.[164] Some of the methods recommended to reduce the likelihood of developing intestinal include eating a diet high in fiber, avoiding alcohol, not smoking, exercising regularly, and losing weight.[165]

Physical Therapy Intervention. Physical therapy intervention is not indicated for intestinal polyps.

Irritable Bowel Syndrome

Irritable bowel syndrome (IBS) is a common, nonspecific intestinal condition. Unlike some of the other bowel diseases, this condition does not damage the intestines, so it does not precede serious diseases such as cancer. As many as 20% of adult Americans have symptoms of IBS, and for some people, the condition can be sufficiently debilitating to interfere with work and leisure activities. The condition usually starts before age 35, with more women affected than men.[166]

Etiology. No specific cause is known for IBS. Stress seems to be the main factor that increases symptoms of this syndrome. Some research indicates that this may be an immune condition that makes the colon more sensitive to both stress and certain foods. The peristalsis (normal muscular contraction of the intestines) may be either reduced or not working, although the reason for this is not known. Some people with IBS have a reduced number of serotonin receptors in the internal wall of the intestines, which results in a buildup of serotonin levels within the intestines and a resultant increased sensitivity of the intestines. Certain people may have IBS after a severe bacterial infection of the intestines such as gastroenteritis.[167]

Signs and Symptoms. The characteristic signs and symptoms of IBS are bouts of alternating diarrhea and constipation and intermittent abdominal pain.[168] The abdominal pain has to be experienced for at least 12 weeks out of a 1-year period to be considered IBS. Other symptoms may include urgency of bowel movements, mucus in the stool, and abdominal bloating. Some of the factors that may increase these symptoms are eating larger than usual meals; drinking a lot of caffeinated beverages such as tea, coffee, and soda; and certain medications. Depression may either be the cause of increased symptoms of IBS or may be caused by the condition.[169]

Prognosis. Although there is no known cure, the prognosis for people with IBS is good. The syndrome does not cause serious disease or permanent damage to the intestines. Most people can control the symptoms through a combination of dietary modifications and stress reduction activities.

Medical Intervention. When people are diagnosed with IBS several screening procedures may be used, including a barium enema and colonoscopy. The exclusion of other more serious conditions may need to be confirmed before a diagnosis of IBS is determined. However, guidelines published by physicians in the January 2009 edition of the *American Journal of Gastroenterology* suggested that extensive medical testing for people without signs of intestinal bleeding was not recommended for people suspected of having IBS.[170] The most commonly suggested treatments include the use of over-the-counter fiber supplements, laxatives, or antidiarrheal medications depending on the symptoms. When diarrhea is a major problem and does not respond to over-the-counter medications, a prescription medication, alosetron hydrochloride (Lotronex) is prescribed. Other treatment suggestions are increased fiber in the diet, stress reduction, eating smaller and more frequent portions of food, regular exercise such as walking, and getting sufficient sleep.[171]

Physical Therapy Intervention. Physical therapy intervention may be indicated for people with IBS to teach relaxation exercises and provide an exercise program within the capabilities of each person.

Ischemic Bowel Disease. Ischemic bowel disease is the term used for a group of ischemic bowel diseases caused by lack of blood supply to the walls of the large or small intestines. These ischemic conditions are more common in people over age 50, and become gradually more prevalent as age increases. The three main types of ischemic bowel disease are acute mesenteric ischemia, chronic mesenteric ischemia, and ischemic colitis.[172]

Etiology. Ischemic bowel disease is usually associated with other diseases such as atherosclerosis or heart diseases such as myocardial infarction, congestive heart failure (CHF), aortic aneurysm, or venous thrombosis.[173] The condition results from reduced or complete lack of blood flow through the mesenteric arteries that supply the tissue of the intestines. The blockage of the blood vessels may be caused by emboli. The ischemia may be acute or chronic. Acute mesenteric ischemia results in the passage of bacteria from the intestines to healthy tissues and inflammation of the intestines, the surrounding tissues, and often the whole body.[174] Chronic mesenteric ischemia is usually the result of chronic atherosclerosis of the mesenteric arteries, which in turn causes fibrosis of the intestinal walls. Ischemic colitis is ischemia specific to the colon and may be caused by cocaine abuse, heart arrhythmias, trauma, or thrombosis and emboli in the blood vessels.[175]

Signs and Symptoms. The characteristic signs and symptoms associated with any ischemic bowel diseases consist of abdominal pain, changes in bowel habits, weight loss, difficulty passing a bowel movement, blood passed with feces, nausea, vomiting, and loss of appetite. Ischemic colitis and acute mesenteric ischemia are also associated with a low-grade fever.[176]

Prognosis. Acute intestinal ischemia and ischemic colitis can cause gangrene of the intestines. If no treatment is provided gangrene can result in death. Some people with ischemic colitis can develop perforation of the colon with severe blood loss, which can be life threatening. In rare instances, ischemic colitis can lead to colon cancer.[177]

Medical Intervention. Acute mesenteric ischemia is considered a medical emergency. The administration of heparin, intravenous fluids, and oxygen to save life, and a surgical angioplasty of the superior mesenteric artery to restore blood supply to the intestines are usually required. If gangrene is present, a bowel resection to remove the affected area of intestine will also be performed. People with chronic mesenteric ischemia undergo surgery for endarterectomy of the celiac or superior mesenteric artery. Because the chronic ischemia is an intermittent problem, the surgery is not usually an emergency procedure.[178]

Physical Therapy Intervention. People recovering from surgery who are lacking mobility may require ambulation, mobility, strengthening, endurance, and functional activities training to return them to presurgical functional status.

Peritonitis

Peritonitis, as the name suggests, is inflammation of the peritoneum. Most peritonitis has an acute onset. Several types of peritonitis are recognized. Spontaneous peritonitis is usually related to bacterial infection or associated with liver of kidney disease.[179] Secondary peritonitis is inflammation of the peritoneum resulting from another condition.[180] Dialysis-associated peritonitis occurs during kidney dialysis procedures.[181] The general incidence of peritonitis is low, but within the population undergoing regular peritoneal kidney dialysis, the incidence is much higher. People undergoing kidney dialysis are anticipated to have a peritoneal infection once each year.[182,183] However, new machinery and procedures are reducing this incidence.[184]

Etiology. Peritonitis is usually caused by infection. Spontaneous peritonitis is frequently associated with liver or kidney failure. This type of peritonitis may also be caused by alcoholic cirrhosis of the liver, and viral hepatitis B or C.[185] Secondary peritonitis may be caused by infection from an intestinal condition such as a perforated intestine, a ruptured appendix, a stomach ulcer, perforated colon, pancreatitis, or infection of the fallopian tubes or ovaries. Post–abdominal surgery peritonitis may also occur as a result of irritation from the chemicals used during surgery.[186] Dialysis-associated peritonitis is caused by infection that enters the peritoneum through the peritoneal catheter used in peritoneal kidney dialysis. The cause of this is usually *Staphylococcus aureus* or *Staphylococcus epidermis* skin bacteria, or fungi.[187]

Signs and Symptoms. The characteristic signs and symptoms of peritonitis are ascites (fluid buildup within the peritoneum), sharp and severe abdominal pain with tenderness over the involved area of the abdomen, abdominal muscle spasms, fever, joint pains, nausea and vomiting, and reduced urine output.[188]

Prognosis. The mortality rate from peritonitis depends on the cause of the peritonitis. Peritonitis may result in sepsis, which is life threatening. Other complications of the disease include abdominal abscess and intestinal scarring with adhesions formation between layers of the intestines resulting in ileus (intestinal obstruction).[189]

Medical Intervention. People with spontaneous peritonitis are usually hospitalized. The testing for diagnostic purposes involves taking samples of the abdominal fluid for culture and chemical analysis to determine the bacteria responsible and blood cultures. People are placed on antimicrobial medications, and intravenous fluids for rehydration.[190] Once the cause of the peritonitis is determined, surgery may be performed to remove infected fluid and repair the defect causing the peritonitis.

Physical Therapy Intervention. As with other intestinal diseases and abdominal surgery, people may require rehabilitation for ambulation, bed mobility, strengthening, endurance, and functional activities to restore their prior level of function.

Rectal Prolapse

Rectal prolapse is the protrusion of rectal tissue beyond the opening of the anus. The condition is seen mainly in the elderly population with a weak pelvic floor musculature. ⊛ Children may also have rectal prolapse. Rectal prolapse is not common. The incidence increases in people in their 40s and 70s. Approximately 80% to 90% of rectal prolapses occur in women. [191,192]

Etiology. Rectal prolapse may start as hemorrhoids. Factors that contribute to the development of a rectal prolapse are usually related to increased intra-abdominal pressure combined with a weak pelvic floor musculature. These factors may include constant straining to pass stools over a prolonged period of time, chronic diarrhea, and chronic coughing caused by infectious diseases such as pertussis or diseases such as chronic obstructive pulmonary disease (COPD). Other diseases that can result in rectal prolapse include cystic fibrosis, parasitic diseases affecting the intestines, and neurological conditions such as cauda equina syndrome, spinal tumors, multiple sclerosis, and trauma to the low back or pelvis that have resulted in nerve damage to the pudendal nerve that supplies the anus and distal colon mucosa.[193]

Signs and Symptoms. The anal sphincter may become damaged, and fecal incontinence is common. Other characteristic signs and symptoms include bleeding and discharge of mucus from the anus and extrusion of soft tissue from the anus.[194]

Prognosis. Most people with rectal prolapse have a good prognosis. People with severe rectal prolapse who require surgery may or may not have a good outcome from surgery.[195]

Medical Intervention. The diagnosis of the cause of the rectal prolapse may involve a sigmoidoscopy, a barium enema, and an ultrasonography. People with underlying causes may require surgery. The rectal tissue can often be pushed back without surgery. If the rectal tissue becomes permanently prolapsed, surgery is required for excision of the affected rectum, or a procedure to tighten the anal opening. Advice on appropriate diet and exercise is helpful to reduce the problems of constipation or diarrhea.[196] A referral may be made to a dietician. For further information on fecal incontinence, please refer to Chapter 14.

Physical Therapy Intervention. Physical therapy intervention may include pelvic floor muscle reeducation through exercises and biofeedback, and electrical stimulation.

Diseases of the Liver and Gallbladder

This section includes noninfectious diseases and conditions of the liver and gallbladder. Many of the infectious diseases related to the liver such as various types of hepatitis are described in Chapter 10.

The general characteristic signs and symptoms related to disease of the liver are **jaundice** or **icterus.** Jaundice is a condition in which the skin, connective tissues, whites of the eyes, and mucosa become yellowish in color. This yellowing is caused by hyperbilirubinemia (an increase in blood bilirubin levels above that of normal) when the liver fails to function correctly. Under normal circumstances, the liver and spleen break down the old red blood cell hemoglobin into heme and globin. The heme is further broken down into a yellow substance called bilirubin. The liver then combines the bilirubin with glucuronide, which is secreted into the intestines through the bile duct to assist with the digestion of fats. Some of the bilirubin is eliminated from the body in urine, giving the urine its yellow coloration, but some is reabsorbed back into the body and returns to the liver to be recycled. When the liver fails to function correctly, the normal cycle is interrupted and bilirubin builds up in the blood and becomes toxic to the body, causing the skin and connective tissues to turn yellow. An excess of bilirubin in urine may cause the urine to turn brown. Jaundice can be caused by an obstruction of the normal secretion of bile from the bile duct in such conditions as gallstones, or tumors, which block the bile duct. Obstructive tumors may be located either in the bile duct itself or in the small intestine close to the opening of the bile duct into the duodenum. Other causes of jaundice may be hepatitis or liver disease such as cirrhosis. When jaundice occurs as the result of a viral infection, the yellowing is usually only temporary, but in some chronic liver diseases, the jaundice may last for prolonged periods.

Cholelithiasis and Choledocholithiasis

Cholelithiasis (gallbladder stones/gallstones) and choledocholithiasis (common bile duct stones) are common throughout the world. Gallstones are more common in females than males and more prevalent in Caucasians, Hispanics, and Native Americans than African Americans. The incidence of cholelithiasis increases after age 40.[197] More than 20 million adults in the United States have gallstones (between 10 and 20%), and each year a further 1% to 3% of people develop them.[198]

Etiology. A genetic predisposition to developing gallstones exists. Gallstones can be formed from excessive amounts of cholesterol or bilirubin in bile or insufficient bile salts. When the gallbladder does not fully empty its contents into the duodenum, this may also cause development of stones.[199] Other risk factors for the development of gallstones include Crohn's disease, diabetes, obesity, cirrhosis of the liver, major trauma, and prolonged stays in the intensive care unit.[200] Many gallstones are composed of cholesterol or bilirubin, but some are made up of calcium and carbonates. Cholesterol stones are usually white, whereas the others are dark brown or black. The gallstones may block the common bile duct, preventing the passage of bile, and the gallbladder may then become gangrenous. If the gallbladder ruptures, it can cause peritonitis as described earlier in this chapter. In most cases of gallstones, the gallbladder will become inflamed, a condition called cholecystitis. Cholangitis is another type of gallbladder inflammation caused by bile duct infection.

Signs and Symptoms. Some gallstones do not cause any symptoms. The characteristic signs and symptoms of acute cholelithiasis, in which the stone blocks the common bile duct, include severe bouts of pain in the central or upper right side of the abdomen. Other symptoms may include fever, jaundice, indigestion, acid reflux, and excessive amounts of intestinal gas. Pain may also be felt in the upper back or near the scapulae.[201]

Prognosis. Diseases of the gallbladder result in approximately 10,000 deaths per year in the United States. Of these, 7,000 are due to complications such as acute pancreatitis, and another 2,000 or more to cancer of the gallbladder. Cholecystectomy is such a commonly performed surgery that several hundred deaths occur each year as a result of surgery.[202]

Medical Intervention. The medical tests used to determine the existence or extent of the gallstones may be x-rays, an ultrasound scan, or CT scan of the abdomen or an endoscopic retrograde cholangiopancreatography (ERCP). The ERCP is an examination of the bile ducts via an endoscope passed through the mouth into the duodenum. A catheter is inserted through the endoscope into the bile ducts and dye is injected. A radiograph is then taken of the bile ducts, which identifies any narrowing of the ducts or blockage from gallstones or a tumor.[203] The medical management for symptomatic cholecystitis may be cholecystectomy (removal of the gallbladder). This may be achieved through a laparoscope or may require conventional surgery. In some cases, the gallstones can be dissolved with the use of medications, or lithotripsy, the use of electricity to dissolve the stones.[204]

Physical Therapy Intervention. Although no physical therapy is indicated for people with cholelithiasis, of particular note for the PTA is that gallbladder pain can mimic the symptoms of a heart attack.

Cirrhosis of the Liver

Liver cirrhosis is a chronic fibrosis of the liver which may lead to complete liver failure. Cirrhosis affects slightly more men than women. Approximately 400,000 people in the United States have liver cirrhosis.[205] Of the people with cirrhosis of the liver, 5% develop liver cancer.[206] The number of deaths per 100,000 of the population associated with chronic liver diseases was 9.3 in 2005 (most recent statistics available at time of publication).[207] Inflammation causes the liver to become enlarged at first, but then it starts to reduce in size as a result of the fibrosis. The liver loses its functional abilities to detoxify the body. Scar tissue replaces the liver tissue and the liver is unable to replace its own damaged cells. When the liver is cirrhosed, it can be palpated as a hardened structure through the abdominal wall. Cirrhosis of the liver causes many other systems in the body to fail including the kidneys, pancreas, lungs, and circulatory system.

Etiology. The etiology of liver cirrhosis can be as a result of heavy alcohol consumption over a prolonged period of time. The by-products of alcohol actually cause toxicity to the liver cells. Cirrhosis may also be caused by obesity; chronic hepatitis B, C, or D infection; autoimmune hepatitis; immune disorders such as cystic fibrosis or Wilson disease (copper metabolism disorder); nonalcoholic fatty liver disease (NAFLD); and primary biliary cirrhosis, which causes inflammation and destruction of the bile duct. Other types of toxicity that cause cirrhosis include exposure to toxic chemicals or drugs and parasitic infections.[208]

Signs and Symptoms. The characteristic signs and symptoms of liver cirrhosis include poor digestion of foods, diarrhea, malnutrition resulting from malabsorption, fatigue, ascites (abdominal edema and inflammation), splenomegaly (enlarged spleen), reduced blood clotting abilities with people easily becoming bruised and bleeding, iron deficiency, jaundice, inability to secrete ammonia and drugs or medications resulting in medications staying in the body longer than usual, and portal hypertension with the associated generalized body edema. Other side effects may include resistance to insulin; liver cancer; an increased risk of infections; varices (distended blood vessels) in the esophagus and/or stomach which can result in severe bleeding; hepatic encephalopathy resulting in reduced mental functions, confusion, personality changes, memory loss, sleep disturbances, and even coma; and kidney and lung failure.[209] All of these signs and symptoms result from the lack of function of the liver, which normally acts as the detoxification center for the body.

Prognosis. After cirrhosis has destroyed liver tissue, the body is unable to eliminate waste products and toxins. Liver cirrhosis and liver disease is the twelfth leading cause of death in the United States and was responsible for 29,165 deaths in 2007 (most recent statistics available before publication of this book).[210]

Medical Intervention. The diagnosis of liver cirrhosis involves a detailed medical history to determine whether there is alcohol or illicit drug use and the use of CT scan, ultrasound, MRI, or liver scans to detect the status of the liver. A staging method for severe end-stage liver disease called "model for end-stage liver disease" (MELD) predicts the likelihood of a 90-day survival. This model requires the results of three tests: the international normalized ratio (INR), which measures clotting factors, a blood bilirubin test, and a creatinine blood test for kidney function. Scores on the MELD range from 6 to 40 with the lower number indicating a better chance of a 90-day survival.[211] Medical treatment includes instructions to avoid alcohol and illicit drugs and eat a healthy diet, avoiding raw seafoods, which may contain bacteria and increase the possibility of infections. Aspiration of ascites from the abdomen may also be necessary. The prescribed medications may include diuretic medications to stimulate removal of fluids from the body, antimicrobial medications to combat infections, antiviral medications for hepatitis, corticosteroid medications for autoimmune hepatitis,[212] and beta blockers for portal hypertension. In recent years, transplant surgery has become an option, but the need for transplant organs is much greater than the availability of these organs. People in need of liver transplant are screened carefully to ensure the benefits of such a surgery.[213] People with the early stages of cirrhosis should also have preventive measures such as annual screening of the liver with abdominal CT scans or ultrasound, a vaccination for pneumococcus, annual influenza vaccinations, and osteoporosis screening to detect the early signs of long-term problems associated with cirrhosis.[214]

Physical Therapy Intervention. Physical therapy intervention for people with end-stage liver disease may be indicated to help improve mobility. Intervention will have no effect on the disease itself, but some improvement in functional independence and quality of life may be achieved. Physical therapy interventions may include ambulation, bed mobility, transfers, strengthening and endurance exercises, and home exercise programs.

CARCINOMA OF THE GALLBLADDER

Primary (originating in the gallbladder) cancerous tumors of the gallbladder and bile duct are comparatively rare. Estimates from the American Cancer Society for 2010 were of 9,760 people newly diagnosed and 3,320 deaths from the disease.[215] The average age of diagnosis of gallbladder cancer in the United States is 73 years.[216]

Etiology. The etiology of gallbladder carcinoma is unknown. However, women and Native Americans have a higher risk for developing gallbladder cancer.[217]

Signs and Symptoms. In the early stages of gallbladder carcinomas, there may be no discernible signs and symptoms. The characteristic signs and symptoms of later stage carcinomas of the gallbladder are similar to those previously described for liver and other intestinal diseases including jaundice, pain in the upper abdomen, fever, nausea and vomiting and bloating of the abdomen.[218]

Prognosis. If gallbladder cancer is diagnosed in the early stages when a cholecystectomy is possible, the prognosis is good. However, the prognosis for people with carcinoma of the gallbladder that has metastasized is usually comparatively poor, because symptoms only become apparent during the later stages of the disease when treatment interventions are less likely to be effective.[219]

Medical Intervention. The diagnosis of gallbladder carcinoma is difficult because there may be no early signs or symptoms of the disease. Diagnostic procedures may include physical examination by a physician; blood tests for liver function; imaging techniques such as ultrasound of the abdomen, CT scan, MRI, or a percutaneous transhepatic cholangiography in which an x-ray is taken of the liver and bile ducts after injection with a dye, a biopsy, and a laparoscopic examination.[220] The staging of gallbladder carcinoma follows the same pattern used for other carcinomas with grading I through IV. The most invasive and metastatic tumors are Stage IV. The preferred medical management for gallbladder carcinoma is with cholecystectomy (removal of the gallbladder). If cholecystectomy is not possible, the alternatives are a percutaneous transhepatic biliary drainage to drain bile from the gallbladder and prevent jaundice, a surgical biliary bypass to form a new tube between the gallbladder and intestine to allow bile drainage when the bile duct is obstructed by a tumor, and an endoscopic stent placement within the bile duct to open the duct and allow bile drainage. Radiation therapy and chemotherapy are usually used after surgery. New trials are underway to test radiosensitizer medications, which make tumor cells more sensitive to radiation therapy and enhance the effects of the treatment.[221]

Physical Therapy Intervention. As with other types of end-stage carcinomas, people with gallbladder carcinoma may benefit from endurance and mobility exercise routines to improve the quality of life. Education of the family and care providers is also of primary importance to assist with transfers, and reduce the risk of injury to those assisting with patient care. Most of the physical therapy intervention is provided during hospice care within the patient's home.

Liver Diseases and Conditions Caused by Drugs, Medications, and Toxins

Liver disease can be caused by any number of over-the-counter and prescription medications as well as vitamin supplements, herbal remedies, illicit drugs, and chemical toxins.[222] Estimates are that more than 1,000 prescribed and over-the-counter medications are capable of inducing liver damage.[223] In some cases, a combination of over-the-counter and prescription medications taken at the same time may cause damage. Some of the more commonly used medications that can adversely affect the liver include NSAIDs such as aspirin, acetaminophen (Tylenol), indomethacin (Indocin), ibuprofen (Motrin), naproxen (Naprosyn), piroxicam (Feldene), and nabumetone (Relafen). Many of these medications taken in more than the recommended dose in a 24-hour period can result in liver damage.[224] This is particularly disturbing because the use of these medications is commonplace in Western countries. Other fairly commonly prescribed medications that can damage the liver include cholesterol-lowering medications, such as the statins and nicotinic acid (Niacin); heart rhythm regulators such as amiodarone (Cordarone) prescribed to control atrial fibrillation and ventricular tachycardia; methotrexate when taken in high doses, used for the treatment of arthritic-associated conditions such as Crohn's disease, psoriasis, psoriatic arthritis, and rheumatoid arthritis; Tacrine (Cognex prescribed for people with Alzheimer's disease); vitamin A supplements taken in more than the required dose over prolonged periods; and several types of antimicrobial medications. Anabolic steroids, taken illegally by athletes and body builders, can cause liver toxicity and liver tumors.[225,226] People who have to be prescribed these medications for prolonged periods of time are monitored closely for liver enzyme levels, and removed from the medication if there are signs of changes in liver status.[227]

Estrogens may affect the mechanism responsible for the secretion of bile and cause gallbladder disease and liver disease.[228] Allopurinol, used to treat gout, can cause liver and gallbladder conditions in rare instances.[229] Still other medications such as corticosteroids may cause liver, kidney, and gallbladder problems when taken over a prolonged period of time. As new medications are developed, it is important for pharmaceutical companies, physicians, and the U.S. Food and Drug Administration to monitor these closely for side effects and the companies must place warnings on packages regarding the likely side effects of taking these medications. The physical therapist and PTA should reiterate to patients that they should not take any over-the-counter medications if they are taking prescription medications or have any illness such as liver disease without first consulting their doctor or pharmacist.

In some cases, cirrhosis of the liver is brought on by hemochromatosis. This hereditary disease causes the body to store too much iron in the liver, heart, and pancreas, which becomes toxic to the body. The conditions and characteristic signs and symptoms associated with hematochromatosis include diabetes, arthritis, a bronze skin discoloration, cardiomegaly (cardiac enlargement), cardiac disease, thyroid deficiency, male incontinence and impotence, and damage to the adrenal glands and pancreas, often causing diabetes. The medical treatment for hemochromatosis involves taking a pint of blood once or twice per week until the iron levels are reduced and then continuing to take blood regularly to keep the levels down. People with the disease have to avoid alcohol and iron and vitamin C supplements.[230] Wilson's disease is another hereditary autosomal recessive disorder that prevents the liver eliminating copper. The resultant buildup of copper in the body, especially in the brain, cornea of the eyes, liver, and kidneys, causes toxicity to the tissues resulting in psychiatric and behavioral problems, personality disorders, and basal ganglia damage with associated tremors and speech problems. The medical treatment for Wilson's disease is with the use of chelating medications (combine with metals) such as zinc salts or penicillamine, which allow the copper to be excreted in urine. Patients must also maintain a diet low in copper. High levels of copper are found in organ meats such as liver, kidneys, heart, shellfish, nuts, mushrooms, chocolate, and certain legumes (vegetables) such as beans.[231]

Infectious hepatitis is covered in Chapter 10, but another type of hepatitis known as autoimmune hepatitis is of note. Usually diagnosed in young females, the disease may follow an infection such as measles or be the result of a drug or medication reaction. The characteristics of the disease are many and include skin rashes and skin conditions such as acne; Sjögren's syndrome (dry eyes); arthritis; ulcerative colitis; thyroiditis (inflammation of the thyroid) and glomerulonephritis (inflammation of the kidney); Graves' disease; Type I diabetes; nausea, vomiting, anorexia, dark-colored urine, and pale-colored feces; abdominal pain; and jaundice. People with severe disease may also have ascites (abdominal edema) and mental confusion. Treatment for the disease is with immune system depressants such as corticosteroids or azathioprine (Imuran).[232]

Carcinoma of the Liver—Primary

Primary liver carcinoma, also called hepatocellular carcinoma or hepatoma, is cancer of the tissue of the liver, which is closely linked with chronic infection with hepatitis B. Metastases from cancers of the breast, colon, lung, pancreas, and stomach may occur in the liver, but these tumors do not originate in the actual cells of the liver. Worldwide, primary liver carcinoma is the fifth most common cancer. This type of cancer is common in areas of Southeast Asia and southern Africa and among Native Alaskans; in these populations, the incidence of hepatitis B is high, with a prevalence rate of 20 people for every 100,000 of the population. In the United States and Europe, the cancer is less prevalent, with only 5 people per 100,000 affected.[233] In areas of the world where hepatitis B is prevalent, men with liver carcinoma outnumber women more than 4:1.[234] According to the National

Cancer Institute 2007 statistics (most recent available), 27,753 were living with liver or hepatic bile duct carcinoma in January 2007, with more than a 2:1 ratio for men to women, and the median age at diagnosis of 64 years of age. The lifetime risk of developing liver carcinoma for all people in the United States is 0.76%, or a 1 in 132 chance for the total population. Based on 2003–2007 data, each year approximately 6.9 people of every 100,000 of the population will develop liver carcinoma.[235]

Etiology. The main known cause of primary liver carcinoma is chronic infection with hepatitis B. The genetic code of the virus invades the genes of the liver cells resulting in mutations of the cells that become cancer. Infection with hepatitis C is also associated with the disease but usually in association with liver cirrhosis, chronic alcohol use, and hepatitis B infection. People with cirrhosis of the liver are at higher risk of developing liver carcinoma, especially those who are chronic alcohol users. Some other factors increase the risk of developing liver carcinoma, such as exposure to toxins such as aflatoxin B1, a toxin found in *Aspergillus flavus* mold that grows on foods such as rice, soybeans, corn, and wheat stored in hot and humid conditions; the use of estrogens and anabolic (protein-building) steroids; chemical exposure to vinyl chloride used in the plastic industry; and hemochromatosis (a genetic disease which causes excess amounts of iron to buildup in the body).[236]

Signs and Symptoms. In the United States and Europe, cancerous tumors of the liver are usually diagnosed in the early stages. The tumors tend to be slow growing and cause minimal symptoms in the early stages. If liver carcinoma has reached an advanced stage before diagnosis, the signs and symptoms may include abdominal pain, unexplained weight loss and fever, ascites (abdominal edema), jaundice, muscle atrophy, esophageal varices that can result in bleeding, tenderness on palpation over the area of the liver, and the sound of hepatic bruit in the liver when examined with a stethoscope. Metastases from carcinoma of the liver tend to settle in the lungs, and occasionally in the bones or brain.[237]

Prognosis. The detection of liver cancer in many areas of the world where health care and preventive screening is not available is frequently not early enough to provide a good prognosis for people with the disease, making the prognosis for people with liver carcinoma poor. Only approximately 5% of people have a 5-year survival rate. Most people with the disease live up to 1 year after diagnosis.[238] However, in the United States and Europe the diagnosis of liver carcinoma is usually made in earlier stages and the outcome is generally better. People who have a tumor less that 1 cm have a 50% chance of surviving 3 years even without any treatment. In people with advances stages of the disease the 1-year survival rate is 30%, and the 5-year survival rate is zero. With treatment the outlook improves for those with a tumor under 3 cm in size to 90% survival for 1 year, 50% survival for 3 years, and 20% for 5 years. [239]

Medical Intervention. The diagnosis of primary liver carcinoma is through blood testing, physical examination for tenderness over the area of the liver, and imaging with ultrasound, CT scan, or MRI.[240] Physicians who are aware that a person has cirrhosis will take additional steps to screen for carcinoma. Standard blood screening tests for the liver do not usually indicate problems. The detection of high levels of alpha-fetoprotein in the blood over 500 ng/mL, is the most common diagnostic finding. The usual level of alpha-fetoprotein is below 5 ng/mL of blood. Other factors that may indicate liver carcinoma are hypercalcemia (high levels of calcium in the blood), hypoglycemia (low blood sugar levels), and hypercholesterolemia (high levels of cholesterol). However, these findings are also indicative of many other diseases and conditions.[241] The medical treatment for liver carcinomas varies according to the physician and the stage of the cancer. Treatment intervention may include chemotherapy and radiation therapy, although few trials have been done to indicate the effectiveness of these techniques. In most people with liver carcinoma, surgical resection of the lobe of the liver affected or a total liver transplant is performed.[242,243] Liver transplant is only beneficial for those people who have localized tumors of the liver that have not metastasized.[244] An alternative treatment for some people with liver carcinoma is radiofrequency ablation of the tumor. In this procedure, a needle electrode is inserted into the tumor using ultrasound, CT scan, or MRI as a guide, and a high-frequency electric current is passed into the tumor to kill the cells.[245,246] A comparatively new treatment for liver carcinoma called transarterial chemoembolization (TACE) is still in the trial stages but is showing promise of improvement for people not eligible for liver transplant. Tiny beads coated with anticancer medications are inserted into the blood vessels supplying the tumors. This intervention has a double effect of attacking the cancerous cells with the medications, and blocking off the blood supply to the tumor effectively preventing the tumor increasing in size.[247]

Physical Therapy Intervention. As with other chronic conditions, physical therapy intervention focuses on improvement of the physical impairments of people with the disease. Treatment sessions will most likely be directed toward bed mobility exercises, transfer training, ambulation activities, strengthening and endurance programs, and general improvement of the quality of life. Home physical therapy under hospice management may be provided for end-of-life care with the associated education for family and care providers for the use of lifts and transfer techniques.

Diseases of the Pancreas

The two diseases of the pancreas described in this section are acute and chronic pancreatitis and pancreatic cancer. Both of these conditions can result in general debility, which is an indication for physical therapy interventions.

Acute and Chronic Pancreatitis

Pancreatitis is inflammation of the pancreas. The disease may occur in early adulthood, although the peak of incidence occurs after age 55. The incidence of the diseases depends on the etiology. A total of 210,000 people per year are admitted to hospital with acute pancreatitis.[248]

Etiology. Pancreatitis is thought to be the result of the digestive enzymes produced by the pancreas, such as amylase, lipase, and trypsin, actually attacking and digesting the tissue of the pancreas itself, causing severe inflammation and eventual destruction.[249] Many people with chronic pancreatitis (inflammation of the pancreas) use alcohol heavily. However, the condition is also prevalent in people with cystic fibrosis, may occur in people with severe cases of cholelithiasis (gallstones), can be caused by trauma, may be the result of hypercalcemia (excess calcium in the blood), hyperlipidemia (high levels of cholesterol/fat in the blood), or hypertriglyceremia (high triglyceride levels) and is suspected to be hereditary in some people.[250] Other causes of acute pancreatitis may be the use of medications such as estrogen, corticosteroids, or diuretics; viral infections such as mumps; pneumonia caused by mycoplasma pneumonia;[251] or infection with campylobacter (a bacteria that causes food poisoning);[252] and as a result of surgery to the pancreas.[253] Children with pancreatitis usually have cystic fibrosis or the hereditary form of the disease.[254] 🖐 Numerous bouts of acute pancreatitis may occur before the onset of the chronic stage of the disease. Many people with chronic pancreatitis develop diabetes as a result of interference with the islet of Langerhans production of insulin and other digestive enzymes.[255]

Signs and Symptoms. The main characteristic of pancreatitis is pain in the left upper quadrant of the abdomen. In people with pancreatitis caused by cholelithiasis, the pain usually occurs after a meal. In those who abuse alcohol, the pain often occurs after a drinking session and may last several hours or even days.[256] Other symptoms may include nausea, vomiting, diarrhea, or constipation, fever, mild jaundice, weakness, weight loss, feces containing a lot of fat, ascites (abdominal edema), and severe abdominal pain that can radiate into the upper back.[257] If hemorrhage occurs in the pancreas there may also be signs of systemic shock such as hypotension (low blood pressure), dehydration, rapid pulse, and sweating.[258]

Prognosis. Many people with pancreatitis have acute symptoms that resolve when the cause of the condition is treated. However, pancreatitis can cause heart, lung, or kidney failure and lead to death.[259]

Medical Intervention. The diagnosis of pancreatitis involves determining the cause of the disease. Blood tests for raised levels of the digestive enzymes amylase, lipase, and trypsin produced by the pancreas, may indicate the presence of pancreatitis. Other diagnostic tools are an ultrasound scan to identify gallstones and a CT scan of the pancreas. The medical treatment for people with pancreatitis includes advice on cessation of alcohol intake, a diet high in carbohydrates and low in fats, pancreatic enzyme substitutes before meals, the use of insulin for those with diabetes, and analgesic medications to reduce pain. Surgical resection of the pancreas is not commonly used but may be an option if cysts exist.[260,261]

Physical Therapy Intervention. The physical therapy intervention for people with chronic pancreatitis follows the same pattern as for other chronic digestive diseases. Treatment sessions will most likely be directed toward bed mobility exercises, transfer training, ambulation activities, strengthening and endurance programs, and general improvement of the quality of life.

Carcinoma of the Pancreas

Malignant neoplasms of the pancreas are the fourth leading form of cancer deaths in the United States.[262] Pancreatic cancer is more common in African Americans, although it can occur in both males and females of any ethnic or cultural background. Age onset is mainly after 50, with the highest incidence of the disease in people between the ages of 60 and 80.[263] The National Cancer Institute estimated that 43,140 people would be newly diagnosed with pancreatic cancer in 2010, and 36,800 people would die as a result of the condition.[264]

Etiology. The incidence of pancreatic carcinoma is thought to be higher in people who use tobacco products and in those with a history of previous intestinal surgery, diabetes, or chronic pancreatitis.[265]

Signs and Symptoms. The characteristic signs and symptoms of pancreatic cancer may include abdominal and/or thoracic and lumbar back pain, diarrhea, jaundice, nausea, anorexia, weight loss, abdominal ascites with abdominal bloating, inflammation of the gallbladder, and deep venous thrombosis (DVT). In many people, once the symptoms are severe, the cancer has progressed into its late stages.[266]

Prognosis. The prognosis for pancreatic neoplasm is generally poor.[267] The early diagnosis of people with a family history of the disease can greatly improve the prognosis. Many people with Stage III or IV pancreatic cancer survive for less than a year.[268]

Medical Intervention. The diagnosis of pancreatic cancer involves the use of several tests, including CT scan or MRI; abdominal ultrasonography (US to the abdomen); endoscopic retrograde cholangiopancreatography (ERCP) in which an endoscope is passed into the duodenum via the esophagus and a small catheter is passed through the endoscope to the common bile duct where dye is injected and radiographs taken to identify obstructions; endoscopic ultrasound (an US probe attached to the end of an endoscope); a PET scan to identify cancer cells that absorb more of the injected radioactive glucose; and angiography (injection of contrast medium into the arteries before taking a radiograph to observe blockages or excessive blood vessels associated with malignant tumors).[269] The medical management for people with cancer of the pancreas includes resection of the pancreas, radiation, and chemotherapy. However, the uses of radiation and chemotherapy are still controversial as a result of the lack of benefits cited from clinical studies. Specific new chemotherapy treatments are undergoing clinical trials in the United States and Europe.[270] The use of gemcitabine (a chemotherapy medication) has shown promise in lengthening the survival time for people with early stage pancreatic cancer who have had surgery.[271] In many people, by the time the neoplasm is diagnosed, the cancer has metastasized into the surrounding abdominal cavity. Analgesic medications are prescribed to reduce pain. Early detection of pancreatic cancer may be possible for those with a family history of the disease who undergo regular screening tests.

Physical Therapy Intervention. Physical therapy intervention may be indicated as part of hospice management to improve the quality of life by increasing bed mobility and ambulation. Instruction on the use of a Hoyer lift for family and care providers is frequently part of the physical therapy intervention.

Why Does the Physical Therapist Assistant Need to Know About the Anatomy and Physiology of the Urinary System?

Knowledge of the anatomy and physiology of the urinary system is essential for the understanding of the pathological mechanisms of diseases of the urinary system. The normal functioning of the urinary tract is a complex system that can be affected by diseases of the urinary system itself or by diseases of other parts of the body.

The Anatomy and Physiology of the Urinary System

The urinary system is dependent on the interaction of multiple body systems to maintain the fluid balance in the body. However, for the purposes of this chapter, the urinary system will be described as the structures including the kidneys, adrenal glands, renal blood supply, urinary bladder, and the ureters. The urinary system serves as an eliminator of waste substances and toxins from the body in conjunction with the intestinal system. The urinary system achieves this by the passage of fluids and substances dissolved in those fluids. Each kidney filters approximately 1,700 liters of blood per day.[272]

The two kidneys are situated high up in the abdominal cavity on either side of the spine. They lie adjacent to the diaphragm, and are protected by the lower ribs (see Fig. 12-6). Renal fascia encloses the kidneys, which serves both to protect and to position the kidneys. Each kidney is the shape of a kidney bean with the hilus on the medial aspect, where the renal artery enters the kidney and the renal vein and ureter exit. The ureters are the tubes that carry urine from the kidneys to the bladder.[273]

Internally, the kidneys are complex. Each kidney consists of three regions, the renal cortex or outer layer, the renal medulla or central area, and a cavity known as the renal pelvis. The functional units of the kidney are called nephrons. The renal cortex contains the tight networks of capillaries called the glomeruli and the Bowman's capsules, which surround and protect these capillaries. The glomeruli and Bowman's capsules are collectively called the renal corpuscle. The convoluted tubules of the nephron are also contained within the renal cortex. The medulla consists of the renal pyramids. These triangular-shaped areas consist of

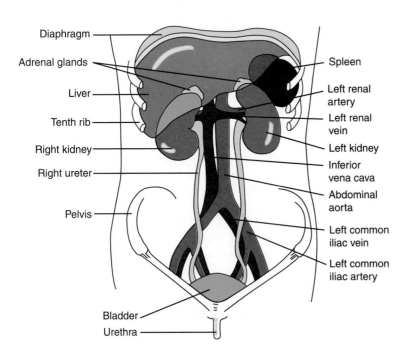

Diaphragm
Adrenal glands
Liver
Tenth rib
Right kidney
Right ureter
Pelvis
Bladder
Urethra

Spleen
Left renal artery
Left renal vein
Left kidney
Inferior vena cava
Abdominal aorta
Left common iliac vein
Left common iliac artery

FIGURE 12.6 Anterior view of the urinary system.

the collecting tubules and the loops of Henle of the nephron. The renal pelvis is an area where the ureter passes into the kidney forming a cavity and the parts of the renal pelvis called calyces (single: calyx) surround the narrow ends of the renal pyramids (see Fig. 12-7).

The actual working unit of the kidneys is the nephron. Approximately 1 million nephrons are enclosed within each kidney. Urine is formed within the nephrons and then passed through the ureter to the bladder. Each nephron is composed of a renal corpuscle, and renal tubule, with an associated network of small blood vessels. The renal corpuscle is further divided into the glomerulus, a network of capillaries, and the Bowman's capsule, which is part of a renal tubule that surrounds the glomerulus. The internal layer of the Bowman's capsule is porous and allows fluid to enter the area between the internal and external layers, where it will become urine. No leakage occurs from the external layer because it is not porous. The renal tubule is made up of the proximal convoluted tubule, the loop of Henle, and the distal convoluted tubule. The convoluted tubules are meandering tubules that end in a collecting tubule. These collecting tubules combine to form a papillary duct that ends within the renal pelvis. The renal artery, a branch of the abdominal aorta, enters the kidney and branches into smaller arterioles, which enter the glomerulus. Capillary exchange takes place within the glomerulus between the arterioles and the venules, and waste products are filtered out into the Bowman's capsule together with plasma, through a process called glomerular filtration. The blood cells remain in the blood vessels for recirculation round the body via the renal vein.

Urine is formed in the glomerulus as renal filtrate within the Bowman's capsule. Approximately 25% of the blood that enters the glomerulus is turned into renal filtrate, and the quantity of fluid formed is termed the **glomerular filtration rate (GFR)** or estimated glomerular filtration rate (eGFR). The GFR is defined as the amount of renal filtrate produced by the kidneys in 1 minute. The usual volume of GFR is between 90 and 120 milliliters per minute (mL/min). As people age, the normal GFR reduces slightly. When chronic kidney disease exists the GFR reduces to below 60 mL/min, and if kidney failure occurs the GFR is below 15 mL/min.[274] The GFR is dependent on the amount of blood flow to the kidneys. Because removal of waste substances is dependent on the mechanism of the GFR, when the GFR is reduced or stops, there is a buildup of waste products in the circulatory system. The waste products remain in the renal vein and are transmitted round the body. Although only about 1% of the renal filtrate becomes urine, a reduction in the GFR can stop urine output altogether. The other 99% of the renal filtrate is reabsorbed back into the body by tubular reabsorption through the renal tubules. Out of approximately 175 liters of renal filtrate processed in a day, only about 1 or 2 liters become urine. Several reasons exist why urine output may be reduced or stopped. Problems may occur with the amount of blood flow into the kidneys as the result of a heart attack or severe hemorrhage, or there may be a kidney infection, which shuts down the mechanisms of the kidney. In some cases, as described in Chapter 11, benign prostatic hyperplasia may constrict the ureter and prevent urination. In severe cases in which the kidney fails to return to normal function, kidney failure occurs, and the individual requires hemodialysis to remove the waste products from the body. Kidney transplantation is becoming increasingly successful for those patients with nonfunctioning kidneys.

Several hormones influence the rate of output of urine from the kidneys. If the blood potassium levels are elevated or the sodium levels are lowered, the adrenal cortex secretes aldosterone, which has the effect on the kidneys of reducing urine output. This allows the volume of blood to remain higher and thus less concentrated. Conversely, atrial natriuretic hormone (ANH), also known as atrial natriuretic factor or atrial natriuretic peptide, is a protein and vasodilator produced by the heart in response to either hypertension or an increased blood volume. This protein causes the kidneys to secrete more renal filtrate, resulting in more urine output, an increased elimination of sodium in the urine, and a reduction in blood pressure.[275] The antidiuretic hormone (ADH), synthesized in the

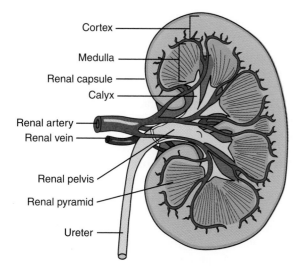

Cortex
Medulla
Renal capsule
Calyx
Renal artery
Renal vein
Renal pelvis
Renal pyramid
Ureter

FIGURE 12.7 The kidney showing internal structure.

hypothalamus and released by the posterior pituitary gland in response to reduced water content in the body, reduces the output of urine to prevent dehydration. In such cases of poor hydration, the urine becomes concentrated with waste products. After sufficient fluids are restored to the body, the kidney function usually returns to normal.[276]

Other functions of the kidney include the maintenance of the normal pH of blood and body fluids. The pH value is a measure of the hydrogen ions in the blood. The normal pH of blood is between 7.35 and 7.45. A pH of over 7.0 is considered alkaline or basic.[277] If the blood and body fluids become too acidic (pH values fall below 7.35), the kidneys allow more hydrogen ions (H+) to pass into the renal filtrate and prevent the bicarbonate ions (HCO3) from being excreted. This allows the pH to return to a more alkaline state. The opposite occurs if the blood and body fluids become too alkaline. The kidneys also assist in the regulation of blood pressure. The arterioles surrounding the kidneys secrete renin, an enzyme that stimulates the adrenal cortex to secrete aldosterone. Together, these two substances assist in raising blood pressure. This mechanism is particularly important when blood volume drops as a result of hemorrhage. The kidneys also function to increase the levels of oxygenation of blood by the secretion of erythropoietin. The erythropoietin stimulates red bone marrow to produce more red blood cells (RBCs) in an attempt to increase oxygen uptake into the RBCs. The kidneys also convert vitamin D into calciferol, which improves the absorption of calcium and phosphates by the intestine.

The urinary bladder is a sac that serves as a reservoir for the collection of urine from the kidneys (see Fig. 12-6). The urinary bladder is situated in the lower abdomen and is connected to the kidneys by a ureter from each kidney. The ureters are tubes with smooth muscle walls able to propel the urine from the kidneys to the bladder. The bladder's position inferior to the uterus in women makes it susceptible to pressure from the enlarged uterus during pregnancy. Contraction of the bladder and elimination of urine through the urethra is accomplished by the **detrusor muscle**, a smooth muscle within the wall of the bladder. The detrusor muscle also forms the internal urethral sphincter. This sphincter is not under voluntary control. The internal wall of the bladder is composed of transitional epithelium tissue that stretches according to the volume of urine within the bladder. The walls have ridges called rugae, which increase the surface area of the inside of the bladder, allowing it to expand. The urethra is a tube passing from the bladder to the external opening in the pelvic floor in a woman, and the end of the penis in the male. The urethra contains the external urethral sphincter,

which is composed of skeletal muscle. This external sphincter is under voluntary control. The length of the urethra in females is approximately 1.5 inches and exits the peroneal wall of the pelvis anterior to the vaginal opening. In males the urethra is longer, approximately 8 inches, because it extends through the penis. In males, the urethra provides passage for the semen, as well as urine.

Micturition, the elimination of urine from the bladder, is controlled by a reflex from the spinal cord that can be influenced by voluntary control. The reflex is stimulated by a stretching of the detrusor muscle by the quantity of urine within the bladder. Although the bladder is capable of holding up to as much as 800 mL of urine without rupture, the reflex is usually triggered well before that time. When approximately 200 to 400 mL of urine builds up in the bladder the reflex is triggered and the internal urethral sphincter relaxes. The external urethral sphincter may be relaxed, or contracted, because it is under voluntary control. For urine to flow from the bladder and into the urethra, the pressure within the bladder has to overcome the pressure within the urethra. However, if the volume of urine builds up too much in the bladder, the body's defense mechanism is to protect the bladder from injury, and the external sphincter can no longer be controlled voluntarily.[278] The normal urine output per person during a 24-hour period is approximately 1 to 2 liters. Urine is usually clear and yellow. The intensity of the color depends on the concentration of the urine, the more concentrated being a deeper yellow. Oliguria (reduced urine output) will occur if there is loss of fluid through other means from the body such as sweating or diarrhea. Conversely polyuria (increased urine output) will occur if excess fluids are taken into the body. See Table 12-3 for the details of normal and abnormal urine.

Diagnostic Tests and Procedures for the Urinary Tract

Some of the more commonly seen diagnostic tests and procedures for the urinary tract are included in this section. These tests are often referred to in the patient chart.

BLOOD TESTS

BUN test: A blood urea nitrogen (BUN) test detects the levels of urea and nitrogen in blood. The range of normal values for the BUN test for adults is between 6 and 20 mg/dL, and for people over 60 years of age ranges from 8 to 23 mg/dL.[279] High levels on a BUN test may indicate reduced kidney function. BUN levels may be high under many circumstances, including intestinal bleeding, congestive heart failure, systemic shock, immediately after

Table 12.3 Normal and Abnormal Constituents and Characteristics of Urine

	NORMAL URINE	ABNORMAL URINE
Appearance	Clear Yellow/amber	Cloudy – indicates infection (Bacteriuria) Brown/red tones – indicates presence of blood or bile pigment (liver disease) Green – bile pigment present in urine indicating jaundice (liver disease)
Creatinine clearance	100-140 ml/minute	Increased in kidney disease
Hematuria (blood in the urine)	0 – 2 red blood cells	3 or more red blood cells – indicates urinary tract infections, trauma, malignancy, polycystic kidney disease
Odor	Slight	Acetone odor – diabetes ketosis Unusual or unpleasant odor – possible infection
Output	1 to 2 liters per day	Anuria (no urine output) Dysuria (painful urination) Frequency (frequent urination) Nocturia (night-time urination) Oliguria (reduced urine output) Polyuria (increased urine output) Urgency (inability to control the need to urinate)
pH	4.6 – 8.0 (Slightly acidic)	Below 4.6 or above 8.0
Proteinuria	10 – 150 mg/day	30—300 mg/day may indicate diabetes mellitus or hypertension glomerular problems Above 300 mg/day indicative of kidney failure, or kidney damage
Specific gravity (Density)	1.010 – 1.025 (a lower number indicates less concentrated urine)	Above 1.025 (indicates very concentrated urine)
Waste products	Creatinine Ketones – small amounts normal Urea Uric acid	Bacteriuria (presence of bacteria) Glucosuria (presence of glucose as in diabetes) Hematuria (presence of blood) Ketonuria (presence of high levels of ketones due to high protein diet or diabetes) Proteinuria (presence of protein) Pyuria (presence of pus) Urinary casts (microscopic particles) – indicates inflammation of kidney tubules
Water	95%	

Partially adapted from *Taber's Cyclopedic Medical Dictionary,* 20th edition, Philadelphia: F. A. Davis Company, p. 2276. Used with permission.

myocardial infarction, in people with severe burns, dehydration, and may be normal during pregnancy.[280]

Creatinine clearance: A creatinine clearance blood test detects whether the kidney can effectively remove creatinine from the blood and excrete it in the urine. The test involves the analysis of a 24-hour urine collection and blood tests at the beginning and end of the period. The patient ingests creatinine, and the blood is tested after intake. If high levels of creatinine remain in the blood, and lower levels of creatinine are detected in the urine, it indicates the kidneys are not functioning well. Creatinine is a normal by-product of muscle work and the results of the creatinine clearance test results are dependent on the muscle mass, age, and physical activity of the patient. Low creatinine clearance results may also be evident in people with congestive heart failure (CHF) and those with kidney disease or kidney failure. Increased creatinine clearance values may be noted during pregnancy, after exercise, and in people who consume large quantities of meat.[281]

CATHETERIZATION OF THE BLADDER

Catheterization of the bladder is used for several reasons. In people who are unable to void the bladder, a catheter is inserted through the urethra into the bladder to enable emptying of the bladder. Aneuria, or the inability to urinate, can occur after abdominal surgery, or in several types of neurological conditions. The bladder may also need to be emptied before some medical procedures, and catheterization is often performed during labor before the birth of the infant. In some cases, medications may be introduced directly into the bladder using a catheter. Several types of catheter can be used for various reasons. A short catheter may be used to drain the bladder. This type of in-and-out catheter is removed immediately after drainage of the bladder. If the catheter is to remain in place for a while, such as after surgery or as a result of incontinence, it is called an **indwelling catheter**. These catheters, often called **Foley catheters**, have an inflatable balloon at the end. The catheter is inserted through the urethra into the urinary bladder, and once in place, the catheter balloon is inflated to ensure it remains in place inside the bladder. A **Texas catheter** is a type used with men. This catheter is attached to the penis with a condom-type mechanism. This type is less likely to cause infection, but PTAs needs to be aware that it will become dislodged easily when the person is performing exercises or activities. A suprapubic catheter is one inserted surgically through the wall of the lower abdomen, usually after surgery on the urinary tract, to allow the area to heal. This may or may not be reversed after recovery. All catheters have urine collection mechanisms that may be a leg bag that attaches to the leg or a larger collection device that is either attached to the bed or placed on the floor. Urine collection devices must be placed below the level of the urethra so that the urine cannot flow back into the bladder and cause infection. Some of the complications of using a catheter for prolonged periods of time may include septicemia (infection of the blood), hematuria (blood in the urine), urethral injury, urinary tract or kidney infections, and the development of kidney stones or bladder cancer.[282] PTAs should be aware that the indwelling catheter can provide a portal of infection for the patient, and strict hand washing should be practiced before and after any handling of catheters. When working with patients who are catheterized, care must be taken to prevent backflow of urine into the bladder. When moving the collection bag higher than the patient's urethra for brief periods, the catheter tube should be constricted to prevent any backflow of urine.

CYSTOSCOPY

The use of a cystoscope (a fiberoptic scope) to observe the inside of the urethra and the bladder may be used for diagnosis of bladder conditions. Cystoscopes may be of a rigid or flexible type of tubing with a camera on the end. The cystoscope enables the physician to take a tissue biopsy or in some cases to actually crush calculi (stones) within the bladder or urethra. This technique cannot be used for the kidney.[283]

RADIOLOGICAL TESTS

Several radiological tests can be performed to detect kidney abnormalities. The **intravenous pyelogram (IVP)** is commonly used. In this test, a dye is injected into the blood and highlights the urinary tract so that an x-ray can detect any obstruction or abnormality.[284] The kidneys-ureter-bladder (KUB) test is an x-ray of the abdomen that can detect some urinary tract abnormalities.[285] In a cystogram dye is inserted directly into the bladder using a catheter. CT and MRI may also be used to detect abnormalities of the kidney.

RENAL BIOPSY (KIDNEY BIOPSY)

A renal biopsy may be performed using a biopsy needle inserted through the skin directly into the kidney. Ultrasound or CT scan imaging is used to determine the area of the kidney for biopsy. A sample of tissue is taken for laboratory analysis. The skin in the area is injected with local anesthetic to reduce the pain. Another method of renal biopsy, called a transjugular biopsy, is performed using a catheter biopsy tube passed through the jugular vein in the neck to the kidney.[286]

RENAL DIALYSIS

Renal dialysis is used extensively in the United States and throughout the world to remove waste products from people whose kidneys do not function. Many patients are unable to urinate or may have a reduced ability to do so. In all cases, the kidneys do not function correctly, and waste products build up in the body to toxic levels. Some patients have acute renal failure, which may recover, whereas others have end-stage renal disease. Some of the latter may be candidates for renal transplant and may receive dialysis while waiting for a donor kidney. Of note is that people can function well with only one kidney or even only part of a kidney. Placing people on a kidney dialysis machine acts similarly to the kidney. The blood is shunted from the patient via a catheter in the arm to a dialysis machine, which filters the blood and removes waste products from the blood and then returns the blood to the body. The procedure has to be repeated two or three times a week and lasts for several hours each time. Strict adherence to a specified diet is necessary, and fluid intake is greatly restricted because the kidneys are unable to process the fluid. **Hemodialysis** is performed in a hospital or outpatient setting, whereas peritoneal dialysis may be completed at home.[287] **Peritoneal dialysis** is also called continuous ambulatory peritoneal dialysis (CAPD). For peritoneal dialysis, catheters are implanted in the peritoneal cavity, and the process is performed every day when the patient is sleeping. This type of dialysis takes several hours but tends to be less traumatic for the patient than hemodialysis. The catheter implanted for peritoneal dialysis tends to increase the chance of infections as it acts as a portal for infections. However, the possibility of infection is a complication for any patient receiving dialysis, and antimicrobial medications are used when infection is detected.[288]

URINALYSIS

Urinalysis is performed to determine the presence of infection or disease of the kidneys. A urine sample is provided and tested using a variety of methods. Direct observation of the urine sample can provide information about the color of the urine. The normal color of urine is pale yellow. If the urine is dark-colored, it could indicate concentrated urine. Blood in the urine may also be apparent from observation. Normal urine is also clear, and the presence of cloudiness may indicate infection. The evaluation of pH levels, protein levels, specific gravity (concentration) readings, glucose detection, ketones (byproducts of fat metabolism), and blood cell detection are all possible through a dipstick urinalysis. Detection of bilirubin in the urine may indicate liver disease. Further examination of urine samples using the microscope can identify bacteria, cell debris, and urine crystals.[289]

URINE CULTURE AND SENSITIVITY (C & S)

This test is used if there is an abnormal urinalysis result and an infection is suspected. The urine sample is spun in a centrifuge to separate out the cells and other particles. A culture of the urine sample may be able to identify the bacteria to provide effective treatment with medications specifically targeting the infective organism. A positive test result is considered to be the presence of more than 10,000 colony count of one specific type of bacteria.[290] A midstream urine sample may be requested. This is one in which the person has to stop the urine stream and then

void into a sterile container. The theory is that the initial urine cleans the internal surface of the urethra, and then the sample will be less likely to be contaminated. However, some people with weak pelvic floor musculature have difficulty cutting off the flow of urine in midstream. In some cases, a sterile catheter may be inserted to obtain a clean sample.

Terms Associated With Urinary Disease

The PTA should be familiar with the different terms that are associated with urinary diseases to understand the patient chart. A basic understanding of these terms enables the PTA to communicate more effectively with patients, physicians, and other health care providers and determine the contraindications and precautions associated with physical therapy interventions when working with people with urinary tract diseases.

DIURETIC MEDICATIONS

Diuretic medications, commonly known as water pills, cause the kidneys to excrete more water and sodium in the urine and act to increase the elimination of water from the body. Diuretics are used to treat hypertension, glaucoma, edema, kidney disease, congestive heart failure, and pulmonary edema. Three types of diuretic include thiazide diuretics such as chlorothiazide (Diuril), loop diuretics such as the commonly prescribed furosemide (Lasix), and potassium sparing such as spironolactone (Aldactone). Diuretics increase the frequency of **micturition** (urination). Some of the side effects of using diuretics include hyponatremia (low amounts of blood potassium) with loop diuretics, hypernatremia (increased amounts of potassium) with potassium sparing diuretics, increased cholesterol levels, and gout.[291]

NEUROGENIC BLADDER

The term **neurogenic bladder,** or spastic bladder, applies to a bladder that has an interrupted nerve supply. This is caused by lack of nerve supply from the sacral nerves, which supply the detrusor muscle of the bladder and affect the reflex mechanism loop for micturition. A neurogenic bladder occurs in people with spinal cord injuries, tumors of the spine affecting the spinal nerves, Alzheimer's disease, multiple sclerosis, and neuropathy. A neurogenic bladder can lead to disorders such as overflow incontinence, reduced bladder capacity, the inability to contract and empty the bladder, urinary retention, and the inability to detect when the bladder is full (see Table 12-4). All of these conditions can lead to an increased risk of urinary tract infections (UTIs), kidney calculi, and kidney disease.[292]

RENAL TRANSPLANT

Kidney transplant is performed on individuals with renal failure. The kidney donor is usually a close relative who donates one kidney if his or her immune system is compatible with the patient's. Donations may also be received from recently deceased people who agree to donate their kidneys. According to the Scientific Registry of Transplant Recipients for the period between January 1, 2009, and December 31, 2009, there were 80,559 people on the waiting list in the United States for kidney transplant at the beginning of the period and 86,071 at the end. During this period, 34,091 new patients were registered to receive kidney transplant, 10,442 people received transplants from deceased donors, and 6,388 people received renal transplants from living donors. The adult patient survival rate after renal transplant was 96.9% and that of children 98.96% in the 2009 reporting period. Approximately 6% of people died waiting for a renal transplant in the second half of 2009.[293] The recipient of a kidney transplant must receive immunosuppressive drugs to prevent rejection of the new kidney. The new kidney is transplanted into the pelvic cavity of the recipient and not into the original location of the kidney. Recipients of kidneys need to continue the immunosuppressive medications, which may make them susceptible to infections. An additional problem is that the original disease process may also affect the transplanted kidney. According to a study by Liem and Weimer, evidence is emerging that performing kidney transplant on people before they have been on dialysis for prolonged periods improves the outcome.[294]

Why Does the PTA Need to Know About Urinary Tract Diseases?

The PTA will be involved with the treatment of people with end-stage renal disease and many other chronic kidney conditions described in this chapter. When treating people who are receiving dialysis, the PTA should be aware that the monitoring of vital signs and checking for signs of dehydration is important. The overexertion of patients with end-stage renal disease should be avoided. Fluid intake is often restricted with these patients, and any fluid input must be well documented by the PTA in the patient chart with the exact quantity of fluid noted. All physician orders regarding fluid intake must be followed closely. In many cases, the PT intervention will be directed at improving mobility, ambulation, and functional abilities, as well as increasing muscle strength and endurance. Postural education may also be indicated. Physical therapy intervention can assist in raising the quality of life for these patients. Remember that people with end-stage renal disease may be lethargic, weak, and also confused or disoriented as a result of the metabolic imbalances caused by the disease process. Patients with different types of incontinence may be treated for pelvic floor reeducation exercises and biofeedback modalities to assist with the control of sphincters. An awareness of some of the pathologies associated with incontinence in its many forms is essential for the PTA working with this population.

Diseases of the Urinary Tract

Several general characteristic signs and symptoms exist that occur with diseases of the urinary tract. These are detailed in Table 12-4. Pain can be elicited for several reasons. Some pain is localized to the area of the problem, whereas other pain is classified as referred pain from the local area to a distant site, dependent on the dermatome distribution of nerves. A dermatome is an area of skin supplied by a particular nerve root. The nerve that supplies the internal organ also supplies an area of skin, and the pain may be felt in that area of skin. Renal pain is often felt in the low back and may radiate into the umbilicus area and the groin of the same side as the kidney involved.[295] Blockage of the ureter may cause pain in the male scrotum or female labium. Acute bladder urinary retention causes pain in the suprapubic area. Prostate pain is often felt in the pelvic floor area, or the lumbosacral spine.

Urinary tract infections (UTIs) are common, resulting in approximately 8.3 million visits to the physician each year in the United States.[296] Infections may be acute or chronic. *Escherichia coli* is the most common causative bacterium of urinary tract infections. The *E. coli* bacteria are found in the colon and cause infections when they migrate to the urinary tract. Nosocomial infections of the urinary tract are often the most serious because they are contracted within a hospital setting where the bacteria may be virulent. Refer to Chapter 10 for further information about nosocomial infections.

Table 12.4 General Characteristic Signs and Symptoms of Urinary Tract Diseases and Conditions

CHARACTERISTICS	LIKELY CAUSE/MANIFESTATION/DESCRIPTION
Aneuria	Inability to urinate May be a sign of urinary tract problem, prostate condition, or may take place temporarily after abdominal surgery
Dysuria (pain on micturition)	Painful urination may indicate many types of urinary tract disease, or uterine, or prostate problems May also indicate inflammation, or infection of the urethra, bladder, or kidney
Fever/malaise	May indicate infection or buildup of toxins resulting from poorly functioning kidneys
Frequency of micturition	Frequent need to urinate May be the result of a variety of urinary tract conditions
Hematuria	Blood in the urine may indicate a renal infection, or other renal or bladder condition
Hesitancy of micturition	Delay in starting to urinate May be caused by a blockage in the urethra
Intermittency/postvoid dribbling	Interruption in urine flow, or lack of fully emptying the bladder May be the result of an obstruction of the urethra
Nocturia	Nighttime need to urinate that disturbs sleep May be caused by a variety of urinary tract conditions
Oliguria	Reduced urine output
Overflow incontinence	Chronic bladder urinary retention often causes overflow incontinence when the bladder can no longer hold the amount of urine
Pain in low back	May indicate renal or bladder infection
Stress incontinence	Leakage of urine when an increase in intra-abdominal pressure occurs such as with exercising, coughing, sneezing, or laughing May be the result of weakness of pelvic floor musculature, or a sign of other urinary conditions.
Urgency of micturition	The need to urinate immediately Lack of ability to control the urge to urinate May be caused by weakness of pelvic floor musculature or the result of other urinary tract conditions
Urge incontinence	Inability to hold urine when the urge to urinate occurs
Voiding problems	May be the result of renal or bladder pathology or prostate problems in men

Those infections that affect the kidneys are potentially dangerous, because they can damage the kidney and result in reduced kidney function. The main cause of UTI in women is through sexual intercourse. The external opening of the urethra lies close to the vagina and bacteria from the vagina may enter the urethra. The urethra is much shorter in women than men, and thus bacteria can more easily enter the bladder and be transmitted up to the kidney via the ureter.[297] In addition, the use of spermicidal (birth control by killing sperm) creams in the female alters the normal flora of the area and may increase the risk for UTI.

Diseases of the Bladder

The two diseases of the bladder included in this section are those most commonly seen in physical therapy practice. People with the effects of bladder cancer and cystitis may benefit from physical therapy interventions.

"It Happened in the Clinic"

A 60-year-old female patient with end-stage renal disease was referred to physical therapy for mobility training and strengthening. Evaluation by the physical therapist revealed that the patient was very weak with overall strength 3+/5 in upper and lower extremities and was unable to rise from a chair without assistance. She required moderate assistance to transfer from bed to chair and was unable to ambulate independently. Physical therapy intervention by the PTA included ambulation training with a wheeled walker because the patient was unable to lift an ordinary walker. The patient continued to find ambulation difficult even with a wheeled walker so forearm supports were attached to the walker and the patient was able to ambulate independently for up to 100 feet using this assistive device. The patient did not have stairs at home, so stair climbing was not attempted. A higher chair seat was used for the patient, and she was able to rise independently, although slowly, using this. A chair insert was ordered for home use to raise the level of the chair seat. Strengthening exercises were provided for upper and lower extremities. The goal for this patient was to improve the quality of life by increasing the level of independence and enabling the patient to return home. These goals were achieved.

Bladder Cancer

The majority of bladder cancers are located in the epithelium of the bladder. Staging of the cancer is similar to that related to other cancers already described in this book using the TNM system. The T stands for the actual location and depth of the tumor, the N relates to the spread to lymph nodes, and the M relates to any metastases. The T stage, or 0 stage refers to a carcinoma in situ (early stage); T1 or Stage I locally invasive; progressing through to T4b or Stage IV in which there is invasion of the cancer into the pelvic wall.[298] The estimates for 2010 from the American Cancer Society were 70,530 new diagnoses and 14,680 deaths from the disease.[299] Bladder cancer occurs three times more frequently in men than women and is one of the more common cancers of the urinary tract. The prevalence of bladder cancer is greater for Caucasian people than for African American, Hispanic, or Asian people. The incidence of bladder cancer increases after age 50 with as many as 90% of people with bladder cancer being over age 55. The lifetime risk of developing bladder cancer is 1 in 26 for men and 1 in 84 for women.[300]

Etiology. The causes of bladder cancer are largely unknown. However, some known risk factors for the development of bladder cancer include cigarette smoking and exposure to industrial carcinogenic solvents.[301]

Signs and Symptoms. The characteristic signs and symptoms of bladder cancer include hematuria (blood in the urine), and changes in bladder habits such as urinary frequency or urgency, and dysuria (painful urination). In advanced stages of bladder cancer lymphedema of the legs may occur.[302]

Prognosis. The early detection of bladder cancer allows for a better prognosis. The 5-year survival rate for people with Stage 0 bladder cancer is 98%, and for Stage IV, the survival rate drops to 15%.[303]

Medical Intervention. The medical management of bladder cancer requires the diagnosis and staging of the cancer. Many of the tests described earlier in this chapter may be used for diagnosis including cystoscopy, urine cytology including tumor marker studies for NMP22, urine culture, biopsy, intravenous pyelography, retrograde pyelography, CT scan, MRI, ultrasound, bone scans, and PET scans.[304] The medical treatment may include chemotherapy, applied directly into the bladder through a catheter, and/or radiotherapy. **Transurethral resection (TUR)** of the affected area of the bladder may be performed. In this procedure, cancerous cells are removed by passing a resection instrument through the urethra into the bladder. A cystectomy is surgical removal of all or part of the bladder.[305]

Physical Therapy Intervention. Some patients who have debility as a result of the bladder cancer may require general strengthening, endurance training, and functional ADL interventions.

Cystitis

Cystitis is inflammation of the bladder, and sometimes the urethra, usually as the result of an infection. Sometimes the condition is called interstitial cystitis or painful bladder syndrome (PBS) when there is no apparent known bacterial cause for the bladder inflammation.[306] Women are more than 10 times more susceptible to cystitis than men because of the position of the external urethral opening, which lies adjacent to the vagina and close to the anus. The prevalence of cystitis in women is estimated to be between 0.16 and 12.6%. Between 1988 and 1994 (most recent available) over 1.3 million adults over age 20 years were diagnosed with interstitial cystitis.[307]

Etiology. When the cause of the condition is bacterial, the causative bacteria are often either *E. coli* or *Pseudomonas*. The infection is termed ascending because it enters the bladder by ascending through the urethra. Infections are either nosocomial (acquired in a hospital setting) or community acquired. Causes of noninfectious cystitis include drug induced as a result of chemotherapy, radiation induced from radiation therapy to the pelvic area, or immune-mediated sensitivity to products such as bubble bath or other bathing products.[308] Risk factors that contribute to the development of infective cystitis may include an enlarged prostate or bladder calculi (stones); changes in the body's immune system as a result of diabetes mellitus, HIV infection, or chemotherapy treatment for cancer; or the use of a bladder catheter for long periods of time.[309]

Signs and Symptoms. The characteristic signs and symptoms of cystitis may include dysuria (pain on voiding); frequency or urgency of micturition; pain in the lower abdomen during voiding; hematuria (blood in the urine); passing frequent, small quantities of urine; strong-smelling urine; and a low-grade fever in the presence of bacterial infection. [310]

Prognosis. Most people with infective cystitis have no long-term effects, although kidney infections can result from untreated bladder infections. People with interstitial cystitis can have chronic complications that lead to urgency and frequent pain with urination and can interfere with leisure and work activities. The need to urinate during the night can lead to sleep deprivation and depression.[311]

Medical Intervention. A urinalysis is performed to identify the bacteria responsible for the infection and then an appropriate antimicrobial medication is prescribed. In the absence of bacterial cause for the condition, a cystoscopy or ureteroscopy may be required (see the section earlier in the chapter for the description of a cystoscopy).[312] According to the Interstitial Cystitis Association, plans are underway to standardize the treatment for interstitial cystitis. Currently, a combination of treatments is provided, including modification of the diet to exclude or reduce the amount of acid intake, and medications such as pentosan polysulfate sodium (Elmiron) to heal the internal surface of the bladder and reduce pain, low doses of tricyclic antidepressants to reduce pain, antihistamines, and some analgesics.[313]

Physical Therapy Intervention. Physical therapy intervention for pelvic floor dysfunction to help relax the pelvic floor musculature is often beneficial for people with interstitial cystitis.[314]

Diseases of the Kidney
The diseases described in this section all affect the function of the kidneys. Some kidney diseases are the result of other conditions, whereas others are primary conditions of the kidneys.

Glomerulonephritis

Glomerulonephritis is inflammation of the glomerulus of the nephron in the kidney (see Fig. 12-8). The condition may be either acute or chronic. The term is used to cover many inflammatory and infectious diseases of the kidney. If the condition remains untreated over a prolonged period, there may be permanent damage to the kidney leading to end-stage renal disease. Acute glomerulonephritis usually occurs in children between the ages of 5 and 15, with males affected twice as often as females. Acute glomerulonephritis accounts for approximately 10% to 15% of all glomerular diseases.[315]

Etiology. The causes of acute glomerulonephritis include bacterial infections such as *Streptococcus* and *Staphylococcus*: viruses such as cytomegalovirus, Epstein-Barr virus, hepatitis B, rubella, and mumps; fungal and parasitic infections such as plasmodium malariae (malaria), filariasis, trichonosis, and trypanosomes; renal disease; vasculitis; systemic lupus erythematosus; polyarteritis nodosa; and drug reactions mainly from gold or penicillamine therapy.[316] The reactions from any of these causative factors result in the development of immune complexes within the kidneys that enlarges the kidneys up to 50%.

Signs and Symptoms. The characteristic signs and symptoms of both acute and chronic glomerulonephritis include edema of the scrotum and periocular tissues (round the eyes), anasarca (general body edema), hypertension, headaches, fever, weakness, abdominal pain, dyspnea, and malaise.[317]

Prognosis. The prognosis for people with acute glomerulonephritis is generally good with only 1% to 3% of cases leading to chronic renal failure. Some of the other rare complications resulting from the condition may include hypertensive retinopathy (eye) and hypertensive encephalopathy (inflammation of the brain).[318]

Medical Intervention. The diagnostic procedures performed for glomerulonephritis are many. A complete blood

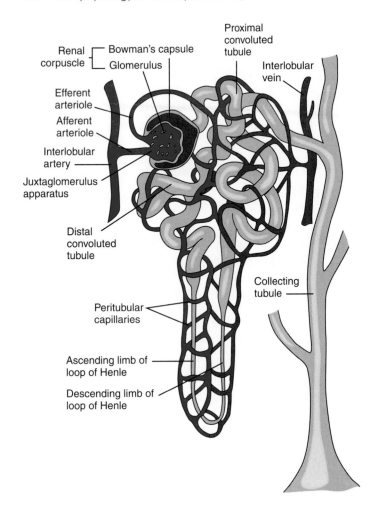

Renal corpuscle ⎡ Bowman's capsule
               ⎣ Glomerulus

Proximal convoluted tubule

Interlobular vein

Efferent arteriole

Afferent arteriole

Interlobular artery

Juxtaglomerulus apparatus

Distal convoluted tubule

Collecting tubule

Peritubular capillaries

Ascending limb of loop of Henle

Descending limb of loop of Henle

FIGURE 12.8 A nephron.

count (CBC) with a BUN and creatinine test is usually performed with a creatinine test of more than 40 considered positive. Urinalysis may determine dark urine with an increased specific gravity concentration, proteinurias (protein in the urine) and red blood cells in the urine. The erythrocyte sedimentation rate (ESR) is usually raised. Radiographs of the chest and abdomen, an echocardiogram, renal ultrasound, and renal biopsy may also be performed.[319] The medical management of glomerulonephritis may include a restricted fluid intake, antimicrobial medications to treat infection, a reduced sodium intake in the diet, the use of diuretic medications for the reduction of edema, and the use of corticosteroid medications to reduce inflammation. The medical intervention is entirely dependent on the cause of disease process.[320]

Physical Therapy Intervention. Physical therapy intervention may be indicated for people who have weakness

as a result of the disease process. Generally, people with acute glomerulonephritis will not require physical therapy intervention.

Kidney Stones

Kidney stones are also known as urinary stones, calculi, urolithiasis, or nephrolithiasis (see Fig. 12-9). Calculi may be composed of calcium phosphate, oxalate, uric acid, cystine (an amino acid), or struvite (large stones otherwise called staghorn stones or calculi). The calcium phosphate types are the most common. Calculi are mainly located in the renal pelvis of the kidney or in the bladder. The incidence of kidney calculi is high in the United States with approximately 1 million people affected each year. The prevalence of kidney stones is 1 in 272 people or 0.37% of the population. Each person has a 10% lifetime risk of developing kidney stones.[321] Approximately

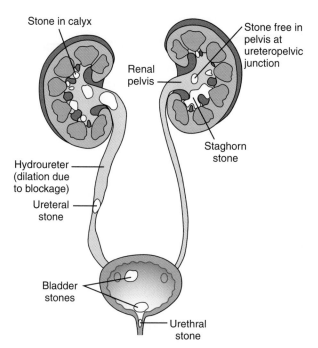

Stone in calyx

Stone free in pelvis at ureteropelvic junction

Renal pelvis

Staghorn stone

Hydroureter (dilation due to blockage)

Ureteral stone

Bladder stones

Urethral stone

FIGURE 12.9 Diagram of various locations of calculi (stones) in the urinary tract.

half a million people go to the emergency room with kidney stones each year in the United States. Men are affected more than women, and Caucasians are affected more than African Americans. The age of onset is mainly between the ages of 30 and 40 years, and the incidence increases with age.[322]

Etiology. For many people who develop kidney stones there is no known cause. Many different possible causes of kidney calculi exist. A family history may cause a predisposition to develop kidney stones. They may develop after prolonged periods of immobilization as a result of injury, be precipitated by dehydration, or form as a result of gout, hyperparathyroidism, cystic kidney disease, or a rare condition of renal tubular acidosis.[323] UTIs may also predispose people to the formation of calculi. Excessive amounts of calcium intake and vitamin D may be also be causative factors in some people.[324]

Signs and Symptoms. The characteristic signs and symptoms of kidney calculi include sudden pain in the abdomen that often occurs during the night and awakens the person, sweating, nausea, and vomiting. If a stone is passed through the ureter, pain may be referred to the testis or labium, and there may be intense urgency or frequency of micturition, particularly if the stone becomes

lodged in the ureter. However, many small calculi are passed in the urine and cause no problems.[325]

Prognosis. The prognosis for those with kidney stones is usually good. Most kidney stones are passed out of the body through the urinary system without any medical or surgical intervention. However, once people have had kidney stones, they are more likely to develop further stones.

Medical Intervention. The diagnosis of kidney stones is often only achieved after onset of severe pain when a stone attempts to pass through the urinary system. Investigatory procedures for severe abdominal pain such as radiographic images, CT scans, and intravenous pyelogram (IVP) often reveal the kidney or ureteral stones. Laboratory tests for the acidic content of the urine may provide further clues to the cause of the stones. The medical management of calculi usually includes advice on adequate fluid intake, especially drinking plenty of water. In many cases, flushing out the urinary system with adequate amounts of water resolves the problem and the stones are passed in the urine. Medications such as allopurinol may be prescribed to reduce the development of crystals in the kidneys to reduce the risk of developing further calculi. Medical procedures used to remove kidney calculi include a comparatively new treatment intervention called extracorporeal shock wave lithotripsy (ESWL), which may be effective in dissolving the stones with shock waves, or breaking large stones into smaller units that can be passed in the urine. Some people with large-sized calculi may require surgery. Percutaneous nephrolithotomy is a direct surgical technique in which the surgeon enters the kidney through the skin in the back. Alternatively, stones in the ureter can be removed using a uteroscope passed through the urethra and bladder and into the ureter.[326]

Physical Therapy Intervention. No physical therapy intervention is indicated for people with kidney stones.

Nephrosclerosis

Nephrosclerosis, or hypertensive nephrosclerosis, is a complication resulting from chronic hypertension and is more commonly seen in people who are diabetic. The condition leads to renal insufficiency and is responsible for between 25% and 33% of the people with end-stage kidney disease who require hemodialysis. The condition is more common in African Americans than in Caucasians.[327] The condition is more easily understood as a syndrome of specific problems including left ventricular heart hypertrophy, proteinuria (blood in the urine), retinopathy of the eye caused by hypertension, and renal insufficiency.[328]

Etiology. No specific cause for nephrosclerosis is known. Family history plays a role in the development of the condition and a genetic marker is suspected. People with the condition all have a history of long-standing hypertension, which is thought to cause ischemia in the glomerulae of the kidneys and a reduction of renal blood flow.[329]

Signs and Symptoms. The signs and symptoms associated with nephrosclerosis are associated with the syndrome of chronic hypertension, retinal changes in the eye, renal insufficiency, and left ventricular hypertrophy.

Prognosis. Most people with nephrosclerosis develop end-stage renal disease and are placed on hemodialysis or have a renal transplant. The mortality rate for people on dialysis is relatively high at 23.3% annually.[330]

Medical Intervention. The diagnosis of nephrosclerosis involves eliminating other kidney diseases. A complete blood count (CBC), creatinine levels, electrolytes levels, and urinalysis are all used as diagnostic tests. An echocardiogram may be performed to observe the left ventricle of the heart to determine whether hypertrophy is present. A renal biopsy is the most conclusive diagnostic procedure but may not be performed on older people.[331] The medications prescribed for people with nephrosclerosis include antihypertensives and diuretics. Dietary advice with modification of eating habits and increased amounts of exercise also assist in controlling hypertension.[332]

Physical Therapy Intervention. Physical therapy intervention for those with the condition may help to reduce hypertension by improving aerobic capacity and endurance to activity. However, the chronic nature of the hypertension in people with nephrosclerosis makes the reduction of hypertension more difficult.

Pyelonephritis

Pyelonephritis is an inflammation of the kidney caused by an infection. More than 250,000 people are diagnosed with the condition each year in the United States, and of those a high proportion are hospitalized.[333]

Etiology. Pyelonephritis is inflammation of the kidney caused by bacterial infection involving the renal pelvis

(see Fig. 12-10). The most common causative bacteria of pyelonephritis are *E. coli*. This is another example of an ascending infection because bacteria usually ascend to the kidney from the lower sections of the urinary tract. The risk of infection is increased with the use of a catheter, which can act as a portal of infection. Other risk factors include cystoscopic procedures to examine the bladder and ureters, surgery on the urinary tract, abnormalities of the urinary tract, and the presence of kidney stones, or prostate enlargement that may interfere with the passage of urine.[334] People in hospital or a nursing home are more at risk of developing infections, as are those with spinal cord injuries, HIV/AIDS, chronic diabetes, and people who are taking immunosuppressive medications after organ transplant.[335]

Signs and Symptoms. The characteristic signs and symptoms of pyelonephritis may include nausea and vomiting; diarrhea; fever; pain in the abdomen, groin, back, or flank (side of the abdomen); urgency and frequency of micturition with pain on urination; dysuria (inability to urinate) or urinary retention; and pus or blood in the urine.[336]

Prognosis. Most people with pyelonephritis recover fully after treatment. If infections of the kidneys recur, or become chronic, the result can be permanent damage to the kidney and the development of chronic renal disease. In rare instances, sepsis (generalized infection of the body) can occur.[337]

Medical Intervention. The medical intervention for pyelonephritis may require hospitalization for people with severe disease. Catheterization may be needed if urinary

Normal-size kidney with some scarring

Kidney with pyelonephritis scarred and shrunken

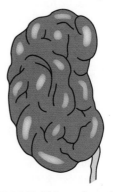 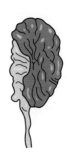

FIGURE 12.10 Kidney of a patient with chronic pyelonephritis compared with a normal-sized kidney with some scarring.

retention is present. Antimicrobials are started intravenously in many cases, and after laboratory identification of the bacteria involved, these may be adjusted to ensure the most effective medication is used. A regimen of several weeks of oral antimicrobials may be required after the completion of the intravenous antimicrobials.[338]

Physical Therapy Intervention. No physical therapy intervention is indicated for people with pyelonephritis.

Renal Carcinoma

Cancer of the kidney is one of the less common cancers, accounting for about 2% of all cancers in the United States. Each year approximately 20,000 men and 12,000 women are diagnosed with renal cancer. Of these, about one third will result in death. Renal carcinoma is more common in males than females in a 2:1 ratio and mainly occurs after age 40.[339] Several different types of renal cancer exist. Renal cell cancer, the most common, is also called adenocarcinoma or hypernephroma. Transitional cell carcinoma is more rare and occurs in the renal pelvis. Wilms' tumor is a special kind of renal cancer occurring in children. Wilms' tumor is described separately later in this chapter.

Etiology. The cause of renal cancer is unknown. The risk factors associated with the development of renal cancer include cigarette smoking; hypertension; long-term renal dialysis; people who work with chemicals and industrial substances such as asbestos, cadmium, or coke (a derivative of coal); and obesity.[340]

Signs and Symptoms. The characteristic signs and symptoms of renal carcinoma may include hematuria (blood in the urine); lateral abdominal pain and occasionally a palpable mass in the abdomen, although this is rare; weight loss; fever; and fatigue and general feelings of being unwell.[341]

Prognosis. If the cancer is isolated to the kidney the prognosis is good with appropriate treatment. As with all types of carcinoma, the further advanced the tumor is, the less favorable is the outcome. The staging of renal carcinoma is based on Stages I through IV, with Stage IV the most advanced.[342]

Medical Intervention. The diagnosis of renal carcinoma includes a variety of tests. A physical examination, blood tests for kidney function, an intravenous pyelogram, a CT scan or MRI, an ultrasound scan, and a needle biopsy of the kidney are all possibilities. The medical treatment is usually with a nephrectomy (removal of the kidney). A radical nephrectomy involves removal of the kidney, the adrenal gland, and the surrounding tissue. A simple nephrectomy involves removal of the kidney, and in a partial nephrectomy, the tumor is removed with part of the kidney. The choice of surgery depends on the staging and size of the tumor. Other treatment options include chemotherapy, radiation therapy, or biological therapy. The biological therapy stimulates the body's own immune system to fight the carcinoma. An infusion of interleukin-2 or interferon alpha into the bloodstream.[343]

Physical Therapy Intervention. Physical therapy intervention is not usually indicated for people with renal carcinoma. However, intervention may be required for people with general debility associated with the disease. The PTA may also be involved with hospice care interventions to help to improve the quality of life for patients and their families.

Renal Cystic Disease

Cysts or cavities within the kidney are defined as renal cystic disease. Estimates are that over half of people over age 50 have at least one cyst in their kidney. Several types of renal cystic disease exist. The disease in general is more common in white males and African Americans. The most common type of cystic disease is simple cysts thought to be present in 5% of the general population over age 50 years. Other types such as autosomal dominant polycystic kidney disease (ADPKD) and autosomal recessive kidney disease (ARPKD) are genetically based and rare, occurring in only 1 in 1,000 to 4,000 live births.[344] Systemic diseases such as tuberous sclerosis (TS) and Von Hippel-Lindau syndrome also result in kidney cysts. Inherited forms of cystic kidney disease are less common, and acquired cystic kidney disease is found only in people with kidney failure and who are on dialysis. Acquired cystic kidney disease occurs in 8% to 13% of people with chronic renal failure before they start dialysis, and the incidence increases for each year of dialysis until after 10 years on dialysis 90% of people have the condition.[345]

Etiology. Developmental forms of cystic kidney disease are the result of abnormal development of the renal tubules. The autosomal dominant form of the disease is the result of mutations on the PKD1 and PKD2 genes. Tuberous sclerosis is caused by mutations of the TSC1 and TSC2 genes. No known cause exists for the development of simple kidney cysts. The mechanism for the development of acquired cystic kidney disease in people with chronic renal failure is not fully understood, but one theory is that it results from blockage of the renal tubules with fibrous tissue or crystals of oxylate as part of the kidney dysfunction.[346] Medical research has identified a protein called mTOR that precipitates the development of cysts in the kidneys in cystic kidney disease.[347]

Signs and Symptoms. The general signs and symptoms of cystic kidney disease may involve lateral abdominal pain, hematuria (blood in the urine), and palpable renal masses resulting from the increased size of the kidneys. People with acquired disease or simple cysts may have no symptoms at all. Those with autosomal dominant polycystic kidney disease may also develop renal infections, hypertension and chronic renal failure by age 40, hepatic cysts (liver), pancreatic cysts, cerebral aneurysms, cardiac mitral valve prolapse, and end-stage renal disease by aged 50. Autosomal recessive polycystic kidney disease (ARPKD) has more severe symptoms and results in renal insufficiency, developmental and growth retardation in 25% of children, and end-stage renal disease within the first 10 years in 50% of children.[348] 🌐 Tuberous sclerosis (TS) is a systemic genetic disease that results in renal cysts, mental retardation, cardiac problems, and epilepsy.

Prognosis. Acquired cystic kidney disease, autosomal dominant polycystic kidney disease, and autosomal recessive polycystic disease are the main causes of end stage renal disease, leading to 10% of all cases. Approximately 50% of people with autosomal recessive polycystic kidney disease require a kidney transplant by the time they are 20 years old. In addition, between 5% and 25% of people with acquired cystic kidney disease develop renal cell carcinoma, which is responsible for an increased mortality rate.[349]

Medical Intervention. Acquired cystic kidney disease tends to resolve after kidney transplantation. The medical intervention for people with genetically or inherited disease consists of increased liquid intake, control of hypertension with antihypertensive medications such as angiotensin-converting enzyme (ACE) inhibitors or calcium channel blockers, prevention of infection, and the treatment of infections with prolonged courses of antimicrobial medications. Because medical research has identified a protein called mTOR that precipitates the development of cysts in the disease, trials are underway to control mTOR biochemically.[350]

Physical Therapy Intervention. Physical therapy intervention is likely to be directed towards people with end-stage renal disease who have reduced physical and ADL function. Interventions are likely to include a team of health care providers and family members. The focus of physical therapy interventions will be improvement of ambulatory status, ADL, aerobic endurance and conditioning, and flexibility and strengthening exercises.

Renal Failure—Acute and Chronic

Acute renal failure, now often called acute kidney injury (AKI), results in sudden loss of function of the kidneys and a change in the body's electrolyte and fluid balance, causing multiple symptoms.[351] Chronic kidney failure is defined according to criteria developed by the National Kidney Foundation in the Kidney Disease Outcomes Quality Initiative of February 2002 as a glomerular filtration rate of less than 15 mL/min/1.73 m² (normal level is over 90 mL/min/1.73 m²).[352] In chronic renal failure, the damage to the kidney is the result of prolonged disease from such conditions as diabetes mellitus, glomerular disease, or polycystic kidney disease. Another term used for chronic renal failure is end-stage renal disease (ESRD). Chronic renal disease is now such a widespread health issue that the U.S. Surgeon General included a chapter about the disease in the Healthy People 2010 report.[353] The prevalence of chronic kidney disease in adults in the United States is 11% with 19.2 million people affected. Over 300,000 (0.2%) are classified as having renal failure.[354]

Etiology. Acute renal failure may be caused by the reduced blood flow to the kidneys as a result of reduced cardiac output with associated hypotension; internal hemorrhage; extensive burns; dehydration; infections; urinary tract obstruction; trauma; or renal blood vessel clotting resulting from blood transfusion reactions, malignant hypertension (uncontrolled), systemic diseases such as scleroderma, or childbirth problems such as placenta previa or abruptio placenta.[355] If a urinary tract obstruction is not removed, the tubules of the kidney may be destroyed, resulting in a condition called tubular necrosis. Chronic renal failure can be caused by multiple factors. The risk factors for development of chronic renal failure include chronic hypertension, proteinuria (protein in the urine), hyperlipidemia (high cholesterol levels), and smoking. Major causative factors include glomerular disease of the kidneys; vascular diseases; several diseases that cause glomerular filtration problems such as diabetes mellitus, systemic lupus erythematosus (SLE), hepatitis B and C; untreated syphilis; HIV/AIDS; connective tissue and autoimmune diseases such as rheumatoid arthritis, and scleroderma; the use of medications such as penicillamine, gold, and allopurinol; illicit drug use of heroin; and urinary tract obstructions resulting from benign prostatic hyperplasia, tumors, or a neurogenic bladder.[356]

Signs and Symptoms. The characteristic signs and symptoms of acute renal failure are multiple and may include general malaise and weakness; changes in mental status including disorientation, mood changes, seizures, and even coma; nausea and vomiting; oliguria (reduced urine output), anuria (no urine output), and unusual or excessive nighttime urination; abdominal pain; weight loss; anasarca (generalized body edema) and lower extremity edema; reduced sensation in the hands and feet; reduced appetite, a metallic taste in the mouth, bad breath, and unusual hiccups; blood in the stool; and easily bruised skin.[357] The characteristic signs and symptoms of chronic renal failure follow a progressively worsening pattern as the acute kidney failure resulting in anuria and buildup of toxic substances in the body. The symptoms can progress to severe anemia; hyperparathyroidism; severe fatigue with reduced exercise tolerance; impaired cognitive function; peripheral neuropathy and encephalopathy that can lead to coma; malnutrition exacerbated by anorexia, nausea, vomiting, and diarrhea; sexual dysfunctions including amenorrhea (cessation of menses) and erectile dysfunction; and renal bone disease caused by dysfunction of the blood platelets.[358]

Prognosis. Chronic renal failure is the ninth leading cause of death in the United States.[359] People with chronic liver failure have a better chance of survival after a kidney transplant than if they are on long-term kidney dialysis. Estimates are that approximately 1% of people admitted to hospital have acute kidney failure and that during the course of hospitalization the incidence is between 2% and 5%. The mortality rates for people with acute renal failure vary between 25% and 90%, with the hospital mortality rate between 40% and 50%, and intensive care rates between 70% and 80%.[360] Many people with acute renal failure recover in weeks or months once the cause is resolved. However, this may not be possible, and renal dialysis or renal transplantation may be required if chronic renal failure occurs. Most fatalities for people with acute renal failure are the result of comorbid diagnoses such as trauma, cardiac or pulmonary disease, cerebrovascular accident, or extreme blood loss.[361]

Medical Intervention. The diagnosis of acute renal failure involves laboratory blood tests for the presence of raised levels of serum creatinine, BUN, and serum potassium, and metabolic acidosis. Urinary obstructions and levels of renal blood flow are determined with the use of abdominal ultrasound scans, CT scans, MRI, or radionuclear scans.[362,363] The medical management for acute renal failure is to treat the underlying cause with the use of antimicrobial medications for infections, diuretics to reduce the edema, and intravenous calcium and glucose or insulin to prevent the accumulation of high levels of potassium in the body. Temporary renal dialysis may be necessary until the kidneys recover.[364] People with chronic renal disease and failure are managed medically with control of hypertension, diabetes, and hyperlipidemia, advice on smoking cessation, and dietary advice regarding reduced levels of protein, potassium, sodium, and water. Dialysis is started as soon as possible and patients are placed on the waiting list for transplant surgery.[365]

Physical Therapy Intervention. Physical therapy intervention is usually indicated to improve mobility, flexibility, strength, and endurance for people with end stage kidney disease.

GERIATRIC CONSIDERATIONS

Many elderly people with chronic digestive or urinary tract diseases may be referred to physical therapy with musculoskeletal problems. Reduced levels of independence and reduced functional activity are the usual precursors to physical therapy referral. The PTA should use the *Guide to Physical Therapist Practice* and remember that it is not the disease that is to be treated in physical therapy but the manifestation of the disease that is causing the musculoskeletal problem. Elderly patients with chronic internal diseases may be very debilitated and unable to tolerate lengthy physical therapy sessions. Treatment interventions will have to be adapted to the tolerance level of the individual patient, and the patient monitored for changes in vital signs, fatigue levels, and signs of dehydration.

Wilms' Tumor ☻

Wilms' tumor, also called nephroblastoma, is a genetic, malignant childhood tumor involving one or both kidneys. The tumor is usually diagnosed in children under age 6, but on average affects boys and girls equally at age 3.

Wilms' tumors account for approximately 5% of all childhood cancers, with 500 new cases diagnosed each year in the United States.[366]

Etiology. The majority of Wilms' tumors are of no known cause. Some Wilms' tumors are linked with genetic mutations on chromosome 11 with genes WT1 or WT2, or on the X chromosome with the WTX gene. Some children with other genetic birth defects also develop Wilms' tumors.[367]

Signs and Symptoms. The characteristic signs and symptoms of the condition may include an abdominal mass, abdominal pain, hematuria (blood in the urine), fever, and nausea.[368]

Prognosis. The prognosis for children with Wilms' tumor depends on the stage of the tumor. Most Wilms' tumors respond well to treatment, and 90% of them are curable.[369] If the tumor has expanded beyond the kidney the prognosis is not as good.

MEDICAL INTERVENTION

A diagnosis of Wilms' tumor usually results from parents bringing the child to a physician with the signs and symptoms associated with the condition. Radiographic tests such as ultrasonography, CT scan, or MRI are used for diagnosis. However, a biopsy of the kidney is the only definitive method of diagnosing the condition. Surgery is usually performed to remove the affected kidney.[370]

Physical Therapy Intervention. Physical therapy intervention is not usually indicated for children with Wilms' tumor.

CASE STUDY 12.1

An 80-year-old woman with end-stage renal disease has been referred for physical therapy interventions. The physical therapist has evaluated the patient and determined that she has overall debility resulting from general muscle weakness that reduces her ability to perform ambulation, bed mobility activities including getting in and out of bed independently, and climbing stairs. The patient has reduced endurance to activity with a maximum tolerance of 20 minutes of physical therapy at any one time. Her hope is to return home to a two-story house where her bedroom is upstairs. She lives with her daughter and her husband. Her husband is 82 years old and in good health. To be able to return home, she has to become more independent in bed mobility, rising from a chair, ambulation, and stairs. The physical therapist has asked you as the PTA to work with the patient on ambulation with an appropriate assistive device for distances up to 50 feet, bed mobility exercises and sit to stand activities, general strengthening exercises for the lower extremities within the patient's tolerance to activity, and stair climbing of 10 steps. The patient has a hand rail on both sides of the stairs at home and a relative is looking into having a stair lift installed in the home before her return.

1. How would you ensure that the patient does not become too fatigued during treatment?

2. How will you structure the treatment sessions to meet the goals determined by the PT with the patient tolerance to activity at 20 minutes?

3. What kind of an assistive ambulatory device do you think might be most appropriate for this patient? Think about her low level of tolerance to activity.

4. Describe the lower extremity exercises you think might be appropriate for this patient to increase strength in the major muscle groups and make a list of these for a home exercise program.

5. What advice might you provide to the daughter and husband in preparation for the patient returning home?

STUDY QUESTIONS

1. List the parts of the digestive system.

2. Describe the process of digestion from entry of food into the mouth to elimination of feces from the rectum.

3. List six enzymes that assist in digestion and state where they are produced.

4. Describe a colonoscopy in terms that a patient would understand.

STUDY QUESTIONS (continued)

5. List four common signs and symptoms of most digestive disorders.

6. Describe the etiology, incidence, characteristics, and possible PT intervention for gastritis.

7. Describe which parts of the intestine are affected by Crohn's disease and ulcerative colitis.

8. Describe the etiology, incidence, characteristics, medical treatment, and PT intervention for carcinoma of the stomach.

9. What part of the digestive system is affected by Whipple's disease?

10. Define the term ileus.

11. Name three locations of possible hernias.

12. Name three possible causes of peritonitis.

13. Describe the possible physical therapy intervention for rectal prolapse.

14. Provide the medical terms for gallbladder stones and common bile-duct stones.

15. List the parts of the urinary system.

16. What is the purpose of glomerular filtration?

17. Describe three tests performed to detect abnormalities of the urinary tract.

18. What is the purpose of renal dialysis?

19. Name a patient condition that would require renal dialysis.

20. What is a UTI?

21. Name two other terms for kidney stones.

22. Describe the etiology, incidence, characteristics, and likely medical treatment for kidney stones.

23. Discuss with a fellow student how you would monitor a patient with end-stage renal disease during physical therapy intervention. What types of patient response to treatment would make you decide to seek help from the supervising PT? (This question requires some critical thinking to apply content of this chapter to a real patient situation).

⬤ USEFUL WEB SITES

American Association of Kidney Patients
http://www.aakp.org/

American Cancer Society
http://www.cancer.org

American Liver Foundation
http://www.liverfoundation.org

American Society of Transplantation
http://www.a-s-t.org

American Urological Association Foundation
http://www.auafoundation.org and http://www.UrologyHealth.org

Celiac Sprue Association
http://www.csaceliacs.org/

Emedicine Health
http://www.emedicinehealth.com

Hepatitis Foundation International
http://www.hepfi.org

MedicineNet
http://www.medicinenet.com

National Cancer Institute
http://www.cancer.gov

National Institute of Dental and Craniofacial Research
http://www.nidcr.nih.gov

National Kidney Foundation
http://www.kidney.org

WebMD
http://www.webmd.com

● REFERENCES

[1] Bollinger, R. R., et al. (2007). Biofilms in the large bowel suggest an apparent function of the human vermiform appendix. *J Theoretical Biol* 249:826–831. An Elsevier On-Line Journal at http://www.sciencedirect.com/science

[2] Papachrysostomou, M., & Smith, A. N. (1994). Effects of biofeedback on obstructive defecation—reconditioning of the defecation reflex? *Gut* 35:252–256. PMCID: PMC1374503

[3] Smith, M. W. (2008). Human anatomy: the liver. *WebMD*. Retrieved 6.18.09 from http://www.webmd.com/a-to-z-guides/human-anatomy-the-liver?page=2

[4] Asenjo, B. (2002). Liver information on Healthline. Retrieved 6.18.09 from http://www.healthline.com/galecontent/liver/4

[5] Stone, C. (2008). Gallbladder disease. *Medline Plus Medical Encyclopedia*. Retrieved 6.18.09 from http://www.nlm.nih.gov/medlineplus/ency/article/001138.htm

[6] Pancreas. (1999). *MedicineNet.com*. Retrieved 6.18.09 from http://www.medterms.com/script/main/art.asp?articlekey=4743

[7] Digestive disorders health center: barium enema. (2007). *WebMD*. Retrieved 6.18.09 from http://www.webmd.com/digestive-disorders/barium-enema

[8] Lower gastrointestinal series (barium enema). (2009). *MedicineNet.Com*. Retrieved 11.27.10 from http://www.medicinenet.com/barium_enema/article.htm

[9] Hoffman, M. (2008). Diagnosing acid reflux disease. *WebMD*. Retrieved 6.18.09 from http://www.webmd.com/heartburn-gerd/diagnosing-acid-reflux-disease

[10] Dugdale, D. C., III. (2008). CBC. *Medline Plus Medical Encyclopedia*. Retrieved 6.19.09 from http://www.nlm.nih.gov/medlineplus/ency/article/003642.htm

[11] Lehrer, J. K. (2007). Bilirubin. *Medline Plus Medical Encyclopedia*. Retrieved 6.19.09 from http://www.nlm.nih.gov/medlineplus/ency/article/003479.htm

[12] Levin, M. (2007). Partial prothrombin time (PPT). *Medline Plus Medical Encyclopedia*. Retrieved 6.19.09 from http://www.nlm.nih.gov/medlineplus/ency/article/003653.htm

[13] Lee, D. (2007). Fecal occult blood test. *MedicineNet.com*. Retrieved 6.19.09 from http://www.medicinenet.com/fecal_occult_blood_tests/article.htm

[14] Hitti, M. (2008). New colon cancer screening guidelines. *MedicineNet.com*. Retrieved 6.19.09 from http://www.medicinenet.com/script/main/art.asp?articlekey=87690

[15] Lee, E. (2005). Colonoscopy. *MedicineNet.com*. Retrieved 6.19.09 from http://www.medicinenet.com/colonoscopy/article.htm

[16] Anand, B. (2007). Flexible sigmoidoscopy. *MedicineNet.com*. Retrieved 6.20.09 from http://www.medicinenet.com/flexible_sigmoidoscopy/article.htm

[17] Lee, E. Ibid.

[18] Stone, C. (2008). Digital rectal exam. *Medline Plus Medical Encyclopedia*. Retrieved 6.20.09 from http://www.nlm.nih.gov/medlineplus/ency/article/007069.htm

[19] Lehrer, J. K. (2007). Endoscopy. *Medline Plus Medical Encyclopedia*. Retrieved 6.20.09 from http://www.nlm.nih.gov/medlineplus/ency/article/003338.htm

[20] Dugdale D. C. III, (2008). Esophageal pH monitoring/esophageal acidity test. *Medline Plus Medical Encyclopedia*. Retrieved 6.20.09 from http://www.nlm.nih.gov/medlineplus/ency/article/003401.htm

[21] Cowles, R. A. (2007). Laparoscopy. *Medline Plus Medical Encyclopedia*. Retrieved 6.23.09 from http://www.nlm.nih.gov/medlineplus/ency/article/007016.htm

[22] Dugdale, D. C. III. (2010). Arteriogram. *Medline Plus Medical Encyclopedia*. Retrieved 11.27.10 from http://www.nlm.nih.gov/medlineplus/ency/article/003327.htm

[23] Mayo Clinic Staff. (2008). CT scan. Retrieved 6.21.09 from http://www.mayoclinic.com/health/ct-scan/MY00309

[24] Bentley-Hibbert, S. (2007). Liver scan. *Medline Plus Medical Encyclopedia*. Retrieved 6.22.09 from http://www.nlm.nih.gov/medlineplus/ency/article/003825.htm

[25] Dugdale, D. C., III. (2009). Bone scan. *Medline Plus Medical Encyclopedia*. Retrieved from http://www.nlm.nih.gov/medlineplus/ency/article/003833.htm

[26] Bentley-Hibbert, S. (2007). PET scan. *Medline Plus Medical Encyclopedia*. Retrieved 11.27.10 from http://www.nlm.nih.gov/medlineplus/ency/article/003827.htm

[27] Dugdale, D. C., III. (2008). MRI. *Medline Plus Medical Encyclopedia*. Retrieved 6.22.09 from http://www.nlm.nih.gov/medlineplus/ency/article/003335.htm

[28] National Cancer Institute. (2010). Esophageal cancer prevention (PDQ®): summary of the evidence. Retrieved 11.28.10 from http://www.cancer.gov/cancertopics/pdq/prevention/esophageal/healthprofessional

[29] National Cancer Institute. (2009). A snapshot of esophageal cancer: incidence and mortality rate trends. Retrieved 11.27.10 from http://www.cancer.gov/aboutnci/servingpeople/snapshots/esophageal.pdf

[30] National Cancer Institute. (2010). Esophageal cancer. Retrieved 11.27.10 from http://www.cancer.gov/cancertopics/types/esophageal/

[31] National Cancer Institute. (2010). Esophageal cancer prevention PDQ(r): evidence of benefit: tobacco, alcohol, and dietary factors. Retrieved 11.27.10 from http://www.cancer.gov/cancertopics/pdq/prevention/esophageal/HealthProfessional/page3

[32] National Cancer Institute. (2008). Esophageal cancer: treatment option overview. Retrieved 6.24.09 from http://www.cancer.gov/cancertopics/pdq/treatment/esophageal/HealthProfessional/page5

[33] American Cancer Society. (2009). Signs and symptoms of esophageal cancer. Retrieved 6.5.09 from http://www.cancer.org/docroot/cri/content/cri_2_4_3x_how_is_esophagus_cancer_diagnosed_12.asp?sitearea=cri

[34] National Cancer Institute. (2008). Esophageal cancer: stage information: TNM definitions. Retrieved 6.5.09 from http://www.cancer.gov/cancertopics/pdq/treatment/esophageal/HealthProfessional/page4

[35] National Cancer Institute. (2008). Esophageal cancer treatment: general overview. Retrieved 6.5.09 from http://www.cancer.gov/cancertopics/pdq/treatment/esophageal/HealthProfessional/page2

[36] American Cancer Society. (2009). Signs and symptoms of esophageal cancer. Retrieved 6.6.09 from http://www.cancer.org/docroot/cri/content/cri_2_4_3x_how_is_esophagus_cancer_diagnosed_12.asp?sitearea=cri

[37] National Cancer Institute. Esophageal cancer: treatment option overview. Ibid.

[38] American Cancer Society. (2009). Surgery. Retrieved 5.7.10 from http://www.cancer.org/docroot/ETO/content/ETO_1_2X_Surgery.asp

[39] Nguyen, N. T., et al. (2008). Minimally invasive esophagectomy: lessons learned from 104 operations. *Ann Surg* 248:1081–1091.

[40] Marks, J. W. (2008). Gastroesophageal reflux disease (GERD, acid reflux, heartburn). *MedicineNet.com*. Retrieved 6.27.09 from http://www.medicinenet.com/gastroesophageal_reflux_disease_gerd/page3.htm

[41] Marks, J. W. (2008). How is GERD diagnosed and evaluated? *MedicineNet.com*. Retrieved 6.27.09 from http://www.medicinenet.com/gastroesophageal_reflux_disease_gerd/page5.htm

[42] Zieve, D., et al. (2007). Gastroesophageal reflux disease. *Medline Plus Medical Encyclopedia*. Retrieved 6.27.09 from http://www.nlm.nih.gov/medlineplus/ency/article/000265.htm

[43] Marks, J. W. How is GERD diagnosed and evaluated? Ibid.

[44] Ibid.

[45] Zieve, D., et al. Ibid.

[46] American Cancer Society. (2010). What are the key statistics about oral cavity and oropharyngeal cancers? Retrieved 11.27.10 from http://www.cancer.org/Cancer/OralCavityandOropharyngeal

Cancer/DetailedGuide/oral-cavity-and-oropharyngeal-cancer-key-statistics

[47] American Cancer Society. (2010). Oral cavity and oropharyngeal cancer: causes, risk factors and prevention topics. Retrieved 11.27.10 from http://www.cancer.org/Cancer/OralCavityand OropharyngealCancer/DetailedGuide/oral-cavity-and-oropharyngeal-cancer-risk-factors

[48] Kadkade, P., & Hale, K. L. (2005). Cancer of the mouth and throat. *eMedicineHealth.* Retrieved 6.27.09 from http://www.emedicinehealth.com/cancer_of_the_mouth_and_throat/article_em.htm

[49] Uppaluri, R. (2007). Sialadenitis. *Medline Plus Medical Encyclopedia.* Retrieved 6.27.09 from http://www.nlm.nih.gov/medlineplus/ency/article/001041.htm

[50] Kadkade, P., & Hale, K. L. Cancer of the mouth and throat. *eMedicineHealth.* Ibid.

[51] American Cancer Society. Oral cavity and oropharyngeal cancer: causes, risk factors and prevention topics. Ibid.

[52] Ibid.

[53] Kadkade, P., & Hale, K. L. (2005). Mouth and throat cancer causes. *eMedicineHealth.* Retrieved 5.6.08 from http://www.emedicinehealth.com/cancer_of_the_mouth_and_throat/page2_em.htm

[54] Ibid.

[55] Ibid.

[56] Kadkade, P., & Hale, K. L. (2005). Cancer of the mouth and throat: exams and tests. *eMedicineHealth.* Retrieved 5.6.08 from http://www.emedicinehealth.com/cancer_of_the_mouth_and_throat/page5_em.htm

[57] Kadkade, P., & Hale, K. L. (2005). Mouth and throat cancer treatment. *eMedicineHealth.* Retrieved 5.6.08 from http://www.emedicinehealth.com/cancer_of_the_mouth_and_throat/page6_em.htm

[58] National Institute of Dental and Craniofacial Research. (2008). Temporomandibular dysfunction. *MedlinePlus Medical Encyclopedia.* Retrieved from http://www.nlm.nih.gov/medlineplus/temporomandibularjointdysfunction.html

[59] Hampton, T. (2008). Improvements needed in management of temporomandibular joint disorders *JAMA* 299:1119. Retrieved 1.31.09 from ProQuest Health and Medical Complete Database (Document ID: 1456860111).

[60] Buescher, J. J. (2007). Temporomandibular joint disorders. *Am Fam Physician* 76:1477–1482. Retrieved 1.31.09 from ProQuest Health and Medical Complete Database (Document ID: 1392565441).

[61] Mannheimer, J. S. (2007). Limited evidence to support the use of physical therapy for temporomandibular disorder. *Evid Based Dent* 8:110–111. Retrieved 1.31.09 from ProQuest Health and Medical Complete Database (Document ID: 1403262781).

[62] Buescher, J. J. (2007). Ibid.

[63] Cancer Survival rates. (2010). Basic things you must know about stomach cancer. Retrieved 11.27.10 from http://www.cancersurvivalrates.net/stomach-cancer-survival-rates.html

[64] National Cancer Institute. (2010). Stomach (gastric) cancer. Retrieved 11.27.10 from http://www.cancer.gov/cancertopics/types/stomach/

[65] National Cancer Institute. (2009). A snapshot of stomach (gastric) cancer: incidence and mortality rate trends. Retrieved 11.27.10 from http://www.cancer.gov/aboutnci/servingpeople/snapshots/stomach.pdf

[66] Stomach cancer: risk factors. (2008). *MedicineNet.com.* Retrieved 1.30.09 from http://www.medicinenet.com/stomach_cancer/page4.htm

[67] Stomach cancer: symptoms. (2008). *MedicineNet.com* Retrieved 1.30.09 from http://www.medicinenet.com/stomach_cancer/page3.htm

[68] National Cancer Institute. (2008). *Gastric cancer treatment: prognosis.* Retrieved 1.30.09 from http://www.cancer.gov/cancertopics/pdq/treatment/gastric/HealthProfessional/page2

[69] Stomach cancer: staging. (2008). *MedicineNet.com.* Retrieved 1.30.09 from http://www.medicinenet.com/stomach_cancer/page4.htm

[70] National Cancer Institute. (2008). Stomach (gastric) cancer: treatment option overview. Retrieved 1.30.09 from http://www.cancer.gov/cancertopics/pdq/treatment/gastric/HealthProfessional/page5

[71] Shayne, P. (2008). Gastritis and peptic ulcer disease. *eMedicine from WebMD.* Retrieved 2.3.09 from http://emedicine.medscape.com/article/776460-overview

[72] Mulkherjee, S., Sepulveda, A., Dore, M. P., & Bazzoli, F. (2009). Gastritis, chronic. *eMedicine from WebMD.* Retrieved 4.6.10 from http://emedicine.medscape.com/article/176156-overview

[73] Lehrer, J. K. (2007). Gastritis. *Medline Plus Medical Encyclopedia.* Retrieved from http://www.nlm.nih.gov/medlineplus/ency/article/001150.htm

[74] Mulkherjee, S., Sepulveda, A., Dore, M. P., & Bazzoli, F. Gastritis, chronic. *eMedicine from WebMD.* Ibid.

[75] Shayne, P. Ibid.

[76] Lehrer, J. K. Ibid.

[77] Mulkherjee, S., Sepulveda, A., Dore, M. P., & Bazzoli, F. Gastritis, chronic: Treatment and medication. *eMedicine from WebMD.* Ibid.

[78] National Institute of Diabetes and Digestive and Kidney Diseases. (2009). Gastroenteritis. *Medline Plus Medical Encyclopedia.* Retrieved 4.6.10 from http://www.nlm.nih.gov/medlineplus/gastroenteritis.html#cat1

[79] Ibid.

[80] Gardiner, J., & Brown, C. (2008). Gastroenteritis, causes. *eMedicine Health.* Retrieved 1.30.09 from http://www.emedicinehealth.com/gastroenteritis/page2_em.htm

[81] National Institute of Diabetes and Digestive and Kidney Diseases. Gastroenteritis. *Medline Plus Medical Encyclopedia.* Ibid.

[82] Stool culture. (2008). *Lab Tests Online.* Retrieved 1.30.09 from http://www.labtestsonline.org/understanding/analytes/stool_culture/test.html

[83] National Digestive Diseases Information Clearinghouse. (2008). *Appendicitis.* Retrieved 1.30.09 from http://digestive.niddk.nih.gov/ddiseases/pubs/appendicitis/

[84] Society of American Gastrointestinal and Endoscopic Surgeons. (2004). Patient information for laparoscopic appendectomy from SAGES. Retrieved 1.30.09 from http://www.sages.org/publications/publication.php?id=PI08

[85] Symptoms of appendicitis. (2009). Appendicitis statistics. Retrieved 11.28.10 from http://www.symptomsofappendicitis.org/Appendicitis-Statistics.html

[86] Lee, D. (2007). Appendicitis and appendectomy. *MedicineNet.com.* Retrieved 1.30.09 from http://www.medicinenet.com/appendicitis/article.htm

[87] Lee, D. (2007). Appendicitis and appendectomy: what are the symptoms of appendicitis? *MedicineNet.com.* Retrieved 1.30.09 from http://www.medicinenet.com/appendicitis/page2.htm

[88] National Digestive Diseases Information Clearinghouse. *Appendicitis.* Ibid.

[89] Lee, D. Appendicitis and appendectomy. Ibid.

[90] Rybkin, A. V., & Thoeni, R. F. (2007). Current concepts in imaging of appendicitis. *Radiol Clin North Am* 45:411–422, vii.

[91] Brown, M. A. (2008). Imaging acute appendicitis. *Semin Ultrasound CT MR* 29:293–307.

[92] Lee, D. (2007). Appendicitis and appendectomy: how is appendicitis diagnosed? *MedicineNet.com.* Retrieved 1.30.09 from http://www.medicinenet.com/appendicitis/page2.htm

[93] Ibid.

[94] Marks, J. W. (2010). Celiac disease (gluten enteropathy). *MedicineNet.* Retrieved 11.28.10 from http://www.medicinenet.com/celiac_disease/page9.htm

95 Wehbi, M., Yang, V. W., & Rutherford, R. E. (2005). Celiac sprue. *eMedicine Health*. Retrieved 1.30.09 from http://www.emedicinehealth.com/celiac_sprue/article_em.htm

96 Marks, J. W. (2010). Celiac disease (gluten enteropathy). *MedicineNet*. Retrieved 11.28.10 from http://www.medicinenet.com/celiac_disease/page9.htm

97 Lee, D., & Marks, J. W. (2008). Celiac disease: what causes celiac disease? *MedicineNet*. Retrieved 2.2.09 from http://www.medicinenet.com/celiac_disease/page2.htm

98 Lee, D., & Marks, J. W. (2008). Celiac disease: signs and symptoms of malabsorption. *MedicineNet*. Retrieved 2.2.09 from http://www.medicinenet.com/celiac_disease/page3.htm

99 Lee, D., & Marks, J. W. Celiac disease: what causes celiac disease? Ibid.

100 Symith, D. J., Plagnol, V., Walker, N. M., et al. (2008). Shared and distinct genetic variants in type 1 diabetes and celiac disease. *New Engl J Med* 26:2767.

101 Brottveit, M., & Lundin, K. E. (2008). Cancer risk in celiac disease. *Tidsskr Nor Laegeforen*, 20:2312–2315.

102 Lee, D., & Marks, J. W. (2008). Celiac disease: signs and symptoms of malnutrition. *MedicineNet*. Retrieved 2.2.09 from http://www.medicinenet.com/celiac_disease/page3.htm

103 Wehbi, M., Yang, V. W., & Rutherford, R. E. (2005). Celiac sprue. *eMedicine Health*. Retrieved 1.30.09 from http://www.emedicinehealth.com/celiac_sprue/article_em.htm

104 Lee, D., & Marks, J. W. (2008). Celiac disease: how is celiac disease diagnosed? *MedicineNet*. Retrieved 1.30.09 from http://www.medicinenet.com/celiac_disease/page6.htm

105 Lee, D., & Marks, J. W. (2008). Celiac disease: what is the treatment of celiac disease? *MedicineNet*. Retrieved 1.30.09 from http://www.medicinenet.com/celiac_disease/page9.htm

106 Mukharjee, S., et al. (2008). Ileus. *eMedicine from WebMD*. Retrieved 2.2.09 from http://emedicine.medscape.com/article/178948-overview

107 Nobie, B. (2007). Obstruction, small bowel. *eMedicine from WebMD*. Retrieved 2.2.09 from http://emedicine.medscape.com/article/774140-overview

108 Nobie, B. Obstruction, small bowel. *eMedicine from WebMD*. Ibid.

109 Juhn, G., Eltz, D. R., & Stacy, K. A. (2007). Intestinal obstruction. *Medline Plus Medical Encyclopedia*. Retrieved 2.2.09 from http://www.nlm.nih.gov/medlineplus/ency/article/000260.htm

110 Juhn, G., Eltz, D. R., & Stacy, K. A. Intestinal obstruction. Ibid.

111 Nobie, B. Obstruction, small bowel. *eMedicine from WebMD*. Ibid.

112 Juhn, G., Eltz, D. R., & Stacy, K. A. Intestinal obstruction. Ibid.

113 Nobie, B. Obstruction, small bowel. *eMedicine from WebMD*. Ibid.

114 Juhn, G., Eltz, D. R., & Stacy, K. A. Intestinal obstruction. Ibid.

115 Nobie, B. Obstruction, small bowel: treatment and medication. *eMedicine from WebMD*. Ibid.

116 Alghafeer, I. S., & Sigal, L. H. (2002). Rheumatic manifestations of gastrointestinal diseases. *Bull Rheum Dis* 51:1–3.

117 National Digestive Diseases Information Clearinghouse. (2004). Whipple's disease. Retrieved 2.2.09 from http://digestive.niddk.nih.gov/ddiseases/pubs/whipple/

118 Ibid.

119 Ibid.

120 Colorectal cancer. (2009). *MedlinePlus Medical Encyclopedia*. Retrieved 4.6.10 from http://www.nlm.nih.gov/medlineplus/colorectalcancer.html

121 Ibid.

122 National Cancer Institute. (2010). Colon and rectal cancer. Retrieved 11.28.10 from http://www.cancer.gov/cancertopics/types/colon-and-rectal

123 McKeever, K. (2009). Genetic data may predict colon cancer odds. *Medline Plus Medical Encyclopedia*. Retrieved 4.6.10 from http://www.nlm.nih.gov/medlineplus/news/fullstory_73922.html

124 Colorectal cancer. *Medline Plus Medical Encyclopedia*. Ibid.

125 Ibid.

126 National Cancer Institute. (2008). *Rectal cancer treatment: general information*. Retrieved 2.3.09 from http://www.cancer.gov/cancertopics/pdq/treatment/rectal/patient/

127 Centers for Disease Control and Prevention. (2008). *Colorectal cancer*. Retrieved 2.4.09 from http://www.cdc.gov/cancer/colorectal/

128 American Cancer Society. (2008). *Colon and rectum cancer: how is colorectal cancer staged? AJCC (TNM) staging system*. Retrieved 2.4.09 from http://www.cancer.org/docroot/CRI/content/CRI_2_4_3X_How_is_colon_and_rectum_cancer_staged.asp

129 Colorectal cancer. Ibid.

130 National Digestive Diseases Information Clearinghouse. (2008). *Diverticulosis and diverticulitis*. Retrieved 4.6.09 from http://digestive.niddk.nih.gov/ddiseases/pubs/diverticulosis/

131 Ibid.

132 Ibid.

133 Makola, D. (2007). Diverticular disease: evidence for dietary intervention? *Practical Gastroenterol* 31:38–46.

134 Jacobs, D. O. (2007). Diverticulitis. *New Engl J Med* 357:2057–2066.

135 National Digestive Diseases Information Clearinghouse. (2008). *Diverticulosis and diverticulitis*. Ibid.

136 White, J. A. (2006). Probiotics and their use in diverticulitis. *J Clin Gastroenterol* 40:S145–S149.

137 Mayo Clinic Staff. (2008). Probiotics: what are they? Retrieved 4.6.09 from http://www.mayoclinic.com/health/probiotics/AN00389

138 Frattini, J., & Longo, W. E. (2006, Aug). Diagnosis and treatment of chronic and recurrent diverticulitis. *J Clin Gastroenterol* 40:S145–S149.

139 National Digestive Diseases Information Clearinghouse. (NDDIC) (2010). *Hemorrhoids*. Retrieved 11.27.10 from http://digestive.niddk.nih.gov/ddiseases/pubs/hemorrhoids/#prevented

140 Marks, J. W. (2010). Hemorrhoids (piles). *MedicineNet*. Retrieved 11.27.10 from http://www.medicinenet.com/hemorrhoids/article.htm

141 National Digestive Diseases Information Clearinghouse. (2010). *Hemorrhoids*. Ibid.

142 Ibid.

143 Marks, J. W. Ibid.

144 Marks, J. W. Ibid.

145 National Digestive Diseases Information Clearinghouse (NDDIC). Hemorrhoids. Ibid.

146 Centers for Disease Control and Prevention. (2010). Inflammatory bowel disease (IBD). Retrieved 11.27.10 from http://www.cdc.gov/ibd/

147 Lashner, B. A. (2010). Inflammatory bowel disease. Cleveland Clinic. Retrieved 11.27.10 from http://www.clevelandclinicmeded.com/medicalpubs/diseasemanagement/gastroenterology/inflammatory-bowel-disease/

148 Hugot, J-P., et al. (2007). Prevalence of CARD15/NOD2 mutations in Caucasian healthy people. *Am J Gastroenterol* 102:1259–1267.

149 Brant, S. R., et al. (2007). A population-based case-control study of CARD15 and other risk factors in Crohn's disease and ulcerative colitis. *Am J Gastroenterol* 102:313–323.

150 Sasaki, M., et al. (2007). Invasive *Eschericia coli* are a feature of Crohn's disease. *Lab Invest* 87:1042–1054.

[151] Dohi, T., & Fujihashi, K. (2006). Type 1 and 2 T helper cell-mediated colitis. *Curr Opin Gastroenterol* 22:651–657.

[152] Arthritis and Rheumatism Research News Alert. (2007). Evidence of a common genetic background for ankylosing spondylitis and inflammatory bowel disease. *Arthritis Rheum* 56:2633–2639.

[153] Kriok, K. L., & Lichtenstein, G. R. (2003). Nutrition in Crohn's disease. *Curr Opin Gastroenterol* 19:148–153.

[154] Inflammatory bowel disease: symptoms. *WebMD.* (2006). Retrieved 2.2.09 from http://www.webmd.com/ibd-crohns-disease/inflammatory-bowel-syndrome?page=2

[155] Ibid.

[156] Ibid.

[157] Jess, T., et al. (2007). Risk factors for colorectal neoplasia in inflammatory bowel disease: a nested case-control study from Copenhagen County, Denmark and Olmsted County, Minnesota. *Am J Gastroenterol* 102:829–836.

[158] How is Crohn's disease diagnosed? (n.d.). *WebMD.* Retrieved 2.2.09 from http://www.webmd.com/ibd-crohns-disease/crohns-disease-diagnosed

[159] Inflammatory bowel disease: surgery. (2006). *Web MD.* Retrieved 2.4.09 from http://www.webmd.com/ibd-crohns-disease/inflammatory-bowel-syndrome?page=6

[160] Stone, C. (2008). Colorectal polyps. *Medline Plus Medical Encyclopedia.* Retrieved 2.6.09 from http://www.nlm.nih.gov/medlineplus/ency/article/000266.htm

[161] Ibid.

[162] National Digestive Diseases Information Clearinghouse. (2008). *What I need to know about colon polyps.* Retrieved 2.6.09 from http://digestive.niddk.nih.gov/ddiseases/pubs/colonpolyps_ez/

[163] Stone, C. Colorectal polyps. Ibid.

[164] Ibid.

[165] National Digestive Diseases Information Clearinghouse. *What I need to know about colon polyps.* Ibid.

[166] National Digestive Diseases Information Clearinghouse. (2007). *Irritable bowel syndrome.* Retrieved 4.8.09 from http://digestive.niddk.nih.gov/ddiseases/pubs/ibs/

[167] Ibid.

[168] Lehrer, J. K. (2006). Irritable bowel syndrome. *MedlinePlus Medical Encyclopedia.* Retrieved 4.8.09 from http://www.nlm.nih.gov/medlineplus/ency/article/000246.htm

[169] National Digestive Diseases Information Clearinghouse. *Irritable bowel Syndrome.* Ibid.

[170] New guidelines for the management of IBS. (2008). *MedlinePlus Medical Encyclopedia.* Retrieved 4.9.09 from http://www.nlm.nih.gov/medlineplus/news/fullstory_72968.html

[171] National Digestive Diseases Information Clearinghouse. *Irritable bowel syndrome.* Ibid.

[172] Knott, L. (2007). Bowel ischaemia. *PatientPlus, UK.* Retrieved 4.10.2009 from http://www.patient.co.uk/showdoc/40024694/

[173] Khan, A. N., et al. (2008). Colitis, ischemic. *eMedicine from WebMD.* Retrieved 3.2.09 from http://emedicine.medscape.com/article/366808-overview

[174] Knott, L. Ibid.

[175] Ibid.

[176] Mayo Clinic Staff. (2008). *Ischemic colitis: symptoms.* Retrieved 4.11.09 from http://www.mayoclinic.com/health/ischemic-colitis/DS00794/DSECTION=symptoms

[177] Mayo Clinic Staff. (2008). Ischemic colitis: complications. Retrieved 4.11.09 from http://www.mayoclinic.com/health/ischemic-colitis/DS00794/DSECTION=complications

[178] Knott, L. Ibid.

[179] Lehrer, J. K. (2006). Peritonitis—spontaneous. *Medline Plus Medical Encyclopedia.* Retrieved 4.11.09 from http://www.nlm.nih.gov/medlineplus/ency/article/000648.htm

[180] Lee, J. A. (2006). Peritonitis—secondary. *Medline Plus Medical Encyclopedia.* Retrieved 4.11.09 from http://www.nlm.nih.gov/medlineplus/ency/article/000651.htm

[181] Levy, D. (2008). Peritonitis—dialysis associated. *Medline Plus Medical Encyclopedia.* Retrieved 4.12.09 from http://www.nlm.nih.gov/medlineplus/ency/article/000652.htm

[182] Keane, W. F., et al. (2000). *Peritoneal dialysis related peritonitis treatment recommendations: 1996 update.* Retrieved 5.3.09 from http://www.ispd.org/guidelines/articles/newkeane/keanall.html

[183] Goldie, S. J., et al. (1996). Fungal peritonitis in a large chronic peritoneal dialysis population: a report of 55 episodes. *Am J Kidney Dis* 28:86–91.

[184] Keane, W. F., et al. Ibid.

[185] Lehrer, J. K. Ibid.

[186] Lee, J. A. Ibid.

[187] Levy, D. Ibid.

[188] Lee, J. A. Ibid.

[189] Lehrer, J. K. Ibid.

[190] Ibid.

[191] Flowers, L. K. (2009). Rectal prolapse. *eMedicine from WebMD.* Retrieved 11.27.10 from http://emedicine.medscape.com/article/776236-overview

[192] Peritz, L. (2010). Rectal prolapse. *eMedicine from WebMD.* Retrieved 11.27.10 from http://emedicine.medscape.com/article/196411-overview

[193] Flowers, L. K. Ibid.

[194] Peritz, L. Ibid.

[195] Peritz, L. (2010). Rectal prolapse: treatment. *eMedicine from WebMD.* Retrieved 11.27.10 from http://emedicine.medscape.com/article/196411-treatment

[196] Flowers, L. K. Ibid.

[197] Vorvick, L. (2009). Gallstones. *Medline Plus Medical Encyclopedia.* Retrieved 11.27.10 from http://www.nlm.nih.gov/medlineplus/ency/article/000273.htm

[198] Chiang, W. K., Lee, F. M., & Santen, S. (2010). Cholelithiasis. *eMedicine from WebMD.* Retrieved 11.27.10 from http://emedicine.medscape.com/article/774352-overview

[199] Vorvick, L. Ibid.

[200] Chiang, W. K., Lee, F. M., & Santen, S. Ibid.

[201] Vorvick, L. Ibid.

[202] Heuman, D. M., et al. (2006). Colelithiasis: overview. *eMedicine from WebMD.* Retrieved 4.10.09 from http://emedicine.medscape.com/article/175667-overview

[203] Stone, C. (2008). ERCP. *Medline Plus Medical Encyclopedia.* Retrieved 4.10.09 from http://www.nlm.nih.gov/medlineplus/ency/article/003893.htm

[204] Chiang, W. K., Lee, F. M., & Santen, S. (2010). Cholelithiasis: treatment and medication. *eMedicine from WebMD.* Retrieved 11.27.10 from http://emedicine.medscape.com/article/774352-treatment

[205] Taylor, C. R. (2009). Cirrhosis. *eMedicine from WebMD.* Retrieved 6.7.10 from http://emedicine.medscape.com/article/366426-overview

[206] Cirrhosis. (2010). *Medline Plus Medical Encyclopedia.* Retrieved 11.27.10 from http://www.nlm.nih.gov/medlineplus/cirrhosis.html

[207] DeFrances, C. J., Cullen, K. A., & Kozak, L. J. (2007). National hospital discharge survey: 2005 annual summary with detailed diagnosis and procedure data. *Vital Health Statistics* 13(165).

[208] National Digestive Diseases Information Clearinghouse. (2008). Cirrhosis. Retrieved 6.7.09 from http://digestive.niddk.nih.gov/ddiseases/pubs/cirrhosis/

[209] Ibid.

[210] Xu, J., et al. (2010). Deaths: final data for 2007. National vital statistics report, Vol 58, # 19. Retrieved 11.27.10 from http://www.cdc.gov/nchs/data/nvsr/nvsr58/nvsr58_19.pdf

[211] National Digestive Diseases Information Clearinghouse. Cirrhosis. Ibid.

[212] Luxon, B. A. (2008). Diagnosis and treatment of autoimmune hepatitis. *Gastroenterol Clin North Am* 37:461–478.

[213] National Digestive Diseases Information Clearinghouse (NDDIC). (2008). Cirrhosis. Ibid.

[214] Taheri, M. R., & Riley, T. P (2008, May). Preventive approaches in chronic liver diseases part II: compensated liver cirrhosis. *Practical Gastroenterol* 32:49–60.

[215] American Cancer Society. (2010). *What are the key statistics about gallbladder cancer?* Retrieved 11.27.10 from http://www.cancer.org/Cancer/GallbladderCancer/DetailedGuide/gallbladder-key-statistics

[216] American Cancer Society. (2010). What are the risk factors for gallbladder cancer? Retrieved 11.27.10 from http://www.cancer.org/Cancer/GallbladderCancer/DetailedGuide/gallbladder-risk-factors

[217] National Cancer Institute. (2008*). Gallbladder cancer treatment: general information about gallbladder cancer.* Retrieved 4.12.09 from http://www.cancer.gov/cancerinfo/pdq/treatment/gallbladder/patient/#Keypoint1

[218] Ibid.

[219] National Cancer Institute. (2008). *Gallbladder cancer treatment (health professional section).* Retrieved 4.12.09 from http://www.cancer.gov/cancertopics/pdq/treatment/gallbladder/HealthProfessional/page2

[220] National Cancer Institute. Gallbladder cancer treatment: general information about gallbladder cancer. Ibid.

[221] National Cancer Institute. (2008) Gallbladder cancer treatment: treatment option overview. *National Institutes of Health.* Retrieved 4.12.09 from http://www.cancer.gov/cancertopics/pdq/treatment/gallbladder/Patient/page4

[222] Lee, D. (2006). Drug induced liver disease. *MedicineNet.com.* Retrieved from http://www.medicinenet.com/drug_induced_liver_disease/article.htm

[223] Palmer, M. (2004). *Medications and the liver/hepatitis.* Retrieved 6.9.09 from http://www.liverdisease.com/medications_hepatitis.html

[224] Lee, D. (2006). Drug induced liver disease. *MedicineNet.com.* Retrieved 6.9.09 from http://www.medicinenet.com/drug_induced_liver_disease/page8.htm

[225] Kuipers, H. (1998). Anabolic steroids: side effects. In: T. D. Fahey, editor. *Encyclopedia of sports medicine and science.* Internet Society for Sport Science. Retrieved 5.16.09 from http://sportsci.org

[226] National Institute on Drug Abuse. (2008). *NIDA infofacts: steroids (anabolic-Androgenic).* Retrieved 5.16.09 from http://www.nida.nih.gov/Infofacts/steroids.html

[227] Lee, D. Drug induced liver disease. Ibid.

[228] U.S. Food and Drug Administration. (2004). *Questions and answers for estrogen and estrogen with progestin therapies for postmenopausal women (updated).* Retrieved 5.16.09 from http://www.fda.gov/Cder/Drug/infopage/estrogens_progestins/Q&A.htm

[229] Allopurinol side effects. (2008). *Drugs.com* Retrieved 5.16.09 from http://www.drugs.com/sfx/allopurinol-side-effects.html#professional_Allopurinol

[230] National Digestive Diseases Information Clearinghouse. (2007). *Hemochromatosis.* Retrieved 5.16.09 from http://digestive.niddk.nih.gov/ddiseases/pubs/hemochromatosis/

[231] National Institute of Neurological Disorders and Stroke. (2007). *NINDS Wilson's disease information page.* Retrieved 5.16.09 from http://www.ninds.nih.gov/disorders/wilsons/wilsons.htm

[232] National Digestive Diseases Information Clearinghouse. (2008). *Autoimmune hepatitis.* Retrieved 5.17.09 from http://digestive.niddk.nih.gov/ddiseases/pubs/autoimmunehep/index.htm

[233] Stuart, K. E. (2010). Hepatocellular carcinoma. *MedicineNet.com.* Retrieved 11.27.10 from http://www.medicinenet.com/liver_cancer/article.htm

[234] Stuart, K. E. (2010). Hepatocellular carcinoma: page 2. *MedicineNet.com.* Retrieved 11.27.10 from http://www.medicinenet.com/liver_cancer/page2.htm

[235] National Cancer Institute. (2010). *Surveillance epidemiology and end results: SEER stat fact sheets: liver and intrahepatic bile duct cancer.* Retrieved 11.27.10 from http://seer.cancer.gov/statfacts/html/livibd.html

[236] Stuart, K. E. Hepatocellular carcinoma: page 2. Ibid.

[237] Stuart, K. E. (2010). Hepatocellular carcinoma: what are liver cancer symptoms and signs? Page 3. *MedicineNet.com.* Retrieved 11.27.10 from http://www.medicinenet.com/liver_cancer/page3.htm

[238] Stuart, K. E. (2010). Hepatocellular carcinoma. *MedicineNet.com.* Retrieved 11.27.10 from http://www.medicinenet.com/liver_cancer/article.htm

[239] Stuart, K. E. (2010). Hepatocellular carcinoma: what is the natural history of liver cancer? Page 7. *MedicineNet.com.* Retrieved 11.27.10 from http://www.medicinenet.com/liver_cancer/page7.htm

[240] Stuart, K. E. (2010). Hepatocellular carcinoma: Imaging studies. Page 5. *MedicineNet.com.* Retrieved 11.27.10 from http://www.medicinenet.com/liver_cancer/page5.htm

[241] Stuart, K. E. (2010). Hepatocellular carcinoma: how is liver cancer diagnosed? Page 4 *MedicineNet.com.* Retrieved 11.27.10 from http://www.medicinenet.com/liver_cancer/page4.htm

[242] Stuart, K. E. (2010). Hepatocellular carcinoma: what are the treatment options for liver cancer? Page 8. *MedicineNet.com.* Retrieved 11.27.10 from http://www.medicinenet.com/liver_cancer/article.htmhttp://www.medicinenet.com/liver_cancer/page8.htm

[243] Liver cancer. (2008). *MedlinePlus Medical Encyclopedia.* Retrieved 5.17.09 from http://www.nlm.nih.gov/medlineplus/livercancer.html

[244] Stuart, K. E. (2010). Hepatocellular carcinoma: liver transplantation. *MedicineNet.com.* Retrieved 11.27.10 from http://www.medicinenet.com/liver_cancer/page12.htm

[245] Radiological Society of North America. (2008). *Radiofrequency ablation of liver tumors.* Retrieved 5.18.09 from http://www.radiologyinfo.org/en/info.cfm?pg=rfa

[246] Lau, W. Y., & Lai, E. C. (2009, Jan). The current role of radiofrequency ablation in the management of hepatocellular carcinoma: a systemic review. *Ann Surg* 249:20–25.

[247] McKeever, K. (2009). Tiny chemo beads boost liver cancer outcomes. *MedlinePlus Medical Encyclopedia.* Retrieved 6.7.10 from http://www.nlm.nih.gov/medlineplus/news/fullstory_74016.html

[248] Pancreatitis. (2010). *MedicineNet.com.* Retrieved 11.27.10 from http://www.medicinenet.com/pancreatitis/article.htm

[249] Ibid.

[250] Ibid.

[251] Bono, M. J. (2008). Pneumonia, mycoplasma. *eMedicine from WebMD.* Retrieved 6.7.10 from http://emedicine.medscape.com/article/807927-overview

[252] Centers for Disease Control and Prevention (2008). *Campylobacter.* Retrieved 6.7.10 from http://www.cdc.gov/nczved/dfbmd/disease_listing/campylobacter_gi.html

[253] Stone, C. (2008). Acute pancreatitis. *Medline Plus Medical Encyclopedia.* Retrieved 12.3.08 from http://www.nlm.nih.gov/medlineplus/ency/article/000287.htm

[254] Pancreatitis. *MedicineNet.com.* Ibid.

[255] National Digestive Diseases Information Clearinghouse. (2008). *Pancreatitis.* Retrieved 12.3.08 from http://digestive.niddk.nih.gov/ddiseases/pubs/pancreatitis/index.htm#hope

[256] Pancreatitis. *MedicineNet.com.* Ibid.

[257] Dugdale, D. C. & Longstreth, G. F. (2008). Pancreatitis. *Medline Plus Medical Encyclopedia.* Retrieved 12.3.08 from http://www.nlm.nih.gov/medlineplus/ency/article/001144.htm

[258] Pancreatitis. *MedicineNet.com.* Ibid.

[259] Stone, C. (2008). Chronic pancreatitis. *Medline Plus Medical Encyclopedia.* Retrieved 12.3.08 from http://www.nlm.nih.gov/medlineplus/ency/article/000221.htm

[260] Pancreatitis. *MedicineNet.com*. Ibid.

[261] Stone, C. Chronic pancreatitis. Ibid.

[262] National Cancer Institute. (2008). Pancreatic cancer treatment: health professional version. Retrieved 12.3.08 from http://www.cancer.gov/cancertopics/pdq/treatment/pancreatic/HealthProfessional/page2

[263] Johns Hopkins Medicine. (n.d.). What are the risk factors for pancreatic cancer? Retrieved 12.3.08 from http://pathology.jhu.edu/pancreas/BasicRisk.php?area=ba

[264] National Cancer Institute. (2010). Pancreatic cancer. Retrieved 11.27.10 from http://www.cancer.gov/cancertopics/types/pancreatic

[265] National Cancer Institute. (2008). Pancreatic cancer treatment: health professional version. Retrieved 12.3.08 from http://www.cancer.gov/cancertopics/pdq/treatment/pancreatic/HealthProfessional/page5

[266] Pancreatic cancer. (2009). *Medline Plus Medical Encyclopedia*. Retrieved 2.5.10 from http://www.nlm.nih.gov/medlineplus/pancreaticcancer.html#cat5

[267] National Cancer Institute. *Pancreatic cancer treatment: health professional version*. Ibid.

[268] National Cancer Institute. (2008). *Pancreatic cancer treatment: Stage III pancreatic cancer*. Retrieved 12.3.08 from http://www.cancer.gov/cancertopics/pdq/treatment/pancreatic/Health Professional/page7

[269] American Cancer Society. (2008). *Detailed guide: pancreatic cancer*. Retrieved 12.3.08 from http://www.cancer.org/docroot/cri/content/cri_2_4_3x_how_is_pancreatic_cancer_diagnosed_34.asp?sitearea=cri

[270] National Cancer Institute. (2008). Pancreatic cancer treatment: Stage I and II pancreatic cancer. Retrieved 12.3.08 from http://www.cancer.gov/cancertopics/pdq/treatment/pancreatic/Health Professional/page6

[271] National Cancer Institute. (2009). *Gemcitabine after pancreatic surgery improves survival*. Adapted from NCI Cancer Bulletin, 5(12). Retrieved 2.2.10 from http://www.cancer.gov/clinicaltrials/results/gemcitabine-pancreatic0608

[272] Sherman, N. D. (2006). Injury—kidney and ureter. *Medline Plus Medical Encyclopedia*. Retrieved 12.3.08 from http://www.nlm.nih.gov/medlineplus/ency/article/001065.htm

[273] Sherman, N. D. Ibid.

[274] Zieve, D. (2007). Glomerular filtration rate. *Medline Plus Medical Encyclopedia*. Retrieved 12.3.08 from http://www.nlm.nih.gov/medlineplus/ency/article/007305.htm

[275] *Taber's cyclopedic medical dictionary*, 20th edition (2001). Philadelphia: F. A. Davis.

[276] Antidiuretic hormone. (2006–2008). *ClinLab Navigator*. Retrieved 12.3.08 from http://www.clinlabnavigator.com/Tests/AntidiureticHormone.html

[277] Arterial blood gases. (2008). *WebMD*. Retrieved 12.4.08 from http://www.webmd.com/a-to-z-guides/arterial-blood-gases

[278] Rackley, R., & Vasavada, S. P. (2006). Neurogenic bladder. *eMedicine from WebMD*. Retrieved 12.3.08 from http://emedicine.medscape.com/article/453539-overview

[279] Burtis, C. A., Ashwood, E. R., & Bruns, D. E., editors. (2006). *Tietz textbook of clinical chemistry and molecular diagnostics*, 4th edition. New York: Elsevier.

[280] American Association for Clinical Chemistry. (2009). BUN. *Lab Tests Online*. Retrieved 3.2.10 from http://www.labtestsonline.org/understanding/analytes/bun/test.html

[281] American Association for Clinical Chemistry. (2005). Creatinine clearance. *Lab Tests Online*. Retrieved 12.3.08 from http://www.labtestsonline.org/understanding/analytes/creatinine_clearance/test.html

[282] Gilbert, S. M. (2008). Urinary catheters. *Medline Plus Medical Encyclopedia*. Retrieved 12.3.08 from http://www.nlm.nih.gov/MEDLINEPLUS/ency/article/003981.htm

[283] Gilbert, S. M., & Zieve, D. (2008). Cystoscopy. *Medline Plus Medical Encyclopedia*. Retrieved 2.2.09 from http://www.nlm.nih.gov/medlineplus/ency/article/003903.htm

[284] Bentley-Hibbert, S. (2006). Intravenous pyelogram. *Medline Plus Medical Encyclopedia*. Retrieved 12.4.08 from http://www.nlm.nih.gov/medlineplus/ency/article/003782.htm

[285] Van Vorhees, B. J. (2007). Abdominal film. *Medline Plus Medical Encyclopedia*. Retrieved 12.4.08 from http://www.nlm.nih.gov/medlineplus/ency/article/003815.htm

[286] Mushnick, R. (2007). Renal biopsy. *Medline Plus Medical Encyclopedia*. Retrieved 12.4.08 from http://www.nlm.nih.gov/medlineplus/ency/article/003907.htm

[287] Patel, P. (2008). Dialysis. *Medline Plus Medical Encyclopedia*. Retrieved 12.4.08 from http://www.nlm.nih.gov/medlineplus/ency/article/003421.htm

[288] Shiel, W. C. (2006). Dialysis: what are the advantages of the different types of dialysis? *MedicineNet.com* Retrieved 12.4.08 from http://www.medicinenet.com/dialysis/page4.htm

[289] Nabili, S., & Shiel, W. C. (2008). Urinalysis. *MedicineNet.com* Retrieved 12.4.08 from http://www.medicinenet.com/urinalysis/page5.htm

[290] Urine culture. (2005). *Lab Tests Online*. Retrieved 12.5.08 from http://www.labtestsonline.org/understanding/analytes/urine_culture/test.html

[291] Mayo Clinic Staff. (2008). *High blood pressure (hypertension): diuretics*. Retrieved 2.2.09 from http://www.mayoclinic.com/health/diuretics/hi00030

[292] Dugdale, D. C., III. (2008). Neurogenic bladder. *Medline Plus Medical Encyclopedia*. Retrieved 2.2.09 from http://www.nlm.nih.gov/MEDLINEPLUS/ency/article/000754.htm

[293] Arbor Research Collaborative for Health with the University of Michigan. (2010). *Scientific Registry of Transplant Recipients: National report: KI: Kidney*. Oversight by Health Resources and Services Administration. Retrieved 11.27.10 from http://www.ustransplant.org/csr/current/nationalViewer.aspx?o=KI

[294] Liem, Y. S., & Weimer, W. (2009). Early living-donor kidney transplantation: a review of the associated survival benefit. *Transplantation* 87:317–318

[295] *Kidney diseases: kidney pain*. (2009). NetWellness. Retrieved 5.3.10 from http://www.netwellness.org/healthtopics/kidney/faq3.cfm

[296] National Kidney and Urologic Diseases Information Clearinghouse. (2005). *Urinary tract infections in adults*. Retrieved 12.5.08 from http://kidney.niddk.nih.gov/Kudiseases/pubs/utiadult/

[297] Rahn, D. D. (2008). Urinary tract infections: contemporary management. *Urol Nurs* 28:333–341.

[298] American Cancer Society (2009). *Detailed guide: bladder cancer. How is bladder cancer staged?* Retrieved 11.27.10 from http://www.cancer.org/docroot/CRI/content/CRI_2_4_3X_How_is_bladder_cancer_staged_44.asp

[299] American Cancer Society. (2010). *Detailed guide: bladder cancer. What are the key statistics about bladder cancer?* Retrieved 11.27.10 from http://www.cancer.org/Cancer/BladderCancer/DetailedGuide/bladder-cancer-key-statistics

[300] American Cancer Society. *Detailed guide: bladder cancer. What are the key statistics about bladder cancer?* Ibid.

[301] Ibid.

[302] American Cancer Society. (2009). *Detailed guide: bladder cancer. How is bladder cancer diagnosed?* Retrieved 12.4.09 from http://www.cancer.org/docroot/CRI/content/CRI_2_4_3X_How_is_bladder_cancer_diagnosed_44.asp?rnav=cri

[303] American Cancer Society. *Detailed guide: bladder cancer. How is bladder cancer staged?* Ibid.

[304] American Cancer Society. *Detailed guide: bladder cancer. How is bladder cancer diagnosed?* Ibid.

[305] American Cancer Society. (2009). *Detailed guide: bladder cancer surgery*. Retrieved 12.4.09 from http://www.cancer.org/docroot/CRI/content/CRI_2_4_4X_Surgery_44.asp?rnav=cri

306 National Institute of Diabetes and Digestive and Kidney Diseases. (2009). Interstitial cystitis. *Medline Plus Medical Encyclopedia*. Retrieved 12.4.09 from http://www.nlm.nih.gov/medlineplus/interstitialcystitis.html

307 National Kidney and Urologic Diseases Information Clearing House. (2008). *Kidney and urologic disease statistics for the United States*. Retrieved 6.5.09 from http://kidney.niddk.nih.gov/kudiseases/pubs/kustats/

308 Mayo Clinic Staff. (2008). *Cystitis: causes*. Retrieved 6.5.09 from http://www.mayoclinic.com/health/cystitis/DS00285/DSECTION=causes

309 Mayo Clinic Staff. (2008). *Cystitis: risk factors*. Retrieved 6.5.09 from http://www.mayoclinic.com/health/cystitis/DS00285/DSECTION=risk-factors

310 Mayo Clinic Staff. (2008). *Cystitis: symptoms*. Retrieved 6.5.09 from http://www.mayoclinic.com/health/cystitis/DS00285/DSECTION=symptoms

311 Mayo Clinic Staff. (2008). *Interstitial cystitis: complications*. Retrieved 6.5.09 from http://www.mayoclinic.com/health/interstitial-cystitis/DS00497/DSECTION=complications

312 National Kidney and Urologic Diseases Information Clearing House. (2005). *Cystoscopy and ureteroscopy*. Retrieved 6.5.09 from http://kidney.niddk.nih.gov/kudiseases/pubs/cystoscopy/

313 Interstitial Cystitis Association. (2009). *Treatment guidelines*. Retrieved 3.2.10 from http://www.ichelp.org/PatientInformation/TreatmentOptions/ICATreatmentGuidelines/tabid/85/Default.aspx

314 Ibid.

315 Papanagnou, D., & Kwan, N. S. (2008). Glomerulonephritis, acute: overview. *eMedicine from WebMD*. Retrieved 12.5.08 from http://emedicine.medscape.com/article/777272-overview

316 Ibid.

317 Ibid.

318 Papanagnou, D., & Kwan, N. S. (2008). Glomerulonephritis, acute: follow-up. *eMedicine from WebMD*. Retrieved 12.5.08 from http://emedicine.medscape.com/article/777272-followup

319 Papanagnou, D., & Kwan, N. S. (2008). Glomerulonephritis, acute: differential diagnosis and work-up. *eMedicine from WebMD*. Retrieved 12.5.08 from http://emedicine.medscape.com/article/777272-diagnosis

320 Papanagnou, D., & Kwan, N. S. (2008). Glomerulonephritis, acute: treatment and medication. *eMedicine from WebMD*. Retrieved 12.5.08 from http://emedicine.medscape.com/article/777272-treatment

321 Prevalence and incidence of kidney stones. (2008). *CureResearch.com*. Retrieved 6.8.09 from http://www.cureresearch.com/k/kidney_stones/prevalence.htm

322 National Kidney and Urologic Diseases Information Clearing House. (2007). *Kidney stones in adults*. Retrieved 7.2.2009 from http://kidney.niddk.nih.gov/Kudiseases/pubs/stonesadults/

323 Ibid.

324 Wedro, B. C. (2007). Kidney stones: causes. *eMedicineHealth*. Retrieved 12.5.08 from http://www.emedicinehealth.com/kidney_stones/article_em.htm

325 National Kidney and Urologic Diseases Information Clearing House. Kidney stones in adults. Ibid.

326 Ibid.

327 Fervenza, F. C., Textor, S. C., & Rosenthal, D. (2008). Nephrosclerosis. *eMedicine from WebMD*. Retrieved 12.5.08 from http://emedicine.medscape.com/article/244342-overview

328 Ibid.

329 Ibid.

330 Ibid.

331 Ibid.

332 Ibid.

333 Shoff, W. H., et al. (2010). Pyelonephritis, acute. *eMedicine from WebMD*. Retrieved 11.27.10 from http://emedicine.medscape.com/article/245559-overview

334 National Kidney and Urologic Diseases Information Clearing House. (2007). *Pyelonephritis in adults*. Retrieved 12.5.08 from http://kidney.niddk.nih.gov/kudiseases/pubs/pyelonephritis/index.htm

335 Di Leo Thomas, L., & Olshaker, J. (2007). Urinary tract infection causes. *eMedicineHealth*. Retrieved 12.6.08 from http://www.emedicinehealth.com/urinary_tract_infections/page2_em.htm

336 National Kidney and Urologic Diseases Information Clearing House. (2007). *Pyelonephritis in adults*. Ibid.

337 Ibid.

338 Ibid.

339 Kidney cancer. (2006). *MedicineNet.com*. Retrieved 6.9.09 from http://www.medicinenet.com/kidney_cancer/page2.htm

340 Kidney cancer: who's at risk? (2006). *MedicineNet.com*. Retrieved 12.6.08 from http://www.medicinenet.com/kidney_cancer/page2.htm

341 Ibid.

342 Dugdale, D. C., III. (2009). Renal cell carcinoma. *Medline Plus Medical Encyclopedia*. Retrieved 2.5.10 from http://www.nlm.nih.gov/medlineplus/ency/article/000516.htm

343 Kidney cancer: methods of treatment. (2006). *MedicineNet.com*. Retrieved 2.5.10 from http://www.medicinenet.com/kidney_cancer/page5.htm

344 Trout, A. T., Siegal, J., & Corman, J. M. (2006). Cystic diseases of the kidney. Overview. *eMedicine from WebMD*. Retrieved 12.6.08 from http://emedicine.medscape.com/article/453831-overview

345 Ibid.

346 Trout, A. T., & Siegal, J., & Corman, J. M. (2006). Cystic diseases of the kidney: Overview. *eMedicine from WebMD*. Retrieved 12.6.08 from http://emedicine.medscape.com/article/453831-overview

347 Mostov, K. E. (2006). mTOR is out of control in polycystic kidney disease. *Proc Natl Acad Sci U S A* 103:5247–5248.

348 Trout, A. T., & Siegal, J., & Corman, J. M. Ibid.

349 Ibid.

350 Shillingford, J. M., et al. (2006). The mTOR pathway is regulated by polycystin–1, and its inhibition reverses renal cytogenesis in polycystic disease. *Proc Natl Acad Sci U S A* 103:5466–5471.

351 Charytan, D. M. (2006). Acute kidney failure. *MedlinePlus Medical Encyclopedia*. Retrieved 12.6.08 from http://www.nlm.nih.gov/medlineplus/ency/article/000501.htm

352 Arora, P., & Verrelli, M. (2008). Chronic renal failure. *eMedicine from WebMD*. Retrieved 12.6.08 from http://emedicine.medscape.com/article/243492-diagnosis

353 Ibid.

354 Ibid.

355 Charytan, D. M. (2006). Acute kidney failure. *MedlinePlus Medical Encyclopedia*. Retrieved 12.6.08 from http://www.nlm.nih.gov/medlineplus/ency/article/000501.htm

356 Arora, P., & Verrelli, M. Ibid.

357 Charytan, D. M. Ibid.

358 Arora, P., & Verrelli, M. Ibid.

359 Ibid.

360 Agraharkar, M., et al. (2007). Acute renal failure: overview. *eMedicine from WebMD*. Retrieved 12.6.08 from http://emedicine.medscape.com/article/243492-overview

361 Charytan, D. M. Ibid.

362 Ibid.

363 Agraharkar, M., et al. Ibid.

364 Charytan, D. M. Ibid.

365 Arora, P., & Verrelli, M. Ibid.

[366] American Cancer Society. (2010). *Detailed guide: Wilms' tumor: what are the key statistics about Wilms' tumor?* Retrieved 11.27.10 from http://www.cancer.org/Cancer/WilmsTumor/DetailedGuide/wilms-tumor-key-statistics

[367] American Cancer Society. (2008). *Detailed guide: Wilms' tumor: Do we know what causes Wilms' tumor?* Retrieved 12.7.08 from http://www.cancer.org/docroot/CRI/content/CRI_2_4_2X_Do_we_know_what_causes_Wilms_tumor.asp?rnav=cri

[368] Wilm's tumor. (2009). *MedlinePlus Medical Encyclopedia.* Retrieved 11.25.10 from http://www.nlm.nih.gov/medlineplus/wilmstumor.html

[369] American Cancer Society. (2008). Detailed guide: Wilms' tumor: What is Wilms' tumor? Retrieved 12.7.08 from http://www.cancer.org/docroot/CRI/content/CRI_2_4_1x_What_is_wilms_tumor_46.asp?sitearea=

[370] American Cancer Society. *Detailed guide: Wilm's tumor: How is Wilm's tumor diagnosed?* Ibid.

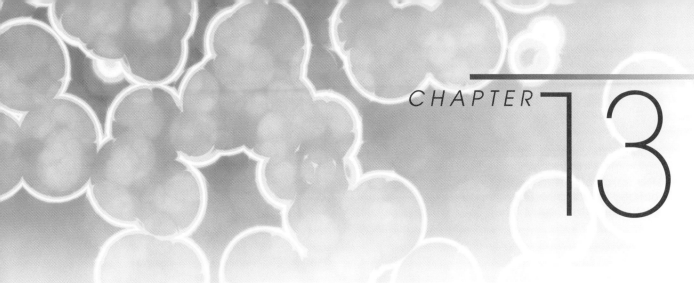

CHAPTER 13

Intensive Care

LEARNING OBJECTIVES

After completion of this chapter, students should be able to:

- List the commonly occurring diagnoses of patients who require care in the intensive care unit
- Describe the machines and monitors commonly used on the intensive care unit
- Determine the impact on physical therapy interventions for patients attached to multiple machines in the intensive care unit
- Discuss the general contraindications and precautions for physical therapists and physical therapist assistants treating patients in the intensive care unit
- Analyze the contraindications and precautions specific to diagnoses for physical therapists treating patients in the intensive care unit
- Delineate physical therapy interventions for patients in the intensive care unit
- Apply the specific considerations for physical therapists treating patients in the pediatric intensive care unit

KEY TERMS

Assist-control ventilator

Bilevel positive airway pressure (BIPAP)

Continuous positive airway pressure (CPAP)

Coronary care unit

Electrocardiogram monitor (ECG)

Intensivist

Intermittent pneumatic compression pump/external sequential compression device

Intracranial pressure (ICP)

Intrinsic PEEP

Pressure-control ventilator (PCV)

Pressure-support ventilator (PSV)

Pressure-cycled ventilator

Pulse oximeter

Synchronized intermittent mandatory ventilator (SIMV)

Volume cycled ventilator

CHAPTER OUTLINE

Introduction
The Intensive Care Unit
    General Precautions and Recommendations for Treating Patients in the ICU
    Equipment Used in the ICU
    What Causes a Patient to Be Placed in the ICU?
Physical Therapy Interventions Used for Patients With Specific Diagnoses on the ICU
    Burns
    Cerebrovascular accident (CVA)
    End-Stage Renal Failure

Introduction

This chapter differs from the previous chapters in both design and format. The intent is to provide an overview of the intensive care unit (ICU) for the physical therapist assistant. Sections include the general precautions and recommendations when working in the ICU, equipment used on the ICU, the reasons for placing people on the ICU, and some of the PT interventions used for people with the most commonly observed diagnoses on the ICU. The physical therapy approaches to treatment of people on the ICU may differ from other areas of practice and thus the precautions and considerations specific to the ICU setting for physical therapy intervention are included. A description of the pediatric intensive care unit (PICU) is also provided. The chapter concludes with the prevention of pressure ulcers and some of the legal and ethical areas of concern when working in the ICU. An understanding of some of the differences inherent in working with people in the ICU may help to relieve anxiety about working in this acute care, hectic setting.

Why Does the Physical Therapist Assistant Need to Know About the Intensive Care Unit?

Working in the ICU is part of acute care physical therapy practice in the hospital setting. Special considerations are needed when working with patients as a result of their serious medical conditions. In addition to existing medical problems patients may develop ICU-acquired weakness (ICUAW), which can be addressed with physical therapy intervention. ICUAW results in disuse atrophy of muscles with decreased muscle mass and reduced protein synthesis. Insulin resistance occurs within a few days, as demonstrated by studies regarding normal healthy people who are on bed rest for 5 days.[1] ICUAW is particularly prevalent in people with multiorgan failure or general sepsis.

The Intensive Care Unit

Physical therapy intervention in the acute care hospital is a specialty area of practice compared with even 10 years ago when the majority of physical therapy interventions were performed in the hospital setting. Physical therapists and physical therapist assistants (PTAs) have to be able to think on their feet and adapt rapidly to changing environments and situations. Clinicians involved in this area of practice can have an exciting practice experience. The presence of comorbid diagnoses often is a reason for admittance to the ICU. Many patients have multiple diagnoses commonly referred to as an "alphabet soup" of diagnoses, placing them at a higher risk of mortality and thus requiring admittance to ICU for minor surgery or injury. The alphabet soup may consist of many of the conditions previously described in this book such as chronic obstructive pulmonary disease (COPD), myocardial infarction (MI), peripheral vascular disease (PVD), and congestive heart failure (CHF). Because many patients are managed on an outpatient surgery basis (less than 24 hours stay in the hospital), only extremely sick patients are admitted as inpatients in the hospital, and the most sick are admitted to the ICU.

The ICU can be a frightening place for physical therapist assistant students and new graduates. The ICU is a place of intensive activity, as well as intensive patient care. The nurse-to-patient ratio is higher in the ICU than on any other hospital unit. The other unit with a high nurse-to-patient ratio is the **coronary care unit** (CCU), which is devoted solely to those patients with cardiac pathologies. The CCU may be called the critical care unit.

Although this chapter is mainly related to the patient population in the ICU, relevance and reference to the CCU will be noted. Working in the ICU is a specialized area of practice within physical therapy. PTAs working in the ICU need more supervision from the physical therapist than may be necessary in other health care settings. Nevertheless, working in the ICU can be rewarding both as a physical therapist (PT) and a PTA. In preparation for working with people in the ICU, the PT and PTA need to be able to reference the normal blood, plasma, and urine laboratory tests and results to read patient charts and understand the condition of patients. Tables 13-1, 13-2, and 13-3 provide some of the more common normal laboratory values for urine and blood constituents.

Table 13.1 Normal Laboratory Values of Blood, Plasma, and Serum

BLOOD, PLASMA, AND SERUM CONTENTS	NORMAL VALUE	NORMAL VALUES IN SI UNITS (INTERNATIONAL SYSTEM OF UNITS)
Bilirubin	Up to 1.0 mg/100 mL	Up to 17 μmol/L (μ = micron, mol = mole or amount of a substance)
Blood volume	8.5–9.0% of body weight in kg	80–85 mL/kg (kg = kilogram)
Calcium	8.5–10.5 mg/100 mL	2.1–2.6 mmol/L
Copper	100–200 μg/100 mL (μg = microgram)	16–31 μmol/L
Creatine kinase (CK)	10–79 U/L in females 17–148 U/L in males	167–1317 nmol/sec/L 283–2467 nmol/sec/L
Creatinine	0.6–1.5 mg/100 mL	53–133 μmol/L
Ethanol	0 mg/100 mL	0 mmol/L
Glucose (fasting)	70–110 mg/100 mL	3.9–5.6 mmol/L
Iron	50–150 μg/100 mL (slightly more in males)	9.0–26.9 μmol/L
Lactic acid	0.6–1.8 mEq/L (mEq = milliequivalent)	0.6–1.8 mmol/L
Lead	50 μg/100 mL or less	Up to 2.4 μmol/L
Lipids Cholesterol (fasting)	<200 mg/dL	<5.18 mmol/L
Triglycerides (fasting)	40–150 mg/100 mL	0.4–1.5 g/L
PCO2	35–45 mm Hg	4.7–6.0 kPa (k = kilo, Pa = pressure)
pH	7.35–7.45	7.35–7.45
PO2	75–100 mm Hg	10.0–13.3 kPa
Potassium	3.5–5.0 mEq/L	3.5–5.0 mmol/L
Protein: total Albumin Globulin	6.0–8.4 g/100 mL 3.5–5.0 g/100 mL 2.3–3.5 g/100 mL	60–84 g/L 35–50 g/L 23–35 g/L
Sodium	135–145 mEq/L	135–145 mmol/L
Uric acid	3.0–7.0 mg/100 mL	0.18–0.42 mmol/L
Vitamin A	0.15–0.6 μg/mL	0.5–2.1 μmol/L

Compiled from *Taber's Cyclopedic Medical Dictionary*, 20th edition, Philadelphia: F. A. Davis, 2001, pp. 2431–2434.
Used with permission.

Table 13.2 Normal Laboratory Values of Urine

URINE CONTENTS	NORMAL VALUE IN CONVENTIONAL UNITS	NORMAL VALUES IN SI UNITS (INTERNATIONAL SYSTEM OF UNITS)
Calcium	300 mg/day or less	7.5 mmol/day or less
Creatine	Under 100 mg/day or less than 6% of creatinine	<0.75 mmol/day
Creatinine	15–25 mg/kg of body weight/day	0.13–0.22 mmol/kg/1 day
Protein	<150 mg/24 hr	<0.15 g/day
Sugar (glucose)	0	0

Compiled from *Taber's Cyclopedic Medical Dictionary,* 20th edition. Philadelphia: F. A. Davis, 2001, pp. 2435–2436. Used with permission.

Table 13.3 Normal Laboratory Hematological Values

HEMATOLOGICAL CONTENTS	NORMAL VALUE (CONVENTIONAL VALUES)	NORMAL VALUES IN SI UNITS (INTERNATIONAL SYSTEM OF UNITS)
Coagulation factors		
Factor I (fibrinogen)	0.15–0.35 g/100 mL	4.0–10.0 µmol/L
Factor II (prothrombin)	60%–140%	0.60–1.40 µmol/L
Factor V (accelerator globulin)	60%–140%	0.60–1.40 µmol/L
	70%–130%	0.70–1.30 µmol/L
Factor VII–X	70%–130%	0.70–1.30 µmol/L
Factor X (Stuart factor)	50%–200%	0.50–2.0 µmol/L
Factor VIII (antihemophilic globulin)	60%–140%	0.60–1.40 µmol/L
Factor IX (plasma thromboplastic cofactor)	60%–140%	0.60–1.40 µmol/L
	60%–140%	
Factor XI (plasma thromboplastic antecedent)		0.60–1.40 µmol/L
Factor XII (Hageman factor)		
Thrombin time	Control ± 5 seconds	Control ± 5 seconds
Complete Blood Count (CBC) values		
Hematocrit	Male 45%–52%	Male 0.45–0.52
	Female 37%–48%	Female 0.37–0.48
Hemoglobin	Male 13–18 g/100 mL	Male 8.1–11.2 mmol/L
	Female 12–16 g/100 mL	Female 7.4–9.9 mmol/L
Erythrocyte sedimentation rate (ESR)	Male 1–13 mm/hour	Male 1–13 mm/hr
	Female 1–20 mm/hr	Female 1–20 mm/hr
Iron (Ferritin serum)		
Iron deficiency (borderline deficiency)	0–12 ng/mL (13–20 ng/mL)	0–4.8 nmol/L (5.2–8 nmol/L)
		>160 nmol/L
Iron excess	>400 ng/L	

Table 13.3   Normal Laboratory Hematological Values (continued)

HEMATOLOGICAL CONTENTS	NORMAL VALUE (CONVENTIONAL VALUES)	NORMAL VALUES IN SI UNITS (INTERNATIONAL SYSTEM OF UNITS)
Leukocyte count	4,300–10,800/mm³	4.3–10.8 X 10 to power of 9/L
Erythrocyte count	4.2–5.9 million/mm³	4.2–5.9 X 10 to power of 12/L
Mean corpuscular volume (MCV)	86–98 μm³/cell	86–98 fl
Mean corpuscular hemoglobin (MCH)	27–32 pg/RBC	1.7–2.0 pg/cell
Platelet count	150,000–350,000/ mm³	150–350 X 10 to power 9/L
Folic acid (Borderline)	>3.3 ng/mL (2.5–3.2 ng/mL)	> 7.3 nmol/L (5.75–7.39 nmol/L)
Vitamin B12 (Borderline)	205–876 pg/mL (140–204 pg/mL)	150—674 pmol/L (102.6–149 pmol/L)

Compiled from *Taber's Cyclopedic Medical Dictionary,* 20th edition. Philadelphia: F. A. Davis, 2001, pp. 2442–2445. Used with permission.

PTA students should try not to panic the first time they enter the ICU. The best advice for PTAs walking into the ICU is to remember that they are there to help patients become more mobile, stronger, and independent, just as with patients with any condition. The PTA should stand at the foot of the patient's bed and observe the machines and lines attached to the patient. PTAs should not initiate treatment without surveying the surroundings. PTAs should speak to the patient, introduce themselves, and create a pleasant atmosphere for the patient. Universal Precautions are important for all patient care situations but are paramount in the ICU to protect both the patients and the PTAs. PTAs must remember to wash their hands before and after seeing patients. Gloves should be donned when the possibility of contact with body fluids exists. PTAs must follow specific instructions for isolation or barriers precautions. The procedures may involve wearing gloves, mask, gown, and even a waterproof apron. PTAs are part of a team together with the physicians, nurses, dieticians, occupational therapists, respiratory therapists, social workers, pharmacists, and the patients and their family. Physical therapy intervention should be scheduled in accordance with other patient procedures. Communication, verbal and written, between all parties involved is of the utmost importance and provides the greatest benefit to patients.

A specialist physician in the ICU is called an **intensivist.** This comparatively new specialty area of medical practice is becoming common in the ICU of many hospitals. These specialists are able to identify warning signs of difficulties for patients on the ICU, such as changes in blood pressure that could cause kidney failure. Other advantages exist to having an intensive care physician on staff. The intensivists can be available in the ICU at all times. Some patients are in ICU after surgery, and the surgeon may remain in the operating room with another patient. If something starts to go wrong with a patient postoperatively, the surgeon may not be available to attend to the patient as a result of being in surgery, whereas the intensivist physician is available for prompt consultation. The disadvantage of having intensivists is that they are not necessarily familiar with each patient. Because intensivist is a comparatively new area of specialization, the statistics are not sufficient to determine whether the presence of an intensivist on the hospital staff can save lives. Many other health care providers work in the ICU and specialize in the field of intensive care medicine, including nurses, respiratory therapists, physical therapists, and social workers.

Intensive care unit rooms always contain a lot of equipment. Such equipment may include intra-arterial lines, automatic blood pressure monitors, electrocardiogram monitors, intracranial pressure monitors, intravenous infusion (IV), lower extremity compression devices, mechanical ventilators, oxygen supply, postsurgical drains, pulse oximeters, suctioning devices, and urinary catheters. All of these items of equipment are explained later in this chapter. The electrocardiogram (ECG) monitor, with moving lines of different colors and alarms, resembles a television set. Patients will be connected to the machine by several electrodes and wires attached to the chest wall. Patients may have an oxygen mask either in place over the nose and mouth or attached to a tracheostomy (a tube surgically inserted into the trachea to assist breathing). Patients may be on a respirator, a machine that assists breathing when the patient is unable to do so independently. Drainage tubes arising from the surgical site may be evident with a drainage container containing a mixture of fluids including blood by the bed. This procedure is normal postoperatively to drain excess blood away from the surgical site and to prevent buildup of the fluids internally. The physician or surgeon removes drainage tubes when the bleeding post-surgery has stopped or diminished. Other tubes may include a catheter tube with a catheter bag to drain urine to allow for accurate measurement of urine output and keep the patient dry to prevent skin breakdown. An intravenous (IV) almost certainly will be attached to the patient. The IV allows for the administration of hydration fluids and medications to be injected directly into the blood stream. Some situations require the insertion of a central line, a device inserted directly into a vein that remains in place. A central line is used for constant or extensive IV access and when the veins are at risk of collapse, preventing insertion of an IV. The central line may predispose the patient to danger of infection so standard precautions are essential. Blood gases may be monitored through a central line. A feeding tube may be in place through the nose for nutrition if patients are unable to feed themselves by mouth or for those who may choke by trying to feed by mouth. A feeding bag setup is attached above the patient or to an intravenous pole (IV pole). In some cases, a gastric feeding tube may be surgically inserted into the stomach via the abdominal wall, which is also attached to a pole or an overhead mechanism.

Compression devices are attached to the lower extremities to assist with circulation and prevent deep venous thrombosis (blood clots). The compression devices must be removed when transferring patients, performing sitting balance activities, or executing bed mobility exercises. The devices should be reapplied after treatment is completed.

PTAs should peruse the room before moving any equipment and initiating treatment. The furniture and equipment should be left as they were found at the conclusion of the treatment session. PTAs should be conscious of possible safety issues such as the possibility of needles inadvertently left on the beds or hanging from IV poles. PTAs should follow the guidelines of the institution carefully, seek help from the supervising physical therapist, and inform the risk manager or designated hospital person in the event of a needle stick. Student PTAs should follow the protocol established by their PTA program in addition to the institutional procedures.

General Precautions and Recommendations for Treating Patients in the ICU

1. Enhance patient care through team work by getting to know the nurses in the ICU.
2. Speak to the nurse assigned to the patient before initiating treatment to ensure the patient is stable and that the orders have not changed.
3. Read the patient chart carefully before initiating treatment. Contact the supervising PT for changes in the patient's status or physician's orders.
4. Observe the equipment attached to patients as well as the location of the equipment and furniture before initiating treatment.
5. Introduce yourself to the patient and any family in the room. Explain who you are, why you are there, and what you plan to do.
6. Treat the patient as you would any other patient.
7. Check vital signs before initiating any treatment. A record of vital signs will probably be situated at the end of the patient's bed. Vital signs are taken frequently on ICU. If in doubt, ask the nurse.
8. Wash hands before and after treating patients.
9. Follow Standard (Universal) Precautions for all patients.
10. Close the curtains while performing exercises, transfers, or bed mobility to protect the patient's dignity and privacy. Have patients wear undergarments or shorts when possible.
11. Move any mobile equipment such as chairs and tables out of the way before commencing treatment. If a chair will be needed for transfers, ensure it is placed in the appropriate position before proceeding.

12. Ask the nurse to provide a longer oxygen tube to enable ambulation, or request a mobile oxygen unit or cart with an oxygen cylinder if necessary.
13. Ensure that the brakes on the bed are in the locked position before moving patients. Push the bed against a wall if the brakes do not work well.
14. Apply a gait belt or similar device for safety before transfers and ambulation.
15. Utilize walking socks or shoes for transfers or ambulation. Provide adequate coverage with hospital gowns or robes to prevent exposure of patients during the activity to maintain patient privacy.
16. Move all tubes and equipment such as catheters, IVs, and oxygen tubes to the side of the bed the patient will exit to prevent pulling on the tubes. If an ECG machine is in use ask the nurse whether the ECG electrode leads need to be moved before ambulation.
17. Avoid raising the catheter bag above the pelvis to prevent backflow of urine.
18. Check all tubes for kinks that may impede flow.
19. Ask the nurse to detach the gastric feeding tube from the machine before physical therapy is initiated, especially if the patient is to be moved extensively. Pulling on the gastric feeding tube could result in peritonitis, a serious condition, as well as possible surgery to reattach the tube into the stomach.
20. Check the IV before initiating treatment to ensure that it is secure. Contact the nurse if the IV appears at risk of dislodging, if it dislodges, or if the IV stops dripping during PT treatment. A second person may be necessary to assist with the IV and other tubes to reduce this risk.
21. Check to determine whether an electrode has been dislodged if the ECG/EKG monitor alarms sounds. Most likely the nurse will come to the room promptly at the sound of an alarm; if not, call the nurse on the intercom. An alarm could indicate that the patient is going into distress, in which case stop treatment immediately and call the nurse.
22. Leave the patient and the room as found.
    a. Make patients comfortable on completion of the physical therapy session ensuring they are in a good position and can reach their essentials easily, such as the emergency call button, the telephone, and the television remote control.
    b. Raise the bed rails after treatment if they were in place before treatment.
    c. Follow all specified recommendations regarding patient position change to prevent pressure ulcers. Place patients in the same position after treatment.

Ask the nurse about positioning before finishing treatment. Document any changes in position.
    d. Document the volume of any fluids issued to the patient during treatment since fluid intake and output is monitored when patients are in the ICU.
    e. Inform anyone who was asked to leave the room during physical therapy that they may return.
23. Any change in patient status should be discussed with the supervising PT. Defer treatment if necessary.
24. Follow all institutional and PT and PTA program protocols in the event of a needle stick.

Equipment Used in the ICU

Some of the equipment used on the intensive care unit is specific to this unit. Other pieces of the equipment such as the electrocardiogram unit may also be found on the Coronary Care Unit and in other areas of acute care. The use of multiple monitoring devices with many leads and tubes attached to patients can make the ICU a daunting place to work. Gaining an understanding of the types of equipment used on the ICU will help to alleviate some of the anxiety for the PTA.

ARTERIAL LINES AND INTRA-ARTERIAL LINES

Intra-arterial lines may be inserted into the radial or axillary artery of the upper extremity or the femoral or pedal artery of the lower extremity. The procedure for insertion of the line is similar to that used for the placement of an IV, except that the line is usually sutured to the skin to prevent it from moving. The line has to be less than 120 cm in length and of a rigid consistency so that it will not compress during the pulsating of blood.[2] The line is attached to an arterial blood pressure monitor usually located at the head of the bed. The insertion of an arterial line allows a constant measurement of the blood pressure for people who require close monitoring of their vital signs. The line also enables frequent arterial blood sampling for the measurement of blood gases and other laboratory testing without the need for the insertion of multiple needles.[3]

BLOOD PRESSURE

Monitoring of the blood pressure (BP) is essential for patients in the ICU. BP is taken by the nurse every hour and recorded on a chart so that any patterns of BP change can be observed. In some cases, an automatically timed BP unit is attached to the patient by a cuff on the arm over the brachial artery and takes the BP readings at specific, preset times. Most BP charts have a graph, which helps to demonstrate the rise and fall of the BP over a period of hours. Even in the age of computers, a visual record of the changes in vital signs readily available for all of the health care team is helpful.

ELECTROCARDIOGRAM MONITOR

The **electrocardiogram** (ECG) monitor is a machine that is connected to the patient by electrodes and leads attached to the chest wall (see Fig. 13.1). The machine monitors the heart rate and rhythm of the heart by sensing the bioelectric current of the heart muscle. (See Chapter 3 for further details about the electrocardiogram.) This machine should be left turned on during PT treatment. The alarm on the machine is set for each patient. The machine is set to alarm if the heart rate goes above or below a predesignated level determined by the physician. The electrocardiogram looks like a television monitor with sets of wires. The machine may be sitting on a bracket attached to the wall or on a mobile cart and is located in the patient's room at the head of the bed where it can readily be observed by any health care worker attending to the patient. The machine is connected to a monitor located in the nurse's station for continuous monitoring of the patient. Other types of ECG machines are portable, about the size of a large cell phone, for use at home during ambulation, or held in a sling round the person's neck for 24-hour heart monitoring. ECG reading is covered in Chapter 3 of this book.

INTRACRANIAL PRESSURE MONITOR

Patients with head injuries, brain tumors, or other neurological conditions affecting the brain are at risk for increased **intracranial pressure (ICP)** that can build up and cause further damage to the brain. Increased pressure cannot escape within the skull and thus the pressure is forced back into the brain tissue.[4] (See Chapter 7 for further details about intracranial pressure.) Monitoring of the ICP in these patients is important. If the pressure builds up to a dangerous level, surgery may have to be performed to release the pressure from the brain. A probe for an ICP monitor is surgically implanted through the skull into the subarachnoid space and attached to the monitor by a lead.[5] A monitor is located at the head of the bed for observation of the pressure. The clinical signs that may indicate an increase in pressure, and the need for pressure monitoring, include changes in BP, pulse, levels of consciousness, and any abnormal muscular activity. An abnormal CT scan may also indicate the potential for an elevated ICP. A normal ICP is between 5 and 15 mm Hg in adults.[6] Levels can rise in people with head injury and may be considered acceptable within the 0 to 20 mm Hg range. The determination of safe levels of ICP for individual patients must be determined by the physician. The risk levels for people with a raised ICP are exacerbated with a reduction in the cerebral perfusion pressure. If the rate of perfusion of the brain tissue is low, the oxygenation of the brain tissue may be impaired and result in further damage.[7] Therefore, when the ICP is higher than usual and the patient also has hypotension, the need for monitoring is more important. The PT and PTA need to be aware that physical therapy interventions may raise the ICP levels, so clinicians should consult with the nurse before initiating physical therapy.

INTRAVENOUS INFUSION (IV)

Intravenous infusion (IV), also called parenteral (nonoral) therapy, an IV drip, or a peripheral intravenous line, is an integral part of patient treatment in the ICU. These tubes either have a plastic or metal needle that is inserted directly into a vein. The vein may be located in the arm, the hand, or occasionally the leg. The needle insert is secured to the body part with tape. The insert may be closed off when not in use and periodically flushed with a saline solution by the nurse to prevent blood from clotting and blocking the flow of fluids. When the IV is in use a bag of fluids is attached via a plastic tube to the IV insertion point. The tube is either free-flowing into the patient or runs through a machine that controls the rate of delivery of the fluid to the patient. The IV allows blood, plasma, and medications to be quickly administered to the patient as well as fluids for hydration and nutrition.[8] During physical therapy intervention the PTA should be careful to avoid pulling on the IV insertion as this may dislodge the mechanism. When the IV is pulled out of the patient a new insertion site must be found by the nurse. In people who are in the ICU for prolonged periods of time, this can be uncomfortable as well as difficult if the person's veins are

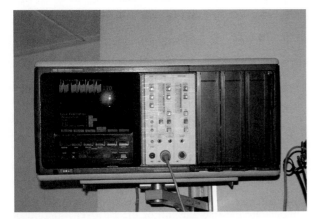

FIGURE 13.1 An electrocardiogram monitor.

fragile. Often the alarm on the IV machines sounds during physical therapy intervention, and the nurse must be called to remedy the situation. IVs may act as a portal of entry for infections and care must be taken to use Standard (Universal) Precautions when handling any part of the mechanism. Guidelines from the Centers for Disease Control and Prevention indicate that peripheral IV catheters should be changed every 72 to 96 hours to reduce the risk of infections.[9] If inflammation of the skin is noted at the site of the IV insertion, the nurse should be informed.

LOWER EXTREMITY COMPRESSION DEVICES

During periods of immobility, patients are at risk for poor circulation, particularly in the lower extremities. In the ICU, and with people who have just had surgery in the general hospital setting, the use of compression devices is common. These devices include an **intermittent pneumatic compression pump** also called an **external sequential compression device,** attached to plastic sleeves placed over the lower extremities (see Fig. 13-2). The pressure sleeve acts as an external pump for the venous system to stimulate the circulation at a time when patients are not using the muscles sufficiently. The external pumping device helps to reduce swelling and minimize the possibility of a deep venous thrombosis (DVT) developing by increasing the velocity of the peak venous flow of blood

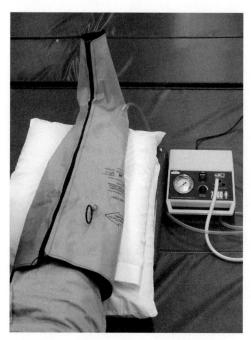

FIGURE 13.2 A lower extremity compression device.

and the volume of blood pumped by the veins.[10] When patients are more mobile, the pump may be used at night exclusively. During the day, patients may use compression stockings (support hose) to create an external pressure to assist venous return. These stockings may be below or above the knee. The patient may be sent home with a pair of custom-fitted support hose (stockings). Elastic compression stockings help to reduce the risk of DVT and also prevent further damage to the veins in patients who have had a DVT.[11]

MECHANICAL VENTILATORS

Mechanical ventilators are one of two main types, either cycled by air volume or pressure. Mechanical ventilators deliver a mixture of oxygen and air through an endotracheal tube of a tracheostomy or via a variety of masks that may cover the nose and mouth. The pressures and volumes associated with respiration are closely linked and interrelated and can be graphed with a pressure-volume curve. See Chapter 4 for further details. All mechanical ventilators are used to provide assistance with breathing and gaseous exchange at the alveolar level for patients unable to breathe sufficiently for adequate oxygenation of the cells and tissues. Typically a mechanical ventilator is used when a person cannot keep the oxygen saturation level at more then 90% for prolonged periods of time. A high respiratory rate with associated shallow breaths may be one cause of low oxygen saturation levels. The physician determines whether to place a person on a mechanical ventilator after observing all of the clinical findings.

During normal inspiration, or inhalation, the expansion of the chest cavity creates a negative intrapleural pressure and air rushes in from the atmosphere to even out the pressure. When a mechanical ventilator is used, this pressure difference is created by increased pressure produced by the ventilator. Resistance to inhalation is created by decreased elasticity of the lung tissue. Additionally, the machine tubes and endotracheal tubing used with ventilator assisted respiration increase the resistance. During the normal final stage of exhalation, the pressure within the alveoli is the same as that of the atmospheric pressure. People with respiratory conditions often have airways that are blocked with secretions or spasm of the bronchi, resulting in the incomplete emptying of the alveoli. This end-expiratory pressure may be higher than that of the atmosphere. This condition of positive end-expiratory pressure is known as **intrinsic PEEP** or **autoPEEP.**[12]

Volume-cycled ventilators deliver tidal volume of air to patients specific to the individual's needs determined by the respiratory team. Two main types of volume controlled ventilator include the **assist-control (A/C) ventilator** and the **synchronized intermittent mandatory ventilator (SIMV)**. With an A/C ventilator, the machine assists with each breath and is set to detect when the patient is having difficulty inhaling which triggers the machine to deliver a preset tidal volume of air to the lungs. If the respiration rate is too low, the machine also delivers the tidal volume of air to make sure the respiratory rate is maintained at a minimum required level. The SIMV also relies on the volume of air with a preset respiratory rate and volume set for the patient. However, with the SIMV the machine does not deliver air if the patient manages to inhale sufficient air. The other main type of mechanical ventilator is **pressure-cycled**. These machines deliver air to a preset pressure through **pressure-control ventilation (PCV)** or **pressure-support ventilation (PSV)**. These machines deliver a preset pressure of air to the lungs, and because the resistance of the lung tissue and the respiratory system as a whole varies, the volume of air changes. The PCV ventilator delivers the full amount of preset pressure and maintains a minimum respiratory rate similar to the A/C ventilator. The PSV is controlled by the depth and length of the inhalation of the patient. Because no respiratory rate is set the patient is in control of the rate of respiration. The deeper the patient breathes, the quicker the machine shuts off.

Several noninvasive types of positive pressure ventilation are possible, with the delivery of air via a mask that covers the nose and mouth. These machines are used for people who can breathe on their own but may not be getting sufficient oxygenation of their tissues and need supplementary oxygen. One more commonly used is the **continuous positive airway pressure (CPAP)** machine. These machines help people to maintain a constant amount of pressure throughout the respiratory cycle and are often used at night by people with sleep apnea. The **bilevel positive airway pressure (BIPAP)** ventilator is also used for people with sleep apnea, although less frequently, and is set for both inhalation and exhalation pressures. People who use the BIPAP machine have to be cognitively aware as a result of the possibility of aspiration of fluids into the lungs.[13]

OXYGEN

Oxygen use is common in the ICU to maintain normal oxygen saturation levels in the arterial blood. The oxygen is usually delivered from a unit at the head of the bed and is pumped directly from pipes in the wall from a central location in the hospital. A valve is located in the wall at the head of the bed for each bed in the ICU. Occasionally oxygen cylinders are used, but this is unusual because of the risks of using oxygen cylinders. If oxygen is inadvertently allowed to escape at a rapid rate from a cylinder, it can turn the cylinder into a missile that can penetrate walls.

The patient is attached to the oxygen supply via tubing attached to an oxygen mask that covers the nose and mouth or a divided nasal tube, or through a tube attached to a tracheostomy tube surgically inserted in the patient's throat. Various types of oxygen masks are available. The nasal tube can become uncomfortable both where it inserts into the nose and where it passes over the ears. Close attention should be given to prevent skin breakdown at these sites. The levels of oxygen prescribed for the patient depend on the physician and the patient's oxygen saturation levels. In some cases, the physician may prescribe a slightly higher level of oxygen during and immediately after physical therapy intervention if there is evidence that oxygen saturation levels are reduced during treatment sessions. The PTA should not increase the concentration of oxygen for a patient during physical therapy intervention unless specifically ordered by the physician or the physical therapist. The PTA needs to read the patient's chart carefully for any instructions regarding oxygen use during activity. If patients appear cyanotic or breathless during physical therapy interventions, the PTA should contact the nurse immediately and the physical therapist for advice. The use of a pulse oximeter during physical therapy intervention is strongly advised to ensure oxygen saturation levels are maintained within acceptable levels.

POSTSURGICAL DRAINS

Postsurgical drains are used in different types of surgery, including cardiac, pulmonary, and orthopedic. Drains may be used in surgery to drain excess blood from the surgery site after the patient is returned to the room or to prevent the wound from closing when infection is present. These drains are tubes that drain fluid and blood into water in a sealed container that is placed by the side of the bed. Usually in the ICU the drainage system is a chest tube used to drain fluids and air after open-heart surgery. This system is called a Hemovac (see Fig. 13-3). The PTA should observe the location of wound drainage systems when working with patients in the ICU. If it is necessary to move the drain reservoir, care should be taken to ensure the container is not lifted too high. The reservoir container must be kept below the level of the entry of the tube into the patient to prevent backflow of the drained fluids. The use of surgical drains after surgery is controversial. Research studies have shown that the need for blood transfusions after surgery may be increased with the use of surgical

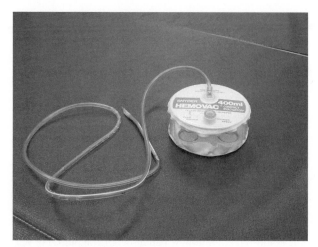

FIGURE 13.3 A Hemovac.

drains.[14] Other studies have shown that the use of a drain does not make any difference to the rate of healing of post-surgical orthopedic wounds.[15,16]

PULSE OXIMETER

The **pulse oximeter** measures the amount of oxygen saturation of hemoglobin in arterial blood, also called arterial saturation (SaO2) or peripheral oxygen saturation (SpO2). Some machines also measure the pulse rate in beats per minute. Pulse oximetry machines may be small and portable, or larger and free-standing. The patient is attached to the machine with a probe that has two parts, light emitting diodes (LEDs), and a light detector. The probe is attached by a small clip to the end of a finger, toe, or to the ear lobe (see Fig. 13-4). Some pulse oximeters have a finger cuff that can be placed on the finger like a glove. Light from the probe shines through the tissues from one side of the probe to the other and is absorbed by the tissues and blood in the body part. The blood absorbs the light depending on the hemoglobin saturation of the blood. The microprocessor in the machine calculates the oxygen saturation level and displays the reading on the monitor.[17] The accuracy of the pulse oximeter reading may be affected if the body part is cold or is moving rapidly in the presence of tremors or shivering, if the room lighting is very bright, or if the person has severe hypotension (low blood pressure).

The oximeter can be left in place during physical activity to monitor the oxygen saturation level of the arteries and ensure it does not fall below a safe level. The normal SaO2 in healthy people is between 95% and 100%, but in many patients with cardiac conditions, it can fall below 90%. When levels of oxygen saturation fall below 94%, the person is considered hypoxic (too little oxygen

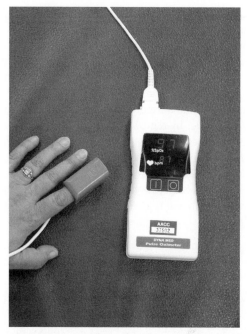

FIGURE 13.4 A pulse oximeter.

to the tissues), and a reading below 90% is considered a clinical emergency.[18] If the level falls below a specified level determined by the physician, such as 95%, then the patient may not be safe to perform physical therapy. In some cases, physical therapy may be possible with adequate use of oxygen during treatment procedures. The effectiveness of the physical therapy intervention has to be weighed against the possible effects of reduced oxygen and fatigue. If the patient is unstable, the PTA may not be the appropriate person to treat the patient and the patient should be referred back to the PT for assistance.

SUCTIONING DEVICES

Suctioning devices are attached to a vacuum system located in the wall of the ICU room. The settings on the vacuum device can be adjusted. The PTA will not be directly involved with suctioning although the PT who specializes in respiratory care may perform suctioning. Most suctioning is performed on patients with a tracheostomy to maintain a clear airway and keep the tracheostomy clear of fluids and secretions. The nurse or PT may perform this suctioning under sterile procedure. A thin tube attached to the suctioning device is inserted into the opening in the tracheostomy and passed down the trachea. In most cases, a cough will be stimulated once the tube reaches the carina, the bifurcation point of the trachea. After a cough is stimulated the suction can assist with removal of the secretions. Suction is applied while the tube is slowly withdrawn from the trachea after the cough. Suctioning may be used on patients in a coma or who are unable to cough and expel secretions for themselves, including infants in the neonatal intensive care unit (NICU). In such instances, the suction catheter can be passed down the trachea either via the nose or the mouth. Suctioning may be performed either by removing patients from the mechanical ventilator or leaving the ventilator in place.[19] Care must be taken to prevent the catheter from entering into the stomach. Exceptions to the rule exist, but in most cases, the PT or respiratory therapist can facilitate an adult patient to cough and rule out the need for suctioning.

URINARY CATHETERS

Indwelling urinary catheters, also called Foley catheters, are common in the ICU. The urinary catheter is described in more detail in Chapter 12. Keeping patients dry is essential for the prevention of pressure sores and skin breakdown. In patients who are immobile, a catheter may be required for a few days or more (see Fig. 13-5). Catheters are inserted during surgical procedures and may be removed within 24 hours or after a few days when the patient is able to be more mobile. Patients who are immobile and very ill may require the continued use of a catheter. The PTA is reminded that an indwelling catheter may act as a portal of infection into the bladder, and care should be taken when handling the catheter tubing to make sure hands are washed and gloves are used to reduce the risk of infection for the patient. The location of the urine collecting bag should be noted and care taken to avoid raising the

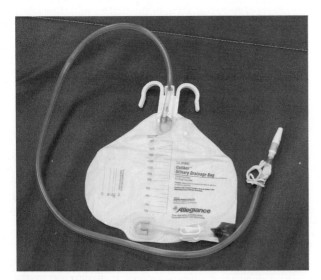

FIGURE 13.5 A catheter tube and bag.

bag above the level of the insertion point in order to prevent backflow of urine into the bladder. Creating a bend in the catheter tube is acceptable short-term to prevent backflow of urine when moving the catheter bag. Maintaining a free flow of urine through the catheter is essential, and the PTA should make sure the catheter tubing is unrestricted at the conclusion of treatment.

What Causes a Patient to Be Placed in the ICU?

The attending physician decides when to place a patient in ICU. Many factors may be taken into consideration. In some cases, a surgeon may decide that a patient needs to be in the ICU for monitoring after a major surgery. This decision would be likely if the patient has a respiratory or cardiac comorbid condition. A patient would be placed in ICU or CCU immediately following open-heart surgery. The ICU enables close monitoring of vital signs and the ability to place the patient on respiratory support easier than in a standard patient room. The ICU is an ideal place to monitor a patient who is medically unstable because the ratio of nurses to patients is higher. After surgery, the stay in the ICU may be for a short time. Then the patient may be moved to a stepdown unit, when medically stable, where the nursing care is still intensive but not as restrictive. Visitors may be restricted in the ICU to reduce the effects of patient fatigue. Return to a standard hospital room enables more visitors and an improvement of patient morale.

Other patients placed in the ICU include individuals who have experienced a myocardial infarction, cerebrovascular accident (CVA), head injury, trauma, extensive burns, general surgery, end-stage renal disease, and persons in respiratory distress or who require close monitoring as a result of uncontrolled high blood pressure or electrolyte imbalances. Patients who are dying may be placed on the ICU. In many cases patients may have multiple diagnoses such as cardiovascular disease combined with respiratory problems and then experience a CVA or a head injury. This combination of diagnoses and comorbidities makes a patient unstable and the close monitoring of vital signs and blood chemistry is required. The multiple diagnoses is often referred to as "alphabet soup," because of the acronyms used to describe the diseases. An individual patient may be described in the patient chart as having a combination of such disorders as COPD, CVA, CHF, ASHD, PVD, and IDDM. Sometimes reading the patient chart is like entering another world and can be difficult for the student and recent graduate. Refer to a medical dictionary for any unfamiliar acronyms. Sometimes individual hospitals have a list of accepted acronyms for specific medical terms to use in patient charts at that institution. In some cases, medical personnel may use acronyms that are not appropriate but are commonly used in the hospital. HA is one example of an abbreviation with multiple meanings. This abbreviation is confusing because some medical personnel use it to describe a headache, whereas others may use it to describe a heart attack. Using abbreviations for multiple meanings poses great danger to the patient because of the risk of the term being misinterpreted. The advice to the PTA is to use abbreviations and acronyms sparingly. Always remember that people reviewing and reading the patient chart may not be familiar with the acronyms used in physical therapy. When reviewing the chart before treating the patient do not be afraid to ask the nurse about unfamiliar terms. Asking for clarification of terms is better than guessing at the meaning and being wrong. Patient safety is of the utmost importance and must be the primary consideration.

Physical Therapy Interventions Used for Patients With Specific Diagnoses on the ICU

The role of the PTA in the ICU will vary according to the hospital and the relationship between the PT and PTA. The supervising PT needs to have sufficient confidence in the PTA's ability to respond to changing circumstances. The patient also needs to be sufficiently medically stable so that constant reevaluation is unnecessary. In some cases, the PTA will assist the PT with the patient intervention, and in others, the PT may treat the patient in the morning to determine the medical status, and the PTA will do a follow-up treatment in the afternoon. One of the most difficult issues to determine when working in the ICU is how much to push and challenge the patient during physical therapy interventions. Many patients decline therapy and will need encouragement to participate. How does the PTA decide whether patients are depressed and unwilling to participate, as opposed to whether they truly are too sick to perform the physical therapy? The status of the patient can be difficult to determine. Often the nurse is a valuable source of information. Perhaps the patient did not sleep well and is fatigued, has just had a bed bath, or recently returned from x-ray and is exhausted. Sometimes the PTA may have to return to see patients after they have rested. Patients have the right to refuse treatment so the PTA cannot force them to participate. Often explaining why patients should participate in physical therapy and discussing their fears will help to encourage them. Try returning to see the patient at a later time and remember to document in the patient chart that the patient declined

treatment, and provide the possible reason. Also document that you have spoken to the nurse and state any additional information received regarding the refusal.

Burns

The management of patients with burns is covered in Chapter 8. However, some specific issues related to patients with burns on the ICU need to be discussed. A patient with extensive burns may be admitted to the ICU in a hospital that does not have a specific burn unit. In many cases, a patient with severe burns will be airlifted to a burn unit hospital; however, in some cases, this is not possible. After being admitted to the ICU, the initial management is to save life. Prevention of infection is important once the patient is stable.

Physical Therapy Intervention. The role of the PT and PTA may include pulmonary PT, wound care, positioning, range of motion exercises, bed mobility, transfer assistance, and ambulation as possible. Washing hands regularly, wearing gloves and gowns, and following all Standard Isolation Precautions are essential to protect the patient from infection.

PRECAUTIONS AND CONSIDERATIONS FOR PHYSICAL THERAPY INTERVENTION

Several general precautions and considerations beyond those listed at the beginning of the chapter are required when working with patients with burns in the ICU:

1. Most people with extensive burns will be placed on a special pressure-relief hospital bed. Use of these special beds is awkward for physical therapy intervention because they often have solid sides that limit the ability to reach patients.
2. Care must be taken when handling patients to minimize the contact time with the areas burned to reduce pain.
3. The repositioning of patients after physical therapy intervention is essential to prevent contracture of limbs. Patients should be positioned after treatment as they were found before treatment. Do not be afraid to ask for assistance if needed.
4. The physical therapist may be involved with wound care. Bedside wound care using the pulsatile lavage unit, electrical stimulation, or ultrasound are all possible. A certain amount of planning is necessary when transporting electrical units to the bedside. The bedside environment is always a challenge for setting up a sterile field.
5. If a full-body whirlpool tank is needed, patients may be transported to the physical therapy department on a

stretcher. A whirlpool tank stretcher hoist is used to transfer the patient into the tank.

Cerebrovascular Accident (CVA)

Patients with a cerebrovascular accident (CVA), also known as a stroke, or more recently as a brain attack, may require a period of time in the ICU after onset of the condition. The full description about CVA is provided in Chapter 7.

Physical Therapy Intervention. Physical therapy intervention for patients with CVA who are on the ICU may include bed mobility exercises and positioning, range of motion of the affected limbs, active assisted exercises for the affected limbs, and active exercises for the unaffected limbs. The PT and PTA are involved with assisted transfers from bed to chair, and ambulation as possible and as allowed by the physician. Encouragement may be needed to help patients turn to the affected side if they have neglect caused by the CVA. If family members are present, the PTA should demonstrate exercises or allow them to watch the treatment. However, if the patient is distracted and unable to concentrate, the family may need to leave the room during the treatment. The PT and PTA should decide the best course to follow with this matter. In the later stages of rehabilitation, family may be asked to be present during treatment. Patients may be on oxygen, be attached to the electrocardiogram monitor, have an indwelling catheter, and have a nasogastric feeding tube if they have problems with swallowing as a result of the CVA. Patients may be mentally disoriented or confused and unable to understand instructions or concentrate on the directed activities.

PRECAUTIONS AND CONSIDERATIONS FOR PHYSICAL THERAPY INTERVENTION

Several general precautions and considerations are required when working with patients with CVA in the ICU beyond those listed at the beginning of the chapter:

1. Observe the patient closely during treatment for signs of changes in vital signs, as well as discoloration of lips or ears for signs of cyanosis.
2. Observe the patient closely for signs of fatigue.
3. Observe the patient closely for any signs of increased weakness or changes in speech such as slurred speech, which might indicate a further CVA. If in any doubt, call the nurse and contact the supervising physical therapist.
4. If the patient is on a thickened liquids diet due to swallowing problems, do NOT give water to drink. The possibility exists that the patient might aspirate (take liquid into the lungs).
5. Stand on the side of the bed close to the affected side to encourage patients to turn the head to their affected side.
6. Speak to the patient and explain exactly who you are and what you are going to work on.
7. Keep instructions to simple one-word commands or short sentences.
8. Be encouraging and assist as needed, but make patients do as much as possible for themselves.
9. Keep treatments fairly short to prevent undue patient fatigue. Sessions may be up to 15 minutes at a time in the initial stages.
10. Remember that patients status post-CVA may not tolerate more than a few exercises the first few days. Getting patients into a chair may be the most they can tolerate in one session.
11. Ask for assistance to perform transfers, particularly for the first attempt.
12. Avoid discussions with the family regarding prognosis. Prognosis is the role of the physician and the PT. Keep discussion to current treatment issues and how the family can help the patient during recovery.

End-Stage Renal Failure

Patients with end-stage renal disease may be placed in the ICU. (See Chapter 12 for further details about kidney diseases.) These patients may be awaiting renal transplant or they may be in the terminal stages of the disease.

Physical Therapy Intervention. Patients with end-stage renal failure fatigue very rapidly, are likely to be on oxygen therapy, and have IV nutritional supplements as well as catheters and ECGs. People with end-stage renal failure have a restricted fluid intake and may not be allowed to have water to drink, although in some cases they may be allowed to suck an ice cube. Physical therapy intervention may include bed mobility, an exercise program to maintain strength and function, assistance with transfers, and possibly some minimal ambulation.

PRECAUTIONS AND CONSIDERATIONS FOR PHYSICAL THERAPY INTERVENTION

Specific precautions for the PTA when treating the patient with end-stage renal disease include all those identified at the beginning of the chapter, plus:

1. Follow all specified recommendations regarding patient position change to prevent pressure ulcers.

2. Observe the patients closely during treatment for signs of changes in vital signs, as well as discoloration of lips or ears for signs of cyanosis. Be sure that the oxygen attachment is maintained during treatment.

3. Observe patients closely for signs of fatigue and be careful not to fatigue patients.

4. Use short-sentence instructions as patients with end-stage renal failure may be disoriented and require similar strategies as those used with patients with a CVA. Keep treatments fairly short to prevent undue patient fatigue. Sessions may be up to 15 minutes at a time in the initial stages.

5. Remember that patients may not tolerate more than a few exercises the first few days. Transfers into a chair may be the most they can tolerate in one session.

6. Any discrepancies between the description of the physical therapist's prior treatment and the current treatment should be discussed with the supervising PT. Defer treatment if necessary.

Myocardial Infarction

People who have had a myocardial infarction (MI) are placed either in the ICU or the cardiac care unit (CCU). Individuals who have had a severe MI are likely to be in the ICU. The goal is to monitor the heart and preserve life. See Chapter 3 for further details about heart diseases.

Physical Therapy Intervention. Physical therapy intervention is indicated once people with an MI have become stable with their vital signs and no further evidence of MI is identified. Possible interventions include bed mobility exercises, strengthening of the upper and lower extremities, and transfers in and out of bed once cleared by the physician. Ambulation may be possible at bedside when the vital signs have stabilized.

PRECAUTIONS AND CONSIDERATIONS FOR PHYSICAL THERAPY INTERVENTION

Specific precautions and considerations for PT intervention for the patient who has experienced a myocardial infarction include all those listed at the beginning of the chapter, plus:

1. Close monitoring of patients for vital signs and any indication of physical stress with exercises.

2. Caution when transferring patients out of bed to ensure the blood pressure remains within acceptable limits. Patients often are in denial after an MI and may not describe increased symptoms when performing activities.

3. The presence of another person during physical therapy intervention is recommended to assist with transfers and ambulation.

4. The PTA may not see patients after an MI as a result of the unstable nature of the vital signs. However, the PTA may accompany the physical therapist to ensure patient safety.

Near-Drowning

Working in the ICU may involve rehabilitation of patients who survive after a near-drowning incident. Patients who have experienced near-drowning are often in a serious and life-threatening state upon admission to the ICU. Many of the individuals who survive near-drowning accidents are aged under 15 years and male. The degree of anoxia of the brain and pulmonary damage resulting from near-drowning depends on the length of time the person was in the water.

Physical Therapy Intervention. Physical therapy intervention primarily is focused on the neurological rehabilitation of patients who survive the first few days after a near-drowning incident. Intervention is focused on the return of functional movement and neurodevelopmental treatment techniques described in Chapter 7. Patient positioning to prevent pressure ulcers is important as well as treatment of the associated impaired respiratory function.

PRECAUTIONS AND CONSIDERATIONS FOR PHYSICAL THERAPY INTERVENTION

Specific precautions and considerations for PT intervention for the patient who has experienced a near-drowning incident include the following:

1. Read patient charts carefully before treatment. Pay particular attention to the physical therapist evaluation and plan of care. Also note the level of consciousness as indicated on the Glasgow Coma Scale (see Chapter 7 for further details and Table 13-4).

2. Do not wear brightly colored clothing because this may overstimulate the sensory pathways and cause the patient distress.

3. Check with the nurse before treatment. When possible schedule the physical therapy session by coordinating with the nursing staff ahead of time so that other patient procedures do not coincide with the physical therapy.

4. Check to see if fluids are allowed to be given to the patient. An "NPO" (*non per os*) sign is placed over the head of the bed if no oral fluids are allowed, with clear documentation noted in the patient chart. If fluids are

Table 13.4 **Glasgow Coma Scale**

EYE OPENING (E)	SCORE
Spontaneous	4
To speech	3
To pain	2
Nil	1

BEST MOTOR RESPONSE (M)	SCORE
Obeys	6
Localizes	5
Withdraws	4
Abnormal reflex	3
Extensor response	2
Nil	1

VERBAL RESPONSE (V)	SCORE
Oriented	5
Confused conversation	4
Inappropriate words	3
Incomprehensible sounds	2
Nil	1
	Coma score = (E + M + V) = 3 to 15

allowed, document the volume of any drink given to the patient during treatment because fluid intake and output is monitored in the ICU.

5. Speak to the patient and explain exactly who you are and what you are going to work on. People who have experienced near-drowning may be in a semiconscious state. Although patients may seem unresponsive, they may hear everything that is said. Be careful to speak to the patient and not to someone else. Also do not talk across patients to another person, because they may be aware of everything that is going on around them.

6. Be encouraging but make patients do as much as possible for themselves.

7. Observe the patient closely during treatment for signs of changes in vital signs, as well as discoloration of lips or ears for signs of cyanosis. A tracheostomy probably will be in place with the oxygen attached. Make sure the oxygen tube remains in place during the physical therapy intervention.

8. People who have experienced near-drowning may be unable to tolerate more than a few minutes intervention at a time, so several short visits during the day may be required.

Surgery—Cardiac, Orthopedic, and Major Internal Surgery

Many patients are placed in the ICU immediately after surgery. The patients admitted to the ICU may include the following:

1. Patients after open heart surgery.
2. Patients after orthopedic surgeries such as total hip replacement.
3. Patients after any major surgery who require constant monitoring of vital signs, respiration assistance, artificial feeding, or who have comorbid diagnoses, such as heart disease or kidney disease.
4. Patients after surgery to correct major traumatic injury.
5. Patients suspected of having a myocardial infarction (MI) or a cerebrovascular accident (CVA).
6. Patients who require an individual room as a result of a compromised immune system.

The length of stay in the ICU varies according to the patient diagnosis. Some patients may be in the ICU for 24 hours after surgery and then be moved to a stepdown unit such as a coronary care unit where the monitoring continues but the patient is not in immediate danger. Some patients with extensive trauma or severe coronary diagnoses may remain in the ICU for several days.

Physical Therapy Intervention. Physical therapy intervention may be indicated for people who are in the ICU after surgery. The reason for the ICU stay may be to ensure close monitoring of vital signs for the first 24 hours after surgery. The physical therapy intervention may include postural drainage and pulmonary hygiene techniques, bed mobility exercises, active assisted exercises for the lower and upper extremities, transfers, and sometimes ambulation particularly if patients remain in the ICU for more than 24 hours. The precautions are the same as for other conditions already noted when working with patients who have had major surgery.

Trauma—Treat the Essential First

When patients with severe trauma resulting from an accident are admitted to the hospital or shock trauma unit the most immediate problems are attended to first. Preservation of life is most important. The triage nurse may direct the initial screening evaluation toward breathing difficulties or loss of blood. The vital signs need to be stabilized and the patient placed on life supporting regimens. Many of the minor issues such as fractured bones are secondary and have to wait to be addressed until the patient is stable. In some cases, fractures are missed in the initial evaluation when the focus is on saving life. An intravenous hookup is started, and oxygen may be required. Blood tests are performed to check electrolytes and blood gases. A magnetic resonance imaging (MRI) scan may be performed to determine whether the person has any brain injury. After the patient is stabilized the cuts, abrasions, and possible fractures are addressed. Surgery to fixate fractures may be delayed until the patient is stable enough to undergo surgery. Internal bleeding may be suspected, in which case immediate surgery is performed to locate the problem and attempt to repair any internal organ damage. In the case of gunshot wounds, surgery may be necessary to remove the projectile. In knife wounds, repair of any injured areas may be necessary. Extensive blood loss must be stopped and blood transfusion may be required. Some patients with fractures of the spine may require traction. Cervical spine fractures may be managed with halo traction surgically attached through the skull.

Physical Therapy Intervention. Patients with cervical spine fractures managed with halo traction may have specific precautions and contraindications indicated by the evaluating physical therapist and the physician. These patients may not be able to get out of bed. However, some patients retain a halo in place for the entire time it takes for the fracture to heal and may return home. Patients with halo traction in place may be seen as outpatients in the physical therapy clinic. The initial physical therapy intervention for patients with severe trauma may involve postural drainage positioning and pulmonary hygiene techniques. Breathing exercises are indicated to improve general circulation and ensure the lungs remain patent. After the life-threatening results of the trauma are stabilized, the physical therapy interventions may include bed mobility exercises, progressive strengthening exercises, endurance activities, stretching exercises, transfer training in and out of bed, and ambulation with an appropriate assistive device depending on the orthopedic injuries sustained in the trauma. Patients with lower extremity fractures and an upper extremity injury may require specialized assistive devices. For example, a rolling walker with a forearm support or crutches with a forearm support may be helpful for people with lower extremity fractures and a sprained wrist. Some patients may require a wheelchair for mobility if both lower extremities are fractured. Weight bearing on both lower extremities may be prohibited for 6 to 12 weeks until the fractures have healed sufficiently. In such instances, wheelchair mobility training is essential.

PRECAUTIONS AND CONSIDERATIONS FOR PHYSICAL THERAPY INTERVENTION

Specific precautions for the PTA when treating patients who have experienced severe trauma include all those indicated at the beginning of the chapter, plus the following:

1. Read patient charts carefully before treatment. Note any of the surgeries performed on patients and read the physical therapist's initial evaluation carefully to determine the plan of care. Pay particular attention to weight-bearing status for the lower extremities. Also check for new physician orders to ensure no change. When changes are indicated contact the physical therapist for a reevaluation of the patient and possible update of the goals.
2. Check with the nurse before treatment. When possible schedule the physical therapy session by coordinating with the nursing staff ahead of time so that other patient procedures do not coincide with the physical therapy.
3. Patients who are on bed traction will not be able to get out of bed but may be able to perform exercises for the uninvolved extremities, as well as some limited bed mobility exercises. Instructions for pressure relief movements may be beneficial. An overhead pulley may be in use to allow patients to raise up in the bed and relieve pressure on bony prominences.
4. Do not allow patients to become overfatigued. Remember that initial intervention sessions may be fairly short.
5. Be encouraging, but make patients do as much as possible for themselves.
6. Observe the patient closely during treatment for signs of changes in vital signs, as well as discoloration of lips or ears for signs of cyanosis. If oxygen is in use, make sure that the attachment is maintained during treatment.
7. Remember that treatment sessions may be limited to a few exercises and breathing exercises with patients in the ICU the first few days. Performing bed mobility exercises or transferring patients into a chair may be the most they can tolerate in one session.
8. Observe all weight-bearing status instructions. Be sure to select the appropriate assistive device for ambulation. Be aware of multiple trauma problems.

Traumatic Brain Injury

Traumatic brain injury (TBI) or head injury (HI) is an external injury to the head that causes damage to the tissue of the brain. Depending on the area of the brain affected, head injury may result in various neurological manifestations. Patients with a TBI serious enough to be admitted to the ICU are usually in an unconscious or semiconscious state. The monitoring of these patients includes all of the machines for blood pressure, urinary catheters, arterial lines or IVs, electrocardiogram, and perhaps a tracheostomy with attached oxygen. In addition, the intracranial pressure may be monitored for signs of increased pressure on the brain that could exacerbate the damage to the neural tissues. See Chapter 7 for further details about traumatic brain injury.

Physical Therapy Intervention. The PT and PTA are involved in a team approach for the care of patients with TBI in the ICU. The members of the team involved in the acute care stage may include the physician, physician assistant, nurse practitioner, nurse (RN), social worker, occupational therapist (OT), certified occupational therapy assistant (COTA), and the speech and language pathologist in addition to the physical therapist and physical therapist assistant. Although the physical therapy intervention is largely directed toward improvement of the motor deficits resulting from TBI, the cognitive level of the patient also must be taken into consideration. The person with a brain injury may be unable to learn new motor skills or understand simple instructions. In the acute care environment, the physical therapy intervention depends on the length of time the patient remains in the ICU. If the patient is on a respirator as a result of damage to the brain stem, the PT intervention may include bed and chair positioning for prevention of contractures and pressure ulcers, postural drainage and pulmonary hygiene techniques, active assisted exercises, bed mobility exercises, and even ambulation. The PT and PTA may be asked to instruct the staff in the ICU in range of motion exercises.

PRECAUTIONS AND CONSIDERATIONS FOR PHYSICAL THERAPY INTERVENTION

Precautions and considerations for PT intervention for patients with TBI in the ICU involve all those previously stated for other conditions, plus the following:

1. Check with the nurse before initiating physical therapy to determine the status of the patient.
2. Check vital signs and intracranial pressure levels before working with the patient.
3. Do not wear brightly colored clothing because this may overstimulate the sensory pathways and cause the patient distress or precipitate a seizure.
4. Speak to the patient and explain what you are doing in simple, short statements, even if the person appears to be in a coma. The person may be able to hear you, and the stimulation may assist with return to consciousness.

5. Observe the patient in a coma carefully for responses to movement such as eye flutter, pupil dilation, withdrawal responses of limbs, or any movement previously not noted. Any changes noted should be reported to the nurse and the PT and documented in the patient chart.
6. Keep treatment times short and visit the patient twice a day or as requested by the physical therapist or physician.
7. Involve the family in the intervention by explaining to them the reason for the intervention and the goals. However, provide these explanations away from the patient to avoid overstimulation of the patient. The family may not be able to participate in the treatment in the ICU setting. When the patient is moved to a subacute setting, the family will be able to increase their involvement.
8. Document the PT intervention carefully and objectively in the patient's chart. Be sure to note the length of time of the intervention and any response to treatment noticed.
9. Keep in communication every day with the supervising physical therapist because patient status is likely to change quite rapidly in some cases, and the plan of care may need to be updated by the physical therapist.

Prevention of Pressure Ulcers

When people remain in bed for any length of time and are relatively immobile, consideration must be given to prevention of pressure ulcers. The PT and PTA are involved with the positioning of patients to ensure they do not remain in one position for more than 2 hours. The preferred turning schedule is once an hour, especially for patients at high risk for developing pressure areas, such as the frail elderly, people with reduced nutritional status, people who are immunosuppressed, and patients with reduced mobility. If physical therapy intervention is performed with patients in the ICU, the treating therapist must comply with the prescribed turning schedule. The physician and nursing staff develop the turning schedule, and all others need to follow it to protect the patients. At the conclusion of the physical therapy intervention, the PT/PTA should either leave patients in the position they found them or ask the nurse whether to turn them on the other side. The nurse may be grateful for assistance with the turning schedule but needs to know the patient position is altered.

Pressure ulcers are described in Chapter 8 of this book. Some specific considerations need to be addressed for prevention of pressure ulcers for patients in the ICU. Patients in the ICU are at risk for pressure ulcers primarily because they are immobile and more sick than patients on other floors in the hospital.

The management of any person immobilized in bed for prolonged periods of time is always a challenge. The prevention of pressure ulcers is difficult and is exacerbated when the person has a severe medical condition. Special beds may be used in the ICU, and in other areas of the hospital, to help to reduce the risk of the development of pressure ulcers. A variety of pressure relief devices are available, including air and water mattress beds or air and water mattress overlays to use on standard hospital beds, memory foam mattress overlays, alternating pressure pads with an electric pump, low air loss beds, motor-driven beds that can be raised and lowered at the foot and head to reposition people, foam mattress overlays with egg-crate design padding. Some beds will rotate laterally as well as adjust at the head and feet. The choice of pressure relief device depends on the individual needs of the patient. Some countries, such as the United Kingdom, have developed guidelines for the use of these pressure-relieving devices.[20] In the United States, statistics are published regarding the incidence of pressure ulcers, but the majority of these data relate to patients in nursing homes. The high-risk factors for pressure ulcers in nursing homes are correlated with recent weight loss of the resident, high levels of immobility, and recent incontinence.[21] Although these factors are specific to the people within nursing homes, the same statistics could be relevant for people who are in the ICU for prolonged periods of time.

Legal and Ethical Issues

The legal and ethical issues for the PT and PTA working in the ICU are the same as for any other practice setting. Each patient deserves the best treatment intervention that the therapist can provide. Issues of end-of-life rights and the right to refuse treatment may become more immediate in this setting. Accurate, objective patient performance and functionally focused documentation is always extremely important regardless of the treatment setting. Patient refusal of PT intervention must be tempered by qualifiers such as "patient very fatigued and unable to participate in PT today" or "patient just returned from medical testing and is too fatigued for PT." Treatment notes may be subpoenaed, therefore accuracy is essential.

Many patients treated in the ICU may have a poor prognosis and may not survive. The PT and PTA who work in the ICU must be prepared to confront death and be able to offer comfort to relatives and accept that death is an integral part of life. Showing compassion for dying patients and their family, as well as respecting their wishes is important. Always remember to keep speaking to patients who are dying as hearing is thought to be the last sense to diminish. Keep orienting patients to the time of year, day of the week, time of day, and the date so they feel a part of life until the end.

Pediatric Intensive Care Unit ☻

The treatment of children in a specialized PICU requires the same considerations as those detailed for adults in the ICU. Multiple tubes and attachments always seem worse when seen on a small infant or child. The PTA needs to be prepared. Exhibiting confidence when working with children in the PICU is important so both the child and the parents will feel comfortable. The PT and PTA need to remember that children may be frightened and uncooperative because they are unable to understand why they have to undergo certain treatments. Infants in an incubator may require physical therapy for pulmonary function and to encourage movement of the limbs. All functional movements require the ability to be able to cross the hands past midline of the body. If a premature baby lies on his or her back, the shoulders lie in a retracted position, and the hands are unable to touch each other. This position causes problems in development and tightness in the shoulder girdle muscles. Physical therapy intervention can enhance normal development and assist the functional movement of the upper and lower extremities. Chest physical therapy may be performed in the PICU. Infants and small children can be placed on the knee of the therapist for postural drainage positioning and percussion.

CASE STUDY 13.1

A 60-year-old female patient in the ICU who underwent open heart surgery for replacement of the mitral valve 2 days ago has been referred to physical therapy for postural drainage, pulmonary hygiene techniques, and bed mobility exercises. The supervising physical therapist is going to perform the initial evaluation and requests the presence of the PTA. Assistance may be needed during the evaluation, and all or some of the care may be delegated to the PTA after the evaluation. The patient has chest drainage tubes in place, is receiving oxygen via a face mask, has an indwelling catheter, an IV in the left arm immediately distal to the antecubital fossa, compression devices on both legs, and dressings over the midsternal incision and is attached to a cardiac monitor and automatic blood pressure device (not an intra-arterial line). The PTA has never treated a patient in the ICU before and is rather daunted by the sight of all the tubes and equipment surrounding the patient.

1. List some of the considerations for the PTA before entering the patient's room.

2. Describe the infection control precautions.

3. Identify the appropriate action of the PTA if the cardiac monitor electrodes displace during treatment and the alarm sounds on the monitor.

4. Explain the physical therapy procedures to the patient.

STUDY QUESTIONS

1. Identify the medical diagnoses of patients in the ICU.

2. List the types of medical equipment likely to be encountered on the ICU.

3. Describe intracranial pressure (ICP).

4. Indicate the normal value range for ICP in the adult.

5. Describe two types of ventilator.

6. Discuss five specific precautions when providing physical therapy intervention for patients in the ICU.

7. Describe three specific precautions when treating a patient with a traumatic brain injury in the ICU.

8. Discuss with another student or PTA concerns you may have about treating a patient in the ICU for the first time.

9. Describe how postural drainage might be performed on an infant.

10. Explain how you will help to prepare yourself to work on the ICU.

● USEFUL WEB SITES

European Society of Intensive Care Medicine
http://www.esicm.org

International Federation of Infection Control
http://www.theific.org

Morbidity and Mortality Weekly Report (CDC)
http://www.cdc.gov/mmwr

National Guideline Clearinghouse, US Department of Health and Human Services
http://www.guideline.gov

Society of Critical Care Medicine
http://www.icu-usa.com

Trauma.org
http://www.trauma.org

World Federation of Societies of Anaesthesiologists
http://totw.anaesthesiologists.org

● REFERENCES

1 Stein, T. P., & Wade, C. E. (2005, July). Metabolic consequences of muscle disuse atrophy. *J Nutr* 135:1824–1828.

2 Turner, K. (2008). *Arterial blood pressure monitoring: an introduction.* St. Vincent's Hospital, Australia. Retrieved 3.22.09 from http://www.clininfo.health.nsw.gov.au/hospolic/stvincents/stvin99/Karen2.htm

3 Society of Critical Care Medicine. (2004). Arterial line. *ICU-USA, Inc.* Retrieved 12.3.08 from http://www.icu-usa.com/tour/equipment/aline.htm

4 Kaups, K. L., Parks, S. N., & Morris, C. L. (1998). Intracranial pressure monitor placement by midlevel practitioners. *J Trauma* 45:884–886.

5 Nucleus Medical Art. (2009). Brain surgery—placement of intracranial pressure monitor—medical illustrations, human anatomy drawing. Retrieved 11.28.10 from http://catalog.nucleusinc.com/ generateexhibit.php?ID=9919&ExhibitKeywordsRaw=&TL=&A=2

6 Neurotrauma—intracranial pressure. (2000). *Trauma.org.* Retrieved 12.3.08 from http://www.trauma.org/archive/neuro/icp.html

7 Ibid.

8 International Federation of Infection Control. (2008). *Education programme for infection control: prevention of IV device-associated infection.* Retrieved 11.29.10 from http://www.theific.org/basic_concepts/ppt_pdf/13.pdf

9 Grady, N. P., et al. (2002, Aug 9). Guidelines for the prevention of intravascular catheter-related infection. *Morb Mortal Wkly Rep* 51(RR10):1–26. Retrieved 12.3.08 from http://www.cdc.gov/mmwr/preview/mmwrhtml/rr5110a1.htm

10 Markel, D. C. (2002). Effect of external sequential compression devices. *J South Orthopaed Assoc* 11:2–8.

11 Prandoni, P., et al. (2004). Below knee elastic compression stockings to prevent the post-thrombotic syndrome: a randomized, controlled trial. *Ann Int Med* 141:249–256.

12 Gehlbach, B. K., & Hall, J. (2007). Overview of mechanical ventilation. *The Merck Manual Online Medical Library, The Merck Manual for Healthcare Professionals.* Retrieved 3.22.09 from http://www.merckmanuals.com/professional/sec06/ch065/ch065b.html

[13] Gehlbach, B. K., & Hall, J. Overview of mechanical ventilation. *Merck Manuals Online Medical Library for Healthcare Professionals.* Ibid.

[14] Gaines, R. J., & Dunbar, R. P. (2008). The use of surgical drains in orthopedics. *Orthopedics* 31:702.

[15] Ibid.

[16] Hadden W. A., & McFarlane A. G. (1990). A comparison study of closed-wound suction drainage vs no drainage in total hip arthroplasty. *J Arthroplasty,* 5(suppl):S21–S24.

[17] Wilson, I. (2009). Pulse oximetry—part 1. *Anaesthesia Tutorial of the Week, World Federation of Societies of Anaesthesiologists.* Retrieved 7.28.09 from http://totw.anaesthesiologists.org/2009/03/03/pulse-oximetry-part-1-123/

[18] Ibid.

[19] Pogson, G. G., & Shirley, P. J. (2002). Hyperoxaemia during tracheal suctioning: comparison of closed versus open techniques at varying PEEP. *Crit Care* 6(suppl 1): 30.

[20] National Guideline Clearinghouse. (2010). Pressure ulcer prevention and treatment. Health care protocol. London: National Health Service. Retrieved 11.29.10 from http://www.guideline.gov/content.aspx?id=16004&search=pressure+relief+devices+and+pressure+ulcer+prevention

[21] Park-Lee, E., & Caffrey, C. (2009). *Pressure ulcers among nursing home residents: United States 2004.* NCHS Data Brief, no. 14. Hyattsville, MD: National Center for Health Statistics.

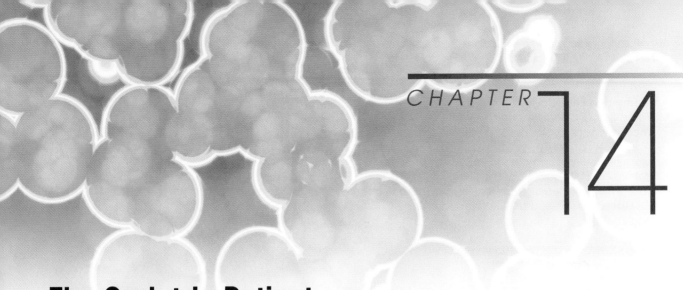

The Geriatric Patient

LEARNING OBJECTIVES

After completion of this chapter, students should be able to:

- Describe definitions of the terms *geriatrics, geriatric medicine,* and *gerontology*
- Name theories related to the aging process
- Determine the issues related to the association of aging and altered balance abilities
- Discuss the major challenges faced by people as they age
- Consider the appropriate and inappropriate use of restraints and restraint alternatives
- List some commonly occurring diagnoses in older people
- Determine the physical therapy interventions used for older people with specific diagnoses
- Apply ideas to enhance communication with older people who are hearing-, sight-, or cognitively impaired
- Describe factors that increase the risk of malnutrition in the older population
- Apply some special concepts of physical therapy interventions for end-of-life care
- Determine venues for physical therapy intervention for elderly people

KEY TERMS

Acoustic neuroma

Age-related macular degeneration (ARMD)

Ageism

Benign paroxysmal positional vertigo (BPPV)

Brandt-Daroff exercises

Cataract

Dix-Hallpike test

Epley maneuver

Exudative retinal detachment

Geriatrics/gerontology/ geriatric medicine

Glaucoma

Neurofibromatosis

Phacoemulsification

Rhegmatogenous

Tractional retinal detachment

CHAPTER OUTLINE

Introduction
Overview of Geriatrics
Physiological Effects of Aging
   Effects of Age on the Skin
   False Assumptions About the Elderly
Psychological Effects of Aging
Specific Diseases Prevalent in the Elderly Population

C H A P T E R   O U T L I N E (continued)

Introduction

This chapter covers the various aspects of aging and geriatrics relevant to the physical therapist assistant (PTA). Although most of the diseases discussed in this chapter have been described elsewhere in this book, the specific interventions and considerations when working with older people with these conditions are delineated in this chapter. New content for this chapter is the anatomy of the eye and ear, as well as the associated pathological conditions. The reason for inclusion of these conditions in this chapter is that many of the diseases and conditions of the eye and ear are either part of, or made worse by, the aging process.

Overview of Geriatrics

The terms **geriatrics, gerontology,** and **geriatric medicine** apply to the field of medicine involved with treatment of problems caused by aging. Geriatrics is not strictly related to those individuals aged over 65 years, but many problems associated with aging are generally applied to the over-65 age group. For example, the field of athletics has a different definition of what is "old" compared with that of internal medicine or cardiac medicine. People in their 30s and 40s are considered "old" in football, and even in professional tennis, people over 35 are classed in the

veterans group. Despite these classifications, some people continue to play sports into their 70s and 80s and are classified as very fit for their age. According to the Centers for Disease Control and Prevention (CDC) and the Merck Company Foundation "State of Aging and Health in America 2007" report, by 2030, there will be 71 million Americans over age 65, representing 20% of the total population.[1] The report also stated that the cost of providing health care to older Americans is approximately 3 to 5 times greater than the cost for those people under age 65. In addition, more than 35% of deaths in the United States for older Americans is attributed to smoking, poor nutrition, or lack of physical activity.

Other statistics indicate that the birth rate in the United States is declining while the life expectancy is increasing. The 2007 birth statistics indicated a birth rate of 14.3 per 1,000 of the population.[2] The CDC reported that the mortality rate in 2006 was 810.4 per 100,000 of the population with the highest number of deaths attributed to heart disease, followed by cancer, and then cerebrovascular accident. The average life expectancy for Americans was 77.7 years with women tending to live slightly longer than men.[3] The numbers of people over 65 at a given time depend on the birth rate, immigration numbers, health issues, and the death rate, among others. Most sources agree that there are an increasingly higher proportion of people over 65, and the trend is likely to continue. Projections are that by 2050, the life expectancy for men in the United States will increase to 81.2 and for women to 86.7 years.[4]

Another factor to take into consideration with the older population is the socioeconomic status. Many older Americans live close to or beneath the poverty line, which presents its own challenges to the health care system. Health care for the elderly is going to be a major aspect of politics in the United States over the next decades. An increased need for rehabilitation services including physical therapy will be apparent. Discussion regarding who will pay the costs is a controversial issue. Medicare is currently available for people over the age of 65, but it is known that the Medicare funds are dwindling and the future of the program is in doubt. What will happen to the millions of Americans who rely on Medicare for health care is a definite concern. Over time, the ratio of working people to retired people is going to decline, and this poses problems for the funding of health care. This topic is one that this book cannot hope to solve, but all people in the health care field need to be aware of the prospective problems of the coming decades associated with the rise in numbers of the elderly population.

Why Does the Physical Therapist Assistant Need to Know About Geriatrics and the Effects of Aging?

As the proportion of people over age 65 continues to grow, the field of geriatric medicine is going to become more important, and the number and need for physical therapists (PTs) and PTAs involved with the treatment of the geriatric population is likely to grow. More people are living into their 90s, and many people live to be more than 100 years. As people age, their physical status may decrease, making them more dependent on others. The importance of maintaining mobility and independence for the elderly cannot be overemphasized. Physical therapy can play an important part in educating older people how to keep themselves fit and active. The ability to remain in their own home or in a senior apartment and maintain their independence gives people a better quality of life. In addition, people who are able to look after themselves are able to keep down the cost of living and stay in better health. Reports from the CDC recognize the role exercise plays in reducing the risk of falls in the older population. Exercise can reduce the risk of falls by 12% and the number of falls by 19% with the use of exercise modalities such as Tai Chi, gait and balance training, and muscle strengthening.[5] All of these exercises can be initiated by physical therapy.

Physiological Effects of Aging

A decline in functional activity is not necessarily the result of aging. However, a direct correlation has been identified between neurological performance and age. Many older people retain good function. A decline in function is mainly related to pathology and disease. Most cells in the body, such as those of the skin and blood, retain the ability to regenerate themselves, whereas some cells, once mature, do not have the ability to reproduce themselves, such as those cells in the nerves and muscles. Scientists do not have a definite theory about aging. Many factors exist that are responsible for the increased life expectancy of humans. Some of these factors include genetics, environment, advances in technology such as immunization against diseases, development of better sanitary living systems, and the development of medications to fight disease. However, some theories state that there may be a preprogrammed life expectancy of certain cells or that the loss of production of certain hormones may influence cell health. Another theory states that the reduction in numbers of immune system cells such as T cells causes an inability to fight off the effects of disease, thus increasing the effects of aging. Another factor of major importance for cell health is sleep. While the body sleeps, it heals itself, and thus sleep deprivation is detrimental to health.

Physiologically, parts of the body tend to alter with chronological time. Unless there is a disease process present, the changes associated with aging occur gradually over many years. At the cellular level, changes occur in the ability of cells to produce energy and to reproduce themselves as a result of changes in the mitochondria and chromosomes. Changes occur in the organs of the body with the aging process that interfere with the functioning of the organ. In the heart and blood vessels, age-related changes may include thickening of the arteries and capillaries, loss of elasticity of vessels, collagen deposition in the walls of the blood vessels, a decreased cardiac output, and an increased systolic blood pressure. Changes in the lungs include a reduction in elasticity of the lung tissue itself, as well as a reduced excursion of the ribs and thus a reduction in vital capacity. This alteration in lung tissue results in less efficiency of the pulmonary system in providing oxygen to the tissues. Skeletal muscles are also affected by the aging process. Connective tissue becomes more inelastic, and fibrous tissue tends to replace some of the muscle tissues and surrounding matrix. The amount of fat in relation to muscle also tends to increase with age and inactivity. Muscle mass also decreases, resulting in a reduction in both the size of the muscles and the number of muscle fibers, and this problem is compounded by the reduced activity level of older people. The loss of bone mass in osteoporosis is discussed in Chapter 5. As previously described, many people with osteoporosis are over 65. The nervous system is affected by age with a reduction of brain size and reduced numbers and function of the neurological cells. The rate of transmission of the nervous impulses slows down, and this results in a slower response rate to changes in the environment that require a muscular response. The resulting loss of balance leads to an increased incidence of falls. The body becomes less resilient to extremes of temperature with increasing age. The hypothalamus is thought to become less reactive to changes in the environment both outside and inside the body, resulting in overheating or underheating effects on the body. Older people are thus more in danger of hypothermia (body too cold) or hyperthermia (overheating of the body) because the body is unable to adapt sufficiently to environmental temperature changes. Added to all these changes are the sensory changes associated with aging, such as loss or reduction of vision, reduced or lost hearing, reduced tactile sensation in the skin, and reductions in proprioceptive and kinesthetic awareness.

Effects of Age on the Skin

The skin alters with age, and exposure to the sun speeds the normal aging process. Some of the changes in the skin include the following:

- Reduced nutrition and hydration
- Reduced elasticity and flexibility
- Bruising more easily to relatively minor trauma
- Reduced circulation
- Thinning of the dermis, epidermis, and subcutaneous layers
- Thinning of the subdermal fat layer
- Alteration of the connective tissue in the dermal layers
- Reduced ability of the nerve endings in the skin to detect heat and cold, touch, and pressure
- Reduced proprioceptive sensation
- Wrinkling of the skin in response to dehydration and loss of elasticity
- Dryness, scaling, and itching
- Loss of body hair

The effects of aging on the skin make the skin more likely to break down in response to pressure and trauma. Several factors increase the incidence of pressure ulcers in the elderly. The highest risk is found in those who are immobile and confined to bed or wheelchair. Weight loss also increases the risk because the body fat is reduced and therefore protective padding of muscle is reduced. Weight loss may also be accompanied by dehydration, which further reduces the flexibility of the skin and predisposes the skin to breakdown. In addition, circulatory problems reduce the nutrition to skin and cause it to be less resilient to damage and more easily bruised. The dermis and epidermis layers of the skin tend to thin with the normal aging process and the connective tissue network starts to alter resulting in an overall loss of elasticity of the skin. The outward effects include wrinkles and dryness of the skin. The sensitivity of the skin to pressure, touch, and temperature tends to reduce with aging, as well as proprioception and kinesthetic sensation. Add to all of these factors prolonged pressure over a bony prominence, and the result is a pressure sore or ulcer, also known as a decubitus (see Chapter 8 for details of ulcers).

False Assumptions About the Elderly

All of the following statements are generally untrue. Many elderly people participate in sports and continue to be sexually active.

1. Overweight individuals are not mobile and cannot do things for themselves.
2. Elderly people do not have sex and are not interested in sex.
3. Most old people are senile.
4. Most old people are inactive.

Psychological Effects of Aging

Many of the psychological problems associated with aging may be related to the reduced level of function, mental capacity, and the resultant depression in certain individuals. Many psychological theories are related to social and psychological development such as those of Erikson and Jung. The relationship of reduced levels of function to the role of the PT and PTA cannot be overemphasized. Older adults may become isolated as a result of the loss of ability to travel in public transport or drive a car; the loss of cognitive abilities, resulting in socially unacceptable behaviors; or the lack of a supportive mechanism to assist with socialization. As people age, their friends and family die, and they may tend to become isolated if they do not seek new methods of enlarging their circle of friends. All of these factors are magnified in people with chronic disease and dementia states. However, it would be wrong to assume that all older people are isolated in this way. The majority of older people lead full, active, and social lives. The term **ageism** was described by Butler in 1968 to delineate the myths surrounding aging and the resultant attitude of people toward the elderly. Ageism is a form of discrimination because it stereotypes older people. Ageism has a huge negative effect, particularly in health care. The PT and PTA must have a positive attitude toward the elderly and encourage activity in older patients by assisting them to return to full function. Depression and anxiety disorders also play a part in isolating the older patient. Some of the signs and symptoms associated with depression include fatigue, changes in sleep pattern, weight change, weakness, lack of concentration, lack of ability to make decisions, fear, loneliness, and anger. If the PTA notes a variety of these changes in the elderly patient, the PT and the physician should be consulted. In some cases, the depression may be directly related to lack of independence, resulting from a physical illness or injury. People go through a grieving process whether they lose a person close to them or lose their independence. The type of depression caused by reduction in independence may be alleviated when people are rehabilitated to former independence levels. In other people, there may be no apparent reason for the depression. In either case, medical advice should be sought.

Why Does the Physical Therapist Assistant Need to Know About Specific Diseases Prevalent in the Elderly Population?

A large part of physical therapy practice is involved with treatment of the elderly. Whether working in the acute care, home health, outpatient, rehabilitation, or skilled nursing facility settings, the majority of patients are likely to be over 65 years of age. Because the general needs of older people may change the interventions provided as a result of hearing or sight dysfunction or multiple comorbid diagnoses such as diabetes mellitus, some consideration must be given to specific physical therapy intervention strategies when working with this population. Although the following diseases are described elsewhere in this book, a review of the specific considerations when working with the elderly patient is provided in this section.

Specific Diseases Prevalent in the Elderly Population

As people age, the number of chronic diseases tends to be greater. By the time people enter their 90s, these conditions may be multiple. Many people have an accumulation of conditions such as arthritis, cardiopulmonary diseases, and neurological conditions. When combined with the general aging process, these conditions have an impact on the function of people to perform activities of daily living (ADLs). Many of the diseases prevalent in the elderly are described elsewhere in this book. Some of these include the following:

- Heart diseases, such as congestive heart failure (Chapter 3)
- Pulmonary diseases such as chronic obstructive pulmonary disease, pneumonia, and obstructive airways diseases (Chapter 4)
- Osteoarthritis and gout (Chapter 5)
- Bone disorders, including osteoporosis and Paget's disease (Chapter 5)
- Rheumatoid-related forms of arthritis (Chapter 6)
- Neurological diseases such as cerebrovascular accident (CVA), Parkinson's disease, amyotrophic lateral sclerosis, multiple sclerosis, and various types of dementia including Alzheimer's (Chapter 7)
- Diabetes mellitus (Chapter 9)

The impact of these conditions on the elderly population are discussed later in this chapter as it pertains to physical therapy interventions. This chapter also includes sections on disorders of the eyes and the ears, which have not been covered previously in this text. They are included in this chapter on the geriatric patient because many of them either first manifest in elderly patients or progress as a result of the aging process.

Anatomy and Physiology of the Eye

In addition to other pathologies, older people must overcome problems with impaired vision. Loss of vision and hearing presents many problems for the older population because it can increase the likelihood of falls, reduce independence, and make the individual feel isolated, resulting in withdrawal from society. Elderly people are encouraged to have their eyes tested every 2 years, or more often if changes are noted in vision. As the eye ages, the pupils become slower to react to changes in light intensity, and the lens is less able to alter in shape to focus the vision. Many adults have "floaters" in the eye, resulting from the breakdown of the vitreous body, which causes shadows to fall on the retina giving the impression of floating specks in the field of vision.[6] No known long-term effects of these floaters exist. Some more serious eye problems include cataracts, detached retina, glaucoma, and macular degeneration.

The two eyes serve to change incoming light into neurological signals for transmission via the optic nerve to the visual centers in the brain, where they translate into a visual image. Having two eyes allows for a three-dimensional (3D) vision and depth perception as a result of the various angles at which light enters the eyes. People with the use of one eye lose depth perception and the 3D effect. Each eye is protected by the bone of the orbital fossa and is roughly spherical in shape (see Fig. 14-1). From the external surface inward, the covering of the eye is the cornea. This clear layer is lubricated with tears and starts to focus light as it enters the eye. Immediately posterior to the cornea, the aqueous humor is a liquid that circulates throughout the anterior portion of the eye and maintains a constant eye pressure. The iris is the colored section of the eye, and its pupil dilates and contracts in response to light to change the amount of light passing through to the retina. The lens lies directly posterior to the pupil of the iris. The lens focuses light and is able to change shape for focus on close or distant objects. The inside of the eye is filled with a clear, viscous liquid called vitreous humor. Within the interior of the eye, the retina is a smooth layer that acts like the film in a camera to capture images. Several layers comprise the retina. The first is a layer of highly sensitive photoreceptor cells consisting of the rods and cones. The cones are responsible for perception of color, and the rods are able to detect minute amounts of light, especially useful for night vision. Within the photoreceptor layer of the retina, the light images are converted to electrochemical signals for transmission via the optic nerve to the brain. The macula is a specialized area of the retina lying close to the entry of the optic nerve that is responsible for clarity of detail of vision. This area has a high concentration of photoreceptors with a central fovea, which provides sharp vision. The macula as a whole serves to provide the central vision of the eye. Immediately deep to the photoreceptor layer lies the retinal pigment epithelium (RPE), which absorbs any excess light and provides nutrition for the photoreceptor layer of the retina. Bruch's membrane separates the RPE from the deeper choroid layer of blood vessels that supplies the retina with oxygen and nutrients. The sclera is the white outer covering of the eye.[7,8]

Pathological Conditions of the Eye

This section discusses pathological conditions of the eye. Many of these are the result of the aging process.

Cataracts

A **cataract** is a condition in which the lens of the eye becomes opaque. The condition tends to develop slowly and is usually bilateral. Approximately 50% of Americans over age 80 either have or have had cataracts.[9]

Etiology. Most cataracts are caused by the normal aging process of the lens of the eye in people over age 60. The lens consists of water and proteins and is usually clear to allow light through to the retina. When the protein in the lens coagulates, it creates an area of cloudiness that interferes with the passage of light. Cataracts also may develop as a result of trauma to the eye, radiation treatment, diabetes mellitus, the use of steroid medications, or after other eye problems such as **glaucoma**. Congenital cataracts may be seen in infants who are born with the defect or develop it within a few months of birth.[10] Risk factors for the development of cataracts include smoking, alcohol use, and exposure to direct sunlight, which can be avoided by wearing sunglasses and a hat.

Signs and Symptoms. The usual signs and symptoms of cataracts may include reduced clarity of vision often described as blurring of vision, a fading of colors, an increased glare from headlights noticed when driving at night or a halo effect around light sources, a reduction in

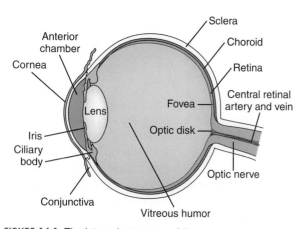

FIGURE 14.1 The internal structures of the eye.

Anterior chamber
Cornea
Iris
Ciliary body
Conjunctiva
Lens
Fovea
Optic disk
Vitreous humor
Sclera
Choroid
Retina
Central retinal artery and vein
Optic nerve

night vision, double vision, or an increased need for changes in the prescription of eyeglasses.[11]

Prognosis. Although cataracts can prevent people from reading, driving, and hobbies such as needlework most people can have surgical intervention to remove the cataracts and improve their vision.

Medical Intervention. The detection of cataracts by the ophthalmologist is performed through use of a visual acuity test with an eye chart, an examination of the retina and internal parts of the eye after dilation of the pupils with eyedrops, and tonometry testing for the presence of increased intraocular pressure. The early symptoms of cataracts may be improved by using antiglare sunglasses and higher magnification eyeglasses. When the vision is impaired sufficiently, surgery can be performed to remove the opaque part of the lens. The surgical procedure more frequently used is **phacoemulsification** in which a tiny ultrasound probe is inserted into the eye through a small opening in the cornea and the ultrasound is used to break up the lens. The pieces of lens are then suctioned out, and an artificial lens is inserted. The less common approach to surgery is extracapsular surgery in which a larger incision is made in the cornea and the lens is removed in one piece.[12] People are given a sedative during the surgery and eyedrops that numb the eye to prevent discomfort. In the majority of cases of cataract removal, the vision is greatly improved after surgery.

Physical Therapy Intervention. Physical therapy intervention is not indicated for people who have cataract surgery. People who have the surgery may not be able to attend physical therapy for several days afterward.

Detached Retina/Retinal Detachment

The retina lines the posterior internal surface of the eye and is light sensitive. Visual data is transmitted through the retina via the optic nerve to the brain. Retinal detachment can occur at any age but is more commonly diagnosed in people over age 40. The condition is a medical emergency that requires immediate evaluation by a physician.

Etiology. Retinal detachment can occur suddenly for no reason or can be a result of trauma to the eye. The condition occurs more frequently in people with a family history of detached retina, those who have had previous cataract surgery in the same eye, those with other eye

diseases, and more frequently in men than women.[13] Three main types of retinal detachment are recognized. **Rhegmatogenous** occurs when there is a tear or small break in the retina that allows fluid from the eye to pass between the retina and its pigment epithelial membrane layer, causing the retina to separate from its nutritional supply. **Tractional retinal detachment** occurs when scar tissue forms on the retina and pulls the retina away from the pigment epithelial layer. After trauma to the eye, inflammation may occur, causing **exudative retinal detachment** when fluid leaks between the retina and the pigment epithelial layer.[14]

Signs and Symptoms. The signs and symptoms of a detached retina are variable. Some people experience a sudden onset of symptoms, whereas for others the onset is slow. Some of the characteristic symptoms include an increase in the number of floaters noted in the eye or a curtain effect across the vision.

Prognosis. Detachment of the retina is considered a medical emergency and can cause permanent vision loss. Although 90% of retinal reattachments are successful prompt treatment of retinal detachment produces a better outcome.[15]

Medical Intervention. Immediate treatment is required for retinal detachment. In some cases, rest in a supine position may allow the retina to become reattached, but in others surgery may be required. Surgery may be performed with a laser to seal the torn part of the retina back in place or with cryopexy that uses extreme cold to fuse the retina back into place.

Physical Therapy Intervention. No physical therapy is indicated for retinal detachment. People who have had eye trauma may be required to rest for several days in a supine position. Eye injuries can occur within the physical therapy department, and extreme caution should be practiced when using Theraband or Theratubing products for resisted exercise to ensure the tubing or band does not recoil into the eye. Goggles should be used by both patients and therapists if any danger of loose objects flying into the eye exists.

Glaucoma

Glaucoma may be acute or nonacute. Acute glaucoma, also called closed-angle glaucoma can occur at any age, but nonacute or open-angle glaucoma tends to occur in people over age 40 years. The people most at risk for glaucoma are those over age 60 and African Americans over age 40 who are at 6 to 8 times more risk than Caucasians. In the United States, more than 4 million people are estimated to have glaucoma, half of whom do not know they have the condition. Worldwide more than 65 million people have glaucoma. The condition accounts for between 9% and 12% of all blindness in the United States, or approximately 120,000 people.[16]

Etiology. People with a thinner cornea are considered to be at higher risk of developing glaucoma.[17] People with a family history of glaucoma and those with diabetes are also more likely to develop the condition.[18] In acute or closed-angle glaucoma, the normal drainage system (drainage angle) of the eye that allows circulation of the aqueous humor becomes either partially or completely blocked causing an increase in the intraocular pressure (IOP). The more commonly occurring open-angle glaucoma is caused by slowing of the drainage of the eye, causing a gradual and more chronic increase in IOP.[19]

Signs and Symptoms. Acute closed-angle glaucoma is of sudden onset and is characterized by severe ocular pain, redness of the eye, blurred vision, halos around lights, headaches, and even nausea and vomiting.[20] In the over-40 age group, open-angle glaucoma tends to be a slowly developing condition with no pain and gradual loss of peripheral vision. An increase of pressure within the eye (IOP) can damage the optic nerve.

Prognosis. Nonacute, open-angle glaucoma is more dangerous because the effects may become severe before a diagnosis is made. Because acute, closed-angle glaucoma is accompanied by severe pain and a sudden onset of blurred vision, people tend to seek help immediately, and the IOP can be relieved. Glaucoma is a leading cause of blindness.

Medical Intervention. No cure exists for glaucoma, but the progression of the condition can be slowed or halted with appropriate intervention. According to the Glaucoma Research Foundation the best way to prevent the effects of glaucoma is through regular eye examinations. Recommendations are for an eye test every 2 to 4 years before age 40, every 1 to 3 years between 40 and 54, every 1 to 2 years between 55 and 64, and every 6 to 12 months after age 65.[21] Regular eye tests include the use of tonometry to measure the intraocular pressure and ophthalmoscopy using a magnifying device to observe the optic nerve. Specific tests for glaucoma are a visual field test called perimetry to determine the extent of the peripheral

vision and gonioscopy to check the angle of the meeting point of the cornea and iris, which may indicate increased IOP. Pachymetry to measure the thickness of the cornea may be performed as a thinner cornea increases the risk of developing glaucoma. Other computerized tests include imaging of the optic nerve. Scanning laser polarimetry (GDx) measures the thickness of the optic nerve; confocal laser ophthalmoscopy (Heidelberg Retinal Tomography or HRT) scans the eye and creates a 3D image of the retina and optic nerve; and optical coherence tomography (OCT) scans with light beams and creates a contour map of the optic nerve fibers. All these tests provide a record that can be compared over time to note the possible decline in thickness of the optic nerve.[22]

Several treatment options are available for people with glaucoma. A variety of oral medications and eyedrops are prescribed to both reduce the production of intraocular fluid and increase the drainage of fluid from the eye. A combination of oral medications and eyedrops may be used. Beta blockers and carbonic anhydrase inhibitors reduce the production of eye fluid, and cholinergics, prostaglandin analogs, and alpha agonists all reduce the production of intraocular fluid.[23] People with acute glaucoma or more advanced disease may require surgical intervention. Argon laser trabeculoplasty (ALT) is used for open-angle glaucoma by treating the trabecular meshwork of the eye to increase the drainage of the aqueous humor and lower the intraocular pressure (IOP).[24] Cyclophotocoagulation is used for advanced or aggressive glaucoma and consists of laser surgery to reduce the amount of fluid that enters the eye and thus reduce the intraocular pressure.[25] Glaucoma filtration surgery or trabeculectomy is a procedure that creates a pocket in the sclera (white of the eye) to collect the excess aqueous humor from the eye to keep the IOP within acceptable levels.[26] A laser iridotomy is used for people with closed-angle glaucoma and creates a small hole in the iris of the eye to enable drainage of the aqueous humor and reduce IOP.[27]

Physical Therapy Intervention. No physical therapy intervention is recommended for glaucoma, but physical therapists and PTAs should be aware of the condition so that they can recommend people to see their ophthalmologist if symptoms of blurred vision or pain in the eye are noted.

Macular Degeneration

Macular degeneration, or **age-related macular degeneration (ARMD),** is an acquired, progressive, and often irreversible loss of central vision and one of the main causes of vision loss in the United States, with vision of 20/200 or worse. Approximately 16,000 new cases of ARMD are diagnosed each year.[28] ARDM usually occurs after age 50, and the incidence increases with age. The risk factors include smoking and a family history of the condition. Types of macular degeneration are exudative (wet) or nonexudative (dry). The dry kind accounts for approximately 90% of all cases. Both types tend to progress, causing a central vision loss, but peripheral vision often remains intact. More than 750,000 Americans have vision loss of 20/200 or worse resulting from ARMD, and approximately 20% to 30% of people over age 75 have some form of ARMD. Men are affected slightly more than women with 25% of females over age 75, and 33.3% of males having some form of ARMD.[29]

Etiology. The cause of macular degeneration is not understood, although vitamins and minerals seem to reduce the progression of the condition in some people. The condition results from deterioration of the macular, a section of the retina of the eye close to the entry of the optic nerve responsible for clear vision. In nonexudative ARMD, there is breakdown of the retinal pigment epithelium, which provides nutrition to the retina that occurs together with a loss of photoreceptors. The exudative form of the condition causes blood leakage into the macular, which directly damages the retina. Risk factors for development of the condition include age over 50 years; Caucasian race; hereditary, with a strong possibility of close family members with the condition; cardiovascular diseases, such CVA, arteriosclerosis, angina, and heart attack; smoking; and exposure to too much UV light.[30]

Signs and Symptoms. The signs and symptoms of macular degeneration depend on the type. Exudative (wet) macular degeneration can occur suddenly and cause disruption in vision. The nonexudative (dry) type of ARMD tends to progress over a series of months or years and is characterized by reduced clarity of vision, gradual loss of color vision, and an empty area in the central field of vision that progressively becomes larger.[31]

Prognosis. The exudative (wet) type of macular degeneration may require laser surgery and tends to progress more rapidly than the nonexudative (dry) type. People with either type of macular degeneration can become legally blind.

Medical Intervention. The diagnosis of macular degeneration is achieved through specific eye tests. Some of these, such as visual acuity, tonometry, and ophthalmoscopy, are described under glaucoma. An Amsler grid can be used to detect deterioration in vision for people with ARMD (see Figs. 14-2 and 14-3). Other tests more specific to macular degeneration include stereoscopic fundus examination with the pupils dilated to observe the whole of the retina, a macular function assessment with photosensitivity and contrasting light, testing of color vision, perimetry of the central vision, and photography of the retina.[32]

The exudative type of macular degeneration may be treated with laser surgery to cauterize the leaking blood vessels causing the problem. No known treatment is available for the dry type of macular degeneration. Measures to slow down the progression of the condition include using sunglasses that filter out ultraviolet rays and blue light and nutrition that includes plenty of green, leafy vegetables containing antioxidants. The use of mineral and vitamin supplements is still under investigation for efficacy, but general guidelines include the use of supplemental vitamins C and E, beta-carotene, selenium, and zinc.[33] People with advanced stages of ARMD are referred to low-vision specialists who can provide advice regarding vision aids, such as mobile magnification devices, large-screen magnification readers for home use,

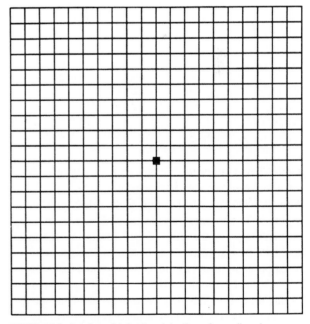

FIGURE 14.2 Amsler grid, for the detection of eye disorders, especially age-related macular degeneration. This image depicts a normal eye. (Courtesy of the National Eye Institute, National Institutes of Health.)

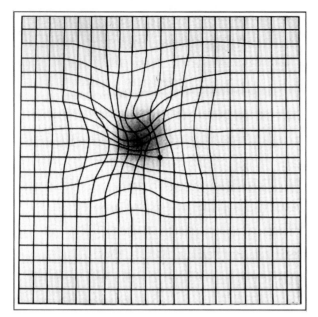

FIGURE 14.3 Amsler grid as it would appear to someone with age-related macular degeneration. (Courtesy of the National Eye Institute, National Institutes of Health)

and computer programs to enhance the visual display and read text.

Physical Therapy Intervention. No physical therapy intervention is indicated for people with ARMD. However, knowledge about ARMD helps the PT and PTA to provide optimal intervention for people in the clinic with this condition. Home exercise programs need to be in an enlarged format (larger drawings) than usual, and an enlarged font should be used for any written materials. Patient forms and information may need to be read to people, and patient data forms may need to be filled out by staff for people who cannot see to write.

IMPLICATIONS OF VISION LOSS AND LOW VISION FOR PHYSICAL THERAPY INTERVENTION

When providing physical therapy to the elderly patient, it is important to take into consideration all factors that may have an impact on the effect of the intervention. If patients have reduced vision, they may be unable to read a home exercise program materials unless the type and diagrams are enlarged enough for them to see. Some elderly patients may be unwilling to admit they cannot see the handout they were given. People may appear uncooperative and not following through with the home program, when they are actually unable to read the handout. Vision loss is also a good reason to take up loose rugs and minimize clutter in the

house to prevent accidental falls. Some people lose depth perception even if they can see quite well, and they may underestimate the height of curbs and steps. Loss or reduction of vision is also psychologically devastating to patients and can make them aggressive. People go through the grieving process with any functional loss and the PT and PTA should bear this in mind.

If the patient has reduced vision, reduced hearing, and is also confused, then the instructions given should be simple and the exercises repeated more often than usual to emphasize the program. Remember that people who have low vision or who are blind or are deaf are not necessarily confused. Another factor to take into consideration is that some people are unable to read or write and may not wish to let you know this. Thus, when providing home exercise programs, the use of drawings is helpful.

Anatomy and Physiology of the Ear

The ear consists of three sections, the outer or external ear, the middle ear, and the inner or internal ear. The outer ear consists of the pinna, the visible part of the outer ear, and the external auditory canal. The pinna is the amplifying and collecting vessel for sound waves to travel from the environment via the external auditory canal to the tympanic membrane before transmission to the middle ear. The external ear also protects the tympanic membrane and middle ear from injury. The middle ear is enclosed within the temporal bone and consists of the tympanic membrane (the ear drum), the three auditory ossicles malleus (hammer), incus (anvil), and stapes (stirrup), the middle ear cavity, and the eustachian tube. The three ossicles are named for the shape of the bones. The malleus attaches to the tympanic membrane, the stapes connects with the fenestra ovalis (oval window) to the inner ear, and the incus connects the malleus and stapes (see Fig. 14-4). A fenestra cochlea (round window) passes from the middle ear to the cochlear of the inner ear. When sound waves hit the tympanic membrane, the ossicles vibrate against each other to transmit sound waves to the inner ear. Approximately 36 mm long, the eustachian tube passes in a downward, forward, and medial direction to connect with the posterior part of the nasal cavity at the nasopharynx. This tube is enclosed for part of its length by cartilage and partly by bone.[34] The eustachian tube serves to equalize air pressure in the middle ear with the outside atmosphere, hence the "popping" sound when someone goes to high altitudes. The inner ear, sometimes called the labyrinth, is made up of the semicircular canals, the cochlea, the vestibular cochlear nerve, and the auditory nerve. The two parts of the inner ear are the bony labyrinth consisting of the vestibule, semicircular canals, and cochlea, all containing a liquid called perilymph, and the membranous labyrinth, which contains endolymph fluid. The acoustic nerve endings are situated in the walls of the membranous labyrinth. The three semicircular canals are tubes curved in a rounded shape, situated at right angles to each other, each approximately 0.8 mm in diameter, which provide vestibular (balance) feedback to the brain. Each canal has a more dilated section at the end called an ampulla and is situated in a different plane. The superior canal is 15 to 20 mm in length and points in a vertical direction. The posterior canal is 18 to 22 mm in length and points in a vertical and posterior direction. The lateral semicircular canal is 12 to 15 mm in length and points in a horizontal, posterior, and lateral direction.[35] Each canal has sensory hair cells that are activated by movement of the inner ear fluid when the head changes position. The nerve impulses from the hair cells are transmitted to the vestibular portion of cranial nerve VIII and then to the brainstem and the cerebellum. In this way, the semicircular canals enable the brain to determine the orientation of the head in space and enable the body to maintain balance. The membranous labyrinth consisting of the utricle and saccule are connected to the semicircular canals and provide feedback to the brain when the head is not moving. They act as a baseline feedback system.[36]

The cochlea is the portion of the inner ear that processes sound. This structure looks like a snail shell and is approximately 5 mm in height and 9 mm in width. Vibrations from the ossicles of the middle ear are translated into mechanical movement of the stapes within the oval window that compresses the fluid of the inner ear. The sound waves are detected by a variety of hair cells in the organ of Corti of the cochlear depending on the frequency of the sound. These signals are transmitted via the acoustic nerve (cranial VIII) to the cochlear nucleus of the midbrain and then to the auditory cortex of the brain. Each hemisphere of the brain receives impulses from both ears.[37]

Pathological Conditions of the Ear

This section presents common pathological conditions of the ear. Many of these conditions develop or progress as a result of the aging process.

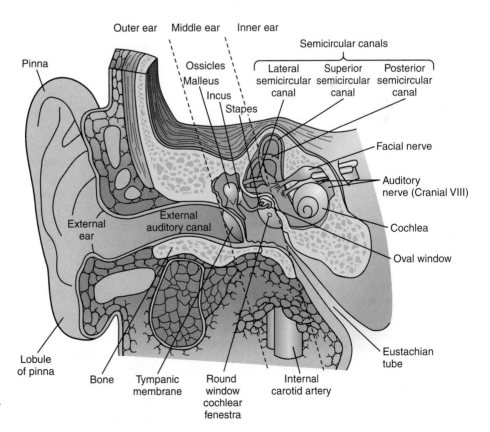

FIGURE 14.4 The internal structures of the ear.

Acoustic Neuroma

An **acoustic neuroma** is a rare, benign (noncancerous) tumor of the eighth cranial nerve located within the internal auditory canal. The tumor is slow growing, and the incidence is 2 in 100,000 people. A specific genetic disorder called **neurofibromatosis (NF2)** causes bilateral acoustic neuromas at an incidence of between 1 in 30,000 and 1 in 50,000 births.[38]

Etiology. The cause of acoustic neuroma is not known. In a few cases, the cause may be genetic.

Signs and Symptoms. The signs and symptoms of acoustic neuroma may be subtle, making diagnosis difficult. The most common signs and symptoms are reduced hearing in the affected ear, a ringing or tinnitus in the ear, a feeling of fullness in the ear, and some problems with balance. In rare incidences, facial numbness may occur as a result of pressure on the trigeminal nerve. Large tumors may press on the brainstem causing headaches, confusion, and increased intracranial pressure.[39]

Prognosis. Large tumors that press on the brainstem may increase the intracranial pressure and become life threatening, but this is rare. Tumors that block the internal auditory canal cause deafness and even with surgical removal there may be hearing loss in the affected ear. Many acoustic neuromas are small and, because they grow slowly, may only cause a reduction in hearing.[40]

Medical Intervention. The diagnosis of acoustic neuroma is usually made with a magnetic resonance imaging (MRI) scan using gadolinium for a contrast medium. An audiogram may be performed to check hearing loss. The treatment for acoustic neuroma may be to monitor the growth of the tumor with periodic scans for small tumors. Microscopic surgical excision through a hole made in the cranium posterior to the mastoid bone may be partial or total. Another option is the use of radiation therapy to shrink or stop the growth of the tumor. A focused radiation is usually performed using a Gamma knife, CyberKnife, or linear accelerator. All these methods of radiation use multiple beams of radiation that intersect at the area of the tumor and do not irradiate the surrounding area.[41]

Physical Therapy Intervention. No physical therapy intervention is indicated for acoustic neuroma. However, people may seek the help of physical therapy if they have balance problems or vertigo, and physical therapy diagnosis may indicate referral to a physician for further medical evaluation.

Benign Paroxysmal Positional Vertigo

Benign paroxysmal positional vertigo (BPPV) is a fairly common vestibular disorder. The prevalence of people having the condition in their lifetime is estimated to be 2.4%. Between 8% and 20% of people who complain of dizziness or vertigo have BPPV, and in older people, the condition is the cause of at least 50% of complaints of dizziness.[42,43]

Etiology. In approximately 50% of people with BPPV, the cause is unknown. Of the other 50%, a head injury, inner-ear infection, or auditory surgery may precipitate the symptoms, or the onset may be associated with migraines. The mechanism of BPPV is associated with a buildup of crystals of calcium carbonate called otoconia or canalith in the inner ear, which becomes lodged in the wrong, semicircular canal, causing incorrect positional information to be transmitted to the brain.[44,45]

Signs and Symptoms. The main signs and symptoms of BPPV are dizziness and vertigo (loss of balance) with a change in position of the head. This occurs most typically when rolling over in bed, getting out of bed, or extending the head posteriorly. Other symptoms may include nausea and vomiting with vertigo.[46] The symptoms of dizziness and vertigo often only last for a minute or less.

Medical Intervention. The diagnosis of BPPV involves hearing tests to rule out other inner-ear disorders because BPPV does not cause hearing loss. An MRI or computed tomography (CT) scan may be performed to rule out possible brain involvement. Electrical recording of involuntary eye movements (nystagmus) with electronystagmography using facial electrodes and the **Dix-Hallpike test** can determine whether the vertigo is likely to be caused by problems with the inner ear or the brain.[47] BPPV may resolve in several weeks without any intervention. The medical management of BPPV may consist of **Brandt-Daroff exercises** or Semont and **Epley maneuvers,** both of which are designed to move the canaliths in the semicircular canals of the inner ear. Medications such as antihistamines or sedatives may also be prescribed to reduce the vestibular symptoms but these medications may prolong the symptoms of vertigo. If people have nausea and vomiting with the vertigo, antiemetic medications may be prescribed.[48]

Physical Therapy Intervention. The details of specific treatment techniques for BPPV are beyond the scope of this book. Physical therapists effectively treat people with BPPV. A full physical evaluation is performed and specific testing for BPPV is undertaken to determine which of the semicircular canals is affected. A positive vertebral artery insufficiency test, extending the head backward in a supine position with rotation that causes dizziness or light headedness, indicates other causes of inner ear problems. The Dix-Hallpike maneuver helps to determine the location of the problem using a series of positions held for 45 seconds each. A variety of techniques may be used to reposition the canaliths within the semicircular canals after a specific diagnosis has been made. These exercises include canalith repositioning exercises also known as the Epley Maneuver,[49] the Liberatory maneuver (also called the Semont maneuver),[50] Brandt-Daroff exercises, and home exercise programs for canalith repositioning. After successful repositioning of the canaliths, patients are instructed to sleep in an upright position for up to the next 48 hours, use two pillows for up to a week, and avoid lying on the affected side or using rapid change of positions to prevent the canaliths from returning to their problem state.[51]

Labyrinthitis and Vestibular Neuritis

Labyrinthitis is an inflammation of the inner ear that may be either bilateral (both ears) or unilateral (one ear). Vestibular neuritis is inflammation of the vestibular nerve. Both of these conditions cause similar signs and symptoms. The incidence of labyrinthitis is approximately 1 in 10,000 people and occurs most frequently in people between the ages of 30 and 60.

Etiology. Labyrinthitis can be caused by either viral or bacterial infections. More frequently the cause is viral. These infections may be localized to the inner ear or result from systemic infections. Some of the bacteria responsible for labyrinthitis include *Streptococcus*, *Staphylococcus*, and *Haemophilus influenzae*. In many cases, labyrinthitis and vestibular neuritis follow an upper respiratory tract viral infection. Some of the causative viruses for these conditions include cytomegalovirus, varicella zoster, rubeola, rubella, and influenza. A specific type of labyrinthitis called herpes zoster oticus or Ramsay-Hunt syndrome is caused by a reoccurrence of the herpes zoster virus several years after initial infection.[52]

Signs and Symptoms. Viral labyrinthitis causes a sudden loss of hearing with vertigo and often nausea and vomiting. Nystagmus of the eyes (rapid involuntary eye movement) may also be present. People with herpes zoster oticus also experience weakness of the facial muscles and have pain and a rash in the outer ear and external auditory canal. In vestibular neuritis, the symptoms are sudden vertigo without hearing loss.[53]

Prognosis. The symptoms of vertigo, nausea, and vomiting resolve after appropriate treatment. However, some hearing loss may be permanent, especially for people who have bacterial infections.

Medical Intervention. The diagnosis of labyrinthitis may be difficult if the cause is viral. A sample of the cerebrospinal fluid may be taken if the physician suspects the person has meningitis. Other tests include a complete blood count (CBC) for detection of possible bacterial infection, audiography to determine hearing loss, vestibular testing for the presence of nystagmus, and an MRI scan specifically focused on the inner ear.[54] The usual treatment for people with viral labyrinthitis is bed rest and plenty of fluids. Anti-inflammatory medications such as steroids help to reduce the risk of edema in the inner ear, antihistamines reduce vertigo symptoms, and antiemetics reduce nausea and vomiting. Some physicians may prescribe antiviral medications. Bacterial labyrinthitis is treated with antimicrobial medications specific to the infective organism.[55]

Physical Therapy Intervention. No physical therapy intervention is indicated for viral or bacterial labyrinthitis or vestibular neuritis unless people have problems with balance after resolution of the infection. Balance exercises and vestibular exercises can be helpful if the problem persists.

Ménière's Disease

Ménière's disease is a disorder of the inner ear that affects approximately 0.2% of the population. The condition usually starts with unilateral involvement and may progress to become bilateral over a number of years.[56]

Etiology. The specific cause of the disease in most cases is not known. The symptoms arise as a result of blockage of the endolymphatic duct of the ear (the drainage system of the ear) and a subsequent buildup of fluid in the inner ear. Some of the causes are thought to be viral infections, head injuries, and allergic reactions; in some cases, a link to genetic factors is thought to be responsible.[57]

Signs and Symptoms. The signs and symptoms of the disease appear suddenly lasting for up to several hours and tend to reoccur. Some people have episodes every few days, whereas others only experience problems occasionally. The main symptoms are dizziness, vertigo with loss of balance, intermittent hearing loss, and pressure and pain in the affected ear.[58] People with severe disease may experience sudden falls, also called drop attacks or "otolithic crisis of Tumarkin," which may result in injury. During these episodes, people feel they are tilted and make corrections in their balance, which result in falls.[59] A side effect of the disease is neck stiffness created by people trying to stabilize the body against the effects of vertigo.

Prognosis. Ménière's disease is not curable but can be managed with the use of medications and diet.

Medical Intervention. The diagnostic tests used for Ménière's disease include the audiometry testing used for other vestibular and hearing problems, electronystagmography (ENG) to measure the nystagmus in the eyes that often accompanies vestibular problems, and a specific test for Ménière's disease called electrocochleography, which is a hearing test that records the electrical responses of the brainstem.[60] The treatment of the disease includes the use of medications such as sedatives, antihistamines, and anti-inflammatories, as previously described for other vestibular conditions. In addition, the use of diuretics may be indicated. A Meniett device that sends pulsed pressure into the external auditory canal may help to reduce symptoms. This can be used at home several times a day. Control of diet seems to help many people. Suggestions include avoidance of excessive salt and sugar, caffeine, monosodium glutamate, and aspirin and NSAIDs that cause fluid retention; limiting alcohol intake; and drinking plenty of fluids. Some of the known migraine-triggering foods such as red wine, smoked meats, and citrus fruits should also be avoided.[61] All of these dietary strategies are thought to help to keep the body fluids in balance and prevent an increase in the fluid pressure within the inner ear that causes the symptoms of Ménière's disease.[62]

Physical Therapy Intervention. People with Ménière's disease may benefit from activities to generally improve the balance so that when they have an episode the effects may not be as severe. Instruction in injury avoidance in case of falls and how to get up off the floor after a fall is also useful. People with neck problems resulting from the condition can also be helped with physical therapy intervention.[63] Vestibular rehabilitation therapy may also be used which involves a combination of balance, head and neck exercises, eye positioning, and body movements to reeducate the vestibular system.[64]

Otosclerosis

Otosclerosis is a hearing disorder affecting the middle ear. Usually the stapes bone is affected. The condition affects approximately 10% of people in the United States, although only 1% of the population has clinical symptoms of deafness caused by the disease.[65,66] Caucasian women over age 30 are most at risk of having the condition.

Etiology. The cause of otosclerosis is not always known. A strong hereditary, autosomal dominant genetic component exists because the incidence of the condition is higher when a family member has the disease. Other causative factors may include viral infections, particularly measles. The pathological cause of the problem is an abnormal growth of bone in the middle ear, usually affecting the stapes bone. The normal vibration of the stapes is affected by the bone growth preventing transmission of sound waves to the inner ear and resulting in deafness.[67]

Signs and Symptoms. Progressive, gradual hearing loss in the affected ear occurs. Occasionally people may experience dizziness, balance problems, and tinnitus (a ringing sound in the ears).

Prognosis. Gradual hearing loss occurs with otosclerosis, but surgery may be able to correct the problem.

Medical Intervention. Diagnosis of otosclerosis is achieved with an audiogram to test hearing sensitivity and a tympanogram to check the ability of the middle ear to conduct sound. A CT scan of the ear may also be used to detect the bone growth. A hearing aid may be supplied to amplify sound and improve hearing. Surgical intervention involves a stapedectomy performed by an otolaryngologist or an otologist. Two types of stapedectomy are possible. In one, the stapes bone is removed and replaced with a prosthetic device to allow the sound waves to bypass the faulty stapes bone and enter the inner ear.[68] In the other type of stapedectomy, a hole is made in the stapes bone, and the prosthesis is inserted into the hole.[69]

Physical Therapy Intervention. Physical therapy intervention may be indicated for people who have balance disorders associated with the otosclerosis.

IMPLICATIONS OF HEARING LOSS FOR PHYSICAL THERAPY INTERVENTION

Loss of hearing has many implications for therapeutic intervention. Patients may become isolated very easily when they are deaf. Hearing aids may not work well, or the batteries may be difficult to replace without fine motor dexterity. When treating a patient who is deaf, the therapist should make sure they are facing the person and demonstrate exercises clearly or write them down. Never speak to the patient and turn away at the same time. Instead of just speaking loudly, the PTA should concentrate on making the voice deeper and lower in tone because most people who are deaf lose the ability to hear upper levels of tones first. Speaking a little more slowly may also help. Because many elderly patients have hearing impairments, the PT and PTA should remember to:

- Speak in a lower tone of voice (high-pitched sounds are often out of the range of hearing)
- Raise the volume of the voice while lowering the tone
- Slow down speech
- Enunciate words clearly and do not mumble
- Do not speak to the patient and walk away at the same time
- Use short sentences
- Demonstrate exercises
- Provide written instructions for exercise home programs in large font type
- Communicate with family/care providers regarding exercise programs and advice

Other Conditions or Disorders Related to Aging

Many older people have several physical and/or psychological complaints. People who have had a cerebrovascular accident (CVA) may already have severe arthritis in the knees and hips that made walking difficult even before they had the CVA. These problems may also be compounded by pulmonary diseases such as asthma, COPD, or other obstructive airways diseases that reduce endurance to activity. Diabetes mellitus is another medical problem that affects many older people that also reduces endurance levels and may reduce the skin sensation in the lower extremities. When working with people who have had a CVA, it is important to bear in mind that other medical problems may be inhibiting progress in functional activities as well as the direct results of the CVA. Sometimes it is difficult for the evaluating physical therapist to gain an adequate medical history of the person without involving other family members. In many cases, no family members are available, and friends are unable to provide adequate information about the medical history of the person. This means that the treating therapist must rely on the physical evaluation for much of the information.

This section looks at the physical therapy interventions for other disorders that are commonly associated with aging. These disorders have been previously described in other chapters, but the focus here is on the significance of these conditions on the older population and the impact on physical therapy interventions.

Amputation

Elderly patients who have an amputation in the lower extremity have some special needs. Because many amputations are performed as a result of diabetes mellitus and other circulatory problems, the healing process is slower than in younger people. Patients must be taught to inspect the skin at the amputation site to ensure there are no pressure areas. Healing must be complete before a fitting can be performed for a prosthesis. After a prosthesis fitting is done and a prosthesis is provided, the skin checks must be continued. The prosthesis may not be worn for prolonged periods to begin with because of the risk of skin break down. It is also important to train patients to check the uninvolved extremity to ensure that the prosthesis is not injuring the other leg.

Arthritis

Statistics from the American Society on Aging indicate that more than 21.4 million older Americans have arthritis and that it is a leading cause of disability among people over age 65.[70] Many older people who are hospitalized for medical conditions also have arthritis. When immobility is enforced on people as a result of illness, the arthritic condition may be exacerbated. Stiffness of joints, pain, and muscle weakness may all occur. This can lead to the loss of independence, reduced mobility, and reduced ability to perform ADLs such as getting in and out of a bathtub or climbing stairs. This makes it important for people to be out of bed as soon as possible. Early intervention by the PT and PTA can greatly improve the long-term rehabilitation of the person. Keeping joints mobile and muscles as strong as possible can make the difference between people being able to return home or entering a nursing home or an assisted living center.

Balance Problems, Falls, and Immobility

Falls and the fear of falling are a very real problem in the over-65 age group. According to the "state of aging and health in America 2007 report," in 2004, falls were the leading cause of injury deaths among older adults, accounting for 14,900 or 43% of all "unintentional injury deaths in this age group" (p. 27).[71] In 2004 (most recent statistics available), more than 1.8 million older Americans were treated for fall injuries in emergency rooms across the country. The rate of falls was 4 to 5 times higher for those people over age 85 than for those between the ages of 65 and 74.[72] In the United States falls in the elderly lead to many accidental deaths, and it is estimated that many of the elderly reduce activity levels due to the fear of falling. Some of the medical problems associated with falls include hip and wrist fractures; however, only a small proportion of those who fall actually sustain a fracture. The risk of fracture is increased in the presence of osteoporosis (see Chapter 5). Estimates are that 60% of women between the ages of 70 and 79, and 84% of women over age 80 have osteoporosis.[73] The risk for falls is increased by multiple factors. According to many studies, neurological performance reduces with age as a direct result of muscle weakness. Because maintaining balance requires moving the line of gravity over the base of support after movement, muscle weakness has a direct effect on the inability to restore this balance. This problem is magnified when climbing stairs or curbs because the person has to balance on one leg longer than when walking. Many people with reduced balance widen their base of support to increase stability as well as slowing down and taking smaller step lengths. In addition to weakness, the general aerobic capacity is reduced in many older people causing reduced endurance to activity. Impaired vision causes reduction in sight, depth perception and the ability to see in three dimensions. If one eye is blind, the depth perception and 3D issues become worse. In addition, sight problems associated with aging tend to affect the night vision. Dark hallways, dimly lit rooms, going from a brightly lit area to one with less lighting, and going outside in the dark all present extra challenges for elderly people. Hearing problems may also be accompanied by vestibular deficits, which increase the risk of falls. If a person needs to get out of bed at night to go to the bathroom, he or she may have reduced balance upon awakening. People should be encouraged to sit on the edge of the bed for a few minutes before standing up so that they can make sure they are awake and get

their balance before walking. Unfamiliar surroundings may further disorient the patient who is slightly confused to begin with and increase the risk of falling. Contributing factors to falls may also include generalized weakness, reduced activity levels, reduced proprioception in the feet due to less activity, reduced kinesthetic and proprioception due to injury, and wearing badly fitting or inappropriate footwear. Many people wear slippers that provide no support for the feet, and if the slippers are too large, they may cause people to trip. The PT and PTA can recommend suitable footwear and try to discourage the use of slippers. Some of the other pathological conditions that increase the risk of falls include Parkinson's disease, dementia including Alzheimer's disease, CVA, vertebral artery insufficiency, which causes dizziness and light-headedness, hypotension, and cardiac diseases. All these conditions can cause a transient loss of balance, dizziness, or light-headedness, resulting in a fall. Ramps are particularly difficult and challenging to balance. Negotiating a ramp requires a good range of motion at the ankle in both dorsiflexion and plantarflexion. Because many older people lose range at the ankle, walking on ramps becomes extremely difficult. Another difficult activity is standing still, which can cause balance difficulties and create edema in the lower extremities as a result of poor circulation. Added to all these factors is the use of multiple medications among older people. In particular, the use of sedatives and antidepressant medications is known to increase the risk of falls.[74]

Physical therapy intervention for helping patients to reduce the risk of falls can include balance reeducation, proprioceptive training, strengthening exercises for the lower extremities with a suitable home exercise program, and use of an assistive device if the patient is able to cope with one. Patients who are very confused do not do well with assistive devices in general because they do not use them correctly and are more likely to fall over the device.

If elderly patients are on bed rest for prolonged periods, they rapidly become weak. Elderly people take considerably longer to return to their prior level of function after prolonged inactivity than younger people. Keeping elderly people immobilized for the minimal necessary time helps to avoid this complication. Some good results for improved balance have been obtained through exercise programs that use concepts of Tai Chi and yoga because these rely on balance and endurance principles. Other interventions are more conservative and include balance exercises such as walking on uneven surfaces, standing and throwing a ball, side-stepping, backward walking, walking in place, high knee stepping, deep knee bends, kicking a ball, and reaching exercises. A controversial activity is teaching patients to get up off the floor so that they will be less fearful of falling. If patients have poor balance, it is probably a good idea to teach this, but sometimes it can increase anxiety levels. The PTA should be aware that adaptations need to be made to exercise programs for elderly patients with balance problems. Sitting exercises for strengthening of the upper and lower extremities and trunk to prepare patients for balance activities may be helpful. Group exercise sessions can assist in developing confidence levels and may be especially helpful for patients with cognitive deficits. The PT and PTA working with the elderly need to be creative, open-minded, and retain respect for the individual patient.

Bowel and Bladder Dysfunction

Bowel and bladder dysfunction is common in both female and male elderly people. As described in Chapter 12, weakness of the pelvic floor musculature is responsible for many cases of incontinence. Various types of incontinence are detailed in Chapter 12. Rectal prolapse is also responsible for some cases of bowel incontinence and may require surgical intervention. Many older people have stress incontinence. This type of incontinence becomes a problem when people cough, sneeze, laugh, or physically exert themselves. Strengthening of the pelvic floor muscles can help to reduce this type of incontinence. Although stress incontinence is not unique to older people and can occur in young people who exercise strenuously, it can be a major source of embarrassment. Physical therapy intervention with biofeedback training for the pelvic floor muscles using a vaginal or rectal electrode and visual display or an insert with a tab that moves when the muscles are contracted correctly can help to increase strength of the pelvic floor muscles and reduce the symptoms. Special weighted vaginal and rectal inserts are available for resisted exercises of the pelvic floor muscles and can be effective in strengthening these muscles and reducing incontinence. In the very sick elderly patient, incontinence can become a problem because of dampness of bed linens, resulting in an environment conducive to skin breakdown. Bed linen must be changed regularly to prevent rubbing of the skin. The use of protective pads and diapers may not be possible because the skin may be too sensitive to tolerate the material of the protective device. The use of indwelling catheters is rarely an option because this can make the patient more susceptible to bladder infections. Bowel incontinence can be a problem for the PT and PTA when treating patients because it can disrupt treatment sessions and embarrass the patient. PTAs must treat people with respect and preserve their dignity if this occurs. Although it may not always be possible to help people clean up, patients should be returned to their room and the nursing staff notified. Setting up a protocol to have patients visit the toilet before PT sessions is helpful in reducing the risk of incontinence incidents. In some cases when bowel and bladder incontinence is an issue, the PT may request a physician order for use of a diaper during PT sessions so that maximal therapeutic effect can be achieved. However, this is only done in extreme cases. Regular scheduled visits to the toilet and appropriate pelvic floor muscle rehabilitation can educate people to manage their condition.

Dementia

Dementia is not a normal part of aging. Many types of dementia exist including senile dementia, vascular dementia (reduced oxygen to the brain), Lewy body dementia associated with the elderly population, and Alzheimer's disease, discussed in Chapter 7. Other causes of dementia include other diseases discussed in Chapter 7, such as Huntington's disease, Creutzfeldt-Jakob disease, brain tumors, Parkinson's disease, endocrine imbalances, infections, and anoxia or hypoxia.[75] Dementia as part of a disease process is a progressive, nonreversible problem that increases in severity over time. The effects of other causes of dementia, confusion states, or delirium such as infections, poisons, endocrine problems, and operable brain tumors may be reversed with treatment. Alzheimer's disease ranks number 7 in the leading causes of death in the United States, and approximately 16% of nursing home residents have the disease.[76] Because more than 5.3 million people are estimated to be affected by Alzheimer's disease in the United States (2009 figures), many elderly people seen by physical therapists and PTAs will have the disease. Approximately 13% of people over age 65 in the United States have Alzheimer's disease, and 14% of people over age 71 have some form of dementia, with prevalence greater in women than men.[77] Many elderly people experience some lapses in recent memory and difficulty retrieving words thought to be part of the normal aging process. Dementia is, however, a progressive condition that makes the person incapable of functioning independently. People with dementia may exhibit times when they have moments of clarity or lucidity and then lapse back into the demented state. Many elderly people suffer from depression, and if this remains undiagnosed and untreated, the person may appear to be confused or demented. In some cases, there are other causes for confused states such as vitamin B_{12} deficiency, adverse reactions to drugs, and thyroid disease. If patients take too many prescription drugs that are not monitored closely, there is a risk of drug interactions that can also cause confusion and depression. Other factors that should not be overlooked in the elderly are the use of alcohol and illicit drugs, which may result in confusion, depression, and suicidal ideation.

The diagnosis of people who are confused is important for the PT. People with transitory confusion resulting from medication reactions or acute pathological conditions must be encouraged to remain active so that they do not become too weak. Some people who are confused tend to wander and may become fatigued. Regular exercise routines help to fatigue muscles and reduce the incidence of aimless wandering. However, people who wander should not be too discouraged by care providers because this wandering maintains their mobility. Many people who live in group homes or assisted living facilities are limited to their access to the outside if they have dementia. If allowed to wander outside they may walk into the road and be in danger. Dementia causes cognitive problems but may also interfere with physical activity levels. People with Alzheimer's disease may become dependent for activities of daily living such as bathing, feeding, and dressing as well as physically inactive. Physical therapy may entail working with the patient to encourage activity levels, work on balance reeducation, strengthening and mobility exercises, and modalities as necessary for pain management. If the cognitive impairment is too great, the PT/PTA may work with the patient in a group setting with general exercises. Preventing a patient from walking around is usually not the answer, unless the patient is at severe risk of falls because it reduces overall mobility levels and may cause anger. When speaking to anyone with dementia, the PT/PTA should use simple short commands and be sure to use the person's name. Advice and education of caregivers is extremely important so that a consistency of approach to people is achieved. People may require assistance with transfers and ambulation and must be supervised when performing exercise programs. Group exercise programs can be helpful with the confused elderly because encouragement from others in the group is beneficial, and no one person is singled out and made to feel he or she is inadequate. Becoming impatient and annoyed with confused people does absolutely no good. Impatience does not facilitate a therapeutic response, nor does it help the patient to become more functional. Although it is not possible to help all patients, many elderly confused people will respond to gently persistent, repetitive exercise programs.

Other considerations when working with people who are confused entail the use of assistive devices for ambulation. Although some people may require assistive devices for safety, the cognitive level of the person must be considered. Many people with dementia carry around the assistive device rather than using it correctly. An alternative may be to install railings along corridors of the home or assisted living facility, in bathrooms, and around the bed area and to ensure railings exist on both sides of stairs. Another factor is that providing an assistive device to people who are confused and possibly lose their temper easily is to place a weapon in their hands! The safety of the person must be tempered by the knowledge of the cognitive abilities to use an assistive device effectively.

Diabetes Mellitus

Elderly people with diabetes must be particularly careful to avoid trauma and pressure to their lower extremities. Because diabetes causes polyneuropathy and reduced circulatory function, especially in the lower extremities, patients with the disease are at a high risk for skin breakdown and pressure ulcers. These patients should be taught how to do a daily self-inspection of the feet and lower extremities with use of a long-handled mirror when necessary. They should also be advised to see a podiatrist or other foot care specialist to have their toenails cut to avoid trauma to the toes, which could become infected. Shoes should be well fitting with plenty of depth at the toes to allow unrestricted movement and prevent rubbing. Shoes should also be inspected before putting feet into them to ensure nothing has fallen into the shoe that could rub the foot. Many patients are unable to feel pressure on their feet because of polyneuropathy, and by the time they take their shoes off, the damage has been done. Some patients with poor sensation may get their feet too close to a heat source and sustain a burn. As patients with diabetes get older and more immobile, the risks of skin breakdown become greater and the ability to do self-checks diminishes, requiring the intervention of a care provider.

Malnutrition

Poor nutritional status in the elderly can precipitate disease and reduce the ability to fight off disease. Some of the normal effects of aging may interfere with people's ability to eat a healthy diet. The overall reduction in sensory abilities such as changes in taste, smell, and vision may have the effect of making food unpalatable or tasteless. Vision problems may interfere with the ability to cook food. The loss of teeth can cause a change in the type of diet chosen to enable people to eat without a lot of chewing. The aging effects on the digestive system may include reduced absorption of minerals and vitamins through the wall of the intestines and reductions in peristaltic muscle action, causing changes in bowel function. All of these changes can result in a reduced nutritional status of elderly patients. Reduced levels of nutrition affect all body systems and can increase the incidence of disease. If a chronic disease process is added to the normal effects of aging, the resulting reduction in nutritional status may be amplified. A person with dementia may forget to eat, or someone with severe arthritis may not be able to get to the shops to buy food. Some patients may have diseases caused by the direct effects of a reduced nutritional status. Such diseases include osteoporosis, heart disease, and diabetes mellitus. However, it cannot be emphasized sufficiently that all body systems rely on adequate nutrition including the muscles and that reduced nutrition will have an effect on the whole body. Some physicians now prescribe a multivitamin supplement for all older patients in an attempt to ensure the adequate presence of vitamins and minerals for body functions. (Refer to Table 9-8 for dietary daily intake of vitamins and minerals and Table 9-9 for vitamin functions and deficiencies.) One of the myths of aging was that older people did not need as much vitamin and mineral intake as younger people. Overall, it has been shown that the elderly require approximately the same amount of vitamins and minerals as people in their middle years. An additional factor is the use of medications by the elderly. Both over-the-counter and prescription medications can interfere with the absorption of nutrients by the intestinal tract or cause increased elimination of nutrients though the bowel and bladder. Alcohol intake can also be detrimental to the elderly, especially if alcohol replaces a balanced diet.

Malnutrition in the elderly population is not just the result of reduced food, vitamin, and mineral intake but also due to the level of absorption of these substances and distribution to body cells, tissues and organs. Many factors can contribute to malnutrition and malabsorption. Some of these are weight changes due to thyroid dysfunction, reduced ability to fight off infection due to the immunological deficiencies of aging, and impaired circulation that is unable to deliver nutrients to body structures. Other contributing factors to malnutrition include the following:

- Poor oral function with loss of teeth and inability to chew food or eat solid food (The bone loss due to aging affects the mandible resulting in loosening of teeth, and gum disease causes loss of teeth.)
- Swallowing disorders are common in the elderly, with esophageal reflux one of the main culprits
- Alcoholism in which patients spend money on alcohol rather than food

- Addiction to smoking when people spend money on cigarettes rather than food
- Severe depression or loneliness causing lack of desire to eat
- Loss of the functional ability to cook and prepare food
- Loss or reduction of sensory functions such as smell and taste, which normally stimulate appetite (Some of this is the normal response of aging, and some is due to illness.)
- Inability to eat sufficient food due to feelings of being full very rapidly
- Poverty causing inability to purchase sufficient food (Some elderly patients may have to choose between buying an expensive medication and buying food.)
- Medications causing a reduction in appetite or a reduction in the ability to absorb nutrients from food (Taking diuretic drugs to stimulate fluid output can increase the excretion of potassium, and thus more potassium needs to be taken in the diet. Taking antacids on a regular basis can reduce the production of acid within the stomach and in turn cause malabsorption of calcium, iron, and vitamin B_{12}. Many elderly patients take more than three prescription medications, which in turn can affect the appetite.)
- Diseases such as cancer or infections that prevent the body absorbing nutrients

Parkinson's Disease

The movement and behavior dysfunctions associated with Parkinson's disease impact people's independence. (Refer to Chapter 7 for more information regarding Parkinson's disease.) Many people with Parkinson's disease attend the physical therapy clinic. The characteristic "pill rolling" resting tremor of Parkinson's, in which the thumb constantly rolls across the fingers, can be disturbing to many people, even though in many instances, the tremor is reduced or absent when performing specific tasks. The cogwheel rigidity of the muscles can make ordinary, everyday tasks, such as reaching into cupboards or cleaning the house, difficult. The bradykinesia (slowness of movement) and akinesia (inability to move) create challenges for ADL. The shuffling gait, muscle rigidity, and the retropulsion (leaning backward) make ambulation more difficult and often result in falls because people are unable to pick up their feet to clear obstacles or walk on uneven surfaces. The usual aging process involving reduced balance is thus further affected by the Parkinson disease process. The masklike face caused by muscle rigidity prevents people from showing emotion and can cause social isolation. Eating can be made difficult by poor control of the muscles of mastication, and swallowing may be affected. Speech can also be affected and make people unable to communicate effectively. In addition to all these motor deficits, many people who are in the later stages of Parkinson's disease have cognitive impairments. When coupled with the memory problems associated with aging, these cognitive impairments can create a need for constant care or admission to a nursing home facility. The role of physical therapy is to help people maintain and improve independent function for as long as possible. Many people with Parkinson's disease manage to remain in their own homes despite considerable physical and mental limitations.

Pressure Ulcers

Approximately 20% of patients who develop pressure ulcers do so at home. The presence of pressure ulcers in patients has a direct impact on the length of hospital stays, increasing them up to 5 times as long as would normally be necessary. Patients at risk for pressure ulcers are also at risk for nosocomial infections, and thus keeping them in hospital longer for management of pressure ulcers increases the risk of them developing a nosocomial infection. The financial cost for treating pressure ulcers is huge; estimates put the price at several billion dollars per year in the United States. One of the keys to prevention of pressure ulcers is good skin care and nursing care. Regular turning of patients to prevent prolonged periods of pressure on bony areas reduces the risk of developing pressure ulcers. Control of incontinence and regular changing of bed linens to keep patients dry is essential in the overall management of elderly, immobile people. Patients should be checked regularly to ensure they do not have areas of skin that are red and showing signs of trauma. When moving people in the bed, care should be taken not to drag their skin across the bed because this can cause a shearing force on the skin that leads to skin breakdown. A patient's position in bed should be checked frequently to ensure there is no sliding down the bed, which could cause a shearing force on the skin overlying the sacrum. If the bed is wet, the skin becomes wet, and the effects of dragging or sliding down the bed are amplified. The presence of infection in patients appears to also increase the risk of developing pressure ulcers. Many nursing homes and hospitals and even home health situations may use waterbeds, egg-crate mattresses, or special air mattresses to prevent skin breakdown. Prevention of pressure areas is much easier than having to treat pressure ulcers. Healing of pressure ulcers takes time and resources, and they are uncomfortable for the patient. (Refer to Chapter 1 for healing of pressure ulcers.) In some people who are extremely debilitated and sick, prevention of pressure ulcers may not be possible. In these individuals, the skin is so fragile that it tears and breaks down easily. Despite taking every precaution to prevent skin breakdown, the skin may not be able to tolerate even 15 minutes of pressure. In many cases, pressure ulcers in these people will not fully heal because of poor nutritional status and illness. Patients with diabetes mellitus are particularly at risk for pressure ulcers as a result of the effects of the disease and poor circulatory and nutritional status.

The role of the PT and PTA in management and prevention of pressure ulcers can be extensive. The PT and PTA should:

- Teach wheelchair and bed positioning to the patient and care providers to minimize pressure
- Ensure a pressure-relieving cushion is placed in the wheelchair for those patients who spend a lot of time in the chair
- Teach patients how to relieve pressure on bony prominences while sitting in a chair for prolonged periods by shifting weight and changing position
- Teach care providers how to assist the patient with position change
- Teach patients and care providers how to use heel supports and other pressure-relieving devices
- Be aware of patient positioning after physical therapy intervention
- Participate on the wound-care team
- Provide physical therapy intervention for wound care as needed and prescribed

Terminal Illness

Working with the dying patient can be both challenging and rewarding. The PT and PTA have to be emotionally prepared to deal with death as a part of life and not become too depressed while maintaining objectivity and the ability to assist the patient and family through a difficult time. Most elderly patients die as a result of chronic illness rather than traumatic injury. Although many people die in hospitals and nursing homes, there is a trend toward allowing people to die at home in the company of their loved ones and with the assistance of hospice programs that provide help from nurses and other health care personnel. Hospice programs allow patients to die with dignity and respect without the encumbrance of multiple machines to maintain life support. The patient may be cared for at home or in a hospice facility. In most cases, to be eligible for hospice care, the physician has to certify that the patient has less than 6 months left to live. Hospice workers such as nurses, social workers, and occupational and physical therapists may assist the family with day-to-day care of the patient. The five Kübler-Ross stages of dying include denial and isolation, anger, bargaining, depression, and acceptance. These stages represent the feelings that a dying person may go through, but each person may not go through all stages or in this order. Thoughts on dying will vary depending on the spiritual beliefs of the patient, cultural beliefs regarding death and the dying process, and family relationships and individual situations.

The role of the PT and PTA with the dying patient may be as a member of the hospice team or as an individual therapist when hospice is not involved. Goals of treatment are to enhance the quality of life as much as possible and to assist the care providers with functional activities and reducing discomfort for the patient. Intervention may include assistance with bed mobility exercises, range of motion and strengthening exercises, transfers including the use of a mechanical lift to reduce stress for patient and care providers, ambulation, and a home exercise program to maintain activity levels as long as possible to ensure quality of life.

End-of-life decisions regarding how and where people wish to die if they have a choice are important. These choices need to be made when people are able to be objective and under discussion with the rest of the family. A living will or a durable power of attorney signed while people are well and able to make decisions can be helpful for the family and the person. These documents can state specific information about whether the person wishes to be placed on life support and under what circumstances. If the person only wishes to be placed on life-support machines if there is a good chance of survival and good quality of life, this can be specified. Specific information can be provided pertaining to artificial feeding, respiratory support, and blood transfusions. The documents release the family from making decisions at times that are stressful and difficult for all concerned. When patients enter a hospital or nursing facility, they are required to sign a document indicating whether they want to be "No Code." This means that they would not be placed on life support or resuscitated in circumstances of cardiac arrest or other life-threatening situations. Patients are also offered a copy of a living will or durable power of attorney to complete. Many families are torn apart because they cannot agree on the action to be taken whether to place a relative on life support and when to remove them from the support. Signing a living will or durable power of attorney form reduces this conflict and helps the physician and family to make a decision that follows the patient's wishes.

Special Issues Related to Geriatric Patients

The physical therapist assistant must be aware of two issues that are unique when assisting geriatric patients. These include elder abuse and the use of restraints and restraint alternatives.

Elder Abuse

Elder abuse is unfortunately a common problem in the United States and throughout other parts of the world. This can take place in a person's own home or within a hospital, nursing home, or the community. State laws exist for the protection of elderly people from abuse. Any situation that places an elderly person at risk of harm is classified as abuse. Several aspects of abuse are recognized. The most direct is that which results in physical, sexual, or emotional abuse of the elderly person. Neglecting or deserting an elderly person by his or her care provider is another type of abuse. The taking of money or property belonging to an elderly person is also classified as elder abuse.[78]

More than 2.1 million older Americans are victims of elder abuse every year, and this estimate is thought to be grossly underestimated. This abuse is most common within families precipitated by stressful changes in living conditions that can create an environment that leads to abuse. The abuse may be inadvertent. Warning signs of elder abuse are similar to those for other types of abuse. Unexplained bruising on arms and neck may be cause for concern, although elderly people do tend to bruise easily. Signs of marks on wrists and ankles that may indicate the use of ropes or chains to tie people down may be noted. Repetitive, unexplained injuries of the elderly person, with reluctance on the part of the care provider to take the person to the emergency room may also indicate a problem. Sometimes people will be very thirsty or hungry, show signs of severe weight loss, or suddenly develop pressure ulcers. Abuse may come from family members, care providers, home health aides, or cleaning staff. Many instances of elder abuse are unintentional.[79] In some cases, the abuse is a continuation of an abusive relationship that has existed for many years within the family.

The prevention of elder abuse can be improved with education programs to raise awareness of the problem. Many health care providers are not aware of the extent of elder abuse and unable to recognize the warning signs.[80] The use of respite care can help to alleviate stress. The ability of care providers to go out for a few hours or the elderly person to be admitted to a home for a short time to allow family to go on vacation can reduce stress to a manageable level. Day-care centers for the elderly within the community can provide socialization for the person as well as respite for the care providers. The National Center on Elder Abuse section of the Administration of Aging can be contacted with suspected cases of elder abuse, or people can call 911.[81] The main thing for PTAs to remember is that all people deserve to be treated with respect, and if they suspect abuse is occurring, they need to talk to the physical therapist, physician, or health care social worker about the problem. If a person is in immediate danger, 911 should be called.

RESTRAINTS AND RESTRAINT ALTERNATIVES

The use of restraints, particularly in the hospital and nursing home settings, has long been controversial. The Omnibus Budget Reconciliation Act (OBRA) of 1987 states, "a patient has the right to be free from any physical or chemical restraints imposed for purposes of discipline or convenience, and not required to treat the resident's medical symptoms." Physicians have to sign an order stating that the restraint is necessary for medical management of the patient and has to update the order regularly. People cannot be restrained just because they may be in danger of falling and thus need to be strapped into the wheelchair or bed. A restraint can be defined as a device that is unable to be removed by the patient. If a strap is used to tie a person into a wheelchair and it is fastened behind the chair out of reach of the patient, this would be a restraint. If the strap had a Velcro closure or buckle that fastened in the front and could be released by the patient, this would be considered a restraint alternative. Restraint alternatives may be very helpful in providing good positioning and safety for patients and acting as a reminder to be careful when they get up out of a chair. Consideration always has to be given to the danger of a fall versus the dangers of imposed immobility on a person. By law, any restraint has to be the least restrictive possible and only used in specific conditions in which a person is at severe risk and no alternative is possible. Restraints have been responsible for serious accidents to residents and patients in nursing home and long-term care facilities. In addition, the psychological reactions to being tied down are detrimental to patients. Some helpful restraint alternatives include the following:

- Using a wedge-shaped cushion in the chair to improve posture and prevent patients sliding forward in the chair

- Using alarm systems that can be attached to beds, so that if patients get out of bed, the alarm goes off to alert staff
- Ensuring beds are low enough to the ground to allow safe, independent transfers
- Using half bed rails rather than full rails to enable patients to get out of bed without getting tangled in bed rails
- Locking outside doors of buildings
- Using rails along the walls of corridors to assist with balance

In many nursing homes and residential care facilities, various strategies must be used to ensure the safety of residents. Some confused and disoriented patients tend to wander constantly and may be at risk of falls. Such patients may become fatigued and unable to determine when they require a rest. In cases in which residents wander through corridors, the staff should ensure that the halls are clear of objects that may cause patients to trip. Loose rugs should be removed from corridors or rooms because these tend to cause people to trip. Strategically placed chairs in corridors can provide resting places for patients. The use of restraints for patients who wander is unacceptable because enforced immobility may cause permanent immobility and reduction in functional walking and transfers. Regular group exercises for people who wander constantly can reduce the incidence of wandering and falling. Providing a structured environment with exercise can help to fatigue the patient while strengthening muscles for increased functional activity and increasing and maintaining joint mobility.

In the home setting, advice on the environment to increase the safety of patients and reduce the risk of falls is essential. Maintaining a balance between suggesting that all loose rugs are removed and clutter is kept to a minimum, and being cognizant of the feelings of the home owners is always difficult. Many elderly people become protective of their environment and do not want to take up rugs. People may remove rugs when the therapist is in the home and put them back down again when the therapist has left. Also when suggesting strategies for improving sitting balance and safety, some families may not wish to comply with recommendations because they are frightened that the patient may fall. A large, deep, low chair may be difficult for the patient to get out of independently, and that may be exactly how the family wishes it to remain because they are worried that if the patient is independent, falls are more likely. In all settings, there is a fine line between independence and the risk of falls, and we must be careful not to be overprotective because this reduces independence and mobility.

CASE STUDY 14.1

An 89-year-old patient with multiple diagnoses is a resident in a nursing home to which the PTA is assigned. The patient's diagnoses include dementia, COPD, CHF, long-standing diabetes mellitus, and a recent fall in which she sustained extensive bruising of the right hip but no fracture. The fall occurred when the patient rose from her chair to go to the bathroom and she lost balance. The patient has physician orders for physical therapy to work on ambulation training, with no restrictions for weight bearing and balance reeducation to try and minimize future falls. The PT has evaluated the patient and determined that the patient has poor balance, general lower extremity strength of 3+/5, and range of motion that is within normal limits in all extremities. The patient is able to follow simple commands and is cooperative. She has low endurance to activity and becomes short of breath if she walks more than 50 feet. The PT states that the patient is at risk for further falls. The patient does not currently use any ambulatory assistive device. The PT plan of care includes ambulation with or without an assistive device, transfer training, balance activities to improve standing and walking balance,

and general lower extremity strengthening exercises. Therapy is to be performed twice daily with plenty of rest periods to ensure the patient is not overfatigued. The PTA is designated to perform the day-to-day treatment of the patient in the nursing home.

1. Discuss how to communicate with the patient so that she understands commands.

2. Discuss whether use of an assistive device is a good idea considering the patient's level of dementia.

3. What assistive device might be suitable for this patient and why?

4. Develop a balance exercise program for the patient.

5. Develop strategies for teaching the care providers how to ensure the patient wears shoes during ambulation.

6. Describe whether a restraint alternative could be an option for this patient and if so, what type.

7. Because of the patient's multiple diagnoses, what particular precautions would the PTA need to take when treating this patient?

STUDY QUESTIONS

1. Describe two specific characteristics of Alzheimer's disease that set it apart from other types of dementia.

2. Describe some of the physiological effects of aging.

3. Describe some of the psychological effects of aging.

4. List four conditions of impaired vision in the elderly.

5. Describe how to help a person with impaired vision reduce the risk of falls in the home setting.

6. Discuss how to prepare the nursing home setting for patients who have dementia and tend to wander the corridors all day.

7. Prepare a group activity class for patients in a nursing home to include range of motion exercises and lower and upper extremity strengthening exercises (consult an exercise book for assistance with this task).

8. Define a restraint and a restraint alternative.

9. A patient who is at high risk for falls is strapped into her chair with a strap that fastens behind the chair,

and she is unable to undo the strap herself. The patient is cognitively alert.
   a. What type of device is the strap?
   b. Describe how this device could be altered.
   c. Discuss the implications for use of such a device.

10. List five reasons for reduced nutritional status in an elderly person.

11. What are the skin changes that occur due to aging?

12. Describe risk factors for skin breakdown in the elderly immobile patient.

13. List three strategies to reduce the risk of pressure ulcers in a nursing home.

14. What are the five Kübler-Ross stages of dying?

15. Describe how the PTA might be involved in treatment of the dying patient.

⬤ USEFUL WEB SITES

Acoustic Neuroma Association
http://www.acausa.org

Administration on Aging
http://www.aoa.gov

Alzheimer's Association
http://www.alz.org

American Hearing Research Foundation
http://www.american-hearing.org

American Optometric Association
http://www.aoa.org

The Foundation of the American Academy of Ophthalmology
http://www.eyecareamerica.org

Glaucoma Research Foundation
http://www.glaucoma.org

National Center on Elder Abuse
http://www.ncea.aoa.gov

National Eye Institute
http://www.nei.nih.gov

National Institute on Deafness and Other Communication Disorders
http://www.nidcd.nih.gov

Vestibular Disorders Association
http://www.vestibular.org

⬤ REFERENCES

[1] Centers for Disease Control and Prevention and the Merck Company Foundation. (2007). *The state of aging and health in America 2007 report.* Whitehouse Station, NJ: The Merck Company Foundation.

[2] Centers for Disease Control and Prevention. (2007). *Births and natality.* Retrieved 11.20.10 from http://www.cdc.gov/nchs/fastats/births.htm

[3] Centers for Disease Control and Prevention. (2007). *Faststats: deaths and mortality.* Retrieved 11.20.10 from http://www.cdc.gov/nchs/fastats/deaths.htm

[4] Federal Interagency Forum on Aging Related Statistics. (2009). *Prepublication version: data sources on older Americans 2008.* Retrieved 4.6.10 from http://www.agingstats.gov/agingstatsdotnet/main_site/Announcements/documents/Pre-Publication_Version_Data_Sources_on_Older_Americans_2008.pdf

[5] Centers for Disease Control and Prevention and the Merck Company Foundation. Ibid., p. 29.

[6] Mayo Clinic Staff. (2010). *Eye floaters.* Retrieved 11.19.10 from http://www.mayoclinic.com/health/eye-floaters/ds01036

[7] Szaflarski, D. M. (2009). How we see: the first steps of human vision. *Access Excellence Classic Collection.* Retrieved 4.4.10 from http://www.accessexcellence.org/AE/AEC/CC/vision_background.php

[8] National Eye Institute. (2009). *Photos, images, and videos of eye disorders.* Retrieved 4.4.10 from www.nei.nih.gov/photo/

[9] National Eye Institute. (2009). *Cataract.* Retrieved 4.9.10 from http://www.nei.nih.gov/health/cataract/cataract_facts.asp

[10] Ibid.

[11] Ibid.

[12] Ibid.

[13] National Eye Institute. (2010). *Retinal detachment.* Retrieved 11.20.10 from http://www.nei.nih.gov/health/retinaldetach/index.asp

[14] Ibid.

[15] Ibid.

[16] Glaucoma Research Foundation. (2009). *Glaucoma facts and stats.* Retrieved 5.6.10 from http://www.glaucoma.org/learn/glaucoma_facts.php

[17] American Optometric Association. (2009). *Glaucoma.* Retrieved 6.12.10 from http://www.aoa.org/Glaucoma.xml

[18] Glaucoma. (2010). *MedlinePlus Medical Encyclopedia.* Retrieved 11.20.10 from http://www.nlm.nih.gov/medlineplus/glaucoma.html

[19] American Academy of Ophthalmology. (2004). *Laser iridotomy.* Retrieved 9.9.09 from http://www.medem.com/?q=medlib/article/ZZZXI9SSSEE

[20] Ibid.

[21] Glaucoma Research Foundation. (2009). *Glaucoma diagnostic tests.* Retrieved 4.4.10 from http://www.glaucoma.org/learn/diagnostic_test.php

[22] Ibid.

[23] Glaucoma Research Foundation. (2009). *Glaucoma medications.* Retrieved 3.12.10 from http://www.glaucoma.org/treating/medication.php

[24] The Glaucoma Foundation. (2010). *How glaucoma is treated.* Retrieved 11.19.10 from http://www.glaucomafoundation.org/info_new.php?id=220

[25] The Foundation of the American Academy of Ophthalmology. (2007). *Cyclophotocoagulation.* Retrieved 5.5.09 from http://www.eyecareamerica.org/eyecare/treatment/cyclophotocoagulation/index.cfm

[26] The Foundation of the American Academy of Ophthalmology. (2007). *Glaucoma filtration surgery.* Retrieved 4.9.09 from http://www.eyecareamerica.org/eyecare/treatment/glaucoma-filtration/index.cfm

[27] American Academy of Ophthalmology. (2004). *Laser iridotomy.* Retrieved 5.5.09 from http://www.medem.com/?q=medlib/article/ZZZXI9SSSEE

[28] Cavallerano, A. A., et al. (2004). *Optometric Clinical Practice Guideline: care of the patient with age-related macular degeneration.* American Optometric Association, Consensus Panel on Care of the Patient with Age-related Macular Degeneration, p. 3.

[29] Ibid., p. 8.

[30] Ibid., p. 8–10.

[31] American Optometric Association. (2009). *Age-related Macular degeneration.* Retrieved 4.6.10 from http://www.aoa.org/Macular-Degeneration.xml

[32] Cavallerano, A. A., et al. Ibid., p. 19–20.

[33] Ibid., p. 18.

[34] The middle ear or tympanic cavity. (2000). *Gray's anatomy.* Bartleby.com. Retrieved 4.4.09 from http://education.yahoo.com/reference/gray/subjects/subject/230

[35] The internal ear or labyrinth. (2000). *Gray's anatomy.* Bartleby.com. Retrieved 4.4.09 from http://education.yahoo.com/reference/gray/subjects/subject/232

[36] American Speech-Language-Hearing Association. (2009). *How hearing and balance work.* Retrieved 11.20.10 from http://www.asha.org/zpublic/hearing/How-Our-Balance-System-Works/

[37] Ibid.

[38] Acoustic Neuroma Association. (2008). *What is acoustic neuroma?* Retrieved 9.9.09 from http://www.anausa.org/what_acoustic_neuroma.shtml

39 Acoustic Neuroma Association. (2008). *Symptoms of acoustic neuroma*. Retrieved 9.9.09 from http://www.anausa.org/symptoms.shtml

40 Ibid.

41 Acoustic Neuroma Association. (2008). *Treatment options*. Retrieved 9.9.09 from http://www.anausa.org/treatment_options.shtml

42 Von Brevern, M., et al. (2007). Epidemiology of benign paroxysmal positional vertigo: a population based study. *J Neurol Neurosurg Psychiatry Pract Neurol* 78:663.

43 Vestibular Disorders Association. (2010). *Benign paroxysmal positional vertigo*. Retrieved 11.20.10 from http://www.vestibular.org/zvestibular-disorders/specific-disorders/bppv.php

44 Ibid.

45 Benign paroxysmal positional vertigo. (2008). *WebMD*. Retrieved 11.20.10 from http://www.webmd.com/brain/tc/benign-paroxysmal-positional-vertigo-bppv-topic-overview

46 Benign paroxysmal positional vertigo: symptoms. (2008). *WebMD*. Retrieved 9.9.09 from http://www.webmd.com/brain/tc/benign-paroxysmal-positional-vertigo-bppv-symptoms

47 Benign paroxysmal positional vertigo: exams and tests. (2008). *WebMD*. Retrieved 9.9.09 from http://www.webmd.com/brain/tc/benign-paroxysmal-positional-vertigo-bppv-exams-and-tests

48 Benign paroxysmal positional vertigo: treatment overview. (2008). *WebMD*. Retrieved 9.9.09 from http://www.webmd.com/brain/tc/benign-paroxysmal-positional-vertigo-bppv-treatment-overview

49 Epley, J. M. (1992). The canalith repositioning procedure: for treatment of benign paroxysmal positional vertigo. *J Otolaryngol* 8:151–158.

50 Semont, A., Freyss, G., & Vitte, E. (1989). Benign paroxysmal positional vertigo and provocative maneuvers. *Ann Otolaryngol Chir Cervicofac* 106:473–476.

51 Li, J. C., & Epley, J. (2010). Benign paroxysmal positional vertigo: medication and treatment. *eMedicine from WebMD*. Retrieved 11.20.10 from http://emedicine.medscape.com/article/884261-treatment

52 Boston, M. E., Strasnick, B., & Steinberg, A. R. (2010). Labyrinthitis. *eMedicine from WebMD*. Retrieved 11.20.10 from http://emedicine.medscape.com/article/792691-overview

53 Ibid.

54 Ibid.

55 Ibid.

56 Hain, T. C. (2008). *Ménière's disease*. Retrieved 9.9.09 from http://www.american-hearing.org/disorders/menieres-disease/

57 Ibid.

58 Ménière's disease. (2010). *MedlinePlus Medical Encyclopedia*. Retrieved 11.20.10 from http://www.nlm.nih.gov/medlineplus/menieresdisease.html

59 Hain, T. C. Ménière's disease. Ibid.

60 Hain, T. C. (2004). *Vestibular testing*. Retrieved 11.20.10 from http://www.american-hearing.org/disorders/vestibular-testing/

61 Vestibular Disorders Association. (2010). *Meniere's disease: dietary considerations*. Retrieved 11.20.10 from http://www.vestibular.org/vestibular-disorders/treatment/diet.php

62 Hain, T. C. Ménière's disease. Ibid.

63 Hain, T. C. (2008). Physical therapy for Ménière's disease. *Dizziness and balance.com*. Retrieved 6.4.09 from http://www.dizziness-and-balance.com/treatment/menieresPT.html

64 Vestibular Disorders Association. (2010). Vestibular rehabilitation therapy (VRT). Retrieved 11.20.10 from http://www.vestibular.org/vestibular-disorders/treatment/vestibular-rehab.php

65 Lipkin, A. (2010). Otosclerosis. *MedlinePlus Medical Encyclopedia*. Retrieved 11.20.10 from http://www.nlm.nih.gov/medlineplus/ency/article/001036.htm#top

66 Roland, P. S. (2008). Otosclerosis. *eMedicine from WebMD*. Retrieved 9.9.09 from http://emedicine.medscape.com/article/994891-overview

67 National Institute on Deafness and Other Communication Disorders. (2008). *Otosclerosis*. Retrieved 9.15.10 from http://www.nidcd.nih.gov/health/hearing/otosclerosis.asp

68 Ibid.

69 Roland, P. S. (2008). Otosclerosis: treatment and medication. *eMedicine from WebMD*. Retrieved 9.15.09 from http://emedicine.medscape.com/article/994891-treatment

70 American Society on Aging. (2006) *CDC encourages older adults to use physical activity and self-management to reduce symptoms of arthritis*. Retrieved 9.15.09 from http://www.asaging.org/media/pressrelease.cfm?id=103

71 Centers for Disease Control and Prevention and the Merck Company Foundation. Ibid., p. 27.

72 Ibid., p. 27.

73 Ibid., p. 29.

74 Ibid., p. 29.

75 National Institute of Neurological Disorders and Stroke. (2010). *NINDS dementia information page*. National Institutes of Health. Retrieved 11.20.10 from http://www.ninds.nih.gov/disorders/dementias/dementia.htm

76 Centers for Disease Control and Prevention (2009). *Alzheimer's disease: Faststats*. Retrieved 9.15.10 from http://www.cdc.gov/nchs/fastats/alzheimr.htm

77 Alzheimer's Association. (2009). *2009 Alzheimer's disease facts and figures*. Retrieved 9.15.10 from http://www.alz.org/national/documents/report_alzfactsfigures2009.pdf

78 Elder abuse. (2010). *MedlinePlus*. Retrieved 11.20.10 from http://www.nlm.nih.gov/medlineplus/elderabuse.html

79 American Psychological Association. (2010). Elder abuse and neglect: in search of solutions. Retrieved 11.20.10 from http://www.apa.org/pi/aging/resources/guides/elder-abuse.aspx

80 Halphen, J. M., Varas, G. M., & Sadowsky, J. M. (2009). Recognizing and reporting elder abuse and neglect. *Geriatrics* 64:13–18.

81 National Center on Elder Abuse. (2010). Administration on Aging Web site. Retrieved 11.20.10 from http://www.ncea.aoa.gov/ncearoot/Main_Site/index.aspx

A

Absolute refractory period: a resting period for a neuron (nerve cell) during which nerve impulses cannot be transmitted.

Acoustic neuroma: a slow-growing, benign tumor of the 8th cranial nerve.

Acromegaly: a condition in adults resulting from the effects of disease such as in hyperpituitarism on growth hormone cells. Characteristics include large hands and feet, enlargement of jaw, nose, and tongue, and general changes in facial appearance. It also causes enlargement of internal organs including the heart and can cause hyperglycemia and hypercalcemia.

Acute on chronic inflammation: When an acute inflammatory process is superimposed over an already chronic inflammation. Such as when an ankle is sprained and healing is not complete, a state of chronic inflammation exists. When a further sprain occurs, the inflammatory process starts again, and acute inflammation is added to the already chronic inflammatory state of the ankle.

Addison's disease: a primary adrenal cortex insufficiency disease. Due to a defect within the structure of the adrenal cortex and thought to have an autoimmune component. Can be due to tuberculosis, hemorrhage in the adrenal glands, infections, such as cytomegalovirus, malignancy or may be precipitated by radiation therapy for malignancy.

Addisonian crisis: An acute adrenal insufficiency episode, results in symptoms such as acute pain in the back, abdomen, or lower extremities, severe vomiting and diarrhea, dehydration, severe hypotension, and, in some cases, loss of consciousness.

Adhesions: a form of scar tissue that connects different kinds of structures together which are not normally linked.

Ageism: a term described by Butler to delineate the myths surrounding aging and the resultant attitude of people toward the elderly regarding physical and mental status.

Age-related macular degeneration (Macular degeneration): an eye disease, mainly of people over 50, causing a loss of central vision.

AIDS/HIV: acquired immunodeficiency syndrome caused by an RNA virus known as the Human immunodeficiency virus (HIV)

AIDS dementia complex: a type of dementia specific to patients with AIDS caused by an encephalopathy associated with AIDS. Consists of a recognized group of signs and symptoms associated with advanced AIDS and may include: encephalitis; behavioral changes; meningitis; a reduction in cognitive function; psychological and neuropsychiatric disorders; central nervous system lymphomas; and brain tumors.

Allograft: a graft from another human, usually a cadaver.

All-or-none response: The response of a neuron to stimulation. Each type of neuron has a different threshold level specific to the purpose of the neuron. This initiation of the action potential is all-or-none, meaning that the stimulus is either large enough to exceed the threshold and stimulate an action potential, or it is not.

Anaphylactic shock: a Type1 hypersensitivity (allergic) reaction characterized by swelling of the mucous membranes causing closing of the trachea and bronchi, and hyperemia of the face, upper trunk and upper extremities. May result in death if not adequately managed.

Anasarca: generalized body edema. May be due to cardiac pathologies.

Angiogenesis: development of a new blood supply to an area. Found in areas of malignant tumors. May also form in response to shutting down of a primary blood supply such as in heart disease, creating an alternative source of blood supply to an area.

Ankylosis: bone formation in a non-bony structure.

Antibiotic resistant bacteria: bacteria that have become resistant to antibiotic medications. Commonly occurring resistant-bacteria include methicillin-resistant **Staphylococcus aureus** (MRSA) and vancomycin-resistant **Enterococcus** (VRE).

Antimicrobial: a medict used to fight infection.

Arterial insufficiency ulcers: a major complication of Peripheral Vascular Disease. These ulcers most frequently occur on the lower leg.

Arthritis mutilans: a disabling form of psoriatic arthritis with severe involvement of the joints of hands and feet. Sacroiliitis may be present.

Ascending spinal tracts: channels of sensory neuron axons taking impulses from the sensory nerve endings in the skin and internal organs to the brain through the white matter of the spinal cord.

Ascites: a type of peritonitis caused by chronic liver disease, or right ventricular cardiac failure, in which there is abdominal edema.

Assist control (AC) ventilation: a type of mechanical ventilation machine, which completely controls breathing with the machine programmed at specific settings. Assisted mechanical ventilation provides a specific delivery of oxygen, but the patient can trigger the machine to work.

Atelectasis: a condition of alveolar collapse in the lungs.

Atherosclerosis: also known as arteriosclerosis and in lay terms hardening of the arteries. It is the narrowing of the lumen of arteries due to deposition of plaques on the interior wall of the artery.

Athetosis: slow, writhing, involuntary movements of the limbs.

Auscultation techniques: auscultation is the act of listening to sounds made by the body, particularly sounds of the heart and lungs. A stethoscope is used to listen to the sounds over the trachea and lung.

Autogenic inhibition: A spinal cord reflex that causes inhibition of neurons that prevents muscles contracting. After motor neuron damage in a cerebrovascular accident (CVA) this reflex is responsible for the sudden release of muscle spasticity during passive motion.

Autograft: a graft performed using the patient's own skin.

Autolytic debridement: a form of self-debridement. The wound is covered with an occlusive (sealing) or semi-occlusive dressing that maintains the moisture in the wound and stimulates the white blood cells to destroy the necrotic tissue.

Autonomic neuropathy: a type of neuropathy that may occur in some patients with diabetes, which can cause general bodily problems such as constipation and/or diarrhea, postural hypotension, impotence and bladder emptying difficulties.

Avascular necrosis: necrosis, usually of bone, caused by cutting off the blood supply to the area of bone.

Axonotmesis: damage to nerves caused by prolonged pressure. Results in atrophy of muscles supplied by the nerve and degeneration of the neuronal axon. The neural sheath remains intact. Damage may be temporary or permanent.

B

Bamboo spine: bamboo appearance on x-ray of the spine of a patient with ankylosing spondylitis.

Barium enema: a medical test performed to detect abnormalities in the wall of the colon. An enema preparation with barium content shows up when the area is x-rayed.

Barium swallow: a medical test performed for upper digestive tract disorders. Sometimes called an upper gastrointestinal series (UGI). The patient swallows a barium mixture solution and x-rays are taken as the liquid enters the stomach and the small intestine. A physician can detect irregularities in the contours of the areas outlined by the barium liquid.

Becker's muscular dystrophy (BMD): a type of muscular dystrophy caused by an X-linked recessive chromosomal trait affecting the production of the protein dystrophin, which is responsible for normal muscle function.

Benign paroxysmal positional vertigo (BPPV): a vestibular condition of the inner ear in which change of position causes vertigo.

Bilevel positive airway pressure (BIPAP): These machines are used for people who can breathe on their own but may not be getting sufficient oxygenation of their tissues and need supplementary oxygen. These machines help people to maintain a constant amount of pressure throughout the respiratory cycle and are often used at night by people with sleep apnea. The machine is set for both inhalation and exhalation pressures. People who use the BIPAP machine have to be cognitively aware as a result of the possibility of aspiration of fluids into the lungs.

Blood-brain barrier: a combination of the arachnoid layer of the meninges covering the brain, the blood and cerebrospinal fluid, and the selectively permeable endothelial cell layer of the cerebral capillaries. This barrier prevents the passage of bacteria and medications into the tissues of the brain.

Body Mass Index (BMI): A value considered to be a fairly accurate measurement for determining body fat levels. It is calculated by dividing the body weight measured in kilograms by the height in meters squared.

Bouchard's nodes: a characteristic of osteoarthritis (osteoarthrosis) in which nodules composed of cartilage or bone are found on the proximal interphalangeal joints of the hands. These nodes can be tender.

Boutonnière's deformity: a characteristic deformity of rheumatoid arthritis in which there is flexion of the PIP and hyperextension of the DIP joint of the fingers.

Brandt-Daroff exercises/maneuvers: a system of exercises and maneuvers used to treat benign paroxysmal positional vertigo.

Braxton-Hicks uterine contractions: uterine contractions often experienced throughout pregnancy.

Broad-spectrum antibiotic: a drug used to destroy a wide range of types of bacteria.

Brodmann's area: the motor cortex of the cerebrum in the brain.

Bronchiectasis: dilation of part of a bronchus with infection distal to the dilated portion. Usually caused by a lung abscess draining pus into the bronchi and forming a blockage of the bronchi. Occurs more commonly on the lower lobes of the lungs.

Bronchopneumonia: pneumonia affecting both lungs. Often results from viral interstitial pneumonia.

Bronchopulmonary segments: each lung lobe is divided into bronchopulmonary segments constituting the bronchial tree. There are nine (9) segments in the left lung and ten (10) in the right. (Some sources say there are eight (8) segments in the left lung because they combine the apical and posterior segments of the left upper lobe).

Bursae: sacs that are enclosed and have a small amount of lubricating fluid within them to provide friction reduced movement of structures over one another. They are located wherever a tendon passes over a bone or muscle, a muscle passes over a bone, or a ligament passes over another structure.

C

Calcimimetic medications: molecular agents that reduce the levels of parathyroid hormone release by the parathyroid glands, and reduce the amount of calcium production in primary hyperparathyroidism.

Candidiasis (thrush): a fungal infection normally causing mild symptoms, but can become a severe problem for the patient with AIDS. The fungus can attack the mucous membranes of the mouth, throat, trachea, lungs and genital areas and may be resistant to treatment.

Carcinogenesis: the process of development of a cancerous tumor.

Cardiac output (CO): the amount of blood pumped out by a ventricle in a one-minute period. It is equal to approximately 4900ml. Resting cardiac output is approximately 5 liters per minute expressed in the following equation: CO = SV (Stroke Volume) X HR (Heart Rate) = 70 X 70 = 4900ml

Cardinal signs of inflammation: the four typical tissue reactions to insult or injury. Heat (Latin: *calor*), redness (*rubor*), swelling (*tumor*), and pain (*dolor*) not necessarily in that order.

Cardiomegaly: enlargement of the heart. Usually starts with hypertrophy of the right ventricle.

Cardiomyopathy: a group of diseases affecting the heart in which the myocardium either hypertrophies or dilates. Causes include alcoholism and certain viruses.

Cataract: a condition in which the lens of the eye becomes opaque.

Cellulitis: inflammation in the dermal and subcutaneous layers of the skin.

Cerclage: a suture used in the incompetent cervix to prevent premature delivery or miscarriage of the fetus during pregnancy.

Cesarean section: a surgical procedure used to deliver the fetus from a pregnant woman in cases where a natural delivery is not possible.

Chest excursion: the amount the ribs expand during breathing from maximum inhalation to maximum exhalation. The amount of chest excursion can be measured with a tape measure at various rib levels and compared to future measurements to denote improvement in breathing patterns.

Chlamydia: a sexually transmitted group of parasitic organisms similar to both bacteria and viruses.

Choreiform movements: involuntary body movements associated with Huntington's disease resulting from damage to the basal ganglia.

Chronic inflammatory bowel disease: a group of bowel disorders mostly including Crohn's disease and Ulcerative colitis.

Chronic Myeloid/Myeloblastic Leukemia: a specific type of leukemia due to a genetic abnormality that affects adults 25 to 60.

Chronic obstructive pulmonary disease (COPD): a disease of the lungs such as chronic bronchitis, emphysema, and asthma, which reduces the function of the lungs.

Chyme: the semi liquid breakdown products of digestion.

Cicatrization: healing of an area by scar tissue, which may result in shortening of the scarred structures.

Circle of Willis: a unique system of arterial blood supply to the brain formed by connection between the posterior cerebral artery and the internal carotid artery with the posterior communicating artery.

Clasp-knife effect: sudden release of tone/spasticity during stretching of a muscle.

Clonus: a rapid, intermittent contraction of a muscle in response to a sudden stretch which occurs in upper motor neuron lesions.

Collateral circulation: an alternative set of blood vessels formed when existing blood vessels anastomose. Collateral circulation systems often occur in the heart to provide an alternative supply of blood to heart muscle.

Colonoscopy: a procedure in which a flexible fiberoptic tube is passed via the rectum into the colon and photographs are taken. It is used to detect signs of colon disease including colon cancer.

Complete Blood Count (CBC): a blood test performed to detect the number of red corpuscles and leucocytes per micro liter of whole blood (Taber's 237).

Contact dermatitis (Urticaria or Hives): a skin condition usually resulting from irritation by an external source such as wool, poison ivy or adhesive tape, or internally due to a drug or food allergy, causing a Type 1 hypersensitivity reaction.

Continuous positive airway pressure (CPAP): a type of mechanical ventilation machine used for patients able to perform some ventilation for themselves.

Controlled mechanical ventilation (CMV): a type of mechanical ventilation machine used for a patient unable to perform breathing for themselves, and unable to assist with breathing.

Cor pulmonale: a name given to the condition in which there is hypertrophy of the right ventricle of the heart.

Coronary Care Unit or Cardiac Care Unit (CCU): a specialized unit in a hospital devoted to the care of patients with cardiac diseases.

Corticospinal tract: the main descending motor tract to voluntary muscle in the spinal cord.

Crepitus: a grating noise within the joint due to bone rubbing on bone or cartilage disintegration.

Crohn's disease: a chronic inflammatory bowel disease.

Cushing's disease: a disease characterized by hyper-cortisolism (high levels of cortisol) usually occurring as result of excessive ACTH production by the pituitary, which causes specific effects and characteristics such as "moon face".

Cytomegalovirus (CMV): a virus transmitted through sexual contact, blood products, close personal contact such as in day care centers, through breast milk, or which may be congenital. May cause abnormalities of the fetus if a woman is infected during pregnancy.

D

Debridement: the removal of necrotic tissue in order that the underlying tissue can heal.

Decubitus ulcer: also called a pressure ulcer or sore. A skin defect caused by pressure over a bony prominence, which creates anoxia of the tissues and a break down of the skin.

Deep partial-thickness burn: a burn that destroys the epidermis and damages the dermis down as far as the reticular layer.

Deep tendon reflex: loop reflex within the spinal cord to muscles causing muscles to contract when the tendon is stretched. Also called the stretch reflex.

Dependent edema: edema (swelling) of the legs, ankles and feet evident when the legs are in a dependent (hanging down) position. It is particularly prevalent towards the end of the day when a patient has had the legs in a dependent position for a prolonged period of time.

Dermatome: an area of skin supplied by a specific spinal nerve; an instrument used to remove an area of skin to use as a graft, especially for the treatment of burns; part of the mesoderm of the embryo that develops into the dermis of the skin.

Descending spinal tracts: channels of motor neuron axons taking impulses from the brain to the muscles through white matter of the spinal cord.

Detrusor muscle: s smooth muscle within the wall of the bladder responsible for contracting the bladder to eliminate urine.

Diabetes insipidus: a condition resulting from damage to the posterior pituitary by tumors, trauma to the base of the skull, or infection, causing a reduced production of antidiuretic hormone (ADH) and the production of a lot of urine.

Diabetes mellitus: a chronic metabolic disorder resulting from the lack of production of insulin by the pancreas, or the inability of the body of utilize insulin.

Diabetic neuropathy: a specific type of peripheral neuropathy affecting the lower extremities and occasionally the upper extremities in patients with longstanding diabetes mellitus.

Disuse atrophy: a reduction in size of cells, tissue and organs due to lack of nutrition or reduced usage. Specifically applies to disuse atrophy of muscles seen in physical therapy.

Diverticular disease: a group of diseases characterized by diverticula (pouches) that form within the walls of the intestine where the bands of circular and longitudinal muscles of the wall of the intestine meet to provide passage for blood vessels.

Diverticulitis: a condition caused by inflammation of diverticula (pouches) in the walls of the intestine. Acute attacks can cause severe abdominal pain.

Diverticulosis: the condition of having diverticula (pouches) in the walls of the intestine. There may be no symptoms. May turn into diverticulitis.

Dix-Hallpike test: an observation test for involuntary eye movements used in the assessment of benign paroxysmal positional vertigo.

E

Eburnation: Bone beneath cartilage within a joint that becomes shiny and smooth due to rubbing of bone against bone in an arthritic joint.

Ectopic pregnancy: an implantation of a fertilized ovum somewhere other than the uterus. Most commonly the implantation occurs in the fallopian tube, abdominal cavity or within the ovary itself.

Edema: swelling or tumor.

Electrocardiogram (ECG): a machine that monitors heart rate and rhythm.

Empyema: accumulation of pus in a cavity. Can relate to pus in the space between the pleura of the lungs.

Endarterectomy: the surgical removal and replacement of an artery using a donor vessel. Most often performed on the carotid, femoral or popliteal arteries.

Endogenous opiates: an opiate-like substance produced by the body, which can affect the perception of pain.

Endometriosis: a condition in which endometrial tissue starts to grow in other areas of the internal organs, such as around the ovaries, in the peritoneal cavity, and on the pelvic ligaments.

Endoscopic ultrasound: an ultrasound instrument attached to the end of an endoscope tube. Used in the diagnosis of diseases of internal organs.

Enthesitis: inflammation at the junction of ligaments and bone.

Epinephrine: adrenalin.

Epley maneuver: a maneuver designed to move the canaliths in the semicircular canals of the inner ear for people with benign proxismal positional vertigo.

Epstein-Barr virus (EBV): a virus similar to the herpes virus responsible for a variety of infectious diseases.

Eschar: blackened, thick, necrotic tissue found in a wound.

Escharotomy: surgical removal of eschar from a wound, particularly that of a burn.

Exudative retinal detachment: a retinal detachment in the eye ensuing after trauma to the eye.

Inflammation occurs causing fluid leakage between the retina and the pigment epithelial layer.

F

Felty's syndrome: a serious, sometimes fatal, side effect of rheumatoid arthritis causing splenomegaly (enlargement of the spleen) and leukopenia (reduced white cell count).

Fibrillation: softening, splitting and fragmentation of cartilage within a joint affected by osteoarthritis (osteoarthrosis).

Fibrocystic disease: a disease mainly of the breast in which nodules occur. The nodules may be painful. Also another name for cystic fibrosis, a disease of the pancreas.

First intention healing: healing of a clinical or surgical wound, or of a skin penetrating injury with clear, clean margins that have not become separated, or can be closed using sutures, staples or steristrips. Examples of such wounds might be a knife cut, a paper cut, or a surgical incision.

Forced expiratory volume in one second (FEV1): the volume of air forcibly expired after a maximal inspiration in one second. The FEV1 is normally 80% of the vital capacity (VC). A change in the ratio of VC and FEV1 indicates lung pathology. An FEV1 of 80% of the VC reflects normal, healthy, elastic, lung tissue since it shows that most of the air can be expelled form the lungs quickly.

Full-thickness burn: a burn, which destroys both epidermis and dermis and often the underlying layers of fat tissue.

Full-thickness skin graft: a skin graft that consists of the epidermis and the dermis.

Fusiform-shaped fingers: Also called spindle fingers. A characteristic of rheumatoid arthritis in which effusion in the PIP joint causes fingers to take on the shape of a spindle.

G

Gate Control Theory: a theory of pain utilized to develop PT intervention strategies.

Genu valgus/valgum: a deformity of the knees also called "knock knee".

Genu varum: a deformity of the knees also called "bow legs".

Geriatric medicine: a branch of medicine dedicated to treatment of older people with medical problems.

Geriatric: pertaining to the elderly person, usually over age 65, but often older.

Gerontology: the branch of medicine dedicated to treatment of older people with medical problems.

Gestational diabetes: diabetes that occurs during pregnancy that wa not present before the pregnancy.

Gigantism: a condition in which the long bones grow excessively due to overproduction of growth hormone secondary to hyperpituitarism in the child.

Glaucoma: an acute or non-acute condition of the eye characterized by increased pressure within the eye which can damage the optic nerve and cause severe pain, blurred vision and loss of peripheral vision.

Glomerular filtration rate (GFR): the amount of renal filtrate produced by the kidneys in one minute. Approximately 25% of the blood that enters the glomerulus is turned into renal filtrate. The usual volume is between 100 and 125 milliliters per minute. The rate of GFR is dependent on the blood flow.

Gonadotropin releasing hormone (GnRH): a hormone produced in the hypothalamus, which controls the pituitary gland.

Graded exercise tolerance test (GXTT): a high-level exercise capacity test, or stress test, performed while the patient uses either a treadmill or a cycle ergometer. Used to determine both cardiac and pulmonary status.

Granulation tissue: in an open wound this tissue forms a red dotted effect in the wound bed due to the development of a network of capillaries.

Grave's disease: a hyperthyroid condition due to overproduction of the thyroid hormones.

H

Hallux valgus: a deformity of the great toe also called a bunion.

Hammer toes: a condition of the toes found in cases of arthritis in which the toes are flexed at the distal interphalangeal joints and extended at the metacarpophalangeal joint.

Hantaviruses: hemorrhagic fever caused by inhalation of rodent excreta containing an RNA virus. Several types of hantavirus have been cited in the USA, South America, and parts of Asia.

Heberden's nodes: nodes composed of cartilage or bone found surrounding the distal interphalangeal joints of the hand in osteoarthritis (osteoarthrosis).

Hemarthrosis: bleeding into the joint.

Hemiballismus: flailing movements of one arm or leg associated with subthalamic nucleus damage in the basal ganglia of the brain.

Hemodialysis: removal of waste products from the body in cases of severe kidney failure by use of a machine.

Hemolytic disease of the newborn (HDN): similar to the result of a blood transfusion that is incompatible with the recipient blood type. Occurs in cases where the fetus is positive for rhesus or factor D and the mother is not. The mother develops antibodies to factor D and the next baby born may have hemolytic disease due to the antibodies in the mother attacking the baby's blood.

Hemoptysis: presence of blood in the sputum coughed up from the lungs. May be due to a lesion in the lungs or in the trachea. Blood in the sputum.

Hepatitis B (HBV): a DNA virus transmitted as a blood-borne pathogen through contact with contaminated blood, blood products or through sexual contact. Causes inflammation of the liver. The risk of contracting hepatitis B is extremely high for those with HIV or other immune suppression disorders.

Heterotopic calcification/ossification: the development of bone in areas where it is not normally found, such as in muscles and fascia.

Highly active antiretroviral therapy (HAART): A commonly used combination of medications that both improves the T-cell count, suppresses the replication of the HIV virus, and reduces the incidence of onset of secondary opportunistic infections in people with HIV/AIDS.

HIV/AIDS: Human immunodeficiency virus (HIV) an RNA retrovirus, which causes acquired immunodeficiency syndrome (AIDS).

Homeostasis: Healthy metabolism is characterized by a pH of extracellular fluids between 7.35 and 7.45. The maintenance of this pH is called homeostasis. This state of homeostasis is characterized by optimal functioning of the body.

Human immunodeficiency virus (HIV): an RNA retrovirus, which causes acquired immunodeficiency syndrome (AIDS).

Hydrocephalus: build-up of cerebrospinal fluid in the ventricles of the brain causing increased intracranial pressure and possible damage to brain tissue.

Hypercalcemia: a condition of excessive amounts of calcium in the blood.

Hypercalcuria: a condition of excessive amounts of calcium in the urine.

Hyperglycemia: high levels of glucose in the blood.

Hyperthyroidism: a disease in which the thyroid gland produces too much thyroxine.

Hypertrophic scarring: a scar that is abnormal in appearance, projects beyond the surface of the skin, and may be unsightly. Unlike keloid scarring the hypertrophic scar remains within the boundary of the original wound.

Hyperuricemia: a high level of uric acid in the blood.

Hypotonia: low muscle tone. Also refers to relaxation of the arteries.

I

Icterus (Jaundice): a liver disease characterized by yellowing of the skin and whites of the eyes due to hyperbilirubinemia.

Immune complex reaction: a Type III hypersensitivity reaction.

Immunoglobulins: antibodies. The five types are: IgA, IgD, IgE, IgG, and IgM.

Incompetent cervix: a weak, dilated cervix that can cause premature effacement and labor leading to a premature delivery of the fetus.

Increased intracranial pressure (ICP): an increase in pressure beneath the skull that can cause brain damage since the pressure cannot release. Occurs mainly after closed head injury.

Indwelling catheter/Foley catheter: a catheter that remains in place in the bladder, vein or artery. In PT practice usually pertains to a urinary catheter.

Inflammatory bowel disease (IBD): a generic term for diseases that are characterized by inflammation of the bowel including Crohn's disease and ulcerative colitis.

Inguinal hernia: a herniation of the intestine through the inguinal canal which can cause an obstruction the intestines.

Inosculation: the process of capillaries penetrating a skin graft as part of the healing process.

Intensivist: a physician who specializes in working on the intensive care unit.

Intermittent claudication: a symptom of arterial disease that can be associated with cardiac conditions. This condition occurs most often as a result of disease in the popliteal artery and causes severe pain in the calf during walking activities, exercise, or prolonged standing.

Intermittent pneumatic compression pump/ external sequential compression device: a compression device attached to plastic sleeves placed over the lower extremities. The pressure sleeve acts as an external pump for the venous system to stimulate the circulation at a time when patients are not using the muscles sufficiently. The external pumping device helps to reduce swelling and minimize the possibility of a deep venous thrombosis (DVT) developing by increasing te velocity of the peak venous flow of blood and the volume of blood pumped by the veins.

Intracranial pressure: the pressure within the skull. Monitored in cases of head injury to ensure it does not rise above 20 mm Hg since this can result in severe brain damage.

Intravenous pyelogram (IVP): a radiological test performed by injecting dye into the blood highlighting the urinary tract so that an x-ray can detect any obstruction or abnormality.

Intrinsic PEEP/Auto PEEP: People with respiratory conditions often have airways that are blocked with secretions or spasm of the bronchi, resulting in the incomplete emptying of the alveoli. This end-expiratory pressure may be higher than that of the atmosphere. This condition of positive end-expiratory pressure is known as intrinsic PEEP or auto PEEP.

Irritable bowel syndrome: a non-specific condition that is associated with bouts of alternating diarrhea and constipation, and abdominal pain.

Ischemia: lack of blood supply to an area of tissue or part of an organ that can lead to necrosis.

J

Jaundice (Icterus): a liver disease characterized by yellowing of the skin and whites of the eyes due to hyperbilirubinemia.

K

Keloid: an often unsightly raised area of scar tissue on the skin resulting from the formation of excessive amounts of granulation tissue and, thus, too much collagen.

L

Leiomyomas: common benign tumor of the uterus.

M

Macular degeneration/Age related macular degeneration: an eye disease, mainly of people over 50, causing a loss of central vision.

Malar (butterfly) rash: a butterfly shaped rash on the face located across the bridge of the nose and onto the heeks on both sides of the face. Typically found in patients with systemic lupus erythematosus.

Meningocele: a spinal defect seen in spina bifida in which the meninges (coverings of the brain and spinal cord) protrude through the defect in the vertebra and the skin.

Metabolic equivalent (MET): the data provided by a graded exercise tolerance test (GXTT) is in metabolic equivalent (MET). One MET is the amount of oxygen required with the body at rest in a sitting position. Each MET is equal to about 3.5 milliliters/ Kg/minute.

Micturition: passing urine.

Motor unit: a motor neuron and the muscle fibers it innervates.

Multigravida: a woman who has been pregnant more than once.

Multipara: a woman who has delivered more than one viable fetus.

Myelomeningocele: a form of spina bifida in which both the meninges and spinal cord protrude through a defect in the spine.

Myoclonus: involuntary twitching and spasm of muscles.

Myofascial pain syndrome: a condition of muscle pain characterized by the presence of trigger points in the muscle. When palpated, trigger points can transmit pain to distal areas resulting in diffuse pain.

Myotome: an area of muscle supplied by a nerve root; part of the mesoderm of the embryo that develops into skeletal muscle.

Myxedema (Gull's disease): characteristic of hypothyroidism, which presents as edema of the skin, obesity, intolerance to cold, and lack of energy.

N

Nebulizer: A machine that provides humidification during breathing for treatment of lung pathologies. Liquid medications can be added to the nebulizer for inhalation.

Necrotizing fasciitis: an infection caused by streptococcus bacteria that destroys the deep muscle fascia.

Neonatal intensive care unit (NICU): an intensive care unit in a hospital devoted specifically to the care of newly born infants in need of constant medical attention.

Neonatal respiratory distress syndrome (Pulmonary hyaline membrane disease): A condition caused by lack of surfactant in immature fetal lungs. Infants born prematurely with this problem require an artificial respirator to enable them to breathe until they mature enough to start producing surfactant.

Neurodevelopmental therapy/Training/ Treatment: a treatment system for people with neurological deficits based on the work of physical therapist Berta Bobath (1907-1991) and her physician husband Karel Bobath.

Neuroendocrine releasing factors: substances released by the hypothalamus into the pituitary, which control the functional release of the hormones produced by the pituitary.

Neurofibromatosis: a genetic condition that results in bilateral acoustic neuromas of the 8th cranial nerve.

Neurogenic bladder (spastic bladder): a bladder that lacks nerve supply from the sacral nerves, which supply the detrusor muscle of the bladder, or affect the reflex mechanism loop for micturition. Occurs in spinal cord injuries and tumors of the spine. Can lead to overflow incontinence, reduced bladder capacity, inability to contract and empty, urinary retention, and inability to detect when the bladder is full.

Neurapraxia: temporary damage to a nerve caused by pressure on the axon that does not cause any structural changes.

Neurotmesis: severe damage to axons and axon sheaths of nerves. Usually requires surgical suturing of nerve. Usually results in some permanent paralysis of mucles innervated by the nerve.

Nosocomial infection: an infection acquired in the hospital or health care facility and was not present in the patient prior to the hospitalization.

Nulliparous: a woman who has not had a child.

O

Oliguria: reduced urine output or reduced urine formation.

Opportunistic infections: infections that present little threat to a healthy person that become problematic and even life threatening in the individual with a compromised immune system such as in AIDS and HIV.

Osteoarthrosis: another name for osteoarthritis. A degenerative joint disease.

Osteopenia: a condition of loss of bone.

Osteophytes: bony spurs that develop at the margins of an arthritic joint. These osteophytes may interfere with joint motion, and in some cases may break off and become lodged inside the joint.

Osteotomy: an orthopedic surgical procedure in which a cut is made in the bone. A wedge osteotomy is a wedge shaped cut in the bone.

Oxyhemoglobin dissociation curve: the relationship between hemoglobin in the blood and the release of oxygen from the hemoglobin, is called the oxyhemoglobin dissociation curve.

P

Palpation: sensing changes in tissue density, heat or cold, through touch.

Pannus: a type of granulation tissue that forms along the joint margins in the rheumatoid arthritis joint as a result of chronic inflammation, which destroys the hyaline cartilage and the underlying bone.

Pelvic floor incompetence/weakness: the muscles of the pelvic floor provide support for the sphincters that control the anus and the urethra, so when these muscles become weak through stretching, weakness or lack of use a lack of control of the bladder and bowel results.

Pelvic inflammatory disease (PID): inflammation of the female pelvic contents resulting in internal scarring and sterility in severe cases. Most commonly caused by an infection of the reproductive system due to diseases such as gonorrhoeae, ÿccreteÿa, and streptococcal infections.

Pencil-in-cup deformity: a deformity of bones of the distal interphalangeal joints in psoriatic arthritis. The distal end of the proximal phalanx becomes pointed and the proximal end of the distal phalanx becomes hollowed thus giving the appearance of the "pencil-in-cup".

Peripheral neuropathy: Many neuropathies cause a "stocking" or "glove" paresthesia. This pattern of paresthesia is unique to a peripheral neuropathy. In a neuropahty, the area of involvement is the result of circulatory ad sensory changes and does not follow the dermatome and myotome patterns. The sensory nerves are affected, making the foot and lower leg, or hand and for arm, insensitive to heat, cold, pain, or vibraiton.

Peritoneal dialysis (Continuous ambulatory peritoneal dialysis) (CAPD): a type of renal dialysis that can be performed in the home setting. Catheters are implanted in the peritoneal cavity and the process is performed when the patient is asleep.

Pertussis (Whooping Cough): a highly infectious disease caused by the gram-negative bacteria *Bordetella pertussis*. It occurs mainly in children before the age of two and is characterized by a hacking cough that gives the disease its name.

Pes planus: flat foot.

Phacoemulsification: surgical procedure for cataract removal using an ultrasound probe through a small opening made in the cornea.

Pleural effusion: build up of fluid in the pleural cavity

Pleural rub or friction rub: a squeaking sound within the lung heard through the stethoscope on both inspiration and expiration. This sound may be due to the rubbing together of inflamed pleura in pleurisy or pleuritis, or to the presence of neoplasm in the pleura.

Pneumocystic jiroeci pneumonia: alternative name for pneumocystis carinii, an opportunistic, pneumonia infection commonly found in people with AIDS.

Pneumocystis carinii: an opportunistic, pneumonia infection commonly found in people with AIDS.

Poliomyelitis: a viral infectious disease, affecting the nervous system, transmitted through contact with mouth fluids and stool. Characterized by inflammation of the gray matter of the spinal cord causing muscular weakness and paralysis.

Portal hypertension: increased blood pressure in the portal vein (liver). Occurs in liver diseases such as alcoholic hepatitis.

Positive end expiratory pressure (PEEP) ventilator: a type of respiratory ventilation machine that assists with alveolar gaseous exchange during the end phase of exhalation.

Positive expiratory pressure therapy (PEP): a type of respiratory ventilation machine that resists the exhalation of air from the lungs and helps to keep the airways open. May be used for patients with cystic fibrosis.

Post polio syndrome: occurs in individuals who previously had paralytic poliomyelitis many years ago. It is characterized by the development of new muscle weakness caused by denervation of previously affected motor neurons.

Pre-eclampsia: a condition in pregnancy of maternal hypertension, proteinuria, and peripheral edema, which can in some cases require the performance of an emergency caesarean section.

Premature ventricular contraction (PVC): the most common arrhythmia. It is characterized on the electrocardiogram (ECG) by a premature beat of the ventricle. PVCs are seen within the normal population after use of caffeine, smoking, anxiety, or drinking alcohol. PVCs are also evident on ECG after a myocardial infarction (MI) or in other cardiac conditions that cause ischemia of heart tissue such as coronary artery disease (CAD) or congestive heart failure (CHF).

Premature ventricular contraction: is the most common arrhythmia of the heart and is characterized on the ECG by a premature beat of the ventricle.

Pressure control ventilator: a type of mechanical ventilator which is pressure cycled. These machines deliver a present pressure of air to the lungs, and because the resistance of the lung tissue and the respiratory system as a whole varies, the volume of air changes. The PCV ventilator delivers the full amount of preset pressure and maintains a minimum respiratory rate similar to the A/C ventilator.

Pressure-cycled ventilator: A type of ventilator that delivers air to a preset pressure through pressure control ventilation (PCV) or pressure-support ventilation (PSV). These machines deliver a preset pressure of air to the lungs, and because the resistance of the lung tissue and the respiratory system as a whole varies, the volume of air changes.

Pressure support ventilation (PSV): a type of mechanical ventilation machine, which provides the patient with some control over breathing while ensuring a minimal level of inspiration.

Primigravida: a woman pregnant for the first time.

Pulse deficit: a pulse deficit occurs when there is a different pulse rate detected over the apical pulse (directly over the heart) to that measured at a peripheral pulse such as the radial pulse.

Pulse oximeter: a small portable device that has a sensor that attaches either to a finger or the ear used to estimate/measure the levels of oxygen saturation in hemoglobin (SaO_2).

Pulse pressure: the difference between systolic and diastolic pressure readings.

Pus: a yellow liquid that consists of leukocytes and cell debris. A product of coagulative and liquefactive necrosis.

Pyothorax: a pus filled pleural cavity.

Pyramidal decussation: junction of the spinal cord and the medulla/pons where the spinal tracts cross over. So named because of its pyramid shape.

Q

QRS wave (QRS Complex): the second wave of the electrocardiogram (ECG), which demonstrates ventricular contraction by measuring the large wave of depolarization in the ventricles.

R

Radiculopathy: a disease of the nerve root usually resulting in neurological symptoms in the distribution of the specific nerve root.

Rate of perceived exertion: Perceived rate of exertion (PRE) is a subjective monitoring technique used in cardiac rehabilitation when patients become familiar enough with their response to exercise to be able to determine a safe level of intensity of activity. The PRE is based on a Rating of Perceived Exertion (RPE) developed by Borg.

Rate-pressure product (RPP): the heart rate multiplied by the systolic blood pressure represented by the equation: Rate-Pressure Product (RPP) = HR (Heart Rate) X Systolic BP. This is a five-digit figure with the last two numbers not used. The number gives an indication of the aerobic exercise condition of the patient. As the aerobic fitness of the patient improves, the RPP value is reduced.

Raynaud's phenomenon: a condition involving vasospasm of the hands in which the skin becomes white or blue in response to cold or emotion, and then turns red and painful when the blood returns to the fingers. Often seen in RA.

Reciprocal inhibition: A spinal cord reflex causing the simultaneous relaxation of the antagonist muscles at the same time as contraction of the synergist muscle.

Rectus abdominis diastasis: a separation of the two sides of the rectus abdominis muscle. May occur after childbirth. It is a contraindication to strenuous abdominal exercises.

Referred pain: pain is felt at a site distant to that of the injury within the area of skin supplied by the same nerve root as that supplying the injured muscle or internal organ.

Relative weight (RW): the weight of the individual divided by the optimal weight for the height in inches of the person (as determined by a scale produced by the US Government), multiplied by 100.

Respiratory distress syndrome of the newborn: a lung immaturity resulting from lack of lung surfactant in infants below 34 weeks of gestation, results in the need for a respirator.

Retrolisthesis: a condition of the spinal column in which one vertebra moves posteriorly on another.

Reverse transcriptase: a chemical that enables an RNA retrovirus such as HIV to multiply within the invaded cells.

Reye's Syndrome: a rare condition in children caused by several types of viral infections. Causes encephalopathy and hepatic failure.

Rhegmatogenous: the most common type of retinal detachment in the eye.

Rheumatoid factor (RF): an antibody to IgG, present in the blood and synovial fluid of many patients with arthritic conditions including rheumatoid arthritis. If the factor is present in the blood the patient is said to be sero-positive for this factor.

Rule of Nines: The Rule of Nines is a tool to classify burns according to the size and area of the body covered by the burn. The Rule of Nines simply means the body is divided into nine sections of surface area that are each 9% of the total.

S

Sacroiliitis: inflammation of the sacroiliac joint.

Second intention healing: delayed healing of a surgical wound or healing of a non-surgical wound. It can also include healing of a wound that has a loss of skin or where the subcutaneous tissue has been exposed too long to enable closing of the wound through use of stitches, staples or steristrips.

Semont and Epley maneuvers: a system of maneuvers used to treat benign paroxysmal positional vertigo.

Sinus bradycardia: a heart rate of less than 60 beats per minute (bpm).

Sinus tachycardia: a heart rate of more than 100 beats per minute (bpm).

Sjögren's syndrome: a condition in which the mucous membranes of the mouth and eyes are dry.

Somatic motor system: nervous system to voluntary muscle.

Spina bifida occulta: a genetic defect in the development of the vertebral arch not visible at birth. At birth skin covers the defect and occasionally there is a patch of dark hair over the area of the defect.

Spinal reflex arcs: any of several reflex arcs including deep tendon reflexes, withdrawal reflex, reciprocal inhibition, and autogenic inhibition.

Spindle fingers: a characteristic of rheumatoid arthritis in which effusion in the PIP joint causes fingers to takes on the shape of a spindle.

Split-thickness skin graft: involves partial-thickness removal of epidermis and some dermis using an instrument called a dermatome.

Spondylolisthesis: a spinal condition in which a vertebra superior to the level of a defect in the pars interarticularis of a vertebra starts to slip anteriorly. It is a progression from spondylolysis.

Subdermal burn: a burn that destroys the epidermis, dermis and all underlying tissues including fat, muscle and even bone. Usually caused by a flame or electric shock and requires surgical intervention.

Superficial burn: a burn affecting only the epidermal layer of the skin. This type of burn does not cause scarring of the skin.

Superficial partial-thickness burn: a burn that destroys the epidermis and damages part of the papillary dermal layers of the skin. There is minimal scarring with this type of burn, but there is danger of infection.

Surfactant: the fluid that that is contained between the two layers of pleura of the lungs. It allows the two layers to glide over each other as the lungs expand during breathing.

Swan-neck deformity: a joint deformity of the fingers occurring in rheumatoid arthritis. The DIP joint is held in flexion and the PIP joint in hyperextension.

synchronized intermittent mandatory ventilator (SIMV): a type of Volume-cycled (A/C) ventilator which delivers tidal volume of air to patients specific to the individual's needs determined by the respiratory team. With an A/C ventilator, the machine assists with each breath and is set to detect when the patient is having difficulty inhaling which triggers the machine to deliver a preset tidal volume of air to the lungs.

T

Tabes dorsalis: a specific type of syphilis that affects the spinal cord.

Talipes equinovarus: clubfoot.

Texas catheter: a type of urinary catheter used in men, which is attached to the penis with a condom type mechanism.

Tophi: lumps that develop under the skin of the elbow, hands, ears, and sometimes the knees in cases of gout due to build up of uric acid.

Tractional retinal detachment: occurs when scar tissue forms on the retina and pulls the retina away from the pigment epithelial layer.

Transurethral prostate resection (TURP): surgical removal of part of the prostate in cases of benign prostatic hyperplasia.

Trendelenburg gait: a gait pattern producing a lateral tilt of the pelvis secondary to weakness of the hip abductor muscles. May be unilateral or bilateral.

U

Ulnar drift: a deformity of the hand in rheumatoid arthritis due to disruption of the MCP joints. The fingers "drift" towards the ulnar side of the hand. Sometimes called a "Z" deformity due to the shape the hand adopts.

Unicondylar knee resurfacing: A surgery performed for OA in which only one side of the knee joint is affected by OA. In this surgery a polyethylene tibial component and a metal femoral component are used to replace one side of the knee joint after removal of any diseased bone.

Upper Gastrointestinal series (UGI): a test such as a barium swallow, performed to detect upper digestive tract disorders. X-rays taken as the liquid enters the stomach and the small intestine highlight areas of abnormality.

V

Varicella/Varicella zoster: infection with the *Herpes zoster/Varicella zoster* virus causes both Varicella (chickenpox) in the child or adult and *Varicella zoster/Herpes zoster* (shingles) in the adult. *Herpes zoster* results from an earlier infection with the virus that is stored in the posterior root ganglion of the spinal nerves. In times of stress or illness the virus becomes reactivated and manifests along the dermatome of the involved nerve root causing acute pain and rash.

Venous stasis ulcer: a skin ulcer resulting from poor venous circulation. Patients with venous stasis ulcers have impaired venous circulation and usually have a history of trauma to the area involved, varicose veins, or thrombosis of the deep veins.

Ventilation perfusion ratio (V/Q ratio): the relationship between the amount of oxygen in inhaled air to the ability of the lungs to absorb it. In the normal adult the V/Q ratio is 0.8 or 80%. Perfusion relates to blood in the pulmonary vessels that supplies the lung tissue itself. The effect of gravity tends to make more blood available to supply the lower lobes of the lungs than the upper ones. If perfusion is reduced in an area of lung there will be reduced ability for oxygen to diffuse from the lungs into the blood vessels for transport to tissues.

Volume cycled ventilator: deliver tidal volume of air to patients specific to the individual's needs determined by the respiratory team. Two main types of volume controlled ventilator include the assist-control (A/C) ventilator and the synchronized intermittent mandatory ventilator (SIMV).

W

West Nile Virus (West Nile Encephalitis): an infectious viral encephalitis transmitted to humans by blood sucking insects such as mosquitoes and ticks, which become infected from birds and small mammals.

Withdrawal reflex: a spinal cord protective reflex that causes the limb to withdraw from a potentially dangerous stimulus.

X

Xenograft: a type of skin graft taken from another animal. The skin of the pig is the most histologically compatible with that of a human.

Index

Toe grasp reflex, 267*t*
TOF. *See* Tetralogy of Fallot
Tongue, 123*f*
Tonic labyrinthine reflexes, 266*t*
Tophi, 182
TORCH syndrome, 53
Torticollis, 202–203
Total hip arthroplasty, 184–185
Total joint arthroplasty, 184
Total knee arthroplasty, 186
Total mastectomy, 486*t*
Total shoulder arthroplasty, 187
Toxicity, 7*t*
Toxic megacolon, 542
Toxic shock syndrome, 457–458
Trachea, 123*f*, 524*f*
Tracheotomy, 158
Tractional retinal detachment, 607
Transcutaneous electrical nerve stimulation
    (TENS), 27, 50
Transfer RNA (tRNA), 3
Transient ischemic attack (TIA), 311–312
Transplants
    heart, 106
    lungs, 158–159
    renal, 558
Transurethral resection (TUR), 560
Transverse colon, 524*f*
Trapezius, 284*f*
Trauma, 594–595
Traumatic brain injury (TBI), 328–331,
    595–596
Trendelenburg gait pattern, 175
Tricuspid valve, 79*f*
Trigeminal nerve, 275*t*
Triglycerides, 140*t*, 141
    normal values, 581*t*
tRNA. *See* Transfer RNA
Trochlear nerve, 275*t*
Trypsin, 525*t*
Trypsinogen, 525*t*
TSH. *See* Thyrotropic hormone
Tuberculosis (TB), 8, 12, 39, 152
    in bone, 194
Tumor, 346*t*
Tumor necrosis factor, 244
TUR. *See* Transurethral resection
Turner syndrome, 58, 58*f*
    etiology, 58
    medical intervention, 58
    prognosis, 58
    signs and symptoms, 58
Two-point discrimination, 299
Tympanic membrane, 611*f*
Typhoid fever, 446*t*
Typhus, 442–443

UGI. *See* United Network for Organ Sharing
Ulcer, 346*t*, 347*f*
Ulcerative colitis, 541–542

Ulcerative inflammation, 13*t*
Ulnar artery, 84*f*
Ulnar drift, 218
Ulnar nerve, 285*f*, 287*t*
Ulnar vein, 85*f*
Ultrasound, 14, 22
Ultraviolet radiation, 23
Unicondylar knee resurfacing, 186
Unified Parkinson's Disease Rating Scale
    (UPDRS), 323
United Network for Organ Sharing (UNOS),
    158
UNOS. *See* United Network for Organ Sharing
UPDRS. *See* Unified Parkinson's Disease
    Rating Scale
Upper gastrointestinal series (UGI), 526
Upper limb tension, 296
Upper subscapular nerve, 285*f*
Ureter, 469*f*, 503*f*
Urethra, 469*f*, 470*f*
Urge incontinence, 559*t*
Uric acid
    normal values, 581*t*
Urinalysis, 557
Urinary bladder, 469*f*, 503*f*
Urinary catheters, 590
Urinary system, 552–568
Urinary tract diseases, 558–568
Urine, 555*t*
    calcium in, 582*t*
    creatine in, 582*t*
    creatinine in, 582*t*
    glucose in, 582*t*
Urine culture, 557
Urogenital triangle, 470*f*
Urostomy, 540*t*
Urticaria, 362–363
Uterine prolapse, 482–483
Uterus, 469*f*
    carcinoma of, 478–479
    leiomyoma of, 480–481

VAC. *See* Vacuum-assisted closure
Vaccination, 40
Vacuum-assisted closure (VAC), 23
Vagina, 469*f*, 470*f*
    carcinoma of, 479
Vagus nerve, 276*t*, 284*f*
Valve disease, 105
Vancomycin-intermediate *S. aureus* (VISA), 43
Vancomycin-resistant *Enterococcus* (VRE), 43
Varicella, 452–453
Varicella zoster (VZV), 358
Varicose veins, 112–113
Variola, 458
Vasoconstriction, 10
Vasodilation, 10
Vector-borne diseases, 438–445
Vector-borne skin infections, 360–362
Veins, 84–86. *See also specific types*

Venous disease, 112–113
Venous stasis ulcers, 372–374
Venous ulcers, 368*t*
Ventilation, 127–128
    control, 128–129
    muscles of, 131
Ventilation-perfusion ratio, 130
Ventilators, 163–164
Ventral funiculus, 280*t*
Ventral horn, 280*t*
Ventral root, 281*f*
Ventricular fibrillation, 92
Verbal Selective Reminding Test (VerbalSR),
    297
VerbalSR. *See* Verbal Selective Reminding
    Test
Vermis of cerebellum, 265*f*
Verruca, 360
Vertebral artery, 84*f*
    test, 299
Vesicle, 346*t*, 347*f*
Vesicle with neurotransmitter, 270*f*
Vestibular cochlear nerve, 611
Vestibular neuritis, 613
Vestibular rehabilitation therapy, 614
Vestibular system, 281
Vestibulocochlear nerve, 275*t*
Villus, 523*f*
Vinblastine, 50*t*
Vincristine, 50*t*
VISA. *See* Vancomycin-intermediate *S. aureus*
Visceral branch, 285*f*
Vision loss, 610
Visual Selective Reminding Test (VisualSR),
    297
VisualSR. *See* Visual Selective Reminding Test
Vitamin A, 412*t*, 413*t*
    normal values, 581*t*
Vitamin B$_1$, 412*t*
Vitamin B$_2$, 412*t*
Vitamin B$_4$, 412*t*, 413*t*
Vitamin B$_{12}$, 412*t*, 414*t*
    deficiency, 617
    normal values, 583*t*
Vitamin C, 412*t*, 414*t*, 609
Vitamin D, 343*t*, 412*t*, 414*t*
Vitamin E, 412*t*, 414*t*, 609
Vitamin K, 412*t*, 414*t*
Voiding problems, 559*t*
Volume-cycled ventilators, 587–588
VRE. *See* Vancomycin-resistant *Enterococcus*
Vulva
    carcinoma of, 479–480
VZV. *See* Varicella zoster

Wart, 360
WBCC. *See* White blood cell count
Werdnig-Hoffman disease, 69
Wernicke's area, 277, 278*t*
Westmead Posttraumatic Amnesia Scale, 297